PHYSIOLOGY OF THE GASTROINTESTINAL TRACT

Volume 1

Physiology
of the
Gastrointestinal Tract

Volume 1

Editor-in-Chief

Leonard R. Johnson, Ph.D.
Professor of Physiology
University of Texas Medical School
Houston, Texas

Associate Editors

James Christensen, M.D.
Professor and Director
Division of Gastroenterology-Hepatology
Department of Internal Medicine
University of Iowa Hospitals and Clinics
Iowa City, Iowa

Morton I. Grossman, M.D., Ph.D.
Professor of Medicine and Physiology
University of California School of
Medicine, Los Angeles; and
Director, Center for Ulcer Research
and Education
VA Wadsworth Medical Center
Los Angeles, California

Eugene D. Jacobson, M.D.
Associate Dean, Basic Science and Research
University of Cincinnati
College of Medicine
Cincinnati, Ohio

Stanley G. Schultz, M.D.
Professor and Chairman
Department of Physiology and Cell Biology
University of Texas Medical School
Houston, Texas

Raven Press ■ New York

Raven Press, 1140 Avenue of the Americas, New York, New York 10036

Made in the United States of America

Great care has been taken to maintain the accuracy of the information contained in the volume. However, Raven Press cannot be held responsible for errors or for any consequences arising from the use of the information contained herein.

Materials appearing in this book prepared by individuals as part of their official duties as U.S. Government employees are not covered by the above-mentioned copyright.

Library of Congress Cataloging in Publication Data
Main entry under title:

Physiology of the gastrointestinal tract.

Includes bibliographies and index.
1. Gastrointestinal system. I. Johnson, Leonard R.,
1942-   [DNLM: 1. Gastrointestinal system—
Physiology. WI 102 P578]
QP145.P492   612'.32   79-65145
ISBN 0-89004-440-6   AACR2

This work is dedicated to Morton I. Grossman who has trained many of us and who knows more about gastrointestinal physiology and has done more to further it as a science than anyone else

Preface

As with any publishing venture and especially one of this magnitude, one must first ask, "Why?" The Associate Editors and I were motivated primarily to collect in one set of volumes the most up-to-date and comprehensive knowledge in our field. Nothing comparable has been attempted in the area of gastrointestinal physiology during the past fourteen years. During this time, there has been a rapid expansion of knowledge and many new areas of investigation have been initiated.

More than fifty leading scientists—physiologists, clinical specialists, morphologists, pharmacologists, immunologists, and biochemists—have contributed chapters on their various areas of expertise for these volumes. Our original goal was to review the entire field of gastrointestinal physiology in one work. After examining all of the chapters, however, it was apparent that the final product encompassed more than physiology. The chapters reflect the backgrounds of the authors and the approaches of their different disciplines. As such, these volumes contain information for not only the investigator working in these fields but for the clinician or graduate student interested in the function of the gastrointestinal tract. Anyone involved in teaching gastrointestinal physiology or pathophysiology can readily find the latest and most pertinent information on any area in the discipline.

This work is divided into five sections. The first consists of topics, such as growth, the enteric nervous system and gastrointestinal peptides, each of which relates to all areas of the GI tract. The second section contains material describing smooth muscle physiology and gastrointestinal motility. The third section presents treatment of the functions of the stomach and pancreas. The fourth series of chapters treats the entire field of digestion and absorption. These chapters vary from basic electrophysiology and membrane transport to reviews of mechanisms leading to clinical conditions of malabsorption. The final section contains chapters on areas peripheral to physiology (such as immunology, parasitology, and prostaglandins) yet necessary for a comprehensive understanding of the subject.

No one person can presume to organize and edit a scientific work of this scope. I was fortunate to enlist the aid of four preeminent scientists whose expertises cover the entire field. James Christensen was primarily responsible for the chapters on smooth muscle and motility. Eugene D. Jacobson solicited and edited most of the chapters dealing with secretory mechanisms as well as those covering many of the general topics. Chapters relating to secretory regulation were primarily handled by Morton I. Grossman, and those covering aspects of digestion and absorption were organized and reviewed by Stanley G. Schultz. I am exceedingly grateful to these four men without whom this work would not have been possible.

L. R. J.

Acknowledgments

From the organizational stage to actual production Dr. Alan Edelson and his staff at Raven Press provided much help, many excellent suggestions, and a great deal of support. Their role has certainly been more than that of the usual publishing house, and I express my thanks to them. I am especially grateful to my own secretary, Ms. Barbara Suttle, who handled correspondence, kept track of chapters, contacted authors, and typed numerous chapters.

We as editors are especially grateful to the individual authors who took the time and effort to make their knowledge available. As such, almost all of the chapters are more than reviews of past contributions to a field; they synthesize, criticize, and point out those areas where voids exist in our knowledge. Many of the chapters are superb presentations of information in fields that never have been reviewed comprehensively before.

It is our expectation that in due course, a second edition will encompass what constraint of time has forced us to omit here as well as new advances in this rapidly progressing field.

L. R. J.

Contents

Volume 1

General

Motility

Functions of the Stomach and Pancreas

Volume 2

Digestion and Absorption

General

Contributors

Siamak A. Adibi, *Clinical Nutrition Center, University of Pittsburgh School of Medicine, Gastrointestinal and Nutrition Unit, Montefiore Hospital, Pittsburgh, Pennsylvania 15213*

Adrian Allen, *Department of Physiology Medical School, The University of Newcastle-upon-Tyne, NE1 7RU Newcastle-upon-Tyne, England*

Kathryn W. Ballard, *Department of Medicine, University of California at Los Angeles, Los Angeles, California 90073*

T. Berglindh, *Department of Membrane Biology, University of Alabama at Birmingham, The Medical Center, Birmingham, Alabama 35294*

Henry J. Binder, *Yale University School of Medicine, New Haven, Connecticut 06510*

John H. Bond, *University of Minnesota Medical School, Department of Medicine, Veterans Administration Hospital, Minneapolis, Minnesota 55417*

James Boyer, *Department of Medicine, Yale University School of Medicine, New Haven, Connecticut, 06510*

Roberto Buffa, *Institute of Anatomy, University of Pavia, 27100 Pavia, Italy*

Thomas F. Burks, *Department of Pharmacology, University of Arizona School of Medicine, Tucson, Arizona 85724*

Carlo Capella, *Institute of Anatomy, University of Pavia, 27100 Pavia, Italy*

Gilbert A. Castro, *Department of Physiology, The University of Texas Medical School, Houston, Texas 77025*

James Christensen, *Division of Gastroenterology-Hepatology, Department of Internal Medicine, University of Iowa College of Medicine, Iowa City, Iowa 52242*

Blaine W. Cobb, *Gastroenterology Service, Guthrie Clinic Ltd., Sayre, Pennsylvania 18840; formerly Department of Internal Medicine, University of Texas Health Science Center, San Antonio, Texas 78284*

Alastair M. Connell, *College of Medicine, University of Nebraska Medical Center, Omaha, Nebraska 68105*

John M. Dietschy, *Department of Internal Medicine, University of Texas Health Science Center, Southwestern Medical School, Dallas, Texas 75235*

Robert M. Donaldson, Jr., *Department of Internal Medicine, Yale University School of Medicine, Veterans Administration Medical Center, West Haven, Connecticut 06516*

Mark Feldman, *Department of Internal Medicine, University of Texas Health Science Center, Southwestern Medical School, Dallas, Texas 75235*

Michael Field, *Departments of Medicine and Pharmacological and Physiological Sciences, University of Chicago, Chicago, Illinois 60637*

Roberto Fiocca, *Institute of Anatomy, University of Pavia, 27100 Pavia, Italy*

Gunnar Flemström, *Department of Physiology and Medical Biophysics, University of Uppsala Biomedical Center, S-751 23 Uppsala, Sweden*

David Fromm, *Department of Surgery, State University of New York, Upstate Medical Center, Syracuse, New York 13210*

Giorgio Gabella, *Department of Anatomy, University College of London, London, WC1E6BT, England*

Jerry D. Gardner, *Digestive Diseases Branch, National Institute of Arthritis, Metabolism, and Digestive Diseases, National Institutes of Health, Bethesda, Maryland 20205*

Jean Gonella, *CNRS, Department of Vegetative Neurophysiology, Institute of Neurophysiology and Psychophysiology, 13274 Marseilles, Cedex 2, France*

Sherwood L. Gorbach, *Infectious Disease Section, Department of Medicine, Tufts-New England Medical Center, Boston, Massachusetts 02111*

Frederick S. Gorelick, *Department of Medicine, Yale University School of Medicine, New Haven, Connecticut 06510*

Raj K. Goyal, *Department of Medicine, Division of Gastroenterology, University of Texas Health Sciences Center, San Antonio, Texas 78284*

Gary M. Gray, *Department of Medicine, Stanford University, School of Medicine, Palo Alto, California 94305*

Morton I. Grossman, *Departments of Medicine and Physiology, University of California School of Medicine; and Center for Ulcer Research and Education, Veterans Administration Wadsworth Medical Center, Los Angeles, California 90073*

Paul H. Guth, *Center for Ulcer Research and Education, Veterans Administration Wadsworth Medical Center, Los Angeles, California 90073*

David J. Hartshorne, *Departments of Biochemistry and Nutrition and Food Sciences, University of Arizona, Tucson, Arizona 85721*

Susumo Ito, *Department of Anatomy, Harvard Medical School, Boston, Massachusetts 02115*

Michael J. Jackson, *Department of Physiology, George Washington University Medical Center, Washington, D.C. 20037*

Eugene D. Jacobson, *College of Medicine, University of Cincinnati, Cincinnati, Ohio 45267*

James D. Jamieson, *Department of Cell Biology, Yale University School of Medicine, New Haven, Connecticut 06510*

Robert T. Jensen, *Digestive Diseases Branch, National Institute of Arthritis, Metabolism, and Digestive Diseases, National Institutes of Health, Bethesda, Maryland 20205*

Leonard R. Johnson, *Department of Physiology, University of Texas Medical School, Houston, Texas 77025*

Martin I. Kagnoff, *School of Medicine M-013, University of California, San Diego, La Jolla, California 92023*

Keith A. Kelly, *Section of Surgery, Mayo School of Medicine, Rochester, Minnesota 55901*

Young S. Kim, *Department of Medicine, University of California at San Francisco, Gastrointestinal Research Laboratory, Veterans Administration Medical Center, San Francisco, California 94121*

George A. Kimmich, *Department of Radiation Biology and Biophysics, University of Rochester, School of Medicine and Dentistry, Rochester, New York 14642*

David G. Levitt, *Department of Physiology, University of Minnesota Medical School, Minneapolis, Minnesota 55417*

Michael D. Levitt, *Department of Medicine, Veterans Administration Medical Center, Minneapolis, Minnesota 55417*

Martin Lipkin, *Memorial Sloan-Kettering Cancer Center, New York, New York 10021*

Enzo O. Macagno, *Division of Energy Engineering, Institute of Hydraulic Research, University of Iowa, Iowa City, Iowa 52242*

James L. Madara, *Department of Medicine, Peter Bent Brigham Hospital; and Harvard Medical School, Boston, Massachusetts 02115*

Gabriel M. Makhlouf, *Division of Gastroenterology, Department of Medicine, Medical College of Virginia, Virginia Commonwealth University, Richmond, Virginia 23298*

Juan-Ramon Malagelada, *Gastroenterology Unit, Mayo Clinic and Mayo Foundation, Saint Mary's Hospital, Rochester, Minnesota 55901*

James H. Meyer, *Gastroenterology Section, Veterans Administration Hospital, Sepulveda, California 91343*

Bjarne G. Munck, *Institute of Medical Physiology Department A, University of Copenhagen, The Panum Institute, Copenhagen North, Denmark*

John S. Patton, *Department of Microbiology, University of Georgia, Athens, Georgia 30602*

Richard J. Paul, *Department of Physiology, College of Medicine, University of Cincinnati, Cincinnati, Ohio 45221*

O. H. Petersen, *Department of Physiology, The University of Dundee, Dundee, DD1 4HN Scotland*

Charles T. Richardson, *Department of Internal Medicine, University of Texas Health Science Center, Southwestern Medical School, Dallas, Texas 75235*

André Robert, *Department of Experimental Biology, The Upjohn Company, Kalamazoo, Michigan 49001*

Claude Roman, *Faculty of Sciences, Department of Physiology and Neurophysiology, 13397 Marseilles, France*

Richard C. Rose, *Department of Physiology, Hershey Medical Center, Pennsylvania State University, Hershey, Pennsylvania 17033*

Irwin H. Rosenberg, *Department of Medicine, Gastroenterology Section, University of Chicago Hospitals and Clinics, Chicago, Illinois 60637*

James P. Ryan, *Department of Physiology, Temple University School of Medicine, Philadelphia, Pennsylvania 19140*

George Sachs, *Laboratory of Membrane Biology, University of Alabama in Birmingham, The Medical Center, Birmingham, Alabama 35294*

Irene Schulz, *Max Planck Institute for Biophysics, 6000 Frankfurt a.m. 70, West Germany*

Stanley G. Schultz, *Department of Physiology and Cell Biology, University of Texas Medical School, Houston, Texas 77025*

Fausto Sessa, *Institute of Anatomy, University of Pavia, 27100 Pavia, Italy*

Gary L. Simon, *Infectious Disease Section, Department of Medicine, George Washington University Medical Center, Washington, D.C. 20037; formerly Infectious Disease Section, Department of Medicine, Tufts-New England Medical Center, Boston, Massachusetts 02111*

Enrico Solcia, *Institute of Anatomy, University of Pavia, 27100 Pavia, Italy*

Andrew H. Soll, *Center for Ulcer Research and Education, Veterans Administration Wadsworth Medical Center, and University of California at Los Angeles School of Medicine, Los Angeles, California 90073*

Travis E. Solomon, *Center for Ulcer Research and Education, Veterans Administration Wadsworth Medical Center, and University of California at Los Angeles School of Medicine, Los Angeles, California 90073*

Joseph Szurszewski, *Department of Physiology and Biophysics, Mayo Medical School Rochester, Minnesota 55901*

Barry L. Tepperman, *Department of Physiology, University of Western Ontario Health Sciences Center, London, Ontario, Canada 76A 5C1*

Alan B. R. Thomson, *Division of Gastroenterology, Department of Internal Medicine, University of Alberta, Edmonton, Alberta, Canada*

Jerry S. Trier, *Department of Medicine, Peter Bent Brigham Hospital; and Harvard Medical School, Boston, Massachusetts 02115*

Luciana Usellini, *Institute of Anatomy, University of Pavia, 27100 Pavia, Italy*

W. Allen Walker, *Department of Pediatrics, Harvard Medical School; and Pediatric Gastrointestinal and Nutrition Unit, Massachusetts General Hospital, Boston, Massachusetts 02114*

John H. Walsh, *Department of Medicine, University of California at Los Angeles, Center for Ulcer Research and Education, Veterans Administration Wadsworth Medical Center, Los Angeles, California 90073*

Norman W. Weisbrodt, *Department of Physiology and Pharmacology, The University of Texas Medical School at Houston, Houston, Texas 77030*

Jack D. Wood, *Department of Physiology, School of Medicine Sciences, University of Nevada, Reno, Nevada 89557; formerly Department of Physiology, University of Kansas Medical Center, Kansas City, Kansas 66103*

Physiology of the Gastrointestinal Tract, edited by
Leonard R. Johnson. Raven Press, New York © 1981.

Chapter 1

Physiology of the Enteric Nervous System

J. D. Wood

Langley (104) introduced the term "enteric nervous system" to describe the neural elements that are distributed within the wall of the gastrointestinal tract. Langley coined the term because he believed that the enteric ganglia had unique structural and functional characteristics that distinguished them from autonomic ganglia outside the gut. The results of subsequent histoanatomical and electrophysiological studies have established this concept to the extent that the enteric ganglia are no longer considered to be simple-relay distribution centers where a multitude of parasympathetic postganglionic neurons relay excitatory signals from relatively few vagal or pelvic nerve fibers to the gastrointestinal effector systems. Current concepts regard the enteric nervous system as an independent integrative system with structural and functional properties analogous to the central nervous system. Command signals from the central nervous system are transmitted to the enteric nervous system along sympathetic and parasympathetic pathways; however, this represents only one kind of input to an integrative network that also contains circuitry for processing information supplied by various kinds of sensory receptors along the gut

and synaptic circuitry that generates precise patterns of neural outflow.

The enteric nervous system functions like a "brain" that coordinates and programs gastrointestinal functions. An eminent neurophysiologist once responded to this statement with the frivolous question of what did I consider to be the "smartest" part of the gut. The reversal of the direction of peristaltic propulsion when the advancing bolus encounters an intestinal obstruction (16) immediately came to mind as "smart" behavior, because this involves mechanoreceptor detection of the halt in forward progress of the bolus, processing of the sensory information by internuncial circuitry, and finally neural outflow that coordinates contractile activity of the muscle layers to achieve retropulsion. Nevertheless, with more reflection on the question, it seemed that the stomach and esophagus of raptorial birds must certainly be the "smartest" part of all gastrointestinal tracts. After a great horned owl has ingested a mouse, the neural control system first programs for strong stomach contractions which crush, macerate, and mix the contents with gastric secretions. As digestion proceeds, information on the state of the lumen is furnished by sensory detectors to the integrative networks that interpret the information and command a reduction from strong gastric contractions to gentle mixing waves. The stomach then empties the liquid content into the small bowel and forceful muscular contractions manipulate and compact the remaining bone and hair into a pellet. The final phase of the process is egestion of the pellet by coordinated movements and reverse peristalsis within the esophagus (100). Other gastrointestinal physiologists might justifiably argue for equally sophisticated neural control in specialized alimentary systems such as those of ruminant animals; however, the point is that the enteric nervous system is indeed "smart."

Although the enteric nervous system offers the most accessible source of neurons for biopsy to evaluate certain nervous disorders in humans, the system is deeply embedded within the gut wall and is not readily accessible for experimental purposes. It is apparent, in spite of this, that gastrointestinal function cannot be well understood without understanding the neurophysiology of the enteric nervous system. The most promising way to this understanding is to apply the same neurophysiological principles and techniques of study that are applied to the brain and spinal cord. During the past decade, many of the problems of inaccessibility of the system have been overcome and standard neurophysiological techniques have been utilized to study the functional properties of enteric ganglion cells. The results that have been obtained from electrophysiological studies of enteric neurons and the relevance of this information to gastrointestinal function constitute the remainder of this chapter.

HISTOANATOMY AND NEUROCHEMISTRY

The morphology of the enteric nervous system is described in another section of this volume. The purpose here is to point out that many histoanatomical and histochemical similarities exist between the enteric nervous system and the brain. This is emphasized because it is consistent with the view that information processing and integrative function are developed to a higher degree in enteric ganglia than in other autonomic ganglia.

The first in the series of similarities is the compact organization of neural and glial elements and paucity of extracellular space that are common characteristics of both enteric ganglia and the brain (52). The significance of this with respect to integrative function is unknown; however, there is evidence that close packing of glial and neural elements in the brain may be related to the glial functions of uptake and release of chemical transmitter substances and buffering of extracellular potassium concentration.

A dense synaptic neuropil exists within both enteric ganglia and central nervous systems. This is significant because in all integrative nervous systems, the bulk of

information processing occurs in microcircuits within a synaptic neuropil (146). In invertebrate animals, most of the cell bodies of neurons in the central nervous system do not receive synaptic input and the information handling associated with behavior of the organism occurs within a synaptic neuropil. Axoaxonal and axodendritic synapses occur within the neuropil of enteric ganglia, and an ultrastructural study of this region within myenteric ganglia revealed at least eight morphologically distinct types of axon terminals based on the appearance of the synaptic vesicles (30). Synapses occur also on the somas of enteric neurons, and up to three morphologically distinct kinds of endings have been described at the neuronal soma (52).

Blood vessels do not enter the enteric ganglia, and a blood-ganglion barrier analogous to the blood-brain barrier has been demonstrated in the myenteric plexus (57). This blood-ganglion barrier to date has been demonstrated only for macromolecules. It appears to reside within the capillary endothelial layer and is unlike the blood-brain barrier in this respect. Nevertheless, it is characteristic of the distinction of the enteric nervous system and should be considered by investigators who feel that there is some advantage to close intra-arterial injection of neuroactive drugs in pharmacological experiments on the bowel.

The synaptic chemistry of the enteric nervous system bears a striking resemblance to the neurochemistry of the brain in that most putative neurotransmitters within the brain also have been implicated as enteric neurotransmitters. Below is a list of putative neurotransmitters or neuromodulators that are located in both the central nervous system and the enteric nervous system:

acetylcholine	somatostatin
norepinephrine	vasoactive intestinal peptide
5-hydroxytryptamine	enkephalin
purine nucleotides	substance P
dopamine	bombesin

This lengthy list, which is probably far from complete, suggests that chemical transfer of information in the enteric nervous system utilizes as diverse an array of messenger molecules for chemical transfer of information as the brain. Because chemical transmission is highly vulnerable to malfunction and to interference by exogenous substances, it suggests many sites for disease mechanisms to operate as well as numerous sites at which therapeutic drugs could be designed to operate.

ELECTRICAL PROPERTIES OF ENTERIC GANGLION CELLS

Although reports on the electrophysiology of the enteric nervous system have appeared at an increasing rate over the past decade, relatively few laboratories are involved with this research, and the only region of the gastrointestinal tract that has received extensive study is the small intestine. Studies of the large intestine have been limited to extracellular recording and no work on enteric neurons of the stomach, esophagus, or specialized regions such as sphincters and the cecum has been reported. Consequently, all of the following discussion directly relates only to the small bowel.

Electrophysiological Methods

Important information on properties and functions of enteric neurons has been obtained with both extracellular and intracellular methods of recording neuronal electrical activity. Several different kinds of metal microelectrodes (169,180) and suction electrodes (39,141) for extracellular recording from enteric neurons have yielded essentially similar results. With extracellular recording, the electrode tip may be designed to be small enough to detect the action potential discharge of portions of single neurons (single-unit recording) or the electrode tip may be sufficiently large to obtain "multiunit" recordings. Because the electrode tip is in the extraneuronal space, this kind of recording provides information only on the occurrence of action potentials within a particular time domain. The principal advantage of extracellular recording is that discharge patterns of single units can be studied over prolonged time spans and several units can be recorded simultaneously for analysis of neuronal interactions. Additional information is obtained by testing the effects of pharmacological agents on the neural activity and by comparing neural activity with behavior of the effector system.

Intracellular recording is technically more difficult than extracellular recording, but it yields a greater variety of information about the membrane properties of the neurons. Information on resting membrane potential, membrane constants, synaptic potentials, and changes in ionic conductances can be obtained only by intracellular recording. A significant advantage of intracellular recording is that the experimenter can control the membrane potential of a neuron by injecting electrical current into the cell through the recording microelectrode (Fig. 1). Depolarizing current can be injected to excite the cell or hyperpolarizing current can be used to move the membrane potential away from action potential threshold and to reduce excitability. The amount of injected current and the corresponding change in transmembrane voltage are measurable parameters with which the ohmic equation ($R = V/I$) can be used to compute the electrical resistance of the cell membrane. The resistance of a membrane is determined by its permeability to ions; consequently, changes in ionic conductance of the membrane produced by synaptic transmitter substances, sensory stimuli, drugs, etc.

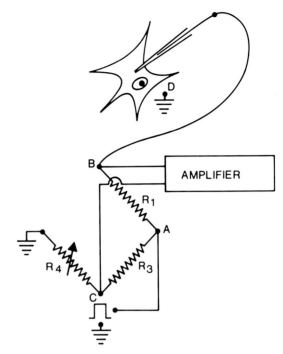

FIG. 1. Wheatstone bridge circuit used to pass electrical current across the membrane of neurons. A single microelectrode is used to inject current into the cell and to record the resulting electrotonic potential across the membrane. The current pulses are passed between points A and D (ground), and the bridge circuit functions to null out the voltage drop that occurs across the resistance of the microelectrode so that only the potential change across the membrane is recorded between points B and C. This is accomplished by adjusting R_4 until the current between A and B equals the current between point B and ground, and the current between A and C equals the current between C and ground. When this is done, the bridge is said to be balanced, and the current pulse between point A and ground does not change the potential between points B and C.

are reflected by changes in membrane resistance. The resistance measured by intracellular current injection is referred to as input resistance because it is not a precise measure of the specific resistance of any given patch of cell membrane. The input resistance is determined not only by the specific membrane resistance, but also by geometric variables such as size of the cell body, number of processes projecting from the cell body, and extent of branching of the processes—all of which are usually unmeasurable. Changes in the electrical characteristics of the microelectrode after impalement of the cell can also distort measurements of input resistance in unpredictable ways. Consequently, most measurements are estimates and only relative changes in input resistance produced by experimental manipulation are of consequence.

Dissection of the gastrointestinal wall is a prerequisite for electrical recording from neurons in the myenteric or submucous plexus (Fig. 2). Two methods are generally used to expose the myenteric plexus for electrical recording. The first method is to strip away the longitudinal muscle coat to expose the plexus on the underlying circular muscle. This preparation has the advan-

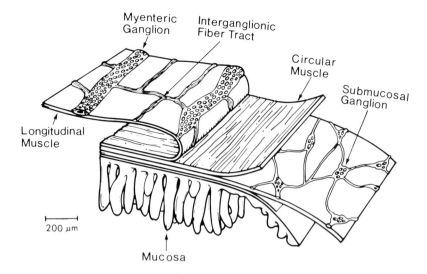

FIG. 2. Schematic drawing of the wall of the small intestine showing the layers which must be removed by microdissection in order to expose the myenteric or submucosal plexus for electrical recording.

tage that Meissner's plexus and its interconnections with the myenteric plexus, as well as any connections be-

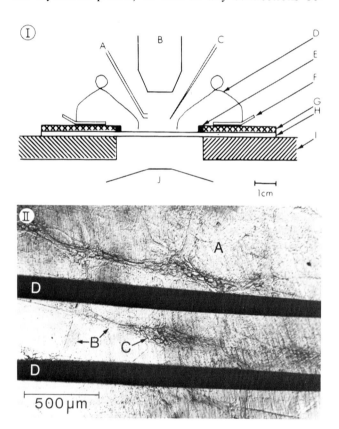

FIG. 3. Method used to record intracellular electrical activity of guinea pig myenteric neurons. I: Schematic drawing of organ chamber. *A:* parallel 100 µm stainless steel wires which are pressed onto the muscle at two sides of the ganglion to immobilize the ganglion. *B:* microscopic objective. *C:* microelectrode. *D:* one of 10 stainless steel wire anchors around perimeter of preparation to hold it flat on bottom of chamber. *E:* Teflon inner ring of organ chamber. *F:* steel base of wire anchors. *G:* rubberized magnetic material cemented to glass slide. *H:* glass slide (7 × 7 × 0.1 cm). *I:* microscope stage. *J:* microscope condenser. II: Photomicrograph of longitudinal muscle-myenteric plexus preparation. *A:* longitudinal muscle layer. *B:* interganglionic fiber tract. *C:* ganglion. *D:* two parallel stainless steel wires pressed onto the muscle to immobilize ganglion. From Wood and Mayer (181).

tween mucosal sensory receptors and the myenteric plexus, remain intact. The two principal disadvantages of the preparation are that disruption of the plexus occurs because some of the plexus adheres to and is removed with the longitudinal muscle; and secondly, the preparations are too thick for transmitted light illumination and usually require vital staining with a dye such as methylene blue in order to adequately visualize the plexus.

The second method, which has been used successfully for the guinea pig bowel, is to open the segment of bowel by cutting along the mesenteric border, pin the tissue flat with mucosal side up, and remove in turn the mucosa and circular muscle layer. The myenteric plexus remains undisrupted on the longitudinal muscle. The preparation is sufficiently translucent to permit transmitted light illumination, and the neurons are readily visualized microscopically for visual control of electrode placement. A major difficulty with this preparation is that spontaneous contractile movements dislodge the microelectrode from an impaled neuron. Figure 3 shows how immobilization is accomplished by pressing L-shaped wires onto the muscle at opposite sides and parallel to the long axis of a ganglion. Guinea pig myenteric ganglia are situated with the long axis perpendicular to the long axis of the longitudinal muscle fibers, and the wires stop muscle movements within their confines apparently by depolarizing the muscle.

Meissner's plexus can be exposed for electrical recording by dissecting the circular muscle from a flat sheet of small bowel wall. Meissner's plexus remains with the submucosa, and transparency of the preparation is increased by scraping the mucosa away with a blunt instrument.

Properties Determined by Extracellular Recording

Both spontaneous and stimulus-evoked patterns of action potential discharge have been recorded from neurons within myenteric and submucosal ganglia of intestinal segments *in vitro* (39,125,141,169,179,180,187,188) and *in vivo* (124). These neurons can be classified into three distinct categories on the basis of the pattern of action potential discharge. The first category of neurons discharges periodic bursts of spikes with silent interburst intervals and is referred to as a "burst-type" neuron. Mechanosensitive neurons, some of which are silent and some of which show ongoing discharge of single spikes, can be induced by mechanical distortion of the ganglionic structure to discharge spikes at increased frequency. These neurons, some of which may be sensory receptors, make up the second category. The third category neurons are called single-spike neurons because they show continuous discharge of action potentials at irregular intervals and are unaffected by mechanical stimulation.

Burst-Type Neurons

The steady, systematic discharge of burst-type neurons (Fig. 4) continues for several hours in segments of intestine *in vitro,* and can be recorded in preparations which have been stored at 5 °C for periods up to 48 hr and then rewarmed to 37 °C. Contrary to some reports (84), enteric neurons are quite resistant to hypoxia as reflected by their ability to discharge action potentials in media with low oxygen partial pressure.

The intervals between bursts of spikes are dependent on the ambient temperature. The duration of the interburst intervals decreases at temperatures above 37 °C and increases below this temperature. The temperature coefficient (Q^{10}) for this effect is 10 to 16 over a temperature range of 32 to 40 °C. This sensitivity to temperature has led to the suggestion that these neurons could function as deep body thermosensors (66). Spontaneous discharge of burst-type units is restricted to a temperature range of 30 to 42 °C. This suggests that the physiological state of the intestine is not the same at temperatures above and below normal body temperature. The neurons continue to respond to pharmacological agents and electrical stimulation at temperatures that are not optimal for spontaneous discharge, and

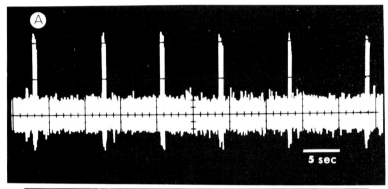

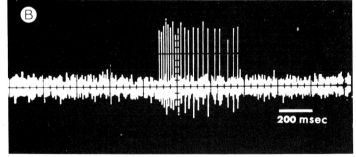

FIG. 4. Discharge of a steady burst-type neuron in the myenteric plexus of cat small intestine. **A:** Burst pattern recorded with a slow time base. **B:** One burst of spikes from the same cell recorded with an expanded time base. **C:** Superimposed traces of 10 consecutive bursts of spikes from the same neuron. Each sweep of the oscilloscope was triggered by the first spike of each burst. Note that variance of interspike interval is least for first interspike interval and increases for subsequent intervals and that spike waveform is bipolar. From Wood (173).

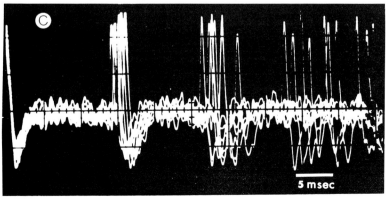

experimental preparations not at optimal temperature may exhibit nerve-mediated motor activity that reflects abnormal physiology. This emphasizes the necessity of taking temperature into account when experiments on the gut are designed and interpreted.

The ongoing discharge of the burst-type neurons represents intrinsic activity that is not due to electrode-induced mechanical irritation. Evidence for this is as follows: (a) the discharge continues unchanged for many hours; (b) distortion of the ganglion produced by movements of the recording electrode does not alter the pattern of discharge; (c) burst activity can be recorded extracellularly with fine tipped (0.5 to 1 µm) NaCl-filled micropipettes; (d) electrical stimulation of synaptic input to the burst neurons elicits bursts of spikes that are similar to the spontaneous bursts of the cell.

Burst-type units are distinguished as either steady bursters or erratic bursters on the basis of the regularity of the interburst time intervals.

Steady bursters (Fig. 5) discharge with relatively low statistical variance of interburst interval. Frequency-distribution histograms for steady bursters are sometimes multimodal, and the secondary peaks on the histograms are distinct multiples of the time interval represented by the primary peak (Fig. 5). This suggests that the timing of the bursts is determined by an oscillatory pacemaker mechanism and that spike generation fails during some cycles of the continuously running oscillator.

The discharge patterns of erratic bursters are characterized by irregular interburst intervals and by periodic conversion to continuous discharge of either single spikes or spike doublets (Fig. 6). Variations in the duration of interburst intervals of some erratic bursters are repeated systematically in cyclical patterns. In these cases, each cycle of activity consists of the following sequential changes in spike discharge: (a) a silent period of relatively long duration; (b) a series of bursts at regular intervals; (c) progressive decrease in intervals separating successive bursts; (d) continuous discharge of spikes (Fig. 6).

The periodic discharge patterns of the burst-type units could be produced by mechanisms either intrinsic or extrinsic to the neuron. Two possible extrinsic mechanisms of burst pattern production are either cyclic bursts of excitatory synaptic input to the neuron or cyclic bursts of inhibitory postsynaptic input that alternate with cyclic bursts of excitatory input. Two possible intrinsic mechanisms are, first, the inherent ability of the ganglion cell membrane to generate cyclic pacemaker potentials that trigger bursts of spikes, as in the parabolic burster of the marine mollusc *Aplysia* (150), or, second, a postinhibitory rebound excitation at the termination of inhibitory synaptic input to the cell. All

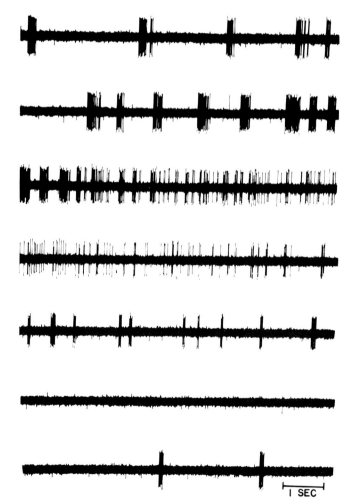

FIG. 6. Discharge of an erratic burst-type neuron in the myenteric plexus of guinea pig small intestine. The discharge pattern shows conversion from a burst pattern to continuous spike discharge and reversion to a burst pattern. The record is continuous from top to bottom. From Wood (172).

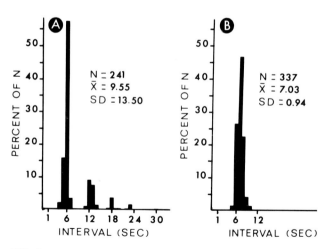

FIG. 5. Histograms of interburst interval distributions of consecutive bursts of spikes from two steady bursters in cat myenteric plexus. The ordinate represents the proportion of the total number of intervals and the abscissa represents the duration of the intervals. Given are number of intervals (N), mean interval (x) and standard deviation (SD). The neuron of histogram A discharged either at intervals of 6 sec or at multiples of this interval. The neuron of histogram B discharged with only small variation around a mean interval of 6 sec. From Wood (173).

of the mechanisms for generation of patterned bursts of spikes, except the endogenous pacemaker mechanism, depend on synaptic input to the neuron. Elevated Mg^{2+} blocks the ongoing activity of the erratic bursters, but not that of the steady bursters *in vitro* (174). It is known from intracellular studies on myenteric neurons, as for other synaptic systems, that elevated Mg^{2+} prevents the release of transmitter substances from presynaptic nerve terminals. Therefore, synaptic mechanisms appear to be required for production of the erratic burst patterns, and burst pattern generation in the steady bursters seems to involve an endogenous pacemaker mechanism.

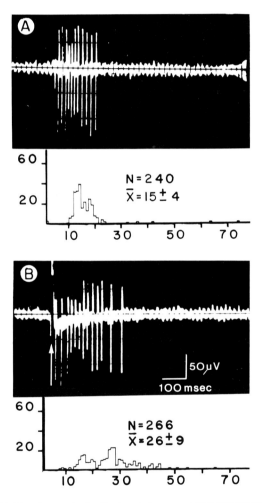

FIG. 7. Stimulus-evoked spike bursts in an erratic burst-type neuron in cat myenteric plexus. **A:** Spontaneously occurring burst of spikes and spike-interval histogram for 24 bursts. **B:** Burst of spikes evoked from the same unit by a single electrical shock *(arrow)* applied to the surface of the ganglion and spike-interval histogram for 22 stimulus-evoked bursts. Ordinate of histograms is number of intervals and abscissa is interval duration in msec. Computer bin width was 1 msec. Given are number of intervals (N) and mean ± SD (x). The spike-interval distributions differed between spontaneous and stimulus-evoked bursts, but the appearance of the spikes and temporal position of small and large spikes were similar within the spontaneous and stimulus-evoked bursts. The recording was made by G. R. Athey.

Focal application of single electrical shocks either to the surface of a myenteric ganglion or to an interganglionic fiber tract to the ganglion evokes a burst of spikes that resembles the spontaneously discharged bursts in erratic bursters (Fig. 7). These stimulus-evoked bursts of spikes appear to be synaptically mediated because they are reversibly blocked in the presence of elevated Mg^{2+}. On the other hand, the stimulus-evoked responses are unaffected by a variety of putative neurotransmitter substances and synaptic blocking drugs which include: curare, hexamethonium, atropine, acetylcholine, norepinephrine, methysergide, 5-hydroxytryptamine, naloxone, and morphine (31). Many different pharmacological agents have been tested on the spontaneously occurring burst discharge (44,126,141,169). In general, only agents that are active at cholinergic synapses seem to alter the ongoing discharge of the erratic bursters. Acetylcholine stimulates some of the units and muscarinic or nicotinic receptor-blocking drugs sometimes halt the discharge of some. No putative neurotransmitters or receptor-blocking drugs have been found to affect the discharge of the steady bursters. From the evidence presently available, it can only be said that the erratic bursters may possess cholinergic receptors and that their discharge is driven by release of an unidentified and uncommon neurotransmitter substance.

The evidence suggests that the steady bursters do not receive synaptic input from other neurons and that they may be continuously running oscillators which synaptically drive the erratic bursters as shown in Fig. 23. Indication of driver-follower coupling has been observed on multiunit records as sequential temporal coupling by a constant time interval of the discharge of two different burst units (Fig. 8). The functional significance of this kind of connectivity will be discussed in a later section on enteric integrative mechanisms.

It would be expected, if the steady bursters are indeed endogenous oscillators, that intracellular recording would detect neurons with rhythmic oscillations of membrane potential. This has never been observed, although rhythmic oscillations can be seen in some myenteric neurons after application of relatively high concentrations of 5-hydroxytryptamine. It could be that the intracellular method has not detected the steady bursters either because the somas are small and difficult to impale or because the oscillatory region of the neuron is morphologically remote from the cell soma. The existence of oscillatory enteric neurons will remain an open question until they can be demonstrated by intracellular recording.

Although none has been found for the steady bursters, a counterpart of the erratic burster has been detected in intracellular studies. The ongoing patterns of spike activity characteristic of the erratic bursters occur in the processes distal to the cell soma, and these spikes electronically invade the soma where they are recorded

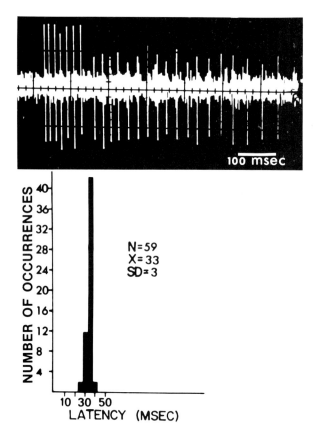

FIG. 8. Driver-follower coupling between burst-type myenteric neurons in cat small intestine. **Top:** Recording of coupled discharge of two different units by the same electrode. **Bottom:** Frequency distribution histogram of the time period between the terminal spike of the first unit to discharge and the initial spike of the follower unit. Given are number of measurements (N), mean ($\bar{x}$), and standard deviation (SD).

by the intracellular microelectrode (Figs. 9 and 10). These are probably the equivalent of dendritic spikes which are triggered by synaptic input within the neuropil of the ganglion. They occur in myenteric neurons that are referred to as AH/type 2 neurons later.

Mechanosensitive Neurons

Extracellular recording from single units within the myenteric plexus reveals three different kinds of units that respond with an increased rate of discharge to mechanical distortion of the ganglion. One kind of mechanosensitive unit behaves like a typical slowly adapting mechanoreceptor (Fig. 11) and another like a fast-adapting mechanoreceptor (Fig. 11). The third kind of mechanosensitive unit is activated by mechanical stimulation to discharge prolonged trains of spikes of up to 40 sec duration (Fig. 11). The discharge frequency of the third kind of unit is independent of the intensity of stimulation, and the discharge continues in a set pattern for many seconds after termination of the mechanical stimulus. These mechanosensitive neurons have been termed "tonic-type" enteric neurons, and evidence presented in a later section of the chapter will suggest that tonic-type neurons of extracellular studies may be the same as AH/type 2 neurons of intracellular studies.

Enteric mechanosensitive units may be activated either by a glass probe pressed onto the surface of the ganglion (169) or by an electrode with a large tip diameter that does not penetrate the periganglionic sheath and so serves as both recording electrode and stimulus probe (107,123).

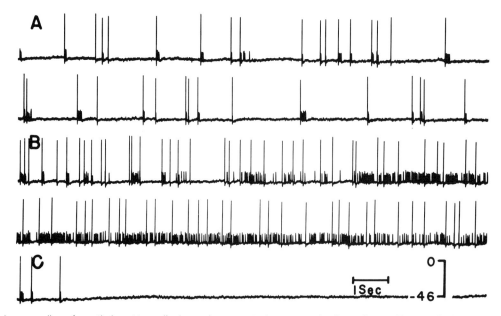

FIG. 9. Intracellular recording of erratic burst-type discharge in a myenteric neuron of guinea pig small bowel. **A:** Continuous record of bursts of low-amplitude potentials accompanied by an occasional action potential. Low-amplitude potentials reflect electrotonic spread of action potentials that originate in the neuropil and propagate to the soma in one of the cell's processes. The cell is an AH/type 2 neuron and only the first electrotonic spike of each burst fires the somal membrane to generate the large-amplitude spikes (refer to Fig. 10). **B:** Progressive decrease in interburst interval and conversion from bursts to trains of low-amplitude potentials. **C:** Long duration silent period of cyclical discharge of the cell. From Wood and Mayer (181).

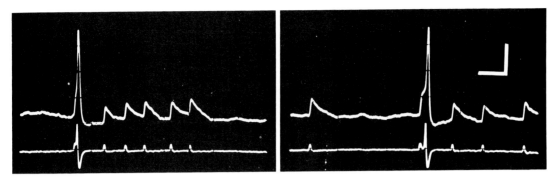

FIG. 10. Intracellular recording of erratic burst-type discharge in a myenteric neuron of guinea pig small bowel. Same neuron as Fig. 9 recorded on an expanded time base. **Left:** Burst of electrotonic potentials during same time period as Fig. 9A. Only first electrotonic potential fires the soma. Postspike hyperpolarization prevents subsequent electrotonic potentials of the bursts from firing the soma. **Right:** Electrotonic potentials and somal spike recorded during continuous activity of Fig. 9B. Upper trace is the transmembrane voltage; lower trace is dV/dt of membrane voltage. Vertical calibration 20 mV; horizontal calibration 10 msec. From Wood and Mayer (181).

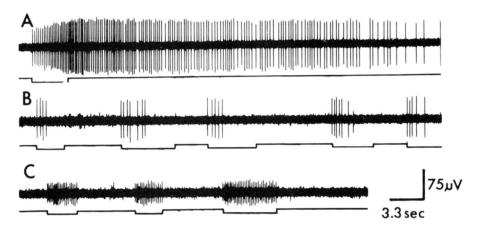

FIG. 11. Examples of the types of mechanosensitive neurons that are detected by extracellular recording electrodes. **A:** Tonic-type mechanosensitive neuron in myenteric plexus of cat small bowel. The unit was activated by transient mechanical deformation of the ganglionic surface (downward deflection of bottom trace) and continued to discharge long after removal of stimulus. Compare with intracellular record of Fig. 17A. **B:** Fast-adapting mechanoreceptor in myenteric plexus of cat small intestine. This unit discharged only at the onset of mechanical distortion of the ganglion indicated by downward deflection of bottom trace. **C:** Slowly adapting mechanoreceptor in myenteric plexus of dog small intestine. This unit discharged throughout mechanical stimulation.

The units that behave like slowly adapting mechanoreceptors (Fig. 11) show sustained discharge without signs of adaption during a stimulus of constant intensity, and the frequency of discharge is directly related to the intensity of stimulation (107). These units may or may not show ongoing discharge prior to stimulation.

The units that behave like fast-adapting mechanoreceptors (Fig. 11) give an intensity-dependent discharge at the onset of the stimulus and quickly fatigue during a sustained stimulus. These units rarely show an "off-discharge" at the termination of stimulation.

Mechanosensitivity is a property of only these three types of units and is not a general property of all myenteric ganglion cells. Other myenteric neurons may show low levels of ongoing discharge of action potentials that may be similar to those of the slowly adapting mechanosensitive neurons, but these units are not excited by the same kind of mechanical stimulation that increases firing rate of the slowly adapting units.

The receptive fields of the slowly adapting mechanosensitive neurons are limited to the region of the ganglion and do not extend to the interganglionic fiber tracts (125). The discharge patterns of both the fast- and slowly adapting mechanosensitive neurons when recorded at the ganglia are similar to patterns of discharge recorded in gastrointestinal afferent fibers within the vagus (35,86) and splanchnic nerves (137). The mechanosensitive units recorded at the myenteric ganglia appear to correspond to the "deep" tension receptors that discharge in vagal afferent fibers, and that were shown by Iggo (86) to be localized within the muscularis externa. The mechanosensitive activity that can be recorded at the myenteric ganglia does not originate from the highly sensitive mechanoreceptors located within the mucosa of the bowel (35,86) because mechanosensitive activity can be recorded from myenteric ganglia situated on the longitudinal muscle layer in isolation from the remainder of the bowel (180). It thus seems that the most probable location of the generator region of the "deep tension receptors" is within the periganglionic connective tissue. Electron microscopic studies of the fine structure of myenteric ganglia show peculiar contacts between neuronal terminals and the intraganglionic surface of the periganglionic sheath that might be sensory structures (52). Light microscopic studies also have shown receptor structures within the connective tissue capsules of myenteric ganglia (114).

The mechanosensitivity of tonic-type enteric neurons is unlike that of intestinal mechanoreceptors and mechanoreceptors elsewhere in the body. These neurons encode neither the static intensity nor the time derivative of the stimulus. Instead, they seem to signal, with a stereotyped train of spikes, only the occurrence of mechanical distortion of the ganglion (107). Once the tonic-type units are activated (Fig. 11), they generate the characteristic train of action potentials independent of the original mechanical stimulus, and when the discharge stops, the units are refractory to activation for 0.5 to 2 min.

Close association between discharge of slowly adapting mechanosensitive neurons and that of the tonic-type neurons has been observed on extracellular records (172). The discharge of the slowly adapting unit always precedes with a constant time interval the discharge of the tonic-type unit, suggesting that the tonic-type neurons may be triggered by input derived from the slowly adapting mechanosensitive units. The synaptic basis for the tonic-type discharge and the serotonergic nature of the synaptic input are presented in the later section of the chapter on synaptic transmission.

The overall behavior of the tonic-type mechanosensitive neurons is not consistent with these units being first-order sensory neurons; it is more likely that they are higher order interneurons. No counterpart of the tonic-type discharge pattern has been observed in centrally directed sensory afferents from the gut.

Single-Spike Neurons

These units continuously discharge action potentials at relatively low frequencies with no consistent pattern to the activity (Fig. 12). The ongoing discharge is sometimes altered but never blocked by elevated Mg^{2+}, indicating that it is not dependent on synaptic input. The most noteworthy characteristic of these cells is that they are sensitive to acetylcholine and other nicotinic-cholinergic agonists (Fig. 12), and the discharge rate is reduced by norepinephrine acting at alpha-adrenergic receptors. This is consistent with these cells receiving nicotinic-cholinergic input because norepinephrine acts presynaptically to prevent release of acetylcholine in myenteric ganglia (see Chemical Neurotransmission section). The pharmacological properties of these cells are significant because they are reminiscent of properties of classic parasympathetic postganglionic neurons.

Intracellular studies reveal that the equivalent of tonic-type neurons sometimes show ongoing, low-frequency discharge of single spikes (see section on Slow Synaptic Excitation). This intracellularly recorded activity reflects a tonic release of the putative neurotransmitter (5-hydroxytryptamine) because continuous electrical stimulation of the interganglionic fiber tracts at low frequencies (0.5 Hz) elicits maintained discharge of single spikes in these cells (181), and application of methysergide, which blocks postsynaptic receptors for 5-hydroxytryptamine, or norepinephrine, which prevents release of 5-hydroxytryptamine, stops the ongoing spike discharge. Intracellular studies also show ongoing discharge of single spikes in neurons that do not receive

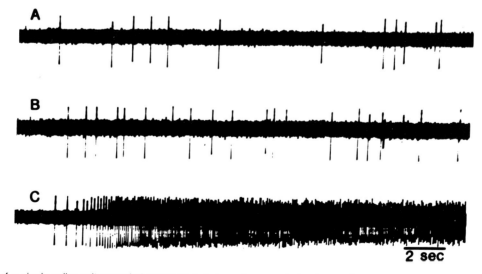

FIG. 12. Example of a single-spike unit recorded extracellularly from the myenteric plexus of cat small intestine. **A:** Ongoing discharge in Tyrode solution. **B:** Same after 5 min in Tyrode solution with an elevated concentration of 10.2 mM Mg^{2+} known to block synaptic transmission within the myenteric plexus. **C:** Same as **B** record begins 12 sec after application of nicotine (1 × 10^{-6} g/ml) in presence of elevated Mg^{2+}. Nicotine acts directly on neuron to increase spike discharge. From Wood (174).

serotonergic input. The conclusion from these observations is that extracellularly recorded single-spike activity probably does not represent a homogenous population of enteric neurons.

Properties Determined by Intracellular Recording

Membrane Properties of Enteric Neurons

The first intracellular studies of enteric neurons were done independently and reported almost simultaneously by Hirst and his associates (72,81) and by North and Nishi (113). The results of these investigations and of subsequent intracellular studies (181) show that there are two distinct types of enteric ganglion cells that are distinguished on the basis of the electrical behavior of the somal membranes (Fig. 13). The first type of ganglion cell was referred to as an AH neuron by Hirst et

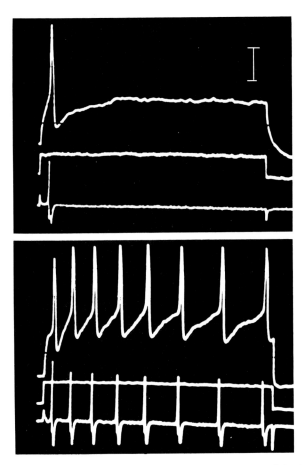

FIG. 13. Comparison of the responses evoked by intracellular injection of depolarizing current in an AH/type 2 neuron and an S/type 1 neuron in myenteric plexus of guinea pig small intestine. **Top:** Injection of a 200-msec duration depolarizing pulse evoked a single spike only at the onset of the current pulse in the AH/type 2 neuron. **Bottom:** Injection of a 200-msec duration depolarizing pulse evoked multiple spike discharges throughout the current pulse in the S/type 1 neuron. Upper trace is transmembrane voltage; middle trace is current; lower trace is dV/dt of membrane voltage. Vertical calibration 20 mV; 1 nA; 60 V/sec.

al. (72) and as a type 2 neuron by Nishi and North (118), and the second type was called an S cell by Hirst et al. and a type 1 neuron by Nishi and North. The terms AH/type 2 and S/type 1 are used here to distinguish the two kinds of ganglion cells. Most of the information of the following discussion has been obtained from guinea pig myenteric neurons; however, preliminary intracellular studies of cat myenteric neurons indicate that the general properties are similar (175).

The distinguishing characteristics of the AH/type 2 neurons are as follows: (a) a high resting membrane potential relative to S/type 1 neurons; (b) low input resistance relative to S/type 1 neurons; (c) discharge of one or two spikes only at the onset of prolonged depolarizing current pulses; (d) no anodal-break excitation at the termination of intracellularly injected hyperpolarizing current pulses; (e) long-duration hyperpolarizing after-potentials associated with action potential discharge; (f) tetrodotoxin-resistant action potentials.

The distinguishing characteristics of the S/type 1 neurons are the following: (a) a low resting membrane potential relative to AH/type 2 neurons; (b) high input resistance relative to AH/type 2 neurons; (c) discharge of spikes throughout a prolonged depolarizing current pulse with frequency of discharge a direct function of current intensity; (d) anodal-break excitation at the termination of intracellularly injected hyperpolarizing current pulse; (e) no hyperpolarizing after-potentials; and (f) tetrodotoxin-sensitive action potentials.

About one-fourth of the neurons of the myenteric plexus display high resting potentials and low input resistance relative to AH/type 2 neurons and cannot be induced to discharge spikes by depolarizing current when initially impaled. This kind of cell was referred to as a type 3 cell by Nishi and North (113) and was presumed to be a glial cell; however, after a 20- to 30-min wait (78) or after treatment with calcium antagonists (see below), many of these initially inexcitable cells turn out to be AH/type 2 neurons. Likewise, myenteric neurons are often encountered that have properties intermediate between the two major types. These neurons usually are found to be AH/type 2 neurons that are partially activated by ongoing release of 5-hydroxytryptamine within the ganglion (see below), because application of methysergide, which blocks serotonergic receptors, and catecholamines, which prevent presynaptic release of serotonin, produces a conversion to typical AH/type 2 behavior. Iontophoretic application of serotonin to AH/type 2 cells replicates this kind of increased excitability. These observations are presented here to point out that care must be exercised in interpreting intracellular recordings from these neurons, and not to suggest that S/type 1 neurons are simply serotonin-activated AH/type 2 neurons. Several lines of evidence discussed in the following sections indicate that the two neuronal types are distinctively different.

The prolonged hyperpolarizing potentials that follow spike discharge in the AH/type 2 neurons have important significance in the neurophysiology of the system. An average of about 35% of the myenteric neurons impaled during the reported studies show the hyperpolarizing after-potentials. AH/type 2 neurons are rare in the submucous plexus. The action potentials have positive after-potentials (hyperpolarizing overshoot of resting potential during the falling phase of the spike), and the prolonged postspike hyperpolarization starts 45 to 80 msec after the membrane potential returns to resting potential from the positive after-potential (Fig. 14). The duration of the hyperpolarizing after-potential can be up to 20 sec. The amplitude of the hyperpolarization summates as a direct function of the number of spikes

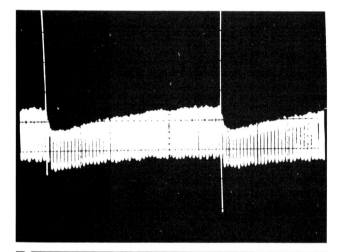

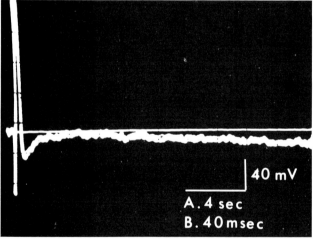

40 mV

A. 4 sec
B. 40 msec

FIG. 14. Intracellular recording of postspike hyperpolarization in an AH/type 2 myenteric neuron of guinea pig small bowel. **Top:** Two action potentials elicited by electrical stimulation of one of the cell's processes were followed by prolonged hyperpolarization of the cell membrane. Decreased amplitude of hyperpolarizing current pulses during hyperpolarization reflects a decrease in input resistance associated with the hyperpolarization. **Bottom:** Action potential and postspike hyperpolarization recorded with expanded time base from same. Note that prolonged hyperpolarization did not begin with the positive after-potential of the spike; its onset was delayed until 133 msec after the spike. From Wood and Mayer (181).

discharged. The input resistance is reduced during the after-hyperpolarization immediately following the spike and it progressively increases to resting level as the membrane depolarizes back to its resting level (Fig. 14). Strong evidence suggests that a calcium-triggered increase in the membrane potassium conductance accounts for the hyperpolarizing after-potentials (77,117). An inward calcium current appears to contribute to the rising phase of the action potential in the cell soma and to trigger the increase in potassium conductance. It is of interest that calcium antagonism by manganese and magnesium ions, but not the organic calcium antagonists D-600 and verapamil, block the calcium-triggered increase in potassium conductance. The functional significance of the postspike hyperpolarization is related to the decreased membrane resistance and hyperpolarization from spike threshold, which decrease the safety factor and probability of repetitive spike discharge by the cell soma.

Topographic Heterogeneity in Enteric Neurons

Unipolar ganglion cells occur within the enteric ganglia, but most of the neurons are multipolar. The results of intracellular studies indicate that the membrane properties and electrical behavior of the multipolar neurons are not the same in all topographic regions of the cell. This is analogous to some of the complexly branched neurons of invertebrate nervous systems where action potentials with different characteristics can originate independently at multiple sites, such as: (a) the cell soma; (b) the axon hillock; (c) a neurite between the axon hillock and axon branch point; (d) the individual axons; (e) the dendrites. It has not been possible, histologically or electrophysiologically, to distinguish between axons and dendrites or to precisely identify axon hillock regions of enteric neurons; nevertheless, the evidence presented below suggests that each multipolar neuron can be a multifunctional integrative unit with distinct kinds of integrative functions occurring in different topographic regions of the same neuron.

The membrane properties of the cell soma and the attached processes of myenteric neurons are distinctly different. The processes are readily excitable, as evidenced by electrotonic invasion of the soma by stimulus-evoked spikes in the processes (see Fig. 21) when the somal membranes are relatively inexcitable. Another indication of these differences is that tetrodotoxin, which specifically blocks sodium-dependent action potentials, always abolishes action potentials in the processes, but often does not block somal action potentials. This is like the ganglion cells of a number of invertebrate species in which the somal spikes are tetrodotoxin insensitive and supported by calcium, and the axon generates the classic sodium spike (164).

The spontaneous occurrence of patterned bursts of electrotonic spike potentials in the cell soma (see Fig. 9) is a reflection of spike activity that originates in regions of the nerve fibers remote from the soma, and is also an indication of multiple sites of spike initiation in these neurons.

There also appear to be topographical differences in excitability between the soma and initial segments of its processes which can be demonstrated by intrasomal injection of depolarizing current. Figure 15 illustrates an experiment in which the initial segment was more readily fired by intrasomal injection of depolarizing current than the soma. This, and the occurrence of spontaneous spikes in the initial segment, but not in the soma, indicated that the initial segment has a much higher safety factor for spike discharge than the somal membrane. In this circumstance, the multipolar soma effectively isolates the initial segments of each of the processes so that action potential discharge by one initial segment does not influence spike activity of another at an opposite pole of the soma. If independent excitatory synaptic input occurred at the initial segments, as indicated by ultrastructural and electrophysiological studies, this would allow independent spike initiation in each of the cell processes. This independence of the cell processes would

be advantageous in terms of neural economy, because one neuron would in effect be acting as several separate neurons depending on the number of processes. However, in specific functional states it might be necessary for all of the processes of the multipolar neuron to fire synchronously. Later discussion of synaptic transmission (see Fig. 21) will show how slow synaptic excitation of the cell soma greatly augments somal excitability and provides for synchronization of the processes by the soma.

CHEMICAL NEUROTRANSMISSION

Ultrastructure and electrophysiology of enteric neurons indicate synaptic mechanisms similar to those of the central nervous system. Both systems utilize many of the same neurotransmitter substances, and in some cases such as the opiate-like transmitter peptides, the enteric nervous system of the guinea pig is the model for the central action of the substances (42,149). The neurochemical similarities between the enteric nervous system and the brain no doubt reflect the neuroectodermal origin of the gut's control systems (133).

Both "fast" and "slow" synaptic potentials occur in enteric ganglion cells. The fast synaptic potentials have

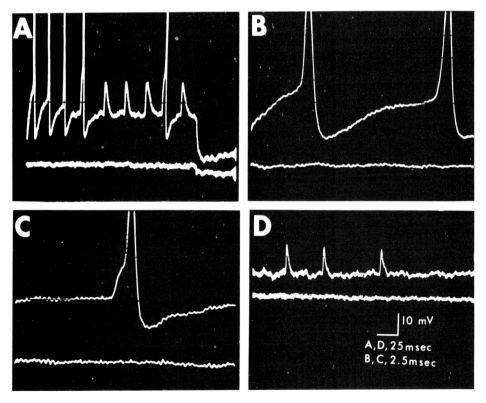

FIG. 15. Intracellular recording showing differential excitability between the membrane of the cell soma and one of its neurites in a guinea pig myenteric neuron. **A:** Intrasomatic injection of a depolarizing current pulse fired both the soma and the neurite; however, the neurite fired more often (low-amplitude electrotonic potentials) than the soma, indicating that the neurite was more excitable than the soma. **B:** Somal spike produced directly by the depolarizing current. **C:** Somal spike produced indirectly by the electrotonic spike spreading into the soma from the neurite during the depolarizing current pulse also indicates lower somal excitability relative to the neurite. **D:** Spontaneously occurring spikes in the neurite spread electrotonically into the soma of the same neuron. Spontaneous discharge of the neurite but not the soma also reflects differential excitability.

short duration less than 50 msec; whereas the slow synaptic potentials last for several seconds. Excitatory postsynaptic potentials (EPSPs) and inhibitory postsynaptic potentials (IPSPs) can be recorded in enteric neurons, and both may occur spontaneously or can be evoked by electrical stimulation of presynaptic fibers.

All of the intracellular studies on enteric synaptic transmission have been done on guinea pig small bowel, with the exception of a few preliminary studies of cat myenteric neurons in my laboratory. Therefore, the bulk of the experimental data, on which the following discussion is based, was obtained from the guinea pig small intestine.

Fast Synaptic Potentials

Fast EPSPs occur in ganglion cells of both the myenteric and submucous plexuses. They are most prominent in S/type 1 neurons, but occur in AH/type 2 neurons also. Earlier workers indicated that fast EPSPs did not occur in AH/type 2 neurons (72,113); however, subsequent studies have shown that AH/type 2 neurons do receive fast synaptic input (61). Fast EPSPs in AH/type 2 neurons usually have smaller amplitudes than the EPSPs in S/type 1 neurons, and computerized signal averaging techniques often are required to demonstrate them (61). Low amplitude of the EPSPs in AH/type 2 neurons probably reflects synaptic input to a region of the cell distal to the recording site within the cell body, perhaps at the cone-like initial segments from which multiple processes are often observed to arise (52).

All of the fast EPSPs that are recorded in somas of cat and guinea pig enteric neurons appear to be mediated by acetylcholine acting at nicotinic-cholinergic receptors. Acetylcholine esterase inhibitors prolong the EPSPs, and nicotinic blocking drugs such as hexamethonium and d-tubocurarine reduce or abolish the EPSPs. Large concentrations of the nicotinic blockers on the order of 1×10^{-4} M are required to significantly reduce the EPSPs. Whether this is related to barriers to entrance of the drugs or to low affinity of the drugs for the ganglionic receptors is unclear.

A noteworthy characteristic of the fast EPSPs is a tendency for the amplitude of the EPSPs to become progressively smaller when they are evoked repetitively by electrical stimulation of the ganglion (Fig. 16). This rundown in amplitude occurs at stimulus frequencies as low as 0.1 Hz, and the rate of rundown is a direct function of stimulus frequency. The mechanism of the synaptic rundown is unclear; a postsynaptic mechanism is not involved because no rundown occurs during repeated iontophoretic applications of acetylcholine. Rundown may be a reflection of presynaptic inhibition of acetylcholine release by additional transmitter substances that are released within the ganglion during electrical stimulation, and so rundown may be only an ex-

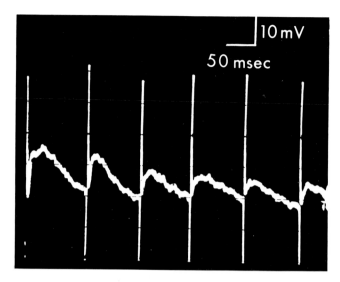

FIG. 16. Rundown in amplitude of fast EPSPs evoked by repetitive stimulation of a presynaptic fiber to a guinea pig myenteric neuron. Vertical transients are stimulus artifacts which are followed by the EPSP.

perimental artifact (see section on presynaptic inhibition). The rate of rundown is often directly related to the strength of the stimulus pulses and sometimes does not occur if the stimulus strength is reduced to just threshold for the EPSP. This is consistent with the idea that the stimulus pulses release additional substances that prevent acetylcholine release from the presynaptic terminals.

Multiple cholinergic inputs converge on the ganglion cells and both spatial and temporal summation of the inputs occur. These inputs appear to be transmitted from widespread sites within the plexus because in some neurons an EPSP can be evoked by electrical stimulation of each of as many as five different interganglionic fiber tracts which enter the ganglion.

Slow Synaptic Excitation

Electrical stimulation of the interganglionic fiber tracts of the myenteric plexus evokes a slow-rising depolarizing potential (slow EPSP) that is prolonged for an average of 88 sec after termination of the stimulus. (Fig. 17). The slow EPSP occurs only in AH/type 2 neurons, and it is associated with increased input resistance and augmented excitability of the somal membrane. The augmented excitability has the following characteristics: (a) the neuron discharges a prolonged train of action potentials that continues for several seconds after termination of the stimulus; (b) intracellular injection of a depolarizing current pulse elicits repetitive spike discharge throughout the current pulse (Fig. 17); (c) electrotonic spike potentials spreading from the processes into the cell soma trigger somal action potentials (see Fig. 21); (d) the characteristic postspike hy-

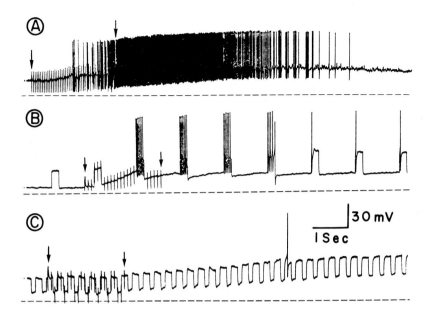

FIG. 17. Slow synaptic excitation in an AH/type 2 myenteric neuron of guinea pig small intestine. **4:** Slow EPSP and spike discharge elicited by electrical stimulation of the interganglionic fiber tract (arrows indicate onset and offset of stimulus pulse train). **B:** Electrical stimulation of the fiber tract caused an increase in excitability as indicated by spike discharge throughout constant current depolarizing pulses of 0.4 nA. **C:** Fiber tract stimulation during repetitive injection of constant-current hyperpolarizing pulses (0.3 nA). Increased input resistance was reflected by increased amplitude of electrotonic potentials following fiber tract stimulation. Membrane potential was held 18 mV more negative than resting potential by steady injection of hyperpolarizing current to prevent spikes at the offset of current pulses. One such spike still occurred.

perpolarizing potentials of AH/type 2 neurons are greatly reduced or abolished (Fig. 18).

The prolonged trains of spikes that occur during the slow EPSP are reminiscent of the spike trains recorded extracellularly in the tonic-type mechanosensitive neurons (Fig. 11) suggesting that the AH/type 2 may be the intracellularly recorded counterpart of the tonic-type units.

Several lines of evidence suggest that the neurotransmitter for the slow EPSP is 5-hydroxytryptamine. The evidence for this can be summarized as follows: (a) Some of the effects of serotonin on contractile activity of the musculature of intestinal segments *in vitro* are blocked by tetrodotoxin, suggesting that these actions are neurally mediated (17,19). (b) Multiunit extracellular records from myenteric neurons show an increase in rate of spike discharge after addition of serotonin to the organ bath (39). (c) Application of serotonin to the myenteric plexus produces an increase in the release of acetylcholine, which is presumably a reflection of increased firing of cholinergic neurons (163). (d) Serotonin, tryptophan hydroxylase, and serotonin binding protein are present within myenteric neurons (45,58,90,153). (e) Myenteric neurons synthesize serotonin from the precursor tryptophan (40). (f) Release of tritium-labeled serotonin and its binding protein occurs during transmural electrical stimulation of intestinal segments *in vitro,* and this release is blocked by tetrodotoxin (89). (g) Microiontophoretic application of

serotonin to the AH/type 2 neurons mimics the stimulus-evoked slow EPSP (183). Both the endogenous transmitter substance and exogenous serotonin produce membrane depolarization, both increase the input resistance of the neuron, both reduce or abolish the hyperpolarizing after-potentials of the spike, and both augment membrane excitability. (h) During tachyphylaxis to excess serotonin in the superfusion solution, the stimulus-evoked slow EPSP is blocked. (i) The serotonin blocking drug, methysergide, prevents both the slow EPSP and the response to exogenous serotonin. (j) A high-affinity uptake mechanism for serotonin, which could accomplish termination of action at the postsynaptic membranes, is associated with myenteric neurons (41).

The mechanism for slow synaptic excitation in the myenteric plexus appears to be a synaptically mediated decrease in the resting membrane conductance for potassium ions that is reflected by an increase in the input resistance of the cell. The reversal potential for the slow EPSP is between −70 and −75 mV, which is near the potassium equilibrium potential. It would be possible also for a transmitter-mediated decrease in chloride conductance to account for the depolarization and increased input resistance of the slow EPSP; however, this possibility is excluded by lack of effect of removal of chloride from the Ringer solution.

The high resting potassium conductance in the AH/type 2 neurons appears to be calcium-dependent, and

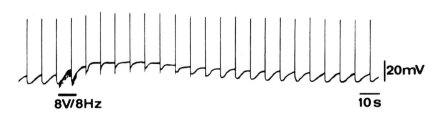

FIG. 18. Reduction of postspike hyperpolarizing potentials during the slow EPSP in AH/type 2 myenteric neuron in guinea pig small intestine. Spikes were elicited continuously by intracellular injection of depolarizing current pulses of sufficiently short duration to elicit only a single spike. Horizontal bar indicates application of stimulus pulse train.

both the neurotransmitter for the slow EPSP and serotonin appear to decrease resting potassium conductance by interfering with the availability of calcium. Accumulated evidence obtained mainly from invertebrate neurons indicates that the resting permeability of some neuronal membranes for potassium is a direct function of the concentration of free calcium in the cytoplasm (28,108). Resting potassium conductance in AH/type 2 neurons appears also to be calcium dependent because application of di- and trivalent cations (e.g., manganese, magnesium, and lanthanum) that impede transmembrane movement of calcium and block calcium-dependent processes mimics the stimulus-evoked slow EPSP and the action of exogenous serotonin (176). The characteristics common to both the slow EPSP and the effects of calcium-antagonistic ions are as follows: (a) depolarization of the membrane potential; (b) increased input resistance; (c) augmented excitability; (d) reduction or blockade of postspike hyperpolarizing potentials; and (e) a reversal potential between −70 and −75 mV. Results of experiments in which the relationship between the extracellular concentration of potassium and the membrane potential were compared in Krebs solution and in Krebs solution with elevated magnesium and reduced calcium are consistent with the calcium-dependent potassium conductance hypothesis (Fig. 19). These results show that at all points on the plots below 50 mM potassium, the slope of the curve in Krebs solution with normal calcium and magnesium is much steeper than the slope of the curve for solution containing elevated magnesium and reduced calcium. This indicates that resting potassium conductance is reduced in elevated magnesium, low calcium solution, and this can account for the increased input resistance that occurs when the neurons are in elevated magnesium solutions.

It is noteworthy that the organic calcium antagonists verapamil and D-600, which block transmembrane calcium fluxes in cardiac and smooth muscles, do not affect the calcium-dependent potassium conductance in myenteric neurons.

Figure 20 shows an equivalent circuit model for the slow EPSP. The somas of AH/type 2 neurons function between extremes of low and high excitability. The low-excitability state is related to high resting membrane conductance for potassium that is dependent on availability of cytoplasmic calcium. The probability of occurrence of an action potential in this state is low; if a spike should occur, additional calcium enters the cell during the rising phase of the action potential and further activates potassium conductance. This in turn produces hyperpolarizing after-spike potentials which restrict repetitive spike discharge. Conversion to high excitability occurs when the chemical transmitter for the slow EPSP reduces the level of free intracellular calcium and secondarily decreases resting potassium conductance. The mechanism by which the chemical transmitter might reduce the concentration of intracellular free calcium is unclear. Both the transmitter and serotonin appear to block the calcium channels that are opened during an action potential, and it may be that they also block channels that in the resting state carry a steady influx of calcium. It might be that only a single calcium channel is involved and because of voltage dependency of the channel, more channels are opened during the action potential. Despite the uncertainty of the cellular mechanisms, it is likely that slow synaptic modulation of excitability is mediated by neurotransmitter or possibly also paracrine suppression of calcium-dependent potassium conductance.

The functional significance of the slow EPSP in AH/type 2 neurons has two major aspects. The first is the

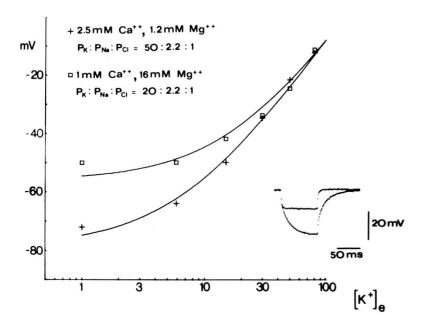

FIG. 19. Relationship between the resting membrane potential of an AH/type 2 myenteric neuron and the logarithm of external potassium concentration in the presence and absence of elevated magnesium. The "constant field" equation was used to fit the solid lines to the data points. The following intracellular ion concentrations (mM) were inserted into the constant field equation: $K^+ = 140$; $Na^+ = 10$; $Cl^- = 10$. The permeability ratios that were used for plotting each curve are given. The *inset* shows superimposed the averaged electrotonic potentials produced by injection of constant-current hyperpolarizing pulses in Krebs solution *(top trace)* and in Krebs solution with elevated Mg^{2+} and reduced Ca^{2+} *(bottom trace).* Increased amplitude of bottom trace indicates increased input resistance which reflects decreased potassium permeability.

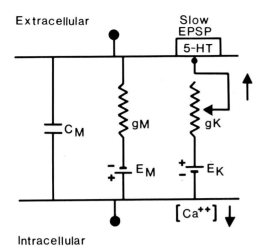

Extracellular

Slow
EPSP

Intracellular

FIG. 20. Equivalent electrical circuit for the slow EPSP in an AH/type 2 myenteric neuron. The high resting potential and low input resistance characteristic of these neurons are reflections of a high potassium conductance (gK) associated with increased levels of free intracellular Ca^{2+}. Activation of the serotonergic receptor decreases free intracellular Ca^{2+}, producing an increase in the resistance of the gK channel, a reduction in gK, and membrane depolarization. C_M is membrane capacitance and gM represents the other ionic conductances of the membrane.

significance intuitively attributed to an excitatory synapse. That is, an increased probability of spike discharge in the postsynaptic neuron, which is then transformed into excitation or inhibition at either the next order neuron or an effector. Intestinal peristalsis, for example, requires sustained discharge by some type of enteric neuron in order to account for the delays of several seconds between stimulus and coordinated responses and to account for sustained neural influence at the effector. The behavior of AH/type 2 neurons during the slow EPSP fits the requirements for a neuronal unit whose functional significance would be production of either prolonged excitation or inhibition at neuronal and neuro-effector junctions within the gut wall. Serotonin stimulates the release of acetylcholine from the myenteric plexus (163), and it is probable that the AH/type 2 neurons either are cholinergic motor neurons or provide synaptic drive to cholinergic motor neurons. Motility studies on isolated segments of guinea pig small bowel indicate that train-like discharge of AH/type 2 neurons is not associated with poststimulus rebound excitation of the circular muscle, and they indicate also that these cells are neither the intrinsic inhibitory neurons (see section on neural control of effectors) nor drivers of the intrinsic inhibitory neuron (161).

The second functional aspect of the behavior of the cell soma of AH/type 2 neurons is provision of a mechanism by which the soma of the multipolar neuron gates or switches the spread of excitation between the processes that arise from opposite poles of the soma (Fig. 21). Intracellular recording from the soma shows that extracellular stimulation of the ganglion cell's processes elicits spikes that electrotonically invade the soma, and also that spontaneously occurring spike patterns in the processes spread electrotonically into the soma (see Fig. 9). The probability that the passive current flow from

FIG. 21. Functional significance of the slow EPSP in an AH/type 2 myenteric neuron. **A–D:** Intracellular recordings of progressive changes in electrotonic potentials within the soma during repetitive stimulation of the fiber tract. Shocks were applied to the fiber tract at a frequency of 1 Hz, and **A** through **D** represent the 1st, 5th, 8th, and 10th stimuli, respectively. Note that the amplitude of the electrotonic potentials increased and the rate of decay decreased as the slow EPSP developed with consecutive stimulus pulses. In **D**, spike threshold was reached and the soma fired a spike. **E:** Diagram of the experiment. An intracellular electrode *(2)* recorded electrical changes within the soma *(1)*. Fiber tract stimulation *(4)* activated both the cell's axon *(3)* and presynaptic fibers to the cell *(5)*. The somal membrane had low resistance due to high resting gK, and antidromic spikes from the axon *(3)* produced only small electrotonic potentials in the soma **(A).** During repetitive stimulation of the presynaptic fiber *(5)*, the slow EPSP and associated increase in resistance and time constant of the somal membrane were reflected by increased amplitude and decreased rate of decay of the electrotonic potentials **(B, C).** These observations suggest that the soma functions as a gate which permits transmission of spike information from its dendrites *(1)* to axons *(3)* only during the slow EPSP. The presynaptic fibers for the slow EPSP project from an adjacent ganglion, and the axon of the AH/type 2 neuron projects to the adjacent ganglion, thereby establishing bidirectional flow of information between the two ganglia. Electrical records were plotted from computer memory. The initial downward deflection is the stimulus artifact. Vertical calibration: 20 mV. Horizontal calibration: 2 msec. From Wood and Mayer (182).

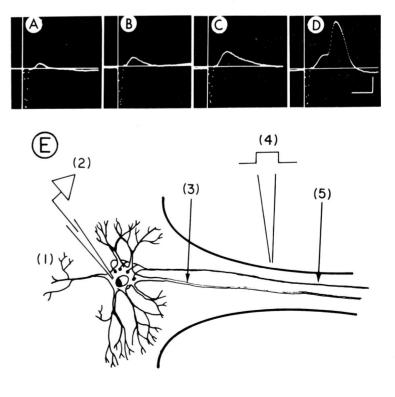

these axonal or dendritic spikes will trigger a somal action potential is low in the absence of the neurotransmitter for the slow EPSP and is increased during the augmented excitability of the slow EPSP. Thus the spike activity associated with information processing in the synaptic neuropil is restricted to single processes of the cell in the absence of the slow EPSP; whereas during the slow EPSP, the soma relays spike information in one neurite to all other neurites arising from other poles of the cell. If the neurons were multiaxonal (this is not known), discharge of all axons would be synchronized during the slow EPSP.

The increase in membrane resistance during the slow EPSP increases the space constant of the somal membrane and facilitates the spread of electrical activity from the processes into the soma. This, and the augmented excitability of the somal membrane, both account for the increased probability of passive current spread from axonal or dendritic spikes triggering a somal spike during the slow EPSP. This may be the mechanism that underlies transfer of information between adjacent ganglia within the neural plexus. The simultaneous occurrence of both the slow EPSP and an electrotonic or initial segment spike in the soma of the neurons during electrical stimulation of an interganglionic fiber tract indicates that the neuron from which the recording is made sends one of its processes in the fiber tract to the adjacent ganglion and, in turn, receives synaptic input from an axon projecting into the same fiber tract from an adjacent ganglion (Fig. 21). This connectivity would enable a neuron in one ganglion to activate the soma of a second neuron in another ganglion to switch ongoing electrical activity in the dendrites of the second neuron to its axon which projects in the fiber tract to the adjacent ganglion. In effect, the specialized properties of the AH/type 2 neurons and their synaptic input provide a mechanism whereby the integrative circuitry of one ganglion can control the information input it receives from an adjacent ganglion. This is probably basic to the regulation of spread of neural information within the plexus and to the behavior of the effectors that the plexus controls.

A few additional points about the slow EPSP and AH/type 2 neurons need to be made before proceeding to other aspects of chemical neurotransmission. These relate to the desensitizing action of relatively low concentrations of serotonin on the neurons and to the action of substance P on the neurons.

Application of substance P to the myenteric neurons mimics the slow EPSP in some aspects (60,92). Substance P depolarizes the neurons and increases the input resistance, but does not reduce the postspike hyperpolarizing potentials in AH/type 2 neurons. Substance P has been detected in myenteric neurons by immunocytochemical techniques (112,132); however, it does not appear to be the neurotransmitter for the slow EPSP

because drugs that block the slow EPSP and the action of serotonin do not affect the action of substance P (60).

The enterochromaffin cells within the intestinal mucosa contain both serotonin and substance P (43,70). The intestine is the source of a large fraction of the substance P in the systemic circulation (54), and levels of serotonin in the venous blood of the hepatic portal system have been reported to reach a concentration of 1 μM after acidification of the duodenum (93,98). This raises the possibility that substance P and serotonin released from mucosal enterochromaffin cells could function as locally acting hormones (i.e., paracrine function). The slow EPSP is blocked by desensitizing concentrations of serotonin (1 μM) that are the same as the levels of serotonin in the portal blood induced by acidification of the duodenum. This suggests that the desensitization phenomenon might have functional significance with important implications for understanding both normal function and pathophysiological states such as carcinoid syndrome in which circulating levels of serotonin and substance P are elevated.

Substance P and serotonin also coexist within the same synaptic vesicles in the brain (25), as well as in enterochromaffin cells of the gut. The functional significance of this close histochemical association between the two substances, like the similarity of action on the myenteric neurons, is unclear. It might be that they modulate neuronal excitability in subtly different ways because serotonin, but not substance P, blocks the postspike hyperpolarizing potentials that limit repetitive discharge. It is known that increased membrane resistance during slow EPSPs in other neuronal systems increases the probability that a fast EPSP will depolarize a neuron to spike threshold (166). Substance P function could be limited to augmentation of the excitability of the initial segments to fast EPSP inputs and could be related to transmission of low-frequency spike discharge by the soma.

A final point about serotonergic desensitization directs attention to the pitfalls of attempting to deduce physiological significance from organ bath pharmacology of contractile responses of segments of bowel in which the neural receptors are "flooded" with putative neurotransmitter substances. Seven years ago, in my laboratory, we screened a number of putative neurotransmitters for effects on extracellularly recorded electrical activity of myenteric neurons and did not detect the action of serotonin on the neurons because the neurons were desensitized by the presence of 1 μM serotonin. Many attempts to understand the role of serotonin in gut function have been unsuccessful and confused also because the exact action of serotonin could not be learned solely from organ bath studies of contractile responses. An example of this is the generally accepted concept that methysergide blocks only serotonergic receptors on the smooth muscle (63); the intracellular studies of myenteric neurons show that this is not the case. Much of the large volume of literature on the pharmacology of gastrointestinal motility is difficult to interpret because the exact sites and kinds of actions of pharmacological agents on enteric neurons and the functional state of the neurons cannot be deduced adequately from contractile responses to drugs. It is historically unfortunate that information on function at the cellular level could not be obtained in parallel with the many descriptive studies that have been made of gastrointestinal motility patterns. Professor Mollie E. Holman, in an earlier review (80), emphasized that techniques are now available for obtaining information at the cellular level, and she encouraged expansion of the application of these techniques for the sake of adequate progress in understanding of gastrointestinal physiology. Presently only a few laboratories around the world are studying the electrophysiology of enteric neurons, and there is a need for expansion of this kind of research.

Inhibitory Postsynaptic Potentials

Inhibitory synaptic potentials (IPSPs) have been recorded in both myenteric and submucosal ganglion cells in guinea pig small bowel (75,181). Electrical stimulation evokes IPSPs in both myenteric and submucosal neurons, whereas spontaneously occurring IPSPs have as yet been reported only for myenteric neurons (181). IPSPs are not often observed in day-to-day intracellular studies of myenteric neurons, whereas about 30% of submucosal neurons show an IPSP when electrical field stimulation is applied.

The characteristics of the IPSP in submucosal neurons are inverse to those of the slow EPSP in myenteric neurons, but the time-related characteristics of the two are similar. Stimulus-evoked IPSPs in submucosal neurons are slowly developing hyperpolarizing potentials which continue for 1 to 5 sec after termination of the stimulus. The IPSPs occur in the equivalent of S/type 1 neurons and result from a single synaptic input to the cell. As in the case of the slow EPSP, "single input" may be a misnomer because these potentials might result from an *en passant* release of transmitter from several synaptic varicosities of a single axon entwined around the cell soma. The stimulus threshold for evoking the IPSP is higher than the threshold for eliciting cholinergic EPSPs in the cells. The IPSPs are associated with a decrease in the input resistance of the cell. The reversal potential for the IPSP is about -86 mV, suggesting that the decrease in input resistance can be accounted for by a transmitter-induced increase in potassium conductance.

The putative neurotransmitter substance for the IPSP is a catecholamine (76). Microiontophoresis of both norepinephrine and dopamine mimics the stimulus-evoked IPSP, but only on the neurons that receive the inhibiting synaptic input. Guanethidine, a drug which prevents release of catecholamines from adrenergic nerve terminals, blocks the IPSP. Both the stimulus-evoked IPSP and the effects of norepinephrine and dopamine are prevented by methysergide. According to Hirst and Silinsky (76), the beta-adrenergic blocking drug propranolol does not affect the action of norepinephrine. There are no reports that alpha-adrenergic blocking drugs have been tested on this preparation. Methysergide does not block mammalian adrenergic receptors, and Hirst and Silinsky are of the opinion that the submucosal neurons may behave like molluscan neurons where methysergide blocks the inhibitory action of dopamine. The IPSP persists in sympathetically denervated loops of intestine, suggesting that if the neurotransmitter for the IPSP is indeed a catecholamine it is released from catecholaminergic fibers intrinsic to the enteric nervous system, rather than from terminals of postganglionic sympathetic neurons. There is no evidence that the cell body of the neuron that releases the inhibitory transmitter is located in the submucous plexus. However, there is evidence that amine-accumulating neurons are located within myenteric ganglia (56).

Serotonin has been ruled out as an inhibitory transmitter in the submucous plexus because its action is always a depolarization associated with decreased input resistance (76).

Hirst and McKirdy (73) have suggested that the functional significance of the IPSP is to delay the onset of descending excitation of cholinergic motor neurons during the peristaltic reflex. Slow synaptic inhibition may function to check the spread of neural information along the plexus; whereas slow EPSPs have the opposite function of facilitating spread of neural signals.

The results of the intracellular studies on submucousal neurons do not support the classic view that the submucous plexus contains only sensory neurons.

Peptidergic Neurotransmission

Immunocytochemical techniques reveal that the peptides substance P, vasoactive intestinal peptide, enkephalin, and somatostatin are present inside enteric neurons. Substance P has been mentioned earlier as a putative neuromodulatory substance, and there is a growing feeling that the latter three peptides also function as chemical messengers in neural control of gut activity.

The action of the enkephalins and somatostatin on the electrical behavior of myenteric neurons has been investigated and will be discussed below. However, before proceeding with this, it is emphasized that the mere presence of an immunoreactive peptide in a neuron should not be construed as evidence of functional significance as a messenger molecule. A variety of peptides that are found in the mammalian brain and gastrointestinal tract (e.g., somatostatin, substance P, and bombesin) are immunologically or chemically similar to peptides in frog skin. Although these occur in abundance in the amphibian skin, they have no effects on skin functions such as melanophore dispersion, mucus secretion, or sodium-potassium ATPase production. Enteric neurons, gastrointestinal endocrine cells, and some of the skin constituents have a common developmental origin from the embryonic neural crest, and the presence of immunologically similar peptides in all of these cell types may reflect only parsimony of genetic templates for protein synthesis. Proof of messenger function for a particular peptide molecule requires evidence that a physiological stimulus releases the peptide and that the peptide is a ligand at a receptor on the target cell.

Enkephalins and Endorphins

Enkephalins and endorphins are endogenous neural peptides that have opioid activity in both the brain and gastrointestinal tract. Opioid activity means that in particular bioassay systems (e.g., guinea pig ileum) these peptides mimic the action of morphine and other active stereoisomers of opiate alkaloids, and that the action is antagonized by pure opiate antagonists such as naloxone. There are two enkephalins and three endorphins, some of which appear to be derived from a common precursor protein.

The enkephalins are pentapeptides. Both enkephalins have the same N-terminal tetrapeptide sequence and vary only by having methionine or leucine in the C-terminal position: hence one is called met-enkephalin and the other leu-enkephalin.

Endorphin is the generic name used for all opioid peptides including the enkephalins. There are three additional opioid peptides which are named α-endorphin, β-endorphin, and γ-endorphin. Respectively, these are composed of amino acid residues 61 to 71, 61 to 91, and 61 to 76 of a 91-residue protein called β-lipotropin. Residues 61 to 65 of β-lipotropin have the same amino acid sequence as met-enkephalin. β-Lipotropin itself has no opioid activity. The β-form appears to be the major endorphin that is stored in neurons. Enkephalins and β-endorphin are present in the brain and gastrointestinal wall but are not present in the same cells. The significance of this is unresolved, as is the question of whether some of the naturally occurring opioid agonists are actually precursors of the "true" agonist molecule. Likewise, little is known about how peptidases might separate a peptide transmitter from its parent molecule and how peptidases terminate the action at the target cell receptors.

The principal action of morphine, met- and leu-enkephalin, and β-endorphin on myenteric neurons of cat and guinea pig small intestine is suppression of electrical excitability of the cell soma (118,120,122,175). Both the probability that a fast EPSP will trigger a spike in the cell soma and repetitive discharge during intracellularly injected depolarizing current are greatly reduced by morphine. This action of opiates and opioid peptides is associated with membrane hyperpolarization that appears to reflect increased membrane conductance for potassium ions. Experimental conditions with blockade of neurotransmitter release show that the action of these substances is directly on the neurons and not mediated by release of an inhibitory transmitter substance or prevention of ongoing release of an excitatory transmitter (38,123,175).

Fast cholinergic EPSPs in myenteric neurons are unaffected by morphine (119,122,175), suggesting that activation of opiate receptors does not directly affect cholinergic synaptic transmission between myenteric neurons. Morphine also does not suppress generation of spikes in the neuronal processes, indicating that the opiate receptors are restricted to or very near to the cell body. The well-known morphine action of prevention of acetylcholine release from the myenteric plexus is probably related to suppression of somal excitability. Nevertheless, the possibility that morphine might act directly on the axon terminals of cholinergic motor neurons to prevent release of acetylcholine cannot be eliminated with the evidence at hand.

The opiate action is most readily demonstrated on the S/type 1 myenteric neurons. It is not yet clear whether the opiate receptors are restricted to this type of neuron. The high resting potentials and low membrane excitability of AH/type 2 myenteric neurons do not appear to reflect action of tonically released opioid peptides because naloxone does not depolarize and increase excitability of this type of neuron. In a few preliminary experiments, we have not observed any depressant action of morphine on the slow EPSP of the AH/type 2 neurons. If this is confirmed, it indicates that antagonistic slow excitatory and inhibitory modulation does not occur on the same neuron. Instead, it suggests that the somas of AH/type 2 neurons normally present a "closed gate" to transmission of information and that the gate is transiently opened during the slow EPSP; whereas S/type 1 neurons normally present an "open gate" to transmission which might be closed by activation of opiate receptors. The opiate antagonist naloxone has not yet been tested for blocking action on spontaneous and stimulus-evoked IPSPs that occur in enteric neurons. A finding of blockade of IPSPs by naloxone would greatly reinforce this concept of gating function.

There is much more to be learned about opioid messenger function within the enteric nervous system, and this deserves concentrated investigation because it is most likely that the constipating changes in intestinal motility produced by morphine and opiate-like agents occur because the substances mimic the neural action of the endogenous opioids (see section on neural control of effectors).

Somatostatin

Somatostatin is a tetradecapeptide which occurs within myenteric neurons and represents another potential transmitter or neuromodulator. The action of somatostatin on electrical behavior of myenteric neurons has been studied only with extracellular recording techniques (167). These studies show that somatostatin suppressed the ongoing spike discharge of most myenteric ganglion cells. The effective concentrations are the same as required for suppression of growth hormone release from pituitary cells. Somatostatin suppresses electrically induced release of acetylcholine from the myenteric plexus (62), and this action does not appear to involve opiate receptors. It has also been reported that somatostatin activates intrinsic inhibitory neurons and relaxes the circular muscle (49). Further study is required to determine if somatostatin functions as a neurotransmitter in the enteric nervous system.

Vasoactive Intestinal Polypeptide

Vasoactive intestinal polypeptide (VIP) is also suspected of being an enteric neurotransmitter. Immunocytochemical studies show intrinsic VIP-containing terminals that appear to innervate ganglion cells in both the myenteric and submucous plexuses (50). The VIP-containing neurons, like the previously mentioned peptidergic neurons, are probably interneurons, although no studies of the effects of VIP on electrical behavior of enteric neurons have been reported. A proposal that VIP is the transmitter released by intrinsic inhibitory neurons at neuromuscular junctions of the gut has been made on the basis of immunocytochemical observations of the distribution of VIP in the gut (13,85). This is unlikely because VIP does not mimic the inhibitory responses in the muscle that are evoked by electrical stimulation of the intrinsic inhibitory neurons (27).

Presynaptic Inhibition

This specialized form of synaptic transmission reflects the inhibition of the release of neurotransmitters by the transsynaptic action of a transmitter released from one axonal terminal acting on another, i.e., axoaxonal synapses. Presynaptic inhibition within myenteric ganglia functions to prevent the release of acetylcholine, serotonin, and perhaps additional unidentified neurotransmitters from their storage depots in presynaptic axonal terminals.

Intracellular recording from guinea pig myenteric neurons shows that application of norepinephrine in the superfusion solution blocks the fast cholinergic EPSPs evoked by electrical stimulation, but does not affect the depolarizing response of the neuron to iontophoretically applied acetylcholine (74,113). Likewise, norepinephrine blocks the stimulus-evoked slow EPSP, but does not affect the action of exogenously applied serotonin (184). This suggests that norephinephrine acts at adrenergic receptors on the cholinergic and serotonergic nerve terminals to prevent release of the respective transmitter substances. This action of norepinephrine is prevented by alpha-adrenergic blocking drugs, suggesting that the presynaptic adrenergic receptors are alpha receptors. Dopamine has the same action as norepinephrine on the serotonergic terminals.

Evidence for presynaptic inhibition within the enteric nervous system has also been obtained by the indirect experimental method of measuring the release of acetylcholine from a segment of intestine *in vitro* (95,144). These experiments show that muscarinic cholinergic agonists (e.g., oxotremorine) reduce the release of acetylcholine, and atropine reverses this effect as well as producing an increase in acetylcholine output. This suggests that released acetylcholine "feeds back" on presynaptic muscarinic cholinergic receptors and reduces further release of acetylcholine.

Purine nucleotides and nucleosides also reduce the release of acetylcholine from the myenteric plexus, and this has prompted the proposal that presynaptic purinergic receptors function to inhibit the release of acetylcholine from axonal terminals (29,68,127,162). The effects of the purine compounds on acetylcholine release are antagonized by theophylline and potentiated by dipyridamole. The action of theophylline is thought to be competitive receptor blockade, and dipyridamole is believed to prevent uptake of adenosine and thus prolong its action at the receptor.

Whether these presynaptic actions of muscarinic agonists and purines occur at neural synapses, at the neuromuscular appositions, or both is unknown. This requires further investigation with direct electrical recording from the ganglion cells to determine if muscarinic agonists and the purines suppress fast cholinergic EPSPs and whether the characteristic "rundown" of the fast EPSP during repetitive stimulation (see earlier section on synaptic transmission) results from presynaptic inhibition produced by endogenous release of these substances.

Presynaptic inhibition demonstrates further the complexity of synaptic interactions within the enteric nervous system. It exemplifies also the futility of attempting to understand the neural mechanisms of control of gastrointestinal motor activity solely on the basis of the usual experimental methods of organ bath pharmacology and transmural electrical stimulation. Complexities arise, for example, with utilization of pharmacological tools such as anticholinesterases which permit accumulation of acetylcholine not only at neuroeffector junctions but also at presynaptic terminals where negative feedback may reduce further release of acetylcholine. Likewise, massive activation of intramural nerve elements with electrical field stimulation no doubt releases a melange of endogenous messenger substances with presynaptic and postsynaptic actions that ultimately produce effector responses that have little relation to normal neurophysiological control.

NEURAL CONTROL OF EFFECTOR FUNCTION

The enteric nervous system can be conceived of as an independent integrative system with neurophysiological properties analogous to those of a central nervous system; especially the "simple" ganglia that control motor behavior of invertebrate animals (173). The enteric nervous system, like the other integrative systems, can be subdivided into three functional divisions for purposes of discussion. Sensory mechanisms constitute the first subdivision. Sensory receptors within the gut transduce changes in mechanical and chemical energy into a steady flow of neural information that is transmitted in the form of coded action potentials along afferent fibers to processing centers within the enteric ganglia and the central nervous system. The second subdivision consists of internuncial circuitry (the central computer) which processes the sensory information and generates appropriate signals for controlling the outflow of commands in motor neurons to the effector systems. Internuncial circuitry also contains neural networks that are programmed to generate cyclical stereotyped patterns of motor behavior that are not built on a series of reflexes. Instead, the role of sensory feedback to these networks is one of adjustment and modulation of the pattern generated by the "hardwired" program. Motor neurons represent the third functional division of an integrative system. Discharge of the motor neurons represents the final decision of the integrative circuitry and the final common pathway from the nervous system to the effector.

The ultimate function of the enteric nervous system is to control and coordinate the activity of the various gastrointestinal effector systems. The nature of the neural control is expected to be dictated by the functional properties of the effector. Consequently, the functional properties of the effectors provide many clues to the mechanisms by which the effector is nervously controlled. The scheme in the remainder of this section will be to discuss first the functional properties of the effector and relate them to neural control and to then consider the three functional subdivisions of the

nervous system. Much will be said about neural control of the gastrointestinal musculature and motor function because considerable information is available. In contrast, knowledge of the neurophysiology of intrinsic control of other gastrointestinal effectors and processes, such as mucosal transport, is meager or nonexistent; and although these represent important functions, not much can be said about them.

Effector Systems

Coordination of secretory activity, mucosal transport, blood flow, and motility is required for efficient progression of the digestive processes, and there are many indications that the enteric nervous system has a major role in unifying these functions. Tactile stimulation of the intestinal mucosa reflexly stimulates both mucus secretion and secretion of fluid into the intestinal lumen (24,105). It is known that putative neurotransmitters (e.g., serotonin, VIP, and acetylcholine) activate various kinds of gastrointestinal secretory cells; however, there is no information on the neurophysiology of the involved circuitry. Likewise, there is suggestive evidence that intrinsic neural networks participate in regulation of ion transport (83) and local blood flow (11,12), but there are no details of neurophysiological mechanisms. It is emphasized that the electrophysiological studies done thus far on enteric neurons did not differentiate association of the neurons with any particular effector system. Although there is a temptation to relate results of enteric neurophysiology to motor function, the neural activity recorded by microelectrodes could just as well be part of the circuitry that controls any of the other effector systems. It may also be that some of the enteric ganglion cells have multifunctional involvement in simultaneous control of more than one kind of effector.

Functional Properties of the Intestinal Musculature

The application of electrophysiological techniques to the study of gastrointestinal muscles has yielded much information on functional properties which provides insight into mechanisms of neural control of this effector system.

The best studied motor effectors of the intestine are the longitudinal and circular muscle layers. These muscle layers of the small intestine differ in both ultrastructural characteristics and mechanisms of neural control. The principal ultrastructural difference is scarcity of nexuses in the longitudinal muscle coat and abundance of nexuses in the circular muscle coat (see Gabella, Chapter 6.) With respect to neural control, contractile responses of the longitudinal muscle *in situ* may be mediated exclusively by neuronal release of acetylcholine because in the absence of the myenteric plexus, strips of longitudinal muscle from both cat and guinea pig cannot be activated by electrical stimulation (131,135). Consistent with this is the observation that the longitudinal muscle layer contains 10 times as many muscarinic cholinergic receptors as the remainder of the gut (186). In contrast, the circular muscle layer is relatively insensitive to acetylcholine (34,67). The longitudinal muscle coat of guinea pig and rabbit small intestine does not show inhibitory junction potentials and does not appear to receive inhibitory innervation (34,73,96). On the other hand, the principal nervous input to the intestinal circular muscle comes from intrinsic inhibitory neurons.

The circular muscle layer possesses two fundamental physiological properties that should be taken into account in any explanation of its neural control. Firstly, the circular smooth muscle from the esophagus to the internal and sphincter behaves as an electrical syncytium. The syncytial properties are conferred by regions of fusion (nexuses) between plasma membranes of contiguous muscle fibers. The nexuses function as intracellular pathways for conduction of excitation between adjacent cells (4,15,111,155). The nexus is the basis for four structural levels of syncytial organization within the muscle: (a) Individual muscle fibers are electrically coupled by the nexus. (b) Many thousands of individual muscle fibers are partitioned into fasciculi approximately 100 μm in diameter by perimysium. These bundles branch and anastomose with other muscle bundles and represent the smallest electrically excitable unit of the muscle (22). (c) Bands of muscle of approximately 1,200 μm diameter separated by connective tissue are probably the neurally controlled contractile units. (d) The whole of the muscle exhibits electrical syncytial properties as a result of electrical coupling between component bands of muscle. In the absence of all nervous influence, the syncytial properties account for the three-dimensional spread of excitation and associated contraction that occurs throughout an intestinal segment when a localized stimulus is applied at any point on the segment. The functional significance of electrical syncytial properties is synchronization of spike discharge in a large population of muscle fibers to produce a coordinated contraction.

The second fundamental functional property of intestinal circular muscle is that organized excitation of the network of electrically coupled muscle cells is initiated by myogenic pacemaker mechanisms (electrical slow waves) in virtually all mammalian species except the guinea pig (see Chapter 58). The electrical slow waves occur in phase around the circumference of the bowel and are out of phase in the longitudinal axis of the bowel; that is, a single slow-wave cycle occurring instantaneously around the bowel appears to travel in the longitudinal direction along the gut. In the absence of neuronal influence, the circular muscle is highly excitable and responsive to the pacemaker so that each electrical slow-wave cycle triggers a synchronous circumferential contraction which propagates along the length of the bowel.

The enteric nervous system functions to control the inherently excitable electrical syncytium. The functional properties of the circular muscle preclude a mechanism of neural control that relies entirely on neuronal excitation for coordination of the contractile pattern of the musculature. Excitatory nerves cannot control the spread of excitation within the muscular syncytium, and observations that excitability of the muscle is greatly increased when neuronal activity is experimentally abolished (see following section on intrinsic inhibitory neurons) indicate that excitatory nerves do not control the responsiveness of the muscle to the pacemaker mechanism. The mechanism for controlling the responsiveness of the muscle to the pacemaker and for control of spread of excitation within the syncytium is neuronal inhibition of the muscle. An inhibitory control mechanism is required to explain: (a) Why each and every electrical slow wave cycle does not trigger action potentials and associated contraction in the circular muscle coat. Only one-third of the slow waves trigger spikes in the circular muscle *in vivo,* and all slow waves trigger spikes after neural blockade. (b) Why each slow wave does not elicit a muscle contraction of maximal strength as is the case after nervous blockade. (c) Why excitation usually does not spread over great extents of the conductile syncytium when spikes occur in a local region as is the case when segmentation patterns of motility predominate in the intestine.

Neuromuscular Transmission

The histoanatomy of neuromuscular transmission in the gut reflects also the specialization required for neural control of a muscular syncytium. Adaptations of neuromuscular transmission that appear to be of functional significance in neuronal control of the musculature are as follows: (a) No specialized neuromuscular junctions occur, and nonlocalized release of neurotransmitter substance from many points along the axons of a relatively small number of neurons produces a diffuse action on many different muscle fibers (8,131,139,154). (b) The transmitter substances persist and exert their effects at the muscle receptors for relatively prolonged periods of time (7,71,102). (c) The space constant of cable-like intestinal muscle is equivalent to 10 to 20 muscle cell lengths, and a junction potential thereby encompasses relatively large areas of the syncytium (155). (d) Since the muscle fibers are electrically coupled, transmitter-induced electrical current of an innervated cell can spread into and affect adjacent muscle fibers that receive no direct nervous influence. (e) Cholinergic junction potentials in the gut musculature have long latencies of 120 to 500 msec that cannot be accounted for by diffusion time and appear to reflect a property of the muscarinic cholinergic receptor (136). This may also be a specialized adaptation of neuromuscular transmission.

The structural and functional characteristics of the innervation of intestinal smooth muscles suggest that the nerves have a diffuse modulatory function rather than providing precise point-to-point excitation as occurs in nervous control of skeletal muscles. Paton and Zar (131) suggested that the lack of anatomically discrete neuroeffector structures is characteristic of a primitive system; on the other hand, it could also represent a specialized mechanism of neural control of an autogenic effector. Observations of gastrointestinal motor function in an evolutionarily specialized invertebrate carnivore favor the latter suggestion (168). The alimentary canal of cephalopods (e.g., squids) evolved in response to selective pressures associated with conversion from a diet of particulate matter to dietary habits similar to those of vertebrate animals, and it is enlightening that physiology of the gut musculature and its nervous control closely resembles that of mammalian species.

Enteric Sensory Receptors

Sensory receptors provide information on the state of the gut to the integrative circuitry of the enteric nervous system, of prevertebral sympathetic ganglia, and of the central nervous system. The receptors transduce changes in both chemical and mechanical energy.

The existence of chemo- and mechanoreceptors within the alimentary canal has been demonstrated by electrical recording from afferent nerve fibers that project to the central nervous system. Tower (158) demonstrated afferent fibers from the intestine in sympathetic nerves of the frog. Gernandt and Zotterman (55) recorded continuous slow discharge of impulses under rest conditions in intestinal afferent fibers in the mesenteric and splanchnic nerves of the cat. Pinching of the gut and peristaltic movements stimulated the receptors at the peripheral terminals of these fibers to fire at a higher frequency. Discharge patterns characteristic of both fast- and slow-adapting mechanoreceptors have been recorded in gastrointestinal afferent fibers within the vagal nerves (35,86,109,128) and splanchnic nerves (137,152). Presumably, as in other better studied sensory systems, slowly adapting receptors function to provide the integrative circuitry with accurate information on the steady-state intensity of stimulus energy and fast-adapting receptors provide information on the rate of change of stimulus energy. The latter form of information is essential for anticipatory control of the effectors by the central processing circuitry.

Stretch receptors have been reported for both stomach (128) and intestine (86). Recordings from single fibers in the vagus show that fibers from stomach and small bowel receptors fire continuously at low frequency and that the frequency increases in direct proportion to increase in distension brought about by inflating a balloon within the lumen of the organ. These receptors also fire at a higher frequency during muscular contraction, which is an indication that these mechanoreceptors are connected "in series" rather than "in parallel" with the contractile units. Paintal (128) described a distension-insensitive mechanoreceptor located in the mucosal region of cat stomach. These receptors appeared to signal movements of the mucosa that resulted from contraction of the muscularis mucosa, as well as the presence and movement of luminal contents. Mechanoreceptors within the distal colon of the guinea pig send afferent fibers in the lumbar colonic nerve to the interior mesenteric ganglion where they provide cholinergic synaptic input to the ganglion cells (152).

Iggo (87) discovered chemoreceptors in the mucosa of the stomach that are innervated by the vagus nerve. These receptors are specifically sensitive to the presence of either acidic or basic solutions on the mucosa and discharge continuously for as long as the stimulus is present. The threshold for initiation of discharge of the acid receptors is about pH 3 and for the alkaline receptors about pH 8. Slowly adapting chemoreceptors that respond specifically to glucose in the small intestine have been recorded in vagal afferent fibers (110) as well as others which respond to hypertonic NaCl or organic acids (26,64,65).

A description of electrical discharge of mechanosensitive neurons that can be recorded extracellularly from myenteric ganglia was given in an earlier section of this chapter. It has been demonstrated that the slowly adapting mechanosensitive units of the extracellular studies discharge during circular muscle contractions (169); nevertheless, these units are not unequivocally identified as mechanoreceptors. In fact, no histological identification of sensory structures nor sensory ganglion cells has been made within the enteric nervous system. Gabella (53) described some muscle cells within the innermost portion of the circular muscle that were much more elongated and had a smaller diameter than the other muscle fibers. The fibers were more electron dense, they had thin processes that surrounded nerve bundles, and, unlike the rest of the muscle, they received a dense innervation and showed some close contacts with nerve boutons. This structure suggested to Gabella that these smooth fibers could function as length detectors whose sensitivity could be preset by nervous input analogous to gamma motor activation of intrafusal skeletal muscle fibers.

It is clear that the electrophysiological work must be done in conjunction with structural studies in order to clarify enteric sensory function. The possibility exists that there are no intrinsic sensory neurons *per se,* rather the multipolar ganglion cells might be multifunctional in that the terminals of some of the cell's processes may be specialized as sensory detectors and others may receive synaptic input and function as dendrites. In this situation, integration of sensory input and synaptic input to the neuron could involve the previously mentioned gating function of the soma.

Final Common Pathways

Motor neurons of the central nervous system receive synaptic input from sensory afferents arising in different parts of the body and from several different interneurons. Discharge of motor neurons represents the final decision of the internuncial integrative circuitry and the final pathway from the nervous system. This concept can be applied to the enteric nervous system from which there are two well-established final pathways: namely, a cholinergic excitatory pathway to the intestinal longitudinal muscle and an inhibitory pathway to the circular muscle.

Electrical field stimulation of myenteric plexus–longitudinal muscle strips from guinea pig and rabbit small bowel releases noncholinergic substances that also contract the muscle. These effects are probably due to overflow of transmitter substance released by the massive electrical stimulation of interneurons, and do not constitute evidence for excitatory motor neurons utilizing a transmitter other than acetylcholine (3).

Cholinergic Motor Neurons

The endings of the cholinergic neurons are at the surface of the myenteric ganglia and interganglionic fiber tracts (52,131); and after release, acetylcholine traverses relatively long diffusion pathways to the longitudinal muscle. Cholinergic junction potentials evoked by electrical field stimulation can also be recorded in some circular muscle fibers but occur less often than in the longitudinal muscle and are species dependent (34). Cholinergic junction potentials seem to be more readily recorded in guinea pig circular muscle than in other mammalian species, and this raises the question, as yet unanswered, of whether the stronger cholinergic excitatory component of the guinea pig circular muscle is related to the absence of the myogenic pacemaker system (electrical slow waves) in the guinea pig.

Intrinsic Inhibitory Neurons

The presence of intrinsic nonadrenergic inhibitory ganglion cells within the enteric nervous system has been confirmed by many different laboratories (20). When the axon terminals of these neurons are activated by electrical field stimulation, they release a transmitter substance which produces an inhibitory junction potential in the muscle (Fig. 22). During electrical stimulation at 1 to 2 Hz, spontaneous muscle spikes are prevented, relaxation of contractile tension occurs, and cholinergic junction potentials cannot be elicited in the muscle by electrical stimulation of cholinergic nerves (47). Appropriate pharmacological experiments show that the inhibitory transmitter substance is not a catecholamine. Several lines of evidence suggest that the transmitter is a purine nucleotide, possibly ATP, and the term "purinergic neuron" has become a synonym for the intrinsic inhibitory neurons (20). The evidence for ATP as the inhibitory transmitter is stronger than the evidence for any other substance (compare 13,27,85); however, the precise identity of the transmitter is still controversial.

Pharmacological evidence suggests that the intrinsic inhibitory neurons possess nicotinic cholinergic receptors because in the presence of atropine, nicotinic agonists (e.g., acetylcholine, DMPP, and nicotine) elicit hyperpolarizing potentials and relaxation of contractile

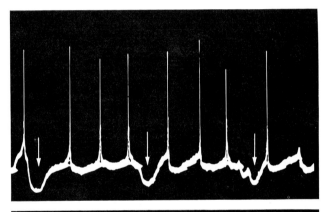
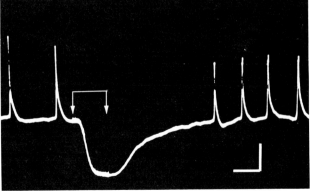

FIG. 22. Inhibitory junction potentials in gastrointestinal smooth muscle. **Top:** Spontaneously occurring inhibitory junction potentials *(arrows)* in guinea pig taenia coli *in vitro* reflect ongoing discharge of intrinsic inhibitory neurons *Vertical calibration:* 15 mV; *horizontal calibration:* 1 sec. Courtesy of C. J. Mayer and J. Riemer, Physiological Institut, Munich. **Bottom:** Inhibitory junction potential in guinea pig taenia coli evoked by electrical field stimulation of the axonal terminals of intrinsic inhibitory neurons. *Arrows* indicate onset and offset of electrical stimulation at 30 Hz. *Vertical calibration:* 11.5 mV; *horizontal calibration:* 0.66 sec. Modified from Bennet and Burnstock (7).

tension in the muscle. The inhibitory action of the nicotinic agonists is blocked by the nicotinic antagonists hexamethonium and curare and by the neurotoxin tetrodotoxin (21,140). Hirst and McKirdy (73) presented direct evidence, obtained by intracellular recording from myenteric neurons, that reflex synaptic excitation of the intrinsic inhibitory neurons in response to stretch is mediated by nicotinic cholinergic receptors.

Pharmacological experiments suggest that somatostatin may activate the intrinsic inhibitory neurons in guinea pig small and large intestine (49). Serotonin appears to activate the inhibitory neurons in the mouse and guinea pig stomach (17), but not in the guinea pig small intestine (161). The problem encountered in interpretation of these kinds of pharmacological results is that one cannot be sure that the drug does not activate intramural neurons that synapse with the inhibitory neurons rather than acting directly at receptors on the inhibitory neurons.

Intracellular electrophysiological studies show that morphine and the opioid peptides directly suppress excitability of myenteric neurons (118,175), and these agents also increase resting tone and phasic contractile activity of circular muscle, suggesting that they act at opiate receptors to remove tonic inhibition from the muscle by suppressing ongoing discharge of the inhibitory neurons (59,147).

The intrinsic inhibitory neurons are ubiquitous at all levels of the gut in all vertebrate species, and there is no doubt that they are of important functional significance in control of the motor activity of the musculature. The evidence presented below suggests that the intrinsic inhibitory neurons are continuously active in nonsphincteric regions of the bowel and that their general function in the intestine is suppression of both the responsiveness of the circular muscle to myogenic pacemaker mechanisms and the three-dimensional spread of excitability within the muscular syncytium.

The first line of evidence for continuous neuronal inhibition of the muscle is that some of the myenteric neurons of dog, cat, guinea pig, and rabbit small intestine show continuous patterned discharge of action potentials (124,125,169,180). This neuronal activity appears to produce continuous inhibition of the autogenous activity of the circular muscle because in segments of intestine *in vitro,* in which neuronal discharge in the myenteric plexus is prevalent, muscle action potentials and associated contractile activity are absent. It is difficult to experimentally evoke a contractile response with electrical stimulation in this circumstance. Myogenic pacemaker potentials (electrical slow waves) in species other than guinea pig are always present, and when the neuronal discharge is blocked experimentally with tetrodotoxin, every cycle of the electrical slow wave triggers intense discharge of action potentials and large-amplitude contractions (10,14,106,156,169,170,177,178).

Following neural blockade, electrical stimulation readily elicits sharp phasic contractions of the muscle (185), and mechanical stimulation as well readily triggers muscle action potentials and waves of contractile activity which may be propagated for distances of several centimeters in either direction along the longitudinal axis of the segment of intestine (170).

Spontaneous inhibitory junction potentials that result from ongoing discharge of the inhibitory neurons can sometimes be recorded from the muscle (Fig. 22); however, in most preparations *in vitro* the ongoing inhibitory activity is manifest in the muscle as steady hyperpolarization and decreased input resistance, both of which reduce the probability of pacemaker electrical current depolarizing the muscle to spike threshold. The steady inhibitory potential probably reflects smoothing of many inhibitory junction potentials due to release of the transmitter from multiple sites during asynchronous discharge of different nerve fibers and to the syncytial properties of the muscle.

As a general rule, any treatment or condition that ablates the intrinsic inhibitory neurons results in tonic contracture and achalasia of the intestinal circular muscle. Following is a list of circumstances that involve functional ablation of the intrinsic inhibitory neurons associated with conversion from a hypoirritable condition of the circular muscle to a hyperirritable state: (a) local anesthetic drugs (170); (b) long periods of cold storage (170); (c) hypoxic vascular perfusion of an intestinal segment (84); (d) surgical ablation (145); (e) congenital absence as in the piebald mouse and Hirschsprung's disease (16,171). All of the evidence suggests that the intrinsic inhibitory neurons are tonically active and that blockade or ablation of these neurons releases the circular muscle from the inhibitory influence permitting excitation and conduction that are mediated by myogenic mechanisms.

If it is true that tonically active inhibitory neurons continuously suppress myogenic activation and conduction of excitation in the circular muscle, then it is implicit that the various patterns of intestinal motor activity are dependent on integrated disinhibition of the muscle. In normal motor function, it is probable that the enteric internuncial circuitry integrates the activity of the inhibitory neurons to control: (a) whether a particular cycle of the electrical slow waves triggers a response in the circular muscle; (b) the number of muscle bundles activated in parallel and consequently the force of the contractile response triggered by a particular slow wave; (c) the distance over which excitation spreads within the syncytium; (d) the direction of spread of excitation within the syncytium.

The general function of intrinsic inhibitory neurons, outside of the various sphincters, appears to be continuous suppression of activity of the inherently excitable musculature. The inhibitory neurons have the additional specific functions of mediating vagally induced relaxation of the lower esophageal sphincter and stomach and of relaxation of tone in other sphincters. These neurons are the terminal ganglion cells of the vagal inhibitory pathways to the upper gastrointestinal tract. Their activation during swallowing relaxes the lower esophageal sphincter (159), and during defecation they relax the internal anal sphincter (138). The major difference between the inhibitory outflow to circular muscle of the intestine and the sphincters is that the inhibitory innervation of the intestine is tonically active, whereas the inhibitory ganglion cells to the sphincters are normally silent. In the intestine, myogenic contractions occur when ongoing discharge of the inhibitory neurons is suppressed by inhibitory synaptic input from internuncial enteric neurons. In the sphincters, myogenic mechanisms maintain contractile tone (e.g., sphincteric muscle is tonically contracted *in vitro* in the absence of extrinsic nervous input and circulating hormones) and the sphincter is relaxed when the normally silent inhibitory neurons are activated by excitatory synaptic input either from internuncial enteric neurons or from preganglionic vagal fibers. This physiology predicts that ablation or malfunction of the inhibitory ganglion cells or of the internuncial circuitry that controls the ganglion cells will lead to spasm of the intestinal circular muscle and to achalasia of the spincteric musculature.

Internuncial Integrative Circuitry

In some parts of the brain, such as the cerebellum, a clear picture of the synaptic connectivity of the identified cell types has been worked out and related to mechanisms of information processing. Our limited knowledge about the circuitry of the enteric nervous system is a sharp contrast to this. Because of the lack of specific information, only general statements about neural mechanisms within the internuncial integrative circuitry of the enteric nervous system will be possible, and these statements will be limited to the intramural nervous system of the intestine.

Peristaltic propulsion of an intraluminal bolus occurs within the isolated intestine without extrinsic innervation *in vitro* (16). Contractile activity persists, but peristaltic propulsion does not occur after blockade of nervous function with tetrodotoxin in the *in vitro* preparations. This indicates that the contractile activity of the intestinal musculature during peristalsis is dependent on intact integrative circuitry within the enteric nervous system and occurs independent of input from the central nervous system. During peristalsis, it can be assumed that intramural sensory receptors supply the integrative circuitry with information on parameters such as bolus size, rate, and direction of bolus movement. The integrative circuitry processes the sensory in-

formation and generates organized excitatory and inhibitory outflow to the musculature in which the same manner as internuncial circuitry within the spinal cord organizes motor outflow during reflex responses.

Reference in the literature to "myogenic" peristalsis is often seen. This is an unfortunate misnomer because it implies that the muscle can accomplish organized propulsion of intraluminal contents in the absence of neural control. Propagated contractile responses, which reflect the functional syncytial properties of the muscle, can be demonstrated after blockade of nervous function; however, these are not propulsive contractions and should not be called peristalsis. The enteric nervous system and the musculature together constitute the functional unit required for physiological motor function.

Although the term "reflex" is often applied to enteric nervous function, reflex circuitry may not be the absolute basis of all neurally controlled motor functions. The gastrointestinal tract is characterized by cyclical stereotyped patterns of motor movement. This is presented here to point out the similarities between neural production of motor movements of the gut and the generation of rhythmic motor behavior by other nervous systems, especially in the invertebrate phyla where one or a few ganglia generate nervous outflow that drives cyclical stereotyped motor patterns of behavior. Three properties are common to these "simple" motor networks. Firstly, the motor outflow patterns consist of rhythmically timed bursts of spikes that either arise from specific connectivity within an ensemble of neurons and cannot be traced to any individual neuron or are derived from endogenous activity of a single neuron. Secondly, the preprogrammed sequence of cyclical motor behavior is triggered by activation of single "command neurons." Thirdly, the motor behavior may be initiated and modulated by sensory input, but the stereotyped sequence of motor events can continue without sensory input. The notion of a motor program, as opposed to motor behavior based on reflex arcs, offers a heuristic concept for the cyclic motor movements of the intestines. Recurrent motor activity in the small intestine occurs in two distinct patterns, with the particular pattern dictated by the intraluminal digestive state. The predominant postprandial motor pattern is segmentation (mixing movements), and the interdigestive pattern is represented by the so-called migrating myoelectric complex (151). Each of these two motor patterns can be thought of as representing the outflow from a "prewired" motor program within the neural circuitry of the enteric nervous system. Sensory input, circulating hormones, and commands from the central nervous system are mechanisms by which one or the other of the motility programs may be selected.

Slow EPSPs, fast EPSPs, hyperpolarizing after-potentials, and the various other distinguishing features of enteric ganglion cells are likely to be of significance in the operation of the internuncial networks, but the precise significance in terms of control and coordination of the effector systems remains unclear. Some insight in this respect can be obtained by associating the electrical behavior of the ganglion cells with particular kinds of abnormal motor function. It is especially interesting to compare the actions of the opioid peptides and serotonin on myenteric neurons with the actions of these agents on intestinal motility.

Morphine and other opiate-like substances increase both phasic contractile activity and contractile tone of the intestinal circular muscle *in situ* (33,160). The action of the opiates is to lock the intestine into a continuous segmentation (mixing) pattern of motility which is nonpropulsive and constipating. The action of morphine on myenteric neurons is suppression of excitability of the somal membranes as discussed earlier in the chapter. This suggests that the action of morphine on the intact bowel is related to decreased release of neurotransmitter substances from the opiate-sensitive neurons. It suggests also that the segmentation pattern of motility is associated with the low excitability state of the somal membranes of the myenteric neurons. That is, a segmentation pattern of motility occurs when the somal gate is closed to interganglionic transfer of neural information (refer to earlier section on slow synaptic excitation). That morphine prevents release of acetylcholine from the myenteric plexus is well established (129), and North and Tonini (121) have argued convincingly that this can be attributed to the hyperpolarizing action of morphine on the myenteric neurons. Suppression of excitability of the intrinsic inhibitory neurons would reduce the tonic release of inhibitory transmitter at the muscle. This would account for the morphine-induced increase in circular muscle contractile activity because decreased inhibition of the muscle would increase its responsiveness to the myogenic pacemaker. It might be concluded that the action of morphine is an exaggeration of the role of an endogenous opioid messenger whose release during the digestive state commands the segmentation motility mode. The endogenous opioid seems to function as a neuromodulator that tones down the activity of both the intrinsic inhibitory neurons to the circular muscle and cholinergic excitatory neurons to the longitudinal muscle during segmentation motility. Contractile activity of the longitudinal muscle probably does not contribute to the mechanical forces required for mixing action; and since acetylcholine release is the principal physiological mechanism for contracting the longitudinal muscle, suppression of acetylcholine release during segmentation motility makes functional sense. Prevention of release of acetylcholine by morphine has received much attention, but this is not the sole factor involved in the constipating action of morphine because certain analogues of morphine (e.g., azedomorphine) reduce the output of acetylcholine from

the myenteric plexus without producing obstipation (97).

Enterochromaffin cell tumors in the gastrointestinal tract and other parts of the body synthesize and release large amounts of serotonin and substance P into the portal and systemic circulations (2,134). The high levels of serotonin and substance P are often associated with increased propulsive motility and diarrhea in people with enterochromaffin cell (carcinoid) tumors. Release of serotonin has also been implicated in postgastrectomy dumping syndrome and other conditions involving hyperpropulsion (165). This raises the question of whether increased propulsive motility of carcinoid syndrome reflects the role of serotonin as the mediator for the slow EPSP in myenteric neurons. Serotonin enhances the excitability of the cell soma and in effect opens the somal gate for interganglionic transfer of neural information. Serotonin is known to lower the threshold for the peristaltic reflex in isolated segments of intestine (18), and it activates the release of acetylcholine from myenteric neurons (163). Prevention of serotonin release from presynaptic terminals by activation of presynaptic alpha receptors with clonidine also produces intestinal pseudo-obstruction (5). In these respects, serotonin has actions opposite to those of the opioid peptides. The suggestion is that serotonin and perhaps substance P transmit the command signal for initiation and maintenance of the propulsive (peristaltic) mode of intestinal motility and that the endogenous opioid peptides command the segmentation motility mode.

Neural Control of Motility Patterns

Ileus, spasm, segmentation, and peristalsis are distinct motility states of the intestinal musculature that can be accounted for by intrinsic neural mechanisms.

Ileus is a state of no motor activity within the intestinal musculature. This state is present in segments of small intestine equilibrated at 37°C *in vitro*. Electrical slow waves, which originate in the longitudinal muscle layer, are present but do not initiate action potentials and associated contractile activity in the circular muscle during this state. Continuous activity of the intrinsic inhibitory neurons accounts for this low responsiveness of the circular muscle to the myogenic pacemaker. The most prominent neural activity during ileus is the ongoing discharge of burst-type neurons, therefore, these are assumed to be the tonically active inhibitory neurons. Electrophysiological studies (see section on burst-type neurons) suggest that the inhibitory neurons may not generate endogenous discharge in the absence of synaptic input. Instead, they appear to be synaptically driven by input from an endogenously active burst-type oscillator. Figure 23 shows hypothetical driver-follower circuitry that is consistent with experimental observa-

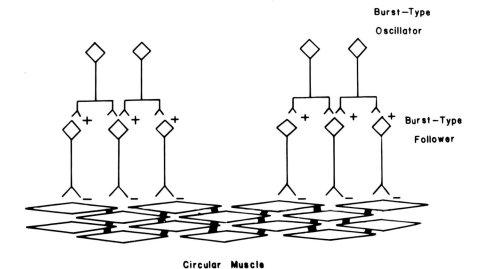

Circular Muscle

FIG. 23. Model of driver-follower circuitry for inhibitory nervous control of intestinal circular muscle. The circular muscle behaves like a functional syncytium that is activated by myogenic mechanisms. Burst-type oscillators discharge continuously and synaptically drive nonspontaneous follower neurons. Burst-type followers are assumed to be the intrinsic inhibitory neurons.

tions and accounts for continuous inhibition of the circular muscle. This two-neuron inhibitory circuit is considered to be the fundamental unit that is modulated by inputs from internuncial integrative circuitry. The driver neuron of this circuit is an endogenous oscillator (steady burster) that runs continuously and synaptically activates the follower cell that is inhibitory to the muscle. Additional synaptic inputs to the follower neuron may be excitatory input that increases the intensity of inhibitory neuron discharge or inhibitory input that decreases follower cell discharge. The former would further reduce the excitability of the muscle and the latter would remove inhibition and permit muscular contractile activity. The transmitter substance that is released by the driver neurons is unknown, but it is likely the same as the transmitter that can be released by focal electrical stimulation of the myenteric ganglia to induce a burst discharge (31).

Ileus in the intact animal is a well-defined entity that is produced by peritoneal irritation and a variety of other causes. Paralysis of the bowel in the intact animal probably also reflects unremitting activity of the intrinsic inhibitory neurons. Furness and Costa (48) have reviewed the literature that suggests that sympathetic reflexes are involved in production of ileus. It seems, however, that factors additional to sympathetic input to the intestine are responsible for postoperative ileus because alpha- and beta-adrenergic blocking drugs do not prevent ileus in either dogs (148) or humans (69). Norepinephrine suppresses both cholinergic and serotonergic synaptic transmission within the enteric internuncial circuitry, and this may lead to ileus by inactivating the networks that synaptically inhibit the tonically active inhibitory neurons. It is unclear whether additional factors also interfere with the circuitry that controls the inhibitory neurons. It is interesting that neither morphine nor naloxone relieves postoperative ileus (82,160).

Spasm

Spasm of the circular muscle is the opposite of ileus: there is no activity of the inhibitory neurons. In this case, the myogenic pacemakers continuously trigger maximal contractile responses which spread within the syncytium and collide with activity from adjacent regions resulting in increased tone and fibrillatory contractions within the affected segment. The model for this is Hirschsprung's disease in humans and aganglionic megacolon in piebald mice where spasm of the aganglionic terminal segment of the large intestine reflects the absence of the intrinsic inhibitory mechanisms (6,46,171). In Hirschsprung's disease, the aganglionic segment behaves like a sphincter without inhibition and with no reflex relaxation.

Loss of enteric ganglion cells can occur after birth. Young rats have more myenteric ganglion cells than older rats, suggesting that myenteric ganglion cells may be lost with advancing age (51). Acquired megacolon associated with disappearance of ganglion cells after birth has been reported (157), and zonal hypoganglionosis also has been reported (91). These observations arouse suspicion that loss of intrinsic inhibitory neurons or malfunction of the neural networks that control these neurons might be involved in the etiology of pathophysiological states associated with spasm. Achalasia in the lower esophageal sphincter and cardia is undoubtedly associated with loss and malfunction of ganglion cells (1).

Segmentation

Segmentation movements accomplish mixing of the intraluminal contents and are characteristic of the digestive state. Segmentation at any moment in time consists of narrow annular contractions interposed between relaxed segments of bowel. Moments later, the contracted annuli relax while previously relaxed intersegments contract. These cycles of reciprocal contraction-relaxation of adjacent segments continue until digestion is complete. Segmentation movements occur at the frequency of the electrical slow waves or at a multiple of the slow wave interval. They occur in the small bowel of all mammals including the guinea pig, an animal that does not exhibit electrical slow waves. As mentioned previously, the longitudinal muscle coat probably does not contract during segmentation motility. The forces for mixing are exerted by the circular muscle.

Segmentation must involve reciprocal neural inhibition and disinhibition of adjacent segments of the muscle; otherwise, excitation of the contracting segment would spread within the syncytium to the adjacent relaxed segment and as a consequence a long length of intestine would contract simultaneously. The system behaves as if the internuncial circuitry periodically turns off the inhibitory neurons to a narrow band of circular muscle, and when this occurs the omnipresent electrical slow waves trigger contraction of the disinhibited band of muscle. The strength of the segmental contraction will depend on the number of muscle fibers in parallel that are disinhibited within the active segment. It is unclear whether cholinergic input to the disinhibited segment of muscle reinforces excitation. This may be true in the guinea pig where there are no electrical slow waves and where cholinergic junction potentials can be evoked in the circular muscle by experimentally distending an adjacent segment (73). On the other hand, the segmentation pattern of motility is enhanced when acetylcholine release from the myenteric plexus is reduced in the presence of morphine.

It is likely, although unproven, that the cyclical inhibition-disinhibition of a given segment of bowel is preprogrammed in the internuncial circuitry of the enteric system, and that the precisely timed discharge of the steady burst-type neurons is the clock for the program.

Previous mention has been made that opiates induce the segmentation motility pattern suggesting the also unproven idea that endogenous opioid peptides might represent the command signal for the segmentation motility pattern.

With respect to the large intestine, it is probable that the haustral movements of the colon are programmed in the same manner as small intestinal segmentation, except that the program is clocked by a slower time base.

Peristalsis

Peristalsis accomplishes mass propulsion of the intraluminal contents of the small and large intestine. Peristalsis can occur in either direction along the bowel, although retroperistalsis is rare and limited to uncommon circumstances such as emesis or in response to a distal obstruction. The occurrence of coordinated retropulsion indicates the existence of neural circuitry that provides appropriate control of the muscular syncytium for production of either forward or reverse peristalsis.

Sequentially timed contractions of the longitudinal and circular muscles appear to be necessary for the peristaltic propulsion, and neural coordination of the musculature is therefore more complex than for segmentation movements. Neurally mediated contraction of the longitudinal muscle and inhibition of the circular muscle occur ahead of the advancing bolus, and circular muscle contraction and longitudinal muscle relaxation occur within the gut segment immediately behind the bolus. Shortening of the longitudinal muscle and relaxation of the circular muscle ahead of the bolus functions to expand the lumen and decrease intraluminal pressure in the path of the forward moving bolus. The gut behaves geometrically as a cylinder with constant surface area; consequently, shortening of the long axis of the cylinder increases the radius and expands the lumen. Inhibition of the circular muscle in the same cylindrical segment ensures that circular muscle contraction does not oppose this action of the longitudinal muscle. Activation of the longitudinal muscle ahead of the advancing bolus is produced by acetylcholine released from the myenteric plexus. Relaxation of the circular muscle results from increased discharge of the intrinsic inhibitory neurons. Contraction of the circular muscle behind the bolus functions to increase intraluminal pressure and propel the bolus forward into the expanded lumen. The mechanism that initiates the circular muscle contraction is unclear and may be species dependent. Activation of the circular muscle could be a myogenic event following neural inhibition of continuously active inhibitory neurons. It could be produced by cholinergic excitatory input to the muscle or both factors could be operative.

Hirst and McKirdy (73) devised an *in vitro* preparation of guinea pig small intestine from which they have obtained additional insight into neural mechanisms of peristalsis and results that support most of the above statements about behavior of the individual muscle layers during peristalsis. The preparation is a 5 cm segment of intestine in continuity with a strip of longitudinal muscle on which the myenteric plexus is exposed by removal of the mucosa and circular muscle. Intracellular microelectrodes are used to record electrical activity in myenteric neurons on the longitudinal strip. Distension of a balloon within the intestinal segment or electrical stimulation of the segment activates neural pathways that project into the myenteric plexus on the strip of longitudinal muscle and initiate synaptic potentials in the neurons. These distension-evoked responses in the neurons can be compared with intracellularly recorded junction potentials in the longitudinal and circular muscle layers.

Distension of the intraluminal balloon elicits two distinct patterns of fast cholinergic EPSPs in the myenteric neurons situated aboral to the distended segment. One group of ganglion cells shows a transient burst of EPSPs which appear within 0.2 to 1.2 sec after balloon distension. A second population of neurons shows EPSPs which appear after a much longer latency of 2 to 11 sec and which persist for the duration of and for some time after distension is terminated. The short-latency EPSPs correspond in time with transient inhibitory junction potentials which appear in the circular muscle after balloon distension. The EPSPs produced by the long-latency descending pathways correspond in time with atropine-sensitive excitatory junction potentials in both longitudinal and circular muscle layers.

Removal of the submucous plexus prevents the distension-evoked descending excitation but does not prevent descending inhibition in the experiments of Hirst and McKirdy; whereas Costa and Furness (32) reported that neither the inhibitory nor the excitatory phase of peristalsis required the presence of the submucous plexus.

Focal electrical stimulation of the processes of the myenteric neurons at various distances from an impaled soma and recording of the spikes that spread into the soma from the activated process indicate that the length of the axons of the descending pathways is less than 2.5 cm. Therefore, these 5- to 7-cm long descending pathways appear to be polysynaptic with each neuron in the pathway receiving several excitatory inputs in cascade arrangement (73). All of the fast EPSPs in these pathways appear to be nicotinic cholinergic.

The suggestion has been made that postinhibitory rebound excitation of the circular muscle could reinforce the contractile response of the circular muscle behind the bolus during peristaltic propulsion (47). Hirst and McKirdy (73) never observed excitatory rebound following distension-evoked inhibitory junction potentials in the circular muscle. Their observations suggest that poststimulus rebound excitation is an experimental artifact that results when large numbers of inhibitory neurons are activated synchronously by electrical field stimulation and that it has no physiological importance in guinea pig small bowel.

Hirst and McKirdy (73) reported that distension-evoked excitatory junction potentials occurred with the same long latency in both the longitudinal and circular muscle coats. This is puzzling because it seems that the two layers should contract out of phase during peristalsis. That is, the longitudinal muscle should contract during the inhibitory phase of the circular muscle. Otherwise, the two layers would produce opposing contractile forces. Contraction of the longitudinal muscle would tend to shorten the cylindrical segment and increase the radius, whereas shortening of the circular muscle decreases the radius and increases the length of the cylinder (185). Electrical recordings from the muscle layers of mouse large intestine and cinéfilms of peristaltic propulsion show that contraction of the longitudinal muscle precedes contractions of the circular muscle (16,171).

Another significant result from the Hirst-McKirdy preparation is that the sequence of neural events is evoked by inflation of a stationary balloon and continuous distension is not required for the sequence to be completed. This indicates that the neural circuitry does not require sensory information on forward movement of the bolus to initiate descending events 5 to 7 cm below the region of stimulation. It is consistent with the idea that the circuitry is "hardwired" for the complete motor sequence, which is analogous to polysynaptic spinal reflex circuitry. The system behaves as if the input from distension receptors constitutes a command that switches on the preprogrammed circuitry for the stereotyped sequence of motor events below the point of stimulation, and once activated, the program continues to completion without further input (refer to internuncial circuitry section).

Although direct neurophysiological studies have provided a wealth of information about the enteric nervous system and a feeling of imminent breakthroughs in understanding prevails, it is still impossible to construct an adequate neural model for peristalsis. One reason for this is that the electrical behavior of single neurons has not with certainty been associated with a particular motility pattern or even a particular effector. Nevertheless, I have attempted in Fig. 24 to construct a simple model that incorporates some of the available information on neurophysiology of the enteric nervous system and the timing of peristaltic motor events.

The fundamental peristaltic circuit is activated by input from stretch receptors that signal radial distension of the muscularis externa. This input acts via cholinergic interneurons to activate inhibitory neurons ahead of the bolus and to inactivate inhibitory neurons behind the advancing bolus. The network that controls the inhibitory neurons is depicted as a cholinergic network based on the observation of a preponderance of fast cholinergic EPSPs in enteric neurons, on blockade of descending inhibition by nicotinic blocking drugs, and on the observation that serotonin or serotonergic antagonists do not affect inhibitory neural activity in guinea pig small bowel (32,161). The cholinergic motor neuron is depicted as an AH/type 2 neuron in which serotonin produces slow synaptic excitation. In this model, the AH/type 2 neuron is illustrated as a multipolar neuron (Dogiel Type II) which has interganglionic processes that project up and down the long axis of the gut. Coordination of contraction of the circular muscle behind the bolus and contraction of the longitudinal muscle ahead of the bolus is achieved in the model by spatial distribution of the processes of the AH/type 2 cell. Dur-

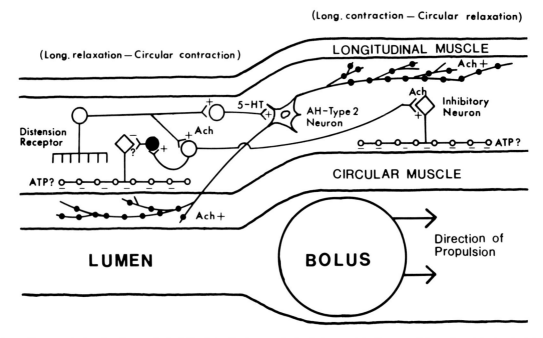

FIG. 24. Schematic neural circuitry for control of the intestinal muscularis during peristaltic propulsion of an intraluminal bolus. Putative neurotransmitters are given; (+) indicates an excitatory synapse; (−) an inhibitory synapse. For details see text.

ing the low excitability state of the cell soma, neural activity would be confined to the individual processes of the cell and peristalsis would not occur. This condition of the cell might correspond to the segmentation motility mode. When serotonin is released by the distension-sensitive pathway, activation of the soma (slow EPSP) synchronizes spike discharge in all processes of the cell that project up and down the long axis of the gut. Circuitry has been included in the model to account for disinhibition of the circular muscle behind the bolus. This model is consistent with the potent acetylcholine releasing effect of serotonin (163) and observations that methysergide and serotonergic desensitization block the excitatory phase of peristalsis. The long time delay for distension-induced excitation in the experimental preparations (32,73) is explained by the slow rise time of the slow EPSP in the AH/type 2 neuron.

Even though radial distension is the stimulus for peristalsis in segments of intestine *in vitro,* it must be considered that the same stimulus may be required for segmentation motility. That is, segmentation occurs in a partly distended intestine. It may be that the particular pattern of motility evoked by the stimulus is determined by the presence of hormonal and/or neuromodulatory factors.

EXTRINSIC NERVOUS INPUT

Parasympathetic Input

Vagal Input

Vagal input to the enteric nervous system originates in the dorsal motor nucleus of the medulla oblongata and

projects as far as the rectum in the cat (142). Experimental stimulation of vagal fibers generally increases contractile activity of the intestinal musculature. However, some of the vagal fibers terminate either on inhibitory ganglion cells or on interneurons of circuitry that activates the inhibitory ganglion cells of the gastric cardia and lower esophageal sphincter. Campbell and Burnstock (23) suggested that the vagal inhibitory pathways to the upper gastrointestinal tract are phylogenetically more primitive than the vagal excitatory pathways. The inhibitory pathways of the vagus transmit information via nicotinic cholinergic synapses and perhaps serotonergic synapses (17,23,159).

The vagi at the level of the diaphragm contain an average of 56,138 afferent fibers and only 1,736 efferent fibers (79). The enteric nervous system in the small intestine contains a minimum of 2×10^7 ganglion cells (143). This great disparity in numbers between preganglionic fibers and enteric ganglion cells brings to question the functional relationship between vagal input and intestinal motor function. Earlier theories invoked the concept of divergence and "mother cells"; however, it is difficult to conceptualize how a divergence ratio of $1:1 \times 10^4$ could accomplish the coordinated control during the motility patterns that are observed along the bowel. A subsequent and more tenable view was that enteric reflex arcs functioned independent of preganglionic parasympathetic fibers (101). A modern proposal, consistent with current neurophysiological concepts, is that the enteric nervous system contains subsets of neural circuits that are preprogrammed for control of distinct intestinal motility patterns and that the preexisting programs receive command inputs that are transmitted from the central nervous system along vagal fibers. This provides an explanation for the potent influence of a small number of vagal efferent fibers on motility over a broad region of bowel, and is analogous to other better-studied neural control systems in which activation of single "command neurons" releases extensive coordinated motor responses (9,94).

Sacral Input

Sacral input to the large intestine is transmitted over pelvic nerves and consists of efferent fibers that synapse within the intramural ganglia of the bowel and within extramural ganglia on the surface of the colon (36). The precise functional significance of the sacral input to the intramural ganglia is unclear. It might also represent command signals to internuncial circuitry of the enteric nervous system. The extramural ganglia function primarily as simple relay-distribution centers (i.e., a classic parasympathetic ganglion) for information arising in the sacral division of the spinal cord (36). Transmission through these ganglia is mediated by nicotinic cholinergic receptors. This system, in the cat, functions to reinforce mass contraction of the terminal large intestine during defecation (37).

Sympathetic Input

Sympathetic pathways transmit command signals from the central nervous system which function to shut down gastrointestinal blood flow and motility. This is well known as a component of the blanket-like response of the sympathetic nervous system to stressful environmental circumstances. Direct electrophysiological study of enteric neurons clearly shows that part of the mechanism of sympathetic shutdown of the bowel is mediated by input that acts on presynaptic terminals to prevent release of excitatory transmitter substances within the enteric nervous system.

Fluorescent histochemical observations suggest that a vast majority of the postganglionic sympathetic fibers to the gut synapse directly with enteric ganglion cells (88,115,116). Stimulation of sympathetic nerves inhibits vagal transmission to the cat small intestine (103), and catecholamines are known to be inhibitors of the release of acetylcholine from enteric neurons (99,130). Intracellular recording shows that norepinephrine blocks the fast cholinergic synaptic potentials induced by electrical stimulation in the guinea pig myenteric plexus, but does not block potential changes produced by exogenous acetylcholine (74,113). Electrical stimulation applied to perivascular nerves of guinea pig intestine also inhibits cholinergic synaptic transmission between myenteric neurons, but does not alter the electrical properties of the postsynaptic neurons (74,81,113). This is an indi-

cation that norepinephrine acts presynaptically to prevent acetylcholine release. Norepinephrine also blocks the slow EPSP and augmented excitability in AH/type 2 neurons, and this action is blocked by the alpha-adrenergic blocker phentolamine (182). Norepinephrine does not affect the action of exogenously applied serotonin, suggesting that this also is presynaptic prevention of serotonin release.

REFERENCES

1. Adams, C. W., Brain, R. H., and Trounce, J. R. (1976): Ganglion cells in achalasia of the cardia. *Virchows Arch. [Pathol. Anta.]*, 372:75–79.
2. Alumets, J., Hakanason, R., Ingemansson, S., and Sundler, F. (1977): Substance P and 5-HT in granules isolated from an intestinal argentaffin carcinoid. *Histochemistry*, 52:217–222.
3. Ambache, N., and Freeman, M. W. (1968): Atropine resistant longitudinal muscle spasm due to excitation of non-cholinergic neurons in Auerbach's plexus. *J. Physiol. (Lond.)*, 199:705–727.
4. Barr, L., Berger, W., and Dewey, M. M. (1968): Electrical transmission at the nexus between smooth muscle cells. *J. Gen. Physiol.*, 51:347–368.
5. Bauer, G. E., and Hellerstrand, K. J. (1976): Pseudoobstruction due to clonidine. *Br. Med. J.*, 1:769.
6. Baumgarten, H. G., Holstein, A. F., and Stelzner, F. (1973): Nervous elements in the human colon of Hirschsprung's disease. *Virchows Arch. [Pathol. Anat.]*, 358:113–136.
7. Bennett, M. R., and Burnstock, G. (1968): Electrophysiology of the innervation of intestinal smooth muscle. In: *Handbook of Physiology, Section 6, Alimentary Canal, Vol. IV*, edited by C. F. Code, pp. 1709–1732. American Physiological Society, Washington, D.C.
8. Bennett, M. R., and Rogers, D. (1967): A study of the innervation of the taenia coli. *J. Cell Biol.*, 33:573–596.
9. Bentley, D. (1977): Control of cricket song patterns by descending interneurons. *J. Comp. Physiol.*, 116:19–38.
10. Biber, B., and Fara, J. (1973): Intestinal motility increased by tetrodotoxin, lidocaine, and procaine. *Experientia*, 29:551–552.
11. Biber, B., Fara, J., and Lundgren, O. (1973): Intestinal vasodilatation in response to transmural electrical field stimulation. *Acta Physiol. Scand.*, 87:277–282.
12. Biber, B., Lundgren, O., and Sovanvik, J. (1971): Studies on the intestinal vasodilatation observed after mechanical stimulation of the mucosa of the gut. *Acta Physiol. Scand.*, 82:177–190.
13. Bloom, S. R., and Polak, J. M. (1978): Peptidergic versus purinergic. *Lancet*, 1:93.
14. Bortoff, A., and Miller, R. (1975): Stimulation of intestinal muscle by atropine, procaine, and tetrodotoxin. *Am. J. Physiol.*, 229:1609–1613.
15. Bozler, E. (1948): Conduction, automaticity and tonus of visceral muscle. *Experientia*, 4:312–318.
16. Brann, L., and Wood, J. D. (1976): Motility of the large intestine of piebald lethal mice. *Am. J. Dig. Dis.*, 21:633–640.
17. Bülbring, E., and Gershon, M. D. (1967): 5-Hydroxytryptamine participation in the vagal inhibitory innervation of the stomach. *J. Physiol. (Lond.)*, 192:823–846.
18. Bülbring, E., and Lin, R. C. Y. (1958): The effect of intraluminal application of 5-hydroxytryptamine and 5-hydroxytryptophan on peristalsis: The local production of 5-HT and its release in relation to intraluminal pressure and propulsive activity. *J. Physiol. (Lond.)*, 140:381–407.
19. Burks, T. F. (1973): Mediation by 5-hydroxytryptamine of morphine stimulant actions in dog intestine. *J. Pharmacol. Exp. Ther.*, 185:530–539.
20. Burnstock, G. (1972): Purinergic neurons. *Pharmacol. Rev.*, 34:509–581.
21. Burnstock, G., Campbell, G., and Rand, M. J. (1966): The inhibitory innervation of the taenia of the guinea-pig caecum. *J. Physiol. (Lond.)*, 182:504–526.

22. Burnstock, G., and Prosser, C. L. (1960): Conduction in smooth muscle: Comparative electrical properties. *Am. J. Physiol.*, 199:553–559.

23. Campbell, G., and Burnstock, G. (1968): Comparative physiology of gastrointestinal motility. In: *Handbook of Physiology, Section 6, Alimentary Canal, Vol. IV,* edited by C. F. Code, pp. 2213–2266. American Physiological Society, Washington, D.C.

24. Caren, J. F., Meyer, J. H., and Grossman, M. I. (1974): Canine intestinal secretion during and after rapid distension of the small bowel. *Am. J. Physiol.*, 227:183–188.

25. Chan-Palay, V., Jansson, G., and Palay, S. L. (1978): Serotonin and substance P coexist in neurons of the rat's central nervous system. *Proc. Natl. Acad. Sci. U.S.A.*, 75:1582–1586.

26. Clarke, G. D., and Davison, J. S. (1974): Vagal afferent nerve endings in the gastric antral mucosa of the rat. *J. Physiol. (Lond.)*, 239:41P.

27. Cocks, T., and Burnstock, G. (1979): Effects of neuronal polypeptides on intestinal smooth muscle; a comparison with non-adrenergic, non-cholinergic nerve stimulation and ATP. *Eur. J. Pharmacol.*, 54:251–259.

28. Connor, J. A. (1979): Calcium current in molluscan neurones: measurement under conditions which maximize its visibility. *J. Physiol. (Lond.)*, 286:41–60.

29. Cook, M. A., Hamilton, J. T., and Okwuasaba, F. K. (1978): Coenzyme A is a purine nucelotide modulator of acetylcholine output. *Nature (Lond.)*, 271:786–791.

30. Cook, R. D., and Burnstock, G. (1976): The ultrastructure of Auerbach's plexus in the guinea-pig. I. Neuronal elements. *J. Neurocytol.*, 5:171–194.

31. Cooke, A. R., Athey, G. R., and Wood, J. D. (1979): Synaptic activation of burst-type myenteric neurons in cat small intestine. *Fed. Proc.*, 28:959.

32. Costa, M., and Furness, J. B. (1976): The peristaltic reflex: An analysis of the nerve pathways and their pharmacology. *Naunyn Schmiedeberg's Arch. Pharmacol.*, 294:47–60.

33. Daniel, E. E., Sutherland, W. H., and Bogoch, A. (1959): Effects of morphine and other drugs on the motility of the terminal ileum. *Gastroenterology*, 36:510–523.

34. Daniel, E. E., Taylor, G. S., Daniel, V. P., and Holman, M. E. (1977): Can nonadrenergic inhibitory varicosities be identified structurally? *Can. J. Physiol. Pharmacol.*, 55:243–250.

35. Davison, J. S. (1972); Response of single vagal afferent fibers to mechanical and chemical stimulation of the gastric and duodenal mucosa in cats. *Q. J. Exp. Physiol.*, 57:405–416.

36. deGroat, W. C., and Krier, J. (1976): An electrophysiological study of the sacral parasympathetic pathway to the colon of the cat. *J. Physiol (Lond.)*, 260:425–445.

37. deGroat, W. C., and Krier, J. (1978): The sacral parasympathetic reflex pathway regulating colonic motility and defecation in the cat. *J. Physiol. (Lond.)*, 276:481–500.

38. Dingledine, R., and Goldstein, A. (1976): Effects of synaptic transmission blockade on morphine action in the guinea-pig myenteric plexus. *J. Pharmacol. Exp. Ther.*, 196:97–106.

39. Dingledine, R. A., Goldstein, A., and Kendig, J. (1974): Effects of narcotic opiates and serotonin on the electrical behavior of neurons in the guinea-pig Auerbach's plexus. *Life Sci.*, 14:2299–2309.

40. Dreyfus, C. F., Bornstein, M. B., and Gershon, M. D. (1977): Synthesis of serotonin by neurons of the myenteric plexus *in situ* and in organotypic tissue culture. *Brain Res.*, 128:125–139.

41. Dreyfus, C. F., Sherman, D., and Gershon, M. D. (1977): Uptake of serotonin by intrinsic neurons of the myenteric plexus grown in organotypic tissue culture. *Brain Res.*, 128:102–123.

42. Ehrenpreis, S., Light, I., and Schonbuch, G. (1972): Use of electrically stimulated guinea-pig ileum to study potent analgesics. In: *Drug Addiction: Experimental Pharmacology,* edited by J. H. Singh, L. H. Miller, and H. Lal, pp. 319–342. Future Pub. Co., Mt. Kisko, New York.

43. Erspamer, F. (1954): Il sistema cellulare entero cromaffine e l'enteramina (5-idrossitriptamine). *Rend. Sci. Farmital.*, 1:1–193.

44. Erwin, D. N., Ninchoji, T. and Wood, J. D. (1978): Effects of morphine on electrical activity of single myenteric neurons in cat small bowel. *Eur. J. Pharmacol.*, 47:401–405.

45. Fehér, E., and Csângi, K. (1953): Ultrastructural effects of parachlorophenylalanine, 5-hydroxytryptamine and the imipramine groups on nerve processes of the small intestine. *Acta Anat. (Basel)*, 100:61–67.

46. Frigo, G. M., Del Tacca, M., Lecchini, S., and Crema, A. (1973): Some observations on the intrinsic nervous mechanism in Hirschsprung's disease. *Gut,* 14:35–40.

47. Furness, J. B., and Costa, M. (1973): The nervous release and the action of substances which affect intestinal muscle through neither adrenoreceptors nor cholinoreceptors. *Philos. Trans. R. Soc. Lond. [Biol.],* 265:123–133.

48. Furness, J. B., and Costa, M. (1974): Adynamic ileus, its pathogenesis and treatment. *Med. Biol.,* 52:82–89.

49. Furness, J. B., and Costa, M. (1979): Actions of somatostatin on excitatory and inhibitory nerves in the intestine. *Eur. J. Pharmacol.,* 56:69–74.

50. Fuxe, K., Hokfelt, T., Said, S. I., and Mutt, V. (1977): Vasoactive intestinal polypeptide and the nervous system. Immunohistochemical evidence for localization in central and peripheral neurones, particularly intracortical neurons of the cerebral cortex. *Neurosci. Lett.,* 5:241–246.

51. Gabella, G. (1971): Neuron size and number in the myenteric plexus of the newborn and adult rat. *J. Anat. (Lond.),* 109:81–95.

52. Gabella, G. (1972): Fine structure of the myenteric plexus in the guinea-pig ileum. *J. Anat. (Lond.),* 111:69–97.

53. Gabella, G. (1974): A special muscle layer in the intestinal muscular coat. *J. Physiol. (Lond.),* 240:1–3P.

54. Gamse, R., Mroz, E., Leeman, S., and Lembeck, F. (1978): The intestine as source of immunoreactive substance P in plasma of the cat. *Naunyn-Schmiedeberg's Arch. Pharmacol.,* 305:17–21.

55. Garnandt, B. Z., and Zotterman, T. (1946): Intestinal pain: electrophysiological investigation of myenteric nerves. *Acta Physiol. Scand.,* 2:56–72.

56. Gershon, M. D., and Altman, R. F. (1971): An analysis of the uptake of 5-hydroxytryptamine by the myenteric plexus of the small intestine of the guinea-pig. *J. Pharmacol. Exp. Ther.,* 179:29–41.

57. Gershon, M. D., and Bursztajn, S. (1978): Properties of the enteric nervous system: Limitation of access of intravascular macromolecules to the myenteric plexus and muscularis externa. *J. Comp. Neurol.,* 180:467–488.

58. Gershon, M. D., Dreyfus, C. F., Pickel, V. M., John, T. H., and Reis, D. J. (1977): Serotonergic neurons in the peripheral nervous system: identification in gut by immunohistochemical localization of tryptophan hydroxylase. *Proc. Natl. Acad. Sci. U.S.A.,* 71:3086–3089.

59. Gillan, M. G. C., and Pollock, D. (1976): Investigation of the effects of drugs on morphine induced contractions of the isolated colon of the rat. *Br. J. Pharmacol.,* 57:444–445P.

60. Grafe, P., Mayer, C. J., and Wood, J. D. (1979): Evidence that substance P does not mediate slow synaptic excitation within the myenteric plexus. Nature (Lond.), 279:720–721.

61. Grafe, P., Wood, J. D., and Mayer, C. J. (1979): Fast excitatory post-synaptic potentials in AH (type 2) neurons of guinea-pig myenteric plexus. *Brain Res.,* 163:349–352.

62. Gullermin, R. (1976): Somatostatin inhibits the release of acetylcholine induced electrically in the myenteric plexus. *Endocrinology,* 99:1653–1654.

63. Gyermak, L. (1961): 5-Hydroxytryptamine antagonists. *Pharmacol. Rev.,* 13:399–440.

64. Harding, R., and Leek, B. F. (1972): Gastroduodenal receptor response to chemical and mechanical stimuli, investigated by a single fibre technique. *J. Physiol. (Lond.),* 222:139–140 P.

65. Harding, R., and Leek, B. F. (1972): Rapidly adapting mechanoreceptors in the reticulo-rumen which respond to chemicals. *J. Physiol. (lond.),* 223:32–33.

66. Hardy, J. D., and Bard, P. (1974): Body temperature regulation. In: *Medical Physiology, 13th Ed., Vol. 2,* edited by B. V. Mountcastle, pp. 1305–1342. C. V. Mosby Co., St. Louis.

67. Harry, J. (1963): The action of drugs on the circular strip from the guinea-pig isolated ileum. *Br. J. Pharmacol.,* 20:399–417.

68. Hayashi, E., Mori, M., Yamada, S., and Kunitomo, M. (1978): Effects of purine compounds on cholinergic nerves. Sepcificity of adenosine and related compounds on acetylcholine release in

electrically stimulated guinea-pig ileum. *Eur. J. Pharmacol.,* 48:297–307.

69. Heimbach, D. M., and Crout, J. R. (1971): Treatment of paralytic ileus with adrenergic neuronal blocking drugs. *Surgery,* 69:582–587.

70. Heitz, P., Polak, J. M., Timson, C. M., and Pearse, A. G. E. (1976): Enterochromaffin cells as the endocrine source of gastrointestinal substance P. *Histochemistry,* 49:343–347.

71. Hidaka, T., and Kuriyama, H. (1969): Responses of the smooth muscle membrane of guinea-pig jejunum elicited by field stimulation. *J. Gen. Physiol.,* 53:471–486.

72. Hirst, G. D. S., Holman, M. E., and Spence, I. (1974): Two types of neurons in the myenteric plexus of duodenum in the guinea-pig. *J. Physiol. (Lond.),* 236:303–326.

73. Hirst, G. D. S., and McKirdy, H. C. (1974): A nervous mechanism for descending inhibition in guinea-pig small intestine. *J. Physiol. (Lond.),* 238:129–144.

74. Hirst, G. D. S., and McKirdy, H. C. (1974). Presynaptic inhibition at a mammalian peripheral synapse. *Nature (Lond.),* 250:430–431.

75. Hirst, G. D. S., and McKirdy, H. C. (1975): Synaptic potentials recorded from neurones of the submucous plexus of guinea-pig small intestine. *J. Physiol. (Lond.),* 249:369–385.

76. Hirst, G. D. S., and Silinsky, E. M. (1975): Some effects of 5-hydroxytryptamine, dopamine and noradrenaline on neurones in the submucous plexus of guinea-pig small intestine. *J. Physiol. (Lond.),* 251:817–832.

77. Hirst, G. D. S., and Spence, I. (1973): Calcium action potentials in mammalian peripheral neurones. *Nature (Lond.),* 243:54–56.

78. Hodgkiss, J. P., and Lees, G. M. (1978): Correlated electrophysiological and morphological characteristics of myenteric neurones. *J. Physiol. (Lond.),* 285:19–20P.

79. Hoffman, H. H., and Schnitzlein, N. N. (1969): The number of vagus nerves in man. *Anat. Rec.,* 139:429–435.

80. Holman, M. E. (1968): An introduction to electrophysiology of visceral smooth muscle. In: *Handbook of Physiology, Section 6, Alimentary Canal, Vol. IV,* edited by C. F. Code, pp. 1665–1708. American Physiological Society, Washington, D.C.

81. Holman, M. E., Hirst, G. D. S., and Spence, I. (1972): Preliminary studies of the neurones of Auerbach's plexus using intracellular microelectrodes. *Aust. J. Exp. Biol. Med.,* 50:795–801.

82. Howd, R. A., Adamovics, A., and Palekar, A. (1978): Naloxone and intestinal motility. *Experientia,* 34:1310–1311.

83. Hubel, K. (1978): The effects of electrical field stimulation and tetrodotoxin on ion transport by the isolated rabbit ileum. *J. Clin. Invest.,* 62:1039–1047.

84. Hukuhara, T., Kotania, S., and Sato, G. (1961): Effect of destruction of intramural ganglion cells on colon motility: Possible genesis of congenital megacolon. *Jpn. J. Physiol.,* 11:635–640.

85. Humphrey, C. S., and Fischer, J. E. (1978): Peptidergic versus purinergic nerves. *Lancet,* 1:390.

86. Iggo, A. (1957): Gastrointestinal tension receptors with unmyelinated afferent fibers in the vagus of the cat. *Q. J. Exp. Physiol.,* 42:130–143.

87. Iggo, A. (1957): Gastric mucosal chemoreceptors with vagal afferent fibers in the cat. *Q. J. Exp. Physiol.,* 42:398–409.

88. Jacobowitz, D. (1965): Histochemical studies of the autonomic innervation of the gut. *J. Pharmacol. Exp. Ther.,* 149:356–364.

89. Jonakait, G. S., Tamir, H., Gintzler, A. R., and Gershon, M. D. (1978): Release of serotonin and its binding protein from enteric neurons. *7th Int. Cong. Pharmacol.,* Paris, P. 737.

90. Jonakait, C. M., Tamir, H. Rapport, M. M., and Gershon, M. D. (1977): Detection of a soluble serotonin binding protein in the mammalian myenteric plexus and other peripheral sites of serotonin storage. *J. Neurochem.,* 28:277–284.

91. Kadair, R. G., Sims, J. E., and Critchfield, C. F. (1977): Zonal colonic hypoganglionosis. *J.A.M.A.,* 238:1838–1840.

92. Katayama, Y., and North, R. A. (1978): Does substance P mediate slow synaptic excitation within the myenteric plexus? *Nature (Lond.),* 274:387–388.

93. Kellum, J. M., Jr., and Jaffe, B. M. (1976): Release of immunoreactive serotonin following acid perfusion of the duodenum. *Ann. Surg.,* 184:633–636.

94. Kennedy, D., Evoy, W. H., and Hannawalt, J. T. (1966): Release of coordinated behavior in crayfish by single central neurons. *Science,* 154:917–919.

95. Kilbinger, H., and Wagner, P. (1975): Inhibition by oxytremorine of acetylcholine resting release from guinea-pig ileum longitudinal muscle strips. *Naunyn-Schmiedebergs Arch. Pharmacol.,* 287:47–60.

96. Kitamura, K. (1978): Comparative aspects of membrane properties and innervation of longitudinal and circular muscle layers of rabbit jejunum. *Jpn. J. Physiol.,* 28:583–601.

97. Knoll, J., Zseli, J., Ronai, A., and Vizi, E. S. (1974): Effect of azidomorphine and related substances on the intestinal motility. *Pharmacology,* 12:283–289.

98. Koren, E., Wapnick, S., Solowiedczyk, M., Pfeifer, Y., and Sulman, F. G. (1976): Serotonin in the portal vein after acidification. *Int. Surg.,* 61:370–371.

99. Kosterlitz, H. W., Lydon, R. J., and Watt, A. J. (1970): the effects of adrenaline, noradrenaline and isoprenaline on inhibitory alpha- and beta-adrenoreceptors in the longitudinal muscle of the guinea-pig ileum. *Br. J. Pharmacol.,* 391:398–413.

100. Kostuch, T. E., and Duke, G. E. (1975): Gastric motility in great horned owls *(Bubo virginianus). Comp. Biochem. Physiol.,* 51A:201–205.

101. Kuntz, A. (1922): On the occurrence of reflex arcs in the myenteric and submucous plexuses. *Anat. Rec.,* 13:193–210.

102. Kuriyama, H., Osa, T., and Toida, N. (1967): Nervous factors influencing the membrane activity of intestinal smooth muscle. *J. Physiol. (Lond.),* 191:251–270.

103. Kwenter, J. (1965); The vagal control of the jejunal and ileal motility and blood flow. *Acta Physiol. Scand. [Suppl.],* 251:3–68.

104. Langley, J. N. (1921): *The Autonomic Nervous System.* Part 1. W. Heffer and Sons.

105. Lent, C. M. (1974): Neuronal control of mucous secretion by leeches: toward a general theory for serotonin. *Am. Zool.,* 14:931–942.

106. Mackenna, B. R., and McKirdy, H. C. (1972): Peristalsis in the rabbit distal colon. *J. Physiol. (Lond.),* 220:33–54.

107. Mayer, C. J., and Wood, J. D. (1975): Properties of mechanosensitive neurons within Auerbach's plexus of the small intestine of the cat. *Pflügers Arch.,* 357:35–49.

108. Meech, R. W. (1974): The sensitivity of *Helix aspera* neurones to injected calcium ions. *J. Physiol. (Lond.),* 237:259–277.

109. Mei, N. (1970): Mechanorecepteurs vagaux digestive chez le chat. *Exp. Brain Res.,* 11:502–514.

110. Mei, N. (1978): Vagal glucoreceptors in the small intestine of the cat. *J. Physiol. (Lond.),* 282:485–506.

111. Nagai, T., and Prosser, C. L. (1963): Electrical parameters of smooth muscle cells. *Am. J. Physiol.,* 204:915–925.

112. Nilsson, G., Larsson, L.-I., Håkanson, R., Brodin, E., Pernow, B., and Sundler, F. (1975): Localization of substance P-like immunoreactivity in mouse gut. *Histochemistry,* 43:97–99.

113. Nishi, S., and North, R. A. (1973): Intracellular recording from the myenteric plexus of the guinea-pig ileum. *J. Physiol. (Lond.),* 231:471–491.

114. Nonidez, J. F. (1946): Afferent nerve endings in ganglia of intermuscular plexus of dog's esophagus. *J. Comp. Neurol.,* 85:177–189.

115. Norberg, R. A. (1964): Adrenergic innervation of the intestinal wall studied by fluorescence microscopy. *Int. J. Neuropharmacol.,* 3:379–382.

116. Norberg, R. A., and Sjogvist, R. (1966): New possibilities for adrenergic modulation of synaptic transmission. *Pharmacol. Rev.,* 18:743–751.

117. North, R. A. (1973): The calcium-dependent slow after-hyperpolarization in myenteric plexus neurons with tetrodotoxin-resistant action potential. *Br. J. Pharmacol.,* 49:709–711.

118. North, R. A. (1976): Effects of morphine on myenteric neurons. *Neuropharmacology,* 15:719–721.

119. North, R. A., and Henderson, G. (1975): Action of morphine on guinea-pig myenteric plexus and mouse vas deferens studied by intracellular recording. *Life Sci.,* 17:63–66.

120. North, R. A., Katayama, Y., and Williams, J. T. (1979): On the mechanism and site of action of enkephalin on single myenteric neurons. *Brain Res.,* 165:67–77.

121. North, R. A., and Tonini, M. (1976): Hyperpolarization by morphine of myenteric neurones. In: *Opiates and Endogenous Opioid Peptides,* edited by H. W. Kosterlitz, pp. 205–212. North-Holland, Amsterdam.

122. North, R. A., and Tonini, M. (1977): The mechanism of action of narcotic analgesics in the guinea-pig ileum. *Br. J. Pharmacol.*, 61:541–549.

123. North, R. A., and Williams, J. T. (1977): Extracellular recording from the guinea-pig myenteric plexus and the action of morphine. *Eur. J. Pharmacol.*, 45:23–33.

124. Nozdrachev, A. D., Katchalov, U. P., and Bnetov, A. F. (1975): Spontaneous discharge of neurons in myenteric plexus of the intestine of rabbits. *Fisiol. Zh. U.S.S.R.*, 61:725–730.

125. Ohkawa, H., and Prosser, C. L. (1972): Electrical activity in myenteric and submucous plexuses of cat intestine. *Am. J. Physiol.*, 222:1412–1419.

126. Ohkawa, H., and Prosser, C. L. (1972): Functions of enteric neurons in enteric plexuses of cat intestine. *Am. J. Physiol.*, 222:1420–1426.

127. Okwuasaba, F. K., Hamilton, J. T., and Cook, M. A. (1978): Evidence for the cell surface locus of presynaptic purine nucleotide receptors in the guinea-pig ileum. *J. Pharmacol. Exp. Ther.*, 207:779–786.

128. Paintal, A. S. (1957): Responses from mucosal mechanoreceptors in the small intestine of the cat. *J. Physiol. (Lond.)*, 139:353–368.

129. Paton, W. D. M. (1957): The action of morphine and related compounds on contraction and on acetylcholine output of coaxially stimulated guinea-pig ileum. *Br. J. Pharmacol. Chemother.*, 12:119–127.

130. Paton, W. D. M., and Vizi, E. S. (1969): The inhibitory action of noradrenaline on acetylcholine output by guinea-pig ileum longitudinal muscle strip. *Br. J. Pharmacol.*, 35:10–28.

131. Paton, W. D. M., and Zar, M. A. (1968): The origin of acetylcholine released from guinea-pig intestine and longitudinal muscle strips. *J. Physiol. (Lond.)*, 194:13–33.

132. Pearse, A. G. E., and Polak, J. M. (1975): Immunocytochemical localization of substance P in mammalian intestine. *Histochemistry*, 41:373–375.

133. Pearse, A. G. E., and Polak, J. M. (1978): The diffuse neuroendocrine system and the APUD concept. In: *Gut Hormones*, edited by S. R. Bloom, pp. 33–39. Churchill Livingstone, New York.

134. Powell, D., Cannon, D., Skrabanek, P., and Kirrane, J. (1978): The pathyphysiology of substance P in man. In: *Gut Hormones*, edited by S. R. Bloom, pp. 524–529. Churchill Livingstone, New York.

135. Prosser, C. L., and Bortoff, A. (1968): Electrical activity of intestinal muscle under *in vitro* condition. In: *Handbook of Physiology, Section 6, Alimentary Canal, Vol. IV*, edited by C. F. Code, pp. 2025–2050. American Physiological Society, Washington, D.C.

136. Purves, R. D. (1974): Muscarinic excitation: A microelectrode study on cultured smooth muscle cells. *Br. J. Pharmacol.*, 52:77–86.

137. Ranieri, F., Mei, N., and Groussilat, J. (1973): Les afferences splanchniques provenant des mechano recepteurs gastrointestinaux et peritoneaux. *Exp. Brain Res.*, 16:276–290.

138. Rayner, V. (1979): Characteristics of the internal anal sphincter and the rectum of the vervet monkey. *J. Physiol. (Lond.)*, 286:383–399.

139. Richardson, K. C. (1958): Electron microscopic observations on Auerbach's plexus in the rabbit with special reference to the problem of smooth muscle innervation. *Am. J. Anat.*, 103:99–136.

140. Rikimura, A., and Suzuki, T. (1971): Neural mechanism of the relaxing response of guinea-pig taenia coli. *Tokohu J. Exp. Med.*, 103:303–315.

141. Sato, T., Tankayanagi, I., and Takagi, K. (1973): Pharmacological properties of electrical activities obtained from neurons in Auerbach's plexus. *Jpn. J. Pharmacol.*, 23:665–671.

142. Satoni, H., Yamamoto, T., Ise, H., and Takatami, H. (1978): Origins of the parasympathetic fibers to the cat intestine as demonstrated by the horseradish peroxidase method. *Brain Res.*, 151:571–578.

143. Sauer, M. E., and Rumble, C. T. (1946): Number of nerve cells in myenteric and submucous plexuses of small intestine of cat. *Anat. Rec.*, 96:373–381.

144. Sawynok, J., and Jhamandas, K. (1977): Muscarinic feedback inhibition of acetylcholine release from the myenteric plexus in the guinea-pig ileum and its status after chronic exposure to morphine. *Can. J. Physiol. Pharmacol.*, 55:909–916.

145. Schiller, W. R., Suriyapa, C., Mutchler, J. H. W., and Anderson, M. C. (1973): Surgical alteration of intestinal motility. *Am. J. Surg.*, 125:122–128.

146. Shepherd, G. M. (1978): Microcircuits in the nervous system. *Sci. Am.*, 238:92–103.

147. Shimo, Y., and Ishii, T. (1978): Effects of morphine on non-adrenergic inhibitory responses of the guinea-pig taenia coli. *J. Pharm. Pharmacol.*, 30:496–497.

148. Smith, J., Kelly, K. A., and Weinshilboum, M. (1977): Pathophysiology of postoperative ileus. *Arch. Surg.*, 112:203–209.

149. Synder, S. H., and Childers, S. R. (1979): Opiate receptors and opioid peptides. *Annu. Rev. Neurosci.*, 2:35–64.

150. Strumwasser, F. (1967): Types of information stored in single neurons. In: *Invertebrate Nervous Systems*, edited by C. A. G. Wiersma, pp. 291–320. University of Chicago Press, Chicago.

151. Szurszewski, J. H. (1969): A migrating electric complex of the canine small intestine. *Am. J. Physiol.*, 217:1757–1763.

152. Szurszewski, J. H., and Weems, W. A. (1976): A study of peripheral input to and its control by postganglionic neurones of the inferior mesenteric ganglion. *J. Physiol. (Lond.)*, 256:541–556.

153. Tafuri, W. L., and Raick, A. (1964): Presence of 5-hydroxytryptamine in the intramural nervous system of the guinea-pig's intestines. *Z. Naturforsch.*, 19:1126–1128.

154. Taxi, J. (1964): Etude, au microscope electronique, de l'innervation du muscle lisse intestinal comparee a' mammiferes. *Arch. Biol. (Liege)*, 75:301–328.

155. Tomita, T. (1970): Electrical properties of mammalian smooth muscle. In: *Smooth Muscle*, edited by E. Bülbring, A. F. Brading, A. W. Jones, and T. Tomita, pp. 197–243. Williams & Wilkins, Baltimore.

156. Tonini, M., Lecchini, S., Frigo, G., and Crema, A. (1974): Action of tetrodotoxin on spontaneous electrical activity of some smooth muscle preparations. *Eur. J. Pharmacol.*, 29:236–240.

157. Touloukian, R. J., and Duncan, R. (1975): Acquired aganglionic megacolon in a premature infant—Report of a case. *Pediatrics*, 56:459–462.

158. Tower, S. S. (1933): Action potentials in sympathetic nerves elicited by stimulation of frog's viscera. *J. Physiol. (Lond.)*, 78:225–245.

159. Tuck, A., and Cohen, S. (1973): Lower esophageal sphincter relaxation: Studies on the neurogenic inhibitory mechanisms. *J. Clin. Invest.*, 52:14–20.

160. Vaughn Williams, E. M., and Streeten, D. H. P. (1950): Action of morphine, pethidine and amidone upon intestinal motility of conscious dogs. *Br. J. Pharmacol.*, 5:584–603.

161. Vermillion, D., Gillespie, J., Cooke, A. R., and Wood, J. D. (1979): Does 5-hydroxytryptamine influence purinergic inhibitory neurons in the intestine? *Am. J. Physiol.*, 237:E198–E202.

162. Vizi, E. S., and Knoll, J. (1976): The inhibitory effect of adenosine and related nucleotides on the release of acetycholine. *Neuroscience*, 1:391–398.

163. Vizi, V. A., and Vizi, E. S. (1978): Direct evidence for acetylcholine releasing effect of serotonin in the Auerbach plexus. *J. Neural Transm.*, 42:127–138.

164. Wald, F. (1972): Ionic differences between somatic and axonal action potentials in snail giant neurones. *J. Physiol. (Lond.)*, 220:267–281.

165. Warner, R. R. (1967): Current status and implications of serotonin in clinical medicine. *Adv. Intern. Med.*, 13:241–282.

166. Weight, F. F., Schulman, J. A., Smith, P. A., and Busis, N. A. (1978): Long-lasting synaptic potentials and the modulation of synaptic transmission. *Fed. Proc.*, 88:2084–2094.

167. Williams, J. T., and North, R. A. (1978): Inhibition of firing of myenteric neurons by somatostatin. *Brain Res.*, 155:165–168.

168. Wood, J. D. (1969): Electrophysiological and pharmacological properties of the stomach of the squid, *Loligo pealii*. *Comp. Biochem. Physiol.*, 30:813–824.

169. Wood, J. D. (1970): Electrical activity from single neurons in Auerbach's plexus. *Am. J. Physiol.*, 219:159–169.

170. Wood, J. D. (1972): Excitation of intestinal muscle by atropine, tetrodotoxin and Xylocaine. *Am. J. Physiol.,* 222:118–125.

171. Wood, J. D. (1973): Electrical activity of the intestine of mice with hereditary megacolon and absence of enteric ganglion cells. *Am. J. Dig. Dis.,* 18:477–488.

172. Wood, J. D. (1973): Electrical discharge of single enteric neurons in guinea-pig small intestine. *Am. J. Physiol.,* 225:1107–1113.

173. Wood, J. D. (1974): Neurophysiology of ganglion of Auerbach's plexus. *Am. Zool.,* 14:973–989.

174. Wood, J. D. (1975): Effects of elevated magnesium on discharge of myenteric neurons of cat small bowel. *Am. J. Physiol.,* 229:657–662.

175. Wood, J. D. (1979): Intracellular study of effects of morphine on electrical activity of myenteric neurons in cat small intestine. *Fed. Proc.,* 38:959.

176. Wood, J. D., Grafe, P., and Mayer, C. J. (1979): Slow synaptic modulation of excitability mediated by inactivation of calcium-dependent potassium conductance in myenteric neurons of guinea-pig small intestine. *Neurosci. Abstr.,* 5:749.

177. Wood, J. D., and Harris, B. R. (1972): Phase relationships of the intestinal muscularis: Effects of atropine and Xylocaine. *J. Appl. Physiol.,* 32:734–737.

178. Wood, J. D., and Marsh, D. R. (1973): Effects of atropine, tetrodotoxin and lidocaine on rebound excitation of guinea-pig small intestine. *J. Pharmacol. Exp. Ther.,* 184:590–602.

179. Wood, J. D., and Mayer, C. J. (1973): Patterned discharge of six different neurons in a single enteric ganglion. *Pflügers Arch.,* 338:247–256.

180. Wood, J. D., and Mayer, C. J. (1974): Discharge patterns of single enteric neurons of the small intestine of the cat, dog and guinea-pig. In: *Proceedings IV International Symposium on Gastrointestinal Motility,* edited by E. E. Daniel, pp. 387–408. Mitchell Press, Vancouver, Canada.

181. Wood, J. D., and Mayer, C. J. (1978): Intracellular study of electrical activity of Auerbach's plexus in guinea-pig small intestine. *Pflugers Arch.,* 374:265–275.

182. Wood, J. D., and Mayer, C. J. (1979): Intracellular study of tonic-type enteric neurons in guinea-pig small intestine. *J. Neurophysiol.,* 42:569–581.

183. Wood, J. D., and Mayer, C. J. (1979): Serotonergic activation of tonic-type enteric neurons in guinea-pig small intestine. *J. Neurophysiol.,* 42:582–593.

184. Wood, J. D., and Mayer, C. J. (1979): Adrenergic inhibition of serotonin release from neurons in guinea-pig Auerbach's plexus. *J. Neurophysiol.,* 42:594–693.

185. Wood, J. D., and Perkins, W. E. (1970): Mechanical interactions between longitudinal and circular axis of the small intestine. *Am. J. Physiol.,* 218:762–768.

186. Yamamura, H. I., and Snyder, S. H. (1974): Muscarinic cholinergic receptor binding in the longitudinal muscle of the guinea-pig ileum with (3H) ouinudidinyl benzilate. *Mol. Pharmacol.,* 10:861–867.

187. Yokoyama, S. (1966): Aktionpotentiale der ganglienzelle des Auerbachschen plexus in kaninchen dundarm. *Arch. Ges. Physiol.,* 288:95–102.

188. Yokoyama, S., and Ozaki, T. (1978): Polarity of effects of stimulation of Auerbach's plexus on longitudinal muscle. *Am. J. Physiol.,* 235:E345–E353.

Physiology of the Gastrointestinal Tract, edited by
Leonard R. Johnson, Raven Press, New York © 1981.

Chapter 2

Endocrine Cells of the Digestive System

Enrico Solcia, Carlo Capella, Roberto Buffa, Luciana Usellini, Roberto Fiocca,
and Fausto Sessa

HISTORICAL BACKGROUND, TERMINOLOGY, AND GENERAL CONCEPTS

Specialized *chromaffin, osmiophilic, basigranular yellow* or *acidophil* cells were described in the gastrointestinal mucosa by a number of histologists from 1870 to the first decade of this century. However, it was only in 1914 that Masson (60) discovered the silver-reducing power of such cells and recognized their endocrine-like nature. The chromaffin and argentaffin product stored in their secretory granules was identified as 5-hydroxytryptamine (5-HT) by Erspamer and associates (28,107).

The presence in the gastrointestinal mucosa of endocrine-like cells lacking 5-HT was repeatedly suggested during the first half of this century. Their morphological and functional independence from 5-HT-storing *argentaffin* or *enterochromaffin* (EC) cells, long disputed, was finally proved by electron microscopy (95) and immunohistochemistry (61). Among these non-EC cells, several morphologically distinct cell types were soon identified and correlated with the production of one or another member of the expanding family of gut endocrine peptides (15,20,33,72,89,106). A series of common histological, histochemical, and ultrastructural properties were found among such cells, which encouraged some authors to group all of them as members of the diffuse endocrine system (DES) (30) and the amine precursor uptake and decarboxylation (APUD) cell system (68).

The possibility that in addition to blood-mediated, truly endocrine effects, such cells display some local modulatory or *paracrine* activity was first suggested by Feyrter (30) and recently supported by finding substances such as somatostatin (27,76) or bombesin (102) in some of these cells. Somatostatin is known to inhibit a number of gut cells, including gastrin, cholecystokinin (CCK), and oxyntic cells, lying in the same epithelia containing somatostatin-producing D cells (70). Apart from direct cell-to-cell contacts through cell bodies or cell prolongations (45), release and diffusion of active products into intercellular spaces (86,87) may provide a morphologic basis of such paracrine function (Figs. 1 and 2). Although some active substances, such as gastrin, glucagon, secretin, CCK, and gastric inhibitory polypeptide (GIP), seem to display mainly endocrine effects and substances such as somatostatin or bombesin might have mainly paracrine functions, much overlapping seems to occur in this field. Thus a clear-cut separation of gut endocrine-paracrine substances and cells into two functional classes is not feasible. On their way to blood capillaries and long-distance targets, the same peptides or amines from gut endocrine-paracrine cells may encounter local targets such as neighboring epithelial cells, subepithelial nerve endings (Fig. 3), and smooth muscle fibers (of the villi, muscularis mucosae, or vessel walls). The functional flexibility of such substances is further exemplified by their occur-

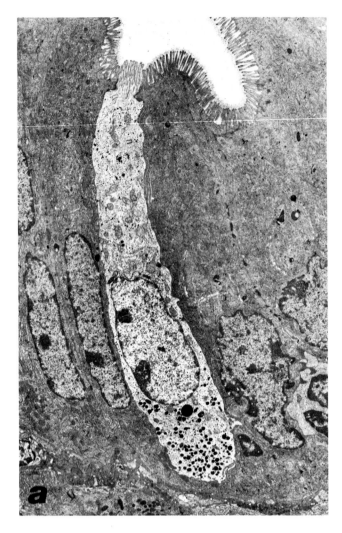

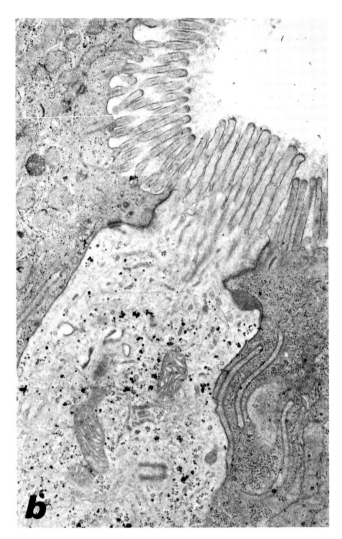

FIG. 1a. S cell of the human jejunum. **a:** In this section the cell extends from the lumen to just above the basal membrane of the epithelium. × 3,510.

FIG. 1b. Enlargement of the luminal ending showing a regular tuft of microvilli, slightly different from those of absorptive cells, elongated cisternae filled with amorphous material, junctional complexes with neighboring absorptive cells, and a centriole. × 19,500.

rence in gut nerves and brain, where they seem to act as neural mediators (35).

Techniques

Recent developments in the field of gut endocrinology have been largely dependent on the application of refined morphologic techniques providing selective detection of the endocrine-paracrine cells scattered in the gastrointestinal mucosa. Techniques staining selectively the secretory granules (as Grimelius', Sevier-Munger's, or Davenport's silver, lead-hematoxylin, and masked metachromasia), histochemical techniques detecting secretory peptides or amines, and electron microscopy have been used for this purpose.

When the whole endocrine cell population of a tissue is to be studied, Grimelius' silver (36) and lead-hematoxylin (88) are the techniques of choice. However, the same techniques are of little help when the exact type of endocrine cell is to be identified. This goal is better

achieved by means of immunoradiochemistry and electron microscopy. Of course, specific antisera and a number of control tests are needed with both immunofluorescence and immunoperoxidase procedures before reasonable confidence can be placed in the demonstration of a hormonal substance. Recently, it has been shown that some endocrine cells of the gut such as gastrin G cells, somatostatin D cells, glucagon A cells, and argentaffin EC cells bind gamma globulins—especially aggregated immunoglobulins—nonspecifically, partly through complement (11). Thus the use of highly dilute, complement-deprived, and aggregate-free sera is mandatory in immunohistochemical tests. Another drawback of immunohistochemical studies is the frequent cross-reactivity among chemically related sequences of peptides. To recognize and prevent it, antibody populations of antihormone sera must be characterized radioimmunochemically as well as immunohistochemically by their incubation with known

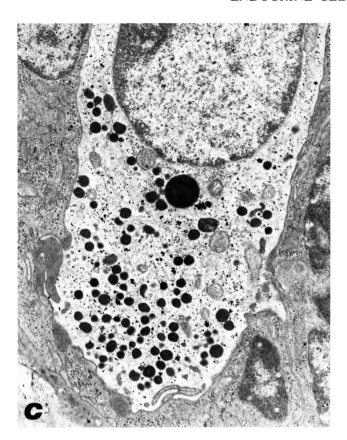

FIG. 1c. Enlargement of the basal part of the cell showing secretory granules. Note accumulation of homogeneous material (secretory products) in the intercellular spaces surrounding the cell × 10,500.

peptide sequences of the hormone-related molecules (13,48).

Amine-storing cells are better shown with fluorescence histochemistry of freeze-dried, vapor-formaldehyde-treated tissues or with immunohistochemistry, although more simple techniques, such as Masson's argentaffin reaction or the diazonium reaction applied to routine paraffin sections, may be helpful for EC cells. Enzyme histochemistry and fluorescence histochemistry of amines resulting from injected precursors (APUD phenomenon) have also been used for the study of gut endocrine cells (39,67). By studying the size, shape, inner structure, osmiophilia, argyrophilia, or argentaffinity of secretory granules, electron microscopists identified different endocrine cell types (15,20,33,89,106). Many of these cell types have been confirmed by subsequent studies coupling immunohistochemistry with electron microscopy, either by means of electron immunocytochemistry or with the consecutive semithin-thin technique (5-7,14,54,99).

GENERAL CYTOLOGY OF THE ENDOCRINE-PARACRINE CELL

Endocrine-paracrine cells are scattered in the epithelium lining the gastric glands, intestinal crypts, and villi.

As a rule, secretory granules are concentrated in the basal part of the cytoplasm, whereas the Golgi complex is supranuclear. In the pyloric and intestinal mucosa, most reach the lumen in a narrow, specialized area showing tufts of microvilli, coated vesicles, and a centriole; likely, this area acts as a receptor surface facing luminal contents (95). Such pattern suggests some functional polarity of the cell (Fig. 1). In the fundic mucosa, endocrine-paracrine cells lack luminal contacts and show less evident polarity (89).

Secretory granules are released at the basal surface of the cell or along the lower part of its lateral surface (43) where intervening cells may form interstitial spaces and canaliculi (Fig. 2). In the upper (juxtaluminal) part of the epithelium, these spaces are closed by junctional complexes with neighboring cells (Fig. 1). Granule release at the luminal surface has never been observed. Smooth vesicles and elongated cisternae are often found just below the luminal surface of the cell or in the supranuclear cytoplasm between the Golgi complex and the luminal endings.

Microtubules, thin microfilaments, and intermediate (100 nm, cytoskeletal) filaments are found in gut endocrine cells. The latter filaments are particularly well developed in some cell types, as in gastric P or D_1 cells and intestinal motilin (Mo) cells, where they may form perinuclear bundles. A mechanical function is to be postulated for such filaments, possibly involved in the reception of mechanical stimuli from the lumen.

Nerves and neurons, which store the same active substances found in endocrine cells [substance P, somatostatin, gastrin, CCK, enkephalin, bombesin, catecholamines; possibly 5-HT, neurotensin, pancreatic polypeptide (PP)] or closely related molecules [vasoactive intestinal peptide (VIP), angiotensin, acetylcholine, and gamma-aminobutyric acid], are widely distributed in the gastrointestinal wall, including the mucosa and submucosa. Small solid granules differing from small empty "cholinergic" and cored "adrenergic" vesicles have been identified ultrastructurally in peptide-storing nerves (Fig. 3). So far, conventional electron microscopy seems of little help in distinguishing nerves storing different peptides. No ultrastructural resemblance has been shown between granules of nerves and those of endocrine cells storing the same peptide. Although lacking direct reciprocal contacts, mucosal nerve endings and endocrine cells might display some functional interaction through release and local diffusion of active amines and peptides. In keeping with Pearse's concept (67), nerves and endocrine cells of the gut should be regarded as two integrated systems modulating digestive functions.

Occasionally, endocrine-like cells resembling P or D_1 cells are found in the lamina propria of the intestinal and gastric mucosa (Fig. 4). These cells may be in contact with nerve endings and Schwann-like cells, thus

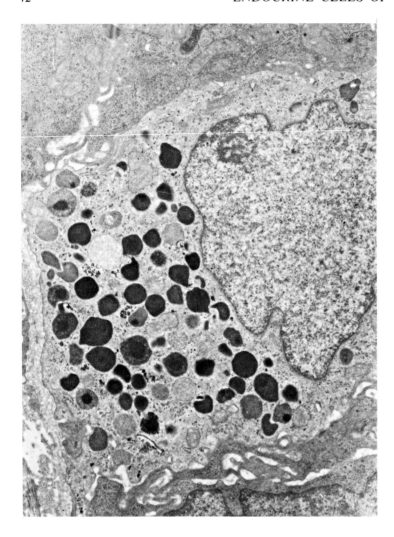

FIG. 2. Basal part of a K cell in the human duodenum. Note large, partly target-like granules and intercellular intraepithelial spaces. × 11,730.

displaying paraganglionic features. Such extraglandular cells are found more frequently in fetal life; they increase dramatically in the inflamed lamina propria of chronic atrophic gastritis.

EMBRYOLOGY AND PHYLOGENESIS

Both endodermal and neuroectodermal origins of gut endocrine-paracrine cells have been considered. Their origin from nervous elements, first put forward by Danisch, has been supported by Pearse and co-workers (67,69,70), who suggested the involvement of neural crest or neurally programmed cells of epiblastic origin. Recent graft experiments accurately performed in embryos (57) suggest that gut endocrine cells are not derived from neural crest or the epiblast. At present, the endodermal theory seems better documented (4,57). Similar conclusions seem valid also for pancreatic endocrine cells (71).

The local modulatory function displayed by paracrine cells through the release of active peptides and amines mimics somewhat the function of the peripheral nerve system. The similarity is strengthened by the fact that most active peptides and amines found in paracrine cells are also present in the peripheral and/or central nervous system and are reputed to act as neurotransmitters (35,70). However, cells of proven neurocrest origin such as adrenal medullary cells, chromaffin cells of sympathetic paraganglia, interneurons, carotid body cells, and other nonchromaffin paraganglionic cells (59) seem functionally and morphologically more related to the nervous system than are paracrine cells. Calcitonin C cells that, despite their neural crest origin (58), are scattered among thyroid endodermal epithelia as are DES cells, are intermediate between paraganglionic and paracrine cells. It is of interest that recently, in addition to the usual C cells, multiple somatostatin-calcitonin immunoreactive cells ultrastructurally indistinguishable from gut D cells have been detected in mammalian thyroid and thyroid medullary carcinoma (10).

In addition to being found in gastrointestinal mucosa and pancreas, some endocrine-paracrine cells are scattered in the lung, trachea, thyroid, thymus, esophagus, biliary system, urethra, prostate, and rabbit vestibulum vaginae, all of which are known to be of endodermal origin or to receive important contributions from the endoderm. Of 17 cell types which may be considered

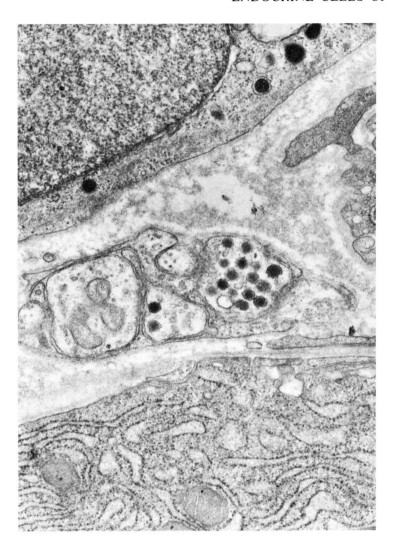

FIG. 3. Nerve ending with peptidergic granules in the lamina propria of the human gastric mucosa, near an ECL cell (*above*) and a peptic cell (*below*). × 29,750.

among DES cells (87), only C cells have been shown to be of neuroectodermal origin. Most of the remaining 16 cell types are likely to come from the endoderm, as do the parathyroid cells.

The amount, type, and distribution of endocrine cells in fetal tissues are often quite different from those of adult tissues. Gastrin cells are known to appear earlier in the duodenum than in the stomach, where they predominate in adult life; moreover, they are present in the fetal and neonatal pancreas of some species, while lacking in adult pancreas of the same species (53). These findings may be relevant in explaining the occurrence of gastrinomas in the pancreas and duodenum more frequently than in the stomach. In both large and small intestine, somatostatin D cells are more numerous during late fetal life than in adult life (3,27). They might contribute to inhibition of intestinal functions which are unnecessary during fetal life. Conversely, gastric ECL cells, likely involved in the local stimulation of acidpeptic secretion, are quite scarce in human fetuses, a finding possibly related with the need to prevent unnecessary gastric secretion (17).

Some cell types, such as gastrin and CCK cells, may have common embryologic and phylogenetic origin (46,49). L (GLI) and glucagon cells are also likely to be related in this respect (31,62,79). A common evolution of all peptides and cells of the glucagon-secretin family, including VIP and GIP, may also be postulated based on the close homology of their molecules and some ultrastructural similarity of related cells. Immunological and biological studies have shown that many of the peptides detected in the endocrine-paracrine cells of mammalian gut have counterparts in lower vertebrates and even in protostomian invertebrates, either in nerves or in epithelial cells (103). The four main hormones of the pancreatic islets first appear in the alimentary canal of invertebrates (protochordates). Studies in cyclostomes and fishes suggest that insulin cells were phylogenetically the first to appear in the islets, followed by somatostatin, glucagon, and, last, PP cells (103). The occurrence of many gut-brain peptides in nerves of protostomian invertebrates, usually lacking corresponding endocrine cells, suggests that the vertebrate hormones may have originated in neural tissue before the

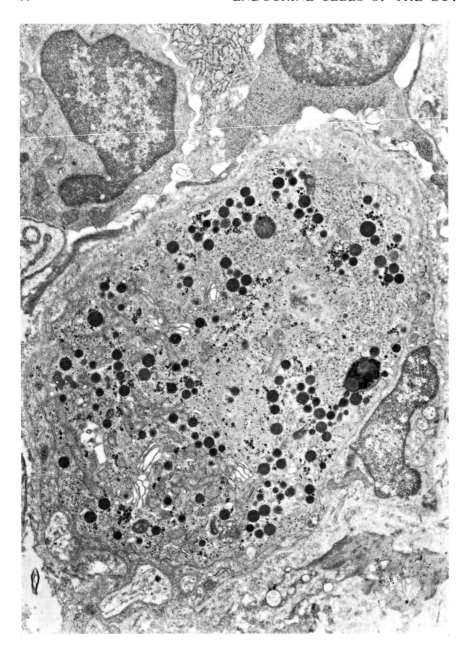

FIG. 4. Endocrine-like, paraganglionic cell in the lamina propria of the human duodenum, enveloped by a Schwann cell showing axons in its cytoplasm. × 9,350.

development of the vertebrate line of evolution (103). The occurrence of such peptides in neurosecretory fibers of coelenterates (82), notoriously lacking a circulatory system, suggests that the neuroparacrine mechanism represents the first form of cell control by extracellular molecular messengers (25).

IDENTIFICATION AND CLASSIFICATION OF CELL TYPES

Criteria to be Followed

Most cytological work done so far in the field of gut endocrinology has been based on the widely held concept "one hormone, one cell." There is increasing evi-

dence, however, that this concept suffers from some limitations. First, instead of just a single peptide hormone, endocrine cells produce a family of biologically and chemically related peptides, which have to be considered in histochemical studies. Second, a peptide and an amine are sometimes produced by the same cell. In this case, it appears that the peptide represents a safer point of reference for cell identification and classification than the amine, which is often found in ultrastructurally different cells that produce different peptide hormones and enter different physiologic reactions. For instance, 5-HT has been found in EC cells producing substance P or enkephalin and also in insulin B cells of the guinea pig, in glucagon A cells of the pig, and in calcitonin C cells of the horse, sheep, and goat (89). As a consequence, the cells so far defined as EC cells due to their 5-HT content are better reclassified on the basis of the peptide they store.

When immunoreactivities with apparently unrelated peptides are detected in the same cell, one has to consider the possibility: (a) of such peptides being part of a bigger precursor molecule, as recently suggested for glucagon and PP occurring together in intestinal L cells (31), (b) of cross-reacting sequences present in yet unknown molecular species of a known hormone, and (c) of a mixed endocrine cell showing different kinds of secretory granules. The ultrastructural evidence suggests that the latter phenomenon occurs seldom in nonpathologic adult gut (21) and more frequently in fetal gut (46).

At any rate, the production of two chemically unrelated, active peptides by the same cell seems possible (10). This may cause difficulties in attempts to introduce a "functional" classification of cells based on the hormones they produce. It seems pertinent to recall that the function of a cell is not defined merely by the nature of its secretory products; its response to physiologic stimuli and the way it releases active substances are also important.

Thus, although in many instances the "one hormone, one cell" concept still works as a basis for cell classification, this rule is not without exceptions and must be followed with caution. Both immunohistochemical and ultrastructural features of the same cell must be considered carefully and compared with the results of radioimmunoassays performed on tissue extracts to discriminate between cells producing the real hormone and cross-reacting cells. For instance, GIP-immunoreactive cells of the dog duodenum correspond to a specific ultrastructural cell type, the K cell (Fig. 2). This cell, whose distribution has been found to match that of GIP-immunoreactivity in tissue extracts, differs ultrastructurally from GIP-immunoreactive cells of the dog pancreas and stomach (to be identified with A cells) or colon, rectum, and terminal ileum (corresponding mostly to L cells), where no or very scarce GIP has been found by radioimmunoassay (84). Anti-GIP sera showing no or weak cross-reactivity with A and L cells have been obtained (7,65). The findings we have obtained with anti-secretin sera are also significant in this respect; only some of them were specific for S cells, while other sera cross-reacted with A and L cells in tissues where no or very scarce secretin has been found by radioimmunoassay (83,84). The use of several anti-hormone sera, directed against different parts of the hormone molecule, should discriminate between immunoreactivities due to appropriate hormones, as a rule reacting with all the antisera available, and those of cross-reacting peptides, often reacting only with some antisera.

The first attempt to classify endocrine cells of mammalian gut was made by Solcia, Forssmann, and Pearse during the Wiesbaden 1969 Symposium, where seven cell types were considered. The Wiesbaden classification was revised during the Bologna meeting in 1973. Two more cell types were added to the gut endocrine cells and these were tentatively compared with pancreatic endocrine cells (91). As many as 15 gastroenteropancreatic (GEP) endocrine cells have been considered in the Lausanne 1977 classification approved by 18 specialists working in the field (93).

This classification, rearranged and improved according to a recent discussion held in Los Angeles (92), is reported in Table 1. It is based on ultrastructural and immunohistochemical studies interpreted in the light of

TABLE 1. *Human GEP endocrine paracrine cells*

Cell	Main product	Pancreas	Stomach Oxyntic	Antral	Intestine Small Upper	Lower	Large
P	Peptides?	a	+	+	+		
D₁	Peptides?	f	+	f	+	f	f
EC	5-HT, peptides	r	+	+	+	+	+
D	Somatostatin	+	+	+	+	f	r
PP(F)	Pancr. peptide	+				b	b
B	Insulin	+					
A	Glucagon	+	a				
X	Unknown		+				
ELC	Unknown (H,5-HT)		+				
G	Gastrin			+	f		
S	Secretin				+	f	
I	CCK				+	f	
K	GIP				+	f	
Mo	Motilin				+	f	
N	Neurotensin				r	+	r
L	GLI				f	+	+

a = fetus or newborn; b = BPP anti serum, mostly GLI cells; f = few; r = rare.

available biochemical data. A concise description of each cell type follows.

Gastrin G Cell, Cholecystokinin I Cell, and Related Cells

The classic gastrin-storing cell of the pyloric mucosa, or *G cell,* is a medium-sized, ovoid to bottle or pear-shaped cell with abundant, slightly eosinophilic, faintly granular cytoplasm and a relatively large, round, clear nucleus. The cell can be distinguished from most surrounding mucous cells even in conventional hematoxylin and eosin preparations. However, in such preparations, activated or immature mucous cells, stem cells with clear cytoplasm, and other types of endocrine-paracrine cells—such as D cells or, in species other than man, EC cells—may be difficult or impossible to distinguish from G cells. Selective detection of G cells without interference of nonendocrine cells can be obtained with Grimelius' silver, lead-hematoxylin, or APUD fluorescence from injected precursors (89). However, EC cells, unless fixed in dichromate-containing fluids, and D cells interfere with the staining of G cells by lead-hematoxylin. With Grimelius' silver, EC cells are stained black, D cells remain practically unstained, and G cells are stained deep yellow to brown as are P and D_1 cells, but these are usually few in the pyloric mucosa. Although Grimelius' silver proved useful in preliminary investigations, especially for the screening of pathological cases, the only reliable technique for G-cell detection and quantitation in the light microscope remains immunohistochemistry (Fig. 5).

Most anti-gastrin sera contain antibody populations directed against the C-terminal part of the molecule, which is in common with CCK (48). When these antisera are used in immunohistochemical tests, staining of both gastrin and CCK cells is obtained (13,48). This cross-reactivity has little impact with studies on normal mammalian stomach, where no CCK cells have been detected so far; however, it is a major drawback when dealing with the small intestine or with pathologic stomachs showing intestinal (small bowel type) metaplasia, where CCK cells occur (52,81). In the latter cases, the use of antibodies directed against the non-C-terminal part of the gastrin molecule, a close comparison with results of CCK-specific antisera and parallel ultrastructural studies are mandatory.

In most species, pyloric G cells are characterized by the presence of vesicular granules with a floccular content, either finely dispersed, as in the rat and rabbit, or aggregated in the relatively dense cores of irregular contours, as in the cat. However, haloed granules with homogeneous, dense core (chicken), relatively compact granules with closely applied membrane (pig, guinea pig), or dense, compact, angular granules (bovine) are prevalent in G cells of some species. These various ultrastructural patterns of granules may coexist in the same species or even in the same cell. In man, the large majority of pyloric G cells display at least a proportion of vesicular granules sufficiently characteristic to allow identification; however, compact granules of various density and round to angular shape are also present in many cells. In a minority of cells, small, round, compact granules prevail; usually these can be identified as G cells because some more characteristic granules are also present (20,33,89,95,104). The functional state of the cell as well as the fixation procedures employed may also modify the ultrastructural appearance of G cell granules.

The G cells so far identified ultrastructurally in the human duodenal mucosa are scarce and disproportionally few in respect to gastrin-immunoreactive cells (51,89) found in the small intestine of man and several other mammals. This discrepancy has been resolved by

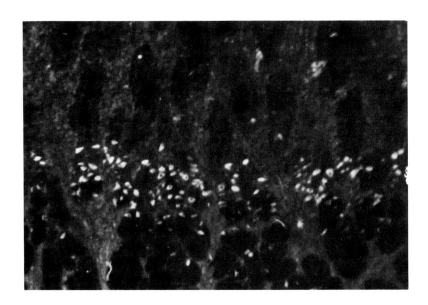

FIG. 5. Gastrin G cells in the human pyloric mucosa. Note their stratification in the deep part of mucous-neck cell zone and upper mucoid cell zone. Immunofluorescence test with anti-human gastrin I serum. × 150.

directly identifying gastrin-immunoreactive cells at the ultrastructural level (intestinal gastrin or IG cells) and finding in many of them small (about 175 nm), solid, round granules differing from those of G cells (8). It remains to be investigated whether the IG cells represent a functional variant of G cells or a distinct population of cells producing somewhat different gastrin-related peptides, including a larger proportion of big gastrin, and responding to different stimuli.

IG cells obviously differ from *CCK cells,* which in the human duodenum and jejunum show larger (about 260 nm) and more dense granules (6). Despite changes in size from one species to another, in all species so far investigated the granules of the CCK cell—corresponding to the I cell of ultrastructural studies—were solid, fairly dense, round, and unreactive with silver techniques (6,18,89). The immunohistochemical identification of this cell type has been obtained by using antibodies directed against the non-C-terminal part of the CCK molecule and lacking reactivity with mammalian G cells (6,13).

By using antisera directed against the C-terminal tetrapeptide of gastrin (and CCK), Larsson and Rehfeld (50) recently found in the pig and monkey intestine a cell (TG) showing granules more solid than those of G cells, less dense than those of CCK cells, and larger than those of IG cells. It remains questionable whether TG cells produce the gastrin-CCK tetrapeptide (50) or a larger molecule somewhat related to gastrin and/or CCK (26).

A further complication in the field comes from the finding in fetal human duodenum of cells with large, irregular granules reacting with C-terminal-specific antigastrin sera (46)—likely corresponding to at least part of the VL cells reported ultrastructurally (86)—and of cells reacting with both anti-gastrin and anti-CCK specific antisera. The latter finding, together with the immunohistochemical behavior of frog antral cells (49), suggest a common phylogenetic and ontogenetic evolution of G cells, CCK(I) cells, and functionally related cells. In a fraction of G cells of some species sequences of peptides other than gastrin and gastrin-related molecules have also been detected immunohistochemically, such as ACTH-like (44) and PP-like peptides (84). Such findings remain of obscure functional and/or evolutionary meaning.

Secretin S Cell, GIP(K) Cell, Glucagon A Cell, and GLI(L) Cell; VIP- and PP-Immunoreactive Cells

The staining of *secretin S cells* in the small intestine of mammals using immunohistochemical techniques has been obtained by several groups (54,73,90). With some antisera, cross-reactivity may occur with cells producing chemically related peptides (84). In these cases addition of glucagon, glicentin, and GIP to the anti-secretin serum is recommended to prevent nonspecific staining of L cells in the small and large intestine, A cells in the pancreas or fundic type gastric mucosa, and K(GIP) cells in the small intestine. When the specificity of the anti-secretin serum is ensured, secretin-immunoreactive cells are detected only in the small intestine, especially in the duodenum and jejunum (90). They are more numerous in the dog, cat, and pig than in man. In our experience secretin immunoreactive cells of the rat and mouse are about equally as numerous in the upper and lower small intestine; moreover, their separation from the intestinal cells producing chemically related hormones seems less obvious than in other mammals.

Ultrastructurally, secretin S cells (Fig. 1) showed round to fairly irregular, slightly haloed, argyrophil, small to medium-sized granules (around 200 nm), mostly grouped at the base of the cell (15,54,89,90).

At least in some mammals such as dog and man, the *GIP*-producing *K cell* has now been characterized both ultrastructurally and histochemically (Figs. 2 and 6). It was first identified ultrastructurally thanks to its large granules, part of which show a target-like pattern with an argyrophil matrix surrounding the argyrophobe core, thus mimicking in part those of pancreatic A cells (12,89). However, K cell granules are often more irregular than alpha granules and may lack any evidence of halo or double structure (18,87). These homogeneous granules are especially prevalent in pig K cells, which may be difficult to distinguish from L cells. In man K cell granules are usually larger than those of L cells; moreover, L cells are practically lacking in the human duodenum where K cells are rather numerous.

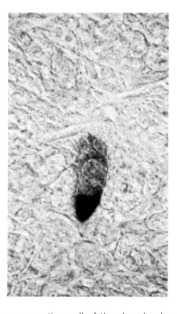

FIG. 6. GIP-immunoreactive cell of the dog duodenum. Note concentration of immunoreactivity in the infranuclear part of the cell where secretory granules are grouped; compare with Fig. 2. Immunoperoxidase using anti-porcine GIP serum (from Dr. V. L. W. Go, Mayo Clinic, Rochester, Minn.). × 1,000.

K cells of the dog and man lack reactivity with anti-glucagon and anti-glicentin sera (84). However, some anti-GIP sera, in addition to K cells, also stain pancreatic or gastric A cells and intestinal L cells (1,84). Cross-reactivity with glicentin or some other component of A and L cells might be the cause of such behavior. Anyway, other anti-GIP sera stain selectively a population of cells peculiar to the upper small intestine, with special reference to deep crypts. Such cells have been shown to correspond ultrastructurally with K cells (7). Thus, at least in some mammals, a specialized GIP-producing cell is present in the small intestine, where it is much better represented in adult than in fetal life. This cell may have a key role in the so-called enteroinsular axis (24).

First suggested by dark-field microscopy and clearly shown by electron microscopy (94), *glucagon A cells* of the fundic-type gastric mucosa have been also detected by immunohistochemistry using non-C-terminal (37) as well as C-terminal (5,99) glucagon antibodies. The same cells also store glicentin or a glicentin-like peptide reacting with Moody's R-64 serum (Fig. 7) (71,84). Gastric A cells are well represented in the dog and cat stomach, but are lacking or scarce in other mammals such as man and pig (89,94). However, they are fairly well represented in the fundic mucosa of human fetuses (17,87).

Secretory granules (alpha granules) of A cells are characterized by a dense, osmiophilic, round core surrounded by a prominent halo separating it from the membrane. With conventional fixation (aldehyde-osmium) and staining (uranyl-lead) techniques in many species the halo is electron lucent; in man it is full of moderately osmiophilic amorphous material, often of

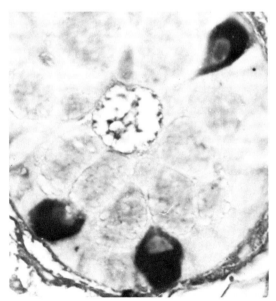

FIG. 7. Three cells of a crypt in the human sigmoid colon stained with anti-glicentin antibodies (Moody's R-64 serum). Resin section; immunoperoxidase. × 1,000.

crescentic shape (Fig. 8, inset). With the aldehyde-silver technique the halo of all species is more (man) or less (dog) full of silver grains (16,37,89). Histochemical tests suggest that some anionic glycoprotein or proteoglycolipid sensitive to lysozyme, neuraminidase, and several proteases is present in the halo of all species (85), more (dog) or less (man) extractable by conventional electron microscopy procedures.

Glucagon is mostly stored in the core of the alpha granule (16,79), which in some fishes shows crystalline patterns reproducing those of glucagon crystals *in vitro* (101). With the indole reagent xanthydrol, glucagon stored in the A cells develops a peculiar blue-gray color, also shown by glucagon crystals *in vitro,* which is not shown by dissolved glucagon (23). This suggests a conformational pattern of glucagon in the alpha granule closely resembling that of crystalline glucagon. Recently, the glicentin-like component of the alpha granule—likely related with proglucagon molecules (62)—has been shown to be mainly associated with the halo (78).

Although a few cells reacting with glucagon-specific C-terminal antibodies have been reported in the intestinal mucosa, ultrastructural evidence for the presence of true A cells at this site is lacking, apart, perhaps, from occasional cells in the upper small intestine. Instead, a large population of cells reacting with antibodies directed against the midpart of the glucagon molecule (37,72,79) as well as antibodies against the nonglucagon part of the glicentin molecule (79,84) have been described which correspond ultrastructurally to a specific type of cell, the *L cell,* clearly differing from the A cell (15,37,79,89). L cells show large (dog) to medium-sized (man), mostly round, solid granules of variable argyrophilia (Fig. 8). Only a few similar granules are found in adult A cells, although they may be numerous in fetal A cells.

It has been shown by Moody et al. (62) that the whole glucagon molecule is present in intestinal glucagon-like immunoreactive peptides (GLI), although in a form leaving the C-terminal part of the molecule inaccessible to specific antibodies. In fact, L cells become reactive with anti-C-terminal glucagon-specific antibodies after treatment with some proteases known to split GLI molecules (78). A GLI molecule of 100 amino acid residues, called glicentin, has been extracted from pig intestine and purified (63). A similar peptide has been extracted from tissues, such as the pancreas and fundic mucosa, producing true glucagon; it has been identified with proglucagon. In keeping with this interpretation, antibodies reacting with the nonglucagon part of the glicentin molecule stained pancreatic and fundic A cells, in addition to intestinal L cells (79,83).

The staining of endocrine cells by some anti-VIP sera has been reported in various sites, including the small and large intestine, stomach, and pancreas. None of

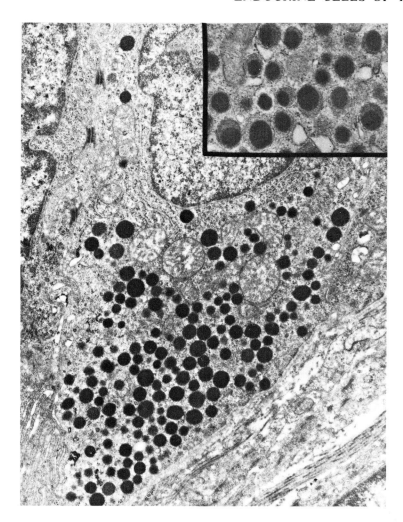

FIG. 8. L cell of human sigmoid colon with homogenous round granules × 14,990. **Inset:** Haloed granules of an A cell in human pancreas. × 23,800.

these cells reacted with all the antisera staining VIP-containing nerves (47). Sometimes the staining of the endocrine cells, unlike that of nerves, was prevented by diluting the anti-VIP serum (9) or by adding it with chemically related peptides such as glucagon, GIP, or secretin or even by removing complement and antibody aggregates from the serum (9,83,84).

VIP-immunoreactive cells lacking cross-reactivity with secretin and glucagon have been reported in the chicken small and large intestine and proventriculus (97). The distribution of this cell closely parallels that of some cells reacting with non-C-terminal glucagon antibodies and glicentin antibodies we have found in the same species and identified ultrastructurally as L cells. Thus, so far, the existence of specialized endocrine VIP cells distinct from L, A, GIP, or S cells is not fully proven. However, the production of VIP-like peptides, distinct from glucagon, secretin, GIP, and neural VIP, by some of the known endocrine cells, with special reference to L cells, remains possible. Such peptides in the chicken might well display a secretin-like influence on the pancreas, whereas in man they would help to explain the occurrence of endocrine tumors producing VIP or VIP-related molecules (so-called vipomas).

No interference with the staining of endocrine cells has been observed by adding the new VIP-like peptide PHI—recently isolated by Tatemoto (100) from pig duodenum—to anti-VIP sera (1 to 50 μg/ml of diluted serum).

Thus present evidence suggests that the L cell should be interpreted as a somewhat primitive form of cell, producing GLI peptides of unknown function containing the glucagon sequence in an inactive, partly reactive form. The possible production of VIP-like peptides by L cells seems in keeping with this interpretation: VIP has been suggested to represent the most primitive molecule of the family (103). In the upper gut (stomach and possibly the duodenum) and its derivatives (pancreas), the A cell evolved from the L cell by acquiring the proteases which split the GLI-proglucagon molecules up to release glucagon. Once released, glucagon molecules are concentrated in the core of the alpha granule—where they undergo conformational changes and even crystallization—leaving proglucagons, the argyrophil material, enzymes, and other components in the peripheral halo.

The recent demonstration of *PP-like sequences* in many L cells (31,83,84) also supports the interpretation of this type of cell as a somewhat primitive precursor cell. Pancreatic PP cells, and possibly rare PP cells of the gastrointestinal mucosa, may well be evolved from such cells. Some structural homology between glucagon and PP, as well as the present failure to identify specific precursors of PP molecules (96), also suggest that a common big proglucagon-PP molecule may exist in the L cell as a phylogenetic, ontogenetic, and biogenetic ancestor to glucagon and PP peptides of pancreatic A and PP cells.

In addition to intestinal L cells and part of gastric A cells, some antral cells have also been found to react with anti-BPP serum. In the dog antrum these cells are fairly numerous and, in our experience, correspond to a fraction of gastrin-immunoreactive cells. Unlike gastrointestinal PP-immunoreactive cells, pancreatic *PP cells* are mostly independent from any other type of pancreatic endocrine cells. In contrast to glucagon A cells they are much more numerous in the splenic part of the pancreas than in the tail (55,66). Ultrastructurally, they correspond to a specific type of cell, although with very different features in different species, from dog F cells with large, irregular, vesicular granules to human D_1-like cells with small, round, solid granules (55). F-like cells have been observed ultrastructurally in the dog antrum, possibly corresponding to PP-immunoreactive cells, although they remain difficult to distinguish from G cells (64). Similar findings have been obtained in *Tupaia belangeri* (97).

Somatostatin D Cell

Somatostatin-immunoreactive cells (Fig. 9) and ultrastructurally identified D cells have been observed along the whole gastrointestinal tract, from cardias to rectum, as well as in the pancreas (3,89,104). Many of these cells show long cell processes (Fig. 10) contacting blood vessels—in the pancreatic islets—or other cell types, including G cells (45). D cell granules are usually round, homogeneous, of low electron density, and with closely fitting membrane; they are large in most mammalian species and relatively small in the rat. Ultrastructural features of D cell granules in different tissues of the same animal species often show consistent changes, suggesting possible changes of somatostatin peptides they produce. D cells are blackened rather selectively with Davenport's alcoholic silver, while failing to react with a number of aqueous silver techniques.

The wide distribution of D cells in several tissues and in close contact with many cells of different function is in keeping with their proposed local modulatory (paracrine) function and the ability of somatostatin to inhibit many endocrine (gastrin, CCK, insulin, glucagon, etc.) and exocrine secretions (pancreatic enzymes, gastric hydrochloric acid, etc.). In particular, pyloric D cells, which have been shown to be stimulated by HCl infusion into the gastric lumen (43), may play an important role in the HCl-mediated feedback mechanism modulating gastrin and gastric acid secretion.

Neurotensin N Cell

Specific neurotensin cells are mostly concentrated in the lower small intestine and correspond ultrastructurally to cells with large, solid granules difficult to distinguish from L(GLI) cells (34,77,98). A few neurotensin cells are scattered in the upper small intestine and, exceptionally, even in the large intestine. The functional meaning of N cells remains obscure, although some (pharmacologic?) action of neurotensin on pancreatic endocrine secretions has been reported.

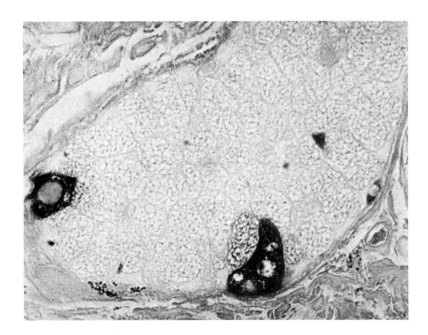

FIG. 9. Two somatostatin cells in a dog pyloric gland. Resin section; immunoperoxidase. × 1,000.

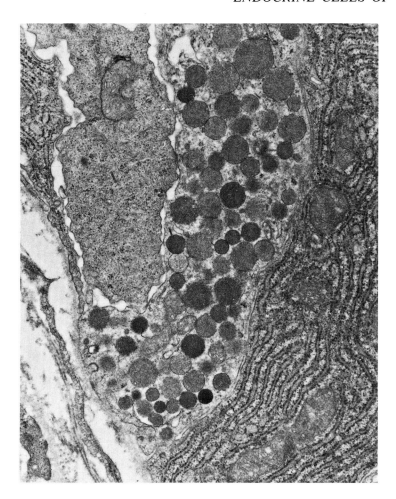

Fig. 10. Cell process of a D cell filled with poorly dense, round, homogeneous granules. × 18,700.

In the chicken antrum neurotensin-immunoreactive cells have been observed (98). No such cells have been found in the mammalian stomach; however, some neurotensin-immunoreactive peptide different from neurotensin has been extracted from the rat stomach (22).

Serotonin EC Cells and Related Cell Variants Producing Substance P (EC₁ Cell) and Enkephalin

Argentaffin or enterochromaffin (EC) cells react with all the histochemical methods detecting 5-HT, including those related to its phenol function and its reducing power, such as chromaffin, diazonium, thioindoxyl, argentaffin, and ferric ferricyanide reactions, and those depending on its pyrrole ring, such as dimethylaminobenzaldehyde-nitrite and xanthydrol reactions (89). Apart from the chromaffin reaction, which requires fixation in dichromate or chromic acid mixtures, the reactions of the first group can be successfully applied to specimens fixed in formaldehyde, glutaraldehyde, acrolein, and glyoxal, or to mixtures of these substances with picric acid, Hg^{2+} and Ca^{2+} salts. Reactions depending on the pyrrole ring require fixation in glutaraldehyde or acrolein solutions; formaldehyde-fixed material is unsuitable for such indole tests, likely because formaldehyde (and glyoxal) blocks C-2 in the pyrrole ring of 5-HT, which must be free to allow this substance to react with dimethylaminobenzaldehyde or xanthydrol. In addition to C-2, formaldehyde also reacts with the amino group, thus giving a new condensation ring involving the lateral chain of 5-HT. This new ring accounts for the strong yellow fluorescence and the Holcenberg-Benditt ninhydrin reaction of formaldehyde-treated EC cells and 5-HT; the last-mentioned reactions are not shown by native 5-HT or unfixed EC cells. Spectrofluorometric analysis of formaldehyde-treated 5-HT and formaldehyde-treated EC cells gives comparable spectra. The reactivity of EC cells with an anti-5-HT serum has also been obtained (29). Thus identification of the chromaffin substance as 5-HT is now fully supported by histochemical tests.

It is well known that, in addition to EC cells, other 5-HT-storing cells react with the above methods under appropriate technical conditions. Among these there are some mast cells of rat, mouse, horse, and dog, as well as thyroid calcitonin (C) cells of horse, sheep, and goat, A cells of pig pancreas, B cells of guinea pig pancreas, some carotid body cells, some ECL cells of cat and rabbit stomach, and bronchial endocrine cells of cat and rabbit (89). Thus cells reacting with 5-HT methods are not necessarily the same as EC cells; not even in the gut mucosa where, in some species, 5-HT-storing mast cells or ECL cells occur in the epithelium.

A more reliable and selective demonstration of EC cells is obtained by directly applying argentaffin or chromaffin reactions in electron microscopy (Fig. 11). In this way EC cells have been directly identified at the ultrastructural level and shown to display granules of peculiar shape, clearly different from those of the non-EC 5-HT-storing cells mentioned above (85,89,104). In thin sections EC granules appear pleomorphic: round, ovoid, oblong, pear-shaped, triangular, kidney-shaped, U-shaped, and so on. EC granules often show heterogeneous internal structure, with highly osmiophilic bodies or particles immersed in a less osmiophilic matrix (Fig. 11).

EC granules of animals treated with an inhibitor of 5-HT synthesis, *p*-chlorophenylalanine, or an inhibitor of 5-HT uptake, reserpine, lose most of their 5-HT content but retain some of their osmiophilia and most of their Grimelius reactivity (20,89). These findings, together with those of a series of histochemical tests (85,89), suggest that, in addition to 5-HT, nonamine components are also present in EC granules, including argyrophilic glycoproteins which may have an important function in the binding mechanism of the amine. Intestinal or pyloric EC cells are much more sensitive to reserpine and *p*-chlorophenylalanine than EC cells of gastric fundic mucosa. Unlike *p*-chlorophenylalanine, reserpine affects mitochondria (which are often swollen and disrupted) and increases the glycogen stores of intestinal EC cells (20). Granule exocytosis seems to be unaffected by both drugs. Intraduodenal HCl and hypertonic glucose infusion has been shown to induce exocytosis of EC granules (43) and 5-HT release, which has been proven to inhibit gastric acid secretion (42).

Apart from relatively few cells occurring in the pancreas and biliary tree, EC cells are mostly distributed in the gastrointestinal tract, especially in the mucosa of the small and large intestine and the pyloric mucosa. In fundic gastric mucosa, the number of EC cells differs markedly according to the animal species. They are numerous in pig, dog, rabbit, and monkey; relatively few occur in guinea pig, cat, and man, and they are practically absent in the rat and mouse.

On ultrastructural grounds, at least three variants of EC cells have been identified in the human gut: the *intestinal* type, with medium-sized pleomorphic, mainly rod-like or biconcave granules; the *duodenal* type, with large, round to irregular granules; and the *gastric* type, with small, mainly oblong granules (18). Recent immunohistochemical findings confirm the heterogeneity of EC cells and their variability in different species. A relatively small fraction of intestinal EC cells (EC$_1$ cells) react with anti-substance P sera (64,68). Other EC cells in the stomach and intestine of several species (pig, rat, mouse, chicken; not man, cat, or guinea-pig) react with anti-enkephalin sera (2).

As producers and releasers of 5-HT, substance P, and enkephalin, EC cells seem well qualified to be modulators of gastrointestinal motility.

Motilin Mo Cell

Motilin immunoreactive cells (Fig. 12) have been found in the duodenal and jejunal mucosa of mammals (70). Although EC cells may be also stained with some anti-motilin sera (40), only a population of nonargentaffin cells reacts with all anti-motilin sera and should be interpreted as a reliable motilin (Mo) cell (41,92). Available information suggests that the Mo cell corresponds ultrastructurally to a cell with small, round, homogeneous granules fitting in the "D$_1$" cell class of the ultrastructural classification (75).

Mo cells, which are often rich in cytoplasmic filaments, might be sensitive to mechanical stimuli coming from the lumen and, by releasing motilin, might play an important part in the modulation of gut motility.

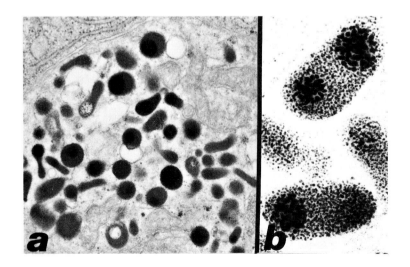

FIG. 11. EC cell of the human stomach with pleomorphic granules, some of which show dense osmiophilic cores **(a)** heavily reacting with the argentaffin test, due to their high 5-HT content **(b)**.
a: × 23,800; **b:** × 85,000.

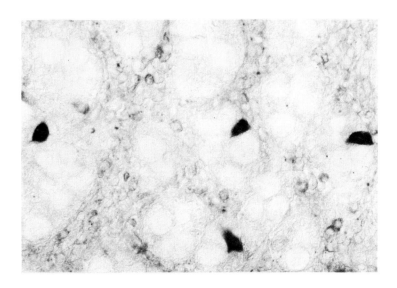

FIG. 12. Four motilin cells in the crypts of pig duodenum stained with immunoperoxidase using anti-porcine motilin serum (from Dr. V. L. W. Go). Note nonimmune staining of some mesenchymal cells, due to endogenous peroxidase activity. The immunoreactive cells proved nonargentaffin. × 380.

Bombesin BN Cell

Bombesin-immunoreactive cells have been detected unequivocally in the chicken (102) and frog (56) stomach. In both species, the immunoreactive cells correspond ultrastructurally to cells with small, round to slightly irregular granules fitting in the D_1 cell class. Ultrastructurally comparable cells have been observed in the mammalian stomach (17). However, so far, immunohistochemical evidence of bombesin endocrine cells in the mammalian gastrointestinal mucosa is lacking or restricted to occasional antisera. Bombesin-immunoreactive nerves might account wholly or in part for the bombesin immunoreactivity detected by radioimmunoassay of mammalian gut extracts (74).

D_1 and P Cells

Pulmonary-type or P cells are small cells with small (from 100 to 140 nm of mean diameter), round granules, often with a thin halo surrounding a moderately electron-dense core. Some vesicular granules may also be present; well-developed reticulum and Golgi, small mitochondria, and numerous microfilaments are regularly found (17).

So-called enterocatecholamine (ECT) cells described in the rat pyloric mucosa (33) are likely to be interpreted as a variant of P cells showing an abundance of vesicular, densely cored granules. Somewhat similar cells have been found in the human, cat, and rabbit stomach (17). In the latter two species P and/or ECT cells might correspond to the dopamine-storing cells shown histochemically by Håkanson et al. (39). Ultrastructurally, ECT cells may be difficult to distinguish from ECL cells. They are distributed in various tissues, especially the upper gut and lung; however, in normal tissues they are never numerous at any site. In the human gut, they are more frequently found in the gastric and duodenal mucosa.

D_1 cells are considered to be all the small cells with round granules of mean diameter from 140 to 190 nm, showing a solid core of moderate osmiophilia with closely applied membranes or a very thin halo (17). We are certainly dealing with a functionally heterogeneous population of cells, among which slight ultrastructural differences have been observed. D_1 cells of the human fundic mucosa are ovoid or dome shaped, with round granules of homogeneous, fairly osmiophilic and argyrophilic core, small, thin, oblong mitochondria, well-developed Golgi and reticulum, and abundant microfilaments. They closely resemble some of the type 3 cells found in human fetal lung (17). D_1 cells of the upper small intestine may be ovoid or elongated; their granules are less osmiophilic and less argyrophilic than those of fundic cells. Hindgut D_1 cells (also called H cells) are elongated cells showing relatively large, ovoid, or cuneiform mitochondria and granules with less dense, sometimes loose core, often with a thin peripheral clear space (9,87). D_1 cells of the human pancreas are scarce, if present at all, when differentiated from islet PP cells (17).

The functions of P and D_1 cells remain partly uncertain. The granules of some P cells resemble closely the neurosecretory granules of nerve endings in the external zone of hypothalamic median eminence; in addition to monoamines, some sort of neuropeptides might well be produced by such cells. In the gastric mucosa and lung, a fraction of D_1 cells might be involved in the production of bombesin-like peptide(s) (108). A relationship between some "D_1 cells" of the human duodenum and jejunum with motilin cells or with intestinal gastrin-immunoreactive cells and some cells present in pancreatic and duodenal gastrinomas is likely (8,105). A relationship of some D_1 cell variant with part of the cells present in VIP-producing tumors of the pancreas also seems possible (19).

ECL Cell

ECL cells are small, irregularly shaped, heavily argyrophilic cells (with Grimelius', Bodian's, and Sevier-Munger's methods) which are scattered in fairly large numbers in fundic gastric glands. Ultrastructurally, they show either vesicular granules with an irregular argyrophilic core eccentrically located in a wide space, or a round, relatively compact (or coarsely granular), argyrophilic core surrounded by a membrane often of wavy appearance and forming a thin clear space (21,89). The argyrophilic histamine-storing cells peculiar to murine fundic mucosa are closely related to ECL cells (21,39,80,89).

In many species, ECL cells of untreated animals are not argentaffin; like other argyrophilic cells, they become argentaffin only after treatment with amine precursors (21,39,85,89). However, ultrastructural findings suggest that some ECL cells of cat and rabbit can display argentaffin granules even under basal conditions (89). Occasional granules of some human ECL cells may also be argentaffin. ECL cells with argentaffin granules differ from argentaffin EC cells in being poorly reactive with the hydrochloric acid-basic dye technique and with lead-hematoxylin.

ECL cells are scattered in the fundic glands, especially in their deep half; very few ECL cells have been found in the neck of the glands, and none in the epithelium covering the luminal surface of the mucosa and the gastric pits. Like other endocrine cells of the fundic mucosa, ECL cells lack any contact with the lumen of the glands, usually being covered by oxyntic or peptic cells (21). No ECL cells have been found in the well developed cardial mucosa of the pig.

ECL cells have been shown to be stimulated by gastrin (38) and to undergo hypertrophic and hyperplastic changes in hypergastrinemic patients suffering from Zollinger-Ellison syndrome (89). They seem likely to take part in the control of acid-peptic secretion.

X Cell

The X cells (Fig. 13) are round to ovoid cells characterized ultrastructurally by their round to slightly irregular, compact, dense, fairly large granules of moderate and diffuse argyrophilia (87,89). In several species they react intensely with acidophilic dyes and are stained deep blue with phosphotungstic hematoxylin, thus suggesting their storage of some basic polypeptide. X cells also react heavily with lead-hematoxylin and the hydrochloric acid-basic dye or "masked metachromasia" technique (20,89). Despite some ultrastructural resemblance with pancreatic A cells (5), X cells fail to react

with anti-glucagon and anti-glicentin sera (79,99). Thus they should not be confused with the A or A-like cells found in the fundic and cardial mucosa of several species and now proven to store glucagon and related peptides.

In several species, as the rat, mouse, and dog, X cells seem to be restricted to the fundic and cardial mucosa. In other species the presence of a few X cells in the pyloric mucosa cannot be excluded. In the pig cardial mucosa X cells account for nearly 50% of the whole endocrine cell population; in the same tissue glucagon and glicentin-immunoreactive cells are quite few. The function of the X cell remains unknown.

ENDOCRINE PROFILE OF THE GUT

In the *pyloric mucosa* of different mammals the proportion of G cells may range from 40 to 60% of the whole endocrine cell population, that of EC cells from 20 to 40%, and that of D cells from 10 to 30%. The remaining cells, including P and D_1 cells, usually account for less than 5% of pyloric endocrine cells.

In all species investigated, ECL cells represent a major fraction of the endocrine cells scattered in the *fundic mucosa*. X cells are also numerous in most species, while being rather few in man. EC cells are about as numerous as ECL cells in the pig, dog, and rabbit, while being relatively few in the guinea pig, cat, and man, and absent in the rat and mouse. D_1 and P cells are consistently represented only in man.

The upper part of the *small intestine* is characterized by S, CCK, GIP, and motilin cells, although EC cells are numerically prevalent. D cells are fairly well represented; L cells are numerous in the whole jejunum and ileum. Only N cells are restricted to the lower small intestine. D and GIP cells are usually concentrated in the deep crypts, while S cells are found in the upper crypts and villi and the remaining cells are scattered in all strata of the mucosa with preference for the crypts.

No endocrine cell is peculiar to the *large intestine*, where EC and L cells account for most of the endocrine cells.

Four cell types have been identified in the *pancreas* of all species so far investigated: insulin B cells, glucagon A cells, somatostatin D cells, and pancreatic polypeptide PP cells. EC cells and a few gastrin cells have been also reported in some species.

In normal conditions, the endocrine-paracrine cells are poorly represented in human biliary ducts, gallbladder, and esophagus. They are scarce also in other endodermal derivatives as the lung, urethra, and prostate.

CONCLUSION

As many as 15 types of endocrine-paracrine cells have been identified in the mammalian gastrointestinal tract,

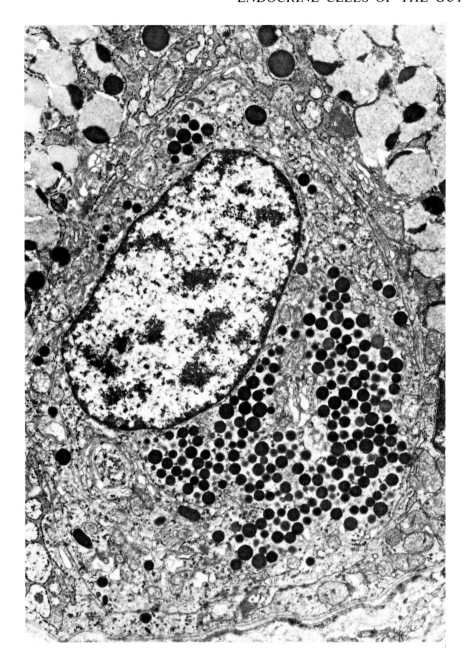

FIG. 13. X cell of the pig cardial gland area, surrounded by mucous cells. × 9,350.

the majority of which have been shown to produce active peptides, and some of them also biogenic amines. Some of these cells seem to display truly endocrine functions through the secretion of gastrin, secretin, cholecystokinin, and GIP; other cells seem to act mainly as local modulators or paracrine cells through the release of somatostatin, VIP, 5-HT, etc. However, secretory products of some cells are still unknown or incompletely identified, and the exact physiological role of many cells—even among the cells whose products have been fully identified—remains uncertain.

Thus considerable work remains to be done in the field of gut endocrinology. The identification of new secretory products, a more precise knowledge of the function and embryology of endocrine-paracrine cells, and a better clarification of neuroendocrine interrelationships are among the main topics awaiting further research. Cytological studies in gut endocrine pathology are at their very beginning. Many more cases are to be carefully investigated in specialized centers before a clear picture of tumor pathology is obtained, including the identification of new types of tumors. Much work remains to be done also on the behavior of endocrine-paracrine cells in a number of digestive diseases, such as peptic ulcer, hyperplastic gastropathy, chronic gastritis, chronic inflammatory diseases of the small and large bowel, acute and chronic pancreatitis, as well as in all functional derangements of digestive processes.

REFERENCES

1. Alumets, J., Håkanson, R., O'Dorisio, T., Sjölund, K., and Sundler, F. (1978): Is GIP a glucagon cell constituent? *Histochemistry*, 58:253-257.
2. Alumets, J., Håkanson, R., Sundler, F., and Chang, K.-J. (1978): Leu-enkephalin-like material in nerves and enterochromaffin cells in the gut. An immunohistochemical study. *Histochemistry*, 56:187-196.
3. Alumets, J., Sundler, F., and Håkanson, R. (1977): Distribution, ontogeny and ultrastructure of somatostatin immunoreactive cells in the pancreas and gut. *Cell Tissue Res.*, 185:465-479.
4. Andrew, A. (1974): Further evidence that enterochromaffin cells are not derived from the neural crest. *J. Embryol. exp. Morphol.*, 31:589-598.
5. Baetens, D., Rufener, C., Srikant, C., Dobbs, R., Unger, R., and Orci, L. (1976): Identification of glucagon-producing cells (A cells) in dog gastric mucosa. *J. Cell Biol.*, 69:455-464.
6. Buchan, A. M. J., Polak, J. M., Solcia, E., Capella, C., Hudson, D., and Pearse, A. G. E. (1978): Electron immunocytochemical evidence for the human intestinal I cell as the source of CCK. *Gut*, 19:403-407.
7. Buchan, A. M. J., Polak, J. M., Solcia, E., Capella, C., and Pearse, A. G. E. (1978): Electron immunocytochemical evidence for the K cell localization of gastric inhibitory polypeptide (GIP) in man. *Histochemistry*, 56:37-44.
8. Buchan, A. M. J., Polak, J. M., Solcia, E., and Pearse, A. G. E. (1979): Localisation of intestinal gastrin in a distinct endocrine cell type. *Nature*, 277:138-140.
9. Buffa, A., Capella, C., Fontana, P., Usellini, L., and Solcia, E. (1978): Types of endocrine cells in the human colon and rectum. *Cell Tissue Res.*, 192:277-240.
10. Buffa, R., Chayvialle, J. A., Fontana, P., Usellini, L., Capella, C., and Solcia, E. (1979): Parafollicular cells of rabbit thyroid store both calcitonin and somatostatin and resemble gut D cells ultrastructurally. *Histochemie*, 62:281-288.
11. Buffa, R., Crivelli, O., Fiocca, R., Fontana, P., and Solcia, E. (1979): Complement-mediated unspecific binding of immunoglobulins to some endocrine cells. *Histochemistry*, 63:15-21.
12. Buffa, R., Polak, J. M., Pearse, A. G. E., Solcia, E., Grimelius, L., and Capella, C. (1975): Identification of the intestinal cell storing gastric inhibitory peptide. *Histochemistry*, 43:249-255.
13. Buffa, R., Solcia, E., and Go, V. L. W. (1976): Immunohistochemical identification of the cholecystokinin cell in the intestinal mucosa. *Gastroenterology*, 70:528-532.
14. Bussolati, G., and Canese, M. G. (1972): Electron microscopic identification of the immunofluorescent gastrin cells in the cat pyloric mucosa. *Histochemie*, 20:198-206.
15. Bussolati, G., Capella, C., Solcia, E., Vassallo, G., and Vezzadini, P. (1971): Ultrastructural and immunofluorescent investigations of the secretin cell in the dog intestinal mucosa. *Histochemie*, 26:218-227.
16. Bussolati, G., Capella, C., Vassallo, G., and Solcia, E. (1971): Histochemical and ultrastructural studies on pancreatic A cells. Evidence for glucagon and non-glucagon components of the α granule. *Diabetologia*, 7:181-188.
17. Capella, C., Hage, E., Solcia, E., and Usellini, L. (1978): Ultrastructural similarity of endocrine-like cells of the human lung and some related cells of the gut. *Cell Tissue Res.*, 186:25-37.
18. Capella, C., Solcia, E., Frigerio, B., and Buffa, R. (1976): Endocrine cells of the human intestine. An ultrastructural study. In: *Endocrine Gut and Pancreas*, edited by T. Fujita, pp. 42-59. Elsevier, Amsterdam.
19. Capella, C., Solcia, E., Frigerio, B., Buffa, R., Usellini, L., and Fontana, P. (1977): The endocrine cells of the pancreas and related tumours. Ultrastructural study and classification. *Virchows Arch. [Pathol. Anat.]*, 373:327-352.
20. Capella, C., Solcia, E., and Vassallo, G. (1969): Identification of six types of endocrine cells in the gastrointestinal mucosa of the rabbit. *Arch. Histol. Jpn.*, 30:479-495.
21. Capella, C., Vassallo, G., and Solcia, E. (1971): Light and electron microscopic identification of the histamine-storing argyrophil (ECL) cell in murine stomach and of its equivalent in other mammals. *Z. Zellforsch.*, 118:68-84.
22. Carraway, R., and Leeman, S. E. (1976): Characterization of radioimmunoassayable neurotensin in the rat. Its differential distribution in the central nervous system, small intestine and stomach. *J.Biol.Chem.*, 251:7045-7052.
23. Cavallero, C., Solcia, E., and Sampietro, R. (1968): Selective histochemistry of glucagon in the A cells of pancreatic islets by indole methods. In: *Pharmacology of Hormonal Polypeptides and Proteins*, pp. 387-395. Plenum Press, New York.
24. Creutzfeldt, W. (1979): The incretin concept today. *Diabetologia*, 16:75-85.
25. Dockray, G. J. (1979): Evolutionary relationships of the gut hormones. *Fed. Proc.*, 38:2295-2301.
26. Dockray, G. J., Vaillant, C., and Hutchison, J. B. (1980): Immunochemical characterization of peptides in endocrine cells and nerves with particular reference to gastrin and cholecystokinin. In: *Cellular Basis of Chemical Messengers in the Digestive System*. Academic Press, New York *(in press)*.
27. Dubois, P. M., and Paulin, C. (1976): Gastrointestinal somatostatin cells in the human fetus. *Cell Tissue Res.*, 166:179-184.
28. Erspamer, V., and Asero, B. (1952): Identification of enteramine, the specific hormone of the enterochromaffin cell system, as 5-hydroxytryptamine. *Nature*, 169:800-801.
29. Facer, P., Polak, J. M., Jaffe, B. M., and Pearse, A. G. E. (1979): Immunocytochemical demonstration of 5-hydroxytryptamine in gastrointestinal endocrine cells. *Histochem. J.*, 11:117-121.
30. Feyrter, F. (1953): *Uber die peripheren endokrinen (parakrinen) Drusen des Menschen*, pp. 1-231. W.Maudrich, Wien-Dusseldorf.
31. Fiocca, R., Capella, C., Buffa, R., Fontana, P., Solcia, E., Hage, E., Chance, R. E., and Moody, A. J. (1980): Glucagon-, glicentin- and pancreatic polypeptide-like immunoreactivities in rectal carcinoids and related colorectal cells. *Am. J. Pathol.*, 100:81-92.
32. Forssmann, W. G., Helmstaedter, V., and Chance, R. E. (1977): Ultrastructural and immunohistochemical demonstration of pancratic polypeptide-containing F-cells in the stomach and pancreas of *Tupaia belangeri*. *Cell Tissue Res.*, 177:481-492.
33. Forssmann W. G., Orci, L., Pictet, R., Renold, A. E., and Rouiller, C. (1969): The endocrine cells in the epithelium of the gastrointestinal mucosa of the rat. *J. Cell Biol.*, 40:692-715.
34. Frigerio, B., Ravazzola, M., Ito, S., Buffa, R., Capella, C., Solcia, E., and Orci, L. (1977): Histochemical and ultrastructural identification of neurotensin cells in the dog ileum. *Histochemistry*, 54:123-131.
35. Furness, J. B., and Costa, M. (1980): Types of nerves in the enteric nervous system. *Neuroscience*, 5:1-20.
36. Grimelius, L. (1968): A silver nitrate stain for α_2 cells in human pancreatic islets. *Acta Soc. Med. Upsala*, 73:243-270.
37. Grimelius, L., Capella, C., Buffa, R., Polak, J. M., Pearse, A. G. E., and Solcia, E. (1976): Cytochemical and ultrastructural differentiation of enteroglucagon and pancreatic-type glucagon cells of the gastrointestinal tract. *Virchows Arch. [Cell Pathol.]*, 20:217-228.
38. Håkanson, R., Larsson, L.-I., Liedberg, G., and Sundler, F. (1976): The histamine-storing enterochromaffin-like cells of the rat stomach. In: *Chromaffin, Enterochromaffin and Related Cells*, edited by R. E. Coupland and T. Fujita, pp. 243-263. Elsevier Scientific Publishing Co., Amsterdam.
39. Håkanson, R., Owman, C. H., Sjoberg, N. O., and Sporrong, B. (1970): Amine mechanisms in enterochromaffin and enterochromaffin-like cells of gastric mucosa in various mammals. *Histochemie*, 21:189-220.
40. Heitz, P. H., Kasper, M., Krey, G., Polak, J. M., and Pearse, A. G. E. (1978): Immunoelectron cytochemical localization of motilin in human duodenal enterochromaffin cells. *Gastroenterology*, 74:713-717.
41. Helmstaedter, V., Kreppein, W., Domschke, W., Mitznegg, P., Yanaihara, N., Wunsch, E., and Forssmann, W. G. (1979): Immunohistochemical localization of motilin in endocrine non-enterochromaffin cells of the small intestine of humans and monkey. *Gastroenterology*, 76:897-902.
42. Jaffe, B. M., Kellum, J. M., Kopen, D. F., and Stechenberg, L. (1978): Release and physiologic action of serotonin. In: *Gut Hormones*, edited by S. R. Bloom, pp. 515-526. Churchill-Livingstone, Edinburgh.

43. Kobayashi, S., and Sasagawa, T. (1976): Morphological aspects of the secretion of gastro-enteric hormones. In: *Endocrine Gut and Pancreas,* edited by T. Fujita, pp. 255–271. Elsevier Scientific Publishing Co., Amsterdam.

44. Larsson, L.-I. (1978): ACTH-like immunoreactivity in the gastrin cell. Independent changes in gastrin and ACTH-like immunoreactivity during ontogeny. *Histochemistry,* 56:245–251.

45. Larsson, L.-I., Goltermann, N., De Magistris, L., Rehfeld, J. F., and Schwartz, T. W. (1979): Somatostatin cell processes as pathways for paracrine secretion. *Science,* 205:1393–1395.

46. Larsson, L.-I., and Mørch Jørgensen, L. (1978): Ultrastructural and cytochemical studies on the cytodifferentiation of duodenal endocrine cells. *Cell Tissue Res.,* 194:79–102.

47. Larsson, L.-I., Polak, J. M., Buffa, R., Sundler, F., and Solcia, E. (1979): On the immunocytochemical localization of the vasoactive intestinal polypeptide. *J. Histochem. Cytochem.,* 27:936–938.

48. Larsson, L.-I., and Rehfeld, J. F. (1977): Characterization of antral gastrin cells with region-specific antisera. *J. Histochem. Cytochem.,* 25:1317.

49. Larsson, L.-I., and Rehfeld, J. F.(1977): Evidence for a common evolutionary origin of gastrin and cholecystokinin. *Nature,* 269:335–338.

50. Larsson, L.-I., and Rehfeld, J. F. (1979): A peptide resembling COOH-terminal tetrapeptide amide of gastrin from a new gastrointestinal endocrine cell type. *Nature,* 277:575–578.

51. Larsson, L.-I., Rehfeld, J. F., and Goltermann, N. (1977): Gastrin in the human fetus. Distribution and molecular forms of gastrin in the antro-pyloric gland area, duodenum and pancreas. *Scand. J. Gastroenterol.,* 12:869–872.

52. Larsson, L.-I., Rehfeld, J. F., Stockbrügger, R., Blohme, G., Schoon, I.-M., Lundqvist, G., Kindblom, L. G., Säve-Söderberg, J., Grimelius, L., and Olbe, L. (1978): Mixed endocrine gastric tumors associated with hypergastrinemia of antral origin. *Am. J. Pathol.,* 93:53–68.

53. Larsson, L.-I., Rehfeld, J. F., Sundler, F., and Håkanson, R. (1976): Pancreatic gastrin in foetal and neonatal rats. *Nature,* 262:609–610.

54. Larsson, L.-I., Sundler, F., Alumets, J., Håkanson, R., Schaffalitzky de Muckadell, O. B., and Fahrenkrug, J. (1977): Distribution, ontogeny and ultrastructure of the mammalian secretin cell. *Cell Tissue Res.,* 181:361–368.

55. Larsson, L.-I., Sundler, F., and Håkanson, R. (1976): Pancreatic polypeptide. A postulated new hormone: Identification of its cellular storage site by light and electron microscopic immunocytochemistry. *Diabetologia,* 12:211–226.

56. Lechago, J., Holmquist, A. L., Rosenquist, G. L., and Walsh, J. H. (1978): Localization of bombesin-like peptides in frog gastric mucosa. *Gen. Comp. Endocrinol.,* 36:553–558.

57. Le Douarin, N. M. (1978): The embryological origin of the endocrine cells associated with the digestive tract: Experimental analysis based on the use of a stable cell marking technique. In: *Gut Hormones,* edited by S. R. Bloom, pp. 49–56. Churchill-Livingstone, Edinburgh.

58. Le Douarin, N., and Le Lièvre, C. (1971): Sur l'origine des cellules à calcitonine du corps ultimo-branchial de l'embryon d'oiseau. *C.R.Assoc.Anat.,* 152:558–568.

59. Le Douarin, N. M., and Teillet, M. A. (1974): Experimental analysis of the migration and differentiation of neuroblasts of the autonomic nervous system and of neuroectodermal mesenchymal derivatives using a biological cell marking technique. *Dev. Biol.,* 41:162–184.

60. Masson, P. (1914): La glande endocrine de l'intestin chez l'homme. *C. R. Acad. Sci. [D] (Paris),* 158:52–61.

61. McGuigan, J. E. (1968): Gastric mucosal intracellular localization of gastrin by immunofluorescence. *Gastroenterology,* 55:315–327.

62. Moody, A. J., Frandsen, E. K., Jacobsen, H., and Sundby, F. (1979): Speculations on the structure and function of gut GLIs. In: *Second International Symposium on Hormonal Receptors in Digestive Tract Physiology,* edited by G. Rosselin. Elsevier, Amsterdam.

63. Moody, A. H., Jacobsen, H., and Sundby, S.(1978): Gastric glucagon and gut glucagon-like immunoreactivity. In: *Gut Hormones,* edited by S. R. Bloom, pp. 369–378. Churchill-Livingstone, Edinburgh.

64. Nilsson, G., Larsson, L.-I., Håkanson, R., Brodin, E., Pernow, B., and Sundler, F. (1975): Localization of substance P-like immunoreactivity in mouse gut. *Histochemistry,* 43:97–99.

65. Orci, L., and Creutzfeldt, W. (1979): Communicated at the "Entero-Insular Axis Symposium," Gottingen, September 1979.

66. Orci, L., Malaisse-Lagae, F., Baetens, D., and Perrelet, A. (1978): Pancreatic-polypeptide-rich regions in human pancreas. *Lancet,* II:1200–1201.

67. Pearse, A. G. E. (1976): Peptides in brain and intestine. *Nature,* 262:92–94.

68. Pearse, A. G. E., and Polak, J. M. (1975): Immunocytochemical localization of substance P in mammalian intestine. *Histochemistry,* 41:373–375.

69. Pearse, A. G. E., and Polak, J. M. (1978): The diffuse neuroendocrine system and the APUD concept. In: *Gut Hormones,* edited by S. R. Bloom, pp. 33–39. Churchill-Livingstone, Edinburgh.

70. Pearse, A. G. E., Polak, J. M., and Bloom, S. R. (1977): The newer gut hormones. Cellular sources, physiology, pathology and clinical aspects. *Gastroenterology,* 72:746–761.

71. Pictet, R. L., Rall, L. B., Phelps, P., and Rutter, W. J. (1976): The neural crest and the origin of the insulin-producing and other gastrointestinal hormone-producing cells. *Science,* 191:191–192.

72. Polak, J. M., Bloom, S., Coulling, I., and Pearse, A. G. E. (1971): Immunofluorescent localization of enteroglucagon cells in the gastrointestinal tract of the dog. *Gut,* 12:311–318.

73. Polak, J. M., Bloom, S., Coulling, I., and Pearse, A. G. E. (1971): Immunofluorescent localization of secretin in the canine duodenum. *Gut,* 12:605–610.

74. Polak, J. M., Buchan, A. M. J., Czykowska, W., Solcia, E., Bloom, S. R., and Pearse, A. G. E. (1978): Bombesin in the gut. In: *Gut Hormones,* edited by S. R. Bloom, pp. 541–543. Churchill-Livingstone, Edinburgh.

75. Polak, J. M., Buchan, A. M. J., Dryburgh, J. R., Christofides, N., Bloom, S. R., and Yanaihara, N. (1978): Immunoreactive motilins? *Lancet,* I:1364–1365.

76. Polak, J. M., Pearse, A. G. E., Grimelius, L., Bloom, S. R., and Arimura, A. (1975): Growth-hormone release-inhibiting hormone in gastrointestinal and pancreatic D cells. *Lancet,* I:1220–1222.

77. Polak, J. M., Sullivan, S. N., Bloom, S. R., Buchan, A. M. J., Facer, P., Brown, M. R., and Pearse, A. G. E. (1977): Specific localisation of neurotensin to the N cell in human intestine by radioimmunoassay and immunocytochemistry. *Nature,* 270:183–184.

78. Ravazzola, M., and Orci, L. (1980): Glucagon and glicentin immunoreactivity are topologically segregated in the α granule of the human pancreatic A cell. *Nature,* 284:66–67.

79. Ravazzola, M., Siperstein, A., Moody, A. J., Sundby, F., Jacobsen, H., and Orci, L. (1979): Glicentin immunoreactive cells: Their relationship to glucagon-producing cells. *Endocrinology,* 105:499–508.

80. Rubin, W., and Schwartz, B. (1979): Electron microscopic radioautographic identification of the ECL cell as the histamine-synthesizing endocrine cell in the rat stomach. *Gastroenterology,* 77:458–467.

81. Russo, A., Buffa, R., Grasso, G., Giannone, G., Sanfilippo, G., Sessa, F., and Solcia, E. (1980): Gastric gastrinoma and diffuse G cell hyperplasia associated with chronic atrophic gastritis. Endoscopic detection and removal. *Digestion,* 20:416–419.

82. Schaller, H. C., Flock, K., and Darai, G. (1977): A neurohormone from hydra is present in brain and intestine of rat embryos. *J. Neurochem.,* 29:393.

83. Solcia, E., Buffa, R., Capella, C., Fiocca, R., Fontana, P., and Crivelli, O. (1979): Immunohistochemical characterization of gastroenteropancreatic endocrine cells and related multihormonal cells: Problems, pitfalls and facts. In: *Gut Peptides. Secretion, Function and Clinicopathology.* edited by A. Miyoshi, pp. 303–309. Kodansha Scientific, Tokyo.

84. Solcia, E., Buffa, R., Capella, C., Fiocca, R., Yanaiyara, N., and Go, V. L. W. (1980): Immunohistochemical and ultrastructural characterization of gut cells producing GIP, GLI, glucagon, secretin and PP-like peptides. *Front. Horm. Res.,* 7:7–12.

85. Solcia, E., Capella, C., Buffa, R., and Frigerio, B. (1976): Histochemical and ultrastructural studies on the argentaffin and

argyrophil cells of the cut. In: *Chromaffin, Enterochromaffin and Related Cells,* edited by R. E. Coupland and T. Fujita, pp. 209–255. Elsevier, Amsterdam.

86. Solcia, E., Capella, C., Buffa, R., Usellini, L., Fontana, P., and Frigerio, B. (1978): Endocrine cells of the gastrointestinal tract: General aspects, ultrastructure and tumour pathology. In: *Gastrointestinal Hormones and Pathology of the Digestive System,* edited by M. Grossman, V. Speranza, N. Basso, and E. Lezoche, pp.11–22. Plenum Press, New York.

87. Solcia, E., Capella, C., Buffa, R., Usellini, L., Frigerio, B., and Fontana, P. (1979): Endocrine cells of the gastrointestinal tract and related tumors. *Pathobiol. Annu.,* 9:163–203.

88. Solcia, E., Capella, C., and Vassallo, G. (1969): Lead-haematoxylin as a stain for endocrine cells. Significance of staining and comparison with other selective methods. *Histochemie,* 20:116–126.

89. Solcia, E., Capella, C., Vassallo, G., and Buffa, R. (1975) Endocrine cells of the gastric mucosa. *Int. Rev. Cytol.,* 42:223–286.

90. Solcia, E., Capella, C., Vezzadini, P., Barbara L., and Bussolati, G. (1972): Immunohistochemical and ultrastructural detection of the secretin cell in the pig intestinal mucosa. *Experientia,* 28:549–550.

91. Solcia, E., Pearse, A. G. E., Grube, D., Kobayashi, S., Bussolati, G., Creutzfeldt, W., and Gepts, W. (1973): Revised Wiesbaden classification of gut endocrine cells. *Rendic. Gastroenterol.,* 5:13–16.

92. Solcia, E., Polak, J. M., Larsson, L.-I., Håkanson, R., Lechago, J., Fujita, T., Rubin, W., Grube, D., Falkmer, S., Greider, M. H., Creutzfeldt, W., and Grossman, M. I. (1980): Human GEP endocrine-paracrine cells: Lausanne 1977 classification revisited. In: *Cellular Basis of Chemical Messengers in the Digestive System.* Academic Press, New York *(in press).*

93. Solcia, E., Polak, J. M., Pearse, A. G. E., Forssmann, W. G., Larsson, L., Sundler, F., Lechago, J., Grimelius, L., Fujita, T., Creutzfeldt, W., Gepts, W., Falkmer, S., Lefranc, G., Heitz, Ph., Hage, E., Buchan, A. M. J., Bloom, S. R., and Grossman, M. I. (1978): Lausanne 1977 classification of gastroenteropancreatic endocrine cells. In: *Gut Hormones,* edited by S. R. Bloom, pp. 40–48. Churchill-Livingstone, Edinburgh.

94. Solcia, E., Vassallo, G., and Capella, C. (1970): Cytology and cytochemistry of hormone producing cells of the upper gastrointestinal tract. In: *Origin, Chemistry, Physiology and Pathophysiology of the Gastrointestinal Hormones,* edited by W. Creutzfeldt, pp. 3–29. Schattauer, Stuttgart.

95. Solcia, E., Vassallo, G., and Sampietro, R. (1967): Endocrine

cells in the antro-pyloric mucosa of the stomach. *Z. Zellforsch.,* 81:474–486.

96. Steiner, D. F. (1980): Synthesis and post-synthesis processing of GEP peptides. In: *Cellular Basis of Chemical Messengers in the Digestive System.* Academic Press, New York *(in press).*

97. Sundler, F., Alumets, J., Fahrenkrug, J., Håkanson, R., and Schaffalitzky de Muckadell, O. B. (1979): Cellular localization and ontogeny of immunoreactive vasoactive intestinal polypeptide (VIP) in the chicken gut. *Cell Tissue Res.,* 196:193–201.

98. Sundler, F., Alumets, A., Håkanson, R., Carraway, R., and Leeman, S. E. (1977): Ultrastructure of the gut neurotensin cells. *Histochemistry,* 53:25–34.

99. Sundler, F., Alumets, J., Holst, J., Larsson, L.-I., and Håkanson, R. (1976): Ultrastructural identification of cells storing pancreatic-type glucagon in dog stomach. *Histochemistry,* 50:33–37.

100. Tatemoto, K. (1980): Chemical assay for natural peptides: Application to the isolation of candidate hormones. In: *Gastrointestinal Hormones,* edited by G. B. J. Glass. Raven Press, New York pp. 975–977.

101. Thomas, N. W. (1970): Morphology of endocrine cells in the islet tissue of the cod *Gadus callarias. Acta Endocrinol. (Kbh),* 63:679–695.

102. Timson, C. M., Polak, J. M., Wharton, J., Ghatei, M. A., Bloom, S. R., Usellini, L., Capella, C., Solcia, E., Brown, M. R., and Pearse, A. G. E. (1979): Bombesin-like immunoreactivity in the avian gut and its localisation to a distinct cell type. *Histochemistry,* 61:213–221.

103. Van Noorden, S., and Falkmer, S. (1980): Gut-islet endocrinology. Some evolutionary aspects. *Invest. Cell Pathol.* 3:21–35.

104. Vassallo, G., Capella, C., and Solcia, E. (1971): Endocrine cells of the human gastric mucosa. *Z. Zellforsch.,* 118:49–67.

105. Vassallo, G., Solcia, E., Bussolati, G., Polak, J. M., and Pearse, A .G. E. (1972): Non-G cell gastrin-producing tumours of the pancreas. *Virchows Arch. [Cell. Pathol.],* 11:66–79.

106. Vassallo, G., Solcia, E., and Capella, C. (1969): Light and electron microscopic identification of several types of endocrine cells in the gastrointestinal mucosa of the cat. *Z. Zellforsch.,* 98:333–356.

107. Vialli, M., and Erspamer, V. (1942): Sulle reazioni chimiche colarate dell'enteramina. I. Ricerche su estratti acetonici di mucosa gastro-intestinale. *Arch. Sci. Biol. (Bologna),* 28:101–121.

108. Wharton, J., Polak, J. M., Bloom, S. R., Ghatei, M. A., Solcia, E., Brown, M. R., and Pearse, A. G. E. (1978): Bombesin-like immunoreactivity in the lung. *Nature,* 273:769–770.

Physiology of the Gastrointestinal Tract, edited by
Leonard R. Johnson. Raven Press, New York © 1981.

Chapter 3

Endocrine Cells of the Digestive System

John H. Walsh

The past decade has brought gastrointestinal endocrinology from the stage of a few well-defined peptides with suspected physiological significance in regulation of gastric and pancreatic secretion and gallbladder contraction (gastrin, secretin, cholecystokinin) to a new stage of complexity. More than a dozen additional peptides have been identified in endocrine cells or nerves and shown to have biological effects on the gut. Several of these peptides exist in multiple molecular forms. Several gut peptides have been identified in the brain and vice versa. Sensitive and specific radioimmunoassays have been developed that have permitted measurement of tissue and circulating concentrations of most of these peptides. However, the physiological roles have been identified for only a few.

In this chapter, I will attempt to present information that is as current as possible and is organized in a similar way for each peptide. Important new papers are being published each month, and some sections will undoubtedly be out of date before they are published. The order of presentation is arbitrary but represents an attempt to discuss more familiar peptides of the gut first and those identified more recently in later sections. The chemical structures of gut peptides have been established principally in the pig, but in some cases structures have been determined for human gut peptides. Table 1 shows the amino acid sequences for many of the peptides discussed in this chapter. Abbreviations of amino acids are listed in Table 2. Insulin and pancreatic glucagon are not discussed.

GASTRIN

Structure

Gastrin was the first gastrointestinal peptide for which the chemical structure was determined. Subsequently it was recognized that there were multiple molecular forms of gastrin that differed among species in substitution of a few amino acid residues and within species in the presence of gastrin molecules that differed in the length of the amino acid chain as well as in the presence or absence of a sulfate group on the single tyrosine residue (34). Gastrin and cholecystokinin (CCK) have identical carboxyl terminal pentapeptide sequences (Table 1). A scheme for consistent naming of the gastrin and CCK peptides has been suggested recently (21). The gastrin peptides for which sequences have been established with some certainty, by Gregory and his co-workers, are shown in Table 3. The presence of G/CCK4 in tissues has been reported on immunochemical grounds (80) but has not yet been proved by direct chemical analysis. The structure shown for human G34 also is deduced from a combination of chemical and immunochemical findings (20,23). The messenger RNA for gastrin is known to be capable of coding for a molecule much larger than G34, and at least three amino acid residues have been identified that could be part of a precursor molecule (77). The precursor forms of gastrin have not been identified chemically, but one form probably corresponds to "Component 1" described on the

TABLE 1. *Structures of some gut peptides*

Peptide	Structure[a]
Cholecystokinin: CCK39 CCK33 CCK8	YIQQARKAPSGRVSMIKNLQSLDPSHRISDRDYMGWMDF# -- --------------------------
Enkephalins: Leu Met	YGGFL ----------M
Gastric inhibitory peptide (GIP)	YAEGTFISDYSIAMDKIRQQDFVNWLLAQQKGKKSDWKHNITQ
Gastrin releasing peptide (GRP)	APVSVGGGTVLAKMYPRGNHWAVGHLM#
Bombesin (frog)	*QQRL-----Q--------------------
Gastrin: hG34 hG17 hG14	*QLGPQGPPHLVADPSKKQGPWLEEEEEAYGWMDF# --- ---------------------------------------
Glucagon	HSQGTFTSDYSKYLDSRRAQDFVQWLMDT
Motilin	FVPIFTYGELQRMQEKERNKGQ
Neurotensin (hNT)	*QLYENKPRRPYIL
Pancreatic polypeptide: pPP hPP	ASLEPVYPGDDATPEQMAQYAAELRRYINMLTRPRY# --P------------BB--------------------D------------------------
Somatostatin	AGCKNFFWKTFTSC
Secretin	HSDGTFTSELSRLRDSARLQRLLQFLV#
Substance P (equine)	RPKPQQFFGLM#
Thyrotropin-releasing hormone (TRH)	*QHP#
Vasoactive intestinal peptide (VIP)	HSDAVFTDNYTRLRKQMAVKKYLNSILN#

[a]Symbols used: *Q, PCA (pyroglutamyl); #, carboxyl terminal amide; Y, tyrosine sulfate; h, human; -, identical to line above.

basis of gel filtration properties of immunoreactive gastrin in plasma (84). *In vitro* studies of gastrin biosynthesis have shown formation of a molecule corresponding to G17 but have not yet delineated the intracellular events after transcription leading to formation of G17 from a precursor or the mechanism for tyrosine sulfation (37). However, it has been demonstrated that hog antral mucosa contains similar amounts of an amino terminal fragment of G34 and of G17 but only small amounts of intact G34, consistent with the intracellular cleavage of G34 to form G17 and a biologically inactive peptide fragment (23).

The presence of large and small forms of gastrin in tissue and blood has been shown by radioimmunoassay of tissue extracts and plasma after separation by chromatography or electrophoresis (2,24,25,84,127). The most abundant forms in human plasma correspond to G34, sulfated (G34s) or nonsulfated (G34), and to G17,

sulfated (G17s) or nonsulfated (G17). A form with apparent molecular weight slightly larger than that of G34 has been identified and named "Component 1" (84), and small amounts of immunoreactive gastrin corresponding to G14 (35) have been found. A peak of immunoreactivity eluting in the position of serum proteins from Sephadex G-50 has been identified and called "big-big gastrin" (127), but it is possible that most of the "big-big gastrin" immunoreactivity is due to nonspecific effects of serum protein (81). The sulfated and nonsulfated forms of gastrin in tissue and blood are present in roughly equal proportions.

Biological Actions

Gastrin has a wide range of actions on epithelial and smooth muscle targets in the gastrointestinal tract, but many of these effects require pharmacologic doses (120).

TABLE 2. *Abbreviations of amino acids*

Amino acid	Abbreviation	
	3-Letter	1-Letter
Alanine	Ala	A
Arginine	Arg	R
Asparagine	Asn	N
Aspartic acid	Asp	D
Asn or Asp	Asx	B
Cysteine	Cys	C
Glutamine	Gln	Q
Glutamic acid	Glu	E
Gln or Glu	Glx	Z
Pyroglutamyl	pGlu	pE
Glycine	Gly	G
Histidine	His	H
Isoleucine	Ile	I
Leucine	Leu	L
Lysine	Lys	K
Methionine	Met	M
Phenylalanine	Phe	F
Proline	Pro	P
Serine	Ser	S
Threonine	Thr	T
Tryptophan	Trp	W
Tyrosine	Tyr	Y
Valine	Val	V

In Vivo

The most apparent action of gastrin *in vivo* is stimulation of acid secretion (69,120). Evidence has accumulated that a substantial fraction of gastric acid response to protein meals is mediated by circulating gastrin (*see,* in this section, Correlation with Physiological Events). Stimulation of acid secretion is associated with increased mucosal blood flow to the acid-secreting portion of the stomach and increased secretion of pepsinogen. It is not known if the stimulation of pepsinogen is primary or is related to increased output of acid, since topical acid also causes increased pepsinogen secretion. Gastrin also causes a modest increase in secretion of intrinsic factor. Other effects of gastrin that have been noted at doses that were submaximal for stimulation of acid secretion include stimulation of antral motility in the dog (100) and modest stimulation of pancreatic enzyme secretion in humans (114). Gastrin is a more effective stimulant of pancreatic enzyme secretion in dog than in humans, and the potencies of exogenous G17 and G34 are not significantly different (115). Evidence has been obtained that gastrin may have a role in regulation of glucose-stimulated insulin release (82). More recently it has been suggested that the C-terminal tetrapeptide of gastrin may

TABLE 3. *Structures of gastrins of various species*

Gastrin	Species	Abbreviation	Structure[a]
Gastrin-34	Human	hG34	pELGPQGPPHLVADPSKKQGPWLEEEEEAẎGWMDF#
("Big")	Porcine	pG34	pELGLQGPPHLVADLAKKQGPWMEEEEEAẎGWMDF#
Gastrin precursor	Porcine		----HRRQLGLQGPPHLVADLAKKQGPWMEE--------
Gastrin-17	Human	hG17	pEGPWLEEEEEAẎGWMDF#
("Little")	Porcine	pG17	pEGPWMEEEEEAẎGWMDF#
	Feline	fG17	pEGPWLEEEEAAẎGWMDF#
	Canine	cG17	pEGPWMEEAEEAẎGWMDF#
	Bovine	bG17	pEGPWVEEEEAAẎGWMDF#
	Ovine	oG17	pEGPWVEEEEAAẎGWMDF#
Gastrin-14	Human	hG14	WLEEEEEAẎGWMDF#
("Mini")	Porcine	pG14	WMEEEEEAẎGWMDF#
1-13 pG17 ("N-terminal fragment")			pEGPWMEEEEEAẎG
C-Terminal tetrapeptide G/CCK4			WMDF#

[a]Symbols used: X, residue different from column above; pE, pyroglutamyl; Ẏ, tyrosine residue either sulfated or nonsulfated.

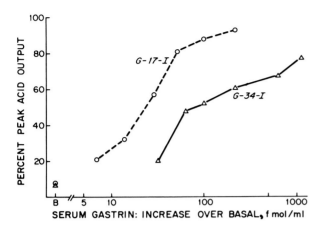

FIG. 1. Increased potency of circulating G17 compared with circulating G34 for stimulation of acid secretion in dogs with gastric fistulas. From Walsh et al. (119).

be important for this function since evidence has been obtained that it occurs in the pancreas and is more potent than G17 for release of pancreatic hormones (80).

Another potentially important role of gastrin *in vivo* is regulation of mucosal growth, especially of the acid-secreting mucosa of the stomach (46). A number of studies have demonstrated that administration of gastrin analogues in rats causes stimulation of DNA, RNA, and protein synthesis in the acid-secreting mucosa and increases the total number of parietal cells. These trophic actions of gastrin analogues are antagonized by secretin (97) and by VIP (47) but not by glucagon. CCK in high doses appears to be a competitive inhibitor of the trophic effects of gastrin in the stomach (47). Trophic effects of gastrin also have been found in the small intestine and colon but not in the esophagus or gastric antrum (47). The trophic effect of gastrin on the pancreas is much less than that of CCK. A comparison of sulfated and nonsulfated G17 and G34 showed that all were effective and that there were no significant differences among these forms of gastrin. Continuous intravenous infusion of gastrin at doses that were submaximal for acid secretion in dogs caused stimulation of DNA synthesis. Also, it has been shown that the gastric atrophy in rats that results from starvation or from parenteral feeding can be prevented partially by concurrent administration of exogenous gastrin (16). The relative importance of gastrin and of other factors such as luminal nutrients and other hormones in regulation of growth of gut tissues has not been established. In humans, it is known that prolonged stimulation of the stomach by gastrin released from gastrin-secreting tumors is associated with gastric mucosal hyperplasia (43), but lesser increases in gastrin that are found after vagotomy do not produce hyperplasia (120).

Gastrin causes contraction of the lower esophageal sphincter and this effect is not antagonized by atropine (45). Doses of G17 and G34 required to produce con-

traction in man produce serum gastrin concentrations higher than those achieved after a meal. Although some early studies suggested that circulating gastrin might be a major regulator of lower esophageal sphincter pressure in man, it was concluded in 1974 that this hypothesis was incorrect (103). More recent studies have shown that there was no correlation between gastrin and sphincter pressure in clinical conditions associated either with hypergastrinemia or with decreased sphincter pressure (67).

Interactions among gastrin, histamine, and acetylcholine are important in determining the overall gastric secretory response to gastrin (94). Cephalic-vagal stimulation enhances the acid stimulation caused by gastrin, and interruption of cephalic-vagal mechanisms by vagotomy or anticholinergic agents decreases the responses. Specific inhibition of H2 histamine receptors with antagonists such as cimetidine also diminishes the acid response to gastrin. The responses to exogenous gastrin also can be inhibited by several peptides including secretin, CCK, GIP, VIP, glucagon, and somatostatin as well as by various prostaglandins.

In Vitro

Gastrin has been shown to stimulate oxygen consumption, aminopyrine accumulation, and morphological transformation of isolated mammalian parietal cells (94). All of these changes are correlated with acid secretion *in vivo*, but none is a direct measure of hydrogen ion secretion. Aminopyrine accumulation occurs in intracellular spaces with pH less than 5 and is presumed to be sequestered in secretory canaliculi of parietal cells under conditions that produce stimulation of the acid secretory process. The stimulatory effect of gastrin alone on isolated canine parietal cells is small compared with the responses obtained with histamine or carbachol (91,92). However, the response appears to be specific since it is not inhibited by antagonists of histamine or acetylcholine. Potentiated responses are obtained with combinations of gastrin with either histamine or carbachol, and the potentiating effects are blocked by specific inhibitors of histamine or carbachol. Histamine appears to act by a mechanism that involves stimulation of parietal cell cAMP, and the potentiating effects of histamine can be mimicked by dibutyryl cAMP. Cimetidine and low concentrations of prostaglandin E_2 prevent histamine stimulation of cAMP and also prevent the potentiating effect of histamine on parietal cell response to gastrin. Neither carbachol nor gastrin stimulates cAMP accumulation in parietal cells. Carbachol appears to act by increasing parietal cell permeability to extracellular calcium, but gastrin action is only moderately impaired by removal of extracellular calcium (93). The secondary mechanisms by which gastrin stimulates parietal cells remain to be defined.

Gastrin has been shown to stimulate acid secretion from isolated gastric mucosa of the amphibian *Necturus* (2). Gastrin and the C-terminal tetrapeptide produced similar maximal responses, but the tetrapeptide appeared to be degraded rapidly by exposure to the tissue. The C-terminal octapeptide of CCK caused less marked stimulation and inhibited the responses to gastrin and to the tetrapeptide.

Two types of radiolabeled gastrin have been used to estimate gastrin receptor binding in rat gastric mucosa. Lewin et al. (61,95) employed tritiated gastrin with a specific radioactivity of 60 Ci/mmol. They demonstrated reversible binding to partially purified plasma membranes or to intact cells that had been separated by pronase digestion that was time and temperature dependent and proportional to cell or membrane concentration. Maximum binding was 50 fmol/mg protein or 12.5 fmol gastrin per 10^6 cells, calculated to be equal to 19,200 binding sites per parietal cell. Binding was proportional to the number of parietal cells rather than to total cell number and was reversed by an excess of pentagastrin or by dilution. The equilibrium constant (K) was calculated to be 0.9×10^{-8}M. Scatchard plot analysis suggested a single class of binding sites. Unfortunately, proportions of specific and nonspecific binding were not calculated. In this preparation there was an increase in cellular adenylate cyclase activity associated with gastrin binding.

Takeuchi et al. (105,106) utilized radioiodinated gastrin with a final specific activity of 2,000 cpm/fmol (about 10^4 higher than the specific activity of tritiated gastrin). Binding was demonstrated in mucosal scrapings of rat gastric mucosa that were centrifuged at 200 × g, homogenized, then centrifuged at 270 × g. The supernatant was recentrifuged at 30,000 × g and the suspended pellet was shown to contain the highest ratio of specific to nonspecific binding. Maximum binding was approximately 4 fmol/mg protein, K_a 2.5×10^{11} M^{-1}, and the equilibrium constant about 4×10^{-10}M. Optimal binding was obtained after 30 min incubation at 30°C at pH 7. Duodenal mucosa also demonstrated considerable binding but little or no binding was obtained in antral mucosa, spleen, kidney, or liver. Competitive inhibition of binding was found for unlabeled gastrin, CCK, cerulein, and pentagastrin over a range that differed by one order of magnitude, whereas secretin produced inhibition of binding that appeared to be noncompetitive. Mucosal binding capacity was decreased in rats that were fasted for 4 days and returned to normal after refeeding. The protein nature of gastrin membrane receptors was shown by a marked decrease in specific binding after pretreatment with trypsin. Gastrin receptor binding also has been assessed in plasma membranes prepared from dog antral smooth muscle (1). Maximal binding was about 50 fmol/mg protein and the K_a was 2×10^9M^{-1}. Pentagastrin was about 1% as potent as gastrin as an inhibitor of binding.

Gastrin effects on smooth muscle *in vitro* include stimulation of muscle contractions and electrical activity. Muscle from the lower esophageal sphincter and antral smooth muscle are especially sensitive. Pentagastrin is about as potent as G17 and G34 on canine antral muscle (72). Although the mammalian gallbladder is much less responsive to gastrin peptides than to CCK, a teleost, the coho salmon, cannot distinguish between sulfated forms of CCK and gastrin, suggesting that receptor selectivity for the two peptides has evolved relatively late (116). In many systems, gastrin appears to act directly on smooth muscle cells to elicit contraction. In dog, antrum pentagastrin stimulates longitudinal muscle partially by release of acetylcholine from nerves whereas it stimulates circular muscle directly (104). In some preparations, there is evidence that it exerts its effect entirely by release of acetylcholine from nervous elements. This is especially evident in guinea pig ileum where contractile responses to both gastrin and CCK peptides are abolished by atropine or tetrodotoxin (118).

In the isolated, perfused porcine pancreas, the C-terminal tetrapeptide amide of gastrin and CCK was found to be a potent stimulant for the release of insulin, somatostatin, glucagon, and pancreatic polypeptide and was more potent than the larger forms of either gastrin or CCK (80).

Structure-Activity Relationships

Tracy and Gregory (34) discovered that the C-terminal tetrapeptide amide of gastrin (G4) possessed the full range of biological effects of G17 although it was less potent on a molar basis. They also established that the sulfated and nonsulfated forms of gastrin had approximately equal potency for stimulation of acid secretion. A series of peptide analogues of G4 was examined for biological activity, and it was found that replacement of the C-terminal amide group with a hydroxyl group (G4 free acid) led to almost complete inactivation (73). N-acylation of the tetrapeptide preserved or enhanced activity. Substitution by D-amino acids virtually abolished activity. Substitutions that preserved activity included norleucine or ethionine for methionine, alterations of the tryptophan ring, and substitution of Tyr-NH$_2$ for Phe-NH$_2$. All changes in the aspartic acid position led to virtually complete inactivation. Subsequently it has been shown that the C-terminal tripeptide retains a small amount of biological activity (64) and that C-terminal desamido G17 is virtually inactive as a stimulant of acid secretion (70). A synthetic 1-15 N-terminal fragment of human G34 was inactive as a stimulant of acid secretion or muscle contraction (87).

The biological potencies of circulating molecular forms of gastrin that differ in chain length are related to both intrinsic activity and differences in rates of clearance. Based on exogenous doses, equimolar infusions of G34, G17, and G14 produce similar rates of acid secretion in dog and humans (11,119,121). The clearance rates of G17 and G14 are similar, but G34 is cleared 6 to 8 times less rapidly from the circulation. The circulating concentrations required to produce equal stimulation of acid secretion are 6 to 8 times higher for G34 than for G17. Therefore the potency of G34 in the circulation is considerably lower than the potency of G17 in the circulation (Fig. 1). Gastrin tetrapeptide and pentagastrin are about one-tenth as potent as G17 as exogenous stimulants of acid secretion. Accurate measurements of these peptides in the circulation are difficult, so it is not known whether the variations in potency are due chiefly to differences in clearance or to differences in intrinsic activity.

Distribution

Cellular

The principal gastrin-containing cell is the G cell, identified easily by immunocytochemical methods in the glands of the antral mucosa (36,68). The granules in these cells vary in size and density, depending on the method of fixation and the functional condition of the cell. In resting cells granules usually are small (200 nm diameter) and electron dense, although they become larger (300 nm) and less dense during stimulation of gastrin release.

The distribution of G cells in the antral glands differs among species. In humans and dog, the cells are localized in a band midway between the neck and base of the glands, whereas in the rat the gastrin cells extend to the base of the glands. Studies with region-specific antisera have shown that both G17 and G34 appear to be located in the same cells in the antrum (113) and that rat, chicken, and frog demonstrate a progressive pattern of decreasing immunochemical identity in the staining reaction with antibodies raised against human G17, retaining at a minimum some reactivity with antibodies that recognize the C-terminal tetrapeptide sequence common to gastrin and CCK (56). Turnover of antral gastrin cells in the mouse has been studied by autoradiography after injection of tritiated thymidine, and the turnover time was estimated to be approximately 40 days (59); recent estimates indicate more rapid turnover, 10 to 15 days, and that gastrin cells originate from ordinary neck cells (33).

Cells that react with antisera to gastrin also have been identified in the fetal and adult small intestine and the fetal pancreas (55,57,58,110). Gastrin cells in the human duodenum can be distinguished from CCK cells by demonstration of specific reactions with antisera directed toward the amino terminal regions of gastrin or CCK and nonspecific staining reactions with antisera directed toward the common amino terminal sequence of gastrin and CCK (4). The intestinal gastrin-containing cells are said to have distinctive differences from antral G cells in the ultrastructural appearance of their secretory granules. Rehfeld et al. (80) also have presented evidence for the presence of the C-terminal tetrapeptide common to gastrin and CCK in both nerves and distinctive cells in the small intestine and pancreas.

Extractable

Highest concentrations of extractable gastrin are present in the antral mucosa of adult mammals, although duodenal gastrin concentration is higher in the fetus (56, 57,110). The adult human duodenum differs from that of other mammals such as dog, cat, and hog because it contains a large amount of gastrin (76). The whole duodenum of humans was estimated to contain approximately the same amount of gastrin as the antrum, whereas the remaining small intestine contained less than 1% of this amount. In dog, cat, and hog neither the duodenum nor the remaining small intestine contains as much as 2% of the antral gastrin content. Recently it has been reported in dogs that resection of the antrum leads to marked increases in the amount of gastrin that can be extracted from canine intestine (74). The above results were obtained by radioimmunoassay of tissue extracts. They agree reasonably well with bioassay results obtained by Lai (52) who found somewhat more total gastrin activity in the whole duodenum of a human subject than in the antrum. Jejunal, ileal, and colonic mucosa had lesser amounts of activity, and none was found in pancreatic extracts.

Molecular forms of gastrin in tissue extracts correspond to those found in the plasma but differ in relative abundance between antrum, duodenum, and blood (3, 19,24,25,84,126). Antral extracts contain predominantly G17 (90%) and the other 10% consists chiefly of G34. In contrast, 50% or more of the gastrin extracted from the duodenal mucosa is G34 and the remaining 50% or less is G17. CCK peptides cross-react with many gastrin antisera, and their presence in duodenal and jejunal extracts may lead to misleading estimates of total gastrin activity when such antisera are used. The most abundant form of gastrin in the blood corresponds to G34 (19,24,25,84,107,126). About 2/3 of circulating gastrin in the basal state and about half in the postprandial state is G34. The remainder is mainly G17 but small amounts are Component 1 and G14. The proportion of G34 and of G17 that is sulfated is approximately half of the total in plasma as it is in tissue (C. B. Lamers, *un-*

published). The amount of G34 found in the peripheral blood is more than would be expected if a pure extract of antral mucosa were infused intravenously, and this implies either that the proportion of G34 released from the antrum and passing the liver is higher than would be expected from tissue extraction studies or that some of the circulating gastrin originates in the small intestine. Biosynthesis of G17 stored in the antrum presumably occurs by synthesis of a precursor that first is converted to G34 and then enzymatically degraded further to G17. Evidence for this pathway is given by the observation that by use of antibodies specific for the N-terminus of G34, amino terminal fragments of G34 can be detected in antral tissue in the same proportion as G17, which is the carboxyl terminal fragment of G34 (23).

Gastrin-like activity has been extracted from tissues other than antrum and small intestine. The nonantral portion of the stomach contains only about 1% the concentration of the antrum, but this is more than other control tissues. Attempts to extract gastrin from the exocrine or whole pancreas have produced mixed results, but evidence was obtained that mouse islets contain gastrin similar to G17 (18). Also there is evidence that a peptide similar to gastrin/CCK tetrapeptide can be extracted from pancreatic tissue (80).

Most of the "gastrin-like" immunoreactivity that has been extracted from the brain corresponds to CCK8 or larger forms of CCK or possibly to the tetrapeptide (see section on CCK). However, Rehfeld (78) used gastrin-specific antibody to identify G17 in the pituitary stalk and anterior and posterior pituitary in pigs. G17-like immunoreactivity also has been extracted from the abdominal portion of the vagus nerve in cats, dogs, and humans (112).

Measurement

Bioassay

Bioassay methods for measurement of gastrin are much less sensitive than radioimmunoassay. They remain useful for monitoring purification of gastrin molecular forms from tissue extracts (34,51,52) and for identification of acid secretagogues in plasma (5,8). Responses most often are measured in anesthetized rats, but cats also have been used. Histamine is present in many tissue extracts and may interfere with gastrin bioassays. The coho salmon gallbladder longitudinal muscle offers a potential system for preferentially measuring sulfated forms of gastrin once they have been separated from CCK peptides (116). CCK may interfere in the bioassay of gastrin, especially when the cat is used to measure acid secretion, since CCK and gastrin produce equal maximal acid responses in this species. A highly sensitive cytochemical assay based on stimulation of carbonic anhydrase in fundus slices has been reported (66).

Radioimmunoassay

Gastrin can be measured by highly sensitive and specific radioimmunoassays, and the characteristics of these assays have been reviewed recently (86). Immunization of rabbits with gastrin conjugated to carrier protein has resulted in production of antibodies with K_a as high as 10^{12} M^{-1} and specific either for the C-terminus or N-terminus of G17 (83) or, rarely, for the entire G17 molecule (22). Antibodies also have been produced that are specific for the amino terminal portion of G34, and one of these antibodies was used to demonstrate immunochemical differences between natural porcine G34 and synthetic porcine G34, leading to a correction in the amino acid sequence (20,22). Radioimmunoassay with sets of antibodies differing in specificity has been used to characterize gastrin and cholecystokinin-like peptides in extracts of gut and brain (23,40,79).

The most common and versatile gastrin radioimmunoassays utilize antibodies specific for the biologically active C-terminus of gastrin that react approximately equally well with G34, G17, and G14, do not distinguish between sulfated and nonsulfated gastrins, and exhibit minimal crossreactivity with CCK peptides (86). These assays measure total carboxyl terminal activity and usually are expressed in terms of a G17 standard. The high affinity of some antibodies permits measurements of physiological concentrations of plasma gastrin in unextracted plasma assayed at dilutions of 1:10 or 1:20. Such dilution minimizes nonspecific inhibition caused by plasma proteins and reveals that normal basal gastrin concentrations are in the order of 10 to 20 pM (20–40 pg/ml G17 equivalent). Further characterization of molecular forms of gastrin in plasma or tissue extracts can be done without further separation by use of G17 specific antibody (23,107). Alternatively, molecular forms of gastrin can be separated by gel filtration (84) or by a combination of affinity chromatography and gel filtration (C. B. Lamers, *unpublished*) and different molecular forms of gastrin can be determined by their characteristic elution position and their reactions with region-specific antisera (19,24,25,40).

Metabolism

The rates at which various forms of gastrin disappear from the circulation and the sites of removal have been studied more thoroughly than the mechanisms for inactivation. In dogs there is good agreement that the disappearance half-time of G17 is approximately 3 min (99, 119) and that the half-time for G34 is between 9 and 15 min. Measurement of disappearance rates of endogenously released gastrin in dogs was consistent with two patterns of disappearance with half-times of 2.8 and 15.4 min (117). In human subjects, the clearance rates of G17 and G34 are about half as rapid as in dogs, and the discrepancy between G17 and G34 is even more apparent with G34 being cleared 7 to 8 times slower than G17 (121). G14 is cleared from the circulation in the dog at a similar rate to G17 (6), and the sulfated and nonsulfated gastrins are cleared at similar rates. The liver does not appear to play a major role in clearance of the forms of gastrin normally present in the circulation, but it removes short gastrin fragments such as the tetrapeptide and pentagastrin almost quantitatively (101). Although the kidney was felt to have a special role in gastrin metabolism, it has been shown that most capillary beds in the body remove similar amounts of G17 leading to venous concentrations about 20 to 25% lower than arterial concentrations (102). It also has been found that some anephric humans have normal serum gastrin and gastrin clearance rates (I. L. Taylor, *unpublished*). The kidney may play a more important role in clearance of G34 but appears to have no special role in G17 clearance. The general arteriovenous (AV) differences found throughout the body explain other reports that small intestine, stomach, and other organs remove gastrin.

Specific mechanisms for gastrin catabolism *in vivo* have not been elucidated. Very little of the gastrin that is filtered by the kidney appears intact in the urine. It was shown that kidney homogenates contain enzymatic activity that cleaves the C-terminal dipeptide amide from gastrin tetrapeptide (122), but it is not known if such an enzyme acts on the larger gastrin molecules. Liver homogenates contain enzymatic activity that leads to deamidation of acylated gastrin tetrapeptide amide, but again the relevance to *in vivo* events is unknown. Intravenous infusion of G34 does not lead to appearance of G17 in the circulation (121). Gastric mucosal cells may degrade radiolabeled gastrin into forms that are unable to bind to antigastrin antibodies or gastrin cell surface receptors (15).

Release

In Vivo

Gastrin is released by peptides, amino acids, and calcium in the gastric lumen, by activation of nervous reflexes, and by circulating catecholamines and bombesin (120). Under some circumstances gastrin release is enhanced by anticholinergic agents. Gastrin release is inhibited by low intragastric luminal pH and by several peptides present in the gastrointestinal tract including somatostatin, as well as by topical administration of certain prostaglandins. The 24-hr circadian pattern of acid secretion, with highest secretion during the evening and lowest in early morning, is not paralleled by changes in immunoreactive serum gastrin in fasting human subjects (71).

Food components, most significantly small peptide and amino acid fragments resulting from digestion of protein (26), are known to cause gastrin release. Glucose and fat do not release easily measurable amounts of gastrin unless protein or amino acids are added (85). Distension of the stomach by liquid or balloon causes minimal gastrin release but does stimulate acid secretion (89, 90). When the effects of distension are taken into account, the amount of gastrin released by intragastric amino acid solution in man is enough to account for the additional increase in acid secretion (31). Furthermore, when graded concentrations of peptone are infused into the stomach at constant pH, there is a strong positive correlation between increase in acid secretion and increase in total serum gastrin and in the specific G17 fraction (53).

Considerable evidence exists that most gastrin released into the circulation by a meal originates from the gastric antrum (120). The human duodenum contains more gastrin than the duodenum in other species, and there is evidence that gastrin may be released from the human duodenum by food after resection of the antrum (98). In dogs, there is some evidence that gastrin can be released into the duodenal vein (65), but perfusion of liver extract into the duodenum of conscious dogs did not lead to an increase in peripheral serum gastrin concentration (48). Protein-rich solutions appear to release some circulating substance distinct from gastrin from dog intestine that augments the acid response to gastrin from vagally denervated (Heidenhain) pouches (10).

Release of gastrin is inhibited by acidification of gastric luminal contents below pH 3 (120,123). This feedback inhibition modulates the amount of gastrin released normally after a meal, since gastric contents commonly are acidified to pH 2 to 3. Maintaining intragastric pH above 3 in the presence of protein or amino acids increases the magnitude and duration of the gastrin response obtained. On the other hand, in the absence of protein or amino acids, neutralization of the gastric contents with solutions of sodium bicarbonate or sodium hydroxide does not cause an acute increase of serum gastrin. Neutralization with calcium carbonate does increase serum gastrin, but this is due to a direct effect of calcium ions on the antral mucosa to release gastrin (60). Prolonged neutralization of the stomach, as found in patients with atrophic gastritis of the acid-secreting gastric mucosa, leads to hyperplasia of gastrin cells and hypergastrinemia by an undefined mechanism.

The effects of vagal and cholinergic stimulation and inhibition on gastrin release are complex. In animals, including dog, activation of vagal-cholinergic reflexes by sham feeding or insulin hypoglycemia causes release of gastrin that can be inhibited by large doses of atropine or antral denervation (9,75,109). The basal gastrin concentration and gastrin response to feeding are increased after truncal vagotomy. Low doses of atropine enhance the gastrin response to feeding in dogs whereas higher doses have little effect (42); after truncal vagotomy atropine has a marked inhibitory effect (13). Reflex release of gastrin initiated by receptors in the stomach can be demonstrated by distension of separated antral pouches, and a crossed oxyntopyloric reflex has been shown in which distension of a fundic pouch caused release of gastrin from the antrum (12). The inhibitory effects of high-dose atropine on some forms of reflex-stimulated gastrin release are compatible with a cholinergic stimulatory mechanism, but the enhancement of gastrin release under other circumstances by lower doses of atropine suggests that some other cholinergic mechanism inhibits the release of gastrin. Increased gastrin release after vagotomy could be the result of removal of a vagal-cholinergic inhibitory mechanism, or to hyperplasia prolonged by hypochlorhydria. Intravenous infusion of cholinomimetic drugs in intact dogs produces weak stimulation of gastrin release and inhibits bombesin-stimulated gastrin release (38,108). Evidence has been obtained that cholinergic suppression of gastrin release depends on vagal fibers that innervate the acid-secreting portion of the stomach (39,88).

In humans, low doses of atropine enhance gastrin release caused by insulin hypoglycemia (27), sham feeding (29), and gastric distension (89) and also prevent the inhibition of gastrin release that normally occurs at low intragastric pH (30). Atropine also enhances the gastrin response to food in humans (124), but this effect is not as great when intragastric pH is maintained constant (28,49). Vagotomy in humans also increases basal and food-stimulated gastrin (120). These data all are compatible with dual vagal-cholinergic mechanisms causing both stimulation and inhibition of gastrin release, presumably by activating separate intermediary mechanisms. A central vagal stimulatory mechanism is supported by small increases in gastrin during sham feeding and abolition of this reponse by a nonsedative neuroleptic drug acting on the hypothalamus (54). The cholinergic-dependent inhibitory factor could be somatostatin, which is present in high concentrations in antral mucosa and whose release is inhibited by atropine (see section on somatostatin), but there is only preliminary evidence for this hypothesis.

Gastrin release from *in vitro* antral organ cultures was stimulated after removal of a protein solution from the medium, suggesting that protein released an inhibitor of gastrin release (63). Vascular perfusion of isolated rat stomach with antibodies to somatostatin markedly increased basal and stimulated gastrin release (see ref. 66, p. 196). Three peptides that are known to inhibit gastrin release—glucagon, secretin, and vasoactive intestinal peptide—produced reciprocal decreases in release of gastrin and increases in release of somatostatin from isolated perfused rat stomach (7). The mechanisms by

which gastrin is released from G cells are not fully characterized, but the intracellular microtubular-microfilament system may be involved (17).

There also is evidence that beta-adrenergic mechanisms may participate in regulation of gastrin release under some circumstances. Intravenous epinephrine caused release of gastrin in humans, and the effect was suppressed by prior administration of a beta-adrenergic blocker (96). Propranolol inhibited gastrin release during insulin hypoglycemia in humans (50). Cutting the sinus nerves in cats resulted in a rapid fall in blood pressure associated with an increase in serum gastrin that was prevented by bilateral adrenalectomy (44). A dopaminergic mechanism for gastrin release was suggested in dogs by experiments that showed release of gastrin by apomorphine injection that was suppressed by prior treatment with haloperidol (111). An effect of oral propranolol to inhibit gastrin release caused by oral acetylcholine in rat suggests that adrenergic and cholinergic mechanisms may interact in the antral mucosa (41).

Certain factors are known to alter antral gastrin stores. Prolonged fasting in rats decreases antral gastrin content and serum gastrin and the decrease is not prevented by a high-bulk non-nutritive diet (62). Chronic administration of hydrocortisone increases serum gastrin response to food in dogs (125) associated with antral gastrin cell hyperplasia (14).

Correlation with Physiological Events

Several attempts to correlate gastric acid secretion with serum gastrin responses yielded equivocal responses, showing general correlation between acid stimulation and release of gastrin but poor relationship between individual gastrin concentrations and secretory rates (32, 85). Distension of the stomach causes moderate stimulation of acid secretion that is not correlated with gastrin release. However, when the effects of distension were taken into effect and individual responses to graded exogenous doses of G17 were measured, it was found that the increase in circulating G17 was sufficient to account for the gastric secretory response to intragastric amino acids (31). More direct evidence for a physiological role of circulating gastrin was obtained by the demonstration that there was a high degree of correlation between serum gastrin and G17 responses to graded intragastric concentrations of peptone (53). G17 is the most potent circulating form of gastrin and it appears to be the most important circulating component in regulation of acid secretion (Fig. 2).

Other physiological effects of circulating gastrin are less well established. There is some evidence that gastrin is one of the important factors regulating growth of the acid-secreting portion of the stomach, since gastrin infusions partially prevent gastric atrophy that results from antrectomy (46,47). Gastrin also may contribute

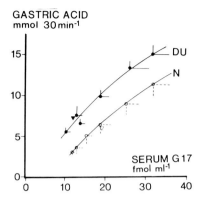

FIG. 2. Relationship between circulating G17 and gastric acid secretion in normal subjects (N) and duodenal ulcer patients (DU) during stimulation with graded concentrations of intragastric peptone. Mean D_{50M} for DU (*closed triangles*) and N (*open triangles*) are also shown. From Lam, et al, ref. 53.

to regulation of antral motor activity (100). There is little evidence that gastrin is a physiological regulator of lower esophageal sphincter pressure in man (103). It has not been established whether the small amounts of gastrin release by sham feeding in man contribute significantly to the acid secretory response.

Effects of Gastrin Excess or Deficiency

Excessive secretion of gastrin in humans due to the presence of a gastrin-secreting tumor (gastrinoma) or more rarely to primary antral G-cell hyperfunction or isolated retained antrum after Billroth II gastrectomy leads to basal acid hypersecretion and hyperplasia of the acid-secreting mucosa (120). The hypersecretory state caused by gastrin excess often is associated with severe peptic ulcer disease and sometimes with diarrhea. On the other hand, hypergastrinemia that occurs in patients with atrophic gastritis of the acid-secreting mucosa appears to have no adverse effects. Hypergastrinemia can be induced in animals by transplantation of the antrum to the colon and causes gastric hypersecretion and hyperplasia of the remaining stomach.

Primary deficiency of gastrin-producing cells has not been reported. It is likely that decreased serum gastrin contributes to the decrease of acid secretory capacity that occurs after antrectomy in humans, but it is difficult to separate the effects of decreased gastrin from other effects of operation including interruption of nervous reflexes and increased reflux of intestinal contents into the stomach.

References

1. Baur, S., and Bacon, V. C. (1976): A specific gastrin receptor on plasma membranes of antral smooth muscle. *Biochem. Biophys. Res. Commun.,* 73:928-933.
2. Berkowitz, J. M., Praissman, M., and LeFevre, M. E. (1976): Effects of peptide hormone structure on H^+ secretion by *Necturus* gastric mucosa. *Am. J. Physiol.,* 231:573-578.
3. Berson, S. A., and Yalow, R. S. (1971): Nature of immunoreactive gastrin extracted from tissues of gastrointestinal tract. *Gastroenterology,* 60:215-222.
4. Buchan, A. M. J., Polak, J. M., Solcia, E., and Pearse, A. G. E. (1979): Localisation of intestinal gastrin in a distinct endocrine cell type. *Nature,* 5692:138-140.
5. Bugat, R., Walsh, J. H., Ippoliti, A., Elashoff, J., and Grossman, M. I. (1976): Detection of a circulating secretagogue in plasma extracts from normogastrinemic patients with acid hypersecretion. *Gastroenterology,* 71:1114-1116.
6. Carter, D. C., Taylor, I. L., Elashoff, J., and Grossman, M. I. (1979): Reappraisal of the secretory potency and disappearance rate of pure human minigastrin. *Gut,* 20:705-708.
7. Chiba, T., Taminato, T., Kadowaki, S. Abe, H., Chihara, K., Goto, Y., Seino, Y., and Fujita, T. (1980): Effects of glucagon, secretin, and vasoactive intestinal polypeptide on gastric somatostatin and gastrin release from isolated perfused rat stomach. *Gastroenterology (in press).*
8. Colin-Jones, D. G., and Lennard-Jones, J. E. (1972): The detection and measurement of circulating gastrin-like activity by bioassay. *Gut,* 13:88-94.
9. Csendes, A., Walsh, J. H., and Grossman, M. I. (1972): Effects of atropine and of antral acidification of gastrin release and acid secretion in response to insulin and feeding in dogs. *Gastroenterology,* 63:257-263.
10. Debas, H. T., Slaff, G. F., and Grossman, M. I. (1975): Intestinal phase of gastric acid secretion: Augmentation of maximal response to Heidenhain pouch to gastrin and histamine. *Gastroenterology,* 68:691-698.
11. Debas, H. T., Walsh, J. H., and Grossman, M. I. (1974): Pure human minigastrin: Secretory potency and disappearance rate. *Gut,* 15:686-689.
12. Debas, H. T., Walsh, J. H., and Grossman, M. I. (1975): Evidence for oxyntopyloric reflex for release of antral gastrin. *Gastroenterology,* 68:687-690.
13. Debas, H. T., Walsh, J. H., and Grossman, M. I. (1976): After vagotomy atropine suppresses gastrin release by food. *Gastroenterology,* 70:1082-1084.
14. Delaney, J. P., Michel, H. M., Bonsack, M. E., Eisenberg, M. M., and Dunn, D. H. (1979): Adrenal corticosteroids cause gastrin cell hyperplasia. *Gastroenterology,* 76:913-916.
15. Del Mazo, J., and McGuigan, J. E. (1976): Degradation of gastrin by gastric mucosal cells. *J. Lab. Clin. Med.,* 88:292-300.
16. Dembinski, A. B., and Johnson, L. R. (1979): Growth of pancreas and gastrointestinal mucosa in antrectomized and gastrin-treated rats. *Endocrinology,* 105:769-773.
17. Deschryver-Kecskemeti, K., Greider, M. H., Rieders, E., and McGuigan, J. E. (1980): Studies on gastrin secretion in vitro from cultures of rat pyloric antrum: Effects of agents modifying the microtubular-microfilament system. *Gastroenterology,* 78:339-345.
18. Dockray, G. J., Best, L., and Taylor, I. L. (1977): Immunochemical characterization of gastrin in pancreatic islets of normal and genetically obese mice. *J. Endocrinol.,* 72:143-151.
19. Dockray, G. J., Debas, H. T., Walsh, J. H., and Grossman, M. I. (1975): Molecular forms of gastrin in antral mucosa and serum in dogs (38848). *Proc. Soc. Exp. Biol. Med.,* 149:550-553.
20. Dockray, G. J., Gregory, R. A., Hood, L., and Hunkapiller, M. (1979): NH_2-terminal dodecapeptide of porcine big gastrin: Revised sequence and confirmation of structure by immunochemical analysis. *Bioorgan. Chem.* 8:465-470.
21. Dockray, G. J., Rehfeld, J. F., and Walsh, J. H. (1979): Naming gastrin and cholecystokinin peptides. In: *Gastrins and the Vagus,* edited by J. F. Rehfeld and E. Amdrup, pp. 95-97. Academic Press, London.
22. Dockray, G. J., and Taylor, I. L. (1977): Heptadecapeptide gastrin: Measurement in blood by specific radioimmunoassay. *Gastroenterology,* 71:971-977.
23. Dockray, G. J., Vaillant, C., and Hopkins, C. R. (1978): Biosynthetic relationships of big and little gastrins. *Nature,* 273:770-772.

24. Dockray, G. J., and Walsh, J. H. (1975): Amino terminal gastrin fragment in serum of Zollinger-Ellison syndrome patients. *Gastroenterology,* 68:222–230.

25. Dockray, G. J., Walsh, J. H., and Passaro, E., Jr. (1975): Relative abundance of big and little gastrins in the tumours and blood of patients with the Zollinger-Ellison syndrome. *Gut,* 16:353–358.

26. Elwin, C. E. (1974): Gastric acid responses to antral application of some amino acids, peptides, and isolated fractions of a protein hydrolysate. *Scand. J. Gastroenterol.,* 9:239–247.

27. Farooq, O., and Walsh, J. H. (1975): Atropine enhances serum gastrin response to insulin in man. *Gastroenterology,* 68:662–666.

28. Feldman, M., Richardson, C. T., Peterson, W. L., Walsh, J. H., and Fordtran, J. S. (1977): Effect of low-dose propantheline on food-stimulated gastric acid secretion. Comparison with an "optimal effective dose" and interaction with cimetidine. *N. Engl. J. Med.,* 297:1427–1430.

29. Feldman, M., Richardson, C. T., Taylor, I. L., and Walsh, J. H. (1979): Effect of atropine on vagal release of gastrin and pancreatic polypeptide. *J. Clin. Invest.,* 63:294–298.

30. Feldman, M., and Walsh, J. H. (1980): Acid inhibition of sham feeding-stimulated gastrin release and gastric acid secretion: Effect of atropine. *Gastroenterology,* 78:722–776.

31. Feldman, M., Walsh, J. H., and Wong, H. C. (1978): Role of gastrin heptadecapeptide in the acid secretory response to amino acids in man. *J. Clin. Invest.,* 61:308–313.

32. Fordtran, J. S., and Walsh, J. H. (1973): Gastric acid secretion rate and buffer content of the stomach after eating. Results in normal subjects and in patients with duodenal ulcer. *J. Clin. Invest.,* 52:645–657.

33. Fujimoto, S., Kimoto, K., Yamashita, S., Kawai, K., Hattori, T., and Fujita, S. (1980): Tritiated thymidine autoradiographic study on origin and renewal of gastrin cells in antral area of hamsters. *Gastroenterology (in press).*

34. Gregory, R. A. (1980): A review of some recent developments in the chemistry of the gastrins. *Bioorgan. Chem. (in press).*

35. Gregory, R. A., Tracy, H. J., Harris, J. I., and Runswick, M. J. (1979): Minigastrin: Corrected structure and synthesis. *Hoppe-Seyler's Z. Physiol. Chem.,* 360:73–80.

36. Greider, M. H., Steinberg, V., and McGuigan, J. E. (1972): Electron microscopic identification of the gastrin cell of the human antral mucosa by means of immunocytochemistry. *Gastroenterology,* 63:572–582.

37. Harty, R. F., Van der Vijver, J. C., and McGuigan, J. E. (1977): Stimulation of gastrin secretion and synthesis in antral organ culture. *J. Clin. Invest.,* 60:51–60.

38. Hirschowitz, B. I., and Gibson, R. G. (1978): Cholinergic stimulation and suppression of gastrin release in gastric fistula dogs. *Am. J. Physiol.,* 235(6):E720–E725.

39. Hirschowitz, B. I., and Gibson, R. G. (1979): Augmented vagal release of antral gastrin by 2-deoxyglucose after fundic vagotomy in dogs. *Am. J. Physiol.,* 236(2):E173–E179.

40. Holmquist, A. L., Dockray, G. J., Rosenquist, G. L., and Walsh, J. H. (1979): Immunochemical characterization of cholecystokinin-like peptides in lamprey gut and brain. *Gen. Comp. Endocrinol.* 37:474–481.

41. Hsu, W. H., and Cooper, C. W. (1977): Serum gastrin in the rat: Cholinergic and adrenergic effects (39680). *Proc. Soc. Exp. Biol. Med.,* 154:401–406.

42. Impicciatore, M., Walsh, J. H., and Grossman, M. I. (1977): Low doses of atropine enhance serum gastrin response to food in dogs. *Gastroenterology,* 72:995–996.

43. Isenberg, J. I., Walsh, J. H., and Grossman, M. I. (1973): Zollinger-Ellison syndrome. *Gastroenterology,* 65:140–165.

44. Jarhult, J., and Uvnas-Wallensten, K. (1979): Reflex adrenergic gastrin relase evoked by unloading of carotid baroreceptors in cats. *Scand. J. Gastroenterol.* 14:107–109.

45. Jensen, D. M., McCallum, R., and Walsh, J. H. (1978): Failure of atropine to inhibit gastrin-17 stimulation of the lower esophageal sphincter in man. *Gastroenterology,* 75:825–827.

46. Johnson, L. R. (1976): The trophic action of gastrointestinal hormones. *Gastroenterology,* 70:278–288.

47. Johnson, L. R. (1977): New aspects of the trophic action of gastrointestinal hormones. *Gastroenterology,* 72:788–792.

48. Kauffman, G. L., and Grossman, M. I. (1979): Serum gastrin during intestinal phase of acid secretion in dogs. *Gastroenterology,* 77:26–30.

49. Konturek, S. J., Biernat, J., Oleksy, J., Rehfeld, J. F., and Stadil, F. (1974): Effect of atropine on gastrin and gastric acid response to peptone meal. *J. Clin. Invest.,* 54:593–597.

50. Kronborg, O., Pedersen, T., Stadil, F., and Rehfeld, J. F. (1974): The effect of beta-adrenergic blockade upon gastric acid secretion and gastrin secretion during hypoglycaemia before and after vagotomy. *Scand. J. Gastroenterol.,* 9:173–176.

51. Lai, K. S. (1964): Studies on gastrin. *Gut,* 5:327–333.

52. Lai, K. S. (1964): Part II. Quantitative study of the distribution of gastrin-like activity along the gut. *Gut,* 5:334–336.

53. Lam, S. K., Isenberg, J. I., Grossman, M. I., Lane, W. H., and Walsh, J. H. (1980): Gastric acid secretion is abnormally sensitive to endogenous gastrin released after peptone test meals in duodenal ulcer patients. *J. Clin. Invest.,* 65:555–562.

54. Lam, S. K., and Lai, C. L. (1976): Inhibition of sulpiride on the cephalic phase of gastric acid and gastrin secretion in duodenal ulcer patients. *Scand. J. Gastroenterol.* 11:27–31.

55. Larsson, L.-I., Hakanson, R., Sjoberg, N.-O., and Sundler, F. (1975): Fluorescence histochemistry of the gastrin cell in fetal and adult man. *Gastroenterology,* 68:1152–1159.

56. Larsson, L.-I., and Rehfeld, J. F. (1977): Characterization of antral gastrin cells with region-specific antisera. *J. Histochem. Cytochem.,* 25:1317–1321.

57. Larsson, L.-I., Rehfeld, J. F., and Goltermann, N. (1977): Gastrin in the human fetus. Distribution and molecular forms of gastrin in the antro-pyloric gland area, duodenum and pancreas. *Scand. J. Gastroenterol.,* 12:869–872.

58. Larsson, L.-I., Rehfeld, J. F., Sundler, F., and Hakanson, R. (1976): Pancreatic gastrin in foetal and neonatal rats. *Nature,* 262:609–610.

59. Lehy, T., and Willems, G. (1976): Population kinetics of antral gastrin cells in the mouse. *Gastroenterology,* 71:614–619.

60. Levant, J. A., Walsh, J. H., and Isenberg, J. I. (1973): Stimulation of gastric secretion and gastrin release by single oral doses of calcium carbonate in man. *N. Engl. J. Med.,* 289:555–558.

61. Lewin, M., Soumarmo, A., Bali, J. P., Bonfils, S., Girma, J. P., Morgat, J. L., and Fromageot, P. (1976): Interaction of ^{3}H-labelled synthetic human gastrin I with rat gastric plasma membranes. Evidence for the existence of biologically reactive gastrin receptor sites. *FEBS Lett.,* 66:168–172.

62. Lichtenberger, L. M., Lechago, J., and Johnson, L. R. (1975): Depression of antral and serum gastrin concentration by food deprivation in the rat. *Gastroenterology,* 68:1473–1479.

63. Lichtenberger, L. M., Shorey, J. M., and Trier, J. S. (1978): Organ culture studies of rat antrum: evidence for an antral inhibitor of gastrin release. *Am. J. Physiol.,* 235(4):E410–E415.

64. Lin, T.-M., Southard, G. L., and Spray, G. F. (1976): Stimulation of gastric acid secretion in the dog by the C-terminal penta-, tetra-, and tripeptides of gastrin and their O-methyl esters. *Gastroenterology,* 70:733–736.

65. Llanos, O. L., Villar, H. V., Konturek, S. J., Rayford, P. L., and Thompson, J. C. (1977): Release of antral and duodenal gastrin in response to an intestinal meal. *Ann. Surg.* 186:614–618.

66. Loveridge, N., Bloom, S. R., Welbourn, R. B., and Chayen, J. (1974): Quantitative cytochemical estimation of the effect of pentagastrin (0.005-5 pg/ml) and of plasma gastrin on the guinea pig fundus *in vitro*. *Clin. Endocrinol.,* 3:389–396.

67. McCallum, R. W., and Walsh, J. H. (1979): Relationship between lower esophageal sphincter pressure and serum gastrin concentration in Zollinger-Ellison syndrome and other clinical settings. *Gastroenterology,* 76:76–81.

68. McGuigan, J. E. (1968): Gastric mucosal intracellular localization of gastrin by immunofluorescence. *Gastroenterology,* 55:315–327.

69. McGuigan, J. E., Isaza, J., and Landor, J. H. (1971): Relationships of gastrin dose, serum gastrin, and acid secretion. *Gastroenterology,* 61:659–666.

70. McGuigan, J. E., and Thomas, H. F. (1972): Physiological and immunological studies with desamidogastrin. *Gastroenterology,* 62:553-557.

71. Moore, J. G., and Wolfe, M. (1974): Circadian plasma gastrin patterns in feeding and fasting man. *Digestion,* 11:226-231.

72. Morgan, K. G., Schmalz, P. F., Go, V. L. W., and Szurszewski, J. H. (1978): Effects of pentagastrin, G_{17}, and G_{34} on the electrical and mechanical activities of canine antral smooth muscle. *Gastroenterology,* 75:405-412.

73. Morley, J. S., Tracy, H. J., and Gregory, R. A. (1965): Structure-function relationships in the active C-terminal tetrapeptide sequence of gastrin. *Nature,* 207:1356-1359.

74. Nilsson, G., and Brodin, K. (1979): Studies on duodenal gastrin concentrations in dogs following antrectomy and total gastrectomy. *Scand. J. Gastroenterol., [Suppl. 54],* 14:84.

75. Nilsson, G., Simon, J., Yalow, R. S., and Berson, S. A. (1972): Plasma gastrin and gastric acid responses to sham feeding and feeding in dogs. *Gastroenterology,* 63:51-59.

76. Nilsson, G., Yalow, R. S., and Berson, S. A. (1973): Distribution of gastrin in the gastrointestinal tract in human, dog, cat and hog. In: *Frontiers in Gastrointestinal Hormone Research.* Proceedings of the 16th Nobel Symposium held July 20-21, 1973, in Stockholm, Sweden, edited by S. Andersson, pp. 95-101.

77. Noyes, B. E., Mevarech, M., Stein, R., and Agarwal, K. L. (1979): Detection and partial sequence analysis of gastrin mRNA by using an oligodeoxynucleotide probe. *Proc. Natl. Acad. Sci. USA,* 76:1770-1774.

78. Rehfeld, J. F. (1978): Localisation of gastrins to neuro- and adenohypophysis. *Nature,* 271:771-773.

79. Rehfeld, J. F., and Kruse-Larsen, C. (1978): Gastrin and cholecystokinin in hyman cerebrospinal fluid. Immunochemical determination of concentrations and molecular heterogeneity. *Brain Res.,* 155:19-26.

80. Rehfeld, J. F., Larsson, L.-I., Goltermann, N. R., Schwartz, T. W., Holst, J. J., Jensen, S. L., and Morley, J. S. (1980): Neural regulation of pancreatic hormone secretion by the C-terminal tetrapeptide of CCK. *Nature,* 284:33-38.

81. Rehfeld, J. F., Schwartz, T. W., and Stadil, F. (1977): Immunochemical studies on macromolecular gastrins: Evidence that "big big gastrins" are artifacts in blood and mucosa, but truly present in some large gastrinomas. *Gastroenterology,* 73:469-477.

82. Rehfeld, J. F., and Stadil, F. (1973): The effect of gastrin on basal- and glucose-stimulated insulin secretion in man. *J. Clin. Invest.,* 52:1415-1426.

83. Rehfeld, J. F., Stadil, F., and Rubin, B. (1972): Production and evaluation of antibodies for the radioimmunoassay of gastrin. *Scand. J. Clin. Lab. Invest.,* 30:221-232.

84. Rehfeld, J. F., Stadil, F., and Vikelsoe, J. (1974): Immunoreactive gastrin components in human serum. *Gut,* 15:102-111.

85. Richardson, C. T., Walsh, J. H., Hicks, M. I., and Fordtran, J. S. (1976): Studies on the mechanisms of food-stimulated gastric acid secretion in normal human subjects. *J. Clin. Invest.,* 58:623-631.

86. Rosenquist, G. L., and Walsh, J. H. (1980): Radioimmunoassay of gastrin. In: *Gastrointestinal Hormones,* edited by G. B. Jerzy Glass, pp. 769-795. Raven Press, New York.

87. Sakagami, M., Shimizu, F., Mochizuki, T., Kubota, M., Mihara, S., Sato, H., Yanaihara, C., and Yanaihara, N. (1978): Syntheses of human gastrin-related peptides and their biological activities. *Peptide Chem.* pp. 177-182.

88. Schafmayer, A., Teichmann, R. K., Swierczek, J. S., Rayford, P. L., and Thompson, J. C. (1978): Influence of vagus on mechanisms for stimulation and inhibition of gastrin release. *Surgery,* 83:711-715.

89. Schiller, L. R., Walsh, J. H., and Feldman, M. (1980): Distention-induced gastrin release in man: Effects of luminal acidification and intravenous atropine. *Gastroenterology,* 78:912-917.

90. Soares, E. C., Zaterka, S., and Walsh, J. (1977): Acid secretion and serum gastrin at graded intragastric pressures in man. *Gastroenterology,* 72:676-679.

91. Soll, A. H. (1978): The actions of secretagogues on oxygen up-take by isolated mammal parietal cells. *J. Clin. Invest.,* 61:370-380.

92. Soll, A. H. (1978): The interaction of histamine with gastrin and carbamylcholine on oxygen uptake by isolated mammal parietal cells. *J. Clin. Invest.* 61:381-389.

93. Soll, A. H., and Grossman, M. I. (1980): Receptors and interactions modulating the function of isolated canine parietal cells. (*in press*).

94. Soll, A. H., and Walsh, J. H. (1979): Regulation of gastric acid secretion. *Annu. Rev. Physiol.,* 41:35-53.

95. Soumarmon, A., Cheret, A. M., and Lewin, M. J. M. (1977): Localization of gastrin receptors in intact isolated and separated rat fundic cells. *Gastroenterology,* 73:900-903.

96. Stadil, F., and Rehfeld, J. F. (1973): Release of gastrin by epinephrine in man. *Gastroenterology,* 65:210-215.

97. Stanley, M. D., Coalson, R. E., Grossman, M. I., and Johnson, L. R. (1972): Influence of secretin and pentagastrin on acid secretion and parietal cell number in rats. *Gastroenterology,* 63:264-269.

98. Stern, D. H., and Walsh, J. H. (1973): Gastrin release in postoperative ulcer patients; evidence for release of duodenal gastrin. *Gastroenterology,* 64:363-369.

99. Straus, E., and Yalow, R. S. (1974): Studies on the distribution and degradation of heptadecapeptide, big, and big big gastrin. *Gastroenterology,* 66:936-943.

100. Strunz, U. T., Code, C. F., and Grossman, M. I. (1979): Effect of gastrin on electrical activity of antrum and duodenum of dogs. *Proc. Soc. Exp. Biol. Med.,* 161:25-27.

101. Strunz, U. T., Thompson, M. R., Elashoff, J., and Grossman, M. I. (1978): Hepatic inactivation of gastrins of various chain lengths in dogs. *Gastroenterology,* 74:550-553.

102. Strunz, U. T., Walsh, J. H., and Grossman, M. I. (1978): Removal of gastrin by various organs in dogs. *Gastroenterology,* 74:32-33.

103. Sturdevant, R. A. L. (1974): Is gastrin the major regulator of lower esophageal sphincter pressure? *Gastroenterology,* 67:551-553.

104. Szurszewski, J. H. (1975): Mechanism of action of pentagastrin and acetylcholine on the longitudinal muscle of the canine antrum. *J. Physiol.,* 252:335-361.

105. Takeuchi, K., Speir, G. R., and Johnson, L. R. (1979): Mucosal gastrin receptor. I. Assay standardization and fulfillment of receptor criteria. *Am. J. Physiol.,* 237(3):E284-E294.

106. Takeuchi, K., Speir, G. R., and Johnson, L. R. (1979): Mucosal gastrin receptor. II. Physical characteristics of binding. *Am. J. Physiol.,* 237(3):E295-E300.

107. Taylor, I. L., Dockray, G. J., Calam, J., and Walker, R. J. (1979): Big and little gastrin responses to food in normal and ulcer subjects. *Gut,* 20:957-962.

108. Taylor, I. L., Walsh, J. H., Carter, D., Wood, J., and Grossman, M. I. (1979): Effects of atropine and bethanechol on bombesin-stimulated release of pancreatic polypeptide and gastrin in dog. *Gastroenterology,* 77:714-718.

109. Tepperman, B. L., Walsh, J. H., and Preshaw, R. M. (1972): Effect of antral denervation on gastrin release by sham feeding and insulin hypoglycemia in dogs. *Gastroenterology,* 63:973-980.

110. Track, N. S., Creutzfeldt, C., Litzenberger, J., Neuhoff, C., Arnold, R., and Creutzfeldt, W. (1979): Appearance of gastrin and somatostatin in the human fetal stomach, duodenum and pancreas. *Digestion,* 19:292-306.

111. Uvnas-Wallensten, K., Lundberg, J. M., and Efendic, S. (1978): Dopaminergic control of antral gastrin and somatostatin release. *Acta Physiol. Scand.* 103:343-345.

112. Uvnas-Wallensten, K., Rehfeld, J. F., Larsson, L.-I., and Uvnas, B. (1977): Heptadecapeptide gastrin in the vagal nerve. *Proc. Natl. Acad. Sci. USA,* 74:5707-5710.

113. Vaillant, C., Dockray, G., and Hopkins, C. R. (1979): Cellular origins of different froms of gastrin. The specific immunocytochemical localization of related peptides. *J. Histochem. Cytochem.* 27:932-935.

114. Valenzuela, J. E., Walsh, J. H., and Isenberg, J. I. (1976): Effect of gastrin on pancreatic enzyme secretion and gallbladder emptying in man. *Gastroenterology,* 71:409-411.

115. Valenzuela, J. E., Bugat, R., and Grossman, M. I. (1978): Effect of big and little gastrins on pancreatic and gastric secretion (40322). *Proc. Soc. Exp. Biol. Med.,* 159:237–238.
116. Vigna, S. R., and Gorbman, A. (1977): Effects of cholecystokinin, gastrin, and related peptides on coho salmon gallbladder contraction *in vitro. Am. J. Physiol.,* 232(5): E485–E491.
117. Villar, H. V., Reeder, D. D., Rayford, P. L., and Thompson, J. C. (1977): Rate of disappearance of circulating endogenous gastrin in dogs. *Surgery,* 81:404–408.
118. Vizi, E. S., Bertaccini, G., Impicciatore, M., Mantovani, P., Zseli, J., and Knoll, J. (1974): Structure-activity relationship of some analogues of gastrin and cholecystokinin on intestinal smooth muscle of the guinea-pig. *Naunyn-Schmiedeberg's Arch. Pharmacol.,* 284:233–243.
119. Walsh, J. H., Debas, H. T., and Grossman, M. I. (1974): Pure human big gastrin. Immunochemical properties, disappearance half time, and acid-stimulating action in dogs. *J. Clin. Invest.* 54:477–485.
120. Walsh, J. H., and Grossman, M. I. (1975): Medical progress: Gastrin. *N. Engl. J. Med.,* 292:1324–1332.
121. Walsh, J. H., Isenberg, J. I., Ansfield, J., and Maxwell, V. (1976): Clearance and acid-stimulating action of human big and little gastrins in duodenal ulcer subjects. *J. Clin. Invest.,* 57:1125–1131.
122. Walsh, J. H., and Laster, L. (1973): Enzymatic deamidation of the C-terminal tetrapeptide amide of gastrin by mammalian tissues. *Biochem. Med.,* 8:432–449.
123. Walsh, J. H., Richardson, C. T., and Fordtran, J. S. (1975): pH dependence of acid secretion and gastrin release in normal and ulcer patients. *J. Clin. Invest.,* 55:462–469.
124. Walsh, J. H., Yalow, R. S., and Berson, S. A. (1971): The effect of atropine on plasma gastrin response to feeding. *Gastroenterology,* 60:16–21.
125. Watson, L. C., Reeder, D. D., and Thompson, J. C. (1974): Hydrocortisone administration and gastrin and gastric secretion in dogs. *Arch. Surg.* 109:547–549.
126. Yalow, R. S., and Berson, S. A. (1970): Size and charge distinctions between endogenous human plasma gastrin in peripheral blood and heptadecapeptide gastrins. *Gastroenterology,* 58:609–615.
127. Yalow, R. S., and Wu, N. (1973): Additional studies on the nature of big big gastrin. *Gastroenterology,* 65:19–27.

CHOLECYSTOKININ

Structure

Cholecystokinin (CCK) and pancreozymin, originally thought to be separate substances, were identified as a single peptide with both gallbladder contracting and pancreatic enzyme secretagogue properties by Mutt and Jorpes (63). This material commonly is called simply cholecystokinin because the gallbladder-stimulating effect was described first. CCK isolated from hog intestine contains 33 amino acid residues, of which the carboxyl terminal pentapeptide amide sequence is identical with that of gastrin (Table 1) (64). In the seventh position from the C-terminus there is a tyrosine O-sulfate residue. A variant form of CCK consisting of 39 amino acid residues also has been isolated from hog intestine. This peptide (CCK39) contains the sequence of cholecystokinin (CCK33) plus an amino terminal hexapeptide extension. The amino terminal group of CCK39 is nonsulfated tyrosine (62). Evidence was obtained for the presence of large amounts of a peptide resembling the C-terminal octapeptide of CCK (CCK8) in brain (13, 61), and this material was purified and found to be identical with CCK8 (17). An enzymatic activity was shown in brain extracts that converted CCK33 to a CCK8-like peptide (86). Immunoreactive material similar to CCK8 has been identified in the small intestine (13), but it is not yet known if the structure is identical to CCK8. Frog skin contains cerulein, a decapeptide with structure and properties very similar to CCK8 (14–16). The gut and brain of the primative vertebrate the lamprey also contain peptides similar immunochemically and in size to CCK8 and cerulein (33).

Recently evidence has been presented that gut tissue also contains a smaller peptide that corresponds immunochemically and by chromatographic elution pattern to the C-terminal tetrapeptide common to gastrin and CCK (50,72). Similar material was found in brain (49). These observations have not yet been confirmed by chemical analysis.

Biological Actions

Pancreatic Secretion

Exogenous CCK is a strong stimulant of pancreatic enzyme secretion *in vivo* but a relatively weak stimulant of water and bicarbonate secretion. When combined with a low dose of secretin, CCK produces marked enhancement of the bicarbonate response in humans (95), dog (57), and cat (43). Similarly, secretin augments pancreatic protein stimulation by CCK. Considerable information regarding the mechanism of action of CCK on the pancreas has been obtained by studies with isolated pancreatic acini and acinar cells. This work has been summarized recently (24). There appear to be two major classes of stimulants of acinar cells. One group causes outflux of cellular calcium and stimulation of cGMP and includes CCK, gastrin, bombesin, substance P, and acetylcholine. The second class causes stimulation of cellular cAMP and includes secretin, VIP, and cholera toxin. Combination of an agent from the first class with an agent from the second class usually causes responses greater than the sum of responses to either agent given alone and may cause maximal responses greater than the maximal responses to either of the individual agents. CCK and cholinergic agents also have been shown to increase the uptake of glucose analogues into isolated mouse pancreatic acini, and this effect appeared to be related to mobilization of cellular calcium (47). Although no peptides have been shown to cause competitive antagonism of CCK action *in vitro,* butyryl derivatives of cGMP and especially dibutyryl cGMP were shown to have the properties of competitive antagonism of CCK action on dispersed guinea pig acini (65) while other cGMP and cAMP analogues had no such effects.

An analogue of the C-terminal pentapeptide of CCK has been prepared with a photoreactive side chain at the amino terminus (23). This compound produced stimulation of acinar enzyme secretion *in vitro* and caused irreversible stimulation of secretion after photolysis in the presence of pancreatic lobules. Use of similar probes may permit direct demonstration of CCK receptors on pancreatic acinar membranes. Direct interaction of ^{125}I-labeled CCK to dispersed acini from guinea pig pancreas has been demonstrated. The binding site was found to be specific for CCK and gastrin peptides, and there was good correlation between occupation of receptor sites and acinar cell function (37).

Biliary Smooth Muscle

CCK peptides are potent stimulants of gallbladder contraction and of relaxation of the sphincter of Oddi (52). *In vitro,* CCK8 was 10 times more potent than CCK33 and 1,800 times more potent than pentagastrin on gallbladder contraction, and the effects of these peptides were not antagonized by atropine or other nerve blockers, suggesting a direct effect on gallbladder muscle (98). More recently, evidence was obtained that blockade of H2 histamine receptors in gallbladder augmented the response to CCK (93).

Other Gastrointestinal Smooth Muscle

CCK causes relaxation of the human lower esophageal sphincter (LES) (73) and has been shown to antagonize the contracting action of gastrin *in vitro* (20). Tetrodotoxin antagonized the inhibitory effects of CCK in cats and produced contraction responses to CCK similar to those obtained with gastrin, suggesting that CCK8 stimulates postganglionic inhibitory neurons which mask direct stimulatory action on the LES (2).

CCK is more potent than gastrin as an inhibitor of gastric emptying of liquids, and significant inhibition is obtained in dogs at doses that are submaximal for stimulation of pancreatic secretion, suggesting that this effect is physiological (10). *In vitro* studies with canine antral smooth muscle suggested that gastrin and CCK act directly on the same muscle receptor rather than through a neural intermediate (19). CCK39, CCK33, and CCK8 all increase contractions and amplitude of action potentials in canine antral circular muscle (59).

CCK analogues markedly increase transit of contrast material through the human small intestine (3,51). CCK causes disruption of the fasting pattern of myoelectric activity in canine intestine, but the stimulation of spike potentials seen is not identical to the pattern that occurs after a meal (60). CCK8 produced contraction of circular muscle and relaxation of longitudinal muscle of dog small intestine that were antagonized by atropine,

tetrodotoxin, and depolarizing concentrations of nicotine, suggesting that CCK8 interacts with a non-nicotinic receptor on postganglionic cholinergic neural elements in intestine (85).

CCK increased the frequency of electrical spike potentials in human colon *in vitro* (84), and *in vitro* muscle contractions of human taenia coli strips during stimulation by CCK8 or CCK were unaffected by atropine or glucagon (18).

Thus CCK has a wide spectrum of actions on intestinal smooth muscle, acting both directly and by neural intermediates.

Other Gut Secretions

CCK peptides cause inhibition of gastric acid secretion and have been considered as possible "enterogastrones." Konturek et al. (42,46) showed that vagal innervation was important for full inhibitory activity against pentagastrin-stimulated secretion in dogs (42, 46). In a recent study, 99% pure CCK33 was found to be only a weak stimulant of gastric secretion and a weak antagonist of gastrin-stimulated acid secretion in humans and dogs (9). The doses required for inhibition were too high to suggest a likely physiological role. Larger effects found earlier with less pure CCK preparations may have been due to contamination with GIP or other peptide contaminants.

CCK infusions have been reported to cause release of a soluble form of enteropeptidase in the intestinal lumen (29).

Trophic Effects on Pancreas

Repeated injections of CCK analogues, especially when combined with secretin, cause marked increases in pancreatic weight, and in DNA, RNA, and protein content in the rat (21,66) accompanied by increased enzyme secretion and trypsin content but without increased lipase content. Repeated injections of CCK caused increased pancreatic insulin and glucagon content (22), and CCK plus secretin injections caused increased somatostatin content (97).

Effects on Satiety

CCK has been proposed as a major mediator of the satiety response that leads to cessation of feeding when food is placed in the stomach or intestine. Gastric administration of phenylalanine and intravenous CCK cause reductions in meal size in monkeys and in sham feeding in rats (25). In humans, either stimulation or inhibition of food intake was observed depending on the dose and duration of administration of exogenous CCK (90). Since CCK is found in the brain and CSF and does not easily cross the blood-brain barrier, it is possible that CCK of central origin might have a role in regulation of food intake. Recently it was reported that injection of picomolar amounts of CCK8 into cerebral ventricles of sheep suppressed feeding (12). Straus and Yalow (89) reported that CCK content in the brains of genetically obese mice was lower than in nonobese littermates and hypothesized a causal relation in production of obesity. Schneider et al. (80a), however, could not demonstrate differences in brain CCK content in similar obese and nonobese strains. The role of CCK in regulation of food intake remains unclear.

Miscellaneous Effects

Stimulation of bile flow in dogs by CCK33 and CCK8 after cholecystectomy has been shown to be independent of clearance of erythritol and probably due to stimulation of a non-bile, salt-dependent ductular mechanism (81).

Effects of CCK on arterial blood flow in various organs in the dog have been determined during intra-arterial injection. Results indicated maximal effects on arterial blood flow to upper small intestine and liver, suggesting that vasodilatation might be a physiologic effect of CCK (8,74). Small doses of CCK8 and histamine produced arteriolar dilatation in the gastric submucosal circulation (30).

Stimulation of release of somatostatin from isolated perfused canine pancreas was reported (36) during CCK infusion, and marked stimulation of trout calcitonin secretion *in vitro* occurred in response to combinations of secretin and CCK8 or gastrin (76).

Some of the biological effects of CCK are summarized in Table 4.

Structure-Activity Relationships

Sulfation of the tyrosine residue in CCK33 and shorter CCK peptides such as CCK8 and cerulein has been shown to be essential for most biological systems to maintain full potency. Major differences in potency have been observed when sulfated and desulfated forms of CCK8 and cerulein were used for stimulation of gallbladder contraction or pancreatic enzyme secretion (39). CCK peptides are only partial agonists of acid secretion in humans and dog but are full agonists in the cat (94) and rat. Sulfated gastrin was reported to be more potent than nonsulfated gastrin as a stimulant of gallbladder contraction (1), and sulfated forms of both gastrin and CCK were more potent than the nonsulfated counterparts as stimulants of coho salmon gallbladder contraction (92). When the C-terminal four to eight amino acid fragments of CCK were compared for effects on bile flow and gastric secretion in dogs, it was

TABLE 4. *Some biological effects of CCK*

Gastrointestinal secretion
Stimulates pancreatic enzyme secretion
Increases acinar cell calcium outflux
Some stimulation of pancreatic volume and bicarbonate (rat)
Pancreatic stimulation inhibited by dibutyryl cGMP
Moderate or weak stimulant of gastric acid secretion
Competitive antagonist of gastrin-stimulated acid (dog, humans)
Causes hypertrophy and hyperplasia of pancreas
Increases intestinal lymph flow
Possibly releases intestinal peptidases

Gastrointestinal motility
Causes gallbladder contraction
Relaxes sphincter of Oddi
Decreases gastric emptying rate
Increases antral smooth muscle contraction
Possibly relaxes fundic smooth muscle
Decreases lower esophageal sphincter pressure
Possibly stimulates contraction of esophageal body
Increases small intestine motility and shortens transit time
Increases colonic motility

Hormone release
Enhances insulin release
Increases pancreatic somatostatin output
Increases pancreatic polypeptide release
Increases GIP release
Releases calcitonin, potentiated by secretin

Food intake
Increases or decreases when given intravenously
Decreases when given centrally (cerebral ventricle)

found that the sulfated hepta- and octapeptides had a high selective potency on bile flow whereas there was no effect of sulfation on acid secretion (41). Analogues of CCK heptapeptide have been synthesized and examined for biological activity. Substitution of serine for tyrosine resulted in a major loss of potency; the sulfated analogue was only slightly more potent than the nonsulfated form. The t-Boc protected CCK heptapeptide was slightly more potent than the unprotected peptide (5). Further modification of CCK heptapeptide by substitution of epsilonhydroxynorleucine O-sulfate for tyrosine O-sulfate resulted in a peptide that was much more potent than the serine O-sulfate compound and only slightly less potent than the unaltered heptapeptide, indicating that the distance of the sulfate ester group from the peptide backbone has a major influence on biological activity of CCK (4). Of the two methionine residues present in CCK8, the one nearest the C-terminus appears more essential for full biological activity (26). Synthetic nonsulfated CCK33 had only 1/250 the potency of natural CCK33 as a stimulant of amylase release from rat pancreas (96). Calculation of the tyrosine-tryptophan distance in CCK heptapeptide provided evidence for some type of folded conformation in this region of the CCK molecule (78). The CCK8-like material extractable from human brain at autopsy was shown to have properties similar to CCK8 (75).

Distribution

Cellular Localization

CCK-containing cells have been identified by immunohistochemical methods in the mucosa of the mammalian duodenum and jejunum (7,69), and further ultrastructural studies revealed that this cell was identical to the intestinal I cell in the human intestine (6). Larsson and Rehfeld (48,50) have reported evidence for a third type of endocrine cell, distinct from gastrin and CCK cells, that appears to contain gastrin CCK tetrapeptide. This cell was identified in gastric antrum as well as in mucosa of the entire small intestine including the ileum. The distribution of CCK peptides in the brain also has been determined by immunohistochemistry. Straus et al. (87) reported staining of cell bodies throughout the cortical gray matter and diffusely in the subcortical white matter with an antibody to CCK8. Innis et al. (35) found extensive distribution of CCK cell bodies and nerve fibers in the rat cerebral cortex, but the densest collections of cells occurred in periaqueductal gray and the dorsomedial hypothalamus. Larsson and Rehfeld (49) reported the occurrence of numerous CCK nerves in guinea pig neocortex, hippocampus, amygdala, hypothalamus, and spinal cord. Evidence has been obtained that immunoreactive CCK is copurified with synaptic vesicles in the rat cerebral cortex (67).

Immunochemical Distribution

Rehfeld (70) reported the distribution of immunoreactive gastrin and CCK in the gut and brain of hog and humans. CCK immunoreactivity was present diffusely throughout the telencephalon and in the thalamus and hypothalamus, whereas gastrin immunoreactivity was found in the posterior pituitary of the hog. Most of the immunoreactive CCK resembled CCK8. Large amounts of CCK immunoreactivity were found in hog and human duodenum and jejunum. Gel filtration revealed peaks corresponding to CCK33 and CCK8 as well as other peaks larger than CCK33, between CCK33 and CCK8 and smaller than CCK8. Similar findings were also reported by Dockray (13). Avian brain and gut also contain substances resembling CCK8 (14), as does the lamprey intestine (33). Different molecular forms of both gastrin and CCK were identified in human cerebrospinal fluid (71) with mean total immunoreactive concentrations of 3.4 and 14 pM, respectively.

Measurement

Radioimmunoassay

Development of sensitive and specific radioimmunoassays for CCK has been more difficult than for several other gut peptides. Preparation of suitable immunoreactive radioiodinated CCK has been a problem in several laboratories. Rehfeld (70) reported that oxidation with small amounts of chloramine T or lactoperoxidase resulted in major losses in immunoreactivity, confirming similar observations made previously that oxidation destroyed biological activity, but he was able to prepare suitable tracer by conjugation with ^{125}I-hydroxyphenyl-propionic acid-succinimide ester. This tracer was used to characterize a series of antibodies raised against CCK33 or gastrin, and evidence was obtained for at least four different patterns of specificity for regions of the CCK molecule. Others have labeled 99% pure CCK33 (28,91) or have utilized CCK39 in order to label the free amino terminal tyrosine residue (79). Two major types of antibody specificity problems have been found. On one hand, antibodies directed at the C-terminal region of CCK often have a high degree of cross-reactivity with gastrin because of the identical C-terminal pentapeptide sequence in the two peptides. On the other hand, antibodies directed against midportion or N-terminal antigenic determinants in porcine CCK often are species specific and detect porcine but not human (28) or canine or monkey CCK (88). An additional potential problem with amino terminal antisera is failure to measure small, biologically active C-terminal fragments of CCK such as CCK8, which is a major form present in gut extracts and is the predominant form present in the brain. Since multiple molecular forms of CCK are present in tissues, it is highly possible that multiple forms also are present in the circulation. Estimates of fasting and food-stimulated CCK concentrations in humans have ranged widely in different assay systems. Schlegel et al. (79,80) reported an increase from 222 to 480 pg/ml in extracted plasma samples. Thompson et al. (91) found increases from about 700 to about 1,200 pg/ml after ingestion of a high-carbohydrate, high-protein meal. Harvey et al. (31) reported increases from basal of 26 pg/ml to more than 8,000 pg/ml after ingestion of one pint of milk. Boiling of serum samples prior to assay was found to increase reproducibility (32).

Half-life of CCK in humans was estimated as approximately 5 to 7 min (31) in one study, whereas another study obtained half-life estimates of about 2.5 min in both humans and dog (91).

Bioassay

The basic unit for biological measurement of CCK is the Ivy dog unit, defined as the amount of material that produces optimal contraction of the canine gallbladder after rapid intravenous injection. The standard method for bioassay of natural CCK is contraction of *in situ* guinea pig gallbladder. Other types of bioassay measurements were reviewed in 1959 (40), and the Ivy unit was considered optimal for dog and humans. It has been shown subsequently that 1 μg of pure porcine CCK33 is roughly equivalent to 3 Ivy dog units (63).

In vitro bioassays have been developed for estimation of CCK activity in human serum. In a modification of an earlier system, Marshall et al. (54) used strips of rabbit gallbladder that were first exposed to normal serum. Responses were compared with standard curves constructed by measurement of contractions induced by addition of graded amounts of CCK. CCK-like activity measured in fasting serum of normal subjects was about 2.4 pmol/ml, and activity approximately doubled after a liquid meal. Aprotinin (Trasylol) decreased the measured activity by 74 to 93%, and extraction with charcoal decreased serum activity to about 0.7 pmol/ml. An earlier bioassay system (38) generated bioassay values that were about threefold higher.

Release of CCK

Most studies of CCK release have involved *in vivo* measurement of pancreatic protein or enzyme secretion and have assumed that the responses obtained were due to circulating CCK (*see* Chapter 32). Fat components appear to be the most potent stimulants of CCK release when introduced into the small intestine. Meyer and Jones (55) found that a fatty acid chain length of nine carbons was the minimum for stimulation, that triglyceride did not stimulate unless subjected to hydrolysis, and the dispersion of fatty acid into micelles by bile acids or by detergents markedly increased stimulating activity. Monolein caused secretion of pancreatic juice similar in composition to that stimulated by CCK, whereas free oleic acid caused secretion of pancreatic juice with higher bicarbonate content than is produced by pure CCK, suggesting that free fatty acids also cause release of secretin or some substance with similar properties. The maximal response to fatty acids was higher pancreatic protein secretion. Meyer found that peptic digestion of albumin markedly increased potency of this protein for stimulation of pancreatic secretion and that undigested albumin was inert. Individual amino acids have been compared in humans and in dog. Go et al. (27) found that only essential amino acids caused stimulation in humans, and of these phenylalanine, methionine, valine, and possibly tryptophan were the most potent. In dog, it was originally reported that many essential and nonessential amino acids stimulated protein secretion, with tryptophan and phenylalanine being the most potent (44). Later studies in dog con-

firmed that phenylalanine and tryptophan were potent stimulants but failed to show release by other amino acids or further augmentation by mixtures of amino acids (56). Evidence has been obtained in dogs that most CCK is released from the proximal half of the small intestine (45). Intraluminal calcium salts may cause release of CCK in man (34), whereas magnesium salts appear to be weak stimulants (53). Chronic consumption of alcohol in dogs did not result in a change in pancreatic response to intraduodenal oleate (77). Release of CCK in humans, as measured by radioimmunoassay, was abolished by intravenous somatostatin (80).

Evidence has accumulated that neural stimulation is an important factor in regulation of pancreatic protein release. It has been known for some time that vagotomy decreases the pancreatic response to endogenous stimulants but not to exogenous CCK (42). This has been taken as evidence that CCK release is dependent on vagal innervation. However, Singer et al. (82) have shown that atropine administration and vagotomy decreased the pancreatic responses to endogenous stimulation of the intact pancreas but had no effect in a transplanted segment of pancreas in the same dogs. Their findings are compatible with the hypothesis that a major part of the pancreatic response to luminal stimulants is mediated by an enteropancreatic cholinergic reflex. Further evidence for such a reflex is offered by the observation that the latency of pancreatic response was shorter with intraduodenal nutrient administration than with intraportal injection of CCK and that both atropine and vagotomy increased the latency period to intraduodenal oleate but not to intraportal CCK (83). A pyloropancreatic reflex for stimulation of exocrine secretion was demonstrated in dogs with innervated pyloric pouches (11). Distension of the pouches with acid caused enzyme secretion without a change in serum gastrin. The stimulation was abolished by atropine or vagotomy. Few of the above observations have been correlated with changes in immunoreactive plasma CCK. In one study it was found that inhibition of pancreatic protein responses to intraduodenal oleate by atropine could not be explained by a decrease in the release of CCK into the circulation (58).

There is little information concerning release of CCK *in vitro*. An increase in CCK immunoreactivity was found when a synaptosome-enriched fraction of rat cerebral cortex was exposed to solutions containing calcium and potassium (68).

Correlation with Physiological Events

Further studies are needed to define the concentrations of various CCK peptides in the circulation during conditions that cause stimulation of pancreatic secretion and gallbladder contraction before firm conclusions can be reached concerning the hormonal nature of this peptide. It is likely from the physiological and pharmacological studies done earlier that small increases in CCK combined with nervous reflex activation and secretin release are sufficient for physiological responses.

Conditions of Excess or Deficiency

No definitive examples of CCK overproduction have been shown. It is possible that decreased pancreatic secretory responses to food in patients with upper intestinal diseases such as celiac disease are due to impaired CCK release.

References

1. Amer, M. S. (1969): Studies with cholecystokinin. II. Cholecystokinetic potency of porcine gastrins I and II and related peptides in three systems. *Endocrinology*, 84:1277.
2. Behar, J., and Biancani, P. (1977): Effect of cholecystokinin-octapeptide on lower esophageal sphincter. *Gastroenterology*, 73(1):57–61.
3. Bertaccini, G., and Agosti, A. (1971): Action of caerulein on intestinal motility in man. *Gastroenterology*, 60:55–63.
4. Bodanszky, M., Martinez, J., Priestley, G. P., Gardner, J. D., and Mutt, V. (1978): Cholecystokinin (pancreozymin). 4. Synthesis and properties of a biologically active analogue of the C-terminal heptapeptide with epsilon-hydroxynorleucine sulfate replacing tyrosine sulfate. *J. Med. Chem.*, 21(10):1030–1035.
5. Bodanszky, M., Natarajan, S., Hahne, W., and Gardner, J. D. (1977): Cholecystokinin (pancreozymin). 3. Synthesis and properties of an analogue of the C-terminal heptapeptide with serine sulfate replacing tyrosine sulfate. *J. Med. Chem.*, 20(8):1047–1050.
6. Buchan, A. M. J., Polak, J. M., Solcia, E., Capella, C., Hudson, D., and Pearse, A. G. E. (1978): Electron immunohistochemical evidence for the human intestinal I cell as the source of CCK. *Gut*, 19:403–407.
7. Buffa, R., Solcia, E., and Go, V. L. W. (1976): Immunohistochemical identification of the cholecystokinin cell in the intestinal mucosa. *Gastroenterology*, 70:528–532.
8. Chou, C. C., Hsieh, C. P., and Dabney, J. M. (1977): Comparison of vascular effects of gastrointestinal hormones on various organs. *Am. J. Physiol.*, 232(2):H103–H109.
9. Corazziari, E., Solomon, T. E., and Grossman, M. I. (1979): Effect of ninety-five percent pure cholecystokinin on gastrin-stimulated acid secretion in man and dog. *Gastroenterology*, 77:91–95.
10. Debas, H. T., Farooq, O., and Grossman, M. I. (1975): Inhibition of gastric emptying is a physiological action of cholecystokinin. *Gastroenterology*, 68:1211–1217.
11. Debas, H. T., and Yamagishi, T. (1978): Evidence for pyloropancreatic reflux for pancreatic exocrine secretion. *Am. J. Physiol.*, 1978, 234(5):E468–E471.
12. Della Fera, M. A., and Baile, C. A. (1979): Cholecystokinin octapeptide: Continuous picomole injections into the cerebral ventricles of sheep suppress feeding. *Science*, 206:471–473.
13. Dockray, G. J. (1977): Immunoreactive component resembling cholecystokinin octapeptide in intestine. *Nature*, 270:357–361.
14. Dockray, G. J. (1979): Cholecystokinin-like peptides in avian brain and gut. *Experientia*, 35:628.
15. Dockray, G. J. (1979): Evolutionary relationships of the gut hormones. *Fed. Proc.*, 38:2295–2301.
16. Dockray, G. J. (1979): Comparative biochemistry and physiology of gut hormones. *Annu. Rev. Physiol.*, 41:83–95.
17. Dockray, G. J., Gregory, R. A., and Hutchison, J. B. (1978): Isolation, structure and biological activity of two cholecystokinin octapeptides from sheep brain. *Nature*, 274:711–713.
18. Egberts, E. H., and Johnson, A. G. (1977): The effect of cholecystokinin on human taenia coli. *Digestion*, 15:217–222.
19. Fara, J. W., Praissman, M., and Berkowitz, J. M. (1979): Interaction between gastrin, CCK, and secretin on canine antral smooth muscle in vitro. *Am. J. Physiol.*, 236(1):E39–E44.
20. Fisher, R. S., DiMarino, A. J., and Cohen, S. (1975): Mechanism of cholecystokinin inhibition of lower esophageal sphincter pressure. *Am. J. Physiol.*, 228:1469–
21. Folsch, U. R., Winckler, K., and Wormsley, K. G. (1978): Influence of repeated administration of cholecystokinin and secretin on the pancreas of the rat. *Scand. J. Gastroenterol.*, 13(6):663–671.
22. Fujita, T., Matsunari, Y., Sato, K., Hayashi, M., and Koga, Y. (1979): Effects of oral administration of trypsin inhibitor and repeated injections of pancreozymin on the insulin and glucagon contents of rat pancreas. *Endocrinol. Jpn.*, 26:35–39.
23. Galardy, R. E., and Jamieson, J. D. (1977): Photoaffinity labeling of a peptide secretagogue receptor in the exocrine pancreas. *Mol. Pharmacol.*, 13:852–863.
24. Gardner, J. D., and Jensen, R. T. (1980): Receptor for secretagogues on pancreatic acinar cells. *Am. J. Physiol.*, 238:63–66.
25. Gibbs, J., and Smith, G. P. (1977): Cholecystokinin and satiety in rats and rhesus monkeys. *Am. J. Clin. Nutr.*, 30:758–761.
26. Gillessen, D., Trzeciak, A., Muller, R. K., and Studer, R. O. (1979): Syntheses and biological activities of methoxinine-analogues of the C-terminal octapeptide of cholecystokinin-pancreozymin. *Int. J. Peptide Protein Res.*, 13:130–136.
27. Go, V. L. W., Hofmann, A. F., and Summerskill, W. H. J. (1970): Pancreozymin bioassay in man based on pancreatic enzyme secretion: potency of specific amino acids and other digestive products. *J. Clin. Invest.*, 49:1558–1564.
28. Go, V. L. W., Ryan, R. J., and Summerskill, W. H. J. (1971): Radioimmunoassay of porcine cholecystokinin-pancreozymin. *J. Lab. Clin. Med.*, 77:684–689.
29. Gotze, H., Gotze, J., and Adelson, J. W. (1978): Studies on intestinal enzyme secretion; The action of cholecystokinin-pancreozymin, pentagastrin and bile. *Res. Exp. Med.*, 173:17–25.
30. Guth, P. H., and Smith, E. (1976): The effect of gastrointestinal hormones on the gastric microcirculation. *Gastroenterology*, 71:435–438.
31. Harvey, R. F., Dowsett, L., Hartog, M., and Read, A. E. (1973): A radioimmunoassay for cholecystokinin-pancreozymin. *Lancet*, 2:826–828.
32. Harvey, R. F., Dowsett, L., Hartog, M., and Read, A. E. (1974): Radioimmunoassay of cholecystokinin-pancreozymin. *Gut*, 15:690–699.
33. Holmquist, A. L., Dockray, G. J., Rosenquist, G. L., and Walsh, J. H. (1979): Immunochemical characterization of cholecystokinin-like peptides in lamprey gut and brain. *Gen. Comp. Endocrinol.*, 37:474–481.
34. Holtermuller, K. H., Malagelada, J. R., McCall, J. T., and Go, V. L. W. (1976): Pancreatic, gallbladder, and gastric responses to intraduodenal calcium perfusion in man. *Gastroenterology*, 70:693–696.
35. Innis, R. B., Correa, F. M. A., Uhl, G. R., Schneider, B., and Snyder, S. H. (1979): Cholecystokinin octapeptide-like immunoreactivity: Histochemical localization in rat brain. *Proc. Natl. Acad. Sci. U.S.A.*, 76:521–525.
36. Ipp, E., Dobbs, R. E., Harris, V., Arimura, A., Vale, W., and Unger, R. H. (1977): The effects of gastrin, gastric inhibitory polypeptide, secretin and the octapeptide of cholecystokinin upon immunoreactive somatostatin release by the perfused canine pancreas. *J. Clin. Invest.*, 60(5):1216–1219.
37. Jensen, R. T., Lemp, G. F., and Gardner, J. D. (1980): Interaction of cholecystokinin with specific membrane receptors on pancreatic acinar cells. *J. Biol. Chem.*, (in press).
38. Johnson, A. G., and McDermott, S. J. (1973): Sensitive bioassay of cholecystokinin in human serum. *Lancet*, 51:589–591.
39. Johnson, L. R., Stening, G. F., and Grossman, M. I. (1970): Effect of sulfation on the gastrointestinal actions of caerulein. *Gastroenterology*, 58:208–216.
40. Jorpes, E., Mutt, V., and Olbe, L. (1959): On the biological assay of cholecystokinin and its dosage in cholecystography. *Acta Physiol. Scand.*, 47:109–114.
41. Kaminski, D. L., Ruwart, M. J., and Jellinek, M. (1977):

Structure-function relationships of peptide fragments of gastrin and cholecystokinin. *Am. J. Physiol.*, 233(4):E286–E292.

42. Konturek, S. J., Radecki, T., Biernat, J., and Thor, P. (1972): Effect of vagotomy on pancreatic secretion evoked by endogenous and exogenous cholecystokinin and caerulein. *Gastroenterology*, 63:273–278.

43. Konturek, S. J., Radecki, T., Mikos, E., and Thor, J. (1971): The effect of exogenous and endogenous secretin and cholecystokinin on pancreatic secretion in cats. *Scand. J. Gastroenterol.*, 6:423–428.

44. Konturek, S. J., Radecki, T., Thor, P., and Dembinski, A. (1973): Release of cholecystokinin by amino acids (37308). *Proc. Soc. Exp. Biol. Med.*, 143:305–309.

45. Konturek, S. J., Tasler, J., and Obtulowicz, W. (1972): Localization of cholecystokinin release in intestine of the dog. *Am. J. Physiol.*, 222:16–20.

46. Konturek, S. J., Tasler, J., and Obtulowicz, W. (1972): Mechanism of the inhibitory action of endogenous cholestokinin and caerulein on pentagastrin-induced gastric secretion. *Scand. J. Gastroenterol.*, 7:657–662.

47. Korc, M., Williams, J. A., and Goldfine, I. D. (1979): Stimulation of the glucose transport system in isolated mouse pancreatic acini by cholecystokinin and analogues. *J. Biol. Chem.*, 254:7624–7629.

48. Larsson, L.-I., and Rehfeld, J. F. (1978): Distribution of gastrin and CCK cells in the rat gastrointestinal tract. *Histochemistry*, 58:23–31.

49. Larsson, L.-I., and Rehfeld, J. F. (1979): Localization and molecular heterogeneity of cholecystokinin in the central and peripheral nervous system. *Brain Res.*, 165:201–218.

50. Larsson, L.-I., and Rehfeld, J. F. (1979): A peptide resembling COOH-terminal tetrapeptide amide of gastrin from a new gastrointestinal endocrine cell type. *Nature*, 277:575–578.

51. Levant, J. A., Kun, T. L., Jachna, J., Sturdevant, R. A. L., and Isenberg, J. I. (1974): The effects of graded doses of C-terminal octapeptide of cholecystokinin on small intestinal transit time in man. *Dig. Dis.*, 19:207–209.

52. Lin, T.-M. (1975): Actions of gastrointestinal hormones and related peptides on the motor function of the biliary tract. *Gastroenterology*, 69:1006–1022.

53. Malagelada, J. R., Holtermuller, K. H., McCall, J. T., and Go, V. L. (1978): Pancreatic, gallbladder, and intestinal responses to intraluminal magnesium salts in man. *Am. J. Dig. Dis.*, 23(6):481–485.

54. Marshall, C. E., Egberts, E. H., and Johnson, A. G. (1978): An improved method for estimating cholecystokinin in human serum. *J. Endocrinol.*, 79:17–27.

55. Meyer, J. H., and Jones, R. S. (1974): Canine pancreatic responses to intestinally perfused fat and products of fat digestion. *Am. J. Physiol.*, 226:1178–1187.

56. Meyer, J. H., Kelly, G. A., Spingola, L. J., and Jones, R. S. (1976): Canine gut receptors mediating pancreatic responses to luminal L-amino acids. *Am. J. Physiol.*, 231:669–677.

57. Meyer, J. H., Spingola, L. J., and Grossman, M. I. (1971): Endogenous cholecystokinin potentiates exogenous secretin on pancreas of dog. *Am. J. Physiol.*, 221:742–747.

58. Modlin, I. M., Hansky, J., Singer, M., and Walsh, J. H. (1979): Evidence that the cholinergic enteropancreatic reflex may be independent of cholecystokinin release. *Surgery*, 86:352–361.

59. Morgan, K. G., Schmalz, P. F., Go, V. L. W., and Szurszewski, J. H. (1978): Electrical and mechanical effects of molecular variants of CCK on antral smooth muscle. *Am. J. Physiol.*, 235(3):E324–E329.

60. Mukhopadhyay, A. K., Thor, P. J., Copeland, E. M., Johnson, L. R., and Weisbrodt, N. W. (1977): Effect of cholecystokinin on myoelectric activity of small bowel of the dog. *Am. J. Physiol.*, 232(1):E44–47.

61. Muller, J. E., Straus, E., and Yalow, R. S. (1977): Cholecystokinin and its COOH-terminal octapeptide in the pig brain. *Proc. Natl. Acad. Sci. U.S.A.*, 74:3035–3037.

62. Mutt, V. (1976): Further investigations of intestinal hormonal polypeptides. *Clin. Endocrinol. (Oxf.) [Suppl.]*, 5:175S–183S.

63. Mutt, V., and Jorpes, J. E. (1968): Structure of porcine cholecystokinin-pancreozymin. *Eur. J. Biochem.*, 6:156–162.

64. Mutt, V., and Jorpes, E. (1971): Hormonal polypeptides of the upper intestine. *Biochem. J.*, 125:57P–58P.

65. Peikin, S. R., Costenbader, C. L., and Gardner, J. D. (1979): Actions of derivatives of cyclic nucleotides on dispersed acini from guinea pig pancreas. *J. Biol. Chem.*, 254:5321–5327.

66. Peterson, H., Solomon, T., and Grossman, M. I. (1978): Effect of chronic pentagastrin, cholecystokinin, and secretin on pancreas of rats. *Am. J. Physiol.*, 234(3):E286–E293.

67. Pinget, M., Straus, E., and Yalow, R. S. (1978): Localization of cholecystokinin-like immunoreactivity in isolated nerve terminals. *Proc. Natl. Acad. Sci. U.S.A.*, 75:6324–6326.

68. Pinget, M., Straus, E., and Yalow, R. S. (1979): Release of cholecystokinin peptides from a synaptosome-enriched fraction of rat cerebral cortex. *Life Sci.*, 25:339–342.

69. Polak, J. M., Pearse, A. G. E., Bloom, S. R., Buchan, A. M. J., Rayford, P. L., and Thompson, J. C. (1975): Identification of cholecystokinin-secreting cells. *Lancet*, 2:1016–1021.

70. Rehfeld, J. F. (1978): Immunochemical studies on cholecystokinin. *J. Biol. Chem.*, 253:4016–4021.

71. Rehfeld, J. F., and Kruse-Larsen, C. (1978): Gastrin and cholecystokinin in human cerebrospinal fluid. Immunochemical determination of concentrations and molecular heterogeneity. *Brain Res.*, 155:19–26.

72. Rehfeld, J. F., and Larsson, L. I. (1979): The predominating molecular form of gastrin and cholecystokinin in the gut is a small peptide corresponding to their COOH-terminal tetrapeptide amide. *Acta Physiol. Scand.*, 105(1):117–119.

73. Resin, H., Stern, D. H., Sturdevant, R. A. L., and Isenberg, J. I. (1973): Effect of the C-terminal octapeptide of cholecystokinin on lower esophageal sphincter pressure in man. *Gastroenterology*, 64:946–949.

74. Richardson, P. D., and Withrington, P. G. (1977): The effects of glucagon, secretin, pancreozymin and pentagastrin on the hepatic arterial vascular bed of the dog. *Br. J. Pharmacol.*, 59(1):147–156.

75. Robberecht, P., Deschodt-Lanckman, M., and Vanderhaeghen, J. J. (1979): Demonstration of biological activity of brain gastrin-like peptidic material in the human: Its relationship with the COOH-terminal octapeptide of cholecystokinin. *Proc. Natl. Acad. Sci. U.S.A.*, 75:524–528.

76. Roos, B. A. (1977): Calcitonin secretion in vitro. III. Synergistic secretory effects of enteric polypeptide hormones. *Endocrinology*, 100(6):1679–1683.

77. Sarles, H., Tiscornia, O., and Palasciano, G. (1977): Chronic alcoholism and canine exocrine pancreas secretion. A long term follow-up study. *Gastroenterology*, 72(2):238–243.

78. Schiller, P. W., Natarajan, S., and Bodanszky, M. (1978): Determination of the intramolecular tyrosine-tryptophan distance in a 7-peptide related to the C-terminal sequence of cholecystokinin. *Int. J. Peptide Protein Res.*, 12(3):139–142.

79. Schlegel, W., Raptis, S., Grube, D., and Pfeiffer, E. F. (1977): Estimation of cholecystokinin-pancreozymin (CCK) in human plasma and tissue by a specific radioimmunoassay and the immunohistochemical identification of pancreozymin-producing cells in the duodenum of humans. *Clin. Chim. Acta*, 80:305–316.

80. Schlegel, W., Raptis, S., Harvey, R. F., Oliver, J. M., and Pfeiffer, E. F. (1977): Inhibition of cholecystokinin-pancreozymin release by somatostatin. *Lancet*, 2(8030):166–168.

80a. Schneider, B. S., Monahan, J. W., and Hirsch, J. (1979): Brain cholecystokinin and nutritional status in rats and mice. *J. Clin. Invest.*, 64:1348–1356.

81. Shaw, R. A., and Jones, R. S. (1978): The choleretic action of cholecystokinin and cholecystokinin octapeptide in dogs. *Surgery*, 84(5):622–625.

82. Singer, M. V., Solomon, T. E., and Grossman, M. I. (1980): Effect of atropine on secretion from intact and transplanted pancreas in dog. *Am. J. Physiol.*, 238:G18–G22.

83. Singer, M. V., Solomon, T. E., Wood, J., and Grossman, M. I. (1980): Latency of pancreatic enzyme response to intraduodenal stimulants. *Am. J. Physiol.*, 238:G23–G29.

84. Snape, W. J., Jr., Carlson, G. M., and Cohen, S. (1977): Human colonic myoelectric activity in response to prostigmin and the gastrointestinal hormones. *Am. J. Dig. Dis.*, 22(10):881–887.

85. Stewart, J. J., and Burks, T. F. (1977): Actions of cholecysto-

kinin octapeptide on smooth muscle of isolated dog intestine. *Am. J. Physiol.*, 232(3):E306–E310.

86. Straus, E., Malesci, A., and Yalow, R. S. (1978): Characterization of a nontrypsin cholecystokinin converting enzyme in mammalian brain. *Proc. Natl. Acad. Sci. U.S.A.*, 75:5711–5714.
87. Straus, E., Muller, J. E., Choi, H.-S., Paronetto, F., and Yalow, R. S. (1977): Immunohistochemical localization in rabbit brain of a peptide resembling the COOH-terminal octapeptide of cholecystokinin. *Proc. Natl. Acad. Sci. U.S.A.*, 74:3033–3034.
88. Straus, E., and Yalow, R. S. (1978): Species specificity of cholecystokinin in gut and brain of several mammalian species. *Proc. Natl. Acad. Sci. U.S.A.*, 75:486–489.
89. Straus, E., and Yalow, R. S. (1979): Cholecystokinin in the brains of obese and nonobese mice. *Science*, 203:68–69.
90. Sturdevant, R. A. L., and Goetz, H. (1976): Cholecystokinin both stimulates and inhibits human food intake. *Nature*, 261:713–715.
91. Thompson, J. C., Fender, H. R., Ramus, N. I., Villar, H. V., and Rayford, P. L. (1975): Cholecystokinin metabolism in man and dogs. *Ann. Surg.*, 182:496–504.
92. Vigna, S. R., and Gorbman, A. (1977): Effects of cholecystokinin, gastrin, and related peptides on coho salmon gallbladder contraction in vitro. *Am. J. Physiol.*, 232(5):E485–E491.
93. Waldman, D. B., Zfass, A. M., and Makhlouf, G. M. (1977): Stimulatory (H1) and inhibitory (H2) histamine receptors in gallbladder muscle. *Gastroenterology*, 72:932–936.
94. Way, L. W. (1971): Effect of cholecystokinin and caerulein on gastric secretion in cats. *Gastroenterology*, 60:560–565.
95. Wormsley, K. G. (1969): A comparison of the response to secretin, pancreozymin and a combination of these hormones, in man. *Scand. J. Gastroenterol.*, 4:413–417.
96. Yajima, H., Kai, Y., Ogawa, H., Kubota, M., and Mori, Y. (1977): Structure-activity relationships of gastrointestinal hormones: Motilin, GIP, and [27-TYR]CCK-PZ. *Gastroenterology*, 72:793–796.
97. Yamada, T., Solomon, T. E., Petersen, H., Levin, S. R., Lewin, K., Walsh, J. H., and Grossman, M. I. (1980): Effects of gastrointestinal polypeptides on hormone content of endocrine pancreas in the rat. *Am. J. Physiol.*, 238:G526–G530.
98. Yau, W. M., Makhlouf, G. M., Edwards, L. E., and Farrar, J. T. (1973): Mode of action of cholecystokinin and related peptides on gallbladder muscle. *Gastroenterology*, 65:451–456.

SECRETIN

Structure

Secretin is a linear peptide containing 27 amino acid residues that has structural similarities with glucagon, vasoactive intestinal peptide, and gastric inhibitory peptide (55) as shown in Table 1. Larger forms of secretin have not been described. A method has been reported for identification of the presence of secretin in a mixture of peptides by analyzing for the presence of the carboxyl terminal valine amide after enzymatic digestion with subtilisins, chymotrypsin, or thermolysin (81). The structure has been determined only in the hog. Partial purification of chicken secretin has been reported (54,56), and it appears to differ significantly from chicken VIP and from porcine secretin. Secretin-like activity has been found in teleost fish extracts, but the pattern of biological responses obtained was more similar to VIP than to secretin (16). Synthetic porcine secretin was found to have full potency and the spectrum of biological actions of natural porcine secretin (57). Secretin

in solution is a basic peptide that forms a helical configuration (4).

Biological Actions

The biological actions of secretin were established in enough detail to permit a thorough review in 1972 (32). This section will not attempt to repeat primary references covered in this review.

Pancreatic Secretion

The primary biological action of secretin, appreciated by Bayliss and Starling in 1902, is stimulation of the pancreas to secrete large volumes of pancreatic juice rich in bicarbonate. The bicarbonate concentration increases in parallel with rate of secretion and reaches a maximum when the secretion rate is about one-third maximal and the chloride concentration of pancreatic juice shows a corresponding fall. The dose required to produce maximal stimulation in humans, dog, or cat is about 1 clinical unit (200 to 250 ng) kg^{-1} given as a single intravenous dose or per hour as a continuous intravenous infusion. Secretin when given alone produces only slight stimulation of pancreatic enzyme secretion. However, there is an important interaction between secretin and CCK given together. A threshold or subthreshold dose of secretin increases the enzyme and bicarbonate responses to exogenous or endogenous CCK more than can be explained by simple additive effects of the two stimulants. In the isolated perfused porcine pancreas, secretin produced significant stimulation of water and bicarbonate secretion at a concentration of 2.8 pM and maximal responses were obtained at a concentration of 92 pM (35). There were no significant effects on insulin and glucagon secretion. Vagotomy and atropine have little effect on the maximal bicarbonate response to exogenous secretin. In the isolated perfused pancreas, cholinergic stimulation with cabamylcholine decreased the D$_{50}$ but had no effect on the maximal response to secretin (85).

Radioiodinated secretin has been found to bind specifically to plasma membranes from cat pancreas with a dissociation constant of 4×10^{-9} M (53). Unlabeled secretin inhibited this binding in the same range of concentrations that caused stimulation of adenylate cyclase. Vasoactive intestinal peptide competed with secretin for binding sites but had 100 times lower affinity. A similar potency ratio between secretin and VIP was found for stimulation of cellular cyclic AMP content in isolated guinea pig acinar cells (23,24). Among the stimulants of pancreatic acinar cells *in vitro*, only secretin, VIP, and cholera toxin, which has a separate receptor, cause stimulation of cyclic AMP. There are four other classes of acinar cell receptors that cause increased calcium outflux and increased cellular cyclic GMP content (25). These receptors are responsive to cholinergic agents, gastrin-CCK peptides, bombesin-like peptides, and substance P-like molecules. Combined stimulation with an agent causing cyclic AMP stimulation and an agent causing calcium outflux leads to true potentiation of responses. The role of cyclic AMP in stimulation of human pancreatic secretion also is supported by closely parallel outputs of bicarbonate and cyclic AMP in pure pancreatic juice obtained during stimulation with graded doses of secretin (18). Although most *in vitro* studies of pancreatic stimulation by secretin have been performed with acinar tissue, there is good evidence that the major fraction of pancreatic bicarbonate secretion originates from duct cells. Selective destruction of acinar tissue in rats reduced the bicarbonate response to secretin by only about 50% but eliminated the response to CCK (22). In this *in vivo* model, atropine had no effect on response to secretin.

Pancreatic Growth

Chronic administration of secretin to rats was shown to cause a small increase in pancreatic weight associated with decreased sensitivity of the pancreas to secretin without any alteration in maximal bicarbonate response (60). More dramatic effects of secretin have been found when it is administered in combination with cerulein (74). Secretin alone produced significant increases in pancreatic weight, RNA, and lipase but not in DNA or other enzymes. Secretin markedly augmented the hypertrophic effects of cerulein without an effect on hyperplasia. Secretin had no trophic effect on the stomach when given alone but inhibited the increase in oxyntic gland DNA and RNA stimulated by pentagastrin (15). Secretin also caused a slight increase in the weight of the proximal duodenum (60). In the rat colon, secretin prevented the increase in mucosal DNA synthesis caused by pentagastrin (36).

Endocrine Pancreas

Much of the interest in secretin as one of the agents responsible for augmentation of insulin release when glucose is administered by mouth or intraduodenally has been diminished by later findings that glucose does not release secretin. Secretin is known to increase plasma insulin concentrations (32); this effect in humans was observed only during stimulation with glucose and not with arginine, isoproterenol, tolbutamide, or glucagon (47). However, it has been shown that intestinal perfusion with acid to release endogenous secretin had no effect on basal or glucose-stimulated insulin concentrations, intraduodenal glucose did not cause an increase in immunoreactive secretin, and exogenous secre-

tin caused enhancement of insulin responses to glucose only when given at a dose that produced plasma secretin concentrations 30 times higher than those achieved with endogenous stimulation (20). Thus the role of secretin on insulin release is not likely to be physiological.

Gastric Function

Secretin stimulates the secretion of pepsin into the gastric juice and inhibits gastric acid secretion, especially during stimulation with gastrin (32). The doses required to inhibit acid secretion are higher than those expected to cause physiological effects, but a combination of secretin and CCK at doses submaximal for pancreatic stimulation caused significant inhibition of pentagastrin-stimulated acid secretion in man (30). However, there is no strong evidence that secretin is a physiologic inhibitor of acid secretion. During pentagastrin stimulation in man, secretin caused no change in intrinsic factor secretion while producing the expected inhibition of acid secretion and stimulation of pepsin secretion (84). Secretin also inhibits gastric emptying (82), and it was found that a dose of secretin half-maximal for stimulation of pancreatic bicarbonate secretion caused a significant decrease in canine gastric pressure (83).

Biliary Function

Secretin causes an increase in biliary output of water associated with increased concentrations of bicarbonate and chloride and decreased concentrations of bile salts (38). This effect appears to be through a ductular mechanism. The effect on bile flow was observed in cholecystectomized monkeys in which the enterohepatic circulation of bile salts was maintained (23). Secretin inhibits water and electrolyte absorption in the gallbladder *in vivo* but has little or no effect on muscle contraction (34) when given alone but may augment contraction caused by CCK. Although intraduodenal acid causes gallbladder contraction, this effect may be explained by release of CCK or by activation of reflexes.

Intestinal Function

Secretin stimulated chloride secretion and inhibited sodium and bicarbonate absorption in the rat (31), but no significant effects on water and electrolyte movement could be demonstrated in dog jejunum (1). Secretin was found to inhibit upper small intestinal motility in humans and to antagonize the stimulation produced by CCK (27). In the dog, secretin produced a dose-dependent decrease in duodenal and jejunal spike activity without significant effect on the frequency of the interdigestive migratory myoelectric complex (89).

Gastrin Release

Secretin decreases serum gastrin concentrations in patients with hypergastremia due to atrophic gastritis or isolated retained antrum but produces an increase in serum gastrin concentrations in patients with gastrin-secretin tumors (86). Secretin also inhibits food-stimulated gastrin release. The decrease in gastrin in pernicious anemia patients was due to decreases in both G17 and G34 forms (75). In patients with gastrinoma, secretin was found to produce increases in gastrin equal to those obtained during calcium infusion (42). In the isolated perfused rat stomach, secretin caused a decrease in gastrin release associated with a parallel increase in somatostatin release (11).

Other Effects

Intravenous secretin decreases lower esophageal sphincter pressure and antagonizes the increase caused by gastrin (32). Secretin also has a diuretic effect. It causes a redistribution of blood flow into the splanchnic circulation without a major change in cardiac output (40). It has a lipolytic effect on fat cells from rat and mouse. Secretin also caused parathyroid hormone release and cyclic AMP accumulation in dispersed bovine parathyroid cells (88).

Structure-Activity Relationships

Secretin has structural similarities to glucagon and VIP and interacts with VIP but not with glucagon receptors (2). Only the whole 27 amino acid peptide has full potency for biological effects, but the 5-27 carboxyl terminal fragment retains some capacity to stimulate pancreatic secretion (50). Substitutions that decreased the helical character of the 5-27 fragment had little effect on biological activity. Replacement of aspartic acid by lysine in position 15 of the 5-27 fragment, so that the molecule was more similar to VIP, resulted in a decrease in secretin-like properties and an increase in VIP-like properties on smooth muscle activity and receptor binding (3).

Distribution

Secretin is found in cells in the small intestine, especially concentrated in the duodenum and jejunum, known as S cells (8,61). These cells are argyrophilic and contain small granules with an average diameter between 150 and 200 nm. When appropriate controls are used, such cells are not demonstrable elsewhere in the adult gastrointestinal tract. A few cells that were immunoreactive with secretin antibody were found in monolayer cultures of fetal rat pancreas (66). Secretin cells also were found in the duodenum of the 17-day-old fetal rat (43). Immunoreactive secretin concentrations in the cat were highest in the duodenum, about one-third as great in the jejunum, and much lower in the ileum (52). In a comparison of immunoreactive secretin distribution among different species, this pattern was found in pig, dog, guinea pig, and monkey, whereas rat ileum contained concentrations of secretin similar to those extracted from the upper small intestine (79). Gel filtration revealed a single peak that coeluted with porcine secretin. No secretin was found in pancreatic extracts.

Measurement

Bioassays for secretin, based on stimulation of pancreatic water and bicarbonate secretion, were used by Bayliss and Starling in the initial identification of secretin and by Jorpes and Mutt to monitor the progress of purification of this peptide. A sensitive bioassay has been described that utilizes the isolated perfused cat pancreas with addition of theophylline to the perfusate (73). Under optimal conditions it was possible to detect secretin concentrations as low as about 100 pM. However, the most sensitive bioassay is about 100 times less sensitive than the best radioimmunoassays.

Radioimmunoassay methods require either labeling of the N-terminal histidine residue of secretin or use of a molecule in which a tyrosine residue has been added because the natural molecule contains no tyrosine. Both methods have been used successfully. Immunization with either unconjugated or conjugated secretin has produced a good yield of high-affinity secretin antibodies (21). Specificity of antisera can be evaluated by comparison of inhibitory potencies of secretin fragments and of structurally related peptides such as glucagon and VIP with pure secretin. Most reported antibodies have had little cross-reactivity with other related gut peptides, possibly because they seem to be directed at antigenic sites in the C-terminal portion of the molecule that has less similarity to other peptides than the N-terminal portion (5,21,90). Substitution by tyrosine at the amino terminus of the secretin molecule appears to result in less loss of immunoreactivity than substitution in position 6 (91). Secretin radioimmunoassay has been used successfully to measure increases in plasma immunoreactivity following acid instillation into the duodenum (5,62). After extraction of plasma to remove interfering factors, fasting secretin concentrations in normal humans were found to average less than 5 pM (67,80).

Metabolism

Disappearance half-time of exogenous secretin in the dog has been found by both bioassay (46) and radioimmunoassay (13) to be between 2.5 and 3 min. Endogenous secretin also was cleared at a similar rate. In anesthetized pigs the half-time was 2.6 min, clearance rate 15 ml min^{-1}kg^{-1}, and space of distribution 64 ml kg^{-1} (19). The half-time in humans was found to be 4.1 min (41). Several studies have indicated that the kidney is a major site for removal of secretin from the circulation. Renal arteriovenous differences during secretin infusion in one study were 52% while no difference was found across the foreleg (19). Exclusion of the kidneys increased plasma secretin concentration and half-time by about 75%. Injection of secretin into the renal artery decreased the biological response by 75% compared with intravenous administration, and ligature of both renal arteries led to an increased biological response and half-life (46). The mass of secretin entering and leaving the liver was the same during secretin infusion while the kidney extracted about 30% (12). Ligation of both ureters had no effect on secretin elimination whereas ligation of the renal vessels increased the half-time by 50% (14). Less than 1% of secretin removed by the kidney appeared in the urine. On the other hand, in a series of patients with severe renal failure secretin was the only one of six gastrointestinal hormones not elevated in the plasma (17). The mechanisms for disposal of secretin after removal from the circulation have not been determined.

Release

There is general agreement that acidification of the duodenum in humans or experimental animals causes release of secretin into the blood in amounts sufficient to explain stimulation of pancreatic bicarbonate secretion. The major controversies related to release of secretin have involved absolute concentrations of immunoreactive secretin as determined by different radioimmunoassay procedures, occurrence of secretin release under physiological stimulation by a meal, and whether or not factors other than acid such as glucose, fatty acids, alcohol, and bile also might stimulate secretin release. It has been demonstrated by *in vivo* bioassay, measurement of pancreatic bicarbonate secretory response, that the volume and bicarbonate response vary directly as a function of the length of proximal small intestine acidified and of the load of acid infused into long segments of intestine (51). When sensitive radioimmunoassay measurement became available, it was shown that secretin was released by intraduodenal HCl but not by intraduodenal glucose (6). Use of the same assay failed to reveal significant increases in immunoreactive secretin in response to a protein meal, oleic acid, or amino acids in dogs (7). In another study, fat added to a protein meal did not cause a significant increase in secretin nor did the meal given without added fat (63).

Alcohol was reported to cause release of secretin in humans (77), possibly by an indirect mechanism involving gastrin release (49). Both of these results were obtained with assays that found high basal secretin concentrations, and the results have not been confirmed with assays that involve extraction of plasma and produce lower results. Intraduodenal infusion of bile was found to release secretin and stimulate pancreatic secretion in humans (58), and sodium taurocholate had a similar effect in cats (29). Secretin release was not produced by vagal stimulation or inhibited by atropine, and acute cervical vagotomy had no effect on the secretin response to intraduodenal acid in anesthetized dogs (44). Similarly, no evidence for vagal control of secretin release was found in humans, since vagotomized patients and duodenal ulcer patients had similar secretin responses to acid (87). Prolonged parenteral feeding in dogs was found to decrease pancreatic bicarbonate and immunoreactive secretin responses to duodenal acidification without a change in response to exogenous secretin, but unexpectedly produced an increase in basal secretin concentrations (37).

Relationship with Physiological Events

It has been shown that progressive acidification of a protein-rich meal in dogs between pH 4.5 and 3.0 leads to progressive augmentation of pancreatic bicarbonate secretion and that the bicarbonate response can be reproduced when the gastric pH is maintained above 4.5 by intravenous infusion of about 0.4 units kg^{-1}hr^{-1} exogenous secretin (26). Since the pH range required to produce stimulation is well within the physiologic range, it would be expected that the pancreatic response should be reflected by increases in circulating secretin concentrations if secretin is the mediator of this effect. The dose required to simulate the response to low pH meals may have been overestimated because a carrier was not added to the secretin solution during infusion and secretin is known to bind to plastic surfaces. A significant increase in immunoreactive plasma secretin was found in dogs when liver extract was administered at pH 2 but not at pH 7 (48), but initial efforts to detect an increase in immunoreactive secretin after a meat meal were unsuccessful in dogs (45) and humans (64) unless the duodenum was also acidified. In these studies the duodenal pH usually remained above 5.0.

Newer information has been obtained that supports a role for secretin in the physiologic regulation of pancreatic bicarbonate secretion after a meal. By use of an extraction procedure for plasma and a sensitive radioimmunoassay, it was shown that basal secretin concentrations were 1.2 pM in normal subjects, 2.5 pM in duodenal ulcer patients, 5.9 pM in gastrinoma patients, and undetectable in achlorhydric patients (68). Insulin hypoglycemia caused a significant increase in secretin values when acid was allowed to enter the duodenum but not during gastric aspiration. After a meal, short-lived increments in plasma secretin were measured that corresponded to brief periods of decreased intraduodenal pH, and these increments were abolished by cimetidine treatment. However, cimetidine had no effect on increments in secretin caused by duodenal acidification. Another investigation was performed to determine whether the low concentrations of secretin detected in plasma could produce measurable pancreatic responses (71). In these studies albumin was added to secretin solutions to prevent losses by adsorption and graded doses were given intravenously. Half-maximal bicarbonate responses were obtained with exogenous dose rates between 2.5 and 8 pmol kg^{-1}h^{-1}, which produced immunoreactive plasma secretin concentrations between 2 and 8 pM. Significant increases in bicarbonate concentration were obtained when plasma secretin increased by 1 to 2 pM (Fig. 3). These values are somewhat lower than the D$_{50}$ for circulating secretin in humans estimated in another study to be 22 pM (28), but both studies indicate that very low concentrations of secretin produce pancreatic responses. Injection of small amounts of HCl in the human duodenum followed by neutralization produced short-lived increases in plasma secretin of about 1 pM (70). Very small bolus injections of secretin in humans (0.1 to 0.5 pmol kg^{-1}) produced increments in plasma secretin between 2 and 6 pM that were associated with increased bicarbonate output (69). After administration of a liquid test meal in man, it was found that plasma secretin increased transiently by 2 to 3 pM during times when duodenal pH decreased below 4 and that bolus in-jections of secretin that produced similar increases in secretin caused stimulation of pancreatic bicarbonate output (59). In another study in man it was found that a meat meal caused an increase in plasma secretin when duodenal pH fell below 4.5 and that this response was eliminated by infusion of bicarbonate solution to maintain intragastric pH above 5.5 (10) (Fig. 4). Prolonged stimulation of plasma secretin and pancreatic bicarbonate were measured in dogs after a meat meal, while duodenal pH remained about 4, and these responses were eliminated by cimetidine treatment (39). More direct evidence was obtained that secretin alone accounted for a major part of the pancreatic bicarbonate response to a meat meal in dogs by demonstrating that administration of antiserum to secretin decreased the response by more than 80% (9) (Fig. 5). Thus it appears clear that secretin can function as a hormonal regulator of pancreatic bicarbonate secretion, but it has not yet been established over what period of time this effect is operative in normal humans.

Conditions of Excess or Deficiency

One case of a pancreatic tumor secreting five different hormones including secretin was reported in a patient who had diarrhea associated with pancreatic hypersecretion, but no cases of isolated production of secretin by a tumor have been found (72). Hypersecretinemia has been found in patients with gastrinoma and gastric acid hypersecretion (78), and it has been suggested that plasma secretin concentrations can be monitored to determine the effectiveness of treatment with drugs that inhibit acid secretion (76,79). Reduced

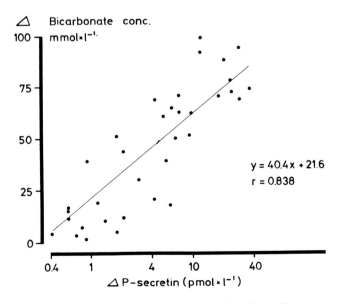

FIG. 3. Duodenal bicarbonate output as a function of increase in plasma secretin concentration in humans during low-dose intravenous infusion of secretin. From Schaffalitzky de Muckadell et al. (71).

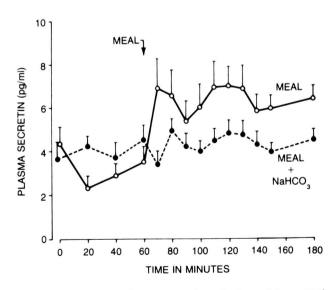

FIG. 4. Plasma secretin response to a test meal in normal human subjects when intragastric pH was allowed to find its normal level or maintained above pH 5.5 by intragastric infusion of bicarbonate. From Chey et al. (10).

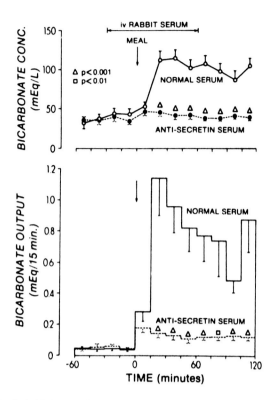

FIG. 5. Inhibition of pancreatic bicarbonate response to a meat meal in dogs by administration of antibody to secretin intravenously. From Chey et al. (9).

release of secretin has been reported in patients with celiac sprue and this may contribute to decreased pancreatic secretion found in these patients (65). The bulk of current evidence suggests that patients with duodenal ulcer have no defect in either secretin release or pancreatic bicarbonate responses to duodenal acidification (33).

References

1. Barbezat, G. O., and Grossman, M. I. (1971): Intestinal secretion: stimulation by peptides. *Science,* 174:422–424.
2. Bataille, D., Freychet, P., and Rosselin, G. (1974): Interactions of glucagon, gut glucagon, VIP and secretin with liver and fat cell plasma membranes. *Endocrinology,* 95:713–720.
3. Bodansky, M., Natarajan, S., Gardner, J. D., Makhlouf, G. M., and Said, S. I. (1978): Synthesis and some pharmacological properties of the 23-peptide 15-lysine-secretin-(5–27). Special role of the residue in position 15 in biological activity of the vasoactive intestinal polypeptide. *J. Med. Chem.,* 21(11):1171–1173.
4. Bodansky, A., Ondetti, M. A., Mutt, V., et al. (1969): Synthesis of secretin. IV. Secondary structure in a miniature protein. *J. Am. Chem. Soc.,* 91:944–949.
5. Boden, G., and Chey, W. Y. (1973): Preparation and specificity of antiserum to synthetic secretin and its use in a radioimmunoassay (RIA). *Endocrinology,* 92:1617–1624.
6. Boden, G., Essa, N., Owen, O. E., and Reichle, F. A. (1974): Effects of intraduodenal administration of HCl and glucose on circulating immunoreactive secretin and insulin concentrations. *J. Clin. Invest.,* 53:1185–1193.
7. Boden, G., Wilson, R. M., Essa-Koumar, N., and Owen, O. E. (1978): Effects of a protein meal, intraduodenal HCl, and oleic acid on portal and peripheral venous secretin and on pancreatic bicarbonate secretion. *Gut,* 19:277–283.
8. Bussolati, G., Capella, C., Solcia, E., Vassallo, G., and Vezzadini, P. (1971): Ultrastructural and immunofluorescent investigations on the secretin cell in the dog intestinal mucosa. *Histochemie,* 26:218–227.
9. Chey, W. Y., Kim, M. S., Lee, K. Y., and Chang, T.-M. (1979): Effect of rabbit antisecretin serum on postprandial pancreatic secretion in dogs. *Gastroenterology,* 77:1268–1275.
10. Chey, W. Y., Lee, Y. H., Hendricks, J. G., Rhodes, R. A., and Tai, H.-H. (1978): Plasma secretin concentrations in fasting and postprandial state in man. *Am. J. Dig. Dis.,* 23:981–988.
11. Chiba, T., Taminato, T., Kadowaki, S., Abe, H., Chihara, K., Seino, Y., Matsukura, S., and Fujita, T. (1980): Effects of glucagon, secretin, and vasoactive intestinal polypeptide on gastric somatostatin and gastrin release from isolated perfused rat stomach. *Gastroenterology,* 79:67–71.
12. Curtis, P. J., Fender, H. R., Rayford, P. L., and Thompson, J. C. (1976): Catabolism of secretin by the liver and kidney. *Surgery,* 80:259–265.
13. Curtis, P. J., Fender, H. R., Rayford, P. L., and Thompson, J. C. (1976): Disappearance half-time of endogenous and exogenous secretin in dogs. *Gut,* 17:595–599.
14. Curtis, P. J., Miller, T. A., Rayford, P. L., and Thompson, J. C. (1977): The effect of nephrectomy on the catabolism of secretin. *Am J. Surg.,* 133:52–54.
15. Dembinski, A. B., and Johnson, L. R. (1980): Stimulation of pancreatic growth by secretin, caerulein, and pentagastrin. *Endocrinology,* 106:323–328.
16. Dockray, G. J. (1976): Comparative studies on secretin and related peptides. *J. Endocrinol.,* 70:4P–5P.
17. Doherty, C. C., Buchanan, K. D., Ardill, J., and McGeown, M. G. (1978): Elevations of gastrointestinal hormones in chronic renal failure. *Proc. Eur. Dial. Transplant. Assoc.,* 15:456–465.
18. Domschke, S., Domschke, W., Rosch, W., Konturek, S. J., Wunsch, E., and Demling, L. (1976): Bicarbonate and cyclic AMP content of pure human pancreatic juice in response to graded doses of synthetic secretin. *Gastroenterology,* 70:533–536.
19. Fahrenkrug, J., Schaffalitzky de Muckadell, O. B., and Holst, J. J. (1978): Elimination of porcine secretin in pigs. *Clin. Sci. Mol. Med.,* 54(1):61–68.
20. Fahrenkrug, J., Schaffalitzky de Muckadell, O. B., and Kuhl, C. (1978): Effect of secretin on basal- and glucose-stimulated insulin secretion in man. *Diabetologia,* 14(4):229–234.
21. Fahrenkrug, J., Schaffalitzky de Muckadell, O. B., and Rehfeld, J. F. (1976): Production and evaluation of antibodies for radioimmunoassay of secretin. *Scand. J. Clin. Lab. Invest,* 36:281–287.
22. Folsch, U. R., and Creutzfeldt, W. (1977): Pancreatic duct cells in rats: Secretory studies in response to secretin, cholecystokinin-pancreozymin, and gastrin in vivo. *Gastroenterology,* 73:1053–1059.
23. Gardiner, B. N., and Small, D. M. (1976): Simultaneous measurement of the pancreatic and biliary response to CCK and secretin. Primate biliary physiology XIII. *Gastroenterology,* 70:403–407.
24. Gardner, J. D., Conlon, T. P., and Adams, T. D. (1976): Cyclic AMP in pancreatic acinar cells: Effects of gastrointestinal hormones. *Gastroenterology,* 70:29–35.
25. Gardner, J. D., and Jensen, R. T. (1980): Receptor for secretagogues on pancreatic acinar cells. *Am. J. Physiol.,* 238:G63–G66.
26. Grossman, M. I., and Konturek, S. J. (1974): Gastric acid does drive pancreatic bicarbonate secretion. *Scand. J. Gastroenterol.,* 9:299–302.
27. Gutierrez, J. G., Chey, W. Y., and Dinoso, V. P. (1974): Actions of cholecystokinin and secretin on the motor activity of the small intestine in man. *Gastroenterology,* 67:35–41.
28. Hacki, W. H., Bloom, S. R., Mitznegg, P., Domschke, W., Domschke, S., Belohlavek, D., Demling, L., and Wunsch, E. (1977): Plasma secretin and pancreatic bicarbonate response to exogenous secretin in man. *Gut,* 18(3):191–195.
29. Hanssen, L. E., Hotz, J., Hartmann, W., Nehls, W., and Goebell, H. (1980): Immunoreactive secretin release following taurocholate perfusions of the cat duodenum. *Scand. J. Gastroenterol.,* 15:89–95.

30. Henriksen, F. W., Jorgensen, S. P., and Moller, S. (1974): Interaction between secretin and cholecystokinin on inhibition of gastric secretion in man. *Scand. J. Gastroenterol.*, 9:735–740.

31. Hubel, K. A. (1972): Effects of secretin and glucagon on intestinal transport of ions and water in the rat (36208). *Proc. Soc. Exp. Biol. Med.*, 139:656–658.

32. Hubel, K. A. (1972): Secretin: A long progress note. *Gastroenterology*, 62:318–341.

33. Isenberg, J. I., Cano, R., and Bloom, S. R. (1977): Effect of graded amounts of acid instilled into the duodenum on pancreatic bicarbonate secretion and plasma secretin in duodenal ulcer patients and normal subjects. *Gastroenterology*, 72:6–8.

34. Jansson, R., Steen, G., and Svanvik, J. (1978): A comparison of glucagon, gastric inhibitory peptide, and secretin on gallbladder function, formation of bile, and pancreatic secretion in the cat. *Scand. J. Gastroenterol.*, 13(8):919–925.

35. Jensen, S. L., Fahrenkrug, J., Holst, J. J., Kuhl, C., Nielsen, O. V., and Schaffalitzky de Muckadell, O. B. (1978): Secretory effects of secretin on isolated perfused porcine pancreas. *Am. J. Physiol.*, 235(4):E381–E386.

36. Johnson, L. R., and Guthrie, P. D. (1978): Effect of secretin on colonic DNA synthesis (40238). *Proc. Soc. Exp. Biol. Med.*, 158: 521–523.

37. Johnson, L. R., Schanbacher, L. M., Dudrick, S. J., and Copeland, E. M. (1977): Effect of long-term parenteral feeding on pancreatic secretion and serum secretin. *Am. J. Physiol.*, 233(6): E524–E529.

38. Jones, R. S., Geist, R. E., and Hall, A. D. (1971): The choleretic effects of glucagon and secretin in the dog. *Gastroenterology*, 60:64–68.

39. Kim, M. S., Lee, K. Y., and Chey, W. Y. (1979): Plasma secretin concentrations in fasting and postprandial states in dogs. *Am. J. Physiol.*, 236(5):E539–E544.

40. Kitani, K., Suzuki, Y., and Miura, R. (1978): Differences in the effects of secretin and glucagon on the blood circulation of unanesthetized rats. *Acta Hepatogastroenterol. (Stuttg.)*, 25(6): 470–473.

41. Kolts, B. E., and McGuigan, J. E. (1977): Radioimmunoassay measurement of secretin half-life in man. *Gastroenterology*, 72: 55–60.

42. Lamers, C. B. H., and Van Tongeren, J. H. M. (1977): Comparative study of the value of the calcium, secretin, and meal stimulated increase in serum gastrin to the diagnosis of the Zollinger-Ellison syndrome. *Gut*, 18:128–135.

43. Larsson, L. I., Sundler, F., Alumets, J., Hakanson, R., Schaffalitzky de Muckadell, O. B., and Fahrenkrug, J. (1977): Distribution, ontogeny and ultrastructure of the mammalian secretin cell. *Cell Tissue Res.*, 181(3):361–368.

44. Lee, K. Y., Chey, W. Y., and Tai, H. H. (1978): Roles of the vagus in endogenous release of secretin and exocrine pancreatic secretion in dog. In: *Gastrointestinal Hormones and Pathology of the Digestive System*, edited by M. Grossman, V. Speranza, N. Basso, and E. Lezoche, pp. 211–216. Plenum Publishing Corp., New York.

45. Lee, K. Y., Tai, H. H., and Chey, W. Y. (1976): Plasma secretin and gastrin responses to a meat meal and duodenal acidification in dogs. *Am. J. Physiol.*, 230(3):784–789.

46. Lehnert, P., Stahlheber, H., Forell, M. M., Fullner, R., Fruhauf, S., Fritz, H., Hutzel, M., and Werle, E. (1974): Studies on the elimination of secretin and cholecystokinin with regard to the kinetics of exocrine pancreatic secretion. *Digestion*, 11:51–63.

47. Lerner, R. L. (1977): The augmentation effects of secretin on the insulin responses to known stimuli: specificity for glucose. *J. Clin. Endocrinol. Metab.*, 45(1):1–9.

48. Llanos, O. L., Konturek, S. J., Rayford, P. L., and Thompson, J. C. (1977): Pancreatic bicarbonate, serum gastrin, and secretin responses to meals varying in pH. *Am. J. Physiol.*, 233(1): E41–E46.

49. Llanos, O. L., Swierczek, J. S., Teichmann, R. K., Rayford, P. L., and Thompson, J. C. (1977): Effect of alcohol on the release of secretin and pancreatic secretion. *Surgery*, 81:661–667.

50. Makhlouf, G. M., Bodanszky, M., Fink, M. L., and Schebalin, M. (1978): Pancreatic secretory activity of secretin 5-27 and substituted analogues. *Gastroenterology*, 75(2):244–248.

51. Meyer, J. H., Way, L. W., and Grossman, M. I. (1970): Pancreatic response to acidification of various lengths of proximal intestine in the dog. *Am. J. Physiol.*, 219:971–977.

52. Miller, T. A., Llanos, O. L., Swierczek, J. S., Rayford, P. L., and Thompson, J. C. (1978): Concentrations of gastrin and secretin in the alimentary tract of the cat. *Surgery*, 83:90–93.

53. Milutinovic, S., Schulz, I., and Rosselin, G. (1976): The interaction of secretin with pancreatic membranes. *Biochim. Biophys. Acta*, 436:113–127.

54. Mutt, V. (1976): Further investigations on intestinal hormonal polypeptides. *Clin. Endocrinol.*, 5:175–183.

55. Mutt, V., Jorpes, J. E., and Magnusson, S. (1970): Structure of porcine secretin: the amino acid sequence. *Eur. J. Biochem.*, 15: 513.

56. Nilsson, A. (1974): Isolation, amino acid composition and terminal amino acid residues of the vasoactive octacosapeptide from chicken intestine. Partial purification of chicken secretin. *FEBS Lett.*, 47:284–289.

57. Ondetti, M., Sheehan, J. T., and Bodanszky, M. (1968): Synthesis of gastrointestinal hormones. *International Symposium on the Pharmacology of Hormonal Peptides*, Milan, 1967, edited by N. Back, L. Martini, and R. Paoletti, pp. Plenum Press, New York, 1968.

58. Osnes, M., Hanssen, L. E., Flaten, O., and Myren, J. (1978): Exocrine pancreatic secretion and immunoreactive secretin (IRS) release after intraduodenal instillation of bile in man. *Gut*, 19(3): 180–184.

59. Pelletier, M. J., Chayvialle, J. A., and Minaire, Y. (1978): Uneven and transient secretin release after a liquid test meal. *Gastroenterology*, 75(6):1124–1132.

60. Petersen, H., Solomon, T., and Grossman, M. I. (1978): Effect of chronic pentagastrin, cholecystokinin, and secretin on pancreas of rats. *Am. J. Physiol.*, 234(3):E286–E293.

61. Polak, J. M., Coulling, I., Bloom, S., and Pearse, A. G. E. (1971): Immunofluorescent localization of secretin and enteroglucagon in human intestinal mucosa. *Scand. J. Gastroenterol.*, 6:739–744.

62. Rayford, P. L., Curtis, P. J., Fender, H. R., and Thompson, J. C. (1976): Plasma levels of secretin in man and dogs: validation of a secretin radioimmunoassay. *Surgery*, 79:658–665.

63. Rayford, P. L., Konturek, S. J., and Thompson, J. C. (1978): Effect of duodenal fat on plasma levels of gastrin and secretin and on gastric acid responses to gastric and intestinal meals in dogs. *Gastroenterology*, 75:773–777.

64. Rhodes, R. A., Tai, H.-H., and Chey, W. Y. (1976): Observations on plasma secretin levels by radioimmunoassay in response to duodenal acidification and to a meat meal in humans. *Am. J. Dig. Dis.*, 21:873–879.

65. Rhodes, R. A., Tai, H.-H., and Chey, W. Y. (1978): Impairment of secretin release in celiac sprue. *Am. J. Dig. Dis.*, 23(9): 833–839.

66. Rufener, C., Amherdt, M., Baetens, D., Yanaihara, N., and Orci, L. (1976): Immunofluorescent localization of secretin in pancreatic monolayer culture. *Histochemistry*, 47:171–173.

67. Schaffalitzky de Muckadell, O. B., and Fahrenkrug, J. (1977): Radioimmunoassay of secretin in plasma. *Scand. J. Clin. Lab. Invest.*, 37(2):155–162.

68. Schaffalitzky de Muckadell, O. B., and Fahrenkrug, J. (1978): Secretion pattern of secretin in man: regulation by gastric acid. *Gut*, 19:812–818.

69. Schaffalitzky de Muckadell, O. B., Fahrenkrug, J., Matzen, P., Rune, S. J., and Worning, H. (1979): Physiological significance of secretin in the pancreatic bicarbonate secretion. II. Pancreatic bicarbonate response to a physiological increase in plasma secretin concentration. *Scand. J. Gastroenterol.*, 14:85–90.

70. Schaffalitzky de Muckadell, O. B., Fahrenkrug, J., and Rune, S. J. (1979): Physiological significance of secretin in the pancreatic bicarbonate secretion. I. Responsiveness of the secretin-releasing system in the upper duodenum. *Scand. J. Gastroenterol.*, 14:79–83.

71. Schaffalitzky de Muckadell, O. B., Fahrenkrug, J., Watt-Boolsen, S., and Worning, H. (1978): Pancreatic response and plasma secretin concentration during infusion of low dose secretin in man. *Scand. J. Gastroenterol.*, 13:305–311.

72. Schmitt, M. G., Jr., Soergel, K. H., Hensley, G. T., and Chey, W. Y. (1975): Watery diarrhea associated with pancreatic islet cell carcinoma. *Gastroenterology,* 69:206–216.

73. Scratcherd, T., Case, R. M., and Smith, P. A. (1975): A sensitive method for the biological assay of secretin and substances with 'secretin-like' activity in tissues and biological fluids. *Scand. J. Gastroenterol.,* 10:821–828.

74. Solomon, T. E., Petersen, H., Elashoff, J., and Grossman, M. I. (1978): Interaction of caerulein and secretin on pancreatic size and composition in rat. *Am. J. Physiol.,* 235(6):E714–E719.

75. Straus, E., Greenstein, A. J., and Yalow, R. S. (1975): Effect of secretin on release of heterogeneous forms of gastrin. *Gut.,* 16:999–1005.

76. Straus, E., Greenstein, R. J., and Yalow, R. S. (1978): Plasma-secretin in management of cimetidine therapy for Zollinger-Ellison syndrome. *Lancet,* 2:73–74.

77. Straus, E., Urbach, H.-J., and Yalow, R. S. (1975): Alcohol-stimulated secretion of immunoreactive secretin. *N. Engl. J. Med.,* 293:1031–1032.

78. Straus, E., and Yalow, R. S. (1977): Hypersecretinemia associated with marked basal hyperchlorhydria in man and dog. *Gastroenterology,* 72:992–994.

79. Straus, E., and Yalow, R. S. (1978): Immunoreactive secretin in gastrointestinal mucosa of several mammalian species. *Gastroenterology,* 75:401–404.

80. Tai, H.-H., and Chey, W. Y. (1978): Rapid extraction of secretin from plasma by XAD-2 resin and its application in the radioimmunoassay of secretin. *Anal. Biochem.,* 87:376–385.

81. Tatemoto, K., and Mutt, V. (1978): Chemical determination of polypeptide hormones. *Proc. Natl. Acad. Sci. U.S.A.,* 75:4115–4119.

82. Vagne, M., and Andre, C. (1971): The effect of secretin on gastric emptying in man. *Gastroenterology,* 60:421–424.

83. Valenzuela, J. E. (1976): Effect of intestinal hormones and peptides on intragastric pressure in dogs. *Gastroenterology,* 71:766–769.

84. Vatn, M. H., Berstad, A., and Myren, J. (1974): The effect of exogenous secretin and cholecystokinin (CCK) on pentagastrin-stimulated intrinsic factor (IF) secretion in man. *Scand. J. Gastroenterol.,* 9:313–317.

85. Vaysse, N., Bastie, M. J., Pascal, J. P., Roux, P., Martinel, C., Lacroix, A., and Ribet, A. (1975): Role of cholinergic mechanisms in the response to secretin of isolated canine pancreas. *Gastroenterology,* 69:1269–1277.

86. Walsh, J. H., and Grossman, M. I. (1975): Gastrin. *N. Engl. J. Med.,* 292:1324–1332.

87. Ward, A. S., and Bloom, S. R. (1975): Effect of vagotomy on secretin release in man. *Gut,* 16:951–956.

88. Windeck, R., Brown, E. M., Gardner, D. G., and Aurbach, G. D. (1978): Effect of gastrointestinal hormones on isolated bovine parathyroid cells. *Endocrinology,* 103(6):2020–2026.

89. Wingate, D. L., Pearce, E. A., Hutton, M., Dand, A., Thompson, H. H., and Wunsch, E. (1978): Quantitative comparison of the effects of cholecystokinin, secretin, and pentagastrin on gastrointestinal myoelectric activity in the conscious fasted dog. *Gut,* 19(7):593–601.

90. Yanaihara, N., Kubota, M., Sakagami, M., Sato, H., Mochizuki, T., Sakura, N., Hashimoto, T., and Yanaihara, C. (1977): Synthesis of phenolic group containing analogues of porcine secretin and their immunological properties. *J. Med. Chem.,* 20:648–655.

91. Yanaihara, N., Sato, H., Kubota, M., Sakagami, M., Hashimoto, T., Yanaihara, C., Yamaguchi, K., Zeze, F., Abe, K., and Kaneko, T. (1976): Radioimmunoassay for secretin using Nα-tyrosylsecretin and [Tyr¹]-secretin. *Endocrinol., Jpn.,* 23(1):87–90.

VASOACTIVE INTESTINAL POLYPEPTIDE

Structure

Vasoactive intestinal polypeptide (VIP) was isolated from hog intestinal extracts after identification of its vasoactive properties in a side fraction obtained during the purification of secretin, and the complete amino acid sequence was determined by Mutt and Said (57). Synthetic VIP was prepared and found to have full biological potency (11). There are a large number of amino acid residue identities in the first 27 residues of VIP, secretin, glucagon, and gastric inhibitory peptide (GIP). The structural similarities can be appreciated by inspection of Table 5. Of the four peptides in this "family," VIP has the greatest number of unique residues (15), followed by GIP (10), secretin (8), and glucagon (7). In the first 16 positions secretin and glucagon have 2 and 4 unique amino acid residues, respectively, whereas VIP has 7 and GIP has 8. All four peptides differ at positions 17 and 19, but only VIP differs from the others at position 18. In positions 20 through 27 VIP and secretin have 5 and 4 unique residues, respectively, whereas glucagon has only one and GIP none. VIP differs completely from the other three peptides in the sequence from position 15 through 22. A peptide similar to porcine VIP has been isolated from chicken intestine and found to differ in 4 amino acid residues (58). Larger or smaller forms of mammalian VIP have not been characterized, but evidence has been obtained for the existence of forms that differ in charge and can be separated by ion-exchange chromatography (19,20).

Biological Actions

Numerous biological responses have been produced by injection or infusion of VIP *in vivo* or by incubation with tissues *in vitro*. The effects reported include actions on vascular, respiratory, and gastrointestinal smooth muscle, blood sugar, hormone release, gastrointestinal secretion, metabolism of liver and fat cells, and actions on the central nervous system. Many effects have been obtained after rapid intravenous injection of large doses of VIP under a variety of experimental conditions, making comparisons of potency difficult.

Cardiovascular and Pulmonary

VIP is a potent vasodilator and hypotensive agent (64). The vasodilatation is found in peripheral, splanchnic, and pulmonary vessels. It also has a positive ionotrophic effect on cardiac muscle and increases cardiac output. VIP relaxes tracheal and bronchial smooth muscle and increases respiratory minute volume. Infusion of VIP in man at doses of 200 and 400 pmol $kg^{-1}hr^{-1}$ produced cutaneous flushing and an increase in pulse rate without a change in blood pressure (46).

Metabolism

VIP stimulates both lipolysis and glycogenolysis (64). These effects are associated with stimulation of cyclic

TABLE 5. *Amino acid sequences of peptides structurally related to VIP (first 27 residues)*

Peptide	Amino acid sequence			
	1	10	20	27
GIP	Yᵃ A E G T F I S D Y S	I A M D K I	R Q Q D F V N W L	L -
Glucagon	H S Q G T F T S D Y S	K Y L D S R R	A Q D F V Q W L	M -
Secretin	H S D G T F T S E L S	R L R D S A R	L Q R L L Q F L	V #
VIP	H S D A V F T D N Y T	R L R K Q M A	V K K Y L N S I	L -

ᵃUnderlined residues differ from each of the other three peptides.

AMP in isolated fat and liver cells, and the VIP receptor in these cells appears to be distinct from either the secretin or glucagon receptor. VIP also caused stimulation of insulin release associated with hyperglycemia in cats and produced a slight increase in serum calcium (53). In the vascularly perfused cat pancreas VIP produced a glucose-dependent increase in insulin response and was even more potent as a stimulant of glucagon release, although the doses required were large (5 μg) (69). Similar effects were obtained in the isolated perfused porcine pancreas, but responses were obtained at VIP concentrations of 30 to 750 pM (38).

Gastrointestinal Secretion

VIP has effects on intestinal, gastric, pancreatic, and biliary secretion. The effect on intestinal secretion is of special interest because of its possible relationship to production of watery diarrhea found in patients with VIP-secreting tumors.

VIP, GIP, and glucagon were shown to produce secretion from intestinal loops in dogs (4). In conscious humans, VIP infused intravenously at doses of 100, 200, and 400 pmol kg^{-1}hr^{-1} caused a dose-dependent increase in transmucosal potential difference, and decreases in water and sodium absorption and chloride secretion from the jejunum (46). Plasma VIP concentrations during these infusions ranged from 40 to 160 pM. VIP resembles cholera toxin and prostaglandin E_1 in its ability to stimulate adenylate cyclase and cyclic AMP accumulation in intestinal epithelial cells (2,42,71), whereas several other peptides that decrease intestinal water and electrolyte absorption do not have similar effects on cyclic AMP. The stimulation of intestinal secretion and cyclic AMP production by VIP in rat intestine were inhibited by somatostatin (17). In anesthetized dogs, it was found that intestinal secretion caused by VIP was associated with decreased absorptive site blood flow and that most of the effects could be reversed by prior treatment with atropine (52).

The effects of VIP on gastric secretion were found to be similar to those of secretin in the inhibition of pentagastrin- and meal-stimulated acid secretion, stimulation of basal pepsin secretion, decrease in mucosal blood flow, and decrease in serum gastrin concentration, but VIP was only about 1/30 as potent on a molar basis (43). VIP differed from secretin in that it was a more effective inhibitor of histamine-stimulated acid secretion and caused decreased pepsin secretion during the concurrent infusion of pentagastrin.

Secretin and VIP have 8 amino acid identities in the first 14 positions in the amino terminal portions of the two molecules, and both cause stimulation of pancreatic water and bicarbonate secretion. However, the maximal responses achieved with VIP in dog and humans are only 15 to 20% as great as the maximal responses to secretin. In the cat VIP is a full agonist (23,45), but the potency is only about 1/15 that of secretin. *In vitro* studies with isolated pancreatic acini and acinar cells have revealed that both VIP and secretin stimulate cellular cyclic AMP content but that each has a separate high-affinity receptor and that the affinity of VIP for the high-affinity secretin receptor is only about 1% (see section on secretin). In the turkey it was found that both porcine VIP and chicken VIP were much more potent stimulants of pancreatic volume secretion than either porcine secretin or chicken secretin, suggesting that VIP may have a more important role than secretin in regulating avian pancreatic secretion (21).

Gastrointestinal Motility

The usual effect of VIP on gastrointestinal smooth muscle is relaxation. Graded doses of VIP produced graded decreases in opossum lower esophageal sphincter pressure, and this effect was not antagonized by tetrodotoxin or by adrenergic antagonists (61). Inhibition of the force of contraction of antral smooth muscle is produced by VIP (56), and the peptide also causes relaxation of the upper stomach *in vivo* (26). VIP also decreases basal and CCK-stimulated tension of guinea pig gallbladder smooth muscle but has no effect on the response to acetylcholine (63,76). In the opossum duodenal muscle, VIP stimulated contraction of longitudinal muscle but inhibited contraction of circular muscle

(3). In conscious rats, VIP markedly decreased transit of a test substance through the small intestine (35).

Other Effects

VIP increases blood flow to the salivary glands in dogs but does not stimulate salivary secretion (72). This effect is not inhibited by atropine. Vasodilatation of the small intestine and colon has been observed during infusion or endogenous release of VIP (26).

Several effects have been reported in the pituitary and central nervous system. Central or peripheral administration of VIP in rats caused release of prolactin that was partially inhibited by naloxone and L-DOPA (40). Ventricular injections of VIP caused release of prolactin, growth hormone, and LH, whereas no stimulation was found during *in vitro* incubation of pituitary tissue with the peptide (78). Injection into the third ventricle also produced hyperthermia in cats (18). Iontophoresis of VIP onto deep cortical motor neurons in rat brain caused excitation that was comparable to the response to substance P (59). Stimulation of adenylate cyclase was found in homogenates of cortical areas of rat brain but not in homogenates of brainstem (13). Specific binding of labeled VIP to receptors in rat brain membranes has been demonstrated (75). These receptors appeared to consist of a single class of high-affinity sites with a K_D of 1 nM and were densest in synaptasomal fractions from cerebral cortex, hippocampus, striatum, and thalamus.

Structure-Activity Relationships

Only the 28 amino acid peptide has been purified from tissues and examined for biological effects, but several synthetic fragments have been prepared and tested in several biological systems. When the C-terminal fragments containing 11, 14, 15, and 22 residues and the N-terminal hexapeptide were compared with the natural and synthetic whole peptide, it was found that the 22 amino acid C-terminal fragment retained about 5 to 10% potency for vasodilatation, tracheal relaxation, and stomach relaxation compared with the whole molecule whereas shorter fragments had little activity (10). Carboxyl terminal fragments of VIP up to the 14–28 fragment had no detectable activity on pentagastrin-stimulated gastric secretion (54). The N-terminal decapeptide had 1:500 potency as a vasodilator compared with the whole molecule (12). When the aspartic acid residue in position 15 of secretin 5–27 fragment was replaced by lysine, which occupies this position in VIP, the analogue showed increased VIP-like activity on smooth muscle and greater affinity for the high-affinity pancreatic VIP receptors than the similar secretin fragment (12).

Distribution

VIP originally was felt to be located in gut endocrine-type cells, but most recent immunohistochemical and extraction data are consistent with a purely neural localization in the gut. VIP also is distributed throughout the brain and in peripheral nerves outside the gut.

Larsson and co-workers (51) first demonstrated convincingly that VIP was localized to peripheral neurons in the gut and also was present in the brain, where it was found in cerebrovascular nerves (49). It was found in nerve fibers and cell bodies throughout the gut, and radioimmunoassay of gut muscle layers revealed concentrations equal to or higher than those found in mucosa plus submucosa. It was suggested that these nerves were intrinsic to the gut since neither vagotomy nor sympathectomy reduced their number. It was shown by electron microscopic immunocytochemistry that VIP granules were present in the terminals of p-type neurons in the colon (48). VIP-containing nerves were found to be abundant in the gallbladder wall (74), in the pancreas (50), and were especially abundant in the region of sphincters including the gastroesophageal junction, pylorus, sphincter of Oddi, and the openings of the ureters, urethra, and vas deferens (1). One group found immunoreactive VIP in cells in the gut mucosa and pancreas that were felt most likely to be D_1 cells (15), but the antiserum used was not completely characterized. Another group initially reported similar findings (60) but later found immunoreactive VIP in both cells and nerves (14) and most recently reported that VIP immunoreactivity in human and rat pancreas was localized entirely to nerve fibers and cell bodies when an antibody with C-terminal specificity was employed (5). They suggested that apparent demonstration of VIP immunoreactivity in endocrine-type cells was due to N-terminal specificity of antibodies used to demonstrate these cells and that there was cross-reactivity with other peptides having similar amino terminal structure. A comparison of immunoreactive VIP measured by radioimmunoassay in hamster intestine epithelial cells and remaining tissue revealed that the cells contained very little peptide and that the remaining tissue had a high concentration, consistent with a completely neural origin (32).

VIP-containing cell bodies and nerve fibers were found to be dense in the celiac-superior mesenteric and the inferior mesenteric sympathetic ganglia (36), and VIP-like immunoreactivity was found in cloned cell lines derived from neuroblastoma and astrocytoma (66). Further evidence that VIP neurons are intrinsic to the gut was obtained when it was shown that nerve fibers were maintained in small intestine organ cultures (70). VIP-containing nerve fibers originating in the guinea pig cecum appear to be derived almost entirely from the submucous plexus, but provide a dense innervation to the myenteric plexus and interact closely with other nerve fibers containing substance P (39).

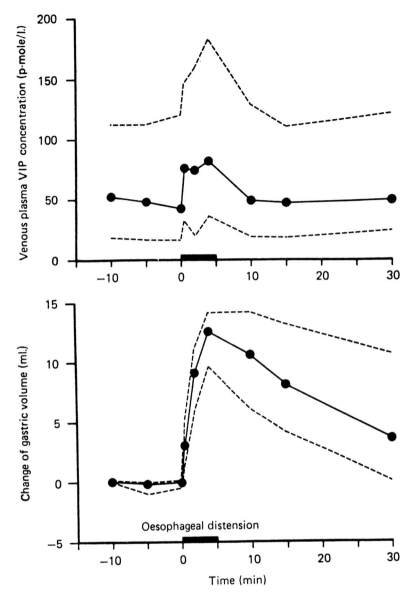

FIG. 6. Increase in gastric volume, indicating relaxation of gastric smooth muscle, and corresponding increase in regional plasma VIP concentration caused by balloon distension of the esophagus. From Fahrenkrug et al. (28).

In the central nervous system, VIP nerve bodies and plexuses are especially dense in parts of the neocortex, in subcortical limbic nuclei, and in some hypothalamic nuclei (31). By radioimmunoassay, all regions of the brain and spinal cord contain VIP, and concentrations are especially high in cerebral cortex and hippocampus (30). High concentrations also were reported in the neurohypophysis and pars intermedia (77). The presence of a VIP-containing pathway was found that appeared to link the amygdaloid complex with the hypothalamus (62). Purification of brain homogenates revealed that VIP activity increased with purification of the synaptosomal fractions and that the peptide could be released by a calcium-dependent mechanism with increased potassium concentrations (34).

Measurement

Bioassays for VIP have been based on smooth muscle relaxation and hypotensive effects, but none can be con-

sidered completely specific (26). Radioimmunoassays have been developed and a few appear to be sensitive enough to permit measurement of VIP concentrations in normal human plasma (16,29,55). The median basal VIP concentrations in normal human subjects were found to be quite low: 1.3, 1.7, and 7.3 pM, respectively. Other assays which employed less sensitive antisera have yielded higher values, but these have often not been corrected for nonspecific plasma effects. Most antisera used for VIP radioimmunoassay are specific for the C-terminus or midportion of the molecule, but varying degrees of cross-reactivity with the N-terminal portion have been reported (19).

Metabolism

During and after constant intravenous infusion of porcine VIP in humans, the disappearance half-time was found to be about 1 min, the clearance rate 9 ml

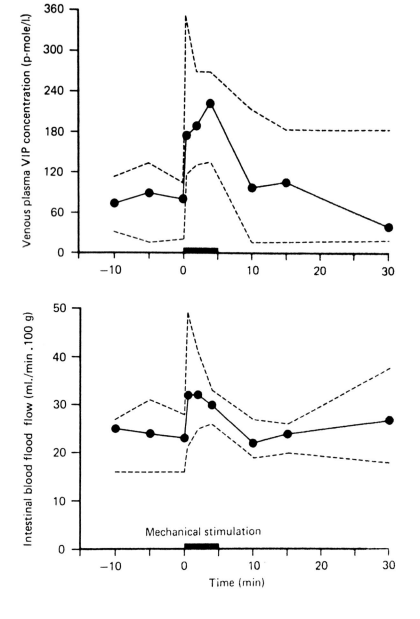

FIG. 7. Simultaneous increase in intestinal blood flow and regional plasma VIP concentration during mechanical stimulation of the mucosa of an intestinal segment. From Fahrenkrug et al. (28).

$kg^{-1}min^{-1}$, and the apparent volume of distribution 14 ml kg^{-1} (22). A significant role for hepatic inactivation was suggested by some studies based on comparison of portal and systemic infusions (24,41), partially confirmed in another study (44), but not supported in another study in conscious dogs with portal-vena caval transposition (73). In this study the disappearance half-time was 3.1 min and was not significantly different after portal or systemic infusions of VIP.

Release

Ingestion of a normal meal in humans did not cause a significant increase in peripheral concentrations of VIP (55), but intraduodenal instillation of hydrochloric acid caused an increase of about 5 pM (7,16). In another study, HCl, fat, and ethanol caused similar increases in plasma VIP in humans, but amino acids, glucose, saline, and mixed meals had no effect (68). Prolonged exercise and fasting but not short-term exercise also caused increases in plasma VIP (33).

Release of VIP from nerves was suggested by the observation that electrical vagal stimulation in pigs caused increased portal and peripheral concentrations (67). This effect was not inhibited by atropine. In calves with cut splanchnic nerves, stimulation of the peripheral ends of the thoracic vagus nerves caused significant increases in arterial and intestinal lymph VIP concentrations (25). In a more extensive study of neural release of VIP, it was shown that neither atropine nor beta-adrenergic blocking agents inhibited VIP release caused by vagus nerve stimulation, but the response was blocked completely by hexamethonium and was enhanced by alpha-adrenergic blockade and by splanchnicotomy (27). VIP also could be released by intra-arterial infusion of acetylcholine but this stimulation was abolished by atropine. Splanchnic nerve stimulation inhibited the response to vagal stimulation and also decreased basal VIP concentrations. These findings suggest that VIP release is due to stimulation of noncholinergic postganglionic vagal fibers by activation of nicotinic receptors and that the final response is modulated by an inhibitory action of alpha-adrenergic fibers.

Relationship with Physiologic Events

Although no physiologic effect of VIP can be said to be established with certainty, experiments performed by Fahrenkrug and co-workers provide good evidence for several possible events mediated by neural release of VIP in the gastrointestinal mucosa and porcine pancreas. Gastric relaxation produced by stimulation of high-threshold vagal fibers to the stomach or by balloon distension of the lower esophagus was associated with a significant increase in venous plasma VIP in blood draining the gastric corpus (28) (Fig. 6). Intestinal vasodilatation produced by mechanical stimulation of the small intestinal mucosa also was accompanied by an increase in venous VIP from the same area (Fig. 7). Finally, stimulation of pelvic nerves produced colonic vasodilatation and local VIP release and both effects were resistant to atropine. All of these effects can be mimicked by local intraarterial infusions of VIP, but specific proof that they are mediated by endogenous VIP will await demonstration that they can be inhibited by some agent that blocks the peripheral effects of VIP specifically. Evidence also has been presented that VIP may mediate the atropine-resistant vagal stimulation of pancreatic bicarbonate secretion in the pig (37). This stimulation was accompanied by increased VIP concentration in pancreatic venous blood (26). Atropine inhibited the pancreatic protein stimulation but not the bicarbonate response during vagal activation, whereas simultaneous stimulation of splanchnic nerves inhibited both responses. These effects may be specific to the pig, since vagal stimulation in dogs causes secretion of protein-rich pancreatic juice rather than bicarbonate. However, there may be a morphological counterpart to the species difference, since VIP-containing nerves appear to innervate acinar cells directly in dogs but to innervate intrapancreatic ganglion cells in the pig (50).

Conditions of Excess or Deficiency

There have been no descriptions of VIP deficiency, but there is strong evidence that overproduction of VIP by endocrine or neuroendocrine tumors may account for many of the manifestations of the pancreatic cholera syndrome (79). Most patients with this syndrome have increased plasma VIP concentrations, and VIP can be

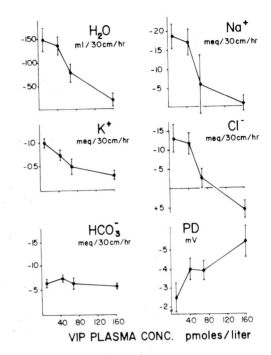

FIG. 8. Relationship between plasma VIP concentration and water and ion movement and PD in human jejunum during intravenous infusion of exogenous VIP (46).

demonstrated in high concentrations in tumors (8,65). These tumors usually originate in the pancreas but may originate in neural crest tissue. Although there is some controversy about the presence of increased plasma VIP concentrations in all patients with this disorder (6,47), the biological actions of this peptide could explain several features of the disease including watery diarrhea due to intestinal secretion, decreased gastric acid secretion, dilatation of the gallbladder, and episodes of flushing. Intravenous infusions of VIP at rates sufficient to produce plasma VIP concentrations similar to those usually reported in patients with pancreatic cholera markedly inhibited intestinal sodium and water absorption and caused net secretion of chloride (46) (Fig. 8). However, these infusions also produced cutaneous flushing that was more pronounced than the occasional flushing reported in patients with pancreatic cholera. Further evidence that VIP is involved in this disease is offered by observations that resection of these tumors alleviates the diarrhea when plasma VIP concentrations return to normal and that in some patients chemotherapy with antitumor agents or steroids has caused parallel decreases in plasma VIP and reduction of diarrhea.

References

1. Alumets, J., Fahrenkrug, J., Hakanson, R., Schaffalitzky de Muckadell, O., Sundler, F., and Uddman, R. (1979): A rich VIP nerve supply is characteristic of sphincters. *Nature*, 280:155–156.
2. Amiranoff, B., Laburthe, M., Dupont, C., and Rosselin, G. (1978): Characterization of a vasoactive intestinal peptide-sensi-

tive adenylate cyclase in rat intestinal epithelial cell membranes. *Biochem. Biophys. Acta,* 544(3):474–481.

3. Anuras, S., and Cooke, A. R. (1978): Effects of some gastrointestinal hormones on two muscle layers of duodenum. *Am. J. Physiol.,* 234(1):E60–E63.

4. Barbezat, G. O., and Grossman, M. I. (1971): Intestinal secretion: stimulation by peptides. *Science,* 174:422–424.

5. Bishop, A. E., Polak, J. M., Green, I. C., Bryant, M. G., and Bloom, S. R. (1980): The location of VIP in the pancreas of man and rat. *Diabetologia,* 18:73–78.

6. Bloom, S. R., and Gardner, J. D. (1978): The VIP controversy, Stephen R. Bloom vs Jerry D. Gardner. *Dig. Dis.,* 23:370–376.

7. Bloom, S. R., Mitchell, S. J., Greenburg, G. R., Christofides, N., Domschke, W., Domschke, S., Mitznegg, P., and Demling, L. (1978): Release of VIP, secretin and motilin after duodenal acidification in man. *Acta Hepatogastroenterol. (Stuttg.),* 25(5)365–368.

8. Bloom, S. R., Polak, J. M., and Pearse, A. G. E., (1973): Vasoactive intestinal peptide and watery-diarrhoea syndrome. *Lancet,* 2:14–16.

9. Bodanszky, M., Henes, J. B., Yiotakis, A. E., and Said, S. I. (1977): Synthesis and pharmacological properties of the N-terminal decapeptide of the vasoactive intestinal peptide (VIP). *J. Med. Chem.,* 20:1461–1464.

10. Bodanszky, M., Klausner, Y. S., and Said, S. I. (1973): Biological activities of synthetic peptides corresponding to fragments of and to the entire sequence of the vasoactive intestinal peptide. *Proc. Natl. Acad. Sci. USA,* 70:382–384.

11. Bodanszky, M., Klausner, Y. S., Yang Lin, C., Mutt, V., and Said, S. I. (1974): Synthesis of the vasoactive intestinal peptide (VIP). *J. Am. Chem. Soc.,* 96:4973–4978.

12. Bodanszky, M., and Natarajan, S. (1978): Synthesis and some pharmacological properties of the 23-peptide 15-lysine-secretin-(5-27). Special role of the residue in position 15 in biological activity of the vasoactive intestinal polypeptide. *J. Med. Chem.,* 21:1171–1173.

13. Borghi, C., Nicosia, S., Giachetti, A., and Said, S. I. (1979): Vasoactive intestinal polypeptide (VIP) stimulates adenylate cyclase in selected areas of rat brain. *Life Sci.* 24:65–70.

14. Bryant, M. G., Polak, J. M., Modlin, I., Bloom, S. R., Albuquerque, R. H., and Pearse, A. G. E. (1976): Possible dual role for vasoactive intestinal peptide as gastrointestinal hormone and neurotransmitter substance. *Lancet,* 1:991–993.

15. Buffa, R., Capella, C., Solcia, E., Frigerio, B., and Said, S. I. (1977): Vasoactive intestinal peptide (VIP) cells in the pancreas and gastro-intestinal mucosa. *Histochemistry,* 50:217–227.

16. Burhol, P. G., Lygren, I., and Waldum, H. L. (1978): Radioimmunoassay of vasoactive intestinal polypeptide in plasma. *Scand. J. Gastroenterol.,* 13:807–813.

17. Carter, R. F., Bitar, K. N., Zfass, A. M., and Makhlouf, G. M. (1978): Inhibition of VIP-stimulated intestinal secretion and cyclic AMP production by somatostatin in the rat. *Gastroenterology,* 74(4):726–730.

18. Clark, W. G., Lipton, J. M., and Said, S. I. (1978): Hyperthermic responses to vasoactive intestinal polypeptide (VIP) injected into the third cerebral ventricle of cats. *Neuropharmacology,* 17:883–885.

19. Dimaline, R., and Dockray, G. J. (1978): Multiple immunoreactive forms of vasoactive intestinal peptide in human colonic mucosa. *Gastroenterology,* 75:387–392.

20. Dimaline, R., and Dockray, G. J. (1979): Molecular variants of vasoactive intestinal polypeptide in dog, rat and hog. *Life Sci.,* 25:1893–1900.

21. Dimaline, R., and Dockray, G. J. (1979): Potent stimulation of the avian exocrine pancreas by porcine and chicken vasoactive intestinal peptide *J. Physiol.,* 294:153–163.

22. Domschke, S., Domschke, W., Bloom, S. R., Mitznegg, P., Mitchell, S. J., Lux, G., and Strunz, U. (1978): Vasoactive intestinal peptide in man: Pharmacokinetics, metabolic and circulatory effects. *Gut,* 19:1049–1053.

23. Domschke, S., Domschke, W., Rosch, W., Konturek, S. J., Sprugel, W., Mitznegg, P., Wunsch, E., and Demling, L. (1977): Vasoactive intestinal peptide: a secretin-like partial agonist for pancreatic secretion in man. *Gastroenterology,* 73:478–480.

24. Ebeid, A. M., Escourrou, J., Soeters, P. B., Murray, P., and

25. Edwards, A. V., Bircham, P. M. M., Mitchell, S. J., and Bloom, S. R. (1978): Changes in the concentration of vasoactive intestinal peptide in intestinal lymph in response to vagal stimulation in the calf. *Experientia,* 34:1186–1187.

26. Fahrenkrug, J. (1979): Vasoactive intestinal polypeptide: measurement, distribution and putative neurotransmitter function. *Digestion,* 19:149–169.

27. Fahrenkrug, J., Galbo, H., Holst, J. J., and Schaffalitzky de Muckadell, O. B. (1978): Influence of the autonomic nervous system on the release of vasoactive intestinal polypeptide from the porcine gastrointestinal tract. *J. Physiol.,* 280:405–422.

28. Fahrenkrug, J., Haglund, U., Jodal, M., Lundgren, O., Olbe, L., and Schaffalitzky de Muckadell, O. B. (1978): Nervous release of vasoactive intestinal polypeptide in the gastrointestinal tract of cats: possible physiological implications. *J. Physiol.,* 284:291–305.

29. Fahrenkrug, J., and Schaffalitzky de Muckadell, O. B. (1977): Radioimmunoassay of vasoactive intestinal polypeptide (VIP) in plasma. *J. Lab. Clin. Med.,* 89:1379–1388.

30. Fahrenkrug, J., and Schaffalitzky de Muckadell, O. B. (1978): Distribution of vasoactive intestinal polypeptide (VIP) in the porcine central nervous system. *J. Neurochem.,* 31:1445–1451.

31. Fuxe, K., Hokfelt, T., Said, S. I., and Mutt, V. (1977): Vasoactive intestinal polypeptide and the nervous system: immunohistochemical evidence for localization in central and peripheral neurons, particularly intracortical neurons of the cerebral cortex. *Neurosci. Lett.* 5:241–246.

32. Gaginella, T. S., Mekhjian, H. S., and O'Dorisio, T. M. (1978): Vasoactive intestinal peptide: quantification by radioimmunoassay in isolated cells, mucosa, and muscle of the hamster intestine. *Gastroenterology,* 74(4):718–721.

33. Galbo, H., Hilsted, J., Fahrenkrug, J., and Schaffalitzky de Muckadell, O. B. (1979): Fasting and prolonged exercise increase vasoactive intestinal polypeptide (VIP) in plasma. *Acta Physiol. Scand.,* 105(3):374–377.

34. Giachetti, A., Said, S. I., Reynolds, R. C., and Koniges, F. C. (1977): Vasoactive intestinal polypeptide in brain: localization in and release from isolated nerve terminals. *Proc. Natl. Acad. Sci. U.S.A.,* 74:3424–3428.

35. Gustavsson, S., Johansson, H., Lundqvist, G., and Nilsson, F. (1977): Effects of vasoactive intestinal peptide and pancreatic polypeptide on small bowel propulsion in the rat. *Scand. J. Gastroenterol.,* 12(8):993–997.

36. Hokfelt, T., Elfvin, L.-G., Schultzberg, M., Fuxe, K., Said, S. I., Mutt, V., and Goldstein, M. (1977): Immunohistochemical evidence of vasoactive intestinal polypeptide-containing neurons and nerve fibers in sympathetic ganglia. *Neuroscience,* 2:885–896.

37. Holst, J. J., Schaffalitzky de Muckadell, O. B., and Fahrenkrug, J. (1979): Nervous control of pancreatic exocrine secretion in pigs. *Acta Physiol. Scand.,* 105:33–51.

38. Jensen, S. L., Fahrenkrug, J., Holst, J. J., Nielsen, O. V., and Schaffalitzky de Muckadell, O. B. (1978): Secretory effect of VIP on isolated perfused porcine pancreas. *Am. J. Physiol.,* 235(4): E387–391.

39. Jessen, K. R., Polak, J. M., Van Noorden, S., Bloom, S. R., and Burnstock, G. (1980): Peptide-containing neurones connect the two ganglionated plexuses of the enteric nervous system. *Nature,* 283:391–393.

40. Kato, Y., Iwasaki, Y., Iwasaki, J., Abe, H., Yanaihara, N., and Imura, H. (1978): Prolactin release by vasoactive intestinal polypeptide in rats. *Endocrinology,* 103(2):554–558.

41. Kitamura, S., Yoshida, T., and Said, S. I. (1975): Vasoactive intestinal polypeptide: Inactivation in liver and potentiation in lung of anesthetized dogs (38469). *Proc. Soc. Exp. Biol. Med.,* 148:25–29.

42. Klaeveman, H. L., Conlon, T. P., Levy, A. G., and Gardner, J. D. (1975): Effects of gastrointestinal hormones on adenylate cyclase activity in human jejunal mucosa. *Gastroenterology,* 68:667–675.

43. Konturek, S. J., Dembinski, A., Thor, P., and Krol, R. (1976): Comparison of vasoactive intestinal peptide (VIP) and secretin in gastric secretion and mucosal blood flow. *Pfluegers Arch.,* 361:175–181.

44. Konturek, S. J., Domschke, S., Domschke, W., Wunsch, E., and

Fischer, J. E. (1978): Hepatic inactivation of vasoactive intestinal peptide in man and dog. *Ann. Surg.,* 188:28–33.

Demling, L. (1977): Comparison of pancreatic responses to portal and systemic secretin and VIP in cats. *Am. J. Physiol.,* 232(2): E156-158.

45. Konturek, S. J., Pucher, A., and Radecki, T. (1976): Comparison of vasoactive intestinal peptide and secretin in stimulation of pancreatic secretion. *J. Physiol.,* 255:497-509.

46. Krejs, G. J., Fordtran, J. S., Bloom, S. R., Fahrenkrug, J., Schaffalitzky de Muckadell, O. B., Fischer, J. E., Humphrey, C. S., O'Dorisio, T. M., Said, S. I., Walsh, J. H., and Shulkes, A. A. (1980): Effect of VIP infusion on water and ion transport in the human jejunum. *Gastroenterology,* 78:722-727.

47. Krejs, G. J., Walsh, J. H., Morawaski, S. G., and Fordtran, J. S., Intractable diarrhea: Intestinal perfusion studies and plasma VIP concentrations in patients with pancreatic cholera syndrome and surreptitious ingestion of laxatives and diuretics. *Am. J. Dig. Dis.,* 22:280-292.

48. Larsson, L.-I. (1977): Ultrastructural localization of a new neuronal peptide (VIP). *Histochemistry,* 54:173-176.

49. Larsson, L.-I., Edvinsson, L., Fahrenkrug, J., Hakanson, R., Owman, C. H., Schaffalitzky de Muckadell, O., and Sundler, F. (1976): Immunohistochemical localization of a vasodilatory polypeptide (VIP) in cerebrovascular nerves. *Brain Res.,* 113:400-404.

50. Larsson, L.-I., Fahrenkrug, J., Holst, J. J., and Schaffalitzky de Muckadell, O. B. (1978): Innervation of the pancreas by vasoactive intestinal polypeptide (VIP) immunoreactive nerves. *Life Sci.,* 22:773-780.

51. Larsson, L.-I., Fahrenkrug, J., Schaffalitzky de Muckadell, O., Sundler, F., Hakanson, R., and Rehfeld, J. F. (1976): Localization of vasoactive intestinal polypeptide (VIP) to central and peripheral neurons. *Proc. Natl. Acad. Sci. USA,* 73:3197-3200.

52. Mailman, D. (1978): Effects of vasoactive intestinal polypeptide on intestinal absorption and blood flow. *J. Physiol.,* 279:121-132.

53. Makhlouf, G. M., and Said, S. I. (1975): The effect of vasoactive intestinal peptide (VIP) on digestive and hormonal function. In: *Gastrointestinal Hormones, A Symposium,* edited by J. C. Thompson. University of Texas Press, Austin.

54. Makhlouf, G. M., Zfass, A. M., Said, S. I., and Schebalin, M. (1978): Effects of synthetic vasoactive intestinal peptide (VIP), secretin and their partial sequences on gastric secretion (40097). *Proc. Soc. Exp. Biol. Med.,* 157:565-568.

55. Mitchell, S. J., and Bloom, S. R. (1978): Measurement of fasting and postprandial plasma VIP in man. *Gut,* 19:1043-1048.

56. Morgan, K. G., Schmalz, P. F., and Szurszewski, J. H. (1978): The inhibitory effects of vasoactive intestinal polypeptide on the mechanical and electrical activity of canine antral smooth muscle. *J. Physiol.,* 282:437-450.

57. Mutt, V., and Said, S. I. (1974): Structure of the porcine vasoactive intestinal octacosapeptide. The amino-acid sequence. Use of Kallikrein in its determination. *Eur. J. Biochem.,* 42:581-589.

58. Nilsson, A. (1975): Structure of the vasoactive intestinal octacosapeptide from chicken intestine. The amino acid sequence. *FEBS Lett.,* 60:322-326.

59. Phillis, J. W., Kirkpatrick, J. R., and Said, S. I. (1978): Vasoactive intestinal polypeptide excitation of central neurons. *Can. J. Physiol. Pharmacol.,* 1978, 56:337-340.

60. Polak, J. M., Pearse, A. G. E., Garaud, J.-C., and Bloom, S. R. (1974): Cellular localization of a vasoactive intestinal peptide in the mammalian and avian gastrointestinal tract. *Gut,* 15:720-724.

61. Rattan, S., Said, S. I., and Goyal, R. K. (1977): Effect of vasoactive intestinal polypeptide (VIP) on the lower esophageal sphincter pressure (LESP) (39740). *Proc. Soc. Exp. Biol. Med.,* 155:40-43.

62. Roberts, G. W., Woodhams, P. L., Bryant, M. G., Crow, T. J., Bloom, S. R., and Polak, J. M. (1980): VIP in the rat brain: evidence for a major pathway linking the amygdala and hypothalamus via the stria terminalis. *Histochemistry,* 65:103-119.

63. Ryan, J. P., and Ryave, S. (1978): Effect of vasoactive intestinal polypeptide on gallbladder smooth muscle in vitro. *Am. J. Physiol.,* 234(1):E44-E46.

64. Said, S. I. (1975): Vasoactive intestinal polypeptide (VIP): current status. In: *Gastrointestinal Hormones, A Symposium,* edited by J. C. Thompson, pp. 591-597. University of Texas Press, Austin.

65. Said, S. I., and Faloona, G. R. (1975): Elevated plasma and tissue levels of vasoactive intestinal polypeptide in the watery-diarrhea syndrome due to pancreatic, bronchogenic and other tumors. *N. Engl. J. Med.,* 293:155-160.

66. Said, S. I., and Rosenberg, R. N. (1976): Vasoactive intestinal polypeptide: abundant immunoreactivity in neural cell lines and normal nervous tissue. *Science,* 192:907-908.

67. Schaffalitzky de Muckadell, O. B., Fahrenkrug, J., and Holst, J. J. (1977): Release of vasoactive intestinal polypeptide (VIP) by electric stimulation of the vagal nerves. *Gastroenterology,* 72(2): 373-375.

68. Schaffalitzky de Muckadell, O. B., Fahrenkrug, J., Holst, J. J., and Lauritsen, K. B. (1977): Release of vasoactive intestinal polypeptide (VIP) by intraduodenal stimuli. *Scand. J. Gastroenterol.,* 12:793-799.

69. Schebalin, M., Said, S. I., and Makhlouf, G. M. (1977): Stimulation of insulin and glucagon secretion by vasoactive intestinal peptide. *Am. J. Physiol.,* 232(2):E197-E200.

70. Schultzberg, M., Dreyfus, C. F., Gershon, M. D., Hokfelt, T., Elde, R. P., Nilsson, G., Said, S., and Goldstein, M. (1978): VIP-, enkephalin-, substance P- and somatostatin-like immunoreactivity in neurons intrinsic to the intestine: immunohistochemical evidence from organotypic tissue cultures. *Brain Res.,* 155(2)239-248.

71. Schwartz, C. J., Kimberg, D. V., Sheerin, H. E., Field, M., and Said, S. I. (1974): Vasoactive intestinal peptide stimulation of adenylate cyclase and active electrolyte secretion in intestinal mucosa. *J. Clin. Invest.,* 54:536-544.

72. Shimizu, T., and Taira, N. (1979): Assessment of the effects of vasoactive intestinal peptide (VIP) on blood flow through and salivation of the dog salivary gland in comparison with those of secretin, glucagon and acetylcholine. *Br. J. Pharmacol.,* 65(4):683-687.

73. Strunz, U. T., Walsh, J. H., Bloom, S. R., Thompson, M. R., and Grossman, M. I. (1977): Lack of hepatic inactivation of canine vasoactive intestinal peptide. *Gastroenterology,* 73:768-771.

74. Sundler, F., Alumets, J., Hakanson, R., Ingemansson, S., Fahrenkrug, J., and Schaffalitzky de Muckadell, O. (1977): VIP innervation of the gallbladder. *Gastroenterology,* 72(6):1375-1377.

75. Taylor, D. P., and Pert, C. B. (1979): Vasoactive intestinal polypeptide: Specific binding to rat brain membranes. *Proc. Natl. Acad. Sci. U.S.A.,* 76:660-664.

76. Vagne, M., and Troitskaja, V. (1976): Effect of secretin, glucagon and VIP on gallbladder contraction. *Digestion,* 14:62-67.

77. Van Noorden, S., Polak, J. M., Bloom, S. R., and Bryant, M. G. (1979): Vasoactive intestinal polypeptide in the pituitary pars nervosa. *Neuropathol. Appl. Neurobiol.,* 5:149-153.

78. Vijayan, E., Samson, W. K., Said, S. I., and McCann, S. M. (1979): Vasoactive intestinal peptide: evidence for a hypothalamic site of action to release growth hormone, luteinizing hormone, and prolactin in conscious ovariectomized rats. *Endocrinology,* 104:53-57.

79. Walsh, J. H. (1978): Pancreatic cholera and related syndromes. In: *Gastrointestinal Disease, Ed. 2,* edited by M. H. Sleisenger and J. S. Fordtran, pp. 1496-1504. W. B. Saunders Co., Philadelphia.

GASTRIC INHIBITORY POLYPEPTIDE

Structure

Gastric inhibitory polypeptide (GIP) was isolated by Brown and co-workers (8) from partially purified porcine CCK and was identified by its inhibitory action on acid secretion from denervated canine gastric pouches during stimulation by pentagastrin. The complete amino acid sequence was published in 1971 (5,6). GIP is a linear chain containing 43 amino acid residues, with a molecular weight of 5,105. It is structurally related to porcine glucagon, with which it has 15 amino acid identities in the first 26 positions, and with porcine secretin, with which it has 9 amino acid identities in the first 26 positions (Tables 1 and 5).

Biological Actions

The major gastrointestinal actions of GIP are inhibition of gastric secretion and stimulation of intestinal secretion (7). GIP is a potent inhibitor of pentagastrin-stimulated acid and pepsin secretion from vagally denervated canine gastric pouches and a less potent inhibitor of histamine-stimulated secretion (33). GIP at high doses also is capable of inhibiting the acid response to insulin hypoglycemia from the innervated stomach. Because fat has been shown to cause release of GIP from the intestine, this peptide has been considered a prime candidate as a major "enterogastrone" that could cause the inhibition of acid secretion observed after ingestion of fat in humans and animals. However, recent evidence suggests that GIP is not likely to have a major function as an enterogastrone. In human subjects with intact stomachs, intravenous infusion of GIP produced only slight inhibition of pentagastrin-stimulated acid secretion when circulating concentrations of GIP were much higher than those achieved by ingestion of a meal or intraduodenal instillation of fat (28) (Fig. 9). In dogs with gastric fistulas, intraduodenal fat caused complete suppression of the acid secretory response to liver extract but caused only modest elevation in plasma GIP concentrations, whereas much higher elevations of plasma GIP during intravenous infusion of GIP caused only 40% inhibition of acid secretion (52).

GIP also inhibits water and electrolyte absorption in the small intestine. An exogenous dose of GIP that produced plasma GIP concentrations in the physiological range found after a meal in human subjects caused net secretion of chloride and reduced absorption of water and sodium in the jejunum (24).

Other gastrointestinal effects that have been observed during administration of exogenous GIP include inhibition of gastric motor activity in the dog (7), inhibition of basal and pentagastrin-stimulated lower esophageal sphincter pressure in cats (41), and reduction of sodium movement from lumen to interstitium in rabbit salivary glands (15).

The other major, and likely most important, biological effect of GIP is enhancement of pancreatic insulin release in the presence of raised concentrations of glucose. It has been suggested that GIP may function as an "incretin" and may be the substance responsible for increased glucose disposal and enhanced insulin responses obtained during intestinal absorption of glucose compared with intravenous administration of glucose (7). Brown has suggested that "glucose-dependent insulinotropic peptide" might be a better name for this substance than "gastric inhibitory polypeptide." When blood glucose was maintained at an increased concentration of 125 mg dl^{-1} by a glucose clamp technique in normal humans, oral administration of glucose produced simultaneous increases in plasma GIP and insulin that were closely correlated (2) (Fig. 10). When normoglycemia was maintained with intravenous insulin, no enhancement of endogenous insulin was caused by oral glucose except in subjects whose plasma glucose increased by 20 mg dl^{-1} or more. It was concluded that the effect of glucose-stimulated endogenous GIP to enhance endogenous insulin release was dependent on some degree of hyperglycemia but was not suppressed by exogenous insulin. This effect was considered likely to be physiological under conditions when blood sugar concentrations were increased. Similar experiments have been carried out during glucose clamping at low, normal, and high plasma glucose concentrations and have examined the effect of GIP released by fat, another GIP releasing substance, on plasma concentrations of insulin C-peptide and glucagon (49) (Fig. 11). Again it was found that consistent enhancement of insulin (C-peptide) was obtained only during hyperglycemic conditions. Plasma glucagon concentrations were not changed during any of the conditions and exogenous insulin did not appear to cause any inhibitory effect on fat-stimulated GIP release.

GIP also has been found to stimulate release of insulin from isolated rat islets (39) or pancreas (34) in a glucose-dependent fashion. In the isolated rat pancreas, GIP also was found to stimulate release of immunoreactive glucagon, but only when glucose concentrations were less than 5.5 mM. GIP also enhanced the stimulation of glucagon by arginine in the presence of low glucose concentrations. Similar results have been obtained in islet cultures (22). Very high concentrations of GIP

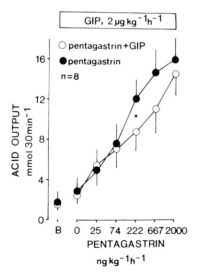

FIG. 9. Effect of GIP infusion on human gastric acid responses to graded doses of pentagastrin. B: basal. From Maxwell et al. (28).

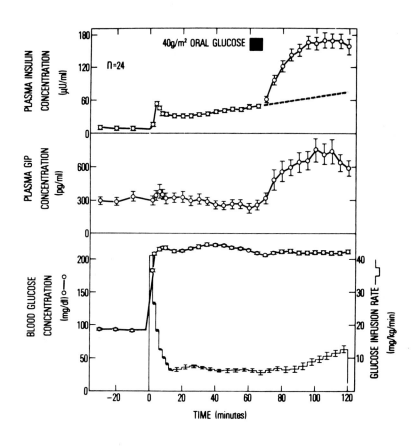

FIG. 10. Simultaneous enhancement of plasma insulin and GIP concentrations caused by administration of oral glucose in human subjects while blood glucose was maintained at a constant hyperglycemic concentration. From Anderson et al. (2).

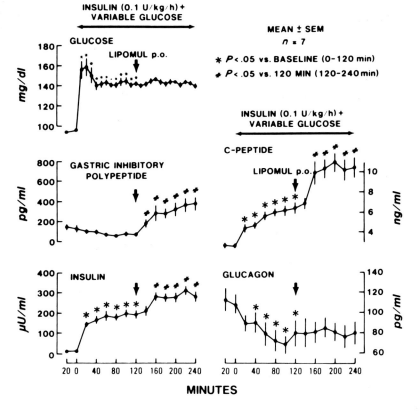

FIG. 11. Hormone responses during hyperglycemic clamp before and after Lipomul (67 g) ingestion. Similar enhancement of plasma insulin and GIP concentrations by fat ingestion in human subjects during constant hyperglycemia. From Verdonk et al. (49).

caused stimulation of insulin release without addition of glucose to the medium. High concentrations of GIP also have been found to cause stimulation of somatostatin release from the isolated perfused dog pancreas (25).

Structure-Activity Relationships

There have been no reports to date of successful synthesis of a peptide with the full acid-inhibitory activity of 43 amino acid GIP. It was reported that a synthetic preparation of the entire 43 amino acid sequence enhanced insulin release in rats and augmented insulin and glucagon secretion from isolated pancreatic islets, whereas the peptide sequences 1–28, 22–43, and 15–43 did not demonstrate these actions (44). The synthetic peptide composed of the 1–38 sequence of GIP was found to have full insulinotropic action but no effect on gastric secretion (30). Another group found that a peptide corresponding to positions 15 through 43 of GIP retained about one-fourth the acid-inhibiting activity of the entire natural molecule while fragments 1–28 and 26–43 were inactive (51). These results are not conclusive but suggest that most of the amino terminal sequence is necessary for insulinotropic action and that most of the C-terminal sequence is necessary for inhibition of gastric acid secretion.

Distribution

Highest concentrations of extractable immunoreactive GIP in canine tissues were found in the duodenum and jejunum, with lower concentrations in the gastric antrum and ileum and no detectable activity in the esophagus, fundus, colon, pancreas, or liver (31,36). This distribution is in agreement with immunocytochemical studies which demonstrated GIP to be located in the K cells of the small intestine of dogs, pigs, and humans (10). These cells are most abundant in the villi and upper crypts and have been identified by immune electron microscopy and found to contain electron-dense granules with a mean corrected diameter of 444 nm (9). There also is some immunocytochemical evidence that alpha cells of the pancreas and glucagon-containing cells of the gut also may contain a peptide with GIP-like immunoreactivity (1,43). Immunoreactive GIP has been detected in the intestine of the fetal rat at the 20th day of gestation, and the concentrations in the duodenum and remaining small intestine increased markedly during the first month of life (23).

Measurement

Suitable bioassays for quantitation of GIP in plasma or tissue extracts have not been reported, but specific radioimmunoassays have been developed that employ antibodies that do not cross-react with other structurally related peptides such as glucagon, secretin, and VIP (27, 29). These assays produced estimates of fasting GIP concentrations in humans of about 200 pg ml^{-1} and were not sensitive enough to detect concentrations below 100 pg ml^{-1} (20 pM) but easily detected increases after stimulation with mixed meals or food components including glucose and fat. More recently an assay has been developed that appears to be more sensitive than several other previous assays (38). With this assay, fasting normal human plasma GIP concentration averaged 9 pM and the peak concentration obtained after ingestion of glucose, fat, or a mixed meal was about 34 pM, compared with stimulated values of 250 to 300 pM reported by others (27,29). There is evidence from gel filtration studies of plasma combined with radioimmunoassay that immunoreactive GIP in the circulation consists of two major forms, one corresponding to 43 amino acid GIP with a molecular weight of approximately 5,000 and another larger form, and that both forms are increased after stimulation by a meal (7,38). Immunoreactive GIP appears to be relatively stable in plasma, and an enzyme inhibitor (aprotinin) did not appear to be necessary for preservation of immunoreactivity in plasma (38).

Metabolism

There is little information available concerning the clearance or metabolic rate of circulating GIP. The half-life of GIP in the circulation was reported informally to be 21 min (7). Basal and food-stimulated serum GIP concentrations were reported to be higher in uremic patients than in normal subjects, and the duration of the food-stimulated response was prolonged (32). Renal arteriovenous gradients also were demonstrated in anesthetized dogs during exogenous GIP infusion, with the maximum gradient being 39%, suggesting a role for the kidney in removal of GIP from the circulation.

Release

GIP is released by several components of normal meals in humans including oral but not intravenous glucose (11), emulsified fat (21), and intraduodenal but not intravenous mixed amino acids (45). Increased serum insulin concentrations were found during enteric administration of glucose or amino acids but not during administration of fat. Intraduodenal administration of a mixture of amino acids including arginine, histidine, isoleucine, leucine, lysine, and threonine caused significant GIP release in humans, whereas administration of a mixture containing methionine, phenylalanine, tryptophan, and valine produced no significant response (47). This study suggests that GIP is released by a different group of amino acids from those that cause most pronounced release of gastrin, CCK, and pancreatic polypeptide. The release of GIP in response to oral glucose in humans was exaggerated in patients with previous vagotomy and pyloroplasty, associated with an exaggerated early increase in plasma glucose that could be explained by enhanced gastric emptying, indicating that the vagus nerve is not an important mediator of GIP release (48). Intraduodenal acidification with hydrochloric acid did not cause release of immunoreactive GIP in the dog (7), but did release GIP in the rat and in humans (18,19).

It is possible that food-stimulated release of GIP is modulated by other gastrointestinal or pancreatic hormones. Exogenous glucagon depresses fasting serum GIP concentrations and markedly inhibits the response to a test meal in humans, similar to its effects on gastrin (16). It is not known whether this effect is exerted directly on the GIP-producing cells or indirectly through some mediator such as somatostatin. In dogs, exogenous glucagon and secretin had no effect on glucose-stimulated GIP release, but gastrin and cholecystokinin caused significant enhancement (42). Exogenous insulin inhibits the GIP response to oral fat (7), and similar inhibition has been observed during intravenous administration of glucose (19). This inhibition appears to be impaired in diabetic subjects and in obese subjects. On the other hand, simultaneous infusion of insulin and glucose to maintain euglycemia failed to alter the basal concentration of GIP in humans (40). It is possible that the inhibition of GIP release attributed to insulin under some conditions is due to prevention of hyperglycemia rather than to a direct effect of insulin on the GIP cell.

Localization of the site of GIP release was studied in humans by perfusion of glucose into the intestine at different sites and measuring GIP responses (46). Duodenal and proximal jejunal perfusion produced larger responses than midjejunal or ileal perfusions, suggesting that the proximal small intestine accounts for a major portion of GIP release. Decreased release of GIP in response to a meal was found in patients with damage to the upper small intestinal mucosa caused by celiac disease, but resection of the pancreas and duodenum did not diminish the GIP response (13).

Relationship with Physiological Events

There is considerable evidence that GIP contributes to the regulation of pancreatic insulin release under conditions in which plasma glucose concentrations are increased and GIP is released by nutrients in the intestine. There is less evidence that GIP has a significant role as an inhibitor of gastric acid secretion (28,52).

Pederson and co-workers (35) demonstrated that similar increases in serum GIP concentrations produced either by oral ingestion of fat or by intravenous GIP infusion in dogs produced similar enhancement of serum insulin responses to intravenous infusion of glucose. These results have been confirmed by experiments in which plasma glucose concentrations have been maintained at constant levels by glucose clamping techniques (2,49) (Figs. 10 and 11) and have demonstrated that some increase in plasma glucose over normoglycemic concentrations is necessary for enhancement of insulin release by GIP. Further evidence for a physiologic role of GIP as an incretin was obtained in rats. It was found that intraduodenal HCl caused an increase in plasma GIP and enhanced glucose-stimulated insulin release and that the enhancement of insulin release was prevented by administration of antiserum to GIP (19).

Conditions of Excess or Deficiency

An initial report that GIP was a probable cause of the pancreatic cholera syndrome in which massive watery diarrhea is associated with a pancreatic islet tumor (20) appeared to be an error due to cross-reactivity of the antiserum used for immunofluorescent localization of tumor cells with VIP. However, mild chronic watery diarrhea has been reported in one patient who had increased plasma GIP concentration and pancreatic islet cell hyperplasia with extractable GIP found in the pancreas of this patient but not in pancreatic extracts from normal subjects (26).

Enhanced release of GIP in response to glucose or fat has been reported in patients with diabetes mellitus (7, 12), obesity (14), chronic pancreatitis (4,17), and duodenal ulcer (3). In obese subjects, the exaggerated responses were reversed by food restriction, suggesting that increased food intake was responsible for the abnormality (50). In the duodenal ulcer patients, increased fasting and food-stimulated GIP concentrations were found mainly in a subgroup of patients with an exaggerated early rise in blood glucose, possibly reflecting abnormally rapid gastric emptying in this subgroup. Although it has been postulated that abnormal GIP release may participate in the pathogenesis of diabetes mellitus (7), no convincing proof has yet been obtained.

References

1. Alumets, J., Hakanson, R., O'Dorisio, T., Sjolund, K., and Sundler, F. (1978): Is GIP a glucagon cell constituent? *Histochemistry*, 58(4):253–257.
2. Anderson, D. K., Elahi, D., Brown, J. C., Tobin, J. D., and Andres, R. (1978): Oral glucose augmentation of insulin secretion. Interactions of gastric inhibitory polypeptide with ambient glucose and insulin levels. *J. Clin. Invest.*, 62:152–161.
3. Arnold, R., Creutzfeldt, W., Ebert, R., Becker, H. D., Borger, H. W., and Schafmayer, A. (1978): Serum gastric inhibitory polypeptide (GIP) in duodenal ulcer disease: Relationship to glucose tolerance, insulin, and gastrin release. *Scand. J. Gastroenterol.*, 13:41–47.
4. Botha, J. L., Vinik, A. I., and Brown, J. C. (1976): Gastric inhib-

itory polypeptide (GIP) in chronic pancreatitis. *J. Clin. Endocrinol. Metab.,* 42:791–797.

5. Brown, J. C. (1971): A gastric inhibitory polypeptide. I. The amino acid composition and the tryptic peptides. *Can. 'J. Biochem.,* 49:255–261.

6. Brown, J. C., and Dryburgh, J. R. (1971): A gastric inhibitory polypeptide. II. The complete amino acid sequence. *Can. J. Biochem.,* 49:867–872.

7. Brown, J. C., Dryburgh, J. R., Ross, S. A., and Dupre, J. (1975): Identification and actions of gastric inhibitory polypeptide. *Recent Prog. Horm. Res.,* 31:487–532.

8. Brown, J. C., Mutt, V., and Pederson, R. A. (1970): Further purification of a polypeptide demonstrating enterogastrone activity. *J. Physiol.,* 209:57–64.

9. Buchan, A. M. J., Polak, J. M., Capella, C., Solcia, E., and Pearse, A. G. E. (1978): Electronimmunocytochemical evidence for the K cell localization of gastric inhibitory polypeptide (GIP) in man. *Histochemistry,* 56:37–44.

10. Buffa, R., Polak, J. M., Pearse, A. G. E., Solcia, E., Grimelius, L., and Capella, C. (1975): Identification of the intestinal cell storing gastric inhibitory polypeptide. *Histochemistry,* 43:249–255.

11. Cataland, S., Crockett, S. E., Brown, J. C., and Mazzaferri, E. L. (1974): Gastric inhibitory polypeptide (GIP) stimulation by oral glucose in man. *J. Clin. Endocrinol. Metab.,* 39:223–228.

12. Creutzfeldt, W., and Ebert, R. (1979): GIP in obesity, diabetes and hyperlipoproteinemia. In: *Lipoprotein Metabolism and Endocrine Regulation,* edited by L. W. Hessel and H. M. J. Krans, pp. 65–73.

13. Creutzfeldt, W., Ebert, R., Arnold, R., Frerichs, H., and Brown, J. C. (1976): Gastric inhibitory polypeptide (GIP), gastrin and insulin: response to test meal in coeliac disease and after duodenopancreatectomy. *Diabetologia,* 12:279–286.

14. Creutzfeldt, W., Ebert, R., Willms, B., Frerichs, H., and Brown, J. C. (1978): Gastric inhibitory polypeptide (GIP) and insulin in obesity: increased response to stimulation and defective feedback control of serum levels. *Diabetologia,* 14:15–24.

15. Denniss, A. R., and Young, J. A. (1978): Modification of salivary duct electrolyte transport in rat and rabbit by physalaemin, VIP, GIP and other enterohormones. *Pfluegers Arch.,* 376(1):73–80.

16. Ebert, R., Arnold, R., and Creutzfeldt, W. (1977): Lowering of fasting and food stimulated serum immunoreactive gastric inhibitory polypeptide (GIP) by glucagon. *Gut,* 18:121–127.

17. Ebert, R., Creutzfeldt, W., Brown, J. C., Frerichs, H., and Arnold, R. (1976): Response of gastric inhibitory polypeptide (GIP) to test meal in chronic pancreatitis—relationship to endocrine and exocrine insufficiency. *Diabetologia,* 12:609–612.

18. Ebert, R., Frerichs, H., and Creutzfeldt, W. (1979): Impaired feedback control of fat induced gastric inhibitory polypeptide (GIP) secretion by insulin in obesity and glucose intolerance. *Eur. J. Clin. Invest.,* 9:129–135.

19. Ebert, R., Illmer, K., and Creutzfeldt, W. (1979): Release of gastric inhibitory polypeptide (GIP) by intraduodenal acidification in rats and humans and abolishment of the incretin effect of acid by GIP-antiserum in rats. *Gastroenterology,* 76:515–523.

20. Elias, E., Bloom, S. R., Welbourn, R. B., Kuzio, M., Polak, J. M., Pearse, A. G. E., Booth, C. C., and Brown, J. C. (1972): Pancreatic cholera due to production of gastric inhibitory polypeptide. *Lancet,* 2:791–793.

21. Falko, J. M., Crockett, S. E., Cataland, S., and Mazzaferri, E. L. (1975): Gastric inhibitory polypeptide (GIP) stimulated by fat ingestion in man. *J. Clin. Endocrinol. Metab.,* 41:260–265.

22. Fujimoto, W. Y., Williams, R. H., and Ensinck, J. W. (1979): Gastric inhibitory polypeptide, cholecystokinin, and secretin effects on insulin and glucagon secretion by islet cultures (40448). *Proc. Soc. Exp. Biol. Med.,* 160:349–353.

23. Gespach, C., Bataille, D., Jarrousse, C., and Rosselin, G. (1979): Ontogeny and distribution of immunoreactive gastric inhibitory polypeptide (IR-GIP) in rat small intestine. *Acta Endocrinol. (Copenh.),* 90(2):307–316.

24. Helman, C. A., and Barbezat, G. O. (1977): The effect of gastric inhibitory polypeptide on human jejunal water and electrolyte transport. *Gastroenterology,* 72(2):376–379.

25. Ipp, E., Dobbs, R. E., Harris, V., Arimura, A., Vale, W., and Unger, R. H. (1977): The effects of gastrin, gastric inhibitory poly-

peptide, secretin, and the octapeptide of cholecystokinin upon immunoreactive somatostatin release by the perfused canine pancreas. *J. Clin. Invest.,* 60(5):1216–1219.

26. Kidd, G. S., Donowitz, M., O'Dorisio, T., Cataland, S., and Newman, F. (1979): Mild chronic watery diarrhea-hypokalemia syndrome associated with pancreatic islet cell hyperplasia. Elevated plasma and tissue levels of gastric inhibitory polypeptide and successful management with nicotinic acid. *Am. J. Med.,* 66(5):883–888.

27. Kuzio, M., Dryburgh, J. R., Malloy, K. M., and Brown, J. C. (1974): Radioimmunoassay for gastric inhibitory polypeptide. *Gastroenterology,* 66:357–364.

28. Maxwell, V., Shulkes, A., Brown, J. C., Solomon, T. E., Walsh, J. H., and Grossman, M. I. (1980): Effect of gastric inhibitory polypeptide on pentagastrin-stimulated acid secretion in man. *Dig. Dis.,* 25:113–116.

29. Morgan, L. M., Morris, B. A., and Marks, V. (1978): Radioimmunoassay of gastric inhibitory polypeptide. *Ann. Clin. Biochem.,* 15(3):172–177.

30. Moroder, L., Hallett, A., Thamm, P., Wilschowitz, L., Brown, J. C., and Wunsch, E. (1971): Studies on gastric inhibitory polypeptide: synthesis of the octatriacontapeptide GIP[1-38] with full insulinotropic activity. *Can. J. Biochem.,* 49:867.

31. O'Dorisio, T. M., Cataland, S., Stevenson, M., and Mazzaferri, E. L. (1976): Gastric inhibitory polypeptide (GIP): intestinal distribution and stimulation by amino acids and medium chain triglycerides. *Dig. Dis.,* 21:761–765.

32. O'Dorisio, T. M., Sirinek, K. R., Mazzaferri, E. L., and Cataland, S. (1977): Renal effects on serum gastric inhibitory polypeptide (GIP). *Metabolism,* 26(6):651–656.

33. Pederson, R. A., and Brown, J. C. (1972): Inhibition of histamine-, pentagastrin-, and insulin-stimulated canine gastric secretion by pure "gastric inhibitory polypeptide." *Gastroenterology,* 62:393–400.

34. Pederson, R. A., and Brown, J. C. (1978): Interaction of gastric inhibitory polypeptide, glucose, and arginine on insulin and glucagon secretion from the perfused rat pancreas. *Endocrinology,* 103(2):610–615.

35. Pederson, R. A., Schubert, H. E., and Brown, J. C. (1975): Gastric inhibitory polypeptide—Its physiologic release and insulinotropic action in the dog. *Diabetes,* 24:1050–1056.

36. Polak, J. M., Bloom, S. R., Kuzio, M., Brown, J. C., and Pearse, A. G. E. (1973): Cellular localization of gastric inhibitory polypeptide in the duodenum and jejunum. *Gut,* 14:284–288.

37. Raptis, S., Dollinger, H. C., Schroder, K. E., Schleyer, M., Rothenbuchner, G., and Pfeiffer, E. F. (1973): Differences in insulin, growth hormone and pancreatic enzyme secretion after intravenous and intraduodenal administration of mixed amino acids in man. *N. Engl. J. Med.,* 288:1199–1202.

38. Sarson, D. L., Bryant, M. G., and Bloom, S. R. (1980): A radioimmunoassay of gastric inhibitory polypeptide in human plasma. *J. Endocrinol.,* 85:487–496.

39. Schauder, P., Brown, J. C., Frerichs, H., and Creutzfeldt, W. (1975): Gastric inhibitory polypeptide: effect on glucose-induced insulin release from isolated rat pancreatic islets *in vitro. Diabetologia,* 11:483–484.

40. Service, F. J., Nelson, R. L., Rubenstein, A. H., and Go, V. L. W. (1978): Direct effect of insulin on secretion of insulin glucagon, gastric inhibitory polypeptide, and gastrin during maintenance of normoglycemia. *J. Clin. Endocrinol. Metab.,* 47:488–493.

41. Sinar, D. R., O'Dorisio, T. M., Mazzaferri, E. L., Mekhjian, H. S., Caldwell, J. H., and Thomas, F. B. (1978): Effect of gastric inhibitory polypeptide on lower esophageal sphincter pressure in cats. *Gastroenterology,* 75:263–267.

42. Sirinek, K. R., Cataland, S., O'Dorisio, T. M., Mazzaferri, E. L., Crockett, S. E., and Pace, W. G. (1977): Augmented gastric inhibitory polypeptide response to intraduodenal glucose by exogenous gastrin and cholecystokinin. *Surgery,* 82:438–442.

43. Smith, P. H., Merchant, F. W., Johnson, D. G., Fujimoto, W. Y., and Williams, R. H. (1977): Immunocytochemical localization of a gastric inhibitory polypeptide-like material within A-cells of the endocrine pancreas. *Am. J. Anat.,* 149(4):585–590.

44. Taminato, T., Seino, Y., Goto, Y., Inoue, Y., and Kadowaki, S. (1977): Synthetic gastric inhibitory polypeptide. Stimulatory ef-

fect on insulin and glucagon secretion in the rat. *Diabetes,* 26(5): 480–484.

45. Thomas, F. B., Mazzaferri, E. L., Crockett, S. E., Mekhjian, H. S., Gruemer, H. D., and Cataland, S. (1976): Stimulation of secretion of gastric inhibitory polypeptide and insulin by intraduodenal amino acid perfusion. *Gastroenterology,* 70:523–527.
46. Thomas, F. B., Shook, D. F., O'Dorisio, T. M., Cataland, S., Mekhjian, H. S., Caldwell, J. H., and Mazzaferri, E. L. (1977): Localization of gastric inhibitory polypeptide release by intestinal glucose perfusion in man. *Gastroenterology,* 72(1):49–54.
47. Thomas, F. B., Sinar, D., Mazzaferri, E. L., Cataland, S., Mekhjian, H. S., Caldwell, J. H., and Fromkes, J. J. (1978): Selective release of gastric inhibitory polypeptide by intraduodenal amino acid perfusion in man. *Gastroenterology,* 74(6):1261–1265.
48. Thomford, N. R., Sirinek, K. R., Crockett, S. E., Mazzaferri, E. L., and Cataland, S. (1974): Gastric inhibitory polypeptide. Response to oral glucose after vagotomy and pyloroplasty. *Arch. Surg.,* 109:177–182.
49. Verdonk, C. A., Rizza, R. A., Nelson, R. L., Go, V. L. W., Gerich, J. E., and Service, F. J. (1980): Interaction of fat-stimulated gastric inhibitory polypeptide on pancreactic alpha and beta cell function. *J. Clin. Invest.,* 65:1119–1125.
50. Willms, B., Ebert, R., and Creutzfeldt, W. (1978): Gastric inhibitory polypeptide (GIP) and insulin in obesity: II. Reversal of increased response to stimulation by starvation or food restriction. *Diabetologia,* 14:379–387.
51. Yajima, H., Kai, Y., Ogawa, H., Kubota, M., and Mori, Y. (1977): Structure-activity relationships of gastrointestinal hormones: Motilin, GIP, and [27-TYR]CCK-PZ. *Gastroenterology,* 72:793–796.
52. Yamagishi, T., and Debas, H. T. (1980): Gastric inhibitory polypeptide (GIP) is not the primary mediator of the enterogastrone action of fat in the dog. *Gastroenterology,* 78:931–936.

ENTEROGLUCAGON

Structure

An extensive review of the possible chemical nature of extrapancreatic glucagon-like molecules was published in 1978 (12), and will serve as the basic reference for work up until that time covered in this section.

The structure of pancreatic glucagon has been known for more than 20 years (4), and recently it has been appreciated that there are a large number of amino acid identities between pancreatic glucagon, GIP, secretin, and VIP (see section on VIP and Table 5). The finding that total pancreatectomy in dogs did not eliminate immunoreactive glucagon from the circulation led to a search for extrapancreatic sources, and glucagon-like immunoreactivity (GLI) was identified in the gastrointestinal tract of dogs (25) and of other species. In the dog, the GLI extracted from the stomach appears to be identical with pancreatic glucagon, whereas other forms have been identified in the intestine. Heterogeneity of pancreatic glucagon also has been found and a larger peptide consisting of 29 amino acid pancreatic glucagon with a carboxyl terminal extension of eight additional amino acids was isolated by Tager and Steiner (27) from a mixture of bovine and porcine crystalline pancreatic glucagon. More recently this group has described an 18,000 molecular weight biosynthetic precursor of glucagon, or proglucagon, in rat islets that could be converted enzymatically to pancreatic glucagon (20).

During pulse-chase and prolonged pulse experiments, intermediate forms were identified with molecular weights of 13,000, 10,000, and possibly 4,500. The 4,500 molecular weight fragment might correspond to the 37 amino acid precursor identified previously as a contaminant of pancreatic glucagon (Fig. 12).

A large form of GLI also has been purified from porcine intestine (26). This peptide contains 100 amino acid residues and has been named glicentin. It exhibits full immunoreactivity with some antisera to porcine glucagon but very little reactivity with antisera that require the free C-terminal region ("pancreatic glucagon-specific antisera"). The two carboxyl terminal residues are Ile-Ala and are identical with the carboxyl terminal residues of the 37 amino acid precursor of glucagon identified by Tager and Steiner, whereas the amino terminal region has no similarity to other known gut peptides. The further analysis of glicentin by chemical, enzymatic, and immunochemical methods supports the concept that glicentin contains the 29 amino acid glucagon sequence in positions 64 through 92 and that the carboxyl terminal octapeptide is identical with that found in the 37 amino acid peptide isolated from the pancreas (17). Immunochemical studies with antibodies specific for the amino terminal portion of glicentin have revealed the presence of immunoreactive material in the pancreatic alpha cell. It is thus possible that the various molecular forms of glucagon in the pancreas and gut share a common precursor and that the differences in structure of peptides isolated from pancreatic and intestinal extracts represent differences in the nature of intracellular processing enzymes present in endocrine cells in the two regions. Although glicentin-like immunoreactivity could not be identified in the larger biosynthetic precursors of rat pancreatic glucagon (20), there could be species differences in the amino terminal regions of porcine and rat glicentin that lead to alterations in immunoreactivity. These questions will not be resolved until further studies have revealed the complete amino acid sequences of large forms of both pancreatic and gut glucagons.

Biological Actions

The general biological and metabolic actions of pancreatic glucagon include glycogenolysis, lipolysis, gluconeogenesis, and ketogenesis and are the subject of an extensive review (29). Exogenously administered glucagon causes inhibition of intestinal motility and of intestinal absorption of water and electrolytes (30), inhibits pancreatic enzyme and bicarbonate secretion (14), inhibits gastric acid secretion (5), inhibits resting and pentagastrin-stimulated lower esophageal sphincter pressure (13), and stimulates hepatic bile flow (7). None of these effects are likely to occur at physiological concentrations of circulating pancreatic glucagon.

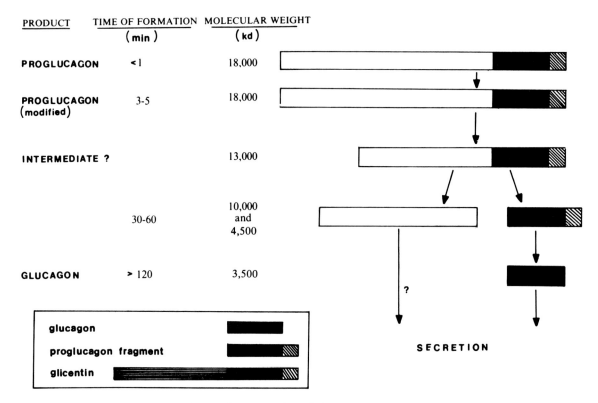

PRODUCT	TIME OF FORMATION (min)	MOLECULAR WEIGHT (kd)	
PROGLUCAGON	< 1	18,000	
PROGLUCAGON (modified)	3-5	18,000	
INTERMEDIATE ?		13,000	
	30-60	10,000 and 4,500	
GLUCAGON	> 120	3,500	

glucagon

proglucagon fragment

glicentin

SECRETION

FIG. 12. Some possible biosynthetic pathways for conversion of glucagon precursors to glucagon. From Patzelt et al. (20).

The biological actions of extrapancreatic glucagons have been difficult to establish except for the immunoreactive material present in dog fundic extracts that appears to be identical with true pancreatic glucagon (12). Extracts of porcine small intestine were found to contain a glucagon-like immunoreactivity with larger apparent molecular weight than pancreatic glucagon that competed with pancreatic glucagon for liver plasma membrane receptors (1). Holst (11) has further purified immunoreactive forms of glucagon in extracts of various regions of the porcine gut and measured the activity of different fractions to inhibit binding of radioiodinated glucagon to porcine liver cell membranes. He found that most tissues contained large and small forms of immunoreactive material that reacted either with antibodies specific for pancreatic-type glucagon or with antibodies specific for enteroglucagon. The form that was similar to true pancreatic glucagon and another form that reacted with enteroglucagon antibodies and had a slightly higher apparent molecular weight both were detected in the radioreceptor assay. Larger immunoreactive forms that were detected with either of the two antibodies had no activity in the radioreceptor system. One of the forms apparently is identical with glicentin. Glicentin itself has not been shown to have any glucagon-like biological activity (17). However, since glicentin apparently contains the entire glucagon sequence, it is possible that partial enzymatic degradation of this molecule in the blood or at tissue receptors could generate biologically active molecules. This may account for the biological activity of smaller forms of gut glucagon-like peptides.

Distribution

Pancreatic glucagon has been demonstrated in the alpha cells of the pancreas and in similar cells in the oxyntic gland mucosa of the dog (15). These cells have similar ultrastructural and staining properties to pancreatic alpha cells (9). Extracts of canine gastric mucosa also contain large amounts of immunoreactive material that reacts with antibodies felt to be specific for pancreatic glucagon and coelutes with pancreatic glucagon on gel filtration columns (15). Much lower concentrations of this pancreatic-type glucagon are present in extracts of pig stomach (11). Glicentin also has been demonstrated by immunocytochemical methods in pancreatic alpha cells (22). The glicentin immunoreactivity appears to be topographically segregated from pancreatic glucagon immunoreactivity in the alpha cell granule (21). The former was localized by immune electron microscopy to the peripheral mantle of the granule, whereas pancreatic-type glucagon was concentrated in the electron-dense core of the granule.

Antibodies that react with both pancreatic glucagon and larger forms present in the gut have been utilized to localize enteroglucagon in the intestine. In most cases, the enteroglucagon content has been estimated as the difference between immunoreactivity measured with such an antibody and the immunoreactivity measured with a pancreatic-glucagon-specific antibody. More recently, antibodies have been developed that are specific for the amino terminal portion of glicentin (17). The majority of muscosal endocrine cells staining with the less specific glucagon antisera in the distal small intestine and colon do not exhibit immunoreactivity with pancreatic-specific antisera (15). These cells have been identified by their silver staining properties and by combined immune and electron microscopy as L cells of the intestine (9). The same cells also can be shown to exhibit immune staining with specific antibodies directed against glicentin (22). The concentration of nonpancreatic glucagon immunoreactivity is highest in the terminal ileum and colon and represents several molecular forms (11). The majority of this immunoreactivity can be accounted for by the content of glicentin in the distal small intestine (17). An earlier study obtained similar results for the distribution of nonpancreatic glucagon in the canine intestine (25) but concluded that this material has a smaller molecular weight than pancreatic glucagon.

Measurement

Glucagon-like immunoreactivity is readily measured by radioimmunoassy, but interpretation of results is complicated by the presence of multiple molecular forms and by differences in antibody specificity (10). Three principal types of antibody specificities have been described. One type is specific for the unblocked carboxyl terminal region of pancreatic glucagon and often is called "pancreatic specific," although it is capable of detecting pancreatic-type glucagon in canine gastric extracts and at least one additional larger molecular form in porcine intestinal extracts (11). The second type has a specificity that is less clearly defined but appears to be directed at a more amino terminal region of pancreatic glucagon, possibly the 11–15 sequence, does not require a free amino or carboxyl terminus, and detects both pancreatic and gastrointestinal forms of glucagon including glicentin. The third type appears to be specific for some amino terminal region of glicentin that is not contained in pancreatic glucagon (17). Most measurements of circulating enteroglucagon have involved use of the second type of antibody to measure total pancreatic plus nonpancreatic immunoreactivity and subtraction of immunoreactivity measured with a pancreatic-specific antibody (11). Such dual assay estimates do not indicate the distribution of molecular forms of circulating enteroglucagon. It should be possible to obtain specific measurements of circulating glicentin by radioimmunoassay with the third type of antibody, but until now such assays have been applied only to tissue

extracts, and molecular forms in plasma samples have been identified by radioimmunoassay of gel filtration fractions.

Release

Although glucose inhibits the release of pancreatic glucagon, oral or intestinal administration of glucose leads to an increase in total glucagon-like immunoreactivity in the plasma, and evidence has been obtained that this response is due to release of a large form of enteroglucagon from the intestine (28). Evidence also has been obtained that intraduodenal administration of fat in dogs leads to release of both pancreatic-type glucagon and enteroglucagon, whereas introduction of fat into the ileum causes release of only enteroglucagon (19). Ingestion of a mixed meal in normal human subjects produced a small increase in plasma enteroglucagon, but patients with impaired upper intestinal absorption due to celiac disease demonstrated an exaggerated response (2). Increased enteroglucagon release also has been reported in patients with reactive hypoglycemia (23). The biological activity of the enteroglucagon released by intestinal stimulation has not been established.

Release of pancreatic-type glucagon from the gastric fundus has been studied in conscious dogs, and it was concluded that the stomach is not a major source of circulating glucagon (18). However, in the isolated perfused dog stomach it was found that glucagon release was minimal under basal conditions but was stimulated by arterial arginine infusion and this response was abolished by somatostatin (16). Gastric glucagon release was not altered by hyperglycemia alone but was significantly inhibited by the combination of insulin and hyperglycemia. Somatostatin also has been shown to decrease plasma glucagon concentrations in the pancreatectomized dog (6).

Relationship with Physiological Events

Possible hormonal effects of enteroglucagon are presently unclear due to the paucity of biological effects found with preparations of gut glucagon fractions that are free from contamination with pancreatic-type glucagon (12). No specific effects on the gut have been identified as being mediated by physiological circulating concentrations of pancreatic glucagon, although there is a suggestion that this hormone may have some inhibitory effect on gastric acid secretion (5). Neutralization of endogenous glucagon with repeated injection of glucagon antibodies in starved rats was found to diminish the augmented intestinal uptake of amino acids that ordinarily accompanies fasting-induced hyperglucagonemia (24).

Conditions of Excess or Deficiency

A single patient has been reported who had an endocrine tumor arising in the kidney that appeared to produce enteroglucagon (8). This patient had marked hyperplasia of the intestinal villi, decreased intestinal transit time, and mild fat malabsorption that were all normalized after tumor resection. A number of patients have been described with pancreatic glucagonoma characterized by hyperglucagonemia, severe dermatitis, weight loss, venous thrombosis, and often diarrhea (16a). These abnormalities were reversed by successful tumor resection. A family has been reported in which macromolecular hyperglucagonemia was inherited in an autosomal dominant manner but produced no apparent clinical or biochemical abnormalities (3). Enteroglucagon deficiency states have not been described.

References

1. Bataille, D. P., Freychet, P., Kitabgi, P. E., and Rosselin, G. E. (1973): Gut glucagon: a common receptor site with pancreatic glucagon in liver cell plasma membranes. *FEBS Lett.,* 30:215–218.
2. Besterman, H. S., Sarson, D. L., Johnston, D. I., Stewart, J. S., Guerin, S., Bloom, S. R., Blackburn, A. M., Patel, H. R., Modigliani, R., and Mallinson, C. N. (1978): Gut-hormone profile in coeliac disease. *Lancet,* 785–788.
3. Boden, G., and Owen, O. E. (1977): Familial hyperglucagonemia—an autosomal dominant disorder. *N. Engl. J. Med,* 296:534–538.
4. Bromer, W. W., Sinn, L. G., Sand, A., and Behrems, O. K. (1957): The amino acid sequence of glucagon. *Diabetes,* 6:45–49.
5. Christiansen, J., Holst, J. J., and Kalaja, E. (1976): Inhibition of gastric acid secretion in man by exogenous and endogenous pancreatic glucagon. *Gastroenterology,* 70:688–692.
6. Dobbs, R. H., Sakurai, H., Sasaki, G., Faloona, I., Valuerde, D., Baetens, L., Orci, L., and Unger, R. H. (1975): Glucagon: role in the hyperglycemia of diabetes mellitus. *Science,* 187:544–547.
7. Dyck, W. P., and Janowitz, H. D. (1971): Effect of glucagon on hepatic bile secretion in man. *Gastroenterology,* 60:400–404.
8. Gleeson, M. H., Bloom, S. R., Polak, J. M., Henry, K., and Dowling, R. H. (1971): Endocrine tumour in kidney affecting small bowel structure, motility, and absorptive function. *Gut,* 12:773–782.
9. Grimelius, L., Capella, C., Buffa, R., Polak, J. M., Pearse, A. G. E., and Solcia, E. (1976): Cytochemical and ultrastructural differentiation of enteroglucagon and pancreatic-type glucagon cells of the gastrointestinal tract. *Virchows Arch. [Cell Pathol.],* 20:217–228.
10. Harris, V., Faloona, G. R., and Unger, R. H. (1979): Glucagon. In: *Methods of Hormone Radioimmunoassay,* edited by B. M. Jaffe and H. R. Behrman, pp. 643–656. Academic Press, New York.
11. Holst, J. J. (1977): Extraction, gel filtration pattern, and receptor binding of porcine gastrointestinal glucagon-like immunoreactivity. *Diabetologia,* 13:159–169.
12. Holst, J. J. (1978): Extrapancreatic glucagons. *Digestion,* 17:168–190.
13. Jaffer, S. S., Makhlouf, G. M., Schorr, B. A., and Zfass, A. M. (1974): Nature and kinetics of inhibition of lower esophageal sphincter pressure by glucagon. *Gastroenterology,* 67:42–46.
14. Konturek, S. J., Tasler, J., and Obtulowicz, W. (1974): Characteristics of inhibition of pancreatic secretion by glucagon. *Digestion,* 10:138–149.
15. Larsson, L.-I., Holst, J., Hakanson, R., and Sundler, F. (1975): Distribution and properties of glucagon immunoreactivity in the digestive tract of various mammals: an immunohistochemical and immunochemical study. *Histochemistry,* 44:281–290.
16. Lefebvre, P. J., and Luyckx, A. S. (1977): Factors controlling gastric-glucagon release. *J. Clin. Invest,* 59:716–721.
16a. Mallinson, C. N., Bloom, S. R., Warin, A. P., Salmon, P. R., and Cox, B. (1974): A glucagonoma syndrome. *Lancet,* 2:1–4.
17. Moody, A. J., Frandsen, E. K., Jacobsen, H., and Sundby, F. (1979): Speculations on the structure and function of gut GLIs. In: *Hormonal Receptors in Digestion and Nutrition,* edited by G. Rosselin, P. Fromgeot, and S. Bonfils, pp. 55–64. Elsevier, Amsterdam.
18. Munoz-Barragan, L., Blazquez, E., Patton, G. S., Dobbs, R. E., and Unger, R. H. (1976): Gastric A-cell function in normal dogs. *Am. J. Physiol.,* 4:1057–1061.
19. Ohneda, A., Yanbe, A., Maruhama, Y., Ishii, S., Kai, Y., Abe, R., and Yamagata, S. (1975): Characterization of circulating immunoreactive glucagon in response to intraduodenal administration of fat in dogs. *Gastroenterology,* 68:715–721.
20. Patzelt, C., Tager, H. S., Carroll, R. J., and Steiner, D. F. (1979): Identification and processing of proglucagon in pancreatic islets. *Nature,* 282:260–266.
21. Ravazzola, M., and Orci, L. (1980): Glucagon and glicentin immunoreactivity are topologically segregated in the α granule of the human pancreatic A cell. *Nature,* 284:66–67.
22. Ravazzola, M., Siperstein, A., Moody, A. J., Sundby, F., Jacobsen, H., and Orci, L. (1979): Glicentin immunoreactive cells: their relationship to glucagon-producing cells. *Endocrinology,* 105:499–508.
23. Rehfeld, J. F., and Heding. L. G. (1970): Increased gut-glucagon release in reactive hypoglycemia. *Br. Med. J.,* 2:706–707.
24. Rudo, N. D., Lawrence, A. M., and Rosenberg, I. H. (1975): Treatment with glucagon-binding antibodies alters the intestinal response to starvation in the rat. *Gastroenterology,* 69:1265–1268.
25. Sasaki, H., Rubalcava, B., Baetens, D., Blazquez, E., Srikant, C. B., Orci, L., and Unger, R. H. (1975): Identification of glucagon in the gastrointestinal tract. *J. Clin. Invest.,* 56:135–145.
26. Sundby, F., Jacobsen, H., and Moody, A. J. (1976): Purification and characterization of a protein from porcine gut with glucagon-like immunoreactivity. *Horm. Metab. Res.,* 8:366–371.
27. Tager, H. S., and Steiner, D. F. (1973): Isolation of a glucagon-containing peptide: Primary structure of a possible fragment of proglucagon. *Proc. Natl. Acad. Sci. U.S.A.,* 70:2321–2325.
28. Unger, R. H., Ohneda, A., Valverde, I., Eisentraut, A. M., and Exton, J. (1968): Characterization of the responses of circulating glucagon-like immunoreactivity to intraduodenal and intravenous administration of glucose. *J. Clin. Invest.,* 47:48–65.
29. Unger, R. H., and Orci, L. (1976): Physiology and pathophysiology of glucagon. *Physiol. Rev.,* 56:778–826.
30. Whalen, G. E. (1974): Glucagon and the small gut. *Gastroenterology,* 67:1284–1286.

SOMATOSTATIN

Structure

The chemical nature of somatostatin was established after purification from ovine hypothalamic tissue (6,9). It was found to be a tetradecapeptide that could exist either as a linear peptide or with a disulfide bridge between cysteine residues in positions 3 and 14 (Table 1). Somatostatin isolated from the pancreatic islet of the teleost fish, anglerfish, had primary structure identical to hypothalamic somatostatin from sheep and pig and pancreatic somatostatin from pigeon (80), suggesting a high degree of evolutionary conservation (52). It has not yet been established whether the structure of immunoreactive peptides demonstrated in reptiles, cyclostomes, and tunicates is identical. However, at least one variant form has been isolated from catfish pancreas (54a) (Table 6). A larger molecular form of somatostatin has been isolated and sequenced from porcine intestine (63). This peptide consists of 28 amino acid residues extended at the amino terminus by the sequence Ser-Ala-Asn-Ser-Asn-Pro-Ala-Met-Ala-Pro-Arg-Glu-Arg-Lys. By analogy to the gastrin and CCK peptides, this larger form of somatostatin could be called SS28 and the smaller form SS14; the use of SS rather than S is to avoid confusion with secretin and its cell of origin the S cell. The structure of SS28 is consistent with a biosynthetic role as a prohormone since it has two consecutive basic residues immediately preceding the SS14 sequence, and these two consecutive basic residues are preceded in the third residue by a proline, a pattern often found in prohormones and possibly providing the structural basis for specificity of activating enzymes. Evidence for the presence of a processing enzyme was obtained in extracts of mouse hypothalamus (42). An activity that eluted with the largest form of immunoreactive SS at an apparent molecular weight of 15,000 caused conversion of larger forms to forms that coeluted with SS14. *In vitro* pulse-chase biosynthesis experiments in anglerfish islets provide additional evidence for intracellular processing of larger to smaller molecular forms of somatostatin (50,51). Progressive conversion of a larger form to a form having the characteristics of SS14 was observed and cell-free supernatant of islet tissue was capable of causing such conversion. A peptide containing 22 amino acid residues has been purified from catfish pancreatic islets and found to have 7 amino acid identities to SS14 in the C-terminal 14 amino acid residues (54a). This peptide had full biological activity for inhibition of growth hormone release from rat anterior pituitary cells but was only about 25% as immunoreactive as hypothalamic somatostatin in the radioimmunoassay system used (54b).

Biological Actions

In Vivo

Although somatostatin originally was isolated and identified by its action to inhibit release of growth hormone from the pituitary, a wide spectrum of gastrointestinal actions has been identified including inhibition of release and peripheral effects of several peptide hormones as well as effects on gut motility and absorption. In the brain, somatostatin inhibits release of growth hormone and TSH from the pituitary (28b), inhibits the hyperglycemic effect produced by intracisternal bombesin (7), and produces a unique pattern of behavioral effects (33a).

The effects of somatostatin on gastric function have been reviewed (18). Intravenous somatostatin inhibits gastric acid and pepsin responses to exogenous and endogenous gastrin and to cholinergic stimulation but produces less marked inhibition of histamine-stimulated secretion. Similar inhibition is obtained after vagotomy. Somatostatin also produces marked inhibition of basal, food-stimulated, and neural-stimulated gastrin release (Fig. 13). In patients with gastrin-secreting tumors, somatostatin infusion markedly decreases acid secretion and produces moderate to marked decreases in serum gastrin as well as inhibition of the increases in gastrin caused by secretin or calcium infusion. All biologically active forms of circulating gastrin appear to be inhibited to a similar extent. In anesthetized pigs, infusion of somatostatin into the arterial blood supply to the antrum prevented the increase in gastrin caused by arterial infusion of calcium, PTH, and acetylcholine (5). Serum gastrin concentrations tend to exhibit a rebound increase after somatostatin infusions are stopped (2) (Fig. 13). Somatostatin also decreases gastrin release caused by electrical vagal stimulation in cats (83).

Effects on gastrointestinal cellular proliferation also have been reported (44). Intravenous infusion of a dose of somatostatin that inhibited 50% the acid response to exogenous gastrin in rats caused a decrease in labeling index, mitotic index, and DNA synthesis in the stomach and less marked changes in intestinal mucosa. Trophic effects of gastrin on the stomach but not on the intestine also were blocked.

Somatostatin has effects on motor activity of the stomach and intestine. Although one study reported that somatostatin increased the myoelectrical activity in fasted dogs and converted the normal response after feeding to a fasting pattern (82), most workers have

TABLE 6. *Structures of hypothalamic somatostatin (SS14), intestinal large somatostatin (SS28), and catfish pancreatic somatostatin (22 residues)*

Somatostatin	Structure
SS28	S A N S N P A M A P R E R K A G C K N F F W K T F T S C
SS14	A G C K N F F W K T F T S C
Catfish	D N T V R S K P L N C M N Y F W K S S T A C

Underlined residues are identical to lines above.

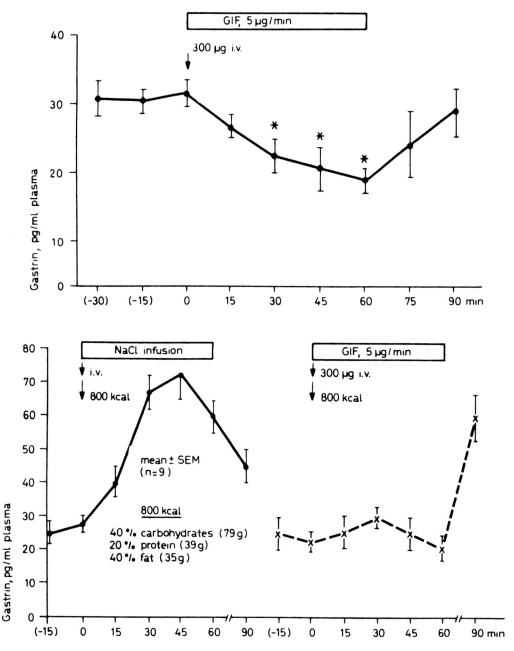

FIG. 13. Inhibition of basal (*top*) and food-stimulated (*bottom*) serum gastrin concentrations in humans by intravenous infusion of somatostatin. From Raptis et al. (63a).

found that somatostatin inhibits the normal occurrence of cyclic interdigestive motor (54) or electrical (61) activity in the stomach and small intestine. Somatostatin also was found to have a direct inhibitory effect on the initiation of myoelectrical activity caused by exogenous motilin, but did not interrupt the distal propagation of activity fronts that already had begun and did not prevent the occurrence of ectopic activity fronts that began in the jejunum (61). Different effects of somatostatin on gastric emptying in human subjects also have been reported. One study reported retardation of gastric emptying (3), whereas another found enhanced gastric emptying of a glucose meal during infusion followed by

slowing of gastric emptying and intestinal transit after the infusion ceased (33).

An inhibitory action of somatostatin on pancreatic exocrine secretion has been found in most mammalian species. In humans, enzyme but not bicarbonate secretion was inhibited in the basal state, and responses to exogenous CCK were inhibited more than the responses to exogenous secretin (19). Similar effects were reported in rat (23). Inhibition of release of immunoreactive secretin and pancreatic bicarbonate responses to intestinal acidification in dogs (4) and of immunoreactive CCK response to olive oil in humans (70) have been found.

Somatostatin also has profound effects on the endocrine pancreas. Acute intravenous infusion in baboons causes a decrease in both insulin and glucagon associated with a decrease in blood sugar during fasting and during arginine stimulation (35). In human subjects similar effects were observed during oral glucose tolerance tests and the rise in plasma glucose was delayed but increased over control values (49). In diabetic subjects, however, somatostatin was found to reduce markedly the blood glucose rise after oral glucose without a change in intravenous glucose tolerance (89). Similar effects were noted on the blood xylose concentrations after oral administration of xylose, suggesting that the major effect of somatostatin on postprandial hyperglycemia in diabetics was due to decreased or delayed carbohydrate absorption rather than a change in carbohydrate disposal. Somatostatin also inhibits release of glucagon-like immunoreactivity from the intestine during stimulation by glucose, amino acids, or fat (68). Prolonged infusions of somatostatin lead to increases in blood glucose despite prolonged suppression of plasma glucagon (79). The complex effects of somatostatin on glucose homeostasis are beyond the scope of this chapter, but many papers on this subject can be found in a recent monograph (24).

In addition to an inhibitory effect on absorption of glucose and xylose, somatostatin also has been shown to inhibit absorption of amino acids in the human small intestine (37a). *In vitro* studies with rabbit small intestine mucosa revealed that somatostatin caused increased ileal mucosal absorption of sodium and chloride (18a) and inhibited the decreased water absorption induced by prostaglandin E_1 in jejunal mucosa (18b).

As additional evidence for the broad spectrum of inhibitory activity of somatostatin on hormone release, it has been shown to inhibit food-stimulated release of pancreatic polypeptide (90) and to inhibit pentagastrin-stimulated release of calcitonin in patients with medullary carcinoma of the thyroid (25). A tonic role for suppression of pituitary and gut hormones but not pancreatic hormones is suggested by the observation that administration of antiserum to somatostatin caused prompt increases in growth hormone and glucagon-like immunoreactivity but not in insulin or pancreatic glucagon (75).

In vitro

Attempts to mimic the *in vivo* effects of somatostatin in *in vitro* systems have not been universally successful. A large number of studies have been performed in isolated pancreatic islets and in pituitary cell cultures (24). Functional receptors for somatostatin have been characterized in rat pituitary cells in culture, and it was found that receptor binding and biological responses had similar dose-response characteristics (71). Receptor binding could not be demonstrated in several nonpituitary cell

lines. Also, TRH enhanced specific receptor binding of somatostatin in pituitary cell lines that possess both types of receptors but had no effect in cell lines that have only receptors for somatostatin (72). Analogues of somatostatin that were more effective for inhibition of insulin release than glucagon release *in vivo* had similar selectivity *in vitro* (81).

Several studies of somatostatin effects have been performed in isolated gastric preparations. Somatostatin inhibited gastric acid secretion in the isolated canine stomach (37). A direct role of somatostatin in the regulation of antral gastrin release is suggested by studies with vascularly perfused rat stomach. Infusion of somatostatin antiserum produced acute increases in venous gastrin concentration (66). A reciprocal relationship has been shown between gastric somatostatin and gastrin release. Infusion of three hormones known to inhibit gastrin release—glucagon, secretin, and VIP—produced the expected inhibition of gastrin release associated with increased somatostatin release in a highly correlated dose-dependent fashion (13). Infusions of methacholine produced increases in gastrin that were highly correlated with decreases in somatostatin, whereas prostaglandin E_2 had an opposite effect (67). Similar observations have been made in anesthetized pigs, in which there was a reciprocal decrease of somatostatin and increase in gastrin concentration in the antral vein during intragastric instillation of bicarbonate or meat extract (28).

Direct effects of somatostatin have been found on short-circuit current of isolated rabbit ileal mucosa (26). Although the effects resembled those produced by alpha-adrenergic agonists, they were not inhibited by phentolamine. Tissue cAMP and cGMP concentrations were not changed. The peptide reduced the short-circuit current response to carbamylcholine but had no effect on responses to VIP, cholera toxin, calcium ionophore, 16,16-dimethyl prostaglandin E_2, theophylline, or 8-bromo-cAMP. The apparent specificity for cholinergic agents is interesting in light of a report that somatostatin inhibits the release of acetylcholine from myenteric plexus of guinea pig ileum (27) and is reminiscent of the dual effects on release and action of peptide hormones. A species difference apparently exists between rabbit and rat ileal mucosa in the effect of somatostatin on VIP-stimulated intestinal secretion. In the rat, somatostatin prevented both the secretion and the stimulation of cellular cAMP caused by VIP but had less marked effects on secretion stimulated directly by cAMP analogues (10).

Structure-Activity Relationships

A large number of synthetic analogues of somatostatin have been prepared and analyzed for biological and immunological activities (87) as well as for molecular conformation (29). Removal of the Ala^1-Gly^2 side chain reduces biological activity (inhibition of growth hormone release *in vitro*) by only 40%, but deletion of any single residue in the 12-membered peptide ring reduces activity by more than 95%. Replacement of L-amino acids by D-amino acids generally reduces activity, but certain analogues including (D-Trp[8]) and (D-Cys[14]) somatostatin have considerably increased activity. Selectivity of action has been demonstrated for certain analogues by simultaneous measurement of inhibition of growth hormone, insulin, and glucagon release. Certain modifications in the 5, 8 and 13 positions singly or combined produced marked increases in selective inhibition of insulin release and caused hyperglycemia associated with hyperglucagonemia. On the other hand, (D-Cys[14]) somatostatin had a higher potency to inhibit glucagon secretion than to inhibit insulin secretion. The role of particular functional side chains on the individual amino acid residues was assessed by selective substitution of each residue by alanine. Replacement of each of the 3 Phe and of the Trp and Lys residues resulted in marked lowering of activity while other replacements were tolerated well. Multiple amino acid deletions also could be tolerated, and a series of hepta- to decapeptides was prepared that had good biological activity. The essential features of these peptides were conservation of critical amino acid residues and the disulfide bridge and one or more spacer amino acids. An octapeptide was prepared that caused prolonged inhibitory activity on secretion of insulin, glucagon, pancreatic polypeptide, and gastrin in human subjects. Tyrosine-containing analogues also have been prepared and used for production of region-specific antibodies and for radioiodination to develop radioimmunoassays. Assays have been developed that are specific either for the amino terminal 4 through 6 residues or for certain residues between positions 5 and 11 in the amino acid ring.

A nonimmunoreactive but biologically active form of somatostatin was utilized to demonstrate a self-inhibiting action of somatostatin on somatostatin release from isolated perfused dog pancreas-duodenum (32). In this bicyclic analogue of somatostatin, a second disulfide bond was created by replacement of the Phe residues in positions 6 and 11 by Cys residues (88). This compound retained high biological activity and provided evidence that these two Phe residues in the native molecule stabilize the molecule but do not interact directly with the receptor. This compound had similar activity relative to SS14 for inhibition of glucagon, insulin, and growth hormone but lesser activity against pentagastrin-stimulated gastric acid secretion. Glycosylation of the Asn residue in position 5 in SS14 markedly decreased biological activity *in vitro* but did not diminish activity *in vivo* (43). Two synthetic analogues of somatostatin—(D-Trp[8]) and (D-Cys[14])—were found to have similar inhibitory activity to SS14 on pentagastric-stimulated acid

secretion and secretin-stimulated pancreatic bicarbonate secretion in dogs (36). Long-acting somatostatin analogues have been used for selective inhibition of glucagon and growth hormone to the experimental treatment of streptozotocin diabetic dogs (45) and for suppression of release of insulin, glucagon, and gastrin from hormone-secreting tumors in man (46). The latter study was done with the cyclic octopeptide: Cys-Phe-Thr-Lys-Trp-Phe-Phe-D-Cys.

These studies indicate significant differences in activity produced by selective amino acid modifications. Similar differences in patterns of activity have not yet been looked for in naturally occurring molecular variants of somatostatin present in gut extracts.

Distribution

Cellular

Somatostatin has been identified in nerves and cell bodies in the central and peripheral nervous system including the autonomic nervous system of the gut and in endocrine-like D cells in the pancreatic islets and the mucosa of the stomach and intestine. Nerve terminals and axons are concentrated in the median eminence and appear to arise from nerve bodies in the nucleus paraventriculus (22). Another dense network of axons and nerve terminals is found within the hypothalamus, but their cellular origin is unknown. Somatostatin immunoreactive small diameter primary afferent neurons have been found with cell bodies in the dorsal root ganglia and central processes that terminate in the substantia gelatinosa of the dorsal horn of the spinal cord. In the gut, somatostatin nerve fibers are most prominent surrounding the ganglion cells of the myenteric plexus in the small intestine. Somatostatin-containing cell bodies also have been demonstrated in prevertebral sympathetic ganglia, and the same cell bodies appear to contain norepinephrine. It has been suggested that somatostatin-containing neurons are interneurons within the enteric nervous system (17). Somatostatin-like immunoreactivity also has been identified in certain populations of amacrine cells in the retina (91).

Endocrine-like cells have been shown to contain somatostatin in the pancreatic islets (20,47) and in all parts of the gut mucosa (62). These cells were identified as D cells by their pattern of distribution and staining characteristics. Within the islets D cells were found to be closely associated with A cells, usually on the periphery of the islet (53). A possible anatomic explanation for local (paracrine) release of somatostatin in the vicinity of other cells in the stomach, including gastrin and parietal cells, is offered by the finding that somatostatin cells have long cytoplasmic processes that terminate near these cells (40).

Immunochemical

Distribution of somatostatin-like activity has been measured by bioassay and by radioimmunoassay and the results are in good general agreement with the distribution found by immunocytochemistry (86). One problem that may be encountered in radioimmunoassay measurements is failure to detect larger molecular forms of somatostatin that have amino terminal amino acid extensions when antisera are employed that are specific for the free amino region of SS14. Somatostatin-like activity has been found in the brain and pancreas of all vertebrates examined and in the gut of all vertebrate species but hagfish (86).

In the brain, somatostatin content is highest in the hypothalamus, particularly the median eminence and arcuate nucleus, although significant amounts are found elsewhere in the brain (8). Molecular heterogeneity of brain somatostatin-like immunoreactivity has been demonstrated (65). SLI purified from different regions of rat brain by immunoaffinity eluted as four distinct peaks on gel filtration, and each was shown to have biological activity that could be removed by absorption with antibodies to somatostatin. SLI was shown to be concentrated in synaptosome fractions in rat brain homogenates (1b). SLI also has been identified in extracts of vagus nerve, especially the abdominal portion, in dog and cat (85).

In the gut, SLI activity is highest in the antral and fundic mucosa of the stomach and in the pancreas, although it can be found throughout the gut (48). Forms of SLI apparently larger than SS14 have been found in extracts of stomach and pancreas, and there is good evidence that the form that elutes at approximately 3,000 daltons is not a disulfide polymer of SS14 (93). In cats SLI content was found to be much higher in the antral mucosa than in mucosa, muscle layer, or parenchyma of other gut organs, but the larger form was relatively more abundant in ileum and cecum (11).

Measurement

Bioassay

The inhibitory properties of somatostatin can be applied to *in vivo* or *in vitro* bioassays. Most commonly the potency of a peptide analogue of somatostatin or of a purified component of tissue extract with somatostatin-like immunoreactivity is assessed for potency compared with synthetic SS14 to inhibit growth hormone release *in vitro* from dissociated rat pituitary cells or to inhibit insulin and glucagon release *in vivo* (43,87). Another bioassay system involves measurement of inhibition of pentagastrin-stimulated gastric acid secretion in rats (93). In general, such bioassay systems produce results that agree well with results obtained by radioim-

munoassay with antibodies directed against the ring structure of the molecule, but marked differences can be obtained when antibodies directed against the amino terminus of SS14 are used and when somatostatin analogues with different patterns of target selectivity are analyzed (87). A radioreceptor assay has been developed that permits analysis of effects of various peptides on the interaction of labeled somatostatin with its receptor on a line of cultured pituitary cells (72). This system was used to demonstrate that TRH modulated the number of receptor binding sites without alteration in affinity for somatostatin.

Radioimmunoassay

A sensitive and specific radioimmunoassay for somatostatin was described by Arimura and co-workers (1,1a). After immunization with somatostatin covalently bound to alpha globulin by glutaraldehyde, rabbits produced antibodies that bound radioiodinated (Tyr[1]) somatostatin with high affinity. Plasma was found to inhibit binding of label to antibody in a nonspecific fashion since this inhibition was not altered by charcoal absorption but could be decreased greatly by acetone extraction. Concentrations of SLI in brain extracts agreed well with estimates of somatostatin content determined by bioassay.

Subsequently several other radioimmunoassay systems have been developed and utilized to measure SLI in tissue extracts and in plasma. Analogues of somatostatin with substitutions of tyrosine for various residues in the molecule have been used to produce region-specific antibodies by selective conjugation through the tyrosine side chains and use of the same analogue to prepare radioiodinated peptide (87). Several antisera were found to be directed at immunological determinants in the ring structure, and one antibody was described with amino terminal specificity when tested against a large number of synthetic analogues. When immunochemical potency and biological potency were compared for these analogues, it was found that those antibodies directed againt ring determinants showed better correlation with inhibition of growth hormone secretion, but that certain substitutions, such as D-Trp for L-Trp at position 8, increased biological activity and abolished immunoreactivity while other substitutions had opposite effects. Similar comparisons have not been made for naturally occurring molecular variants of somatostatin obtained from tissue extracts. The marked variation in biological activity and immunoreactivity for one analogue was used to study the effect of this analogue on release of SLI from dog pancreas by permitting measurement of endogenous SLI in the presence of high concentrations of the nonimmunoreactive analogue (32).

Several studies have reported use of radioimmunoassay to characterize SLI obtained by extraction of mammalian brain and gut tissues. In two studies that utilized antibodies specific for the midportion of the peptide ring, several molecular forms were identified (65,93). Two peaks eluted with higher apparent molecular weight than SS14 and there was another peak that appeared later. On the other hand, in another study that utilized an uncharacterized antiserum, almost all immunoreactivity in human stomach and pancreas extracts was found to coelute with SS14 (48). There is some evidence that that largest apparent molecular form of SLI which coelutes with protein is due to noncovalent binding of somatostatin to protein (21). On the other hand, there is no doubt that a larger form exists, since the structure of SS28 has been determined (63).

Radioimmunoassay for somatostatin in blood has presented some problems. As noted previously, plasma may have nonspecific effects on antibody binding to labeled antigen and there are differences in region specificity among antibodies. Chromatographic analysis of SLI in dog plasma revealed that the major fraction was associated with the plasma proteins and could be separated from the large protein region by affinity chromatography with antibodies directed against the ring structure but not with antibodies directed against the amino terminal region of SS14 (16). Nonspecific effects of plasma could not be abolished by enzyme inhibitors or by use of somatostatin-free plasma for construction of standard curves, but good results were obtained after prior extraction of somatostatin from plasma onto silica glass (60). Under these conditions fasting immunoreactive somatostatin in human subjects ranged from 17 to 81 pg/ml with 78% recovery of somatostatin added to plasma. Prior extraction of rat plasma with acetone (1) or with acid-ethanol (57a) also produced fasting concentrations in peripheral blood that were less than 50 pg ml^{-1}. These results are lower than fasting values of 274 pg/ml obtained in human serum that was not extracted (39). Until more radioimmunoassay systems have been fully characterized as to specificity, nonspecific interference, and recovery of different molecular forms of somatostatin, it is premature to define the "physiological" concentrations in plasma.

Metabolism

The clearance rates of exogenously administered somatostatin have been measured in dog and in humans and found to be rapid. In dog the half-life of immunoreactive somatostatin was 1.8 min and the clearance rate 63 ml min^{-1} (20 kg dogs), whereas suppression of plasma glucagon and insulin lasted for 1.4 and 6.7 min, respectively, after the infusion was stopped (74). In humans there were two components to the disappearance curve: the first component varied from 1.1 to 3.0 min in normal subjects while the second component was much longer (78). The initial half-life was prolonged by

about 50% in patients with severe renal failure. In normal subjects the clearance rate was 1,900 ml min^{-1} or 28 ml min^{-1}kg^{-1}. The metabolic fate of somatostatin after disappearance from the circulation has not been defined.

Release

In vivo

Because of difficulties with radioimmunoassay measurement of somatostatin in plasma, there have been few reports concerning the release of this peptide under physiological conditions. Much of the current information was obtained in anesthetized dogs by selective sampling of venous blood from the pancreas, gastric antrum, and gastric fundus (73,76,77). Intragastric glucose caused SLI release from all three regions whereas intraduodenal glucose produced smaller responses. Intragastric fat produced larger increases in pancreatic and fundic than in antral SLI, while intraduodenal fat produced larger antral and pancreatic than fundic responses. Amino acids in the stomach caused a larger fundic than antral response and an intermediate pancreatic response. Acidification of the gastric lumen caused mainly an increase in antral SLI whereas acidification of the duodenum caused an increase in all three regions. It appeared that gastric acidification caused a decrease in SLI from the fundus. The effects of vagotomy and of atropine on SLI responses to intragastric liver extract were studied when liver extract was introduced at pH 7 or pH 2. Antral SLI release was accentuated at pH 2, and this release was not influenced by vagotomy but was inhibited by atropine. Fundic SLI release was less at pH 2 than at pH 7 before and after vagotomy and actually decreased at the lower pH. Atropine inhibited the rise found at pH 7 and reversed the inhibition found at pH 2, leading to significant stimulation. Pancreatic vein SLI responses were inhibited by atropine but not by vagotomy.

SLI also has been found in the gastric lumen of antral pouches in cats during acute electrical vagal stimulation (85). Intravenous infusion of gastrin caused somatostatin release in anesthetized dogs (28a).

In vitro

Somatostatin release has been demonstrated from various preparations of isolated pancreas and pancreatic islets. In the isolated perfused dog pancreas, perfusion with arginine or glucagon but not with insulin caused increased SLI output (59). In a similar preparation, increases in SLI were observed during infusion of glucose at concentrations above 100 mg/dl, mixed amino acids, CCK, leucine, and tolbutamide (30). Evidence has been obtained for beta-adrenergic stimulation and alpha-adrenergic suppression of SLI release from isolated dog pancreas (69). In monolayer cultures of neonatal rat pancreas, insulin had no effect on SLI release but stimulation was produced by dibutyryl cAMP, theophylline, glucose, arginine, and glucagon (56). Also, somatostatin may exert feedback autoinhibition on release of SLI, since a biologically potent but nonimmunoreactive analogue of somatostatin inhibited the SLI response to CCK and arginine in the isolated perfused dog pancreas (32).

The isolated perfused rat stomach also has been utilized to study release of SLI and the relationships between SLI and gastrin release. Gastric SLI was stimulated by infusions of glucagon, theophylline, or dibutyryl cAMP (12) as well as by secretin, bombesin, and pentagastrin, whereas Met-enkephalin and substance P caused inhibition of SLI and neurotensin had no effect (13,14). A functional relationship between somatostatin and gastrin release was suggested by the high degree of negative correlation between stimulation of SLI and inhibition of immunoreactive gastrin during glucagon, secretin, and VIP infusion (13,14). A similar inverse relationship has been found during methacholine infusion, where stimulation of gastrin and inhibition of somatostatin were closely linked (67) (Fig. 14).

Calcium-dependent release of SLI from rat neurohypophysis *in vitro* has been reported (58). Similar results were obtained in another study where acetylcholine was found to inhibit rat hypothalamic somatostatin release *in vitro* (64).

Alterations in tissue content of somatostatin have been measured in diabetes and after administration of other hormones. Tissue concentration and somatostatin cell number were decreased in the pancreas and stomach but increased in the hypothalamus of dbdb and obob genetically diabetic mice compared with normal littermates (55). On the other hand, somatostatin content of islets increased markedly, associated with increased gastric somatostatin and unchanged hypothalamic concentrations, in rats that had been made diabetic by the administration of streptozotocin (57). These changes were associated with marked decreases in pancreatic insulin and increases in pancreatic glucagon. Chronic administration of secretin plus cerulein or of glicentin to rats caused an increase in pancreatic somatostatin content without a change in D-cell number, whereas administration of GIP or pancreatic polypeptide produced no significant effect (92). These observations are difficult to interpret without further information about rates of synthesis and release.

Relationship with Physiological Events

Other than the studies with rat stomach that show inverse correlation between somatostatin and gastrin release, there are few observations that permit assessment of the possible role of circulating somatostatin. There is not yet any information relating concentrations of different molecular forms of somatostatin in the circulation to physiological events. A tonic inhibitory role of somatostatin for regulation of release of growth hormone and glucagon is suggested by the observation that infusion of antibody to somatostatin caused prompt increase in circulating concentrations of these hormones (75). In a more recent publication (77), the same group observed an increase in insulin, gastrin, and pancreatic polypeptide responses to a meal after administration of somatostatin antiserum. A tonic inhibitory role for gastrin release is suggested by the observation that somatostatin antiserum caused prompt increase in gastrin output from the isolated rat stomach (66) (Fig. 15).

Additional observations that support a reciprocal relationship between release of somatostatin and of other hormones have been made in the pancreas and the hypothalamus. It was found that morphine and beta-endorphin caused an increase in release of insulin and glucagon, preceded slightly by a marked decrease in somatostatin (31). In urethane-anesthetized rats, it was found that immunoreactive somatostatin content was increased in hypophyseal portal blood and that plasma growth hormone concentrations were significantly lowered (15).

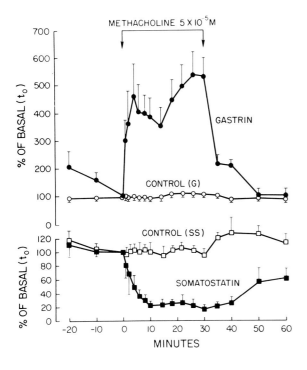

FIG. 14. Reciprocal stimulation of gastrin release and inhibition of somatostatin release from vascularly perfused rat stomach during methacholine infusion. From Saffouri et al. (67).

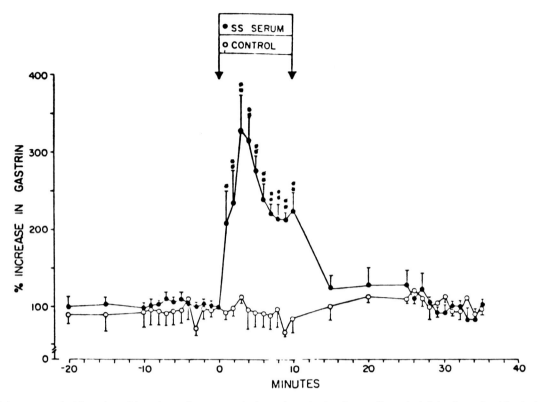

FIG. 15. Enhancement of basal gastrin release from vascularly perfused rat antrum after administration of antibody to somatostatin. From Saffouri et al. (66).

Effects of Excess or Deficiency

Several patients have been discovered to have somatostatin-secreting tumors of the pancreas. One patient was found to have high circulating SLI that could be separated by gel filtration into at least four components, and tumor extracts were shown to inhibit insulin and glucagon release (41). This patient had low acid secretion, steatorrhea, and impaired glucose tolerance. Of six patients reported with this type of tumor, all those tested had diabetes mellitus, steatorrhea, and weight loss and all but one had gallstones. One tumor also produced ACTH and two produced calcitonin. Extensive endocrine and digestive evaluation on one patient revealed several expected findings including decreased growth hormone, insulin, and pancreatic responses to stimuli but an unexpected increase in glucagon response to arginine (38). Other findings included low acid secretion, delayed gastric emptying, increased frequency of interdigestive myoelectric complexes, and steatorrhea.

No primary or secondary causes of somatostatin deficiency have been reported.

References

1. Arimura, A., Lundquist, G., Rothman, J., Chang, R., Fernandez-Durango, R., Elde, R., Coy, D. H., Meyers, C., and Schally, A. V. (1978). Radioimmunoassay of somatostatin. *Metabolism, [Suppl. 1], 27:1139-1144.*

1a. Arumura, A., Sato, H., Coy, D. H., and Schally, A. V. (1975): Radioimmunoassay for GH-release inhibiting hormone (38631). *Proc. Soc. Exp. Biol. Med.,* 148:784-789.

1b. Berelowitz, M., Matthews, J., Pimstone, B. L., Kronhein, S., and Sacks, H. (1978): Immunoreactive somatostatin in rat cerebral cortical and hypothalamic synaptosomes. *Metabolism, [Suppl. 1],* 27:1171-1174.

2. Bloom, S. R., Mortimer, C. H., Thorner, M. O., Besser, G. M., Hall, R., Gomez-Pan, A., Roy, V. M., Russell, R. C. G., Coy, D. H., Kastin, A. J., and Schally, A. V. (1974): Inhibition of gastrin and gastric-acid secretion by growth-hormone release-inhibiting hormone. *Lancet,* 2:1106-1109.

3. Bloom, S. R., Ralphs, D. N., Besser, G. M., et al. (1975): Effect of somatostatin on motilin levels and gastric emptying. *Gut,* 16:834.

4. Boden, G., Sivitz, M. C., Owen, O. E., Essa-Koumar, N., and Landon, J. H. (1975): Somatostatin suppresses secretin and pancreatic exocrine secretion. *Science,* 190:163-165.

5. Bolman, R. M. III, Copper, C. W., and Wells, S. A. (1978): Somatostatin inhibition and reversal or parathyroid hormone-, calcium-, and acetycholine-induced gastrin release in the pig. *Endocrinology,* 103:259-266.

6. Brazeau, P., Vale, W., Burgus, R., Ling, N., Butcher, M., Rivier, J., and Guillemin, R. (1973): Hypothalamic polypeptide that inhibits the secretion of immunoreactive pituitary growth hormone. *Science,* 179:77-79.

7. Brown, M., Rivier, J., and Vale, W. (1978): Somatostatin, central neurosystem (CNS) action on glucoregulation. *Metabolism, [Suppl. 1],* 27:1253-1256.

8. Brownstein, M., Arimura, A., Sato, H., Schally, A. V., and Kizer, J. S. (1975): The regional distribution of somatostatin in the rat brain. *Endocrinology,* 96:1456-1461.

9. Burgus, R., Ling, N., Butcher, M., and Guillemin, R. (1973): Primary structure of somatostatin, a hypothalamic peptide that inhibits the secretion of pituitary growth hormone. *Proc. Natl. Acad. Sci. U.S.A.,* 70:684-688.

10. Carter, R. F., Bitar, K. N., Zfass, A. M., and Makhlouf, G. M.

(1978): Inhibition of VIP-stimulated intestinal secretion and cyclic AMP production by somatostatin in the rat. *Gastroenterology,* 74(4):726–730.

11. Chayvialle, J.-A., Miyata, M., Rayford, P. L., and Thompson, J. C. (1980): Immunoreactive somatostatin and vasoactive intestinal peptide in the digestive tract of cat. *Gastroenterology (in press).*

12. Chiba, T., Seino, Y., Goto, Y., Kadowaki, S., Taminato, T., Abe, H., Kato, Y., Matsukura, S., Nozawa, M., and Imura, H. (1978): Somatostatin release from isolated perfused rat stomach. *Biochem. Biophys. Res. Commun.,* 82:731–737.

13. Chiba, T., Taminato, T., Kadowaki, S., Abe, H., Chihara, K., Goto, Y., Seino, Y., and Fujita, T. (1980): Effects of glucagon, secretin, and vasoactive intestinal polypeptide on gastric somatostatin and gastrin release from isolated perfused rat stomach. *Gastroenterology,* 79:67–71.

14. Chiba, T., Taminato, T., Kadowaki, S., Inoue, Y., Mori, K., Seino, Y., Abe, H., Chihara, K., Matsukura, S., Fujita, T., and Goto, Y. (1980): Effects of various gastrointestinal peptides on gastric somatostatin release. *Endocrinology,* 106:145–149.

15. Chihara, K., Arimura, A., and Schally, A. V. (1979): Immunoreactive somatostatin in rat hypophyseal portal blood: effects of anesthetics. *Endocrinology,* 104:1434–1441.

16. Conlon, J. M., Srikant, C. B., Ipp, E., Schusdziarra, V., Vale, W., and Unger, R. H. (1978): Properties of endogenous somatostatin-like immunoreactivity and synthetic somatostatin in dog plasma. *J. Clin. Invest.,* 62:1187–1193.

17. Costa, M., Patel, Y., Furness, J. B., and Arimura, A. (1977): Evidence that some intrinsic neurons of the intestine contain somatostatin. *Neurosci. Lett.,* 6:215–222.

18. Creutzfeldt, W., and Arnold, R. (1978): Somatostatin and the stomach: Exocrine and endocrine aspects. *Metabolism,* 27:1309–1315.

18a. Dharmsathaphorn, K., Binder, H. J., and Dobbins, J. W. (1980): Somatostatin stimulates sodium and chloride absorption in the rabbit ileum. *Gastroenterology,* 78:1559–1565.

18b. Dharmsathaphorn, K., Sherwin, R. S., and Dobbins, J. W. Somatostatin inhibits fluid secretion in the rat jejunum. *Gastroenterology,* 78:1554–1558.

19. Dollinger, H. C., Raptis, S., and Pfeiffer, E. F. (1976): Effects of somatostatin on exocrine and endocrine pancreatic function stimulated by intestinal hormones in man. *Horm. Metab. Res.,* 8:74–78.

20. Dubois, M. P. (1975): Immunoreactive somatostatin is present in discrete cells of the endocrine pancreas. *Proc. Natl. Acad. Sci. U.S.A.,* 72:1340–1343.

21. Dupont, A., and Alvarado-Urbina, G. (1976): Conversion of big pancreatic somatostatin without peptide bond cleavage into somatostatin tetradecapeptide. *Life Sci.,* 19:1431–1434.

22. Elde, R., Hokfelt, T., Johansson, O., Schultzberg, M., Efendic, S., and Luft, R. (1978): Cellular localization of somatostatin. *Metabolism,* 27:1151–1159.

23. Folsch, U. R., Lankisch, P. G., and Creutzfeldt, W. (1978): Effect of somatostatin on basal and stimulated pancreatic secretion in the rat. *Digestion,* 17:194–203.

24. Gerich, J. E., Raptis, S., and Rosenthal, J. (1978): Metabolism, clinical and experimental. *Somatostatin Symposium [Suppl. 1],* 27:1129–1469.

25. Gordin, A., Lamberg, B. A., Pelkonen, R., and Almqvist, S. (1978): Somatostatin inhibits the pentagastrin-induced release of serum calcitonin in medullary carcinoma of the thyroid. *Clin. Endocrinol.,* 8(4):289–293.

26. Guandalini, S., Kachur, J. F., Smith, P. L., Miller, R. J., and Field, M. (1980): In vitro effects of somatostatin on ion transport in rabbit intestine. *Am. J. Physiol.,* 238:G67–G74.

27. Guillemin, R. (1976): Somatostatin inhibits the release of acetylcholine induced electrically in the myenteric plexus. *Endocrinology,* 99:1653–1654.

28. Gustavsson, S., and Lundqvist, G. (1978): Participation of antral somatostatin in the local regulation of gastrin release. *Acta Endocrinol. (Copenh.),* 88:339–346.

28a. Guzman, S., Lonovics, J., Chayvialle, J.-A., Hejtmancik, K. E., Rayford, P. L., and Thompson, J. C. (1980): Effects of gastrin on circulating levels of somatostatin, pancreatic polypeptide,

and vasoactive intestinal peptide in dogs. *Endocrinology,* 107: 231–236.

28b. Hall, R., Snow, M., Scanlon, M., Mora, B., and Gomez-Pan, A. (1978): Pituitary effects of somatostatin. *Metabolism, [Suppl. 1],* 27:1257–1262.

29. Holladay, L. A., Rivier, J., and Puett, D. (1977): Conformational studies on somatostatin and analogues. *Biochemistry,* 16: 4895–4899.

30. Ipp, E., Dobbs, R. E., Arimura, A., Vale, W., Harris, V., and Unger, R. H. (1977): Release of immunoreactive somatostatin from the pancreas in response to glucose, amino acids, pancreozymin-cholecystokinin, and tolbutamide. *J. Clin. Invest.,* 60: 760–765.

31. Ipp, E., et al. (1978): Morphine and β-endorphin influence the secretion of the endocrine pancreas. *Nature,* 276:190–191.

32. Ipp, E., Rivier, J., Dobbs, R. E., Brown, M., Vale, W., and Unger, R. H. (1979): Somatostatin analogs inhibit somatostatin release. *Endocrinology,* 104:1270–1273.

33. Johansson, C., Efendic, S., Wisen, O., Uvnas-Wallensten, K., and Luft, R. (1978): Effects of short-time somatostatin infusion on the gastric and intestinal propulsion in humans. *Scand. J. Gastroenterol.,* 13:481–483.

33a. Kastin, A. J., Coy, D. H., Jacquet, Y., Schally, A. V., and Plolnikoff, N. P. (1978): Central nervous system (CNS) effects of somatostatin. *Metabolism, [Suppl. 1],* 27:1247–1252.

34. Kayasseh, L., Haecki, W. H., Gyr, K., Stalder, G. A., Rittmann, W. W., Halter, F., and Girard, J. (1978): The endogenous release of pancreatic polypeptide by acid and meal in dogs. Effect of somatostatin. *Scand. J. Gastroenterol.,* 13(4):385–391.

35. Koerker, D. J., Ruel, W., Chideckel, E., Palmer, J., Geodner, C. J., Ensich, J., and Gule, C. C. (1974): Somatostatin: hypothalamic inhibitor of the endocrine pancreas. *Science,* 184:482–484.

36. Konturek, S. J., Tasler, J., Krol, R., Dembinski, A., Coy, D. H., and Schally, A. V. (1977): Effect of somatostatin analogs on gastric and pancreatic secretion (39842). *Proc. Soc. Exp. Biol. Med.,* 155:519–522.

37. Kowalewski, K., Kolodej, A., and Kocylowski, M. (1978): Effect of somatostatin on pentagastrin stimulated secretion by isolated canine stomachs perfused ex vivo with homologous blood. *Digestion,* 17(5):441–444.

37a. Krejs, G. J., Browne, R., and Raskin, P. (1980): Effect of intravenous somatostatin on jejunal absorption of glucose, amino acids, water, and electrolytes. *Gastroenterology,* 78:26–31.

38. Krejs, G. J., Orci, L., Conlon, J. M., Ravazzola, M., Davis, G. R., Raskin, P., Collins, S. M., McCarthy, D. M., Baetens, D., Rubenstein, A., Aldor, T. A. M., and Unger, R. H. (1979): Somatostatinoma syndrome. *N. Engl. J. Med.,* 301:285–292.

39. Kronheim, S., Berelowitz, M., and Pimstone, B. L. (1978): The characterization of somatostatin-like immunoreactivity in human serum. *Diabetes,* 27(5):523–529.

40. Larsson, L.-I., Goltermann, N., de Magistris, L., Rehfeld, J., and Schwartz, T. W. (1979): Somatostatin cell processes as pathways for paracrine secretion. *Science,* 205:1393–1395.

41. Larsson, L.-I., Holst, J. J., Kuhl, C., Lundqvist, G., Hirsch, M. A., Ingemansson, S., Lindkaer Jensen, S., Rehfeld, J. F., and Schwartz, T. W. (1977): Pancreatic somatostatinoma: clinical features and physiological implications. *Lancet,* 666–668.

42. Lauber, M., Camier, M., and Cohen, P. (1979): Higher molecular weight forms of immunoreactive somatostatin in mouse hypothalamic extracts: evidence of processing *in vitro. Proc. Natl. Acad. Sci. U.S.A.,* 76:6004–6008.

43. Lavielle, S., Ling, N., Brazeau, P., Benoit, R., Wasada, T., Harris, D., Unger, R., and Guillemin, R. (1979): Synthesis and biological activity of glycosylated analogs of somatostatin. *Biochem. Biophys. Res. Commun.,* 91:614–622.

44. Lehy, T., Dubrasqeut, M., and Bonfils, S. (1979): Effect of somatostatin on normal and gastrin-stimulated cell proliferation in the gastric and intestinal mucosae of the rat. *Digestion,* 19:99–109.

45. Lien, E. L., Greenwood, J., and Sarantakis, D. (1979): Treatment of streptozotocin-diabetic dogs with a long-acting somatostatin analog. *Diabetes,* 28:491–495.

46. Long, R. G., Adrian, T. E., Brown, M. R., Rivier, J. E., Barnes,

A. J., Mallinson, C. N., Vale, W., Christofides, N. D., and Bloom, S. R. (1979): Suppression of pancreatic endocrine tumour secretion by long-acting somatostatin analogue. *Lancet*, 2:764-767.

47. Luft, R., Efendic, S., Hokfelt, T., Johansson, O., and Arimura, A. (1974): Immunohistochemical evidence for the localization of somatostatin-like immunoreactivity in a cell population of the pancreatic islets. *Med. Biol.*, 52:428-430.

48. McIntosh, C., Arnold, R., Bothe, E., Becker, H., Kobberling, J., and Creutzfeldt, W. (1978): Gastrointestinal somatostatin: Extraction and radioimmunoassay in different species. *Gut*, 19: 655-663.

49. Mortimer, C. H., Carr, D., Lind, T., Bloom, S. R., Mallinson, C. N., Schally, A. V., Tunbridge, W. M. G., Yeomans, L., Coy, D. H., Kastin, A., Besser, G. M., and Hall, R. (1974): Effects of growth-hormone release-inhibiting hormone on circulating glucagon, insulin, and growth hormone in normal, diabetic, acromegalic, and hypopituitary patients. *Lancet*, 1:697-701.

50. Noe, B. D., Fletcher, D. J., Bauer, G. E., Weir, G. C., and Patel, Y. (1978): Somatostatin biosynthesis occurs in pancreatic islets. *Endocrinology*, 102:1675-1685.

51. Noe, B. D., Fletcher, D. J., and Spiess, J. (1979): Evidence for the existence of a biosynthetic precursor for somatostatin. *Diabetes*, 28:724-730.

52. Noe, B. D., Spiess, J., Rivier, J. E., and Vale, W. (1979): Isolation and characterization of somatostatin from anglerfish pancreatic islet. *Endocrinology*, 105:1410.

53. Orci, L., and Unger, R. H. (1975): Functional subdivision of islets of Langerhans and possible role of D cells. *Lancet*, 20:1243-1246.

54. Ormsbee, H. S., Koehler, S. L., and Telford, G. L. (1978): Somatostatin inhibits motilin-induced interdigestive contractile activity in the dog. *Dig. Dis.*, 23:781-788.

54a. Oyama, H., Bradshaw, R. A., Bates, O. J., and Permutt, A. (1980): Amino acid sequence of catfish pancreatic somatostatin I. *J. Biol. Chem.*, 255:2251-2254.

54b. Oyama, H., Hirsch, H. J., Gabbay, K. H., and Permutt, A. (1980): Isolation and characterization of immunoreactive somatostatin from fish pancreatic islets. *J. Clin. Invest.*, 65:993-1002.

55. Patel, Y. (1977): Somatostatin: Widespread abnormality in tissues of spontaneously diabetic mice. *Science*, 198:930-931.

56. Patel, Y. C., Amherdt, M., and Orci, L. (1979): Somatostatin secretion from monolayer cultures of neonatal rat pancreas. *Endocrinology*, 104(3):676-679.

57. Patel, Y. C., Cameron, D. P., Bankier, A., Malaisse-Lagae, F., Ravazzola, M., Studer, P., and Orci, L. (1978): Changes in somatostatin concentration in pancreas and other tissues of streptozotocin diabetic rats. *Endocrinology*, 103:917.

57a. Patel, Y. C., Wheatley, T., Fitz-Patrick, D., and Brock, G. (1980): A sensitive radioimmunoassay for immunoreactive somatostatin in extracted plasma: Measurement and characterization of portal and peripheral plasma in the rat. *Endocrinology*, 107:306-313.

58. Patel, Y. C., Zingg, H. H., and Dreifuss, J. J. (1977): Calcium-dependent somatostatin secretion from rat neurohypophysis *in vitro*. *Nature*, 267:852-853.

59. Patton, G. S., Ipp, E., Dobbs, R. E., Orci, L., Vale, W., and Unger, R. H. (1977): Pancreatic immunoreactive somatostatin release. *Proc. Natl. Acad. Sci. U.S.A.*, 74:2140-2143.

60. Penman, E., Wass, J. A., Lund, A., Lowry, P. J., Stewart, J., Dawson, A. M., Besser, G. M., and Rees, L. H. (1979): Development and validation of a specific radioimmunoassay for somatostatin in human plasma. *Ann. Clin. Biochem.*, 16(1):15-25.

61. Poitras, P., Steinbach, J. H., VanDeventer, G., Code, C. F., and Walsh, J. H. (1980): Motilin independent ectopic fronts of the interdigestive myoelectric complex in dogs. *Am. J. Physiol.*, 239:G215-G220.

62. Polak, J. M., Pearse, A. G. E., Grimelius, L., Bloom, S. R., and Arimura, A. (1975): Growth-hormone release-inhibiting hormone in gastrointestinal and pancreatic D cells. *Lancet*, 1: 1220-1224.

63. Pradayrol, L., Jornvall, H., Mutt, V., and Ribet, A. (1980): N-terminally extended somatostatin: the primary structure of somatostatin-28. *FEBS Lett.*, 109:55-58.

63a. Raptis, S., Dollinger, H. C., von Berger, L. Schlegel W., Schröder, K. E., and Pfeiffer, E. F. (1975): Effects of somatostatin and gastric secretion and gastrin release in man. *Digestion*, 13:15-26.

64. Richardson, S. B., Hollander, C. S., D'Eletto, R., Greenleaf, P. W., and Thaw, C. (1980): Acetylcholine inhibits the release of somatostatin from rat hypothalamus *in vitro*. *Endocrinology*, 107:122-129.

65. Rorstad, O. P., Epelbaum, J., Brazeau, P., and Martin, J. B. (1979): Chromatographic and biological properties of immunoreactive somatostatin in hypothalamic and extrahypothalamic brain regions of the rat. *Endocrinology*, 105:1083-1092.

66. Saffouri, B., Weir, G., Bitar, K., and Makhlouf, G. (1979): Stimulation of gastrin secretion from the perfused rat stomach by somatostatin antiserum. *Life Sci.*, 25:1749-1754.

67. Saffouri, B., Weir, G. C., Bitar, K. N., and Makhlouf, G. M. (1980): Gastrin and somatostatin secretion by perfused rat stomach: functional linkage of antral peptides. *Am. J. Physiol.*, G495-G501.

68. Sakurai, H., Dobbs, R. E., and Unger, R. H. (1975): The effect of somatostatin on the response of GLI to the intraduodenal administration of glucose, protein, and fat. *Diabetologia*, 11:427-430.

69. Samols, E., and Weir, G. C. (1979): Adrenergic modulation of pancreatic A, B, and D cells, alpha-adrenergic suppression and beta-adrenergic stimulation of somatostatin secretion, alpha-adrenergic stimulation of glucagon secretion in the perfused dog pancreas. *J. Clin. Invest.*, 63(2):230-238.

70. Schlegel, W., Raptis, S., Harvey, R. F., Oliver, J. M., and Pfeiffer, E. F. (1977): Inhibition of cholecystokinin-pancreozymin release by somatostatin. *Lancet*, 2:166-168.

71. Schonbrunn, A., and Tashjian, A. H., Jr. (1978): Characterization of functional receptors for somatostatin in rat pituitary cells in culture. *J. Biol. Chem.*, 253:6473-6483.

72. Schonbrunn, A., and Tashjian, A. H., Jr. (1980): Modulation of somatostatin receptors by thyrotropin-releasing hormone in a clonal pituitary cell strain. *J. Biol. Chem.*, 255:190-198.

73. Schusdziarra, V., Harris, V., Conlon, J. M., Arimura, A., and Unger, R. (1978): Pancreatic and gastric somatostatin release in response to intragastric and intraduodenal nutrients and HCl in the dog. *J. Clin. Invest.*, 62:509-518.

74. Schusdziarra, V., Harris, V., and Unger, R. H. (1979): Half-life of somatostatin-like immunoreactivity in canine plasma. *Endocrinology*, 104:109-110.

75. Schusdziarra, V., Rouiller, D., Arimura, A., and Unger, R. H. (1978): Antisomatostatin serum increases levels of hormones from the pituitary and gut, but not from the pancreas. *Endocrinology*, 103(5):1956-1959.

76. Schusdziarra, V., Rouiller, D., Harris, V., and Unger, R. H. (1979): Gastric and pancreatic release of somatostatin-like immunoreactivity during the gastric phase of a meal. *Diabetes*, 28: 658-663.

77. Schusdziarra, V., Rouiller, D., Harris, V., and Unger, R. H. (1980): Splanchnic somatostatin: a hormonal regulator of nutrient homeostasis. *Science*, 207:530-532.

78. Sheppard, M., Shapiro, B., Pimstone, B., Kronheim, S., Berelowitz, M., and Gregory, M. (1979): Metabolic clearance and plasma half-disappearance time of exogenous somatostatin in man. *J. Clin. Endocrinol. Metab.*, 48:50-53.

79. Sherwin, R. S., Hendler, R., DeFronzo, R., et al. (1977): Glucose homeostasis during prolonged suppression of glucagon and insulin secretion by somatostatin. *Proc. Natl. Acad. Sci. U.S.A.*, 74:348-352.

80. Speiss, J., Rivier, J. E., Rodkey, J. A., Bennett, C. D., and Vale, W. (1979): Isolation and characterization of somatostatin from pigeon pancreas. *Proc. Natl. Acad. Sci. U.S.A.*, 76:2974-2978.

81. Taborsky, G. J., Jr., Smith, P. H., and Porte, D., Jr. (1979): Differential effects of somatostatin analogues on α- and β-cells of the pancreas. *Am. J. Physiol.*, 236(2)E123-E128.

82. Thor, P., Krol, R., Konturek, S. J., Coy, D. H., and Schally, A. V. (1978): Effect of somatostatin on myoelectrical activity of small bowel. *Am. J. Physiol.*, 235(3):E249-E254.

83. Uvnas-Wallensten, K., Efendic, S., and Luft, R. (1977): Inhibi-

tion of vagally induced gastrin release by somatostatin in cats. *Horm. Metab. Res.,* 9:120–123.

84. Uvnas-Wallensten, K., Efendic, S., and Luft, R. (1978): The occurrence of somatostatin-like immunoreactivity in the vagal nerves. *Acta Physiol. Scand.,* 102:248–250.

85. Uvnas-Wallensten, K., Efendic, S., and Luft, R. (1978): Release of somatostatin into the antral lumen of cats. *Metabolism,* 27: 1233–1234.

86. Vale, W., Ling, N., Rivier, J., Villarreal, J., Rivier, C., Douglas, C., and Brown, M. (1976): Anatomic and phylogenetic distribution of somatostatin. *Metabolism,* 25:1491–1494.

87. Vale, W., Rivier, J., Ling, N., and Brown, M. (1978): Biologic and immunologic activities and applications of somatostatin analogs. *Metabolism,* 27:1391–1401.

88. Veber, D. F., Holly, F. W., Paleveda, W. J., Nutt, R. F., Bergstrand, S. J., Torchiana, M., Glitzer, M. S., Saperstein, R., and Hirschmann, R. (1978): Conformationally restricted bicyclic analogs of somatostatin. *Proc. Natl. Acad. Sci. U.S.A.,* 75: 2636–2640.

89. Wahren, J., and Felig, P. (1976): Influence of somatostatin on carbohydrate disposal and absorption in diabetes mellitus. *Lancet,* 2:1213–1216.

90. Wilson, R. M., Boden, G., and Owen, O. E. (1978): Pancreatic polypeptide responses to a meal and to intraduodenal amino acids and sodium oleate. *Endocrinology,* 102(3):859–863.

91. Yamada, T., Marshak, D., Basinger, S., Walsh, J., Morley, J., and Stell, W. (1980): Somatostatin-like immunoreactivity in the retina. *Proc. Natl. Acad. Sci. U.S.A.,* 77:1691–1695.

92. Yamada, T., Solomon, T. E., Petersen, H., Levin, S. R., Lewin, K., Walsh, J. H., and Grossman, M. I. (1980): Effects of gastrointestinal polypeptides on hormone content of endocrine pancreas in the rat. *Am. J. Physiol.,* 238:G526–G530.

93. Zyznar, E. S., Conlon, J. M., Schusdziarra, V., and Unger, R. H. (1979): Properties of somatostatin-like immunoreactive polypeptides in the canine extrahypothalamic brain and stomach. *Endocrinology,* 105:1426–1431.

MOTILIN

Structure

Motilin was purified from a side fraction of hog upper intestine extract obtained during the purification of secretin and was characterized by its ability to stimulate gastric motor activity in antral and fundic pouches in dogs and by stimulation of gastric pepsin but not acid secretion (4). The complete amino acid sequence was published in 1972 (Brown) and corrected to include a glutamine residue where a glutamic acid residue was initially found (2,31). It is a linear peptide containing 22 amino acids and has a molecular weight of 2,700. It contains a single tyrosine residue and several acidic and basic residues (Table 1). Synthetic motilin and 13-Leu and 13-Nleu analogues have full biological activity (33, 39).

Biological Actions

Motilin has significant effects on gastrointestinal smooth muscle. Intravenous infusion of motilin in conscious dogs during the interdigestive period initiates myoelectric complexes in the antroduodenal region that are propagated distally in the small intestine and appear identical to the myoelectric complexes that appear spontaneously at 80- to 90-min intervals during fasting (38)

(Fig. 16). However, it has little effect on the postprandial pattern of intestinal activity (16). Motilin also produces strong contractions in the lower esophageal sphincter and stomach in fasting but not in fed dogs (15). The stimulation of canine lower esophageal sphincter contraction by motilin was partially inhibited by atropine and completely abolished by a combination of atropine and hexamethonium, suggesting that it acts by stimulation of preganglionic cholinergic neurons in this muscle (20). The stimulation of canine gastric myoelectric activity (increased frequency of spike potentials on slow waves) was inhibited by secretin, GIP, CCK, and gastrin (5,19a).

Motilin increased the rate of emptying of liquid but not solid meals in dogs, possibly because of its stimulatory action on fundic contraction (8). Antrectomy had little effect on motilin-stimulated emptying, but vagotomy caused a 10-fold decrease in sensitivity to exogenous motilin. In humans, natural motilin increased gastric emptying of a solid meal (7) but slowed emptying of a liquid meal (30) while increasing gastric pepsin output. Motilin had no effect on salivary or pancreatic secretion in man (9).

Motilin also caused contraction of gastric and intestinal muscle strips from human and rabbit *in vitro,* and this stimulation appeared to be direct rather than by neural mediation (35). The stimulation was abolished by the calcium antagonist verapamil. Evidence also was obtained for potentiation of the contractile response of isolated rabbit pyloric sphincter muscle to acetylcholine *in vitro* by addition of subthreshold concentrations of motilin (34). In both these studies the synthetic 13-Nleu analogue of motilin was used.

An extragastrointestinal neural action of motilin was found in rat brain and spinal cord and amphibian spinal cord, characterized by excitation and depolarization of corticospinal neurons and cortical cells (26). The effects were diminished by tetrodotoxin, suggesting a site of action on spinal cord interneurons.

Structure-Activity Relationships

Neither the 1–6 nor the 12–22 amino acid sequences of motilin had any effect on gastric motor activity, whereas the 7–22 amino acid sequence had a weak stimulating activity (18). Replacement of even the first residue in the 22 amino acid sequence caused 300-fold decrease in activity. It was concluded that the entire molecule is necessary for most of the biological activity.

Distribution

Motilin-containing cells have been demonstrated in the mucosa of the upper part of the small intestine in several species, including humans, but the specific cell type has been a matter of some dispute. One group has

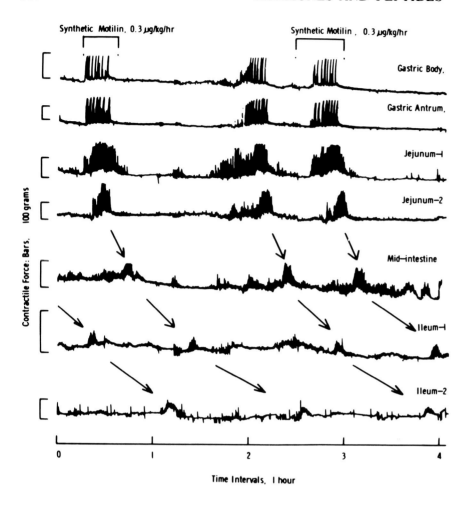

FIG. 16. Induction of premature interdigestive myoelectric complexes in dogs by intravenous infusion of synthetic motilin. From Itoh et al. (16).

reported that motilin-containing cells represent a subpopulation of enterochromaffin cells distinct from enterochromaffin cells that contain substance P (13,25,29). These cells were demonstrated in small intestine and in bile duct epithelium of several species of mammals. The enterochromaffin nature of these cells in human duodenum was confirmed by parallel staining and immunoelectron microscopy of serially sectioned cells (12). Another group, using similar methods, concluded that motilin-containing cells in various mammals including humans were distinct from 5-hydroxytryptamine-containing enterochromaffin cells (11,14). A possible explanation for this discrepancy is that the antibodies used for each of these studies may recognize two distinct molecular forms of motilin-like immunoreactivity that are present in two distinct cell types (28).

Discrepancies also have been reported when tissue distribution of motilin was examined by radioimmunoassay. Using an antiserum that demonstrates motilin in enterochromaffin cells, Bloom and co-workers (1) found very high concentrations in human duodenum (166 pmol/g), decreasing concentrations in jejunum and ileum, a small amount in stomach, and no detectable activity in esophagus, pancreas, colon, liver, or brain. In contrast, Yanaihara and co-workers (40) used an antiserum that demonstrates motilin in nonenterochromaffin cells for radioimmunoassay of extracts from three mammalian species and found widespread distribution of lower concentrations of motilin-like immunoreactivity. In their study, motilin concentrations in various regions of the gut averaged 2 to 20 pmol/g and were not concentrated in the duodenum. They found higher concentrations in some regions of dog brain than dog gut, especially in pituitary and pineal tissue. Again it would appear that two different molecules were being measured, although both groups found that the major peak of immunoreactivity coeluted with synthetic motilin on gel filtration. In the hog, highest concentrations of motilin were found in the jejunum with much less in duodenum and ileum and none in stomach (10).

Measurement

Motilin originally was detected by its ability to stimulate gastric motor activity (4), but all recent measurements of motilin have been performed by radioimmunoassay. Several radioimmunoassays have been reported in some detail (1,10,17,19). In each case, porcine motilin, usually conjugated to bovine serum albumin, was used for production of antisera and also for labeling and as the assay standard. All assays were reported to produce good recovery of motilin added to plasma; in one assay (19) methanol extraction was used with recovery of about 70%. All but one assay were used for measurement of canine motilin-like immunoreactivity; the latter assay was used to measure the peptide in human plasma (1). Regional specificity of motilin antibodies for fragments of the motilin molecule was not reported for most assays, but one antibody was shown to be specific for a C-terminal fragment between 11 and 16 residues long (27).

Metabolism

Pharmacokinetic analysis of motilin disappearance from human plasma after intravenous infusion of synthetic motilin or suppression of endogenous motilin by somatostatin infusion yielded similar estimates of disappearance half-time, about 4.5 min. Apparent volume of distribution during infusion was 49 ml kg^{-1}, and clearance rate was 8 ml kg^{-1}min^{-1} (22). Infusion of exogenous motilin at rates of 36 and 144 pmol kg^{-1}hr^{-1} produced increments in plasma motilin of about 70 and 300 pmol l^{-1}, respectively. The sites of clearance of motilin from the circulation and the mechanisms for inactivation are unknown. Patients with advanced renal failure were found to have elevated plasma motilin concentrations that were not altered by hemodialysis (32). However, peptides with disappearance half-times less than 5 min must be removed by more than one vascular bed

and the kidney cannot account entirely for motilin clearance. In dogs, systemic and portal administration of motilin produced similar effects on intestinal motor activity, suggesting that the liver has a minor role in metabolism of motilin (18).

Release

The least controversial feature of patterns of motilin release is the regular increase in immunoreactive plasma motilin during the fasting state in dogs that corresponds closely and often coincides with the onset of the interdigestive myoelectric complex in the duodenum (17,19,27) at regular intervals of 90 to 120 min (Fig. 17). Plasma motilin concentrations during initiation of the myoelectric complex are two- to threefold higher than during the midpoint of the motility cycle. Failure to take these cyclic variations into account may obscure efforts to release or inhibit the release of motilin. In the dog, intraduodenal infusion of acid or alkali was found to increase plasma motilin (3,19). However, ingestion of a meal prevented the normal cyclic increase in plasma motilin (17,19a,27), and somatostatin infusion decreased motilin below normal fasting values in dog (27) and humans (22). Motilin also was found to be released by acid but not by a meal in the pig (24).

Several studies of the effects of acid, alkali, and nutrients on plasma motilin concentrations have been reported in humans, but these usually have been done without monitoring of the motility cycle and without prolonged

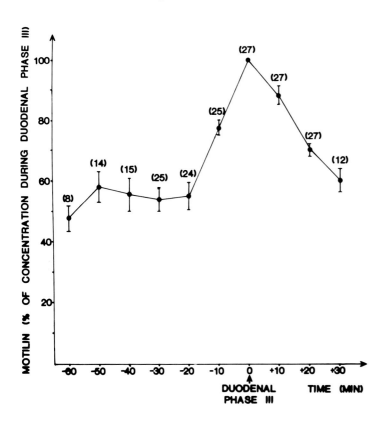

FIG. 17. Peak serum motilin concentration coincides with onset of duodenal phase 3 myoelectric complexes in fasting dogs. Blood samples were taken at 10-min intervals during the interdigestive phase. From Poitras et al. (27).

control periods to monitor the normal cycle of release of motilin. It was concluded that acidification of the duodenum produced a prompt increase in plasma motilin whereas alkalinization produced a small decrease (21). A mixed meal had little effect, but fat increased and glucose slightly decreased plasma motilin. Intravenous glucose and amino acids decreased plasma motilin whereas intravenous fat increased motilin concentrations (6). Intravenous secretin produced dose-related decreases in human plasma motilin (23).

Relationship with Physiological Events

It has been shown clearly in dogs that there is a strong positive correlation between cyclic increases in plasma motilin concentration and the onset of the interdigestive myoelectric complex (17,19,27) (Fig. 17). Furthermore, intravenous infusion of motilin during the quiescent period at rates sufficient to produce similar increases in plasma motilin regularly induces premature onset of the myoelectric complex (19,27) (Fig. 16). It is possible that inhibition of the myoelectric complex observed after ingestion of a meal is due to the inhibition of motilin release that has been found regularly in dogs. In humans, it was found that a rise in plasma motilin also preceded onset of gastroduodenal activity fronts and that intravenous infusions of motilin induced premature onset of fronts, although the plasma motilin concentrations achieved were somewhat higher than those observed normally during fasting (37). In dogs with transplanted, extrinsically denervated pouches of proximal stomach, cyclic increases in intraluminal pressure were closely associated with increases in endogenous plasma motilin (36). Somatostatin infusion in dogs abolished gastroduodenal myoelectric complexes but did not prevent the occurrence of ectopic complexes lower in the small intestine while markedly inhibiting plasma motilin concentrations (27). However, it was found that somatostatin also inhibited the gastroduodenal myoelectric response to exogenous motilin. Thus there is good evidence that cyclic release of motilin could be the initiating factor in production of interdigestive myoelectric complexes, but complete proof of a cause-effect relationship has not been obtained.

Conditions of Excess or Deficiency

There have been no reports of the effects of prolonged administration of motilin, nor have conditions leading to overproduction or underproduction been identified.

References

1. Bloom, S. R., Mitznegg, P., and Bryant, M. G. (1976): Measurement of human plasma motilin. *Scand. J. Gastroenterol.,* 11:47–52.

2. Brown, J. C., Cook, M. A., and Dryburgh, J. R. (1973): Motilin, a gastric motor activity stimulating polypeptide: The complete amino acid sequence. *Can. J. Biochem.,* 51:533–537.

3. Brown, J. C., and Dryburgh, J. R. (1978): Isolation of motilin. In: *Gut Hormones,* edited by S. R. Bloom, pp. 327–331. Churchill Livingstone, Edinburgh.

4. Brown, J. C., Mutt, V., and Dryburgh, J. R. (1971): The further purification of motilin, a gastric motor activity stimulating polypeptide from the mucosa of the small intestine of hogs. *Can. J. Physiol. Pharmacol.,* 49:399–405.

5. Castresana, M., Lee, K. Y., Chey, W. Y., and Yajima, H. (1978): Effects of motilin and octapeptide of cholecystokinin on antral and duodenal myoelectric activity in the interdigestive state and during inhibition by secretin and gastric inhibitory polypeptide. *Digestion,* 17:300–308.

6. Christofides, N. D., Bloom, S. R., Besterman, H. S., Adrian, T. E., and Ghatei, M. A. (1979): Release of motilin by oral and intravenous nutrients in man. *Gut,* 20:102–106.

7. Christofides, N. D., Modlin, I. M., Fitzpatrick, M. L., and Bloom, S. R. (1979): Effect of motilin on the rate of gastric emptying and gut hormone release during breakfast. *Gastroenterology,* 76:903–907.

8. Debas, H. T., Yamagishi, T., and Dryburgh, J. R. (1977): Motilin enhances gastric emptying of liquids in dogs. *Gastroenterology,* 73:777–780.

9. Domschke, S., Domschke, W., Schmack, B., Tympner, F., Junge, O., Wunsch, E., Jaeger, E., and Demling, L. (1976): Effects of 13-nle-motilin on salivary, gastric, and pancreatic secretions in man. *Dig. Dis.,* 21:789–792.

10. Dryburgh, J. R., and Brown, J. C. (1975): Radioimmunoassay for motilin (for dog). *Gastroenterology,* 68:1169–1176.

11. Forssmann, W. G., Yanaihara, N., Helmstaedter, V., and Grube, D. (1976): Differential demonstration of the motilin-cell and the enterochromaffin-cell. *Scand. J. Gastroenterol., [Suppl. 11],* 39:43–45.

12. Heitz, P. U., Kasper, M., Krey, G., Polak, J. M., and Pearse, A. G. E. (1978): Immunoelectron cytochemical localization of motilin in human duodenal enterochromaffin cells. *Gastroenterology,* 74:713–717.

13. Heitz, P., Polak, J. M., Kasper, M., Timson, C. M., and Pearse, A. G. E. (1978): Immunoelectron cytochemical localization of motilin and substance P in rabbit bile duct enterochromaffin (EC) cells. *Histochemistry,* 50:319–325.

14. Helmstaedter, V., Kreppein, W., Domschke, W., Mitznegg, P., Yanaihara, N., Wunsch, E., and Forssmann, W. G. (1979): Immunohistochemical localization of motilin in endocrine nonenterochromaffin cells of the small intestine of humans and monkey. *Gastroenterology,* 76:897–902.

15. Itoh, Z., Aizawa, I., Honda, R., Hiwatashi, K., and Couch, E. F. (1978): Control of lower-esophageal-sphincter contractile activity by motilin in conscious dogs. *Dig. Dis.,* 23:341–345.

16. Itoh, Z., Honda, R., Hiwatashi, K., Takeuchi, S., Aizawa, I., Takayanagi, R., and Couch, E. F. (1976): Motilin-induced mechanical activity in the canine alimentary tract. *Scand. J. Gastroenterol., [Suppl. 11],* 39:93–110.

17. Itoh, Z., Takeuchi, S., Aizawa, I., Mori, K., Taminato, T., Seino, Y., Imura, H., and Yanaihara, N. (1978): Changes in plasma motilin concentration and gastrointestinal contractile activity in conscious dogs. *Dig. Dis.,* 23:929–935.

18. Itoh, Z., Takeuchi, S., Aizawa, I., Takayanagi, R., Mori, K., Taminato, T., Seino, Y., Imura, H., and Yanaihara, N. (1978): Recent advances in motilin research: Its physiological and clinical significance. In: *Gastrointestinal Hormones and Pathology of the Digestive System,* edited by M. Grossman, V. Speranza, N. Basso, and E. Lezoche, pp. 241–258. Plenum Press, New York.

19. Lee, K. Y., Chey, W. Y., Tai, H., and Yajima, H. (1978): Radioimmunoassay of motilin: Validation and studies on the relationship between plasma motilin and interdigestive myoelectric activity of the duodenum of dog. *Dig. Dis.,* 23:789–795.

19a. Lee, K. Y., Kim, M. S., and Chey, W. Y. (1980): Effect of a meal and gut hormones on plasma motilin and duodenal motility in dog. *Am. J. Physiol.,* 238:280–283.

20. Meissner, A. J., Bowes, K. L., Zwick, R., and Daniel, E. E. (1976): Effect of motilin on the lower oesophageal sphincter. *Gut,* 17:925–932.

21. Mitznegg, P., Bloom, S. R., Christofides, N., Besterman, H., Domschke, W., Domschke, S., Wunsch, E., and Demling, L. (1976): Release of motilin in man. *Scand. J. Gastroenterol., [Suppl. 11]*, 39:53–56.

22. Mitznegg, P., Bloom, S. R., Domschke, W., Domschke, S., Wuensch, E., and Demling, L. (1977): Pharmacokinetics of motilin in man. *Gastroenterology*, 72:413–416.

23. Mitznegg, P., Bloom, S. R., Domschke, W., Haecki, W. H., Domschke, S., Belohlavek, D., Wunsch, E., and Demling, L. (1977): Effect of secretin on plasma motilin in man. *Gut*, 18:468–471.

24. Modlin, I. M., Mitznegg, P., and Bloom, S. R. (1978): Motilin release in the pig. *Gut*, 19:399–402.

25. Pearse, A. G. E., Polak, J. M., Bloom, S. R., Adams, C., Dryburgh, J. R., and Brown, J. C. (1974): Enterochromaffin cells of the mammalian small intestine as the source of motilin. *Virchows Arch. [Cell Pathol.]*, 16:111–120.

26. Phillis, J. W., and Kirkpatrick, J. R. (1979): Motilin excites neurons in the cerebral cortex and spinal cord. *Eur. J. Pharmacol.*, 58:469–472.

27. Poitras, P., Steinbach, J. H., VanDeventer, G., Code, C. F., and Walsh, J. H. (1980): Motilin independent ectopic fronts of the interdigestive myoelectric complex in dogs. *Am. J. Physiol.*, 239:G215–G220.

28. Polak, J. M. (1978): Immunoreactive motilins? *Lancet*, 1:1364.

29. Polak, J. M., Pearse, A. G. E., and Heath, C. M. (1975): Complete identification of endocrine cells in the gastrointestinal tract using semithin-thin sections to identify motilin cells in human and animal intestine. *Gut*, 16:225–229.

30. Ruppin, H., Domschke, S., Domschke, W., Wunsch, E., Jaeger, E., and Demling, L. (1975): Effects of 13-Nle-motilin in man—inhibition of gastric evacuation and stimulation of pepsin secretion. *Scand. J. Gastroenterol.*, 10:199–202.

31. Schubert, H., and Brown, J. C. (1974): Correction to the amino acid sequence of porcine motilin. *Can. J. Biochem.*, 52:7–8.

32. Shima, K., Tanaka, A., Sawazaki, N., Hamabe, J., Tanaka, R., Kumahara, Y., and Yanaihara, N. (1979): Hypermotilinemia in chronic renal failure. *Horm. Metab. Res.*, 11:320–321.

33. Shimizu, F., Imagawa, K., Mihara, S., and Yanaihara, N. (1976): Synthesis of porcine motilin by fragment condensation using three protected peptide fragments. *Bull. Chem. Soc. Jpn.*, 49:3594–3596.

34. Strunz, U., Domschke, W., Domschke, S., Mitznegg, P., Wunsch, E., Jaeger, E., and Demling, L. (1976): Potentiation between 13-Nle-motilin and acetylcholine on rabbit pyloric muscle in vitro. *Scand. J. Gastroenterol., [Suppl. 11]*, 39:29–33.

35. Strunz, U., Domschke, W., Mitznegg, P., Domschke, S., Schubert, E., Wunsch, E., Jaeger, E., and Demling, L. (1975): Analysis of the motor effects of 13-norleucine motilin on the rabbit, guinea pig, rat, and human alimentary tract in vitro. *Gastroenterology*, 68:1485–1491.

36. Thomas, P. A., Kelly, K. A., and Go, V. L. W. (1979): Does motilin regulate canine interdigestive gastric motility? *Dig. Dis. Sci.*, 24:577–582.

37. Vantrappen, G., Janssens, J., Peeters, T. L., Bloom, S. R., Christofides, N. D., and Hellemans, J. (1979): Motilin and the interdigestive migrating motor complex in man. *Dig. Dis. Sci.*, 24:497–500.

38. Wingate, D. L., Ruppin, H., Thompson, H. H., Green, W. E. R., Domschke, W., Wunsch, E., Demling, L., and Ritchie, H. D. (1975): 13-Norleucine motilin versus pentagastrin: Contrasting and competitive effects on gastrointestinal myoelectrical activity in the conscious dog. *Acta Hepatogastroenterol. (Stuttg.)*, 22:409–410.

39. Wunsch, E. (1976): Syntheses of motilin analogues. *Scand. J. Gastroenterol., [Suppl. 11]*, 39:19–24.

40. Yanaihara, C., Sato, H., Yanaihara, N., Naruse, S., Forssmann, W. G., Helmstaedter, V., Fujita, T., Yamaguchi, K., and Abe, K. (1978): Motilin-, substance P- and somatostatin-like immunoreactivities in extracts from dog, tupaia and monkey brain and GI tract. In: *Gastrointestinal Hormones and Pathology of the Digestive System*, edited by M. Grossman, V. Speranza, N. Basso, and E. Lezoche, pp. 269–283. Plenum Publishing Corp., New York.

PANCREATIC POLYPEPTIDE

Structure

Pancreatic polypeptide (PP) was isolated from chicken pancreas as a by-product of insulin purification by Kimmel and co-workers (24) and from pancreatic extracts from several mammalian species by Chance et al. (14).

The avian and bovine peptides each contain 36 amino acid residues and have identical residues at 16 positions (Table 7). The molecular weights of the two peptides are 4,240 and 4,226, respectively. Ovine and porcine PP (identical to canine) differ from the bovine peptide by single amino acid substitutions, whereas human PP differs at 2 to 4 positions (Table 7). All pancreatic polypeptides have a carboxyl terminal tyrosine amide, and the avian and mammalian peptides are identical in 4 of the 5 C-terminal positions. There are no obvious structural similarities between pancreatic polypeptide and other gastrointestinal peptides.

Biological Actions

The biological actions of avian PP (aPP) and of bovine PP (bPP) differ significantly. In chickens, aPP is a potent stimulant of acid and pepsin secretion from the proventriculus and these effects are resistant to inhibition by vagotomy or anticholinergics (25). The same doses of aPP had no demonstrable effects on pancreatic secretion or gallbladder contraction. aPP causes a rapid decrease in avian liver glycogen concentration without a change in blood glucose. Plasma glycerol decreases and plasma triglyceride increases while plasma amino acid concentrations, especially alanine, decrease rapidly. These effects are consistent with stimulation of hepatic lipogenesis by aPP in the chicken. Decreased plasma glycerol and free fatty acids following aPP injections are consistent with inhibition of adipose tissue lipolysis, and depression of glucagon-stimulated lipolysis has been demonstrated directly in chicken adipocytes (14). A possible trophic effect of aPP was suggested by the finding that injection of this peptide into fertilized chicken eggs caused stimulation of proventricular protein synthesis (32). Mammalian PP has little effect on any of the secretory or metabolic parameters that are responsive to aPP in the chicken.

The actions of bPP in the conscious dog have been studied by Lin and co-workers (33). bPP is a weak stimulant of acid secretion from vagally innervated gastric pouches and a weaker stimulant in vagally denervated pouches. During stimulation of gastric secretion by pentagastrin, bPP has an inhibitory effect. Lower doses of bPP cause inhibition of basal pancreatic secretion and inhibit the protein and bicarbonate responses obtained during infusion of CCK plus secretin but have less

TABLE 7. *Structures of pancreatic polypeptides*

Pancreatic polypeptides	Abbreviation	Structure			
Avian	(aPP)	GPSQPTYPGDDAPVEDLIRPYDNLQQYLNVVTRHRY#			
Bovine	(bPP)	APLEPQYPGDDATPEQMAQYAAELRRYINMLTRPRY#			
Porcine	(pPP)	V			
Canine	(cPP)	V			
Ovine	(oPP)	S			
Human	(hPP)	V	BB	D	

Underlined residues indicate identities between avian and bovine PP; other residues indicate differences between bovine and other mammalian PP molecules.

marked effects on bicarbonate secretion stimulated by secretin alone. Inhibition of pancreatic secretion also was obtained during endogenous stimulation by intraduodenal infusion of amino acids. bPP has a slight relaxing effect on the gallbladder and a moderate stimulating action on choledochal sphincter tone but no effect on bile flow. The peptide also increased motility in the stomach and intestine and caused increased gastric emptying of a meal and increased rate of intestinal transit. The C-terminal tyrosine amide was found to be essential for these actions, since tryptic removal of this residue abolished the effects on gastric and pancreatic secretion. Intravenous bPP had no effect on blood glucose, electrolytes, or urine flow in dogs (34).

Intravenous infusions of porcine PP (pPP) produced significant inhibition of basal and stimulated (secretin plus cerulein) pancreatic secretion in dogs at doses that caused lower circulating PP concentrations than those achieved after a protein meal (49) (Table 8). Similar inhibitory effects on pancreatic secretion have been reported in humans (17,19). On the other hand, PP had no significant effects in dog (37) or humans (18) on stimulated gastric acid secretion at doses that were near the physiologic range. Large doses of bPP had no effect on intestinal water and electrolyte transport in the rat (55). Graded doses of bPP produced a dose-related increase in lower esophageal sphincter pressure in the opossum that appeared to involve both stimulation of cholinergic nerve fibers and a direct action on the smooth muscle (39). bPP was reported to increase DNA synthesis in the rat pancreas but did not increase or decrease the stimulation produced by CCK (20). An effect on food intake was shown in obese hyperphagic mice (ob/ob) where repeated injections of bPP caused a significant decrease in body weight (36). Effects on satiety have not been reported in other mammalian species, and this author is not aware of studies on hepatic glycogenolysis or lipolysis in mammals.

Structure-Activity Relationships

The C-terminal tyrosine amide is essential for biological activity of bPP (33). The C-terminal hexapeptide was said to possess all the biologic actions of the entire peptide (33). Although there are major differences in effects between avian and mammalian PP, no differences have been reported between different mammalian PP molecules.

Distribution

The pancreas appears to be the major site for production and storage of PP, and release of PP into the blood could not be demonstrated in patients with previous total pancreatectomy (4). PP-containing cells have been demonstrated by immunohistochemical methods in a large number of mammals (29,30). In most species, they

TABLE 8. *Decrease in pancreatic secretion produced by PP infusion in dogs during background stimulation with secretin (41 pmol kg^{-1}hr^{-1}) and cerulein (37 pmol kg^{-1}hr^{-1})*

pPP dose (pmol kg^{-1}hr^{-1})	HCO$_3$ output (% decrease)	Protein output (% decrease)	Plasma PP (pM)
100	35	11	36
200	52	29	73
400	76	45	175
Protein meal	—	—	210

Data from Taylor et al. (49).

occur in islets as well as scattered throughout the exocrine parenchyma and are more abundant in the portion of the pancreas adjacent to the duodenum. The PP cells of dog and cat contain fairly large granules similar to those found in F cells, and the definite identity of these cells as F cells has been confirmed by immune electron microscopy (21). In humans and rat, the PP-containing cells contain small granules, and the cell type in human pancreas was identified by electron microscopy as the D_1 cell (23). Others have found that PP was located in the F cell of the human pancreas (15). The concentration of PP and of PP-containing cells is much greater in the uncinate process and head of the human and canine pancreas than in the body and tail, and this distribution is opposite to that found for glucagon (15). In the rat this distribution corresponds to the region drained by the ventral pancreatic duct, in which the islets contain 14% PP and 1% glucagon cells, contrasted with the body and tail drained by the dorsal pancreatic duct, in which islets contain 15% glucagon cells and less than 1% PP cells (8).

By use of a radioimmunoassay with an antiserum specific for avian PP, aPP-like immunoreactivity could be extracted from the pancreas but no other organs in the bird (27). Similar material was found in several avian species and in the turtle and alligator but not in mammalian or amphibian pancreatic extracts. aPP-containing cells in the chicken pancreas are found predominantly in the exocrine parenchyma and rarely in the islets (31). They are most abundant at about the time of hatching, and at this time they are present in the duodenum. One group has reported that such cells persist in the proventriculus and small intestine after hatching (7).

Measurement

Pancreatic polypeptide initially was isolated by chemical methods, and no bioassay system has been described that is sensitive or specific enough to be useful for its detection. However, measurement by radioimmunoassay has proved to be rather easy. The first RIA method was developed for aPP (27) and was sufficiently sensitive to demonstrate aPP in chick plasma after feeding. The antibody was specific for avian PP and demonstrated no cross-reactivity with mammalian pancreatic extracts. Most of the measurements of mammalian PP have been performed with antibody raised to bPP by Chance et al. (12) and supplied to different research laboratories (42,47,48). This antibody has equal affinity for bovine and human PP and no cross-reactivity with other known gastrointestinal peptides. It does not detect aPP and is not satisfactory for measurement of PP from rat pancreas. The PP concentration in fasting serum from dogs or normal human subjects is about 10 to 30 pM with this assay system. Another radioimmunoassay was developed with antibody raised

against pure human PP and yielded measurements that were comparable in fasting human subjects (4).

Metabolism

The pharmacokinetics of PP have been measured in humans and dog during and after infusion of pure PP intravenously. In humans the disappearance half-time was estimated as 6.9 min, the clearance rate was 5 ml $kg^{-1}min^{-1}$, and the volume of distribution was 51 ml kg^{-1} (6). In dogs the disappearance half-time was 5.5 min, the clearance rate was 26 ml $kg^{-1}min^{-1}$, and the volume of distribution was 209 ml kg^{-1} (49). In both studies, there was a linear relationship between infusion dose and increment in circulating PP. A significant role of the kidney in removal of PP from the circulation was suggested by the finding that patients with advanced renal failure had approximately fivefold elevations in basal PP concentrations (22).

Release

Pancreatic polypeptide is released by protein meals and other nutrients and by cholinergic reflexes, and the release is inhibited markedly by anticholinergic agents. Factors influencing plasma PP concentrations in humans were reviewed by Floyd and co-workers (14). Basal PP concentrations were found to be related to age and increased progressively from about 12 pM to about 50 pM between the third and seventh decades of life. The most potent stimulant for PP release was found to be ingestion of a protein-rich meal. Intravenous infusion of amino acids produced a significant but much smaller response. Fat ingestion produced a small response. Instillation of hydrochloric acid into the duodenum did not cause an increase in plasma PP. Intravenous rapid injection of pentagastrin caused a rapid rise in PP concentration, whereas chronic infusion of somatostatin prevented the increases in PP normally observed after meals during a 24-hr period. Ingestion of glucose produced a small initial increase in PP followed by a large increase 3 to 6 hr later when blood sugar decreased and plasma growth hormone also increased. Intravenous glucose produced suppression of PP concentrations during the infusion. Intravenous insulin infusion produced a large increase in PP during the time of maximal hypoglycemia. During a 72-hr fast the plasma PP concentration increased as blood glucose fell and the increase in PP was accentuated by exercise.

Other workers have reached similar conclusions concerning the effects of nutrients on PP release in humans and in dog. In humans, homogenized food produced a large and prolonged PP response when introduced into the stomach, whereas saline and glucose produced transient small responses (47) (Fig. 18). Sham feeding in humans causes a small increment in plasma PP and sig-

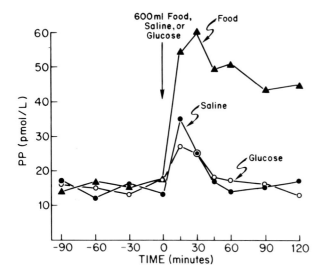

FIG. 18. Pancreatic polypeptide (PP) responses to intragastric administration of saline, glucose, or homogenized food in normal human subjects. From Taylor et al. (47).

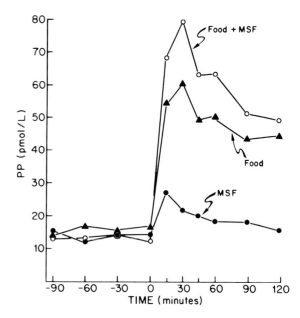

FIG. 19. Pancreatic polypeptide responses to modified sham feeding (MSF), intragastric food, and a combination of the two in normal human subjects. From Taylor et al. (47).

nificantly enhances the PP response in intragastric food (47) (Fig. 19). In dogs, intraduodenal administration of sodium oleate or of mixed amino acids produced an increase in PP only slightly less than that produced by a meal, whereas intraduodenal acid had no effect (54). These responses were abolished by intravenous infusion of somatostatin. Intravenous infusion of amino acids, glucose, or fat failed to produce measurable changes in human PP in another study (2), although significant increases were found after intravenous administration of cerulein and an impure (Boots) preparation of secretin. However, administration of synthetic gastrin (G17) or pure CCK at doses that achieved maximal rates of gastric and pancreatic secretion failed to stimulate human PP release (47).

Vagal cholinergic mechanisms are important in the regulation of PP release. The PP response to insulin hypoglycemia was abolished by prior administration of atropine in humans (42). PP release by sham feeding in humans also is abolished by atropine (13,40,44). PP release also has been demonstrated during balloon distension of the antral or fundic portions of the stomach (41). Electrical stimulation of vagus nerves in anesthetized pigs caused an increase in portal PP concentration that was partially inhibited by atropine and abolished by hexamethonium (42). In the isolated perfused porcine pancreas, acetylcholine caused a dose-dependent stimulation of PP that was completely abolished by atropine (42). Cutting of the splanchnic nerves in calves had no effect on the PP response to a 2-deoxyglucose, but this response was abolished by atropine (10). These studies all demonstrate that vagal cholinergic stimulation leads to PP release and that atropine inhibits the response.

Plasma PP responses to hormonal stimulation also

are inhibited by atropine. Atropine prevented the increases in PP obtained during intravenous administration of cerulein or Boots secretin in human subjects (1). Bombesin was found to be as potent a stimulant of PP release as of gastrin release in dogs, and the stimulation by bombesin was markedly inhibited by atropine (49,51). The maximal response to bombesin was greater than the response to a protein meal. Bethanechol did not enhance the PP response to bombesin although it produced moderate stimulation when administered alone. Since the responses obtained after ingestion of a protein meal are larger and more prolonged than the responses produced by distension of the stomach or sham feeding, it is assumed that additional hormonal mechanisms are involved. These mechanisms also are dependent on cholinergic innervation, since administration of anticholinergics markedly inhibits the total PP response to food in humans (47,48) and dog (48) (Fig. 20). The effects of vagotomy on meal-stimulated PP secretion are not as clear as the results of anticholinergic agents. Patients with vagotomy performed months to years previously had virtually normal responses to a meal but no response to vagal stimulation (2,47). On the other hand, PP responses to food were markedly diminished in patients studied 3 months after truncal vagotomy (43), and similar results were obtained in dogs studied after vagotomy (48). It is possible that these differences are due to the interval between vagotomy and testing and that vagus-dependent factors are regained over time following vagotomy.

Plasma pancreatic polypeptide concentrations were found to fluctuate during fasting over 60- to 90-min periods in patients with duodenal ulcer and normal

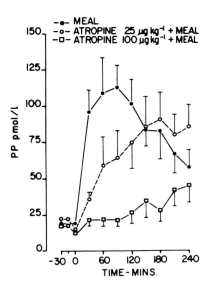

FIG. 20. Dose-dependent inhibition of food-stimulated pancreatic polypeptide release in dogs by atropine. From Taylor et al. (48).

human subjects, and the periods of highest PP concentrations were associated with highest rates of basal acid secretion (40,44,45). Since both acid secretion and plasma PP were suppressed by anticholinergic agents, these data were interpreted as suggesting that PP concentrations were a reflection of abdominal vagal tone. A possible role of adrenergic factors in regulation of PP release was suggested by the observation that alpha-adrenergic blockade increases the PP response to exercise in man whereas beta-adrenergic blockade prevents the increase (9).

The possible hormonal mediators of PP release were assessed in the isolated perfused dog pancreas (5). Significant responses were obtained during infusion of 1 nM concentrations of cerulein, GIP, VIP, and gastrin but not during infusion of secretin, glucagon, bombesin, or epinephrine. None of the responses were as high as those achieved during acetylcholine infusion. In a similar preparation, arginine produced a significant increase in PP but no responses were obtained with glucagon or insulin (53).

The data obtained concerning PP release all are consistent with the idea that cholinergic innervation of the pancreas is necessary for effective release of this peptide and that activation of cholinergic reflexes results in PP release. It also is clear that protein-rich meals activate some factor, possibly a hormone, that causes more exaggerated release of PP, but the nature of this factor has not been defined.

Relationship with Physiological Events

The role of pancreatic polypeptide in regulation of digestion or metabolism has not been established. In-

travenous infusion of PP in dogs at doses that produce serum PP concentrations lower than those found after a protein-rich meal produces significant inhibition of basal pancreatic secretion and of pancreatic secretion stimulated by secretin plus cerulein (49,51) (Table 8). These observations suggest that PP may modulate the pancreatic secretory response to feeding. However, the effects of PP on food-stimulated pancreatic secretion have not been studied directly.

Conditions of Excess or Deficiency

Release of PP is markedly diminished or abolished after total pancreatectomy and in patients with severe pancreatic insufficiency due to chronic pancreatitis (3,52). No specific adverse consequences of PP deficiency have been identified.

Certain endocrine tumors contain PP cells in addition to other hormone-producing cells, and plasma PP concentrations often are increased in such patients (38). This association seems to be greater for tumors that produce VIP than for tumors that produce gastrin (40,41). A few tumors have been identified that appeared to contain exclusively PP cells (11,35). One of these patients had peptic ulcer disease with gastric acid hypersecretion and one had a watery diarrhea syndrome. However, there is no evidence that PP can produce either gastric or intestinal hypersecretion. Hyperplasia of PP cells also has been observed in the remaining pancreas in patients with islet cell tumors (28–30). This hyperplasia may give rise to increased plasma PP concentrations found in some of these patients, but no specific clinical abnormalities have been related to this condition. Studies of pancreatic exocrine secretion apparently have not been performed in such patients. In patients with insulinoma and elevated plasma PP, the PP concentrations often remain elevated after successful tumor resection (14). Increased plasma PP concentrations also have been found in some patients with islet cell carcinomas previously thought to be nonfunctioning (14) and in patients with hyperparathyroidism but no apparent pancreatic tumor from families with type 1 multiple endocrine neoplasia syndrome (26).

Plasma PP concentrations are increased in patients with diabetes mellitus, especially the juvenile-onset type, and there is a positive correlation between PP concentrations and the severity of the diabetes (14). Some apparent increases in plasma PP are due to the presence of circulating antibodies to PP caused by contamination of insulin preparations with this peptide, but the increases in mean PP values in diabetics are still found when these patients are excluded. The pancreatic content of PP and numbers of PP cells per islet were found to be significantly increased in obese-hyperglycemic (ob/ob) mice (16). Repeated injections of PP in rats produced no significant effect on the composition of the exocrine (46) or endocrine (56) pancreas. Suitable assays are not yet available to determine whether chronic administration of hormones influences the PP content of the rat pancreas, since rat PP cross-reacts poorly with antibodies currently available for measurement of mammalian PP by radioimmunoassay. Thus it is not possible to conclude whether changes in pancreatic content and release of PP in diabetic humans and animals are a result of other endocrine or metabolic abnormalities, nor are any data available to suggest that PP may contribute to peripheral insensitivity to insulin.

References

1. Adrian, T. E., Besterman, H. S., and Bloom, S. R. (1979): The importance of cholinergic tone in the release of pancreatic polypeptide by gut hormones in man. *Life Sci.* 24:1989–1994.
2. Adrian, T. E., Besterman, H. S., Cooke, T. J. C., Bloom, S. R., Barnes, A. J., Russell, R. C. G., and Faber, R. G. (1977): Mechanism of pancreatic polypeptide release in man. *Lancet,* 161–163.
3. Adrian, T. E., Besterman, H. S., Mallinson, C. N., Garalotis, C., and Bloom, S. R. (1979): Impared pancreatic polypeptide release in chronic pancreatitis with steatorrhea. *Gut,* 20:98–101.
4. Adrian, T. E., Bloom, S. R., Bryant, M. G., Polak, J. M., Heitz, Ph., and Barnes, A. J. (1976): Distribution and release of human pancreatic polypeptide. *Gut,* 17:940–944.
5. Adrian, T. E., Bloom, S. R., Hermansen, K., and Iversen, J. (1978): Pancreatic polypeptide, glucagon and insulin secretion from the isolated perfused canine pancreas. *Diabetologia,* 14:413–417.
6. Adrian, T. E., Greenberg, G. R., Besterman, H. S., and Bloom, S. R. (1978): Pharmacokinetics of pancreatic polypeptide in man. *Gut,* 19:907–909.
7. Alumets, J., Hakanson, R., and Sundler, F. (1978): Distribution, ontogeny and ultrastructure of pancreatic polypeptide (PP) cells in the pancreas and gut of the chicken. *Cell Tissue Res.,* 194:377–386.
8. Baetens, D., Malaisse-Lagae, F., Perrelet, A., and Orci, L. (1979): Endocrine pancreas: Three-dimensional reconstruction shows two types of islets of Langerhans. *Science,* 206:1323–1325.
9. Berger, D., Floyd, J. C., Jr., Lampman, R. M., and Fajans, S. S. (1979): The effect of adrenergic receptor blockade on the exercise-induced rise in pancreatic polypeptide in man. *J. Clin. Endocrinol. Metab.,* 50:33–39.
10. Bloom, S. R., Edwards, A. V., and Hardy, R. N. (1978): The role of the autonomic nervous system in the control of glucagon, insulin and pancreatic polypeptide release from the pancreas. *J. Physiol.,* 280:9–23.
11. Bordi, C., Togni, R., Baetens, D., Ravazzola, M., Malaisse-Lagae, F., and Orci, L. (1977): Human islet cell tumor storing pancreatic polypeptide: A light and electron microscopic study. *J. Clin. Endocrinol. Metab.,* 46:215–219.
12. Chance, R. E., Moon, N. E., and Johnson, M. G. (1979): Human pancreatic polypeptide (HPP) and bovine pancreatic polypeptide (BPP). In: *Methods of Hormone Radioimmunoassay,* edited by B. M. Jaffe and H. R. Behrman, pp. 657–670. Academic Press, New York.
13. Feldman, M., Richardson, C. T., Taylor, I. L., and Walsh, J. H. (1979): Effect of atropine on vagal release of gastrin and pancreatic polypeptide. *J. Clin. Invest.,* 63:294–298.
14. Floyd, J. C., Jr., Fajans, S. S., Pek, S., and Chance, R. E. (1977): A newly recognized pancreatic polypeptide; plasma levels in health and disease. *Recent Prog. Horm. Res.,* 33:519–570.
15. Gersell, D. J., Gingerich, R. L., and Greider, M. H. (1979): Regional distribution and concentration of pancreatic polypeptide in the human and canine pancreas. *Diabetes,* 28:11–15.
16. Gingerich, R. L., Gersell, D. J., Greider, M. H., Finke, E. H., and Lacy, P. E. (1978): Elevated levels of pancreatic polypeptide in obese-hyperglycemic mice. *Metabolism,* 27(10):1526–1532.
17. Greenberg, G. R., Adrian, T. E., Baron, J. H., McCloy, R. F.,

18. Greenberg, G. R., McCloy, R. F. Adrian, T. E., Baron, J. H., and Bloom, S. R. (1978): Effect of bovine pancreatic polypeptide on gastric acid and pepsin output in man. *Acta Hepatogastroenterol. (Stuttg.),* 25:384–387.
19. Greenberg, G. R., McCloy, R. F., Chadwick, V. S., Adrian, T. E., Baron, J. H., and Bloom, S. R. (1979): Effect of bovine pancreatic polypeptide on basal pancreatic and biliary outputs in man. *Dig. Dis. Sci.,* 24:11–14.
20. Greenberg, G. R., Mitznegg, P., and Bloom, S. R. (1977): Effect of pancreatic polypeptide on DNA-synthesis in the pancreas. *Experentia,* 33:1332–1333.
21. Greider, M. H., Gersell, D. J., and Gingerich, R. L. (1978): Ultrastructural localization of pancreatic polypeptide in the F cell of the dog pancreas. *J. Histochem. Cytochem.* 12:1103–1108.
22. Hallgren, R., Landelius, J., Fjellstrom, K.-E., and Lundqvist, G. (1979): Gastric acid secretion in uraemia and circulating levels of gastrin, somatostatin, and pancreatic polypeptide. *Gut,* 20:763–768.
23. Heitz, Ph., Polak, J. M., Bloom, S. R., and Pearse, A. G. E. (1976): Identification of the D_1-cell as the source of human pancreatic polypeptide (HPP). *Gut,* 17:755–758.
24. Kimmel, J. R., Hayden, L. J., and Pollock, H. G. (1975): Isolation and characterization of a new pancreatic polypeptide hormone. *J. Biol. Chem.,* 24:9369–9376.
25. Kimmel, J. R., Pollock, H. G., and Hayden, L. J. (1978): Biological activity of avian PP in the chicken. In: *Gut Hormones,* edited by S. R. Bloom, pp. 234–241. Churchill Livingstone, Edinburgh.
26. Lamers, C. B., Diemel, J., and Roeffen, W. (1978): Serum levels of pancreatic polypeptide in Zollinger-Ellison syndrome, and hyperparathyroidism from families with multiple endocrine adenomatosis type I. *Digestion,* 18(5-6):297–302.
27. Langslow, D. R., Kimmel, J. R., and Pollock, H. G. (1973): Studies on the distribution of a new avian pancreatic polypeptide and insulin among birds, reptiles, amphibians and mammals. *Endocrinology,* 93:558.
28. Larsson, L.-I. (1977): Two distinct types of islet abnormalities associated with endocrine pancreatic tumours. *Virchows Arch. [Pathol. Anat.],* 376:209–219.
29. Larsson, L.-I., Schwartz, T., Lundqvist, G., Chance, R. E., Sundler, F., Rehfeld, J. F., Grimelius, L., Fahrenkrug, J., Schaffalitzky de Muckadell, O., and Moon, N. (1976): Occurrence of human pancreatic polypeptide in pancreatic endocrine tumors. *Am. J. Pathol.* 85:675–684.
30. Larsson, L.-I., Sundler, F., and Hakanson, R. (1976): Pancreatic polypeptide—A postulated new hormone: Identification of its cellular storage site by light and electron microscopic immunocytochemistry. *Diabetologia,* 12:211–226.
31. Larsson, L.-I., Sundler, F., Hakanson, R., Pollock, H. G., and Kimmel, J. R. (1974): Localization of APP, a postulated new hormone, to a pancreatic endocrine cell type. *Histochemistry,* 42:377–382.
32. Laurentz, D. A., and Hazelwood, R. L., (1979): Does the third pancreatic hormone (APP) play a trophic role in the growth of the embryonic chick proventriculus? (40407). *Proc. Soc. Exp. Biol. Med.,* 160:144–149.
33. Lin, T.-M., and Chance, R. E. (1978): Spectrum of gastrointestinal actions of bovine PP. In: *Gut Hormones,* edited by S. R. Bloom pp. 242–246. Churchill Livingston, Edinburgh.
34. Lin, T.-M., Evans, D. C., Chance, R. E., and Spray, G. F. (1977): Bovine pancreatic peptide: Action on gastric and pancreatic secretion in dogs. *Am. J. Physiol.,* 232(3):E311–E315.
35. Lundqvist, G., Krause, U., Larsson, L.-I., Grimelius, L., Schaffalitzky de Muckadell, O. B., Fahrenkrug, J., Johnson, M., and Chance, R. E. (1978): A pancreatic-polypeptide-producing tumour associated with the WDHA syndrome. *Scand. J. Gastroenterol.,* 13:715–718.
36. Malaisse-Lagae, F., Carpentier, J.-L., Patel, Y. C., Malaisse, W. J., and Orci, L. (1977): Pancreatic polypeptide: A possible role in the regulation of food intake in the mouse. Hypothesis. *Experientia,* 33:915–917.
37. Parks, D. L., Gingerich, R. L., Jaffe, B. M., and Akande, B. (1979): Role of pancreatic polypeptide in canine gastric acid secretion. *Am. J. Physiol.,* 236(4):E488–494.

38. Polak, J. M., Adrian, T. E., Bryant, M. G., Bloom, S. R., Heitz, Ph., and Pearse, A. G. E. (1976): Pancreatic polypeptide in insulinomas, gastrinomas, vipomas, and glucagonomas. *Lancet,* 328–330.
39. Rattan, S., and Goyal, R. K. (1979): Effect of bovine pancreatic polypeptide on the opossum lower esophageal sphincter. *Gastroenterology,* 77:672–676.
40. Schwartz, T. W. (1979): Pancreatic polypeptide (PP) and endocrine tumours of the pancreas. *Scand. J. Gastroenterol.,* [*Suppl. 4*] 53:93–100.
41. Schwartz, T. W., Grotzinger, U., Schoon, I.-M., and Olbe, L. (1979): Vagovagal stimulation of pancreatic-polypeptide secretion by graded distention of the gastric fundus and antrum in man. *Digestion,* 19:307–314.
42. Schwartz, T. W., Holst, J. J., Fahrenkrug, J., Lindkaer Jensen, S. Nielsen, O. V., Rehfeld, J. F., Schaffalitzky de Muckadell, O. B., and Stadil, F. (1978): Vagal, cholinergic regulation of pancreatic polypeptide secretion. *J. Clin. Invest.,* 61:781–789.
43. Schwartz, T. W., Stadil, F., Chance, R. E., Rehfeld, J. F., Larson, L.-I., and Moon, N. (1976): Pancreatic-polypeptide response to food in duodenal-ulcer patients before and after vagotomy. *Lancet,* 1102–1106.
44. Schwartz, T. W., Stenquist, B., and Olbe, L. (1979): Cephalic phase of pancreatic-polypeptide secretion studied by sham feeding in man. *Scand. J. Gastroenterol.,* 14:313–320.
45. Schwartz, T. W., Stenquist, B., Olbe, L., and Stadil, F. (1979): Synchronous oscillations in the basal secretion of pancreatic-polypeptide and gastric acid. Depression by cholinergic blockade of pancreatic-polypeptide concentrations in plasma. *Gastroenterology,* 76:14–19.
46. Solomon, T. E., Petersen, H., Elashoff, J., and Grossman, M. I. (1979): Effects of chemical messenger peptides on pancreatic growth in rats. *Gut Peptides,* 213–219.
47. Taylor, I. L., Feldman, M., Richardson, C. T., and Walsh, J. H. (1978): Gastric and cephalic stimulation of human pancreatic polypeptide release. *Gastroenterology,* 75:432–437.
48. Taylor, I. L., Impicciatore, M., Carter, D. C., and Walsh, J. H. (1978): Effect of atropine and vagotomy on pancreatic polypeptide response to a meal in dogs. *Am. J. Physiol.,* 235(4): E443–E447.
49. Taylor, I. L., Solomon, T. E., Walsh, J. H., and Grossman, M. I. (1979): Pancreatic polypeptide. Metabolism and effect on pancreatic secretion in dogs. *Gastroenterology,* 76:524–528.
50. Taylor, I. L., Rotter, J., Walsh, J. H., and Passaro, E., Jr. (1978): Is pancreatic polypeptide a marker for Zollinger-Ellison syndrome? *Lancet,* 845–848.
51. Taylor, I. L., Walsh, J. H., Carter, D., Wood, J., and Grossman, M. I. (1979): Effects of atropine and bethanechol on bombesin-stimulated release of pancreatic polypeptide and gastrin in dog. *Gastroenterology,* 77:714–718.
52. Valenzuela, J. E., Taylor, I. L., and Walsh, J. H. (1979): Pancreatic polypeptide response in patients with chronic pancreatitis. *Dig. Dis. Sci.,* 24:862–864.
53. Weir, G. C., Samols, E., Loo, S., Patel, Y. C., and Gabbay, K. H. (1979): Somatostatin and pancreatic polypeptide secretion. Effects of glucagon, insulin, and arginine. *Diabetes,* 28:35–40.
54. Wilson, R. M., Boden, G., and Owen, O. E. (1978): Pancreatic polypeptide responses to a meal and to intraduodenal amino acids and sodium oleate. *Endocrinology,* 102:859–863.
55. Wu, Z. C., O'Dorisio, T. M., Cataland, S., Mekhjian, H. S., and Gaginella, T. S. (1979): Effects of pancreatic polypeptide and vasoactive intestinal polypeptide on rat ileal and colonic water and electrolyte transport *in vivo. Dig. Dis. Sci.,* 24:625–630.
56. Yamada, T., Solomon, T. E., Petersen, H., Levin, S. R., Lewin, K., Walsh, J. H., and Grossman, M. I. (1980): Effects of gastrointestinal polypeptides on hormone content of endocrine pancreas in the rat. *Am. J. Physiol.,* 238:G526–G530.

NEUROTENSIN

Structure

Neurotensin is a tridecapeptide originally isolated from bovine hypothalamus (9) and later, in identical form, from bovine intestine (8,17) (Table 1). The amino acid sequence of human intestinal neurotensin was found to be identical to that of bovine neurotensin (15). A minor contaminant of immunoreactive material in bovine intestinal extract appeared to be the N-terminal dodecapeptide and was devoid of hypotensive activity (8). A smaller C-terminal fragment also has been identified in rat stomach (11). Neurotensin is structurally similar to the amphibian skin peptide xenopsin (4).

Biological Activity

Intravenous administration of neurotensin causes a wide range of pharmacologic actions in addition to systemic hypotension, the biological effect used for initial identification and isolation of the peptide (9). These include increased vascular permeability, hyperglycemia (7), hypoinsulinemia, hyperglucagonemia, accentuation of the action of barbiturates, mediation of pituitary growth hormone and prolactin release, and increase in plasma concentrations of ACTH, LH, and FSH (20). Neurotensin also produces hypothermia when injected intracisternally in cold-exposed rats, but is 10^4 times less potent than bombesin for this effect (6). The hyperglycemic effect appears to be mediated by a mechanism that causes depletion of liver glycogen but is distinct from the effect of glucagon and is not prevented by adrenalectomy (7). Neurotensin was ineffective in an *in vitro* liver slice preparation that showed a response to glucagon.

In humans, intravenous infusion of neurotensin at a dose of 144 pmol $kg^{-1}hr^{-1}$ produced approximately 30% inhibition of pentagastrin-stimulated gastric acid and pepsin secretion and significantly delayed gastric emptying of oral glucose (5). In dogs, inhibition of gastric acid secretion was found during stimulation by pentagastrin but not during stimulation by histamine (1). Vagally innervated fundic pouches were more sensitive to inhibition by neurotensin than vagally denervated pouches (3). Canine gastric motor activity also is inhibited by neurotensin at doses lower than those required to produce hypotension or hyperglycemia, and vagally innervated antral pouches are more sensitive to this effect than vagally denervated fundic pouches (2). Infusion of Gln^4-neurotensin in a human subject at a rate of 360 pmol $kg^{-1}hr^{-1}$ led to prompt decrease in lower esophageal sphincter pressure whereas plasma neurotensin concentration increased from about 30 to about 300 pM (27). These values compared with mean basal concentration of 65 pM and peak values of 233 pM obtained in normal subjects after a meal. In isolated smooth muscle preparations from the rat, low concentrations of neurotensin caused contraction of fundic muscle strips, and this effect was not inhibited by atropine, hexamethonium, or methysergide (25). Higher concentrations caused contraction of guinea pig ileum and relaxation of rat duodenum but had no effect on smooth muscle from vas deferens, aorta, or skeletal muscle.

Specific binding of labeled neurotensin has been demonstrated *in vitro*. Binding to rat mast cells was found to be optimal at pH 7 in hypotonic buffers with a K_D of 154 nM (21). Specific binding also has been found to synaptic membranes from rat brain, with K_D between 1 and 2 nM (18).

Structure-Activity Relationships

The C-terminal region of neurotensin appears to contain the determinants of biological activity such as hypotension, vascular permeability, hyperglycemia, and smooth muscle contraction. Partial sequences of the C-terminal portion of the molecule of 5 or more amino acids retained biological activity whereas N-terminal sequences containing up to 10 residues were ineffective (10). Amidation of the C-terminal leucine residue also destroyed activity (13). A series of synthetic analogues was assessed for effects on hypothermia and binding to mast cell receptors (24). It was found that substitutions in positions 1 through 7 had little effect, whereas substitutions in positions 8 through 13 produced marked effects that often were not parallel in the two systems. For example, substitution of D-Tyr or D-Phe in position 11 markedly increased hypothermic activity whereas D-Arg in positions 8 or 9 increased binding affinity to mast cells. The C-terminal penta-and hexapeptides retained binding to mast cells while most substitutions in positions 10 through 13 including C-terminal substitution with N-methylamide markedly decreased binding (22). Similar findings were reported for displacement of labeled neurotensin from rat brain synaptic membranes (18). The C-terminal hexa-, octa-, and decapeptides appeared more potent than neurotensin, whereas the 1–12 sequence was ineffective.

Distribution

Neurotensin has been localized to a specific endocrine cell type, called the N cell, in ileal mucosa of the dog (14) and in humans (23). Highest concentrations of immunoreactive neurotensin were found in human ileal mucosa, with smaller amounts found in jejunal mucosa, stomach, duodenum, and colon (23). In the rat, about 90% of immunoreactive neurotensin is found in the gut and about 10% in the brain (11). When an antibody specific for the whole molecule was used, highest concentrations were found in the jejunum and ileum, while an antibody specific for the C-terminal portion of the molecule detected large amounts of gastric and duodenal immunoreactivity with smaller apparent molecular weight, possibly the C-terminal pentapeptide. Mucosal extracts contained more activity than muscle

extracts, but the latter contained significant amounts suggesting a source other than mucosal cells. In the brain, highest concentrations were found in hypothalamus and pituitary, but some activity was detected throughout the brain. Extracts of rat and bovine plasma were found to contain two forms of immunoreactive neurotensin, corresponding on gel filtration to the whole molecule and to the C-terminal pentapeptide. More detailed analysis of neurotensin distribution in rat brain revealed a wide distribution with highest concentrations in median eminence, medial and lateral preoptic nuclei, and other hypothalamic and preoptic nuclei (19). Neurotensin binding sites in the rat brain were most abundant in the thalamus, followed by the hypothalamus and cerebrum (20).

Measurement

Prior to development of a radioimmunoassay for neurotensin, the content of this peptide in tissue extracts could be estimated only roughly by bioassay because of interfering vasoactive substances. Antibodies with differing regional specificities for neurotensin have been produced by immunization of rabbits with conjugates prepared by coupling to different carrier molecules (12). Antibodies that recognized the whole molecule and others with specificity for C-terminal fragments were obtained. By radioimmunoassay with different antisera and gel filtration of extracts, it was shown that acid/acetone extracts of hypothalamus contained a single form of neurotensin-like immunoreactivity that coeluted with synthetic and natural neurotensin but that acid aqueous extracts appeared to contain multiple forms with C-terminal immunoreactivity. Similar results were obtained with rat brain and intestine, but stomach extracts and blood were found to contain forms that corresponded to the intact molecule and to the C-terminal pentapeptide (11).

Metabolism

The half-life of synthetic Gln^4-neurotensin in one human volunteer after cessation of intravenous infusion was estimated to be 10 min (27). The clearance rate of exogenous neurotensin in humans was about 37 ml kg^{-1} min^{-1} (5).

Release

Limited studies have been performed to date on regulation of neurotensin release. In humans it has been shown that a mixed meal resulted in elevation of plasma neurotensin-like immunoreactivity, measured with an antibody that has N-terminal specificity, and that fat was a potent stimulant whereas glucose, amino acids, and saline caused small and insignificant increases (26). No response was obtained with alcohol, coffee, or heavy exercise. Calcium-dependent release of neurotensin also has been demonstrated *in vitro* from slices of rat hypothalamus (16).

Relationship with Physiological Events

No physiologic role has been shown for neurotensin at normal circulating concentrations.

Conditions of Excess or Deficiency

Such conditions have not been identified other than a demonstration that neurotensin release is increased in patients with rapid gastric emptying (5).

References

1. Andersson, S., Chang, D., Folkers, K., and Rosell, S. (1976): Inhibition of gastric acid secretion in dogs by neurotensin. *Life Sci.,* 19:367–370.
2. Andersson, S., Rosell, S., Hjelmquist, U., Chang, D., and Folkers, K. (1977): Inhibition of gastric and intestinal motor activity in dogs by (Gln⁴) neurotensin. *Acta Physiol. Scand.,* 100:231–235.
3. Andersson, S., Rosell, S., Sjödin, L., and Folkers, K. (1980): Inhibition of acid secretion from vagally innervated and denervated gastric pouches by (Gln⁴)-neurotensin. *Scand. J. Gastroenterol.,* 15:253–256.
4. Araki, K., Tachibana, S., Uchiyama, M., Nakajima, T., and Yasuhara, T. (1975): Isolation and structure of a new active peptide xenopsin on rat stomach strip and some biogenic amines in the skin of *Xenopus laevis. Chem. Pharm. Bull. (Tokyo),* 23:3132–3140.
5. Blackburn, A. M., Bloom, S. R., Long, R. G., Fletcher, D. R., Christofides, N. D., Fitzpatrick, M. L., and Baron, J. H. (1980): Effect of neurotensin on gastric function in man. *Lancet,* 1:987–989.
6. Brown, M., Rivier, J., and Vale, W. (1977): *Science,* 196:998–1000.
7. Carraway, R. E., Demers, L. M., and Leeman, S. E. (1976): Hyperglycemic effect of neurotensin, a hypothalamic peptide. *Endocrinology,* 99:1452–1462.
8. Carraway, R., Kitabgi, P., and Leeman, S. E. (1978): The amino acid sequence of radioimmunoassayable neurotensin from bovine intestine: Identity to neurotensin from hypothalamus. *J. Biol. Chem.,* 253:7996–7998.
9. Carraway, R., and Leeman, S. E. (1975): The amino acid sequence of a hypothalamic peptide, neurotensin. *J. Biol. Chem.,* 250:1907–1911.
10. Carraway, R., and Leeman, S. E. (1975): In: *Peptides: Chemistry, Structure, and Biology,* edited by R. Walter and J. Meinhafer, p. 679., Ann Arbor Science Publishers, Ann Arbor, Michigan.
11. Carraway, R. and Leeman, S. E. (1976): Characterization of radioimmunoassayable neurotensin in the rat: Its differential distribution in the central nervous system, small intestine, and stomach. *J. Biol. Chem.,* 251:7045–7052.
12. Carraway, R., and Leeman, S. E. (1976): Radioimmunoassay for neurotensin, a hypothalamic peptide. *J. Biol. Chem.,* 251: 7035–7044.
13. Folkers, K., Chang, D., Humphries, J., Carraway, R., Leeman, S. E., and Bowers, C. Y. (1976): Synthesis and activities of neurotensin, and its acid and amide analogs: Possible natural occurrence of [Gln⁴]-neurotensin. *Proc. Natl. Acad. Sci. U.S.A.,* 73:3833–3837.
14. Frigerio, B., Ravazola, M., Ito, S., Buffa, R., Capella, C., Solcia, E., and Orci, L. (1977): Histochemical and ultrastructural identification of neurotensin cells in the dog ileum. *Histochemistry,* 54:123–131.
15. Hammer, R. A. (1980): Isolation of human intestinal neurotensin. *J. Biol. Chem.,* 255:2476–2480.
16. Iverson, S. D. (1978): Calcium-dependent release of somatostatin and neurotensin from rat brain *in vitro. Nature,* 273:161–163.
17. Kitabgi, P., Carraway, R., and Leeman, S. E. (1976): Isolation of a tridecapeptide from bovine intestinal tissue and its partial characterization as neurotensin. *J. Biol. Chem.,* 251:7053–7058.
18. Kitabgi, P., Carraway, R., Van Rietschoten, J., Granier, C., Morgat, J. L., Menez, A., Leeman, S., and Freychet, P. (1977): Neurotensin: Specific binding to synaptic membranes from rat brain. *Proc. Natl. Acad. Sci. U.S.A.,* 74:1846–1850.
19. Kobayashi, R. M., Brown, M., and Vale, W. (1977): Regional distribution of neurotensin and somatostatin in rat brain. *Brain Res.,* 126:584–588.
20. Lazarus, L. H., Brown, M. R., and Perrin, M. H. (1977): Distribution, localization and characteristics of neurotensin binding sites in the rat brain. *Neuropharmacology,* 16:625–629.
21. Lazarus, L. H., Perrin, M. H., and Brown, M. R. (1977): Mast cell binding of neurotensin. *J. Biol. Chem.,* 252:7174–7179.
22. Lazarus, L. H., Perrin, M. H., Brown, M. R., and Rivier, J. E. (1977): Mast cell binding of neurotensin. II. Molecular conformation of neurotensin involved in the stereospecific binding to mast cell receptor sites. *J. Biol. Chem.,* 252:7180–7183.
23. Polak, J. M., Sullivan, S. N., Bloom, S. R., et al. (1977): Specific localisation of neurotensin to the N cell in human intestine by radioimmunoassay and immunocytochemistry. *Nature,* 270:183–184.
24. Rivier, J. E., Lazarus, L. H., Perrin, M. H., and Brown, M. R. (1977): Neurotensin analogues. Structure-activity relationships. *J. Med. Chem.,* 20:1409–1412.
25. Rokaeus, A., Burcher, E., Chang, D., Folkers, K., and Rosell, S. (1977): Actions of neurotensin and (Gln⁴)-neurotensin on isolated tissues. *Acta Pharmacol. Toxicol.,* 41:141–147.
26. Rosell, S., and Rokaeus, A. (1979): The effect of ingestion of amino acids, glucose and fat on circulating neurotensin-like immunoreactivity (NTLI) in man. *Acta Physiol. Scand.,* 107: 263–267.
27. Rosell, S., Rokaeus, A., Mashford, M. L., Thor, K., and Folkers, K. (1980): Neurotensin as a hormone in man. In: *Neuropeptides and Neural Transmission, IBRO Volume 7,* edited by C. Ajmone Marsan and W. Z. Traczyk, pp. 181–190.

BOMBESIN-LIKE PEPTIDES

Structure

Numerous biologically active peptides have been isolated from amphibian skin, principally by Erspamer and co-workers (12), and later shown to have structurally similar counterparts in mammalian brain and gut. Two peptides, named bombesin and alytesin for the species of frogs from which they were isolated, have diverse actions on mammalian smooth muscle, blood pressure, urine flow, and acid secretion and were found to be similar in structure to another amphibian peptide, ranatensin (29). The structure of bombesin was confirmed by synthesis (1). Subsequently several other peptides with structures similar to bombesin or to ranatensin have been isolated from other frogs and toads (12) (Table 9). All of these peptides have carboxyl terminal methionine amide. The bombesin-like peptides have a leucine residue preceding the methionine whereas the ranatensin peptides have a phenylalanine residue in this position.

TABLE 9. *Structures of peptides related to bombesin*

Related peptide	Structure[a]
Gastrin releasing peptide (pig)	APVSVGGGTVLAKMYPRGNHWAVGHLM#
Bombesin (*Bombina bombina*) (*Bombina variegata variegata*)	Q̇QRLGNQWAVGHLM#
Alytesin (*Alytes obstetricans*)	Q̇GRLGTQWAVGHLM#
Ranatensin (*Rana pipiens*)	Q̇VPQWAVGHPM#
Litorin (*Litoria aurea*) (*Uperoleia rugosa*)	@ Q̇QWAVGHPM# @ = OMet or OEt also
Ranatensin R (*Rana rugosa*)	SDATLRRYNQWATGHPM#
Ranatensin C (*Rana catesbiana*)	xZTPQWAVGHPM#

[a] ___ , Residue different from line above; #, amide; Q, pyroglutamyl.

More recently, McDonald et al. (22) have isolated a peptide from nonantral gastric tissue and from intestine that has potent gastrin-releasing activity. This gastrin-releasing peptide (GRP) contains 27 amino acid residues, of which 9 of the 10 C-terminal residues are identical to bombesin (22) (Table 9). A peptide with similar size, charge, and immunochemical properties to GRP has been partially characterized after isolation from canine intestinal muscle and appears to differ from porcine GRP in several residues (J. G. Reeve, *unpublished*).

Biological Effects

In Vivo

Bombesin is a potent stimulant of acid secretion in humans, dog, and cat but not in the rat (24). The acid response appears to be secondary to release of gastrin. Bombesin is a potent inhibitor of gastric motor activity in the dog. Similar inhibitory effects have been noted in upper intestinal motility. The interdigestive migratory complex was abolished. Electrical potentials in the upper small intestine show increased frequency and decreased amplitude during bombesin infusion (24). In dog and humans, bombesin stimulates pancreatic enzyme secretion and gallbladder contraction (24). These effects may be direct or may be indirectly mediated by release of CCK (2,25).

Bombesin and its C-terminal nonapeptide are potent stimulants of gastrin release in several species including dog and humans (3). In dogs the threshold dose of stimulation of gastrin is about 100 ng $kg^{-1}hr^{-1}$, and maximal responses are achieved at 500 to 1,000 ng $kg^{-1}hr^{-1}$. The response is moderately decreased by gastric or antral acidification, not inhibited by atropine, but

abolished by antrectomy (19). Partially or highly purified bombesin-like peptides from hog (23), rat (40), or a variety of species (15) have been shown to cause release of gastrin in dog or rat. Bombesin also is an effective stimulant of pancreatic polypeptide in the dog, and the doses required are similar to those that produce stimulation of gastrin release (33) (Fig. 21). The PP response to bombesin is inhibited markedly by atropine but is unaffected by bethanechol, whereas gastrin response is inhibited by bethanechol but not affected by atropine. Fundic vagotomy in dog increases gastrin responses to bombesin but decreases the gastric acid secretory response (18). There is generally good correlation between gastrin release and gastric acid secretion during bombesin infusion at low doses, but there is decreased acid secretion at high doses that may reflect direct or indirect secondary inhibitory effects on the acid-secreting mu-

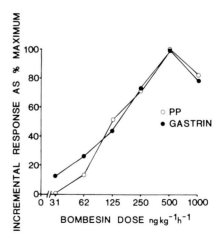

FIG. 21. Dose-response relationship for stimulation of gastrin and pancreatic polypeptide by intravenous bombesin in dogs. From Taylor et al. (33).

cosa (37). Intracisternal administration of bombesin in rats caused release of prolactin (36), but intravenous infusion of bombesin in man failed to alter anterior pituitary hormone release (28).

Brown et al. (6,7) reported that several vasoactive peptides administered intracisternally in rats have the ability to lower core temperature during exposure to a cold environment. Bombesin was 10,000 times more potent than the other peptides tested. The hypothermic effect was markedly decreased by alterations of amino acids at the C-terminus of the molecule but not at the N-terminus (31). Ranatensin was 20% and litorin less than 1% as active as bombesin. The effect of bombesin was reversed by TRF, prostaglandin E_2, and naloxone (7).

Intracisternal administration of bombesin produces hyperglycemia in the rat that is associated with increased plasma glucagon and decreased plasma insulin (8,9). For this effect, bombesin and litorin are equipotent. The mechanism is postulated to be central stimulation of adrenal epinephrine release, which in turn releases pancreatic glucagon. In support of this hypothesis it was shown that concurrent administration of somatostatin prevented both the increase in glucagon and the hyperglycemic response (9).

Intraperitoneal bombesin in a dose range of 1 to 10 nmole caused inhibition of liquid food intake in rats (17). Bombesin was about 10-fold less potent than CCK8.

In most species, especially the dog, bombesin produces arterial hypertension (24). In the monkey bombesin produces hypotension and in humans the effects on blood pressure are minimal. In dogs bombesin produces decreased urine flow associated with vasoconstriction of afferent glomerular arteries.

In Vitro

Bombesin and litorin exhibit a wide spectrum of effects on isolated smooth muscle strips (13). The usual response is muscle contraction, and litorin usually is 2 to 6 times more potent than bombesin except for gallbladder contraction.

In rat pancreatic fragments, bombesin was nearly as potent as CCK8 in stimulation of amylase secretion and calcium efflux and did not stimulate cyclic AMP (10). Litorin was about one-third as potent. The effect of bombesin on rat pancreatic lobules was potentiated by secretin (42). Bombesin and litorin were shown to interact with specific receptors on dispersed guinea pig acini that were distinct from receptors for eledoisin and other pancreatic stimulants. There was close correlation between binding and stimulation of amylase release, and bombesin was 10 times as potent as litorin (20). A direct inhibitory effect of bombesin on release of insulin from isolated pancreatic islets in rats also has been shown (32).

Structure-Activity Relationships

The biological effects of bombesin and a number of naturally occurring and synthetic analogues have been compared in several systems. A comparison of bombesin and litorin revealed that litorin generally was more potent in stimulation of smooth muscle contraction but was less potent in stimulation of gastrin release, pancreatic secretion, and antidiuresis (13). Comparison of a series of synthetic analogues of bombesin for smooth muscle contracting activity revealed that effects began to appear with the C-terminal heptapeptide, increased in the octapeptide, and reached maximal activity with the nonapeptide (24). Bombesin is approximately 10 times as potent as litorin for stimulation of enzyme release from isolated pancreatic acini from the guinea pig (20). Analogues which contain tyrosine substitutions at the amino terminal portion of the molecule retain full biological activity (20,43). The central hypothermic effects of a large number of synthetic bombesin analogues were compared (31). Alterations at the C-terminus markedly decreased activity whereas alterations at the N-terminus were well tolerated. The C-terminal amide was essential for activity. Ranatensin was 20% and litorin less than 1% as potent as bombesin. Similar comparisons have not been made for large and small forms of mammalian bombesin-like peptides, but it was shown that both forms of rat intestinal bombesin-like immunoreactivity (BLI) caused gastrin release in the rat (40). It seems safe to conclude that peptides which contain a carboxyl terminal sequence closely similar to that of bombesin will exhibit similar properties.

Distribution

Cellular

In addition to its localization in amphibian skin, bombesin-like immunoreactivity has been identified in stomach and brain of amphibians (21); esophagus, proventriculus, and brain of birds (15,35); brain and gut of rats (9,39,40); and in the mucosa of the human gastrointestinal tract (30). In the frog stomach (21) and in the avian proventriculus (34,35), BLI has been localized to endocrine-type cells. In contrast, BLI in rat gastrointestinal tissues appears to be confined to nerve fibers in the myenteric and submucous plexuses and mucosal nerve fibers in the stomach (11). Polak et al. originally described cells with bombesin-like immunoreactivity to be distributed widely throughout the human gut (30) but more recently have reported that it is localized mostly in fine varicose nerve fibers in the submucosa and mucosa

(4). Bombesin-containing cells also were reported in human fetal lung but not in adult lung (41). Distribution of bombesin-like peptides in the brain has not yet been described by immunohistochemical localization.

Immunochemical

Mammalian bombesin-like immunoreactivity is extractable mainly from the gut and brain. In the rat, tissue concentrations increase markedly between the first and 16th days of life (40). Gel filtration reveals two major peaks of immunoreactivity, one larger and one approximately the same molecular weight as bombesin. The latter can be resolved further into two peaks by ion-exchange chromatography. In the stomach, BLI is distributed almost equally between mucosa and muscle layers, whereas in the small intestine most of the activity is found in the muscle layer (11). In the brain, highest concentrations of BLI have been found in the hypothalamus (5,26), but lesser amounts are distributed widely throughout the brain except in the cerebellum. Receptors for bombesin were found to parallel the distribution of immunoreactive BLI in the brain except that hippocampus contained a high density of receptors but low content of immunoreactive bombesin (26). Immunoreactive materials similar in size to bombesin (39,40) and with higher apparent molecular weight (38) have been found in brain extracts. BLI was identified in rat plasma after extraction with formic acid (5). Assays used to detect bombesin-like immunoreactivity generally have had low cross-reactivity with ranatensin and litorin. By use of an antibody with a high degree of specificity for ranatensin/litorin, it has been possible to show that both bombesin-like and ranatensin-like peptides occur in the brain of certain frogs (J. H. Walsh and H. C. Wong, *unpublished observations*).

Measurement

Radioimmunoassay

Several radioimmunoassays have been described that are capable of measuring bombesin-like immunoreactivity in tissue extracts (5,39,40). Most antibodies raised against bombesin are directed at the C-terminus and cross-react poorly with ranatensin, litorin, and substance P. These antibodies have been used for measurement of tissue distribution of BLI and for immunocytochemistry. An antibody that had 50% cross-reactivity with ranatensin produced similar values for tissue BLI in the rat to an antibody that was highly specific for bombesin (5). A radioreceptor assay for radioiodinated (Tyr^4) bombesin was used to map receptor sites in the brain and revealed generally good correlation between ability of peptide analogues to inhibit receptor binding and potency to induce hypothermia in the rat (27).

Bioassay

Bioassay methods have been used extensively to monitor purification of bombesin-like and litorin-like peptides in extracts of amphibian skin (14) and amphibian and avian gut (15). Partial characterization of the peptides being isolated has been possible by comparison of effects on a series of smooth muscle preparations. Some fractions obtained resembled litorin more than bombesin. The gastrin-releasing activity in porcine gastric extracts was used to monitor purification of porcine gastrin-releasing peptide (23).

Metabolism

Pharmacodynamics of bombesin in man have been measured by use of radioimmunoassay (24). The disappearance half-time was 5 min, volume of distribution 39 ml kg^{-1}, and clearance rate 5.2 ml kg^{-1}min^{-1}.

Release

Preliminary evidence was reported that bombesin-like immunoreactivity was increased in human plasma following ingestion of a meal (12). Also, vascular perfusion of the isolated rat stomach with cholinergic agents resulted in parallel increase in immunoreactive gastrin and bombesin-like immunoreactivity (G. M. Makhlouf, *unpublished*), and electrical vagal stimulation in the cat resulted in stimulation of bombesin-like immunoreactivity (K. Uvnas-Wallensten, *unpublished*). However, there have been no convincing demonstrations of a relationship between bombesin release and gastrin or other hormone release in intact animals or man.

Relationship with Physiological Events

Lack of suitable measurements of bombesin in blood has precluded correlations between endogenous peptide and biological events. In one recent report it was found that human subjects were extremely sensitive to exogenous bombesin and that gastric acid responses and serum gastrin responses similar to those that were obtained during protein ingestion were achieved at exogenous doses of approximately 3 to 12 pmol kg^{-1}hr^{-1} (37). Circulating bombesin concentrations achieved during these doses were too low to measure with the available radioimmunoassay.

Effects of Hormone Excess or Deficiency

No model for endogenous hormone excess or deficiency has been reported. Chronic exogenous administration of bombesin resulted in pancreatic hyperplasia and increase in antral gastrin content (Solomon, *unpublished*).

References

1. Anastasi, A., Erspamer, V., and Bucci, M. (1972): Isolation and amino acid sequences of alytesin and bombesin, two analogous active tetradecapeptides from the skin of European discoglossid frogs. *Arch. Biochem. Biophys.*, 148:443–446.
2. Basso, N., Giri, S., Importa, G., Lezoche, E., Melchiorri, P., Percoco, M., and Speranza, V. (1975): External pancreatic secretion after bombesin infusion in man. *Gut*, 16:994–998.
3. Bertaccini, G., Erspamer, V., Melchiorri, P., and Sopranzi, N. (1974): Gastrin release by bombesin in the dog. *Br. J. Pharmacol.*, 52:219–225.
4. Bloom, S. R., and Polak, J. M. (1979): Neuropeptides in the gut and other peripheral tissues. In: *Brain Peptides: A New Endocrinology*, edited by A. M. Gotto, Jr., E. J. Peck, Jr., and A. E. Boyd, III, pp. Elsevier/North-Holland Biomedical Press, Amsterdam.
5. Brown, M., Allen, R., Villarreal, J., Rivier, J., and Vale, W. (1978): Bombesin-like activity: Radioimmunologic assessment in biological tissues. *Life Sci.*, 23:2721–2728.
6. Brown, M., Rivier, J., and Vale, W. (1977): Bombesin: potent effects on thermoregulation in the rat. *Science*, 196:998–1000.
7. Brown, M., Rivier, J., and Vale, W. (1977): Actions of bombesin, thyrotropin releasing factor, prostaglandin E_2 and naloxone on thermoregulation in the rat. *Life Sci.*, 20:1681–1688.
8. Brown, M. R., Rivier, J., and Vale, W. W. (1977): Bombesin affects the central nervous system to produce hyperglycemia in rats. *Life Sci.*, 21:1729–1734.
9. Brown, M., Tache, Y., and Fisher, D. (1979): Central nervous system action of bombesin: mechanism to induce hyperglycemia. *Endocrinology*, 105:660–665.
10. Deschodt-Lanckman, M., Robberecht, P., De Neef, P., Lammens, M., and Christophe, J. (1976): In vitro action of bombesin and bombesin-like peptides on amylase secretion, calcium efflux, and adenylate cyclase activity in the rat pancreas. A comparison with other secretagogues. *J. Clin. Invest.*, 58:891–898.
11. Dockray, G. J., Vaillant, C., and Walsh, J. H. (1979): The neuronal origin of bombesin-like immunoreactivity in the rat gastrointestinal tract. *Neuroscience*, 4:1561–1568.
12. Erspamer, V. (1980): Active peptides: from amphibian skin to gastrointestinal tract and brain of mammals. *Trends Pharmacol. Sci.* (in press).
13. Erspamer, V., Falconieri Erspamer, G., Improta, G., Melchiorri, P., Negri, L., and Sopranzi, N. (1975): Parallel bioassay of bombesin and litorin, a bombesin-like peptide from the skin of *litoria aurea*. *Br. J. Pharmacol.*, 55:213–219.
14. Erspamer, V., Falconieri Erspamer, G., Inselvini, M., and Negri, L. (1972): Occurrence of bombesin and alytesin in extracts of the skin of three European discoglossid frogs and pharmacological actions of bombesin on extravascular smooth muscle. *B. J. Pharmacol.*, 45:333–348.
15. Erspamer, V., Falconieri Erspamer, G., Melchiorri, P., and Negri, L. (1979): Occurrence and polymorphism of bombesin-like peptides in the gastrointestinal tract of birds and mammals. *Gut*, 20:1047–1056.
16. Erspamer, V., and Melchiorri, P. (1973): Active polypeptides of the amphibian skin and their synthetic analogues. *Pure Appl. Chem.*, 35:463–494.
17. Gibbs, J., Fauser, D. J., Rowe, E. A., Rolls, B. J., Rolls, E. T., and Maddison, S. P. (1979): Bombesin suppresses feeding in rats. *Nature*, 282:208–210.
18. Hirschowitz, B. I., and Gibson, R. G. (1978): Stimulation of gastrin release and gastric secretion: effect of bombesin and a nonapeptide in fistula dogs with and without fundic vagotomy. *Digestion*, 18:227–239.
19. Impicciatore, M., Debas, H., Walsh, J. H., Grossman, M. I., and Bertaccini, G. (1974): Release of gastrin and stimulation of acid secretion by bombesin in dog. *Rendic. Gastroenterol.*, 6:99–101.
20. Jensen, R. T., Moody, T., Pert, C., Rivier, J. E., and Gardner, J. D. (1978): Interaction of bombesin and litorin with specific membrane receptors on pancreatic acinar cells. *Proc. Natl. Acad. Sci. USA*, 75:6139–6143.
21. Lechago, J., Holmquist, A. L., Rosenquist, G. L., and Walsh, J. H. (1978): Localization of bombesin-like peptides in frog gastric mucosa. *Gen. Comp. Endocrinol.*, 36:553–558.
22. McDonald, T. J., Jornvall, H., Nilsson, G., Vagne, M., Ghatei, M., Bloom, S. R., and Mutt, V. (1979): Characterization of a gastrin releasing peptide from porcine non-antral gastric tissue. *Biochem. Biophys. Res. Commun.*, 90:227–233.
23. McDonald, T. J., Nilsson, G., Vagne, M., Ghatei, M., Bloom, S. R., and Mutt, V. (1978): A gastrin releasing peptide from the porcine non-antral gastric tissue. *Gut*, 19:767–774.
24. Melchiorri, P. (1978): Bombesin and bombesin-like peptides of amphibian skin. In: *Gut Hormones*, edited by S. R. Bloom, pp. 534–540, Churchill-Livingstone, Edinburgh.
25. Miyata, M., Rayford, P. L., and Thompson, J. C. (1980): Hormonal (gastrin, secretin, CCK) and secretory effects of bombesin and duodenal acidification. *Surgery* (in press).
26. Moody, T. W., and Pert, C. B. (1979): Bombesin-like peptides in rat brain: Quantitation and biochemical characterization. *Biochem. Biophys. Res. Commun.*, 90:7–14.
27. Moody, T. W., Pert, C. B., Rivier, J., and Brown, M. R. (1978): Bombesin: Specific binding to rat brain membranes. *Proc. Natl. Acad. Sci. U.S.A.*, 75:5372–5376.
28. Morley, J. E., Varner, A. A., Modlin, I. M., Carlson, H. E., Braunstein, G. D., Walsh, J. H., and Hershman, J. M. (1980): Failure of bombesin to alter anterior pituitary hormone secretion in man. *Clin. Endocrinol.*, 13:369–373.
29. Nakajima, T., Tanimura, T., and Pisano, J. J. (1970): Isolation and structure of a new vasoactive polypeptide. *Fed. Proc.*, 29:282.
30. Polak, J. M., Bloom, S. R., Hobbs, S., Solcia, E., and Pearse, A. G. E. (1976): Distribution of a bombesin-like peptide in human gastrointestinal tract. *Lancet*, 1:1109–1110.
31. Rivier, J. E., and Brown, M. R. (1978): Bombesin, bombesin analogues, and related peptides: effects on thermoregulation. *Biochemistry*, 17:1766–1771.
32. Taminato, T., Seino, Y., Goto, Y., Matsukura, S., Imura, H., Sakura, N., and Yanaihara, N. (1978): Bombesin inhibits insulin release from isolated pancreatic islets of rats in vitro. *Endocrinol. Jpn.*, 25:305–307.
33. Taylor, I. L., Walsh, J. H., Carter, D., Wood, J., and Grossman, M. I. (1979): Effects of atropine and bethanechol on bombesin-stimulated release of pancreatic polypeptide and gastrin in dog. *Gastroenterology*, 77:714–718.
34. Timson, C. M., Polak, J. M., Wharton, J., Ghatei, M. A., Bloom, S. R., Usellini, L., Capella, C., Solcia, E., Brown, M. R., and Pearse, A. G. E. (1979): Bombesin-like immunoreactivity in the avian gut and its localisation to a distinct cell type. *Histochemistry*, 61:213–221.
35. Vaillant, C., Dockray, G. J., and Walsh, J. H. (1979): The avian proventriculus is an abundant source of endocrine cells with bombesin-like immunoreactivity. *Histochemistry*, 64:307–314.
36. Vale, W., Rivier, C., Rivier, J., and Brown, M. (1978): Adenohypophysial and other extracentral nervous system roles of hypothalamic regulatory peptides. In: *Psychopharmacology: A Generation of Progress*, edited by M. A. Lipton, A. DiMascio, and K. F. Killam, pp. 403–421. Raven Press, New York.
37. Varner, A. A., Modlin, I. M., and Walsh, J. H. (1980): Bombesin: High potency in man supports a physiological role in regulation of gastrin release and acid secretion. *Gastroenterology*, 78:1284.
38. Villarreal, J. A., and Brown, M. R. (1978): Bombesin-like peptide in hypothalamus: chemical and immunological characterization. *Life Sci.*, 23:2729–2734.
39. Walsh, J. H., and Wong, H. C. (1979): Bombesin-like peptides. In: *Methods of Hormone Radioimmunoassay*, pp. 581–594. Academic Press, New York.
40. Walsh, J. H., Wong, H. C., and Dockray, G. J. (1979): Bombesin-like peptides in mammals. *Fed. Proc.*, 38:2315–2319.
41. Wharton, J. Polak, J. M., Bloom, S. R., Ghatei, M. A., Solcia, E., Brown, M. R., and Pearse, A. G. E. (1978): Bombesin-like immunoreactivity in the lung. *Nature*, 1978, 273:769–770.

42. Wolpert, D. N. (sponsored by Solomon, T. E.) (1979): Potentiation by secretin of bombesin-stimulated amylase secretion from *in vitro* rat pancreatic lobules. *Gastroenterology,* 76:1308.

43. Yanaihara, C., Inoue, A., Mochizuki, T., Sakura, N., Sato, H., and Yanaihara, N. (1978): Syntheses of bombesin-related peptides and their use for bombesin-specific radioimmunoassay. *Peptide Chem.,* 183–188.

SUBSTANCE P

Structure

Substance P is a peptide composed of 11 amino acid residues with a molecular weight of 1,348. This peptide was identified in 1931 by von Euler and Gaddum (11) as a vasodepressor substance in tissue extracts and later by Leeman and Carraway (29) as a substance that caused salivary flow in anesthetized rats (29). Preparations of substance P purified from bovine hypothalamus (5) and from horse intestine (48) have the same chemical structure (Table 10). Substance P is chemically similar to the amphibian peptides phylasaemin and eledoisin, and four of the five carboxyl terminal residues of each peptide are identical (48). Biosynthesis of substance P has been demonstrated in isolated rat dorsal root ganglia (19).

Biological Actions

The initial effects described for substance P were atropine-resistance decrease in systemic blood pressure, stimulation of smooth muscle contractions, and stimulation of salivary flow (29). Recently considerable attention has been given to the effects of substance P on synaptic transmission (27). The major biological effects of physalaemin and eledoisin in mammals are similar to those of substance P (10). These include (a) potent vasodilating and hypotensive action in most species due to a direct action on vascular smooth muscle, especially the arteries of the limb and the coronary arteries; increased cardiac output associated with decreased peripheral and pulmonary vascular resistance; intense cutaneous erythema; (b) powerful stimulation of salivary secretion similar to that obtained by stimulation of postganglionic nerve fibers and a more potent stimulating effect on myoepithelial cell contraction in the salivary ducts and powerful stimulation of lachrymal secretion, both by direct action on secretory cells; (c) intense smooth muscle contracting activity especially on rabbit large intestine, guinea pig ileum, human Fallopian tube, and rat urinary bladder; contraction of *in situ* dog jejunal loops with a potency greater than that of cholecystokinin; (d) increased capillary permeability associated with pain, local edema, and erythema with intradermal injection. Secretory stimulation of dog pancreas was very weak.

Comparison of substance P with the "tachykinins" eledoisin and phylasaemin for effects on various types of smooth muscle revealed that substance P had greater relative effects on blood pressure whereas the tachykinins were much more potent stimulants of contraction of rat colon, dog urinary bladder, hamster urinary bladder, rabbit uterus, and rat vas deferens (9). Substance P produced dose-related increases in the opossum lower esophageal sphincter pressure that were partially antagonized by atropine but not by other pharmacologic antagonists of nerve transmission or by vagotomy (35).

Substance P also has been found to have effects on gastrointestinal secretions. It inhibited sodium absorption and caused chloride secretion by the *in vitro* rat ileum but did not cause a detectable change in tissue cyclic AMP (53). In the anesthetized dog, substance P inhibited hepatic bile flow under basal conditions and during stimulation by VIP or CCK and produced mild stimulation of pancreatic volume and enzyme secretion (50). Specific receptors have been identified on guinea pig pancreatic acinar cells that interact with substance P, eledoisin, and physalaemin but not with CCK, bombesin, or cholinergic agents (15). Stimulation of these receptors does not cause increased accumulation of cellular cyclic AMP. However, a transient stimulation of intracellular cyclic GMP associated with stimulation of enzyme release has been demonstrated in guinea pig pancreatic lobules (1). In rat parotid gland slices and

TABLE 10. *Structures of peptides related to substance P*

Peptide	Structure[a]
Substance P (Cow)	RPKPQQFFGLM#
Physalaemin (*Physalamus bigilonigerus*) (″ *centralis*) (″ *bresslaui*)	Q̇AD PNKFYGLM#
Uperolein (*Uperoleia rugosa*) (″ *marmorata*)	Q̇PDPNAFYGLM#
Eledoisin (*Eledone moschata*)	Q̇PSKDAFIGLM#

[a] ___, Residue different from line above; #, amide; Q, pyroglutamyl.

acinar cells, substance P stimulated calcium uptake (45) and caused a calcium-dependent release of potassium without a significant stimulation of amylase secretion (13).

Effects of substance P on central nervous system function have been reported. In the rat it was a potent inhibitor of the increased drinking of water elicited by angiotensin (7), whereas in the pigeon it was a weak stimulant of drinking behavior (12). Intravenous substance P was found to lower body temperature and decrease aggressive behavior in mice (52), although intracisternal administration in the rat produced little if any hypothermic response (46).

Considerable evidence has been accumulated that substance P may function as a neurotransmitter or as a modulator of synaptic transmission in the central nervous system, spinal cord, and peripheral autonomic nervous system. In the spinal cord, where substance P is especially concentrated in dorsal root ganglia, electrical stimulation of dorsal roots causes calcium-dependent release of substance P, and application of substance P at concentrations as low as 10^{-7} M causes depolarization of ventral root motoneurons (42). Substance P also modulates synaptic excitability of spinal motoneurons (27) and selectively inhibits nicotinic cholinergic stimulation of Renshaw cells (2). In the central nervous system substance P causes excitatory transmission and stimulates synthesis and utilization of dopamine, norepinephrine, and serotonin (4). Injection of the peptide into the lateral ventricle of rats caused excitatory responses of locomotion and rotary movements. In the myenteric plexus, substance P has a powerful depolarizing action on neurons that suggests a role as a mediator of slow synaptic excitation (25), but some workers have obtained evidence that serotonin is a more likely candidate for this function (16). Substance P also was found to inhibit nicotinic cholinergic release of norepinephrine by adrenal chromaffin cells in culture (30). In cultured neuroblastoma cells, substance P increased cyclic AMP levels and induced neurite extension (36).

Intraarterial infusion of substance P produces marked vasodilatation in the skin and muscle of the human forearm (8). The effect is not blocked by propranolol or indomethacin, and the potency is about 50 times greater than for bradykinin and about equal to that of prostaglandin E_1. Substance P also was found to decrease renin release in anesthetized dogs during renal arterial infusion associated with diuresis and natriuresis and during intravenous infusion when diuresis was not stimulated (17). A potent bronchoconstrictor effect also was found in guinea pigs, with the potency of substance P about 45 times greater than that of histamine (38).

Structure-Activity Relationships

The biologically active region of substance P appears to be contained in the C-terminal hexapeptide amide fragment. Fragments containing this hexapeptide region retain almost full potency for contraction of guinea pig ileum, whereas deletions of substitutions in the C-terminal hexapeptide lead to marked decreases or complete loss of activity (47,57). Similar findings have been obtained with fragments of physalaemin, where full activity was retained in the C-terminal hexapeptide but was almost completely absent in the C-terminal pentapeptide (10). Substance P is relatively more potent than physalaemin and eledoisin in decreasing systemic blood pressure and increasing hepatic arterial and portal vein blood flow, but is less potent in stimulation of most isolated smooth muscles (9,33). There is some evidence that the amino terminal portion of substance P contains information related to neural functions that is not required for stimulation of smooth muscle contraction (41).

Distribution

Substance P has been isolated in pure form from horse intestine, and distribution of immunoreactive substance P (ISP) has been determined by radioimmunoassay in several mammalian species (37). A widespread distribution was found in the gut, with highest concentrations of ISP in the duodenum. The majority of extractable ISP was found in the muscle layers of the gut and only a relatively small amount in the mucosa. By gel filtration and starch gel chromatography, at least three molecular forms were detected in dog duodenal extracts. ISP also is widely distributed in the subcortical areas of the brain with very little material being found in the cerebellum (34).

Most information about ISP distribution has been obtained by immunohistochemical methods. Most of the immunoreactive material has been demonstrated in nerves, but ISP also has been identified in endocrine-like cells of the duodenal and colonic mucosa (39) later shown to be a subpopulation of enterochromaffin cells that also contained 5-HT (49). In the brain, the distribution of ISP has been extensively mapped (31), and cell bodies were identified in more than 30 areas including the spinal cord and many parts of the brainstem. Substance P nerve terminals were closely associated with catecholamine-containing cells (32). Dense concentrations of ISP have been found in dorsal horns of the spinal cord, in spinal ganglia at all levels, and in the nodose and trigeminal ganglia, and ISP-positive nerve fibers have been found in most peripheral tissues (21). ISP also has been found in the human vagus nerve, and fibers containing ISP appear to be more numerous than fibers containing immunoreactive enkephalin or VIP. ISP-positive nerves also have been identified in mammalian lung (55). Within the central nervous system, ISP was concentrated in synaptic vesicles (6) and calcium-dependent release from synaptosomes has been demonstrated.

The possible significance of peptidergic neurons, including those that contain ISP, has been reviewed recently (22). Peptides are contained in large granular vesicles in nerve endings, but are synthesized only in cell bodies and then transmitted by axonal transport. No systems for synthesis and reuptake in nerve endings have been identified for peptides, although such systems are regularly found for "classic" neurotransmitters. The patterns of distribution of individual neuropeptides in the nervous system appear to be unique for each peptide, although two peptides occasionally are found in the same neuron. In the spinal ganglia, ISP is found in three different systems: primary sensory neurons, interneurons, and descending systems. ISP neurons in the autonomic ganglia such as the prevertebral sympathetic ganglia are primarily sensory. In the gastrointestinal tract ISP, immunoreactive VIP, and immunoreactive enkephalin are present in different populations of nerves. In some central nerves, ISP and serotonin have been found in the same neurons. However, there is no example in which all nerves that contain one peptide also contain a certain biogenic amine or vice versa. There is some evidence that substance P may interact with serotonin receptors and that it may block cholinergic receptors, but no specific function has been assigned to these actions. The most likely function for substance P nerves, based on distribution and known properties of substance P, is processing of pain impulses and participation in axon reflexes causing cutaneous vasodilatation. Within the enteric nervous system, there appear to be reciprocal projections between ISP fibers originating in nerve bodies in the myenteric plexus and terminating in the submucous plexus and immunoreactive VIP fibers originating in nerve bodies in the submucous plexus and terminating in the myenteric plexus (23).

Measurement

Biologically active substance P has been detected by use of various bioassay systems including measurement of salivary stimulation in rats, depression of systemic blood pressure, and stimulation of guinea pig ileum smooth muscle contraction (29). Several radioimmunoassays also have been described. Powell and co-workers (44) used an antiserum with an ID_{50} of about 30 pg/tube and minimal cross-reactivity with eledoisin and physalaemin to measure ISP in tissue extracts and biological fluids. Apparent concentrations of ISP in plasma were found to range between 20 and 151 pg ml^{-1}, with occasional higher values. No difference was detected between samples taken in the morning and evening, but marked variations in ISP concentration were found in samples taken every 30 min during sleep. ISP could not be measured in cerebrospinal fluid. Nilsson and co-workers (40) used a similar assay system but with higher

sensitivity and found concentrations of ISP of 3 pM in human cerebrospinal fluid. In this assay, human plasma ISP concentrations averaged 180 pM compared with 88 pM in dogs. Hemolyzed red blood cells markedly increased apparent substance P concentrations. The "true" substance P concentrations in rat and calf plasma were determined by Leeman and Carraway (29) before and after extraction by a method that yielded quantitative recovery of added substance P. This method resulted in a decrease in apparent ISP in calf plasma from 423 to 9 pM. When concentrated extracted plasma was subjected to ion-exchange or gel filtration chromatography, all extracted immunoreactive material coeluted with synthetic substance P. These results indicated that assay of unextracted plasma may produce falsely elevated values. The specificity of one substance P antibody was examined with synthetic fragments of substance P, and it was found that this antibody recognized the C-terminal deca- and nonapeptides equally, had 50% reactivity with the C-terminal octapeptide, but did not detect the C-terminal heptapeptide, physalaemin, or eledoisin (56). On the other hand, we have produced an antiserum that has equal immunoreactivity with substance P and physalaemin (J. H. Walsh and H. C. Wong, *unpublished*).

Metabolism

Hepatic and renal clearance of circulating substance P has been shown by the observations that portal infusion produced much smaller increases in hepatic arterial blood flow than femoral infusion (33), and that there was a significant gradient between arterial and renal venous immunoreactive substance P during intravenous infusion of this peptide in anesthetized dogs (3). During infusion of radioiodinated substance P, a denatured product appeared in the urine.

Enzymatic degradation of substance P has been demonstrated in several systems. Kidney homogenates, especially of renal cortex and purified brush border of proximal tubules, destroyed substance P biological activity more rapidly than extracts of liver, brain, and other organs (54). The activity was greatest in microsomal and plasma-membrane-enriched fractions and appeared to require a metal cofactor. Cleavage of the N-terminal proline dipeptides, Arg-Pro and Lys-Pro, has been demonstrated by dipeptidyl aminopeptidases isolated from rat liver (20) and from human submaxillary gland (26). The latter enzyme did not cleave the N-terminal Arg-Pro from bradykinin. Cultured human endothelial cells also were found to destroy biological activity of substance P (24). Another substance P-inactivating enzyme has been identified in the supernatant fraction of rat brain homogenates (28). This activity was inhibited by the nonapeptide SQ 20881 that was previously described as a specific inhibitor of angiotensin-converting enzyme. The possible contributions of these various enzymes to overall degradation of substance P in the body have not been determined.

Release

There is little information about the factors that regulate circulating concentrations of substance P. Immunoreactive substance P concentrations were increased in the lumen of cats with antral pouches during electrical vagal stimulation (51). An intestinal origin for circulating substance P was supported by experiments in cats where it was shown that evisceration or ligation of intestinal blood vessels markedly decreased extractable immunoreactive substance P in blood plasma (14).

Relationship with Physiological Events

None of the biological effects of substance P are known to be produced by concentrations that are likely to be present in the circulation. It is possible, however, that substance P acts as a transmitter or modulator of nerve impulses (22).

Conditions of Excess or Deficiency

Decreased substance P content has been demonstrated in the aganglionic colon segments in patients with Hirschsprung's disease and in the atrophic areas of the brain in patients with Huntington's chorea, but no pathophysiological relationships have been established (43). Immunoreactive substance P has been demonstrated in some intestinal carcinoid tumors and increased plasma ISP has been found in some patients with this condition (18,43). Again, the pathophysiological significance has not been determined.

References

1. Albano, J., Bhoola, K. D., and Harvey, R. F. (1977): The effect of substance P on cyclic AMP and cyclic GMP levels in actively secreting pancreatic lobules. *J. Physiol. (Lond.),* 275:60 P.
2. Belcher, G., and Ryall, R. W. (1977): Substance P and Renshaw cells: a new concept of inhibitory synaptic interactions. *J. Physiol,* 272:105–119.
3. Campbell, W. B., and Ward, P. E. (1979): Renal metabolism of substance P in the dog. *Life Sci.,* 1979, 24:1995–2002.
4. Carlsson, A., Magnusson, T., Fisher, G. H., Chang, D., and Folkers, K. (1977): Effect of synthetic substance P on central monoaminergic mechanisms. In: *Substance P,* edited by U. S. von Euler and B. Pernow, pp. 201–205. Raven Press, New York.
5. Carraway, R., and Leeman, S. E. (1979): The amino acid sequence of bovine hypothalamic substance P. Identity to substance P from colliculi and small intestine. *J. Biol. Chem,* 254:2944–2945.
6. Cuello, A. C., Jessell, T. M., Kanazawa, I., and Iversen, L. L. (1977): Substance P: localization in synaptic vesicles in rat central nervous system. *J. Neurochem.* 29:747–751.
7. De Caro, G., Massi, M., and Micossi, L. G. (1978): Antidipsogenic effect of intracranial injections of substance P in rats. *J. Physiol.,* 279:133–140.
8. Eklund, B., Jogestrand, T., and Pernow, B. (1977): Effect of substance P on resistance and capacitance vessels in the human forearm. In: *Substance P,* edited by U. S. von Euler and B. Pernow, pp. 275–285. Raven Press, New York.
9. Erspamer, V., Erspamer, F., and Linari, G. (1977): Occurrence of tachykinins (physalemin- or substance P-like peptides) in the amphibian skin and their actions on smooth muscle preparations. In: *Substance P,* edited by U. S. von Euler and B. Pernow, pp. 67–73. Raven Press, New York.
10. Erspamer, V., and Melchiorri, P. (1973): Active polypeptides of the amphibian skin and their synthetic analogues. *Pure Appl. Chem.,* 35:463–494.
11. Euler, U. S. von, and Gaddum, J. H. (1931): An unidentified depressor substance in certain tissue extracts. *J. Physiol. (Lond),* 72:74–87.
12. Evered, M. D., Fitzsimons, J. T., and de Caro, G. (1977): Drinking behaviour induced by intracranial injections of eledoisin and substance P in the pigeon. *Nature.* 268:332–333.
13. Friedman, Z. Y., and Selinger, Z. (1978): A transient release of potassium mediated by the action of substance P on rat parotid slices. *J. Physiol.,* 278:461–469.
14. Gamse, R., Mroz, E., Leeman, S., and Lembeck, F. (1978): The intestine as source of immunoreactive substance P in plasma of the cat. *Arch. Pharmacol.,* 305:17–21.
15. Gardner, J. D., and Jensen, R. T. (1980): Receptor for secretagogues on pancreatic acinar cells. *Am. J. Physiol.,* 238:G63–G66.
16. Grafe, P., Mayer, C. J., and Wood, J. D. (1979): Evidence that substance P does not mediate slow synaptic excitation within the myenteric plexus. *Nature,* 279:720–721.
17. Gullner, H-G., Campbell, W. B., and Pettinger, W. A. (1979): Effects of substance P on renin release and renal function in anesthetized dogs. *Life Sci.,* 24:237–246.
18. Hakanson, R., Bengmark, S., Brodin, E., Ingemansson, S., Larsson, L.-I., Nilsson, G., and Sundler, F. (1977): Substance P-like immunoreactivity in intestinal carcinoid tumors. In: *Substance P,* edited by U. S. von Euler and B. Pernow, pp. 55–58. Raven Press, New York.
19. Harmar, A., Schofield, J. G., and Keen, P. (1980): Cycloheximide-sensitive synthesis of substance P by isolated dorsal root ganglia. *Nature,* 284:267–269.
20. Heymann, E., and Mentlein, R. (1978): Liver dipeptidyl aminopeptidase IV hydrolyzes substance P. *FEBS Lett.,* 91:360–364.
21. Hokfelt, T., Johansson, O., Kellerth, J.-O., Ljungdahl, A., Nilsson, G., Nygards, A., and Pernow, B. (1977): Immunohistochemical distribution of substance P. In: *Substance P,* edited by U. S. von Euler and B. Pernow, pp. 117–145. Raven Press, New York.
22. Hokfelt, T., Johansson, O., Ljungdahl, A., Lundberg, J. M., and Schultzberg, M. (1980): Peptidergic neurons. *Nature,* 284:515–521.
23. Jessen, K. R., Polak, J. M., Van Noorden, S., Bloom, S. R., and Burnstock, G. (1980): Peptide-containing neurons connect the two ganglionated plexuses of the enteric nervous system. *Nature,* 283:391–393.
24. Johnson, A. R., and Erdos, E. G. (1977): Inactivation of substance P by cultured human endothelial cells. In: *Substance P,* edited by U. S. von Euler and B. Pernow, pp. 253–260. Raven Press, New York.
25. Katayama, Y., and North, R. A. (1978): Does substance P mediate slow synaptic excitation within the myenteric plexus? *Nature,* 274:387–388.
26. Kato, T., Naghatsu, T., Fukasawa, K., Harada, M., Nagatsu, I., and Sakakibara, S. (1978): Successive cleavage of N-terminal Arg^1-Pro^2 and Lys^3-Pro^4 from substance P but no release of Arg^1-Pro^2 from bradykinin, by X-Pro dipeptidyl-aminopeptidase. *Biochim. Biophys. Acta,* 525:417–422.
27. Krivoy, W. A., Couch, J. R., Henry, J. L., and Stewart, J. M. (1979): Synaptic modulation by substance P. *Fed. Proc.,* 38:2344–2347.
28. Lee, C. M., Arregui, A., and Iversen, L. L. (1979): Substance P degradation by rat brain peptidases: inhibition by SQ 20881. *Biochem. Pharmacol.,* 28:553–556.

29. Leeman, S. E., and Carraway, R. E. (1977): Discovery of sialogogic peptide in bovine hypothalamic extracts: its isolation, characterization as substance P, structure, and synthesis. In: *Substance P,* edited by U. S. von Euler and B. Pernow, pp. 5–13, Raven Press, New York.

30. Livett, B. G., Kozousek, V., Mizobe, F., and Dean, D. M. (1979): Substance P inhibits nicotinic activation of chromaffin cells. *Nature,* 278:256–257.

31. Ljungdahl, A., Hokfelt, T., and Nilsson, G. (1978): Distribution of substance P-like immunoreactivity in the central nervous system of the rat. I. Cell bodies and nerve terminals. *Neuroscience,* 3:861–943.

32. Ljungdahl, A., Hokfelt, T., Nilsson, G., and Goldstein, M. (1978): Distribution of substance P-like immunoreactivity in the central nervous system of the rat. II. Light microscopic localization in relation to catecholamine-containing neurons. *Neuroscience,* 3:945–976.

33. Melchiorri, P., Tonelli, F., and Negri, L. (1977): Comparative circulatory effects of substance P, eledoisin, and physalemin in the dog. In: *Substance P,* edited by U. S. von Euler and B. Pernow, pp. 311–319. Raven Press, New York.

34. Mroz, E. A., Brownstein, M. J., and Leeman, S. E. (1977): Distribution of immunoassayable substance P in the rat brain: Evidence for the existence of substance P-containing tracts. In: *Substance P,* edited by U. S. von Euler and B. Pernow, pp.147–154. Raven Press, New York.

35. Mukhopadhyay, A. K. (1978): Effect of substance P on the lower esophageal sphincter of the opossum. *Gastroenterology,* 75: 278–282.

36. Narumi, S., and Maki, Y. (1978): Stimulatory effects of substance P on neurite extension and cyclic AMP levels in cultured neuroblastoma cells. *J. Neurochem.,* 30:1321–1326.

37. Nilsson, G., and Brodin, E. (1977): Tissue distribution of substance P-like immunoreactivity in dog, cat, rat, and mouse. In: *Substance P,* edited by U. S. von Euler and B. Pernow, pp.49–57. Raven Press, New York.

38. Nilsson, G., Dahlberg, K., Brodin, E., Sundler, F., and Strandberg, K. (1977): Distribution and constrictor effect of substance P in guinea pig tracheobronchial tissue. In: *Substance P,* edited by U. S. von Euler and B. Pernow, pp. 75–81. Raven Press, New York.

39. Nilsson, G., Larsson, L.-I., Hakanson, R., Brodin, E., Pernow, B., and Sundler, F. (1975): Localization of substance P-like immunoreactivity in mouse gut. *Histochemistry,* 43:97–99.

40. Nilsson, G., Pernow, B., Fisher, G. H., and Folkers, K. (1977): Radioimmunological determination of substance P. In: *Substance P,* edited by U. S. von Euler and B. Pernow, pp. 41–47. Raven Press, New York.

41. Oehme, P., Bergmann, J., Bienert, M., Hilse, H., Piesche, L., Minh Thu, P., and Scheer, E. (1977): Biological action of substance P—Its differentiation by affinity and intrinsic efficacy. In: *Substance P,* edited by U. S. von Euler and B. Pernow, pp. 327–335. Raven Press, New York.

42. Otsuka, M., and Konishi, S. (1977): Electrophysiological and neurochemical evidence for substance P as a transmitter of primary sensory neurons. In: *Substance P,* edited by U. S. von Euler and B. Pernow, pp. 207–216. Raven Press, New York.

43. Powell, D., Cannon, P., Skrabanek, P., and Kirrane, J. (1978): The pathophysiology of substance P in man. In: *Gut Hormones,* edited by S. R. Bloom, pp. 524–529. Churchill Livingstone, Edinburgh.

44. Powell, D., Skrabanek, P., and Cannon, D. (1977): Substance P: Radioimmunoassay studies. In: *Substance P,* edited by U. S. von Euler and B. Pernow, pp. 35–39. Raven Press, New York.

45. Putney, J. W., Jr., VanDeWalle, C. M., and Leslie, B. A. (1978): Receptor control of calcium influx in parotid acinar cells. *Mol. Pharmacol.,* 14:1046–1053.

46. Rivier, J. E., and Brown, M. R. (1978): Bombesin, bombesin analogues and related peptides: Effects on thermoregulation. *Biochemistry,* 17:1766–1771.

47. Rosell, S., Bjorkroth, U., Chang, D., Yamaguchi, I., Wan, Y.-P., Rackur, G., Fisher, G., and Folkers, K. (1977): Effects of substance P and analogs on isolated guinea pig ileum. In: *Substance P,* edited by U. S. von Euler and B. Pernow, pp. 83–88. Raven Press, New York.

48. Studer, R. O., Trazeciak, H., and Lergier, W. (1977): Substance P from horse intestine: its isolation, structure, and synthesis. In: *Substance P,* edited by U. S. von Euler and B. Pernow, pp.15–18. Raven Press, New York.

49. Sundler, F., Alumets, J., and Hakanson, R. (1977): 5-Hydroxytryptamine-containing enterochromaffin cells: storage site of substance P. *Acta Physiol. Scand.,* [*Suppl.*], 452:121–123.

50. Thulin, L., and Holm, I. (1977): Effect of substance P on the flow of hepatic bile and pancreatic juice. In: *Substance P,* edited by U. S. von Euler and B. Pernow, pp. 247–251. Raven Press, New York.

51. Uvnas-Wallensten, K. (1978): Release of substance P-like immunoreactivity into the antral lumen of cats. *Acta Physiol. Scand.,* 104:464–468.

52. Uyeno, E. T., Chang, D., and Folkers, K. (1979): Substance P found to lower body temperature and aggression. *Biochem. Biophys. Res. Commun.,* 86:837–842.

53. Walling, M. W., Brasitus, T. A., and Kimberg, D. V. (1977): Effects of calcitonin and substance P on the transport of Ca, Na, and Cl across rat ileum *in vitro. Gastroenterology,* 73:89–94.

54. Ward, P. E., and Johnson, A. R. (1978): Renal inactivation of substance P in the rat. *Biochem. J.,* 171:143–148.

55. Wharton, J., Polak, J. M., Bloom, S. R., Will, J. A., Brown, M. R., and Pearse, A. G. E. (1979): Substance P-like immunoreactive nerves in mammalian lung. *Invest. Cell. Pathol.,* 2:3–10.

56. Yanaihara, C., Sato, H., Hirohashi, M., Sakagami, M., Yamamoto, K., Hashimoto, T., Yanaihara, N., Abe, K., and Kaneko, T. (1976): Substance P radioimmunoassay using N^α-tyrosyl-substance P and demonstration of the presence of substance P-like immunoreactivities in human blood and porcine tissue extracts. *Endocrinol. Jpn.,* 23(6):457–463.

57. Yanaihara, N., Yanaihara, C., Hirohashi, M., Sato, H., Iizuka, Y., Hashimoto, T., and Sakagami, M. (1977): Substance P analogs: Synthesis, and biological and immunological properties. In: *Substance P,* edited by U. S. von Euler and B. Pernow, pp. 27–33. Raven Press, New York.

ENKEPHALINS

Structure

The two pentapeptides were isolated from pig brain (35) and also from calf brain (81) and were found to have the same amino acid sequences except at the carboxyl terminus: Tyr-Gly-Gly-Phe-Met and Tyr-Gly-Gly-Phe-Leu. These were named methionine-enkephalin and leucine-enkephalin, respectively, based on the carboxyl terminal residue and the previously demonstrated biological property of competing for occupation of opiate receptor sites. The methionine-enkephalin (Met-enkephalin) was about four times more abundant than the leucine-enkephalin (Leu-enkephalin) in pig brain while the reverse was true in the sheep brain. Both peptides had similar or greater potency than morphine for occupation of morphine receptors and producing the biological effects of morphine on smooth muscle, with Met-enkephalin being two to five times more potent than Leu-enkephalin.

The biosynthetic precursor of the enkephalins has not been established. A large precursor with a molecular weight of approximately 30,000 (14) can be processed by pituitary cells to yield ACTH, alpha-MSH, CLIP, beta-lipotropin, beta-endorphin, and other fragments (19). Met-enkephalin is contained as the amino terminal sequence of beta-endorphin (48). Beta-endorphin in turn is the 61–91 fragment of beta-lipotropin, a molecule that contains the ACTH sequence in residues, 1 through 39. Beta-endorphin and other fragments of beta-lipotropin that contain Met-enkephalin as the amino terminal sequence, such as alpha-endorphin (61–76 fragment) and gamma-endorphin (61–77 fragment), also interact with endogenous morphine receptors (53 or 54). A similar biosynthetic process has been demonstrated in the bovine hypothalamus (55). Soluble and particulate enzyme activities have been identified in brain extracts that are capable of cleaving the 61–69 nonapeptide of beta-lipotropin to yield Met-enkephalin (42). Such enzymes could account for some of the Met-enkephalin found in areas of the brain such as hypothalamus, midbrain, and striatum that contain relatively large amounts of beta-endorphin and its precursor molecules. However, there is little evidence that the biosynthetic precursors of beta-endorphin or the beta-endorphin molecule itself exists in other sites that contain large amounts of Met-enkephalin, such as the myenteric plexus of the gut, and the distributions of endorphins and enkephalins in the brain appear to differ significantly. Furthermore, the Leu-enkephalin sequence is not contained in the endorphin molecules. Therefore it seems likely that the enkephalins may originate, at least in part, from other precursors.

Other possible precursors for Leu- and Met-enkephalin have been described recently following the demonstration of large nonendorphin opiate peptides in brain extracts (51). One of these is a pentadecapeptide with the amino terminal sequence Tyr-Gly-Gly-Phe-Leu-Arg-Lys-Arg and has been named alpha-Neo-endorphin (41). This peptide was about five times more potent than Met-enkephalin. An even more potent peptide sequence that contains Leu-enkephalin as its amino terminal portion is dynorphin, a pituitary peptide which has Tyr-Gly-Gly-Phe-Leu-Arg-Arg-Ile-Arg-Pro-Lys-Leu-Lys as its first 13 residues (24). This peptide is more than 500 times more potent than Leu-enkephalin in a guinea pig ileum bioassay. Another possible precursor of Met-enkephalin has been found in acid extracts of porcine hypothalamus and characterized as the hexapeptide Tyr-Gly-Gly-Phe-Met(0)-Arg (33). All three of these sequences contain a basic amino acid, arginine, as the first residue after the enkephalin sequence, consistent with the idea that they are parts of typical prohormones that can be converted into smaller active hormones by the action of trypsin-like enzymes combined with carboxypeptidase B-like enzymes. Sequential digestion with trypsin and carboxypeptidase B was employed to identify a precursor molecule in extracts of bovine adrenal medulla that contained multiple Met-enkephalin and Leu-enkephalin sequences (51a). A large precursor with molecular weight about 50,000 and several smaller fragments were found. Digestion of the large molecule produced both Met-enkephalin in and Leu-enkephalin in a

molar ratio of about 7 to 1. Evidence was obtained from amino acid incorporation that large protein fragments of the 50,000 dalton molecule were biosynthetic precursors of free Met-enkephalin. These studies suggest that both Met- and Leu-enkephalin may be derived from a single large precursor and that the higher relative abundance of free Met-enkephalin in tissue extracts can be explained by the presence of multiple Met-enkephalin sequences but only a single Leu-enkephalin sequence in the precursor.

Adding to the confusion about possible sources of the endorphin-enkephalin peptides was the recent finding that a high molecular weight protein that contained beta-endorphin and ACTH-like immunoreactivities isolated from human placenta was actually the heavy chain of human immunoglobulin class IgG_1 (40). This homology between apparently unrelated proteins should be kept in mind as a caution about interpretation of immunochemical and immunocytochemical results obtained in tissue extracts possibly contaminated with IgG. There also is evidence that other lipophilic and nonpeptide substances that interact with the morphine receptor are present in human blood (68), small intestine (76), and cerebrospinal fluid (78). Such material can be demonstrated by receptor binding assays or by antibodies to morphine but not by antibodies directed against opiate peptides. The nature of this substance or substances has not been determined, but incubation with various proteases has no effect on the biological activity.

Biological Actions

Gastrointestinal

Intravenous infusion of morphine or Met-enkephalin produced a dose-dependent increase in basal, histamine-stimulated, and pentagastrin-stimulated gastric acid secretion in dogs that was strongly inhibited by naloxone (45). In humans, naloxone reduced basal and meal-stimulated acid secretion, presumably by antagonism of endogenous opiates (20). In the dog, vagal innervation of the stomach was not required for this effect, and no significant effects on serum gastrin concentration were measured in either species. The enhanced acid response to naloxone supports a role for endogenous opiates in normal regulation of acid secretion, but it is not known whether this effect is produced by action directly on the parietal cell, indirectly by modulation of the release of some gastrointestinal factor other than gastrin, or through an effect on the central nervous system (83). Local intra-arterial injection of Leu- or Met-enkephalin in anesthetized cats caused contraction of pyloric muscle and relaxation of the stomach, and these effects could be reversed or prevented by naloxone (18). Naloxone also blocked pyloric contraction caused by electrical vagal stimulation that was resistant to adrenergic and cholinergic blocking agents.

Enkephalin and morphine blocked pancreatic secretory responses to exogenous and endogenous secretin and cholecystokinin in conscious dogs (44). In anesthetized rats, methadone inhibited 2-DG-stimulated pancreatic secretion but not responses to secretin or cholecystokinin (73). These effects were more pronounced with intraventricular than with intravenous infusion of the drug. Central injection of beta-endorphin in conscious rats decreased basal gastric and pancreatic secretion, whereas the same doses given intravenously had no effect (74). Central administration of Leu- and Met-enkephalin at similar doses had no effect. Opioids also influence endocrine pancreatic secretion. Beta-endorphin and morphine suppress somatostatin secretion and cause glucose-dependent increases in glucagon and insulin secretion from the isolated perfused dog pancreas (36). Morphine also blocks meal-stimulated release of pancreatic polypeptide release in humans, possibly through an anticholinergic action (20).

Since one of the identifying actions for isolation of the enkephalins was relaxation of ileal muscle, it is not surprising that effects of these agents have been noted on intestinal motility. Enkephalins appear to mimic most of the known actions of morphine on the stomach and small intestine (43).

Central Nervous System

Central administration of endorphin, enkephalins, and enkephalin analogues caused analgesia associated with other behavioral changes (17,37,58,62). Administration of large doses of Met-enkephalin into the third ventricle of cats caused emesis and hyperthermia that were inhibited by naloxone (10). Small doses of naloxone selectively abolished overeating in genetically obese mice and rats, and increased concentrations of beta-endorphin were found in the pituitary and blood of these animals (60).

Pituitary Hormone Release

Many studies have demonstrated that endorphins, enkephalins, and enkephalin analogues influence anterior pituitary secretion when administered either centrally or peripherally and that these effects are blocked by naloxone. The major effects are stimulation of growth hormone and prolactin release and inhibition of release of LH and FSH (16,63,84). TSH is stimulated modestly and ACTH release may be either stimulated or inhibited. In general, effects on fasting concentrations of gastrointestinal hormones are minimal (84). The effects on growth hormone and prolactin cannot be demonstrated on pituitary tissue *in vitro* (77) and may be

mediated by increases in serotonin and decreases in dopamine metabolism (63).

Effects on Neurotransmitters and Cells

Enkephalins have been shown to decrease acetylcholine release from rat cerebral cortex (39). Beta-endorphin inhibited norepinephrine release from rat cerebral cortex, although efforts to demonstrate effects on brain dopamine release have produced mixed results (3). This may be because opiates such as Met-enkephalin cause stimulation of dopamine synthesis in the brain that may mask effects on release (6). No effects on serotonin synthesis have been observed. Enkephalin analogues also were found to inhibit potassium-stimulated calcium-dependent release of substance P from sensory neurons in culture (64). Application of enkephalin to single neurons in the brain depressed spontaneous and glutamate-induced firing (23). Specific inhibition of calcium uptake by brain synaptosomes was produced by low concentrations of beta-endorphin (27). Met-enkephalin caused stimulation of cyclic AMP production by neuroblastoma-glioma hybrid cells, and these cells demonstrated tolerance and dependence to this opiate (46a). It is apparent that endogenous opiates have multiple central effects.

Structure-Activity Relationships

The relationships between structure and biological actions and receptor binding of opiate peptides have been studied extensively. Receptor binding studies have been possible because of the availability of high specific activity ^{3}H ligands for the receptor such as ^{3}H-naloxone and ^{3}H-Leu-enkephalin (59) and more recently ^{3}H-beta-endorphin (47). Specific binding can be determined by incubation in the presence and absence of highly potent morphine antagonists, whereas agonist activity can be estimated by changes in affinity produced by decreasing sodium concentration which selectively decreases binding of agonists (82). Such binding assays have made possible the mapping of distribution of opiate receptors in the central nervous system and estimating the potency of analogues, since close correlations have been obtained between binding affinity and biological activity. Evidence has been obtained that there are at least two classes of binding sites for opioid peptides. For Leu-enkephalin, the two sites have K_D values of about 0.5 and 5 nM (59), whereas for beta-endorphin, the measured K_D values were about 0.8 and 7 nM (47). There also is evidence that receptor populations in the guinea pig ileum and mouse vas deferens are not homogeneous and identical, since relative potencies of beta-endorphin, Met-enkephalin, Leu-enkephalin, and other analogues vary widely in these two tissues (59). Recently it has been shown that an analogue of naloxone, nalox-azone, irreversibly binds to high-affinity opiate receptors but not to low-affinity receptors and blocks the analgesic effects of morphine but does not alter the lethal effects of high-dose morphine (66), suggesting that analgesia is mediated by high-affinity receptors.

Some discrepancies that have been found between receptor binding affinity *in vitro* and biological potency *in vivo* for natural enkephalins, such as relatively low analgesic potency of Met-enkephalin when administered into cerebral ventricles, may be explained by rapid enzymatic degradation. Substitution of D-alanine for glycine in the 2 position of Met-enkephalin either with or without amidation of the C-terminal methionine residue produces a compound that has similar receptor affinity to Met-enkephalin but markedly increased biological potency because of resistance to degradative enzymes that act on the N-terminal tyrosine residue (67, 87). Further modifications of the enkephalin molecule revealed that the C-terminal amino acid is not necessary for biological potency since Tyr-D-Ala-Gly-Phe-NH$_2$ had full analgesic and receptor binding potency in the brain and even the N-terminal dipeptide amide Tyr-D-Ala-NH$_2$ retained significant biological activity (61). Compounds with even greater potency on the guinea pig ileum have been synthesized by reversing the peptide bonds between positions 4 and 5 in the D-Ala^2 Leu- and Met-enkephalinamides (9). Studies with fragments of beta-lipotropin have shown that this molecule has no opioid activity whereas beta-endorphin has typical opioid activity (12) and that Met-enkephalinamide and beta-endorphin have similar potency on guinea pig intestine (54). Modifications at the C-terminus of beta-endorphin have been performed that increased the analgesic effects of beta-endorphin (52).

Some effects of beta-endorphin may be mediated by nonopiate binding sites since specific binding of beta-endorphin to lymphocytes is not affected by enkephalin analogues or by opiate agonists or antagonists (28). Cerebroside sulfate has been identified as a possible anionic site of the opiate receptor (57). The nonsulfated C-terminal heptapeptide of cholecystokinin but not the sulfated peptide has a weak affinity for brain and ileal opiate receptors, being 0.2 to 0.5% as potent as Met-enkephalin (75). This activity can be explained by structural similarities between the two peptides.

Distribution

Enkephalin-like immunoreactivity has been detected in the human gastrointestinal tract by immunocytochemistry and radioimmunoassay with antibodies produced against Met-enkephalin (69). Nerve fibers in the myenteric plexus and endocrine cells in the antrum that appeared to be gastrin cells as well as a few endocrine cells in the duodenum and pancreas were specifically stained. No staining was obtained with antibodies to en-dorphins. Extraction of various gut tissues revealed concentrations of immunoreactive enkephalin in the range of 20 to 50 ng/g tissue throughout the gut except for the fundic mucosa. Endorphin immunoreactivity was not detected. Immunocytochemistry with antibodies to Leu-enkephalin revealed similar distribution of nerve fibers in the myenteric plexus throughout the gut, but endocrine cells containing enkephalin-like material were identified in the pig antrum and duodenum as enterochromaffin cells that also contained 5-HT (2). Especially dense enkephalinergic innervation has been demonstrated in the cat pylorus (18) and in the human esophagus (85) in the circular smooth muscle and myenteric plexus with relatively sparse innervation of the stomach. The inferior mesenteric ganglion has a dense plexus of immunoreactive enkephalin fibers that represent preganglionic neurons (29). In the gut, consecutive staining with different antibodies has revealed that enkephalin is present in nerves that are distinct from those that contain VIP or substance P. Cells in the adrenal medulla contain both enkephalin and epinephrine, and cells in the carotid body contain both enkephalin and dopamine. In the spinal cord, enkephalin nerves have been identified as interneurons in the dorsal horn and may also be present in a descending system that projects to the dorsal horn. Preganglionic localization of Leu-enkephalin has been demonstrated in nerve processes and cell bodies in the sacral autonomic nucleus of the cat spinal cord (23a).

In the brain, Leu- and Met-enkephalins are distributed widely and represent most of the opioid activity, whereas endorphins are the major opioid peptide in the pituitary (34). Although the ratios vary in different regions, Leu-enkephalin is more abundant than Met-enkephalin in the brain, while Met-enkephalin is more abundant than Leu-enkephalin in the ileum. Immunohistochemical mapping of the distribution of enkephalin fibers in the brain revealed distinct localization in multiple discrete regions including the dorsal motor nuclei of the vagus nerve (80). Enkephalin and substance P immunoreactive nerves are found in corresponding but distinct pathways in the brain and spinal cord that could represent pathways regulating pain and analgesia (30). In the pituitary, Met-enkephalin immunoreactivity was found only in growth hormone cells whereas ACTH and endorphin immunoreactivities were found only in a separate cell type, indicating that endorphin is not the precursor to Met-enkephalin even in the pituitary (90). Other studies have revealed separate distribution of nerves containing immunoreactive enkephalin and beta-endorphin (7,89).

Measurement

Specific bioassays for endogenous opiates and for opioid drugs commonly are performed with guinea pig ileum and mouse vas deferens preparations in the presence and absence of naloxone (24). Radioreceptor assays also have been used extensively. Radioimmunoassays also have been developed to distinguish between the enkephalin and endorphin peptides. It has been shown that rapid boiling of tissue samples in 1 M acetic acid is an effective method for extraction and preparation of tissue extracts for either enkephalin or endorphin assay (72). Assays have been described that discriminate Leu- from Met-enkephalin with about 5% cross-reactivity with the other peptide (26). Leu-enkephalin-like immunoreactivity has been detected in dog plasma by radioimmunoassay after prior extraction in the presence of excess antibody to Leu-enkephalin (46). There are several reports of assays that can detect low concentrations of beta-endorphin (2 to 6 pM) in normal human plasma (31,65,88). A radioimmunoassay for gamma-endorphin also has been described (38).

Metabolism

The disappearance half-times of beta-endorphin (21) and of beta-lipotropin (56) in humans are about 37 min. Such data are difficult to obtain for circulating enkephalins since they are degraded rapidly by plasma and have a disappearance half-time less than 4 min in the cerebral ventricle (13). Met-enkephalin is markedly inactivated by hepatic passage (45). Extremely rapid clearance of ^{3}H-Met-enkephalin was found in the rat after intravenous injection (15). Only 5% of total radioactivity was intact peptide in plasma obtained 15 sec after injection, indicating a half-time of about 2 to 4 sec. The first step in degradation appeared to be cleavage of the amino terminal tyrosine residue. Resistance to degradation probably accounts for most of the increased potency obtained with D amino acid analogues of the enkephalins, but other factors such as receptor affinity also are important (4). Spontaneous inactivation of enkephalins can occur in solutions after prolonged storage because of alterations in the tyrosine residue (86). The blood-brain barrier prevents general penetration of enkephalins into the central nervous system from the blood (11), but there is evidence for significant brain uptake during continuous infusions of enkephalin analogues over a period of several minutes (71).

Release

Data on release of enkephalins, especially from the gut, are sparse. Electrical stimulation of the guinea pig ileum causes release of a substance that inhibits longitudinal muscle contraction and this effect is antagonized by naloxone (70). Similar results have been obtained for inhibition of electrically induced contractions of cat esophagus (85) and for electrically induced

contraction of cat pylorus (18). Administration of morphine to anesthetized dogs caused increased Leu-enkephalin-like immunoreactivity in portal and peripheral but not hepatic vein plasma and this effect was antagonized by naloxone (46). Electrical stimulation of periventricular brain sites in patients with chronic pain caused a significant rise in ventricular enkephalin-like material detected by bioassay or receptor binding assays after separation from endorphins by chromatography (1). Immunoreactive beta-endorphin also was released into ventricular fluid during similar stimulation (32). Calcium-dependent potassium-stimulated release of Met- and Leu-enkephalins has been found in pieces of rat brain (5), and similar release of endorphins has been demonstrated in mouse pituitary tumor cells in culture (79).

Relationship with Physiological Events

Neural release of enkephalins may play some role in regulation of gut smooth muscle contraction (18,85) and could contribute to basal stimulation of gastric acid secretion in dogs (45) and humans (20), as well as enhancement of food-stimulated acid secretion. A more important role for endogenous opioids as a modulator of neural transmission, especially as a natural analgesic substance, has been suggested by several studies (22,49), but attempts to demonstrate such a role have not been uniformly successful (25). Some types of painful stimuli appear to activate either opioid or nonopioid analgesia systems depending on the conditions under which pain is produced (50). Beta-endorphin appears to play a role in neuroendocrine regulation, especially of pituitary hormone secretion (8).

Conditions of Excess or Deficiency

No conditions of enkephalin excess or deficiency have been identified in the gastrointestinal tract. There is speculation that alterations in central nervous system opioids may be a factor in pathogenesis of nervous disorders or in sensitivity to pain (8).

References

1. Akil, H., Richardson, D. E., Hughes, J., and Barchas, J. D. (1978): Enkephalin-like material elevated in ventricular cerebrospinal fluid of pain patients after analgetic focal stimulation. *Science*, 201:463–465.
2. Alumets, J., Hakanson, R., Sundler, F., and Chang, K.-J. (1978): Leu-enkephalin-like material in nerves and enterochromaffin cells in the gut. *Histochemistry*, 56:187–196.
3. Arbilla, S., and Langer, S. Z. (1978): Morphine and β-endorphin inhibit release of noradrenaline from cerebral cortex but not of dopamine from rat striatum. *Nature*, 271:559–561.
4. Bajusz, S., Patthy, A., Kenessey, A., Graf, L., Szekely, J. I., and Ronai, A. Z. (1978): Is there correlation between analgesic potency and biodegradation of enkephalin analogs? *Biochem. Biophys. Res. Commun.*, 84:1045–1053.

5. Bayon, A., Rossier, J., Mauss, A., Bloom, F. E., Iversen, L. L., Ling, N., and Guillemin, R. (1978): *In vitro* release of [5-methionine]-enkephalin and [5-leucine]-enkephalin from the rat globus pallidus. *Proc. Natl. Acad. Sci. USA,* 75:3503–3506.

6. Biggio, G., Casu, M., Corda, M. G., Di Bello, C., and Gessa, G. L. (1978): Stimulation of dopamine synthesis in caudate nucleus by intrastriatal enkephalins and antagonism by naloxone. *Science,* 200:552–554.

7. Bloom, F., Battenberg, E., Rossier, J., Ling, N., and Guillemin, R. (1978): Neurons containing β-endorphin in rat brain exist separately from those containing enkephalin: Immunocytochemical studies. *Proc. Natl. Acad. Sci. USA,* 75:1591–1595.

8. Bunney, W. E., Jr., Pert, C. B., Klee, W., Costa, E., Pert, A., and Davis, G. C. (1979): Basic and clinical studies of endorphins. *Ann. Intern. Med.,* 91:239–250.

9. Chorev, M., Shavitz, R., Goodman, M., Minick, S., and Guillemin, R. (1979): Partially modified retro-inverso-enkephalinamides: Topochemical long-acting analogues *in vitro* and *in vivo. Science,* 204:1210–1212.

10. Clark, W. G. (1977): Emetic and hyperthermic effects of centrally injected methionine-enkephalin in cats (39713). *Proc. Soc. Exp. Biol. Med.,* 154:540–542.

11. Cornford, E. M., Braun, L. D., Crane, P. D., and Oldendorf, W. H. (1978): Blood-brain barrier restriction of peptides and the low uptake of enkephalins. *Endocrinology,* 103:1297–1303.

12. Cox, B. M., Goldstein, A., and Li, C. H. (1976): Opioid activity of a peptide, β-lipotropin-(61–91), derived from β-lipotropin. *Proc. Natl. Acad. Sci. USA,* 73:1821–1823.

13. Craves, F. B., Law, P. Y., Hunt, C. A., and Loh, H. H. (1978): The metabolic disposition of radiolabeled enkephalins *in vitro* in *in situ. J. Pharmacol. Exp. Ther.,* 206:492–506.

14. Crine, P., Gianoulakis, C., Seidah, N. G., Gossard, F., Pezalla, P. D., Lis, M., and Chretien, M. (1978): Biosynthesis of β-endorphin from β-lipotropin and a larger molecular weight precursor in rat pars intermedia. *Proc. Natl. Acad. Sci. USA,* 75:4719–4723.

15. Dupont, A., Cusan, L., Garon, M., Alvarado-Urbina, G., and Labrie, F. (1977): Extremely rapid degradation of [^{3}H] methionine-enkephalin by various rat tissues *in vivo* and *in vitro. Life Sci.,* 21:907–914.

16. Dupont, A., Cusan, L., Garon, M., Labrie, F., and Li, C. H. (1977): β-Endorphin: Stimulation of growth hormone release *in vivo. Proc. Natl. Acad. Sci. USA,* 74:358–359.

17. Dutta, A. S., Gormley, J. J., Hayward, C. F., Morley, J. S., Shaw, J. S., Stacey, G. J., and Turnbull, M. T. (1977): Enkephalin analogues eliciting analgesia after intravenous injection. *Life Sci.,* 21:559–562.

18. Edin, R., Lundberg, J., Terenius, L., Dahlstrom, A., Hokfelt, T., Kewenter, J., and Ahlman, H. (1980): Evidence for vagal enkephalinergic neural control of the feline pylorus and stomach. *Gastroenterology,* 78:492–497.

19. Eipper, B. A., and Mains, R. E. (1980): Structure and biosynthesis of pro-adrenocorticotropin/endorphin and related peptides. *Endocrine Rev.,* 1:1–27.

20. Feldman, M., Walsh, J. H., and Taylor, I. (1980): Effect of naloxone and morphine on gastric acid secretion and on serum gastrin and pancreatic polypeptide concentrations in man. *Gastroenterology,* 79:294–298.

21. Foley, K. M., Kourides, I. A., Inturrisi, C. E., Kaiko, R. F., Zaroulis, C. G., Posner, J. B., Houde, R. W., and Li, C. H. (1979): β-Endorphin: analgesic and hormonal effects in humans. *Proc. Natl. Acad. Sci. USA,* 76:5377–5381.

22. Frederickson, R. C. A. (1977): Enkephalin pentapeptides—A review of current evidence for a physiological role in vertebrate neurotransmission. *Life Sci.,* 21:23–42.

23. Frederickson, R. C. A., and Norris, F. H. (1976): Enkephalin-induced depression of single neurons in brain areas with opiate receptors—Antagonism by naloxone. *Science,* 194:440–442.

23a. Glazer, E. J., and Basbaum, A. I. (1980): Leucine enkephalin: Localization in and oxoplasmic transport by sacral parasympathetic preganglionic neurons. *Science,* 28:1479–1481.

24. Goldstein, A., Tachibana, S., Lowney, L. I., Hunkapiller, M., and Hood, L. (1979): Dynorphin-(1-13), an extraordinarily potent opioid peptide. *Proc. Natl. Acad. Sci. USA,* 76:6666–6670.

25. Grevert, P., and Goldstein, A. (1978): Endorphins: naloxone fails to alter experimental pain or mood in humans. *Science,* 199: 1093–1095.

26. Gros, C., Pradelles, P., Rouget, C., Bepoldin, O., Dray, F., Fournie-Zaluski, M. C., Roques, B. P., Pollard, H., Llorens-Cortes, C., and Schwartz, J. C. (1978): Radioimmunoassay of methionine- and leucine-enkephalins in regions of rat brain and comparison with endorphins estimated by a radioreceptor assay. *J. Neurochem.,* 31:29–39.

27. Guerrero-Munoz, F., de Lourdes Guerrero, M., Way, E. L., and Li, C. H. (1979): Effect of β-endorphin on calcium uptake in the brain. *Science,* 206:89–91.

28. Hazum, E., Chang, K. J., and Cuatrecusas, P. (1979): Specific nonopiate receptors for β-endorphin. *Science,* 205:1033–1035.

29. Hokfelt, T., Johansson, O., Ljungdahl, A., Lundberg, J. M., and Schultzberg, M. (1980): Peptidergic neurones. *Nature,* 284: 515–521.

30. Hokfelt, T., Ljungdahl, A., Terenius, L., Elde, R., and Nilsson, G. (1977): Immunohistochemical analysis of peptide pathways possibly related to pain and analgesia: Enkephalin and substance P. *Proc. Natl. Acad. Sci. USA,* 74:3081–3085.

31. Hollt, V., Muller, O. A., and Fahlbusch, R. (1979): β-Endorphin in human plasma: Basal and pathologically elevated levels. *Life Sci.,* 25:37–44.

32. Hosobuchi, Y., Rossier, J., Bloom, F. E., and Guillemin, R. (1979): Stimulation of human periaqueductal gray for pain relief increases immunoreactive β-endorphin in ventricular fluid. *Science,* 203:279–281.

33. Huang, W-Y., Chang, R. C. C., Kastin, A. J., Coy, D. H., and Schally, A. V. (1979): Isolation and structure of pro-methionine-enkephalin: Potential enkephalin precursor from porcine hypothalamus. *Proc. Natl. Acad. Sci. USA.,* 76:6177–6180.

34. Hughes, J., Kosterlitz, H. W., and Smith, T. W. (1977): The distribution of methionine-enkephalin and leucine-enkephalin in the brain and peripheral tissues. *Br. J. Pharmacol.,* 61:639–647.

35. Hughes, J., Smith, T. W., Kosterlitz, H. W., Fothergill, L. A., Morgan, B. A., and Morris, H. R. (1975): Identification of two related pentapeptides from the brain with potent opiate agonist activity. *Nature,* 258:577–579.

36. Ipp, E., Dobbs, R., and Unger, R. H. (1978): Morphine and β-endorphin influence the secretion of the endocrine pancreas. *Nature,* 276:190–191.

37. Jacquet, Y. F. (1978): Opiate effects after adrenocorticotropin or β-endorphin injection in the periaqueductal gray matter of rats. *Science,* 21:1032–1034.

38. Jegou, S., Tonon, M. C., Leboulenger, F., Delarue, C., and Vaudry, H. (1978): Radioimmunoassay for γ-endorphin. *Biochem. Biophys. Res. Commun.,* 83:201–208.

39. Jhamandus, K., Sawynok, J., and Sutak, M. (1977): Enkephalin effects on release of brain acetylcholine. *Nature,* 269:433–434.

40. Julliard, J. H., Shibasaki, T., Ling, N., and Guillemin, R. (1980): High-molecular-weight immunoreactive β-endorpin in extracts of human placenta is a fragment of immunoglobulin G. *Science,* 208:183–185.

41. Kangawa, K., Matsuo, H., and Igarashi, M. (1979): α-Neo-endorphin: A "big" leu-enkephalin with potent opiate activity from porcine hypothalami. *Biochem. Biophys. Res. Commun.,* 86:153–160.

42. Knight, M., and Klee, W. A. (1979): Enkephalin generating activity of rat brain endopeptidases. *J. Biol. Chem.,* 254: 10426–10430.

43. Konturek, S. J., Pawlik, W., Tasler, J., Thor, P., Walus, K., Krol, R., Jaworek, J., and Schally, A. V. (1978): Effects of enkephalin on the gastrointestinal tract. In: *Gut Hormones,* edited by S. R. Bloom, pp. 507–512. Churchill Livingstone, Edinburgh.

44. Konturek, S. J., Tasler, J., Cieszkowski, M., Jaworek, J., Coy, D. H., and Schally, A. V. (1978): Inhibition of pancreatic secretion by enkephalin and morphine in dogs. *Gastroenterology,* 74:851–855.

45. Konturek, S. J., Tasler, J., Cieszkowski, M., Mikos, E., Coy, D. H., and Schally, A. V. (1980): Comparison of methionine-enkephalin and morphine in the stimulation of gastric acid secretion in the dog. *Gastroenterology,* 78:294–300.

46. Laasberg, L. H., Johnson, E. E., and Hedley-White, J. (1980): Effect of morphine and naloxone on leu-enkephalin-like immunoreactivity in dogs. *J. Pharmacol. Exp. Ther.*, 212:496–502.

46a. Lampert, A., Nirenberg, M., and Klee, W. A. (1976): Tolerance and dependence evoked by an endogenous opiate peptide. *Proc. Natl. Acad. Sci. USA*, 73:3165–3167.

47. Law, P. Y., Loh, H. H., and Li, C. H. (1979): Properties and localization of β-endorphin receptor in rat brain. *Proc. Natl. Acad. Sci. USA*, 76:5455–5459.

48. Lazarus, L. H., Ling, N., and Guillemin, R. (1976): β-Lipotropin as a prohormone for the morphinomimetic peptides endorphins and enkephalins. *Proc. Natl. Acad. Sci. USA*, 73: 2156–2159.

49. Levine, J. D., Gordon, N. C., and Fields, H. L. (1978): The mechanism of placebo analgesia. *Lancet*, 2:654–659.

50. Lewis, J. W., Cannon, J. T., and Liebeskind, J. C. (1980): Opioid and nonopioid mechanisms of stress analgesia. *Science*, 208:623–625.

51. Lewis, R. V., Stein, S., Gerber, L. D., Rubinstein, M., and Udenfriend, S. (1978): High molecular weight opioid-containing proteins in striatum. *Proc. Natl. Acad. Sci. USA*, 75:4021–4023.

51a. Lewis, R. V., Stern, A. S., Kimura, A. S., Rossier, J., Stein, S., and Udenfriend, S. (1980): An about 50,000 dalton protein in adrenal medulla: A common precursor of (met)- and (leu)-enkephalin. *Science*, 208:1459–1461.

52. Li, C. H., Yamashiro, D., Tseng, L. F., Chang, W. C., and Ferrara, P. (1979): β-Endorphin: Synthesis of analogs modified at the carboxyl terminus with increased activities. *Proc. Natl. Acad. Sci. USA*, 76:3276–3278.

53. Ling, N., Burgus, R., and Guillemin, R. (1976): Isolation, primary structure, and synthesis of α-endorphin and γ-endorphin, two peptides of hypothalamic-hypophysial origin with morphinomimetic activity. *Proc. Natl. Acad. Sci. USA*, 73: 3942–3946.

54. Ling, N., and Guillemin, R. (1967): Morphinomimetic activity of synthetic fragments of β-lipotropin and analogs. *Proc. Natl. Acad. Sci. USA*, 73:3308–3310.

55. Liotta, A. S., Gildersleeve, D., Brownstein, M. J., and Krieger, D. T. (1979): Biosynthesis *in vitro* of immunoreactive 31,000-dalton corticotropin/β-endorphin-like material by bovine hypothalamus. *Proc. Natl. Acad. Sci. USA*, 76:1448–1452.

56. Liotta, A. S., Li, C. H., Schussler, G. C., and Krieger, D. T. (1978): Comparative metabolic clearance rate, volume of distribution and plasma half-life of human β-lipotropin and ACTH. *Life Sci.* 23:2323–2330.

57. Loh, H. H., Law, P. Y., Ostwald, T., Cho, T. M., and Way, E. L. (1978): Possible involvement of cerebroside sulfate in opiate receptor binding. *Fed. Proc.*, 37:147–152.

58. Loh, H. H., Tseng, L. F., Wei, E., and Li, C. H. (1976): β-Endorphin is a potent analgesic agent. *Proc. Natl. Acad. Sci. USA*, 73:2895–2898.

59. Lord, J. A. H., Waterfield, A. A., Hughes, J., and Kosterlitz, H. W. (1977): Endogenous opioid peptides: multiple agonists and receptors. *Nature*, 267:495–499.

60. Margules, D. L. Moisset, B., Lewis, M. J., Shibuya, H., and Pert, C. B. (1978): β-Endorphin is associated with overeating in genetically obese mice (ob/ob) and rats (fa/fa). *Science*, 202:988–991.

61. McGregor, W. H., Stein, L., and Belluzzi, J. D. (1978): Potent analgesic activity of the enkephalin-like tetrapeptide H-TYR-D-ALA-GLY-PHE-NH$_2$. *Life Sci.*, 23:1371–1378.

62. Meglio, M., Hosobuchi, Y., Loh, H. H., Adams, J. E., and Li, C. H. (1977): β-Endorphin: Behavioral and analgesic activity in cats. *Proc. Natl. Acad. Sci. USA*, 74:774–776.

63. Meites, J., Bruni, J. F., Van Vugt, D. A., and Smith, A. F. (1979): Relation of endogenous opioid peptides and morphine to neuroendocrine functions. *Life Sci.*, 24:1325–1336.

64. Mudge, A. W., Leeman, S. E., and Fischbach, G. D. (1979): Enkephalin inhibits release of substance P from sensory neurons in culture and decreases action potential duration. *Proc. Natl. Acad. Sci. USA*, 76:526–530.

65. Nakao, K., Nakia, Y., Oki, S., Horii, K., and Imura, H. (1978): Presence of immunoreactive β-endorphin in normal human plasma. A concomitant release of β-endorphin with adrenocor-

ticotropin after metyrapone administration. *J. Clin. Invest.*, 62:1395–1398.

66. Pasternak, G. W., Childers, S. R., and Snyder, S. H. (1980): Opiate analgesia: evidence for mediation by a subpopulation of opiate receptors. *Science*, 208:514–516.

67. Pert, C. B., Pert, A., Chang, J-K., and Fong, B. T. W. (1976): [D-Ala^2]-Met-Enkephalinamide: A potent, long-lasting synthetic pentapeptide analgesic. *Science*, 194:330–332.

68. Pert, C. B., Pert, A., and Tallman, J. F. (1976): Isolation of a novel endogenous opiate analgesic from human blood. *Proc. Natl. Acad. Sci. USA*, 73:2226–2230.

69. Polak, J. M., Bloom, S. R., Sullivan, S. N., Facer, P., and Pearse, A. G. E. (1977): Enkephalin-like immunoreactivity in the human gastrointestinal tract. *Lancet*, 1:972–974.

70. Puig, M. M., Gascon, P., Craviso, G. L., and Musacchio, J. M. (1977): Endogenous opiate receptor ligand: Electrically induced release in the guinea pig ileum. *Science*, 195:419–420.

71. Rapoport, S. I., Klee, W. A., Pettigrew, K. D., and Ohno, K. (1980): Entry of opioid peptides into the central nervous system. *Science*, 207:84–86.

72. Rossier, J., Bayon, A., Vargo, T. M., Ling, N., Guillemin, R., and Bloom, F. (1977): Radioimmunoassay of brain peptides: Evaluation of a methodology for the assay of α-endorphin and enkephalin. *Life Sci.*, 21:847–852.

73. Roze, C., Chariot, J., de La Tour, J., Souchard, M., Vaille, C., and Debray, C. (1978): Methadone blockade of 2-deoxyglucose-induced pancreatic secretion in the rat. *Gastroenterology*, 74:215–220.

74. Roze, C., Dubrasquet, M., Chariot, J., and Vaille, C. (1980): Central inhibition of basal pancreatic and gastric secretions by beta-endorphin in rats. *Gastroenterology*, 79:654–664.

75. Schiller, P. W., Lipton, A., Horrobin, D. F., and Bodanszky, M. (1978): Unsulfated C-terminal 7-peptide of cholecystokinin: a new ligand of the opiate receptor. *Biochem. Biophys. Res. Commun.*, 85:1332–1338.

76. Schulz, R., Wuster, M., and Herz, A. (1977): Detection of a long acting endogenous opioid in blood and small intestine. *Life Sci.*, 21: 105–116.

77. Shaar, C. J., Frederickson, R. C. A., Dininger, N. B., and Jackson, L. (1977): Enkephalin analogues and naloxone modulate the release of growth hormone and prolactin—evidence for regulation by an endogenous opioid peptide in brain. *Life Sci.*, 21:853–860.

78. Shorr, J., Foley, K., and Spector, S. (1978): Presence of a nonpeptide morphine-like compound in human cerebrospinal fluid. *Life Sci.*, 23:2057–2062.

79. Simantov, R. (1978): Basal and potassium stimulated, calcium dependent, endorphins release from pituitary cells. *Life Sci.*, 23: 2503–2508.

80. Simantov, R., Kuhar, M. J., Uhl, G. R., and Snyder, S. H. (1977): Opioid peptide enkephalin: immunohistochemical mapping in rat central nervous system. *Proc. Natl. Acad. Sci. USA*, 74:2167–2171.

81. Simantov, R., and Snyder, S. H. (1976): Morphine-like peptides in mammalian brain: Isolation, structure elucidation, and interactions with the opiate receptor. *Proc. Natl. Acad. Sci. USA*, 73:2515–2519.

82. Snyder, S. H. (1977): Opiate receptors in the brain. *N. Engl. J. Med.*, 296:266–271.

83. Solomon, T. E. (1980): Endogenous opiates and gastric acid secretion. *Gastroenterology*, 78:411–413.

84. Stubbs, W. A., Jones, A., Edwards, C. R. W., Delitala, G., Jeffcoate, W. J., and Ratter, S. J. (1978): Hormonal and metabolic responses to an enkephalin analogue in normal man. *Lancet*, 1225–1227.

85. Uddman, R., Alumets, J., Hakanson, R., Sundler, F., and Walles, B. (1980): Peptidergic (enkephalin) innervation of the mammalian esophagus. *Gastroenterology*, 78:732–737.

86. Vogel, Z., Miron, T., Altstein, M., and Wilchek, M. (1978): Spontaneous inactivation of enkephalin. *Biochem. Biophys. Res. Commun.*, 85:226–233.

87. Walker, J. M., Berntson, G. G., and Sandman, C. A. (1977): An analogue of enkephalin having prolonged opiate-like effects *in vivo*. *Science*, 196:85–87.

88. Wardlaw, S. L., and Frantz, A. G. (1979): Measurement of β-endorphin in human plasma. *J. Clin. Endocrinol. Metab.*, 48: 176–180.
89. Watson, S. J., Akil, H., Richard, C. W., and Barchas, J. D. (1978): Evidence for two separate opiate peptide neuronal systems. *Nature*, 275:226–228.
90. Weber, E., Voigt, K. H., and Martin, R. (1978): Pituitary somatotrophs contain [met]enkephalin-like immunoreactivity. *Proc. Natl. Acad. Sci. USA*, 75:6134–6138.

UROGASTRONE

Structure

Urogastrone is a 53 amino peptide containing three disulfide bonds obtained from human urine and purified by monitoring its inhibitory effect on gastric acid secretion (9). This peptide is remarkably similar to epidermal growth factor (EGF) isolated from the submaxillary glands of male mice (4,5) and also composed of 53 amino acid residues. The same amino acid residues occupy 37 of the 53 positions in these two molecules (Fig. 22). The two molecules subsequently have been shown to share several biological properties. Slightly smaller forms of each peptide have been isolated in which the C-terminal amino acid or dipeptide is absent, probably as a result of cleavage during the isolation procedures. These carboxyl terminal amino acids are not required for biological activity. A human epidermal growth factor was purified from urine and was partially characterized as similar to but not identical with urogastrone (3). Urogastrone is relatively resistant to tryptic digestion despite the presence of several basic amino acid residues. Urogastrone-like molecules have been identified in human plasma, saliva, gastric juice, and milk (14,17,18). Larger forms have been found in serum and saliva (14) and in urine (19). The larger urinary form did not appear to be an aggregate and had lower receptor binding activity than the smaller molecule. It was partially converted to a smaller form with increased biological activity by incubation with an arginine esterase from mouse submandibular glands. Trypsin treatment of the larger serum fraction produced a smaller molecule with significant mitogenic activity (14).

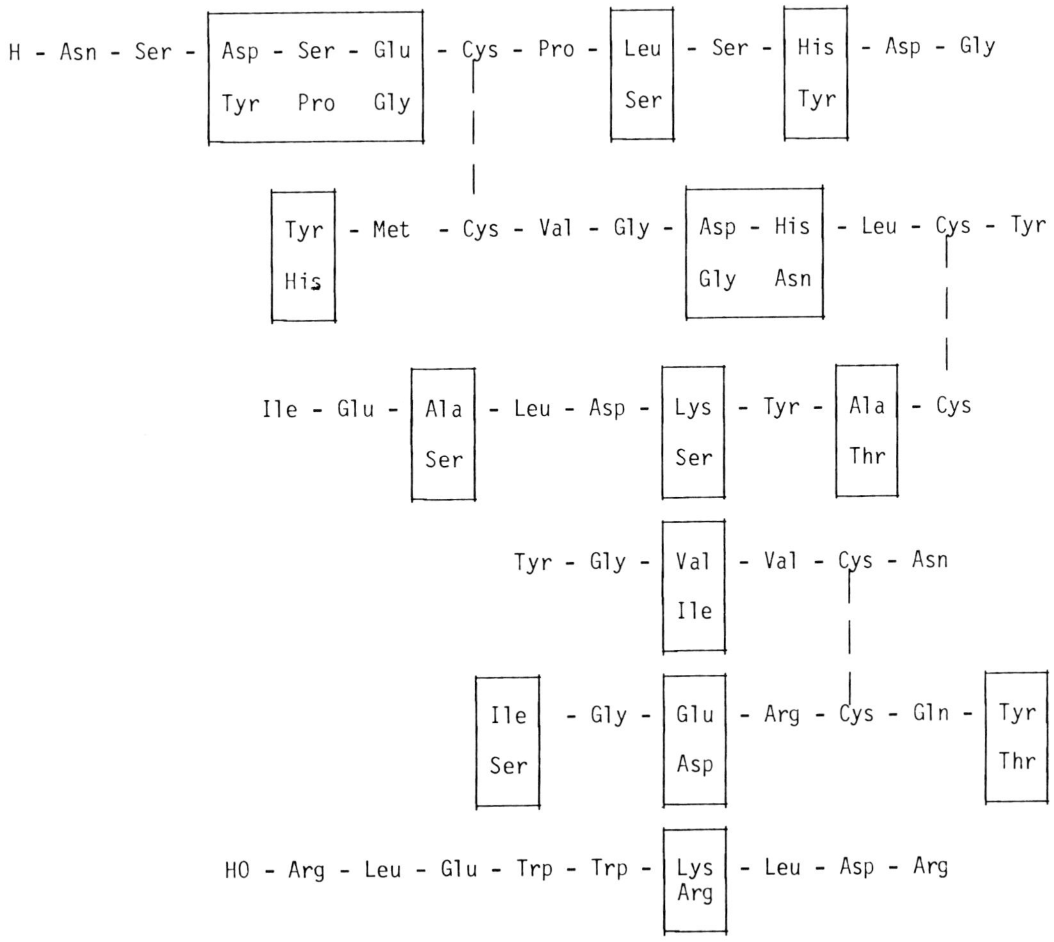

FIG. 22. Amino acid sequence of human urogastrone. Amino acid residues enclosed in boxes are those in which human urogastrone and mouse epidermal growth factor differ. From Gregory and Preston (13).

Biological Actions

The identifying action of urogastrone is inhibition of gastric acid secretion. The inhibition has been found in several mammalian species during stimulation by histamine, pentagastrin, or insulin, and in human subjects with gastrinomas (10). Doses as low as 0.25 μg kg^{-1} suppress basal and stimulated gastric secretion in humans. It appears to have no effect on pancreatic, biliary, or salivary secretion.

Not surprisingly, urogastrone shares many if not all biological actions with the structurally related epidermal growth factor. Urogastrone has the same enhancing effect as EGF on time of eye opening in newborn mice and on tooth eruption (10). Human urogastrone and mouse EGF were found to share a common receptor in cultured human fibroblasts (20). Both stimulate DNA synthesis and amino acid uptake and compete equally for a high-affinity (K_D 0.4 nM) receptor binding site. Epidermal growth factor also is a potent inhibitor of acid secretion (1). No effects on heart rate, blood pressure, respiration, or body temperature have been found.

Enhanced healing of experimental ulcers or prevention of ulcer formation has been reported in rats and guinea pigs (10). There is some evidence that this effect is not due simply to inhibition of acid secretion. EGF induces increased activity of ornithine decarboxylase in the epidermis (22). This enzyme is important in the biosynthesis of polyamines that are associated with tissue growth. Similar stimulatory activity of EGF was found in the stomach, duodenum, small intestine, and colon of mice but not in the heart (8). EGF has been identified as the probable active agent in serum that causes the expression of fibrillar large external transformation-sensitive protein at the surface of cells in tissue culture (2). These effects suggest that urogastrone could contribute to the endogenous regulation of epithelial cell growth.

Distribution

Cells that contain immunoreactive urogastrone have been identified in the human duodenum in Brunner's glands and in the human submandibular gland (7,15). Low concentrations of immunoreactive urogastrone/ EGF were found in extracts of human pancreas, duodenum, jejunum, kidney, submandibular gland, and thyroid but not in a variety of other gastrointestinal and nongastrointestinal tissues when examined by radioimmunoassay after affinity chromatographic concentration (17). Concentrations in these tissues ranged from 1 to 5 ng/g tissue, and the immunoreactive material coeluted with the peptide found in urine. It is difficult to relate these relatively low concentrations in tissues with the high concentrations of urogastrone found in human urine.

Measurement

Measurement of urogastrone in human urine, plasma, and other body fluids has been possible by use of radioimmunoassay with antibodies raised against the pure peptide (6,12). Cross-reactivity with mouse EGF was less than 0.1% in one assay (12) and not reported in the other (6). Cross-reactivity with other peptides could not be demonstrated in either assay.

Concentration in Human Body Fluids

Daily urinary excretion of urogastrone was similar in normal men and women and slightly higher in women when expressed in terms of body weight or daily urinary creatinine excretion (6,10). No consistent changes have been found during the menstrual cycle, in peptic ulcer patients, or in patients with skin diseases or Cushing's disease. No diurnal rhythm or change after meals has been found. Women taking oral contraceptives excreted about 50% more immunoreactive peptide than control female subjects.

Radioimmunoassay of unextracted serum in a sensitive assay that recognizes predominantly a large molecular form of urogastrone yielded average circulating concentrations of about 500 pg ml^{-1} (12). Circulating contrations of urogastrone that were estimated to inhibit acid secretion in humans based on exogenous doses and a measured half-life of about 1.5 min in dogs were about 100 to 150 pg ml^{-1}. However, the acid-inhibiting potency of the large circulating form of human urogastrone has not been determined. In another radioimmunoassay performed after affinity chromatographic concentration of plasma, the major form recovered was a smaller molecule that coeluted with human urogastrone/EGF (16). Mean plasma concentrations were 163 pg ml^{-1} in normal men, 139 pg ml^{-1} in normal women, and 121 pg ml^{-1} in pregnant women. No changes in plasma concentrations could be measured after meals and there was no circadian rhythm. The urinary clearance of urogastrone/ EGF was similar to that of creatinine.

It is not possible at the present time to assign a physiological or pathophysiological role to urogastrone. The most potent known effect of circulating urogastrone is inhibition of acid secretion, but there are no data showing negative correlations between plasma concentrations and acid secretion rates in humans. Since urogastrone also has effects on epithelial cell proliferation and is found in gastric and salivary secretions and breast milk, it is possible that it acts locally in the region of glandular epithelium or topically on epithelial cells.

References

1. Bower, J. M. (1975): The inhibition of gastric acid secretion by epidermal growth factor. *Separatum Experientia,* 31:825–826.

2. Chen, L. B. (1977): Control of a cell surface major glycoprotein by epidermal growth factor. *Science,* 197:776–778.
3. Cohen, S., and Carpenter, G. (1975): Human epidermal growth factor: Isolation and chemical and biological properties. *Proc. Natl. Acad. Sci. USA,* 72:1317–1321.
4. Cohen, S., and Savage, R. C., Jr. (1974): Part II. Recent studies on the chemistry and biology of epidermal growth factor. *Recent Prog. Horm. Res.,* 30:551–574.
5. Cohen, S., and Taylor, J. M. (1974): Part I. Epidermal growth factor: Chemical and biological characterization. *Recent Prog. Horm. Res.,* 30:533–550.
6. Dailey, G. E., Kraus, J. W., and Orth, D. N. (1978): Homologous radioimmunoassay for human epidermal growth factor (urogastrone). *J. Clin. Endocrinol. Metab.,* 46:929–936.
7. Elder, J. B., Williams, G., Lacey, E., and Gregory, H. (1978): Cellular localisation of human urogastrone/epidermal growth factor. *Nature,* 271:466–467.
8. Feldman, E. J., Aures, D., and Grossman, M. I. (1978): Epidermal growth factor stimulates ornithine decarboxylase activity in the digestive tract of mouse (40357). *Proc. Soc. Exp. Biol. Med.,* 159:400–402.
9. Gregory, H. (1975): Isolation and structure of urogastrone and its relationship to epidermal growth factor. *Nature,* 257: 325–327.
10. Gregory, H., Bower, J. M., and Willshire, I. R. (1978): Urogastrone and epidermal growth factor. In: *Growth Factors,* 11th FEBS Meeting, edited by K. W. Kastrup and J. H. Nielsen, pp. 75–84. Pergamon Press, Oxford.
11. Gregory, H., Holmes, J. E., and Willshire, I. R. (1975): Urogastrone—Epidermal growth factor. In: *Methods of Hormone Radioimmunoassay, Ed. 2,* edited by B. M. Jaffe and H. R. Behrman, pp. 927–939. Academic Press, New York.
12. Gregory, H., Holmes, J. E., and Willshire, I. R. (1977): Urogastrone levels in the urine of normal adult humans. *J. Clin. Endocrinol. Metab.,* 45:668–672.
13. Gregory, H., and Preston, B. M. (1977): The primary structure of human urogastrone. *Int. J. Peptide Protein Res.,* 9:107–118.
14. Gregory, H., Walsh, S., and Hopkins, C. R. (1979): The identification of urogastrone in serum, saliva, and gastric juice. *Gastroenterology,* 77:313–318.
15. Heitz, Ph. U., Kasper, M., Van Noorden, S., Polak, J. M., Gregory, H., and Pearse, A. G. E. (1978): Immunohistochemical localisation of urogastrone to human duodenal and submandibular glands. *Gut,* 19:408–413.
16. Hirata, Y., Moore, G. W., Bertagna, C., and Orth, D. N. (1980): Plasma concentrations of immunoreactive human epidermal growth factor (urogastrone) in man. *J. Clin. Endocrinol. Metab. (in press).*
17. Hirata, Y., and Orth, D. N. (1979): Epidermal growth factor (urogastrone) in human tissues. *J. Clin. Endocrinol. Metab.,* 48: 667–672.
18. Hirata, Y., and Orth, D. N. (1979): Epidermal growth factor (urogastrone) in human fluids: size heterogeneity. *J. Clin. Endocrinol. Metab.,* 48:673–679.
19. Hirata, Y., and Orth, D. N. (1979): Conversion of high molecular weight human epidermal growth factor (hEGF)/urogastrone (UG) to small molecular weight hEGF/UG by mouse EGF-associated arginine esterase. *J. Clin. Endocrinol. Metab.,* 49:481–483.
20. Hollenberg, M. D., and Gregory, H. (1976): Human urogastrone and mouse epidermal growth factor share a common receptor site in cultured human fibroblasts. *Life Sci.,* 20:267–274.
21. Starkey, R. H., and Orth, D. N. (1977): Radioimmunoassay of human epidermal growth factor (urogastrone). *J. Clin. Endocrinol. Metab.,* 45:1144–1153.
22. Stastny, M., and Cohen, S. (1970): Epidermal growth factor. IV. The induction of ornithine decarboxylase. *Biochim. Biophys. Acta,* 204:578–589.

CHYMODENIN

Chymodenin is the name applied to a peptide that has been purified and partially characterized from porcine intestinal mucosa (1). Originally it was identified as a factor that liberated enzymes from isolated pancreatic zymogen granules *in vitro* and later as a substance that caused selective secretion of chymotrypsin without stimulation of lipase secretion from the rabbit pancreas *in vitro* and *in vivo*.

Purified chymodenin contains 74 to 76 amino acids and has a molecular weight of approximately 9,000. It contains four cysteine residues and two disulfide bridges, one immediately adjacent to the amino terminal pyroglutamyl residue. A partial sequence analysis of 13 residues revealed a pentapeptide sequence identical to a sequence near the amino terminal region of GIP. The carboxyl terminal amino acid is isoleucine.

A radioimmunoassay has been developed that exhibits a slight cross-reactivity with GIP and insulin. It has not yet been possible to demonstrate chymodenin immunoreactivity conclusively in rat serum. No data have been reported on the concentration and distribution of extractable chymodenin-like immunoreactivity in tissues or on cellular localization.

Further studies are necessary before any conclusions can be reached about a possible role for this peptide in digestive function.

Reference

1. Adelson, J. W., Nelbach, M. E., Chang, R., Glaser, C. B., and Yates, G. B. (1980): Chymodenin: Between "factor" and "hormone." In: *Comprehensive Endocrinology, Vol. 20, Gastrointestinal Hormones,* edited by G. B. Jerzy Glass, pp. 387–396. Raven Press, New York.

THYROTROPIN RELEASING HORMONE

Thyrotropin releasing hormone (TRH) was originally isolated from the hypothalamus by Schally and co-workers as the tripeptide amide pyroGlu-His-Pro-NH$_2$ and was shown to cause release of pituitary thyrotropin. TRH also releases prolactin from the pituitary, and there are reports that it can release FSH, norepinephrine, and growth hormone under some conditions. TRH is widely distributed in neurons and nerve terminals in the brain and spinal cord and has multiple central effects (1). These include excitatory actions, antagonism of sedative drugs, increased synthesis and release of norepinephrine, antagonism of morphine effects and possible modulation of some of the symptoms of morphine withdrawal, and rhythmic changes in concentration in the pineal gland and retina. Peripheral or central administration of TRH produces tachycardia, increased blood pressure, tachypnea, urinary urgency, and increased body temperature.

Immunoreactive and bioactive TRH-like material has been identified in gut extracts and shown to coelute with synthetic TRH in a number of chromatographic systems.

Concentrations are relatively low, 1 to 3 ng/g, with highest amounts found in the pancreas and specifically in the islets. TRH stimulates glucagon release from the isolated rat pancreas and contracts several gastrointestinal smooth muscles *in vitro*. It has been found to inhibit pancreatic polypeptide release. TRH appears to have minimal effects on gastrointestinal secretion when given intravenously but stimulates gastic acid secretion when given intraventricularly (2). The possible function of this peptide in the gut remains to be determined.

References

1. Morley, J. E., (1979): Extrahypothalamic thyrotropin releasing hormone (TRH)—Its distribution and its functions. *Life Sci.*, 25: 1539-1550.
2. Taché, Y., Vale, W., and Brown, M. (1980): Thyrotropin-releasing hormone: central nervous system action to stimulate gastric acid secretion. *Nature*, 287:149-151.

ENTEROOXYNTIN

There is considerable evidence that the presence of food in the intestine augments gastric acid secretion, especially acid secretion stimulated by gastrin from vagally denervated gastric pouches. Recently a peptide was identified in partially purified form that had weak stimulatory action when given alone but significantly enhanced maximal Heidenhain pouch acid responses to pentagastrin in cats (1). This material was contained in porcine intestinal extracts in fractions that did not contain other known gastrointestinal peptides. The pepsin response to pentagastrin also was enhanced by this material.

Reference

1. Vagne, M., and Mutt, V. (1980): Entero-oxyntin: A stimulant of gastric acid secretion extracted from porcine intestine. *Scand. J. Gastroenterol.*, 15:17-22.

Physiology of the Gastrointestinal Tract, edited by
Leonard R. Johnson. Raven Press, New York © 1981.

Chapter 4

Proliferation and Differentiation of Gastrointestinal Cells in Normal and Disease States

Martin Lipkin

The awareness that cells renew rapidly in the gastrointestinal tract has initiated research into many aspects of cell development and function. Important questions that have been considered revolve around processes that initiate and terminate the proliferative cell cycle, and that lead to increased differentiation and functional specialization of the cells; what are the controls governing the maximum number of cells in the mucosa at a specific time and place, which cells normally are responsive to the need for renewal and activation of the renewal process, and how do the mechanisms malfunction during the development of disease states?

HISTORICAL BACKGROUND

Bizzozero (24,25) in the late nineteenth century observed areas of increased mitotic activity in the crypts of the small intestine and gastric pits which he called "regeneration zones." According to his concept regeneration started in the crypts, the cells migrated to the villi and differentiated into columnar and goblet types.

Bensley (21) further reported that mitotic gastric cells moved toward the surface, replacing cells in that location. They also migrated downward, taking the place of chief or mucous cells. Friedman (102) continued this type of analysis using radiation techniques; he noticed how irradiated swollen goblet cells traveled from crypt to villus. Leblond and co-workers (19,168,169), utilizing ³²P, and Quastler (254,255) and others (93–95,139,223, 286), working with tritiated thymidine (³HTdR) carried out the earliest analyses of cell renewal and migration from which were developed the kinetics of proliferation of isotopically labeled cells (255).

With time, cells were considered to have differing degrees of proliferative activity (113), e.g., nondividing neurons were termed "static"; muscle, adrenal medulla, thyroid follicle, liver and kidney cells were termed "expanding"; adult ovary cells were termed "decaying"; and gastrointestinal epithelia, bone marrow, and skin were referred to as "renewing."

Dividing transit cells were those undergoing in-process cell differentiation and division. Simple transit cells maintained a steady population kinetics. Mature cells did not redivide. However, in the early classifications it was recognized that tumor cells and those in tissue culture often divided without reference to the presence of other developing cell populations (15,113,182).

Further observations of major importance to the analysis of cell proliferation described the cell cycle as composed of a series of specific phases. By 1925 Wright (328) had used numerical analysis to estimate mitotic phase duration in chick embryo cells (328). Hoffman's parameters (136) dealt with the rate of cell growth, doubling, and turnover time. The earlier considerations had been concerned with development of the cell and proceeded toward the mitotic process, the critical stage in its life span (36–38). Subsequently, DNA replication in a specific cell cycle phase was described by Howard and Pelc (138), and investigators began to stress the DNA synthetic phase of the cell cycle as well as events prior and subsequent to replication of chromosomes.

Of considerable importance, also, were the studies of molecular events that paralleled these findings: the characterization of DNA and its transmission of genetic information (9); separation of the structure and function of RNA from DNA (262), and of nucleic acids from protein (264); identification of nucleic acid precursor components and sequential steps leading to DNA and RNA synthesis (63,142,309); discovery of the structural components of DNA and RNA (251,311); *in vitro* preparation of polymers associated with DNA (160) and the early analyses of the genetic code (311). It is significant that the greatest utility of cell cycle analysis has been its ability to identify biochemical modifications in the cells in conjunction with events in the cell cycle. This combination of measurements has the greatest potential for elucidating major occurrences in both normally and abnormally functioning gastrointestinal cells.

CELL TYPES AND THEIR LOCATION IN REGIONS OF THE GASTROINTESTINAL TRACT

Esophagus

The epithelium of the esophagus is squamous and, therefore, unlike that in the lower regions of the gastrointestinal tract. The proliferating cells, situated in the basal layer beneath the surface of the mucous membrane, are covered with migrating and nondividing cells. These move toward the lumen and eventually are extruded from the mucosal surface. Human and other mammalian species have cells in this basal layer that are columnar, with ovoid nuclei. Adjacent cells are larger and the nuclei more spherical. Transitional cells are of intermediate type between the two varieties. The surface cells are squamous with flattened nuclei, sometimes degenerated. The deep basal layer alone has cells exhibiting mitotic activity.

Esophageal epithelium is squamous and stratified, penetrated at irregular intervals by the papillae of the lamina propria (205). Mucous glands that resemble cardiac glands of the stomach are found at the cricoid cartilage near the esophageal junction beneath the epithelium. Basal layer cells when labeled with ³HTdR have been shown to proliferate by microautoradiography. All basal layer cells in the rat can be labeled and presumed to proliferate. Like normal stomach cells (187), those synthesizing DNA are seen randomly among the basal layer of esophageal cells (44). Such cells parallel the proliferative crypt cells of the lower intestine, and cells migrating randomly originate from the basal epithelial layer.

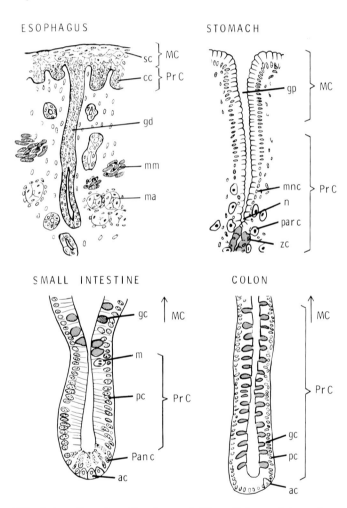

FIG. 1. Location of proliferating and differentiating cell types in esophagus, stomach, and small and large intestine. In all diagrams, MC is area where mature well-differentiated and nonproliferative cells are normally found; PrC, proliferative cell area. Diagram of esophagus shows mucosa containing proliferating and mature cells and glandular duct extending into submucosa. sc, squamous cells; cc, cuboidal cells; gd, glandular duct; mm, muscularis mucosae; ma, mucinous acini. Diagram of stomach shows surface epithelium and a gastric pit extending into deeper portion of glandular area; gp, glandular pit; mnc, mucous neck cell; n, neck region; par c, parietal cell; zc, zymogen cell. In small intestine a complete crypt and lower portion of villus are shown; gc, goblet cell; m, principal cell in mitosis; pc, principal cell; Pan c, Paneth cell; ac, argentaffin cell. Colon diagram shows lower two-thirds of a colonic crypt. Same notations.

Figure 1 illustrates the location of the cell types, proliferative and nonproliferative, in various areas of the gastrointestinal tract. In mice, ^{3}HTdR labeling reveals a replacement rate of approximately 7 days. In the esophagus renewal rates in these cells in humans are slower (20). Since the esophagus is not an absorbing or secreting organ, the epithelial cells function mainly in a protective capacity.

Stomach

On the surface of the body and fundus of the stomach lie mucous-secreting cells, extending down into the gastric pits, beneath which are long glands within the gastric mucosa. These glands are lined by acid and intrinsic factor-secreting parietal cells and pepsinogen-secreting chief cells, which empty into the gastric mucosal pits. The second major type of mucosa is pyloric, located in the antrum of the stomach. Mucous-secreting cells also line the gastric pits, while the glandular cells underneath secrete an alkaline mucous containing pepsinogen. Both types of mucosae contain endocrine cells which secrete various hormones (119,148,216). Mucous neck cells are believed to act as stem cells for the endocrine cells (55, 208). Endocrine cells are intermingled with other mucous cells and are mainly in the midzone of the gastric glands. They synthesize, store, and secrete the various hormones (Table 1). These endocrine cells are believed to have originated from the neural crest, and to respond to autonomic, mechanical, and intraluminal stimuli by discharging their granules into the circulation. Although there appear to be at least 11 different endocrine cell types in the gastrointestinal mucosa, the primary cells in the gastric fundus are the A cell or enteroglucagon-secreting cell, the G-cell or gastrin cell, and the argentaffin cell which secretes serotonin and histamine.

The mucosa of the pyloric antrum has gastric pits deeper than in fundus, and is lined mainly with a cell type similar to the mucous neck cell. In this region also are the parietal acid secretory cell (293) and the G cell which secretes gastrin. The most concentrated G cell population is in the middle third of the antral mucosa.

During embryogenesis the glands first develop mucoid and then parietal and chief cells. In developing and adult stomachs, mucous-containing cells differentiate into the parietal and chief cell types. Transitional cells are also present with characteristics between mucous and other glandular types (294). More rapidly proliferating cells replace those at the gastric mucosal surface during migration and can be found in the isthmus region between the gastric pits and glands, as well as in the mucous neck region of the gastric pits (332). Labeling of these cells with ^{3}HTdR is easily observed after pulse injection; zymogen and parietal cells are replaced by mucous neck cells. In rodent and man parietal and zymogen cells renew more slowly (67,140) than mucous epithelial cells (187,256). Cell renewal in rodents also is more rapid than in humans, and cell renewal rates can vary in different regions of the stomach (169,195,201, 224,225). Parietal cells which appear to originate from undifferentiated stem cells in upper glands (52,256,321) may not undergo cell division, and it is unclear whether stem cells for the parietal cells are the same as the stem cells from which the epithelium originates. Division in chief cells occurs approximately once per month in mice (321). The parietal cells in mice have a 23-day half-life, whereas chief cells can appear 291 days after initial labeling with ^{3}HTdR.

Small Intestine

In the small intestine a single cell thickness epithelial layer lines the crypts and covers the villi (134). Cheng and Leblond (53–57) described small intestinal epithelial cell types as columnar, mucous, Paneth, and enteroendocrine. Columnar cells begin as immature proliferative cells. Starting at the base of the crypts, columnar cells migrate up to the villi, differentiating as they move to-

TABLE 1. *Cell types in regions of stomach*

Region of stomach	Cell type	Function or secretory product
Cardia	Surface mucous	Mucus
	Undifferentiated mucous	Cell renewal
Fundus	Surface mucous	Mucus
	Mucous neck	Cell renewal
	Parietal	HCl, intrinsic factor
	Zymogen or chief	Pepsinogen
	A cell	Enteroglucagon
	G cell	Gastrin
	Argentaffin	Serotonin, histamine, motilin (?)
	Argyrophil	Secretin (?)
Pylorus	Surface mucous	Mucus
	Parietal	HCl
	G Cell	Gastrin

From Deschner and Lipkin (80).

ward the bowel lumen (42,55). The time involved approximates 5 to 6 days (182,188,194,195,201,271) in most of the human small intestine and 3 in the ileum (195). In rodents the process takes 2 to 3 days (55,105, 106,169,225). These variations may result from a normal proximal-distal decrease in villous height (7) as opposed to differences in cell movement rate. Evidence indicates that basal columnar cells in the first four cell positions give rise to the other three types of epithelial cells (55,57).

The two kinds of mucous cells in the small intestine are the immature oligomucous, located in the crypts, and the mature goblet cells (53,223). The immature cells are found exclusively in the crypts while mature cells are located in both upper crypts and villi. These cells migrate along with the columnar cells to the tips of the villi, taking about 3 days in mice (53,170,171).

Paneth cells appear in the small intestinal crypts. Their function may be secretory (2,299). They probably do not divide (39,54,223,301) or migrate, but they eventually degenerate and are phagocytosed by cells at the base of the crypts (54,74). Renewal occurs in the order of weeks (58). The "intermediate"-type cells have features common to Paneth, undifferentiated precursor, and goblet cells and may be transitional between undifferentiated and mature secretory cells.

Enteroendocrine cells also move toward the villous tips, after originating from the crypt-base columnar type. Migration takes approximately 4 days. As the cells differentiate, the number of cytoplasmic granules increases, and the cells can no longer divide.

Large Intestine

The proliferative zone of the large intestine covers the basal three-quarters of the crypts. Cells migrate toward the gut lumen and are extruded from the mucosal surface between crypts. These large intestinal crypts are more closely spaced than either stomach or small intestine and the organ surface is flat.

The colonic epithelial cells, columnar, mucous, and enteroendocrine cells most likely originate in the crypt base (51). Migration takes from 3 to 8 days in man (64, 188,271) and 2 to 3 days in rodents (51,225). Argentaffin (enteroendocrine) cells of the human rectal mucosa undergo slow renewal in 35 to 100 days (77).

PROLIFERATION KINETICS OF NORMAL CELLS IN REGIONS OF THE GASTROINTESTINAL TRACT

Methods of Analysis

The rate of cell loss is equivalent to the rate of cell production in the normal adult gastrointestinal mucosa. Except for a few human investigations, the majority of

studies of proliferation kinetics are based on rodent cell populations. Villus growth is not due specifically to mitosis in the maturing cells, but rather to a rate of cell extrusion lower than the proliferative rate.

Analyses of cell proliferation have been carried out by pulse labeling of proliferating epithelial cells with ^{3}HTdR and detecting ^{3}HTdR-labeled mitoses (221,254, 255) as well as labeled cell distributions (14,41,182,278). Microautoradiography measures the fraction of mitoses labeled with ^{3}HTdR. During DNA synthesis (or S phase) radioactive thymidine is incorporated into DNA. Pulse labeling followed by analysis of the appearance of labeled mitoses indicates the durations of S and mitosis (M) phases, along with the interphase gaps G_1 and G_2 prior and subsequent to DNA synthesis.

Figure 2 illustrates the theoretical uniform distribution of cells in the proliferative cycle in a steady state. Unlabeled mitotic cells pass through G_2 (T_{G_2}) prior to the linear rise from 0 to 1 which signals the duration of mitosis (T_m). Then the distance between the rise and fall of the curve represents the transit time during S phase (T_s). Finally, the interval before the second rise shows the transit time through $G_1 + G_2(T_{G_1} + T_{G_2})$ before the second rise. Estimates of proliferation kinetic parameters throughout the cell cycle have been made because of this type of analysis and can be directly measured from corresponding points on successive curves of labeled mitoses.

In biological systems this theoretical curve (Fig. 2) becomes broadened and bell-shaped with variations indicating desynchronization of the cells and decline in size of the successive cycles that follow. The ascending limb gradually rises when there are variations in T_{G_2}. This may conceal the measurement of T_m. Waves blending into preceding and succeeding ones reflect the frequency distributions of times that have elapsed between the cells leaving S and entering mitosis and vice versa (254,255). After two or three proliferative cycles of gastrointestinal cells, total desynchronization is common. Variations in cell cycle duration are estimated from plotted frequency distributions of the points on the

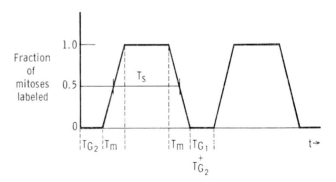

FIG. 2. Fraction of mitoses labeled after a pulse injection of tritiated thymidine, as a function of time, for an ideal steady-state population of identical cells moving uniformly through cell cycle. Symbols defined in text. From Lipkin (182).

curves (14,254), from the 0.5 points on the ascending and descending limbs (254), or within the curves themselves (14,254). Asymmetric labeled mitosis curves show variation in G_2 and S.

The concepts of age and phase distributions of cells after mitosis are important, and these are measured from the end of the previous mitosis. Age measurements are expressed in hours; phase measurements are a fraction of cell cycle duration. As shown in Fig. 3, when death or migration allows for an equivalency between cell loss and production, cells remain in a steady state; or the population may change, usually increasing as when tumors exist, or, ideally, during exponential expansion. In age or phase distribution diagrams (14,277, 278), estimation of the probability of locating cells within the cycle at a time after mitosis in a given age or phase is expressed as the ratio of cells in a particular phase to the total cell population.

Steady-state conditions allow for the number of cells in a given phase to be proportional to the phase duration. New proliferative and nonproliferative cells are produced equally. Ideal steady-state conditions imply $(N_m/N_c) = T_m/T_c$, N_m equalling number of cells undergoing mitosis and N_c, those proliferating, T_m mitotic duration and T_c cell cycle duration. (MI) is mitotic index (N_m/N_c), and (LI) or thymidine (^{3}HTdR) labeling index is (N_s/N_c), observed microautoradiographically with cells in S phase (N_s) and the number proliferative (N_c). An important relationship has been that $(N_s/N_c) = (T_m/T_c)$.

During steady-state conditions, the theoretical possibility of solving for the cell cycle duration (T_c) exists, since microscopic counts can be made for N_m (cells in mitosis), N_s (^{3}HTdR-labeled cells), and N_c (total cells in proliferative region of mucosa). Birth rate (K_b) then equals the mitotic index divided by the mitotic duration ($K_b = MI/T_m$), or the labeling index divided by S phase duration = (LI/T_s), and $K_b = 1/T_c$) the inverse of the cell cycle duration, with all cells proliferating.

Correction factors are often necessary in these estimations when nonproliferating cells are found with proliferating cells in parts of the jejunal and colonic crypts and for maturing cells which can no longer proliferate (278).

The double-label technique allows for estimations of S phase duration and is particularly useful when specimens are limited. The two isotopes first employed were ^{3}HTdR and ^{14}CTdR; then ^{3}HTdR in both weak and heavy dosages was used. S phase duration is estimated from ($H_w/H_h = T/T_s$) where H_w/H_h is the ratio of weak to heavily labeled cells, T being the interval between the pulses. Turnover time of the tissue can then be estimated: ($T = S/LI \times 100$), as carried out in studies of cell proliferation in ulcerative colitis and in familial polyposis (27,87). It is essential here to ensure that nuclei are sufficiently separated so that spread of grains in microautoradiographic preparations does not lead to incorrect measurements.

The stathmokinetic analysis also can be employed *in vivo*, in addition to isotopic techniques where radioactive isotopes localize within DNA in the nucleus. An alkaloid substance (colchicine or vincristine, for example) is given intravenously in the stathmokinetic method. Biopsies are taken several times before and after injection, as carried out for estimates of kinetic parameters in large bowel cancer. The alkaloid blocks the metaphase portion of mitosis which is necessary for the equal distribution of the chromosomes to the two daughter cells. The rate at which metaphases accumulate indicates both the durations of mitosis and the cell cycle (329).

Esophagus

Epithelial cell renewal in rodents occurs approximately every 4 to 5 days in the basal layer, and is slower in humans (20). The entire rodent epithelium renews every 7 to 8 days. Migration is random from basal to epithelial layer, daughter cells migrating separately or conjunctly. As in the rest of the gastrointestinal tract, cells in the esophagus alter their structure after proliferation as they migrate to their new environment. After cell division, two daughter cells may stay basal and re-divide, or one may remain in the basal layer while the other differentiates, or both may leave to differentiate.

Rodents have a 54-hr esophageal proliferative cell cycle with a life span of 80 hr (longer than in lower intestine), whereas in humans the esophageal cell span during migration may be 8 days. Jejunal crypt cells in man proliferate about 3 times more quickly, with the average basal layer cell generation approximately 6 days in the esophagus and 2 in the jejunum (20,187,215,271).

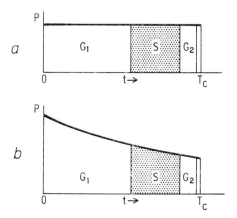

FIG. 3. Age distribution diagrams for ideal populations of cells: a, in steady state with one proliferative and one nonproliferative cell produced; and b, expanding with two proliferative cells produced at each division and no loss of cells. From Steel et al. (278).

Stomach

Gastric cell types renew at varying rates. In rodent and human, migrating mucous epithelial cells moving toward the gastric surface show proliferative parameters similar to those of epithelial cells in the colon and small intestine (182,215,271). Mucous epithelial cells of the stomach do not proliferate as readily as those in the small intestine, and gastric cell proliferation varies in general more than in the small intestine. There is a superimposed circadian rhythm (11,59,187).

Gastric cell migration velocities and cell cycle phase durations in humans are not unlike jejunal and colonic migration rates (20,187,215,271). Mucous epithelial cells proliferating in atrophic gastric mucosa exhibit a more rapid cell cycle than in normal gastric mucosa. The life span is faster and turnover more rapid (20,236). Extensive desynchronization of proliferating cells is in evidence resulting in near random distribution in the gastric mucosa, which in turn acts as a protective influence (187).

Parietal cells, which are replaced in 3 months in rodents (although some survived longer), had a longer replacement duration in humans, and this was similar for zymogen elements also. Parietal and zymogen cells originating from stem cells in the neck and isthmus slowly migrate deeper into the stomach glands (184,321). Cell renewal is slower than in superficial epithelium. In one study (322), peptic cells showed a labeling index suggesting self-renewal in mouse mucosa with the highly specialized parietal cells maintained by differentiation of immature cells.

Table 2 indicates renewal rates of mucosal epithelial cells of gastric mucosa in man using labeling and mitotic data. In the pyloric antrum new DNA synthesis is carried out by more cells than in the fundic mucosa. Analysis of the cardia indicates similar findings compared to the antrum (13.1 to 15.2%) (284). It takes 7 to 10 hr for S phase duration in mucous epithelium of the fundus measured in *in vitro* and *in vivo* methods. The proliferative cell cycle time for gastric mucous epithelial cells is 2 to 3 days, and mucosal replacement takes 4 to 6 days (195,201). The question of variations in diurnal cell renewal was addressed in rodent, canine, and human gastric mucosa. Only in rodents was a circadian rhythm evident (60).

Small Intestine

In the rat the proliferative region contains a crypt length of 36 cell positions (41) with mitotic figures in the low 30s, and a nondividing zone in the upper region where cells leave the proliferative cycle. The cell cycle takes approximately 10 hr, S phase 6.5 hr, G_1 2 hr, and G_2 and M each 1 hr. Proliferating cells incorporated ^{3}HTdR in the crypts and then migrated to the villi.

An area of total cell proliferation was defined from the observation of labeling index which was 60%, similar to the observation of T_s/T_c of 6.5/10; findings were based on the concept of DNA synthesis followed by mitosis and with all cells proliferating. The crypt as a whole showed a 35% labeling index, and the difference between 60% and 35% indicated the nongrowing fraction of cells; values here were comparable for mouse and rat. Rodent cells undergo about 2.2 divisions in the crypt, a 10-hr cycle, and 20 hr migration with about a 1.2 cell positions per hour velocity. It took 4 hr in mice for cells to travel through the maturation compartment to the villi, judging from time of ^{3}HTdR injection to

TABLE 2. *Summary of kinetic parameters in the gastric mucosa of man*

Organ	LI%	MI%	T_{G_2} (hr)	T_S (hr)	T_{G_1} (hr)	T_M (hr)	T_C (hr)	References
Gastric mucosa								
Normal								
Cardia	13.1	1.3						284
Fundus	4.2–14	0.8–1.0	2–4	7.1–10	62		48–72	20,29,49,195,284
Antrum	12.8–15.2	1.4						123,284
Diseased								
Atrophic gastritis								
Fundus	14–19		1–6	16			>30	123,326
Antrum	12.9	2.9						123,175
Gastric cancer								
Cardia	20.1	2.1						284
Fundus	13.4							123,137,284
Antrum	16.2							123,284
Zollinger-Ellison syndrome	15.7	0.8	1	6.7	36		45	49

From Deschner and Lipkin (80).

appearance on villi; 20 to 30 hr is the villus transit time in rodents.

At the bottom of the crypts, daughter cells divide and then redivide, whereas throughout the crypts cell division appears to be asymmetric with only one daughter cell dividing; at the top of the crypts a nondividing cell zone is present. Overall, a steady-state condition is evident; cells in the upper half of the crypts leave the proliferative cell cycle rapidly as DNA synthesis and mitosis fall to zero and normal maturation occurs.

Although labeling and mitotic indices indicate that cell proliferation is most rapid in the small intestine, cell cycle times vary among the various cell types, and even within the same cell type. For example, labeled epithelial cells may remain weeks after injection, which is an indication of a prolonged G_1 phase. A slow renewal rate has been shown for Paneth and argentaffin cells extending to several days. Table 3 shows examples of cell cycle durations in the small intestine.

Large Intestine

The generation time of epithelial cells of mice was 16 hr, DNA synthesis 6.5 hr, G_2 and mitosis 1.5 hr, and G_1 8 hr (.193). Rapid proliferation of some cells in combination with already mature cells took place in the middle one-third of the colonic crypts; in contrast, in jejunum the separation between the proliferative region and nonproliferative was more distinct. Slower division of ^{3}HTdR-labeled epithelial cells, which then stayed in the mucosa longer than jejunum, was observed in the colon of humans and rodents (153,192,193). Diurnal variation was slight in mice and guinea pigs, the latter having a 24-hr generation time for epithelial cells in the colon with velocity greater at the crypt mouth, 0.7 to 0.8 cell widths per hr (261).

The lower three-fourths of human crypt columns contained the ^{3}HTdR-labeled proliferating cells in biopsies, with approximately 15 to 20% of all cells undergoing DNA synthesis. In the upper crypt, less cell proliferation was evident as more cells differentiated, and cells nearing the surface of the colonic crypts ceased proliferative activity (76,78,81,88,188–190,192,271). Slower re-entry of sigmoid colon cells into the cell cycle occurred, compared to cells in other areas, and faster recycling of cells occurred in the jejunum (190). Table 4 gives examples of cell cycle phase durations in rodent and human cells of the large intestine.

PROLIFERATION KINETICS OF GASTROINTESTINAL CELLS IN DISEASE

Esophagus

In patients with reflux esophagitis, organ-cultured biopsies showed more ^{3}HTdR incorporation than in normal patients (196). Observations here further confirmed earlier findings of more frequent appearance of mitotic figures in the basal zone of biopsies of specimens from patients, compared to controls, possibly contributing to a thickened basal layer in the former (145,146).

In a study without controls, cell turnover appeared increased in esophageal biopsies of patients with Barrett's epithelium or columnar-lined esophagus (132). In 3 of 4 patients, labeled cells appeared at the characteristic villus-like base. In this disease, the actual zone of epithelial cell proliferation is not established; however, ^{3}HTdR incorporation occurs in the basal layer similar to normal gastric and small bowel epithelium. Labeled villous and surface cells in noncancerous areas of esophageal tissue were observed in a patient who had multiple foci of carcinoma in situ. Proliferative activity in normal nonproliferating zones near the crypt surface has been observed in histologically normal colonic mucosa adjacent to polyps (28,65,81), hyperplastic mucosa adjacent to rectal carcinoma (179), and atrophic intestinalized gastric mucosa adjacent to gastric carcinoma (326). Thus information concerning Barrett's epithelium also appears to confirm the disease as a premalignant lesion (232).

TABLE 3. *Summary of kinetic parameters in mucosa of small intestine of man*

Organ	LI%	MI%	T_{G_2} (hr)	T_S (hr)	T_{G_1} (hr)	T_M (hr)	T_C (hr)	References
	Small intestine							
Normal								
Duodenum		2.36				1.1	48–54	22,329
Jejunum		1.5				1.1	42–48	20,271,329,330
Diseased								
Duodenum-jejunum		5.1				1.3–1.5	21–22	329
Sprue		5.2						330
Ileum conduit			1–2	11	22	1	24–36	75

From Deschner and Lipkin (80).

TABLE 4. *Summary of kinetic parameters in mucosa of large intestine of man*

Organ	LI%	MI%	T_{G_2} (hr)	T_S (hr)	T_{G_1} (hr)	T_M (hr)	T_C (hr)	Turnover time	References
Normal									
Colon									
in vivo	12–18		1–6	11–20	14	1	40	72–96	188,195
Rectum									
in vivo	18–25		2	9–14			24–48	96–192	64,195,201
in vitro	1–17			7–11			77–130	58–87	28,45,108,274
									26,27,272
Diseased									
Ulcerative colitis									
Active ulcerative colitis	26			9.2				34	27
Remission	7								
Adenomas									81
Rectum									
in vitro	23			7.4–12				32	28
in vitro	2			15				>40	191
Carcinomas									
in vivo	13–23	1.1–2.9		14				26–244	45,137,289
in vitro	4–32	0.3–2.8		19				30–177	26,179

From Deschner and Lipkin (80).

Stomach

Gastric stress erosion as a result of 12-hr restraint and fasting in mice decreased mitoses and ³HTdR-labeled cells (143,156,187). Gastric epithelial cell mitosis was also significantly depressed in mice who were given aspirin orally, although duodenal, jejunal, and colonic mitosis appeared normal (320). The two kinds of mucosal lesions caused by aspirin (331) involved superficial healing in 24 hr and did not extend to the proliferative zones; those entering deep into the zone of proliferative activity and increasing the ³HTdR labeling of cells in adjacent mucosal regions reached their peak 16 to 48 hr after ingestion and healed within 10 days. There was greater migration and proliferation of gastric cells with gastric atrophy in pernicious anemia (20) when cells were labeled with ³HTdR *in vivo*.

In cases of gastritis, G_1 phase appears to be shortest in the atrophic type and longest in the superficial type (48). When *in vitro* radioisotopes were used for labeling, nucleic acid and protein synthesis was shown to be abnormal in atrophic gastritis (82). In normal mucosae, labeling studies showed RNA, protein, and DNA syntheses most active in proliferative areas at the base of the gastric pits. When mild gastritis was present these activities increased in gastric surface cells of histologically normal mucosa. The same was apparent in atrophic gastritis and intestinalized gastric mucosa (82,326), supporting the likelihood that these were precancerous lesions.

In Zollinger-Ellison (ZE) syndrome, chronic gastritis, and pernicious anemia, epithelial cell proliferative activity increases despite a steady state. Double-labeling measurements have shown that ZE patients had a reduction of cell cycle duration (49) of mucous epithelial cells in fundic mucosa, with increased ³HTdR labeling index and decreased G_1 phase. The zone of cell proliferation also expanded. It is likely that parietal cells undergo self-proliferation leading to hyperplasia (235).

Biopsies of fundic mucosa from ZE patients showed an increase in labeled cells when analyzed *in vitro* with ³HTdR. The zone of proliferative activity and number of labeled cells expanded within the gastric pits (49). The cell cycle duration decreased in the ZE gastric biopsies because of a G_1 phase shortening; S, G_2, and M phases remained normal.

In atrophic gastritis, more mitotic activity occurs in intestinal metaplastic glands than in normal gastric pits (175). The mitotic index doubles (1 to 2.3%) and the labeling index increases (123), together with the appearance of small intestinal cells in the stomach. With gastric ulcers increased mitotic activity and labeling indices occur, together with changes in ploidy, suggesting an association with premalignancy. Serum gastrin levels rise in many cases of pernicious anemia (158) as in many forms of chronic gastritis, and simultaneously enhanced gastric cell proliferation occurs. Although (159) this holds true in atrophic gastritis, parietal and peptic cell renewal in rats has been shown to be inhibited by parietal cell and intrinsic factor antibodies in pernicious anemia and chronic gastritis (159,198).

The degree of metaplasia and histological type of cancer in gastric mucosa are generally associated with more differentiated carcinoma occurring with greater metaplasia; poorly differentiated adenocarcinoma occurs with less metaplasia (229). Metaplasia accompanies or precedes adenocarcinoma in 90% of gastric specimens studied. A higher degree of intestinal metaplasia is present in the gastric mucosa of the patient with cancer than with gastric ulcer, which implies that the metaplastic condition is precancerous (229,240,280).

Studies of DNA, RNA, and protein syntheses in biopsies from atrophic gastritis patients (82) revealed that as cells migrated through the gastric pits, cells failed to repress DNA synthesis shown by thymidine incorporation, in contrast to normals. An increase of RNA and protein syntheses occurred in these cells as they demonstrated a metabolic profile of immature cells.

As atrophy increased with immature cuboidal cells replacing surface cells, the pattern continued with increased DNA, RNA, and protein syntheses in the upper region of the gastric pits. With severe intestinal metaplasia two patterns were observed: firstly, increased DNA, RNA, and protein syntheses in the surface region of gastric pits with major activity in the upper two-thirds of the glands, and secondly, the mucosa histologically and biochemically similar to normal small intestinal mucosa (82). Where gastric tissue became highly differentiated into normal appearing small bowel mucosa, the appearance suggested that carcinogens could be absorbed and presumably the cancer risk become greater.

Using *in vitro* autoradiographic techniques, instillation of ethanol into the dog stomach (324) reduced the gastric pit height within 4 hr; within 8 to 20 hr ^{3}HTdR-labeled cells increased; mitotic activity increased between 20 to 24 hr and led to the restoration of normal mucosa. Administration of ethanol to humans was correlated with the DNA content of epithelia shed into gastric washings (69). This method is limited; since the types of cells and their origins are not defined, other cells may contribute DNA, and gastric washing can cause desquamation. More DNA was present in gastric washings after acute ethanol consumption (161), but patients who consumed ethanol regularly did not show the same changes.

Studies in animals and humans have given the impression that either stimulation or decrease of epithelial cell renewal in the stomach can result from mucosal injury of different types. Initial decrease can be followed by compensatory stimulation, and the development of ulceration has been associated with persistent depression of proliferation.

Included in Table 2 is available information on the mitotic and labeling indices of mucous epithelial cells in gastric neoplasms. Malignant nuclei in gastric mucosa are larger than normal, and their size is more variable. The DNA content of gastric cells in normal tissue is less than 10% in the 3N to 4N range, whereas malignant cells show only 30 to 40% of nuclei having 2N or normal diploid DNA according to spectrophotometric measurements (118,236,319).

Small Intestine

Rapid epithelial cell renewal was shown in celiac disease by intracellular DNA loss that exceeded loss in control patients and those on a gluten-free diet. Another study employing organ cultures confirmed the previous findings. The epithelial cell renewal cycle was estimated at one-half of normal duration (68,298,329). Structurally, cells, crypts, and villi can become markedly altered. An increased incidence of carcinomas and lymphomas appears when gluten enteropathy is present. The proliferation rate can triple with proliferation throughout the entire crypt. There may be a loss of villi, enlarged crypts, and an immature mucosal cell lining (8,298). The cell cycle time may decrease to less than 1 day.

In celiac disease, cell loss judged by DNA accumulation was 3 times higher and cell migration 3 times faster than normal (68,298). The celiac crypt can develop 4 times the usual number of cells (330), widening and lengthening (from 780 to 3,050). In these patients a smaller percent of cells renew (0.5 and 0.6%) than in controls (0.8 to 0.7%); however, greater numbers of cells synthesize DNA (e.g., 1,525 to 1,830 as opposed to a normal count of 546 to 624). It takes 22 to 39 hr for epithelial cells to renew in sprue compared to the normal 54 to 58 hr (329). Findings in tropical sprue have not been analyzed completely, but mitotic indices were greater than normal when mild lesions were present, and not when they were severe or atrophic (283).

Therapeutic abdominal irradiation reduces crypt mitosis 25 to 50% (297), shortens villi, and initiates megaloblastosis and megalocytosis of the epithelial cells. Mitotic counts lasted 3 days, and villus structure required 2 weeks to become normal. Proliferation decreased after 1 day of 290 rads in rats, and returned to normal for 4 days afterward despite continued radiation (258). The number of villous cells decreased by the second day, and the proliferative zone expanded in the crypts. One day after cessation of irradiation proliferation increased and villous cell number and expanded proliferation zones became normal. Proliferation varied according to the phase of the renewal cycle of cells when irradiation was given (122). S phase cells resisted treatment more readily than cells in G_2 phase, and the latter were more resistant than G_1, indicating irradiation sensitivity proportional to the number of cells in each phase.

Methotrexate illustrates the effect of one class of chemotherapeutic agents, depressing the mitotic index after injection into patients in 3 hr and nearly eliminating mitosis in 6 to 48 hr. By 96 hr mitotic counts were back to normal (295). Fragmented mitochondria, dilated Golgi and endoplasmic reticulum, and clumped nucleochromatin were visible under the electron microscope (204,295,296). DNA synthesis inhibition is a major effect of methotrexate.

In the case of duodenal ulcer, a single study implied that decreased cell proliferation was associated with causation. A study of *in vitro* biopsies from 5 cases of duodenal ulcer demonstrated less ³HTdR incorporation and less mitosis than in controls, and therefore decreased proliferative activity can be a contributing factor to actual ulceration (334), as occurred in the stomach of rodents under stress (144,156).

In infants in marasmus, the intestinal mucosa becomes thin and mitotic counts decrease even more profoundly than in kwashiorkor (33). Biopsies from adults with untreated pernicious anemia indicated short villi, epithelial cells that were megaloblastic and megalocytic, and a nearly 50% reduction in mitosis (100). Vitamin B₁₂ therapy for 2 weeks increased mitotic counts to normal and 2 months later the structural alterations also returned to normal. Chronic alcoholics with folate deficiency showed similar findings and responses to therapy; in two subjects histologic abnormalities appeared when folate deficiency occurred (133).

Chronic ingestion of ethanol for several weeks has been studied in the rat (13). Crypt and villus cell number decreased in the jejunum, and villi shortened; however, ileal crypts showed increased numbers of cells ³HTdR incorporation, mitosis, and thymidine kinase activity. Villi were of normal size and increased proliferative activity in crypts may have been a response to injury induced by the alcohol.

Several infectious disorders are associated with increased cell proliferation. Rats with *Salmonella typhimurium* and pigs with Nebraska transmissible gastroenteritis virus showed increased proliferation and migration of cells (290,335). Humans with viral gastroenteritis have not been studied, but acute nonbacterial enteritis (Norwalk agent) revealed villous shortening, crypt hypertrophy, and increased mitosis, which could have resulted from increased proliferative activity or mitotic arrest (265). *Strongyloides* infection increased DNA loss into the duodenum; however, patients with hookworm showed no change in DNA loss (70).

Chronically uremic mice showed a lengthened S phase of the proliferative cell cycle (50). Chronic renal failure in mice resulted in a lengthened DNA synthesis phase, mitosis, and a generally longer cell proliferation cycle (212,213). Thus cell proliferation was inhibited, and this was associated with the development of uremic lesions, erosions, and bleeding.

Large Intestine

Studies have now shown that increased proliferation of colonic epithelium occurs prior to development of polyps and malignant tumors. Migrating cells move from the proliferative area toward the mucosal surface, meanwhile undergoing modifications in nucleic acid enzyme activities which differ from those associated with the repression of DNA synthesis normally occurring in mature epithelial cells (143,300). Surface epithelial cells of adenomas and carcinomas show nucleic acid metabolic enzyme patterns characteristic of young proliferative cells (248,300). The proliferative zone in familial polyposis included upper crypt and mucosal surface thymidine labeling (76), also characteristic of colorectal carcinomas where peripheral tumor nodules and mucosa adjacent to tumor showed more labeling in upper crypts near the surface (179). This has been found in normal-appearing mucosa as well (28,65,81), in frequencies similar to those in undifferentiated proliferating cells in the lower crypts. ³HTdR has also been discovered in high frequency in upper crypt regions in rectal mucosa of relatives of familial polyposis patients (79).

The movement of proliferating cells outside the normal proliferative zone into the upper crypt and surface epithelium has been termed "phase 1" of a two-phase theoretical model. In the second abnormal growth phase, cells develop additional properties with the ability to be retained in the mucosa where they accumulate in adenomas and cancers (185,186). Measurements of proliferative rates in these neoplasms have varied. In a patient with limited life expectancy, who had familial polyposis, the labeling index was only 2% (191) in seemingly normal mucosa and adenomas with very slow cell renewal. *In vitro* experiments, however (28), showed 22.3% as opposed to 10.4% labeling of adenoma compared to flat mucosa.

Using double labeling, familial polyposis patients (28) showed normal S phase in adenoma epithelium but a difference of 47 hr between normal mucosa (slower rate of proliferation) and benign adenomatous polyps. These limited analyses (28,191) indicate a need for additional data to evaluate the full range of turnover measurements in the mucosa of normal subjects and during the development of neoplasms. In hyperplastic polyps, the normal pattern of mucosal labeling and mitosis (in lower two-thirds of crypts) are found; such measurements are not indicative of structural changes associated with colonic cancer (164).

Metabolic and histological findings do not always agree in mucosa that is adjacent to polyps. Epithelial cells along the upper portion and surfaces (81) of colonic crypts have been observed to incorporate DNA-labeled precursors (Fig. 4), which indicates a defect in the mechanism regulating DNA synthesis with a failure to terminate DNA synthesis in proliferating cells. Polyp growth, in addition, indicates an imbalance of cell birth and extrusion within the colonic crypts. Cells accumulate on the epithelial surface and adenomas develop (76, 79,81).

DNA synthesis at the surface and upper crypt wall is present not only in patients with adenomas and polyposis but also in their asymptomatic progeny (79,81) and to a lesser extent in normals, and now has been shown to be a marker for high-risk colon cancer-prone populations (185) (Fig. 4).

Colon cancer appears linked to early and continued cell damage and ulceration. *In vitro* labeling has shown a doubling of S phase cells (27,87) in cases of colitis along with an epithelial cell proliferation zone also expanding to the luminal surface of the colonic crypts, and more rapid epithelial cell migration to the upper crypts. Patients with ulcerative colitis had a rapidly renewing colonic mucosa (34 hr compared to 90 in controls) with a constant S phase. Decreased T_c resulted from a G_1 cell cycle phase reduction or from more renewing cells or both. During early colitis, changes in colonic fibroblasts could contribute to the abnormalities in epithelial cells, with defective mesenchymal cells or anoxic environment and depletion of collagen fibers (83,155).

The precancerous nature of ulcerative colitis has been studied using rectal biopsies *in vitro* (27,87). Increased proliferation and faster migration were accompanied by an upward expanded proliferation zone, and these changes are similar to those observed in colonic adenomas. Thus the progression to "phase 1 proliferative lesion" and then a "phase 2" type of lesion occurs in ulcerative colitis.

Irradiation produced cuboidal epithelial cells (110), diminished mitosis, tissue eosinophilia, and eosinophilic crypt abscesses. Normal rectal mucosa regrew a month after treatment. The drug 5-fluorouracil (98,227) affected the mucosa similarly with decreased mitosis (98, 194,227).

In one study of colonic carcinoma, a 6-day sampling of ³HTdR-labeled cell populations in a rectal carcinoma showed a generation time of 26 hr, a labeling index 23.1% higher than usual, and an S phase of 14 hr. This enabled the growth fraction to be estimated, with 43% of tumor cells part of the proliferative pool as a fraction of replacement cells. In a colonic tumor (189) the S phase duration was 12 hr, but the total cell cycle duration was not measurable since the G_1 phase was very variable. This variability limits the utility of cell cycle-specific chemotherapeutic agents.

In Table 4, the range of variability is high because of either *in vitro* technique or the heterogeneous structure of the tumor. For example, one study revealed varying mitotic indices in different parts of the same tumor, and another showed growth fractions varying among proliferative cells in a group of tumors from 20 to 70% (45, 277,289). The stathmokinetic analysis indicated that mitotic durations vary between colonic carcinoma cells and normal cells (45) with values of 2.3 hr for 19 tumors and 1.2 hr for controls when cell cycle durations were

estimated between 159 and 244 hr. In another instance T_c of 26 hr was reported (289). A potential doubling time of 45 days for a rectal carcinoma was computed by Terz et al. (289) using this approach. The problem in this approach has been the discrepancy between the theoretical prediction and direct measurements of the growth of the tumor (314). In one instance, a growth fraction of 50% was noted (289), whereas another study pointed to increased tumor growth rate with small size and slower growth with increased size (163,289).

An additional factor relating to doubling time is the cell loss rate estimated from the equation: $\Phi = 1 - (t/d)$. In Terz's colonic carcinoma, a 39 to 49% cell loss and a 51 to 64% retention of cells were estimated (289). In slowly expanding adenomas, one-quarter of the cells were retained and three-quarters were extruded (191). There appears to be greater cell loss as tumors expand (103) with cell cycle time remaining fairly stable.

REGULATORY CONTROL OF PROLIFERATION AND DIFFERENTIATION OF GASTROINTESTINAL CELLS IN NORMAL AND ABNORMAL STATES

Both intra- and extracellular factors must be considered in normal cell proliferation, migration, and differentiation. During their normal life cycle gastrointestinal cells move through a proliferative phase into cell differentiation and maturation. Studies with *in vivo* and *in vitro* systems on intestinal cells, hepatocytes, lymphocytes, and uterine epithelium have shown common growth characteristics, as well as similar proliferative abnormalities during the transitional states leading to disease. Both extracellular and intracellular environments can further modify gastrointestinal epithelial cell renewal and maturation and regulatory control of the cell cycle phases.

Factors Contributing to Initiation of Cell Proliferation

In earlier work, both hormones (166) and resection (200) of a portion of the intestinal mucosa were noted to induce new cell renewal. Similar findings resulted from inhibition of cholinergic neural activity (183,273). Earlier investigations also indicated a reduction in cell proliferation, and maturation occurred with restraint-stress or inhibition of adrenergic neural activity (156). Additional factors implicated in cell proliferation included serum proteins and enzymes (34,35,90,180,181, 237,241), hormones (47,59,91,128,148,157,166,197, 199,302,303,333), antigens and antibodies (117,266–269), viruses (287,288), and ischemia.

The cellular production of RNA and protein (152) which may result from intra- and extracellular stimu-

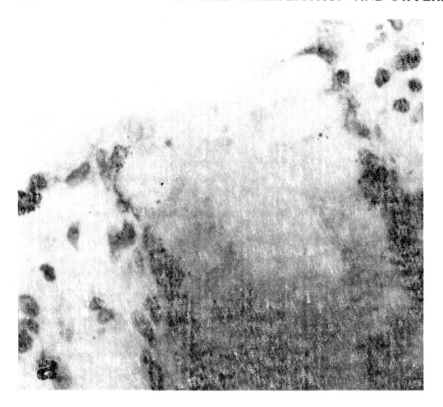

FIG. 4a. [3]HTdR incorporation into surface epithelial cells of flat colonic mucosa near a single villous adenoma.

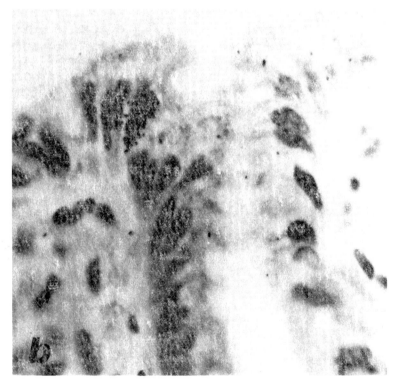

FIG. 4b. [3]HTdR incorporation into surface epithelial cells of flat colonic mucosa of a patient with familial polyposis.

lation contributes to new DNA synthesis. Between the stimulation and the onset of DNA synthesis, ultrastructural changes occur and RNA and protein syntheses increase. Cytoplasmic ribosomes also increase during this lag phase in the liver, uterus, and lymphocytes, implying production of new ribosomal RNA and protein (18,34, 35,107,116,129,230,282); in the intestine, RNA and protein syntheses are greater in proliferating cells (78) than in resting cells. These syntheses must continue for proliferation to take place. Cycloheximide blocks protein synthesis and decreases intestinal cell proliferation (16).

It is likely that additional factors also contribute to the initiation of cell proliferation. Cyclic nucleotides in-

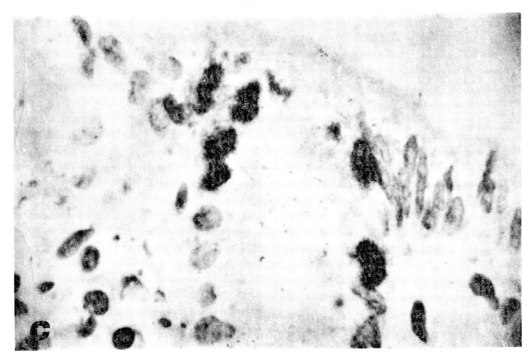

FIG. 4c. Early net retention and accumulation of thymidine-labeled cells in an individual with familial polyposis.

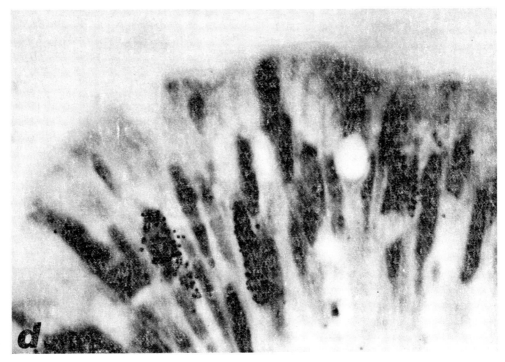

FIG. 4d. Example of ³HTdR incorporation into epithelial cells of an expanding adenomatous polyp, after injection of tritiated thymidine into a subject with familial polyposis and advanced neoplastic disease. From Lipkin (185).

duce modifications in association with increases or reductions of proliferative activity: cyclic AMP generally has been associated with inhibition of epidermal and other cell proliferation (84,252,310), and cyclic GMP has been implicated in proliferation in lymphocytes and other cells (121,317). Small amounts of both cyclic nucleotides can modify proliferation, and modulations among cyclic AMP, GMP, and calcium ions may influence responses of lymphocytes to stimuli inducing proliferation (211,317).

Cyclic nucleotide messenger systems contribute to the phosphorylation of proteins associated with chromosomes (165). These proteins are involved in the expression of portions of the genome, as well as other characteristics of DNA. Nonhistone or acidic chromosomal proteins have been implicated in gene activation and events related to cell proliferation and differentiation (17,270,279).

In the various cell types, a portion of the DNA becomes a template for RNA synthesis, with each cell type transcribing its own region of DNA; control mechanisms determine which genes will be involved in RNA synthesis. Limited regions of DNA are transcribed and repressors function to block transmission of information in neighboring regions of DNA. Specific chromosomal proteins act to recognize nucleotide sequences in DNA that modify template specificity during RNA synthesis by RNA polymerase. Histones, for example, are involved in the recognition of general features of DNA, whereas nonhistones act on gene activation and more closely on proliferative activity (17,270,279).

Cessation of Cell Proliferation

During migration of the gastrointestinal epithelial cells, differentiation continues while new molecular species are synthesized and new structures are developed which are associated with the cessation of DNA synthesis. Nucleic acid precursor enzymes and their templates become modified with changes in stability and life span during important stages of differentiation (144). During the initiation of DNA synthesis and its cessation, complex modifications in metabolic activity occur (12,42,62,92,260).

Precursor nucleic acid enzymes are required at each step in the formation of DNA, and activities of certain of these enzymes increase as proliferative activity begins to take place in intestine, liver, and salivary glands (16, 30,35,180). Thymidine kinase and thymidylate synthetase are examples of nucleic acid precursor enzymes that increase or decrease with proliferative activity of the cells in the resting phase (143,247,300). Inhibition of DNA synthesis with migration of gastric cells was suggested to result from a protein or another differentiation-specific substance (249). Feedback inhibition of overproduction of the four deoxyribonucleotides has also been noted with control of TMP kinase activity believed to be associated with cessation of proliferative activity (31,147,260).

Thus modifications in precursor nucleic acid enzyme activities, variability of enzyme and template stabilities during important stages of cell differentiation, and feedback control of reactions in intermediary metabolism associated with stages of cell differentiation all appear to have a role in regulating the cessation of DNA synthesis in the mid-life of the cell cycle of gastrointestinal cells. Further modifications involved in normal differentiation and maturation of these cells include interaction in the cell membranes with extracellular growth stimuli through specific receptor sites and release of macromolecules modifying gene activation in the nucleus. With further cell differentiation, receptor elements would also change leading to the activation of new genetic material. The implication is that of continued modification of the cells influencing the activation of new genes needed for the next stage of differentiation as influenced by extracellular stimuli.

G_2 and Mitosis Phases

The important events that occur during G_2 and mitotic phases of the cell cycle (36–38,209,210) are still not completely defined. Initiation of mitosis in cultured kidney cells involves the synthesis of RNA and protein during most of the G_2 phase (285). Mitosis also stopped in intestinal crypts within 2 to 3 hr after injecting cycloheximide into rats to inhibit protein synthesis. Cells were affected in late G_1 but not in mitosis (308). Experiments on liver have implicated several proteins produced during G_2 that influence passage of cells into and through mitosis (220).

In both rodent and human gastrointestinal cells, G_2 phase ranges from 30 min to a few hours. During G_2 new metabolic activities are developed bringing the cell into mitosis after DNA synthesis. It has been assumed that cells passed rapidly from G_2 to mitosis, but it now appears cells may remain in G_2 phase for a longer period; experiments on ear epidermis (111,112) and osteogenic tissue (242) reveal cells in G_2 phase for several days. A study in starved chicks involved duodenal and esophageal epithelia, which rapidly and slowly proliferated, respectively. Findings demonstrated that feeding led to mitosis in duodenal cells after DNA synthesis. However, a few esophageal epithelial cells divided immediately after feeding indicating they had been resting in G_2 (43). Tritiated thymidine studies in humans (194) as well as in other species (192,193) have shown colonic epithelial cells to be in resting phases for days after DNA synthesis. Epithelial cells remain in the colon for a longer period than in the small intestine where orderly recycling of cells is more rapid. The recycling of proliferative cells and movement of the cells through the G_2 phase are less orderly in stomach and colon, where most human neoplasms develop (190,192).

Studies of molecular events during mitosis have suggested that cells are programmed to synthesize terminal proteins allowing for the transition from interphase into prophase when the biosynthetic capacity of the cells decreases (292). In the transition from mitosis to G_1, it is unclear whether synthetic activity during interphase preprograms the cells for the completion of mitosis and entrance into G_1 or whether proteins contributing to the movement of cells into G_1 originate during mitosis (292). RNA and protein syntheses decrease during mitosis (253), resulting from lack of DNA in condensed chromosomes available to RNA polymerase or from unavailability of RNA to ribosomes (152).

Dependence of Cell Differentiation on DNA Synthesis

Proliferation of gastrointestinal epithelial cells occurs prior to cell differentiation. Normally before differentiation of gastric progenitor cells into parietal and zymogen cells, DNA synthesis takes place (183,256). However, the transition of the cells through the mucosa is associated with a reprogramming of the cells as they move toward the mucosal surface. Cell migration and differentiation involve changes within the cells essential for the next stages of the cell cycle and differentiation. There is a decrease in important constituents of the cells active in nucleic acid metabolism and necessary for DNA synthesis (e.g., thymidine kinase and thymidylate synthetase.

Proliferation occurs prior to differentiation in other cell systems as well such as embryonic tissues or mammary glands (203,303). Embryonic kidney mesenchyme did not differentiate when DNA synthesis was inhibited, and in adult tissues during hematopoiesis DNA synthesis precedes differentiation (61,62,97). DNA, and then differentiation products myosin and actin are all synthesized in separate muscle cells. Xylem differentiation takes place similarly in plants (101,281).

Therefore, in numerous organ systems DNA synthesis occurs before cell differentiation (120,135,167) leading to a mutually exclusive relationship between proliferation and differentiation. However, some overlap can exist. Pancreatic cells in mitosis have some zymogen, plasma cells may develop antibody before proliferation comes to an end, and collagen and DNA synthesis are found in cell cultures (73,202,316).

Normally this relationship in the intestine is similar to that in other organs, and as protein and other syntheses occur, proliferation slows down or comes to a halt (99,245). In diseased states associated with premalignancy, as noted above, epithelial cells develop morphologic structures similar to those of well-differentiated cells, yet continue to synthesize DNA and enter into mitosis (65,76,78,81,300).

Differentiation and Development of New Metabolic Activities

Regulatory control of cell differentiation and maturation takes place in several stages. These include (a) the transcription of DNA into RNA influenced by the chromosomal proteins; (b) the translation of RNA into protein; and (c) post-transcriptional events involving enzymatic and related steps.

Differentiating gastrointestinal cells have shown variations in the synthesis and degradation of nucleic acid precursor enzymes and templates. For example, adenosine deaminase was quickly synthesized and degraded in differentiating cells after cycloheximide and actinomycin D. This implied that genetic material producing the enzyme was continually used, and that rapid control of the enzyme level occurred during cell differentiation. Purine nucleoside phosphorylase had greater stability (144), whereas thymidine kinase showed a brief half-life. Metabolic pathways are altered rapidly during critical stages of cell differentiation, with differences in rate of replacement of enzymes and templates.

Thus new patterns of enzyme activity develop in an orderly manner during cell differentiation. During migration and differentiation of intestinal epithelium, disaccharide activity increases and alkaline phosphatase isoenzymes are modified (71,228) together with alterations in purine, pyrimidine, and nucleic acid intermediary metabolism.

As cell proliferation ceases, thymidine kinase activity also declines. The enzyme thymidine kinase has a short half-life and is associated with rapid proliferation (62); it acts as a catalyst in the phosphorylation of thymidine to its monophosphate derivative, and is subsequently converted to the triphosphate precursor of DNA. As DNA synthesis ceases and cell differentiation and migration take place, there are other rapid changes in enzymatic activities (143). Numerous synthetic, energy-yielding reactions develop which also include the reutilization of substances from the intestinal lumen. These follow an orderly sequential process as normal cell differentiation proceeds (16).

Influence of Extracellular Factors

In animals raised in a germ-free environment, "physiological inflammation" occurs when bacteria colonize the intestine, leading to higher rates of proliferation and migration of mucous epithelial cells (1,66).

In the fundic mucosa of dogs, although not in human antral or fundic mucosa (124,325), food stimulated cell proliferation. Starved mice had decreased DNA synthesis and diminished proliferation and migration of intestinal cells (32). Starved rats also showed decreased proliferative activity as well as prolongation of the cell renewal cycle (3,6). Refeeding led to reversal of these findings.

Contributing to the interpretation of these findings are recent experiments using intravenous alimentation. In rats, mucosal weight and thickness, protein and DNA content, as well as disaccharidase activity were lower than in orally fed animals (130,149,172). Changes occurred only during the first 3 days of alimentation, whereas continued decreases occurred in starved animals. Proximal intestine was affected more than distal both structurally and functionally, similar to intravenously fed rabbits where proliferative activity decreased (86,130,172).

After Thiry-Vella loops are formed from segments of small intestine without fecal matter passing through, mucosa also becomes hypoplastic and cell renewal decreases, indicating a direct correlation between intraluminal contents and epithelial cell renewal. However, hormonal effects may occur here, since rats with intragastric feeding had less mucosal cell hypoplasia than intravenously fed rats, implying possible hormonal or vascular influences (85,115).

Starvation in rats produced decreased levels of antral and serum gastrin; with a high-bulk, non-nutritive diet this effect continued (177). Although intravenous feeding decreased the antral gastrin levels (149), intravenous pentagastrin equal to half the D_{50} for acid secretion maintained gastrointestinal tissue weight and disaccharidase activity (149,151,177).

The trophic action of gastrin on gastrointestinal tissue has been under study. ZE syndrome is often present in conjunction with gastric mucosal cell hyperplasia, involving the parietal cell mass (250). However, within a year post-antrectomy for duodenal ulcer, atrophic gastritis and a thinner parietal cell region can be observed, possibly related to postoperative serum gastin levels (114,217,218). Similarly in rats after antrectomy parietal cells were decreased but pentagastrin appeared to stimulate parietal cell growth (46). Pentagastrin also was associated with increased proliferation of rat gastric and duodenal epithelial cells *in vitro,* as well as human gastric epithelial cells, DNA synthesis in fundus of stomach, duodenum, and ileum of rat, and increased rat gastric parietal cells (150,178,226,275). On the other hand, secretin can inhibit DNA synthesis and parietal cell production (150,275). The stimulatory effect of gastrin on parietal cell growth appears to develop through DNA synthesis in the progenitor cells of the proliferative region of mouse fundus, increasing the maturation of progenitor cells into parietal cells (322,323). However, gastrin had no effect on mouse chief cells nor pentagastrin on rat antral or esophageal mucosa (151,174, 322). Thus trophic effects of gastrin are believed to be tissue and cell specific.

Further stimulation of epithelial cell proliferation occurs during lactation (40,187) and under the influence of growth hormone (166) and thyroxine; however, hydrocortisone inhibited cell proliferation in rodent gastric and duodenal epithelium, believed to be associated with decreased healing of ulcers (10,162,231). Small amounts of serotonin increased crypt cell renewal but decreased proliferative activity when administered in large doses (305). In addition, α-adrenergic stimulation using norepinephrine and β blockade by propranolol both stimulate cell renewal, and β-adrenergic stimulation with epinephrine or isoproterenol and α blockade by phentolamine work conversely. Surgical sympathec-

tomy and chemical sympathectomy with 6-hydroxydopamine likewise inhibit cell renewal (307).

Increased mitosis followed electrical stimulation of the neurovascular bundle innervating an exteriorized loop of rat jejunum; chemical sympathectomy was ineffectual here, implying that proliferative activity was further influenced by nonadrenergic nerves (306).

The vagus may have a trophic effect in the stomach (174,259). Sectioning the vagus before stimulation inhibits hyperplasia of mucous neck, parietal, and chief cells induced by the anterior hypothalamus (246); however, numbers of parietal cells were the same in postvagotomy patients.

Additional studies on cyclic AMP, which prevents DNA synthesis and proliferation in nonintestinal cells (89,104), have shown a similar effect in colonic mucosa (4); its presumed relationship to calcium in the inhibition of DNA synthesis is not clear in intestinal cells (318). Vitamin D increases cell renewal in the intestine of rachitic rat intestine (23) and may not be associated with calcium transport.

Resection of a portion of the bowel has been used to study regulatory control (176,214,234,238), and is a strong stimulus to epithelial cell renewal (125,126). Resection of the small intestine of rats increases mucosal thickness with expanded villi and deeper crypts, and stimulates pyrimidine biosynthetic enzymes with increased proliferation (127,239). Colonic (238) and gastric (327) epithelial cells also proliferate more rapidly after small bowel resection.

Factors affecting the mechanics of the compensatory response to resection are now known to include the following:

1. Oral food intake contributes to the hyperplasia of intestinal cells. After ileal resection feeding rats spontaneously ate more and exhibited expanded villi and deeper crypts than controls (173,222). Intravenous feeding of jejunectomized dogs for 6 weeks led to reduced villous height compared to that in orally fed dogs (96), and similar results were found in rats.

2. Secretions of the upper bowel may affect compensatory responses to resection as well as maintain normal intestinal mass. Enlarged villi in the ileal mucosa of rats occurred as a result of transplanting duodenal papillae to the ileum. Pancreatic secretions also were associated with greater responses when diverted to an ileal segment (5). The combination of jejunectomy and duodenal papillary transplant into an ileal segment increased mucosal weight as well as protein and DNA content in ileum more than either perturbation alone (131).

3. The amount of excised tissue influences the intestinal compensatory response. Other local and humoral stimuli may be associated with this.

4. Humoral stimulus has been implicated in parabiotic rats, for nonresected parabiotic mates of resected rats exhibited hyperplasia.

5. The fact that more compensatory characteristics

show up in the distal segment when transplanted proximally than is the opposite (315) may have resulted primarily from food ingestion or bowel secretions which contact the distal segment. Mucosal thickness, protein and DNA content, and disaccharidase activity normally decrease from upper jejunum to distal ileum (172). When ileum is transposed to jejunum, villi enlarge, but when jejunal segments are attached to ileum, the transposed villi decrease in size (7).

Additional factors that are likely to assume a more important role in the regulation of epithelial cell renewal in the future include the possible association of intestinal epithelium with mesenchymal tissue (153,154,219, 244). Epithelial cytoplasmic processes have been noted to contact underlying mesenchymal cells in rat duodenum during fetal and early postnatal development (207). The importance of mesenchyme during growth of fetal intestinal epithelium was suggested, since deprivation of cultured or grafted rabbit gastric epithelium of mesenchyme results in impaired development (72).

In normal adult mucosal crypts of large and small bowel, a surrounding sheath of fibroblasts proliferates and appears to migrate to the upper crypts in a manner analogous to epithelial cell migration (206,243,244). Additional study of human colonic adenomas has suggested that neoplastic colonic lesions may be associated with changes in the pericryptal fibroblast sheath (304). Fully differentiated fibroblastic sheaths are apposed to the epithelium in hyperplastic polyps, whereas fibroblasts underlying adenomatous epithelium resemble the adjacent epithelium in these true neoplasms (155,164). Villous cells may also act to influence feedback regulation of crypt cell proliferation. For example, rats recovering from irradiation manifested increased proliferation of crypt cells and fewer villous cells (109,258), whereas germ-free rats recovering from irradiation had slower proliferation with villi having more epithelial cells than normal. Further confirmation of this has been observed by clamping the superior mesenteric artery and vein for 1 hr (257), which led to a reduction of the villous cell population, whereas crypt cells were not affected. When ^{3}HTdR labeling was used, villous cell reduction paralleled the crypt cell increase, and proliferative activity expanded. Thus the decreased villous cell population appeared to stimulate crypt cell proliferation.

Extracts of mucosa, some fractions of which have been termed chalones, also are believed to inhibit mitosis and are considered to contribute to regulation of cell proliferation (37). It has been suggested that stimulating factors may release chalones which could act in negative feedback. In these studies gastric mucosa of chicks inhibited mitosis in cultured chick epithelium; it did not, however, appear to influence developing intestine, skin, or mesenchyme (249). Crypt cell proliferation in small bowel also was inhibited by extracts from rat

small intestinal crypts (304), although neither colonic crypts, esophagus, nor skin was affected.

CONCLUSION

We are beginning to see the application of the preceding findings to several areas of analysis of normal and abnormal gastrointestinal cell function. Cell kinetic measurements have contributed to an improved understanding of the various disease states described. Analyses of the cell cycle have identified biochemical and physiological abnormalities affecting cell development and function, and have provided the beginnings of a basis for understanding malfunctions of cell growth in disease.

Current approaches are continuing to elucidate intracellular abnormalities during the stages of cell proliferation and differentiation in disease states. In recent years studies of extracellular contributions to cell growth and metabolism also have expanded. Of further interest are recent applications of cell kinetic measurements to the identification of individuals at increased risk for gastrointestinal cancer. The modifications in cell proliferation and maturation observed in gastrointestinal epithelial cells of man resemble those that develop in rodents following administration of chemical carcinogens. Quantitations of the abnormalities in cell proliferation and differentiation that develop are underway to improve the surveillance of subjects at increased risk for gastrointestinal cancer. The findings are also being used as a basis for attempts to inhibit the early development of neoplasia.

REFERENCES

1. Abrams, G. D., Bauer, H., and Sprinz, H. (1963): Influence of the normal flora on mucosal morphology and cellular renewal in the ileum. A comparison of germ-free and conventional mice. *Lab. Invest.,* 12:355–364.
2. Ahonen, A. (1973): Histochemical and electron microscopic observations on the development, neural control and function of the Paneth cells of the mouse. *Acta Physiol. Scand. [Suppl.],* 398.
3. Aldewachi, H. S., Wright, N. A., Appleton, D. R., et al. (1975): The effect of starvation and re-feeding on cell population kinetics in the rat small bowel mucosa. *J. Anat.,* 119:105–121.
4. Alpers, D. H., and Philpott, G. W. (1975): Control of deoxyribonucleic acid synthesis in normal rabbit colonic mucosa. *Gastroenterology,* 69:951–959.
5. Altmann, G. G. (1971): Influence of bile and pancreatic secretions on the size of the intestinal villi in the rat. *Am. J. Anat.,* 132:167–178.
6. Altmann, G. G. (1972): Influence of starvation and refeeding on mucosal size and epithelial renewal in the rat small intestine. *Am. J. Anat.,* 133:391–400.
7. Altmann, G. G., and Leblond, C. P. (1970): Factors influencing villus size in the small intestine of adult rats as revealed by transposition of intestinal segments. *Am. J. Anat.,* 127:15–36.
8. Anderson, K. E., Finlayson, N. D. C., and Deschner, E. E. (1974): Intractable malabsorption with a flat jejunal mucosa and selective IgA deficiency: A case report with immunological and autoradiographic studies. *Gastroenterology,* 67:709–716.

9. Avery, O. T. C., MacLeod, M., and McCarty, M. (1944): Studies on the chemical nature of the substance inducing transformation of pneumococcal types. Induction of transformation by a deoxyribonucleic acid fraction isolated from pneumococcus type III. *Exp. Med.*, 79:137–158.

10. Avetisyan, A. A. (1973): Effect of hydrocortisone on the mitotic cycle in mucus-forming cells of the gastric fundus epithelium. *Bull. Eksp. Biol. Med.*, 76:101–103.

11. Baker, B. L., and Clark, R. H. (1961): Influence of hypophysectomy on oxidative enzymes and size of parietal cells in gastric mucosa. *Proc. Soc. Exp. Biol. Med.*, 106:65–67.

12. Balis, M. E. (1968): Antagonists and nucleic acids. In: *Frontiers of Biology, Vol. 10*, edited by A. Neuberger and E. L. Tatum, p. 293. North Holland, Amsterdam.

13. Baraona, E., Pirola, R. C., and Lieber, C. S. (1974): Small intestinal damage and changes in cell population produced by ethanol ingestion in the rat. *Gastroenterology*, 66:226–234.

14. Barrett, J. A. (1966): A mathematical model of the mitotic cycle and its application to the interpretation of percentage labeled mitoses data. *J. Natl. Cancer Inst.*, 37:443–450.

15. Baserga, R. (1965): The relationship of the cell cycle to tumor growth and control of cell division: A review. *Cancer Res.*, 25:581–595.

16. Baserga, R. (1968): Biochemistry of the cell cycle: A review. *Cell Tissue Kinet.*, 1:167–191.

17. Baserga, R., and Stein, G. (1971): Nuclear acidic proteins and cell proliferation. *Fed. Proc.*, 30:1752–1759.

18. Becker, F. F., and Lane, B. P. (1966): Regeneration of the mammalian liver. IV. Evidence on the role of cytoplasmic alterations in preparation for mitosis. *Am. J. Pathol.*, 49:227–237.

19. Belanger, L. F., and Leblond, C. P. (1946): A method for locating radioactive elements in tissues by covering histological sections with photographic emulsion. *Endocrinology*, 39:8–13.

20. Bell, B., Almy, T. P., and Lipkin, M. (1967): Cell proliferation kinetics in the gastrointestinal tract of man. III. Cell renewal in esophagus, stomach, and jejunum of a patient with treated pernicious anemia. *J. Natl. Cancer Inst.*, 38:615–623.

21. Bensley, R. R. (1898): The structure of the mammalian gastric glands. *Q. J. Microsc. Sci.*, 41:361–389.

22. Bertalanffy, F. D., and Nagy, K. P. (1961): Mitotic activity and renewal of the epithelial cells of human duodenum. *Acta Anat. (Basel)*, 45:362–370.

23. Birge, S. J., and Alpers, D. H. (1973): Stimulation of intestinal mucosal proliferation by vitamin D. *Gastroenterology*, 64:977–982.

24. Bizzozero, G. (1888): Ueber die regeneration der elemente der schlauchformigen drusen und des epithels des magendarm kanals. *Anat. Anz.*, 3:781.

25. Bizzozero, G. (1889): Ueber die schlauchformigen drusen des magendarmkanals und die berziehungen inhres epithel zu dem onerflachenepthel der schleimhaut. *Arch. Mikrosk. Anat.*, 33:216–246.

26. Bleiberg, H., and Galand, P. (1976): *In vitro* autoradiographic determination of cell kinetic parameters in adenocarcinomas and adjacent healthy mucosa of the human colon and rectum. *Cancer Res.*, 36:325–328.

27. Bleiberg, H., Mainguet, P., Galand, P., Chreteen, J., and Dupont-Mairesse, N. (1970): Cell renewal in the human rectum: *In vitro* autoradiographic study on active ulcerative colitis. *Gastroenterology*, 58:851–855.

28. Bleiberg, H., Mainguet, P., and Galand, P. (1972): Cell renewal in familial polyposis. Comparison between polyps and adjacent healthy mucosa. *Gastroenterology*, 63:240–245.

29. Bleiberg, H., Mainguet, P., and Vandenhende, J. (1971): Mesure autoradiographic—que de la proliferation cellulaire a differente niveaux du tractus digestif normal et pathologique: Utilisation de biopsies incubees *in vitro*. *Rev. Eur. Etud. Clin. Biol.*, 16:233–239.

30. Bresnick, E. (1965): Early changes in pyrimidine biosynthesis after partial hepatectomy. *J. Biol. Chem.*, 240:2550–2556.

31. Bresnick, E., Thompson, U. B., Morris, H. P., and Liebelt, A. G. (1964): Inhibition of thymidine kinase activity in liver and hepatomas by TTP and dCTP. *Biochem. Biophys. Res. Commun.*, 16:278–284.

32. Brown, H. O., Levine, M. L., and Lipkin, M. (1963): Inhibition of intestinal epithelial cell renewal and migration induced by starvation. *Am. J. Physiol.*, 205:868–872.

33. Brunser, O., Reid, A., Monckeberg, F., et al. (1966): Jejunal biopsies in infant malnutrition: With special reference to mitotic index. *Pediatrics*, 38:605–612.

34. Bucher, N. L. (1963): Regeneration of mammalian liver. *Int. Rev. Cytol.*, 15:245–300.

35. Bucher, N. L. (1967): Experimental aspects of hepatic regeneration. *N. Engl. J. Med.*, 277:686–696, 738–746.

36. Bullough, W. S. (1952): The energy relations of mitotic activity. *Biol. Rev.*, 27:133–168.

37. Bullough, W. S. (1962): The control of mitotic activity in adult mammalian tissues. *Biol. Rev.*, 37:307–342.

38. Bullough, W. S. (1965): Mitotic and functional homeostasis: a speculative review. *Cancer Res.*, 25:1683–1727.

39. Cairnie, A. B. (1970): Renewal of goblet and Paneth cells in the small intestine. *Cell Tissue Kinet.*, 3:35–45.

40. Cairnie, A. B., and Bentley, R. (1967): Cell proliferation studies in intestinal epithelium of the rat: hyperplasia during lactation. *Exp. Cell Res.*, 46:428–440.

41. Cairnie, A. B., Lamerton, L. F., and Steel, G. G. (1965): Cell proliferation studies in the intestinal epithelium of the rat. I. Determination of the kinetic parameters. *Exp. Cell Res.*, 39:528–538.

42. Cameron, I. L. (1972): Cell proliferation and renewal in aging mice. *J. Gerontol.*, 27:162–172.

43. Cameron, I. L., and Clefmann, G. (1964): Initiation of mitosis in relation to the cell cycle following feeding of starved chickens. *J. Cell Biol.*, 21:169–174.

44. Cameron, I. L., Gosslee, D. G., and Pilgrim, C. (1965): The spatial distribution of dividing and DNA-synthesizing cells in mouse epithelium. *J. Cell. Comp. Physiol.*, 66:431–435.

45. Camplejohn, R. S., Bone, G., and Sherne, W. (1973): Cell proliferation in rectal mucosa. A stathmokinetic study. *Eur. J. Cancer*, 9:577–581.

46. Capoferro, R., and Nygaard, K. (1973): Effects of antrectomy on the gastric mucosa of the rat. *Scand. J. Gastroenterol.*, 8:347–352.

47. Carriere, R. M. (1966): The influence of thyroid and testicular hormones on the epithelium of crypts of Lieberkuhn in the rat's intestine. *Anat. Rec.*, 156:523–531.

48. Castrup, H. J., and Fuchs, K. (1974): Cell renewal in inflammatory changes of the gastric mucosa. *Dtsch. Med. Wochenschr.*, 99:892–895.

49. Castrup, H. J., Fuchs, K., and Peiper, H. J. (1975): Cell renewal of gastric mucosa in Zollinger-Ellison syndrome. *Acta Hepatogastroenterol. (Stuttg.)*, 22:40–43.

50. Castrup, H. J., Lohrs, U., and Eder, M. (1970): The origin of changes in the intestinal mucosa in uremia. *Klin. Wochenschr.*, 48:244–245.

51. Chang, W. W. L., and Leblond, C. P. (1971): Renewal of the epithelium in the descending colon of the mouse. I. Presence of three cell populations: vacuolated-columnar, mucous and argentaffin. *Am. J. Anat.*, 131:73–100.

52. Chen, K. Y., and Withers, H. R. (1975): Proliferative capability of parietal and zymogen cells. *J. Anat.*, 120:421–432.

53. Cheng, H. (1974): Origin, differentiation and renewal of the four main epithelial cell types in the mouse small intestine. II. Mucous cells. *Am. J. Anat.*, 141:481–502.

54. Cheng, H. (1974): Origin, differentiation and renewal of the four main epithelial cell types in the mouse small intestine. IV. Paneth cells. *Am. J. Anat.*, 141:521–536.

55. Cheng, H., and Leblond, C. P. (1974): Origin, differentiation and renewal of the four main epithelial cell types in the mouse small intestine. I. Columnar cells. *Am. J. Anat.*, 141:461–480.

56. Cheng, H., and Leblond, C. P. (1974): Origin, differentiation and renewal of the four main epithelial cell types in the mouse small intestine. III. Enteroendocrine cells. *Am. J. Anat.*, 141:503–520.

57. Cheng, H., and Leblond, C. P. (1974): Origin, differentiation and renewal of the four main epithelial cell types in the mouse small intestine. V. Unitarian theory of the origin of the four epithelial cell types. *Am. J. Anat.*, 141:537–562.

58. Cheng, H., Merzel, J., and Leblond, C. P. (1969): Renewal of Paneth cells in the small intestine of the mouse. *Am. J. Anat.,* 126:507–525.

59. Clark, R. H., and Baker, B. L. (1963): Effect of hypophysectomy on mitotic proliferation in gastric epithelium. *Am. J. Physiol.,* 204:1008–1022.

60. Clarke, R. M. (1970): A new method of measuring the rate of shedding of epithelial cells from the intestinal villus of the rat. *Gut,* 11:1015–1019.

61. Clarkson, B. D., Fried, J., Strife, A., Sakal, Y., Ota, K., Ohkita, T., and Masuda, R. (1970): Studies of cellular proliferation in human leukemia. IV. Behavior of normal hematopoietic cells in three adults with acute leukemia given continuous infusions of ³H-thymidine. *Cancer,* 26:1

62. Cleaver, J. E. (1967): Thymidine metabolism and cell kinetics. *Front. Biol.,* 6:43–69.

63. Cohn, W. E. (1949): A simplified procedure for the analytical extraction of lipids. *Science,* 109:377–378.

64. Cole, J. W., and McKalen, A. (1961): Observations of cell renewal in human rectal mucosa in vivo with thymidine-H³. *Gastroenterology,* 41:122–125.

65. Cole, J. W., and McKalen, A. (1963): Studies on the morphogenesis of adenomatous polyps in the human colon. *Cancer,* 16:998–1002.

66. Cook, R. H., and Bird, F. H. (1973): Duodenal villus area and epithelial cellular migration in conventional and germ-free chicks. *Poult. Sci.,* 52:2276–2280.

67. Crean, G. P. (1963): The endocrine system and the stomach. *Vitam. Horm.,* 21:215–280.

68. Croft, D. N., Loehry, C. A., and Creamer, B. (1968): Small-bowel cell-loss and weight-loss in the coeliac syndrome. *Lancet,* 2:68–70.

69. Croft, D. N., Pollock, D. J., and Coghill, N. F. (1966): Cell loss from human gastric mucosa measured by the estimation of deoxyribonucleic acid (DNA) in gastric washings. *Gut,* 7:333–343.

70. Da Costa, L. R. (1971): Small-intestinal cell turnover in patients with parasitic infections. *Br. Med. J.,* 3:281–283.

71. Dahlquist, A., and Nordstrom, C. (1966): The distribution of disaccharidase activities in the villi and crypts of the small intestinal mucosa. *Biochem. Biophys. Acta,* 113:624–626.

72. David, D. (1972): Epithelio-mesenchymal relations during gastric organogenesis in the rabbit fetus. *J. Embryol. Exp. Morphol.,* 27:177–197.

73. Davies, L. M., Priest, S. H., and Priest, R. E. (1968): Collagen synthesis by cells synchronously replicating DNA. *Science,* 159:91–93.

74. Deschner, E. E. (1967): Observations on the Paneth cell in human ileum. *Exp. Cell Res.,* 47:624–628.

75. Deschner, E. E., Goldstein, M. J., Melamed, M. R., and Sherlock, P. (1976): Autoradiographic observations of a nineteen month old ileal conduit. *Gastroenterology,* 71:832–834.

76. Deschner, E. E., Lewis, C. M., and Lipkin, M. (1963): In vitro study of human rectal epithelial cells. I. Atypical zone of H³ thymidine incorporation in mucosa of multiple polyposis. *J. Clin. Invest.,* 42:1922–1928.

77. Deschner, E. E., and Lipkin, M. (1966): An autoradiographic study of the renewal of argentaffin cells in human rectal mucosa. *Exp. Cell Res.,* 43:661–665.

78. Deschner, E. E., and Lipkin, M. (1970): Study of human rectal epithelial cells in vitro. III. RNA, protein, and DNA synthesis in polyps and adjacent mucosa. *J. Natl. Cancer Inst.,* 44:175–185.

79. Deschner, E. E., and Lipkin, M. (1975): Proliferative patterns in colonic mucosa in familial polyposis. *Cancer,* 35:413–418.

80. Deschner, E. E., and Lipkin, M. (1978): Proliferation and differentiation of gastrointestinal cells. In: *Gastrointestinal Tract Cancer,* edited by M. Lipkin and R. A. Good, pp. 3–24, Plenum Medical Book Company, New York.

81. Deschner, E. E., Lipkin, M., and Solomon, C. (1966): In vitro study of human epithelial cells. II. H³ thymidine incorporation into polyps and adjacent mucosa. *J. Natl. Cancer Inst.,* 36:849–857.

82. Deschner, E. E., Winawer, S. J., and Lipkin, M. (1972): Patterns of nucleic acid and protein synthesis in normal human gastric mucosa and atrophic gastritis. *J. Natl. Cancer Inst.,* 48:1567–1574.

83. Donnellan, W. (1966): Early histological changes in ulcerative colitis. *Gastroenterology,* 50:519–540.

84. Duell, W., Voorhees, J. J., Kelsey, W., and Hayes, E. (1971): Isoproterenol-sensitive adenyl cyclase in a particulate fraction of epidermis. *Arch. Dermatol.,* 104:601–610.

85. Dworkin, L. D., Levine, G. M., and Spector, M. H. (1976): Small intestinal mass of the rat is partially determined by indirect effects of intraluminal nutrition. *Gastroenterology,* 71:626–630.

86. Eastwood, G. L. (1976): Small bowel morphology and epithelial proliferation in intravenously alimented rabbits. *Gastroenterology,* 70:882 (abstr.).

87. Eastwood, G. L., and Trier, J. S. (1973): Epithelial cell renewal in cultured rectal biopsies in ulcerative colitis. *Gastroenterology,* 64:383–390.

88. Eastwood, G. L., and Trier, J. S. (1974): Epithelial cell proliferation during organogenesis of rat colon. *Anat. Rec.,* 179:303–310.

89. Eker, P. (1974): Inhibition of growth and DNA synthesis in cell culture by cyclic AMP. *J. Cell Sci.,* 16:301–307.

90. Epstein, L. B., and Stohlman, F. (1964): RNA synthesis in cultures of normal human peripheral blood. *Blood,* 24:69–75.

91. Fahrenkrug, J., Schaffalitsky de Muckadell, O. B., Hornum, I., et al. (1976): The mechanism of hypergastrinemia in achlorhydria. Effect of food, acid, and calcitonin on serum gastrin concentrations and component pattern in pernicious anemia, with correlation to endogenous secretin concentrations in plasma. *Gastroenterology,* 71:33–37.

92. Farber, E., and Baserga, R. (1969): Differential effects of hydroxyurea on survival of proliferating cells in vivo. *Cancer Res.,* 29:136–139.

93. Feinendegen, L. E., and Bond, V. P. (1962): Differential uptake of ³H-thymidine into the soluble fraction of single bone marrow cells, determined by autoradiography. *Exp. Cell Res.,* 27:474–484.

94. Feinendegen, L. E., Bond, V. P., and Hughes, W. L. (1961): RNA mediation in DNA synthesis in HeLa cells studied with tritium labeled cytidine and thymidine. *Exp. Cell Res.,* 25:627–647.

95. Feinendegen, L. E., Bond, V. P., and Painter, R. B. (1961): Studies on the interrelationship of RNA synthesis, DNA synthesis and precursor pool in human tissue culture cells studied with tritiated pyrimidine nucleosides. *Exp. Cell Res.,* 22:381–405.

96. Feldman, E. J., Dowling, R. H., McNaughton, J., et al. (1976): Effects of oral versus intravenous nutrition on intestinal adaptation after small bowel resection in the dog. *Gastroenterology,* 70:712–719.

97. Fitzgerald, P. (1964): The immunological role and long life span of small lymphocytes. *J. Theor. Biol.,* 6:13–25.

98. Floch, M. H., and Hellman, L. (1965): The effect of five-fluorouracil on rectal mucosa. *Gastroenterology,* 48:430–437.

99. Florkin, M., and Stotz, E. H. (1967): Morphogenesis, differentiation and development. *Compr. Biochem.,* 28:276.

100. Foroozan, P., and Trier, J. S. (1967): Mucosa of the small intestine in pernicious anemia. *N. Engl. J. Med.,* 277:553–559.

101. Fosket, D. E. (1968): Cell division and the differentiation of wound-vessel members in cultured stem segments of coleus. *Proc. Natl. Acad. Sci. U.S.A.,* 59:1089–1096.

102. Friedman, N. B. (1945): Cellular dynamics in the intestinal mucosa: The effect of irradiation on epithelial maturation and migration. *J. Exp. Med.,* 81:553–558.

103. Frindel, E., Malaise, E., and Tubiana, M. (1968): Cell proliferation kinetics in five human solid tumors. *Cancer,* 22:611–620.

104. Froehlich, J. E., and Rachmeler, M. (1972): Effect of adenosine 3′-5′-cyclic monophosphate on cell proliferation. *J. Cell Biol.,* 55:19–31.

105. Fry, R. J. M., Lesher, S., Kisieleski, W. E., and Sacher, G. (1963): Cell proliferation in the small intestine. In: *Cell Proliferation,* edited by L. F. Lamerton and R. J. M. Fry, pp. 213–233. F. A. Davis, Philadelphia.

106. Fry, R. J. M., Lesher, S., and Kohn, H. I. (1961): Age effect on cell-transit time in mouse jejunal epithelium. *Am. J. Physiol.*, 201:213–216.

107. Fujioka, M., Koga, M., and Liberman, I. (1963): Metabolism of ribonucliec acid after partial hepatectomy. *J. Biol. Chem.*, 238:3401–3406.

108. Galand, P., Mainguet, P., Arguello, M., Chretien, J., and Douxfils, N. (1968): In vitro autoradiographic studies of cell proliferation in the gastrointestinal tract of man. *J. Nucl. Med.*, 9:37–39.

109. Galjaard, H. N., Meer-Fieggen, W. van der, and Giesen, J. (1972): Feedback control by functional villus cells on cell proliferation and maturation in intestinal epithelium. *Exp. Cell Res.*, 73:197–207.

110. Gelfand, M. D., Tepper, M., Katz, L. A., et al. (1968): Acute irradiation proctitis in man. Development of eosinophilic crypt abscesses. *Gastroenterology*, 54:401–411.

111. Gelfant, S. (1959): A study of mitosis in mouse ear epidermis in vitro. I. Cutting of the ear as mitotic stimulant. *Exp. Cell Res.*, 16:527–537.

112. Gelfant, S. (1963): Patterns of epidermal cell division. *Exp. Cell Res.*, 32:521–528.

113. Gilbert, C. W., and Lajtha, L. G. (1965): The importance of cell population kinetics in determining response to irradiation of normal and malignant tissue. In: *Cellular Radiation Biology*, pp. 474–497. Williams & Wilkins Co., Baltimore.

114. Gjuruldsen, S. T., Myren, J., and Fretheim, B. (1968): Alterations of gastric mucosa following a graded partial gastrectomy for duodenal ulcer. *Scand. J. Gastroenterol.*, 3:465–470.

115. Gleeson, M. H., Cullen, J., and Dowling, R. H. (1972): Intestinal structure and function after small bowel by-pass in the rat. *Clin. Sci.*, 43:731–742.

116. Glinos, A. D. (1958): The mechanism of liver growth and regeneration. In: *The Chemical Basis of Development*, edited by W. McElroy and B. Glass, pp. 813–842. Johns Hopkins Clin. Press, Baltimore.

117. Gowans, J. L., and McGregor, D. D. (1965): The immunological activities of lymphocytes. *Progr. Allergy*, 9:1–78.

118. Grable, E., Zamcheck, N., Janelson, P., and Shipp, F. (1957): Nuclear size of cells in normal stomachs, in gastric atrophy and in gastric cancer. *Gastroenterology*, 32:1104–1112.

119. Greider, M. H., Steinberg, V., and McGuigan, J. E. (1972): Electron microscopic identification of the gastrin cell of the human antral mucosa by means of immunocytochemistry. *Gastroenterology*, 63:572–583.

120. Grobstein, C. (1959): Differentiation of vertebrate cells. In: *The Cell*, edited by J. Brachet and A. E. Mirsky, pp. 437–496. Academic Press, New York.

121. Hadden, J. W., Hadden, L. M., Haddox, M. K., and Goldberg, N. D. (1972): Guanosine cyclic 3′,5′-monophosphate: a possible intracellular mediator of mitogenic influences in lymphocytes. *Proc. Natl. Acad. Sci. U.S.A.*, 69:3024–3027.

122. Hagemann, R. F., and Lesher, S. (1971): Intestinal crypt survival and total and per crypt levels of proliferative cellularity following irradiation: age response and animal lethality. *Radiat. Res.*, 47:159–167.

123. Hansen, P. H., Pedersen, T., and Larsen, J. K. (1975): A method to study cell proliferation kinetics in human gastric mucosa. *Gut*, 16:23–27.

124. Hansen, P. H., Pedersen, T., and Larsen, J. K. (1976): Cell proliferation kinetics in normal human gastric mucosa. *Gastroenterology*, 70:1051–1054.

125. Hanson, W. R., and Osborne, J. W. (1971): Epithelial cell kinetics in the small intestine of the rat 60 days after resection of 70 per cent of the ileum and jejunum. *Gastroenterology*, 60:1087–1097.

126. Hanson, W. R., Osborne, J. W., and Sharp, J. G. (1977): Compensation by the residual intestine after intestinal resection in the rat. I. Influence of amount of tissue removed. *Gastroenterology*, 72:692–700.

127. Hanson, W. R., Osborne, J. W., and Sharp, J. G. (1977): Compensation by the residual intestine after intestinal resection in the rat. II. Influence of postoperative time interval. *Gastroenterology*, 72:701–705.

128. Harding, J. D., and Cairnie, A. B. (1975): Changes in intestinal cell kinetics in the small intestine of lactating mice. *Cell Tissue Kinet.*, 8:135–144.

129. Harkness, R. D. (1957): Regeneration of liver. *Br. Med. Bull.*, 13:87–93.

130. Heird, W. C., Tsang, H. L., MacMillan, R., et al. (1974): Comparative effects of total parenteral nutrition, oral feeding and starvation on rat small intestine. *Gastroenterology*, 66:709 (abstr.).

131. Heller, R., Tawil, T., and Weser, E. (1974): Effect of bile and pancreatic secretions on mucosal hyperplasia after small bowel resection. *Gastroenterology*, 67:568 (abstr.).

132. Herbst, J. J., Berenson, M. M., Wiser, W. C., et al. (1976): Cell proliferation in Barrett's esophageal epithelium. *Clin. Res.*, 24:168A (abstr.).

133. Hermos, J. A., Adams, W. H., Liu, Y. K., et al. (1972): Mucosa of the small intestine in folate-deficient alcoholics. *Ann. Intern. Med.*, 76:957–965.

134. Hermos, J. A., Mathan, M., and Trier, J. S. (1971): DNA synthesis and proliferation by villous epithelial cells in fetal rats. *J. Cell Biol.*, 50:255–258.

135. Herrmann, H., Marchok, A. C., and Baril, E. F. (1967): Growth rate and differentiated function of cells. *Natl. Cancer Inst. Monogr.*, 26:303–326.

136. Hoffman, J. G. (1953): The size and growth of tissue cells. In: *American Lecture Series*, p. 97. Charles C. Thomas, Springfield, Ill.

137. Hoffman, J., and Post, J. (1967): In vivo studies of DNA synthesis in human normal and tumor cells. *Cancer Res.*, 27:898–902.

138. Howard, A., and Pelc, S. R. (1953): Synthesis of desoxyribonucleic acid in normal and irradiated cells and its relation to chromosome breakage. *Heredity [Suppl.]*, 6:261–273.

139. Hughes, W. L., Bond, V. P., Brecher, G., Cronkite, E. P., Painter, R. B., Quastler, H., and Sherman, F. G. (1958): Cellular proliferation in the mouse as revealed by autoradiography with tritiated thymidine. *Proc. Natl. Acad. Sci. U.S.A.*, 44:476–483.

140. Hunt, T. E., and Hunt, E. A. (1961): Thymidine-H³ radioautographs of the gastric mucosa of the rat after stimulation with compound 48/80. *Anat. Rec.*, 139:240–241.

141. Hunt, T. E., and Hunt, E. A. (1962): Radioautographic study of proliferation in the stomach of the rat using thymidine-H³ and compound 48/80. *Ant. Rec.*, 142:505–517.

142. Hurlbert, R. B., Schmitz, H., Brumm, A. F., and Potter, V. R. (1954): Nucleotide metabolism. II. Chromatographic separation of acid-soluble nucleotides. *J. Biol. Chem.*, 209:23–39.

143. Imondi, A. R., Balis, M. E., and Lipkin, M. (1969): Changes in enzyme levels accompanying differentiation of intestinal epithelial cells. *Exp. Cell Res.*, 58:323–330.

144. Imondi, A. R., Lipkin, M., and Balis, M. E. (1970): Enzyme and template stability as regulatory mechanisms in differentiating intestinal epithelial cells. *J. Biol. Chem.*, 245:2194–2198.

145. Ismail-Beigi, F., Horton, P. F., and Pope, C. E., II (1970): Histological consequences of gastroesophageal reflux in man. *Gastroenterology*, 58:163–174.

146. Ismail-Beigi, F., and Pope, CE, II (1974): Distribution of histologic changes of reflux. *Gastroenterology*, 66:1109–1113.

147. Ives, D. H., Morse, P. A., Jr., and Potter, V. R. (1963): Feedback inhibition of thymidine triphosphate. *J. Biol. Chem.*, 238:1467–1474.

148. Johnson, L. R. (1976): The trophic action of gastrointestinal hormones. *Gastroenterology*, 70:278–288.

149. Johnson, L. R., Copeland, E. M., Dudrick, S. J., et al. (1975): Structural and hormonal alterations in the gastrointestinal tract of parenterally fed rats. *Gastroenterology*, 68:1177–1183.

150. Johnson, L. R., and Guthrie, P. D. (1974): Secretin inhibition of gastrin-stimulated deoxyribonucleic acid synthesis. *Gastroenterology*, 67:601–606.

151. Johnson, L. R., Lichtenberger, L. M., Copeland, E. M., et al. (1975): Action of gastrin on gastrointestinal structure and function. *Gastroenterology*, 68:1184–1192.

152. Johnson, T. C., and Holland, J. J. (1965): Ribonucleic acid and protein synthesis in mitotic HeLa cells. *J. Cell Biol.*, 27:565–574.

153. Kaye, G. I., Lane, N., and Pascal, R. R. (1968): Colonic pericrytal fibroblast sheath: Replication, migration, and cytodifferentiation of a mesenchymal cell system in adult tissue. II. Fine structural aspects of normal rabbit and human colon. *Gastroenterology,* 54:852-865.

154. Kaye, G. I., Maenza, R. M., and Lane, N. (1966): Cell replication in rabbit gallbladder. An autoradiographic study of epithelial and associated fibroblast renewal in vivo and in vitro. *Gastroenterology,* 51:670-680.

155. Kaye, G. I., Pascal, R. R., and Lane, N. (1971): The colonic pericryptal fibroblast sheath: Replication, migration, and cytodifferentiation of a mesenchymal cell system in adult tissue. III. Replication and differentiation in human hyperplastic and adenomatous polyps. *Gastroenterology,* 60:515-536.

156. Kim, Y., Kerr, R. J., and Lipkin, M. (1967): Cell proliferation during the development of stress erosions in mouse stomach. *Nature,* 215:1180-1181.

157. Koldovsky, O., Sunshine, P., and Kretchmer, N. (1966): Cellular migration of intestinal epithelia in suckling and weaned rats. *Nature,* 212:1389-1390.

158. Korman, M. G., St. John, D. J. B., and Hansky, J. (1970): Studies on serum gastrin levels in pernicious anemia. *Gut,* 11:981.

159. Korman, M. G., Strickland, R. G., and Hansky, J. (1971): Serum gastrin in chronic gastritis. *Br. Med. J.,* 2:16-18.

160. Kornberg, A. (1960): Biological synthesis of deoxyribonucleic acid. *Science,* 131:1503-1508.

161. Krasner, N., Thomson, T. J., Crean, G., et al. (1974): Gastric epithelial cell turnover after acute and chronic alcohol ingestion. *Gut,* 15:336 (abstr.).

162. Laguchev, S. S., and Avetisyan, A. A. (1972): Effect of hydrocortisone on time parameters of the mitotic cycle of duodenal epithelial cells. *Biull. Eksp. Biol. Med.,* 73:86-88.

163. Lala, P. K., and Patt, H. M. (1966): Cytokinetic analysis of tumor growth. *Proc. Natl. Acad. Sci. U.S.A.,* 56:1742-1753.

164. Lane, N., Kaplan, H., and Pascal, R. R. (1971): Minute adenomatous and hyperplastic polyps of the colon: Divergent patterns of epithelial growth with specific associated mesenchymal changes. *Gastroenterology,* 60:537-551.

165. Langan, T. A. (1970): Phosphorylation of histones in vivo under the control of cyclic AMP and hormones. *Adv. Biochem. Psychopharmacol.,* 3:307-323.

166. Leblond, C. P., and Carriere, R. (1955): The effect of growth hormone and thyroxine on the mitotic rate of the intestinal mucosa of the rat. *Endocrinology,* 56:261-266.

167. Leblond, C. P., Greulich, R. C., and Pereira, J. P. M. (1964): Relationship of cell formation and cell migration in the renewal of stratified squamous epithelia. In: *Advances in Biology of Skin, Vol. 5,* edited by W. Montagna and R. E. Billingham, pp. 39-67. Pergamon Press, New York.

168. Leblond, C. P., and Messier, B. (1958): Renewal of chief cells and goblet cells in the small intestine as shown by radioautography after injection of thymidine-H^3 into mice. *Anat. Rec.,* 132:247-259.

169. Leblond, C. P., and Walker, B. E. (1956): Renewal of cell populations. *Physiol. Rev.,* 36:255-276.

170. Lesher, S., Fry, R. J. M., and Kohn, H. I. (1961): Influence of age on transit time of cells of mouse intestinal epithelium. I. Duodenum. *Lab. Invest.,* 10:291-300.

171. Lesher, S., Fry, R. J. M., and Kohn, H. I. (1961): Age and the generation time of the mouse duodenal epithelial cell. *Exp. Cell Res.,* 24:334-343.

172. Levine, G. M., Deren, J. J., Steiger, E., et al. (1974): Role of oral intake in maintenance of gut mass and disaccharide activity. *Gastroenterology,* 67:975-982.

173. Levine, G. M., Deren, J. J., and Yezdimir, E. (1976): Small-bowel resection. Oral intake is the stimulus for hyperplasia. *Am. J. Dig. Dis.,* 21:542-546.

174. Ley, R., Willems, G., and Vansteenkiste, Y. (1973): Influence of vagotomy on parietal cell kinetics in the rat mucosa. *Gastroenterology,* 65:764-772.

175. Liavag, I. (1968): Mitotic activity of gastric mucosa. *Acta. Pathol. Microbiol. Scand.,* 72:43-63.

176. Liavag, I., and Vaage, S. (1972): The effect of vagotomy and pyloroplasty on the gastrointestinal mucosa of the rat. *Scand. J. Gastroenterol.,* 7:23-27.

177. Lichtenberger, L. M., Lechago, J., and Johnson, L. R. (1975): Depression of antral and serum gastrin concentration by food deprivation in the rat. *Gastroenterology,* 68:1473-1479.

178. Lichtenberger, L., Miller, L. R., Erwin, D. N., et al. (1973): Effect of pentagastrin on adult rat duodenal cells in culture. *Gastroenterology,* 65:242-251.

179. Lieb, L. M., and Lisco, H. (1966): In vitro uptake of tritiated thymidine by carcinoma of the human colon. *Cancer Res.,* 26:733-740.

180. Lieberman, I. (1969): Studies on the control of mammalian deoxyribonucleic acid synthesis. In: *Biochemistry of Cell Division,* edited by R. Baserga, pp. 119-137. Charles C. Thomas, Springfield, Ill.

181. Lieberman, I., Abrams, R., and Ove, P. (1963): Changes in the metabolism of ribonucleic acid preceding the synthesis of deoxyribonucleic acid in mammalian cells cultured from the animal. *J. Biol. Chem.,* 238:2141-2149.

182. Lipkin, M. (1971): The proliferative cycle of mammalian cells. In: *The Cell Cycle and Cancer,* edited by R. Baserga, pp. 6-26. Marcel Dekker, New York.

183. Lipkin, M. (1972): Proliferation and differentiation of mucus containing cells in normal and diseased mucosa. In: *Proc. Int. Congr. Gastroenterol.,* pp. 691-693.

184. Lipkin, M. (1972): Gastric cell regeneration. In: *Archives Francaises des Maladies de l'Appareil Digestif,* p. 500c. Masson et Cie, Paris.

185. Lipkin, M. (1974): Phase 1 and phase 2 proliferative lesions of colonic epithelial cells in diseases leading to colon cancer. *Cancer [Suppl.],* 34:878-888.

186. Lipkin, M. (1974): Proliferative changes in the colon. *Am. J. Dig. Dis.,* 19:1029-1032.

187. Lipkin, M., and Bell, B. (1968): Cell proliferation. In: *Handbook of Physiology, Sec. 6, Vol. V.,* edited by C. F. Code, pp. 2861-2879. American Physiological Society, Washington, D.C.

188. Lipkin, M., Bell, B., and Sherlock, P. (1963): Cell proliferation kinetics in the gastrointestinal tract of man. I. Cell renewal in colon and rectum. *J. Clin. Invest.,* 42:767-776.

189. Lipkin, M., Bell, B., Stalder, G., and Troncale, F. (1970): The development of abnormalities of growth in colonic epithelial cells of man. In: *Carcinoma of the Colon and Antecedent Epithelium,* edited by H. Burdette, pp. 213-221. Charles C. Thomas, Springfield, Ill.

190. Lipkin, M., and Deschner, E. E. (1968): Comparative analysis of cell proliferation in the gastrointestinal tract of newborn hamster. *Exp. Cell Res.,* 49:1-12.

191. Lipkin, M., Lightdale, C., and Deschner, E. E. (1980): Kinetic parameters in the colon of a patient with Gardners' syndrome. In preparation.

192. Lipkin, M., and Quastler, H. (1962): Cell retention and incidence of carcinoma in several portions of the gastrointestinal tract. *Nature,* 194:1198-1199.

193. Lipkin, M., and Quastler, H. (1966): Cell population kinetics in the colon of the mouse. *J. Clin. Invest.,* 41:141-146.

194. Lipkin, M., Sherlock, P., and Bell, B. M. (1962): Generation time of epithelial cells in the human colon. *Nature,* 195:175-177.

195. Lipkin, M., Sherlock, P., and Bell, B. (1963): Cell proliferation kinetics in the gastrointestinal tract of man. II. Cell renewal in stomach, ileum, colon and rectum. *Gastroenterology,* 45:721-729.

196. Livstone, E., Sheahan, D. G., and Behar, J. (1976): In vitro tritiated ^{3}H thymidine uptake by esophageal squamous mucosa from patients with reflux esophagitis. *Gastroenterology,* 70:909 (abstr.).

197. Loehry, C. A., and Creamer, B. (1969): Three-dimensional structure of the rat small intestinal mucosa related to mucosal dynamics. II. Mucosal structure and dynamics in the lactating rat. *Gut,* 10:116-118.

198. Lopes, J. D., Ito, H., and Glass, G. B. J. (1976): Inhibition of parietal and peptic cell proliferation by parietal cell and intrinsic factor antibodies. *Gastroenterology,* 70:910 (abstr.).

199. Loran, M. R., and Carbone, J. V. (1968): The humoral effects of intestinal resection on cellular proliferation and maturation in parabiotic rats. In: *Gastrointestinal Radiation Injury,* edited by M. F. Sullivan, pp. 127-139. Excerpta Medica Foundation, Amsterdam.

200. Loran, M. R., and Crocker, T. T. (1963): Population dynamics of intestinal epithelia in the rat two months after partial resection of the ileum. *J. Cell Biol.,* 19:285–291.

201. MacDonald, W. C., Trier, J. S., and Everett, N. B. (1964): Cell proliferation and migration in the stomach, duodenum, and rectum of man: radioautographic studies. *Gastroenterology,* 46:405–417.

202. Makela, P., and Nossal, G. (1962): Autoradiographic studies on the immune response. II. DNA synthesis amongst single antibody-producing cells. *J. Exp. Med.,* 115:231–244.

203. Malamud, D. (1971): Differentiation and the cell cycle. In: *The Cell Cycle and Cancer,* edited by R. Baserga, pp. 132–141. Marcel Dekker, New York.

204. Margolis, S., Philips, F. S., and Sternberg, S. S. (1971): The cytotoxicity of methotrexate in mouse small intestine in relation to inhibition of folic acid reductase and of DNA synthesis. *Cancer Res.,* 31:2037–2046.

205. Marques-Pereira, J. P., and Leblond, C. P. (1965): Mitosis and differentiation in the stratified squamous epithelium of the rat esophagus. *Am. J. Anat.,* 117:73–90.

206. Marsh, M. N., and Trier, J. S. (1974): Morphology and cell proliferation of subepithelial fibroblasts in adult mouse jejunum. I. Structural features. *Gastroenterology,* 67:622–635.

207. Mathan, M., Hermos, J. A., and Trier, J. S. (1972): Structural features of the epithelio-mesenchymal interface of rat duodenal mucosa during development. *J. Clin. Biol.,* 52:577–588.

208. Matsuyama, M., and Suzuki, H. (1970): Differentiation of immature mucous cells into parietal, argyrophil and chief cells in stomach grafts. *Science,* 169:385–387.

209. Mazia, D. (1961): Mitosis and the physiology of cell division. In: *The Cell,* edited by J. Brachet and A. Mirsky, pp. 77–412. Academic Press, New York.

210. Mazia, D. (1963): Synthetic activities leading to mitosis. *J. Cell. Comp. Physiol., [Suppl. 1],* 62:123–140.

211. McCrery, J. E., and Rigby, P. G. (1972): Lymphocyte stimulation by cyclic AMP, GMP and related compounds. *Proc. Soc. Exp. Biol. Med.,* 140:1456–1459.

212. McDermott, F. T., Dalton, M. K., and Galbraith, A. J. (1974): The effect of acute renal failure on mitotic duration of mouse ileal epithelium. *Cell Tissue Kinet.,* 7:31–36.

213. McDermott, F. T., Galbraith, A. J., and Dalton, M. K. (1974): Effects of acute renal failure on ileal epithelial cell kinetics: autoradiographic studies in the mouse. *Gastroenterology,* 66:235–239.

214. McDermott, F. T., and Roudnew, B. (1976): Ileal crypt cell population kinetics after 40% small bowel resection. Autoradiographic studies in the rat. *Gastroenterology,* 70:707–711.

215. McDonald, W. C., Trier, J. S., and Everett, N. B. (1964): Cell proliferation and migration in stomach, duodenum and rectum of man. *Gastroenterology,* 46:405–417.

216. McGuigan, J. E., and Greider, M. H. (1971): Correlative immunochemical and light microscopic studies of the gastrin cell of the antral mucosa. *Gastroenterology,* 60:223–236.

217. McGuigan, J. E., and Trudeau, W. L. (1970): Serum gastrin concentrations in pernicious anemia. *N. Engl. J. Med.,* 282:358–361.

218. McGuigan, J. E., and Trudeau, W. L. (1972): Serum gastrin levels before and after vagotomy and pyloroplasty or vagotomy and antrectomy. *N. Engl. J. Med.,* 286:184–188.

219. McLoughlin, C. B. (1963): Mesenchymal influences on epithelial differentiation. *Symp. Soc. Exp. Biol.,* 17:359–387.

220. Melvin, J. B. (1967): The effect of actinomycin D on mitosis in regenerating mouse liver. *Exp. Cell Res.,* 45:559–569.

221. Mendelsohn, M. L. (1965): The kinetics of tumor cell proliferation. In: *Cellular Radiation Biology,* pp. 498–513. Williams & Wilkins Co., Baltimore.

222. Menge, H., Grafe, M., Lorenz-Meyer, H., et al. (1975): Influence of food intake on the development of structural and functional adaptation following ileal resection in the rat. *Gut,* 16:468–472.

223. Merzel, J., and Leblond, C. P. (1969): Origin and renewal of goblet cells in the epithelium of the mouse small intestine. *Am. J. Anat.,* 124:281–306.

224. Messier, B. (1960): Radioautographic evidence for the renewal of the mucous cells in the gastric mucosa of the rat. *Anat. Rec.,* 136:242.

225. Messier, B., and Leblond, C. P. (1960): Cell proliferation and migration as revealed by radioautography after injection of thymidine-H³ into rats and mice. *Am. J. Anat.,* 106:247–294.

226. Miller, L. R., Jacobson, E. D., and Johnson, L. R. (1973): Effect of pentagastrin on gastric mucosal cells grown in tissue culture. *Gastroenterology,* 64:254–267.

227. Milles, S. S., Muggia, A. L., and Spiro, H. M. (1962): Colonic histologic changes induced by 5-fluorouracil. *Gastroenterology,* 43:391–399.

228. Moog, F., Etzler, M. E., and Grey, R. D. (1967): The differentiation of alkaline phosphatase in the intestine. *J. Cell Biol.,* 32:Cl.

229. Morson, B. (1955): Carcinoma arising from areas of intestinal metaplasia in the gastric mucosa. *Br. J. Cancer,* 9:377–385.

230. Mueller, G. C. (1971): Biochemical perspectives of the G_1 and S intervals in the replication cycle of animal cells: a study in the control of cell growth. In: *The Cell Cycle and Cancer,* edited by R. Baserga, pp. 269–307. Marcel Dekker, New York.

231. Myhre, E. (1960): Regeneration of the fundic mucosa in rats. V. An autoradiographic study on the effect of cortisone. *Arch. Pathol.,* 70:476–485.

232. Naef, A. P., Savary, M., and Ozzello, L. (1975): Columnar-lined lower esophagus: an acquired lesion with malignant predisposition. Report on 140 cases of Barrett's esophagus with 12 adenocarcinomas. *Thorac. Cardiovasc. Surg.,* 70:826–835.

233. Nagayo, T. (1975): Microscopical cancer of the stomach—a study on histogenesis of gastric carcinoma. *Int. J. Cancer,* 16:52–60.

234. Nakayama, H., and Weser, E. (1975): Pyrimidine biosynthetic enzymes in rat intestine after small bowel resection. *Gastroenterology,* 68:480–487.

235. Newburger, P., Lewin, M., de Recherche, C., and Bonfils, S. (1972): Parietal and chief cell population in four cases of Zollinger-Ellison syndrome. *Gastroenterology,* 63:937–942.

236. Nieburgs, H. E., and Glass, G. B. J. (1963): Gastric-cell maturation disorders in atrophic gastritis, pernicious anemia, and carcinoma. *Am. J. Dig. Dis.,* 8:135–159.

237. Nowell, P. (1960): Phytohemagglutinin: An initiator of mitosis in cultures of normal leukocytes. *Cancer Res.,* 20:462–466.

238. Nundy, S., Malamud, D., Obertop, H., et al. (1977): Onset of cell proliferation in the shortened gut: Colonic hyperplasia after ileal resection. *Gastroenterology,* 72:263–266.

239. Obertop, H., Nundy, S., Malamud, D., et al. (1977): Onset of cell proliferation in the shortened gut: rapid hyperplasia after jejunal resection. *Gastroenterology,* 72:267–270.

240. Oota, K. (1967): Pathohistology. In: *Carcinoma of the Stomach in Early Phase,* edited by T. Kurokawa, T. Kajetani, and K. Oota. Nakayama-Shoten, Tokyo.

241. Oppenheim, J. J. (1968): Relationship of in vitro lymphocyte transformation to delayed hypersensitivity in guinea pigs and man. *Fed. Proc.,* 27:21–28.

242. Owen, M., and MacPherson, S. (1963): Cell population kinetics of an osteogenic tissue. II. *J. Cell Biol.,* 19:33–44.

243. Parker, F. G., Barnes, E. N., and Kaye, G. I. (1974): The pericryptal fibroblast sheath. IV. Replication, migration, and differentiation of the subepithelial fibroblasts of the crypt and villus of the rabbit jejunum. *Gastroenterology,* 67:607–621.

244. Pascal, R. R., Kaye, G. I., and Lane, N. (1968): Colonic pericryptal fibroblast sheath: replication, migration, and cytodifferentiation of a mesenchymal cell system in adult tissue. I. Autoradiographic studies in normal rabbit colon. *Gastroenterology,* 54:835–851.

245. Paul, J. (1968): Molecular aspects of cytodifferentiation. *Adv. Comp. Physiol. Biochem.,* 3:115–172.

246. Pearl, J. M., Ritchie, W. P., Gilsdorf, R. B., et al. (1966): Hypothalamic stimulation and feline gastric mucosal cellular populations. Factors in the etiology of the stress ulcer. *JAMA,* 195:281–284.

247. Peterson, A., and Lipkin, M. (1973): Thymidylate synthetase and thymidine kinase activity in the jejunum of rat. *Fed. Proc.,* 32:321.

248. Peterson, A., and Lipkin, M. (1974): Thymidine kinase and thymidylate synthetase activity in normal intestinal cells and neoplastic lesions of the colon. *Proc. Am. Assoc. Cancer Res.,* 15:28.

249. Philpot, G. W. (1971): Tissue specific inhibition of cell proliferation in embryonic stomach epithelium in vitro. *Gastroenterology,* 61:25–34.

250. Polacek, M. A., and Ellison, E. H. (1966): Parietal cell mass and gastric acid secretion in the Zollinger-Ellison syndrome. *Surgery,* 60:606–614.

251. Potter, V. R. (1960): *Nucleic Acid Outlines, Vol. 1,* pp. 18–19. Burgess, Minneapolis.

252. Powell, J., Duell, E., and Voorhess, J. J. (1971): Beta adrenergic stimulation of endogenous epidermal cyclic AMP formation. *Arch. Dermatol.,* 104:359–365.

253. Prescott, D. M., and Bender, M. A. (1962): Synthesis of RNA and protein during mitosis in mammalian tissue culture cells. *Exp. Cell Res.,* 26:260–268.

254. Quastler, H. (1963): The analysis of cell population kinetics. In: *Cell Proliferation (A Guiness Symposium),* edited by L. R. Lamerton and R. J. M. Fry, pp. 18–34. Blackwell, Oxford.

255. Quastler, H., and Sherman, F. G. (1959): Cell population kinetics in the intestinal epithelium of the mouse. *Exp. Cell Res.,* 17:420–438.

256. Ragins, H., Wincze, F., Lui, S. M., and Dittbrenner, M. (1968): The origin and survival of gastric parietal cells in the mouse. *Anat. Rec.,* 162:99–110.

257. Rijke, R. P. C., Hanson, W. R., Plaisier, H. M., et al. (1976): The effect of ischemic villus cell damage on crypt cell proliferation in the small intestine: Evidence for a feedback control mechanism. *Gastroenterology,* 71:786–792.

258. Rijke, R. P. C., Plaisier, H., Hoogeveen, A. T., et al. (1975): The effect of continuous irradiation on cell proliferation and maturation in small intestinal epithelium. *Cell Tissue Kinet.,* 8:441–453.

259. Roland, M., Berstad, A., and Liavag, I. (1975): A histological study of gastric mucosa before and after proximal gastric vagotomy in duodenal ulcer patients. *Scand. J. Gastroenterol.,* 10:181–186.

260. Roth, J. S. (1970): The phosphorylation of thymidine as a factor controlling cellular proliferation. In: *Protein Metabolism and Biological Function,* edited by E. Bianchi, pp. 141–219. Rutgers Press, Rutgers, N.J.

261. Sawicki, W. J., Rowinski, W., Maciejewski, W., and Kawrecki, K. (1968): Kinetics of proliferation and migration of epithelial cells in the guinea pig colon. *Exp. Cell Res.,* 50:93–103.

262. Schmidt, G., and Thannhauser, S. J. (1945): A method for the determination of desoxyribonucleic acid, ribonucleic acid, and phosphoproteins in animal tissues. *J. Biol. Chem.,* 161:83–89.

263. Schmidt, M., Deschner, E. E., DeHarven, E., and Good, R. A. (1977): Morphological and kinetic features of gastrointestinal cancer xenografts in the nude mouse. *Gastroenterology,* 72.

264. Schneider, W. C. (1945): Phosphorus compounds in animal tissues. I. Extraction and estimation of desoxypentose nucleic acid. *J. Biol. Chem.,* 161:293–303.

265. Schreiber, D. S., Blacklow, N. R., and Trier, J. S. (1973): The mucosal lesion of the proximal small intestine in acute infectious nonbacterial gastroenteritis. *N. Engl. J. Med.,* 288:1318–1323.

266. Schrek, R. (1963): Cell transformation and mitoses produced in vitro by tuberculin purified protein derivative in human blood cells. *Am. Rev. Respir. Dis.,* 87:734–738.

267. Sell, S., and Gell, P. G. H. (1965): Studies on rabbit lymphocytes in vitro. I. Stimulation of blast transformation with an antiallotype serum. *J. Exp. Med.,* 122:423–440.

268. Sell, S., and Gell, P. G. H. (1965): Studies on rabbit lymphocytes in vitro. IV. Blast transformation of the lymphocytes from newborn rabbits induced by antiallotype serum to a paternal IgG allotype not present in the serum of the lymphocyte donors. *J. Exp. Med.,* 122:923–928.

269. Sell, S., Rowe, D. S., and Gell, P. G. H. (1965): Studies on rabbit lymphocytes in vitro. III. Proteins, RNA, and DNA synthesis by lymphocyte cultures after stimulation with phytohaemagglutinin, with staphylococcal filtrate, with antiallotype serum, and with heterologous antiserum to rabbit whole serum. *J. Exp. Med.,* 122:823–839.

270. Shelton, K., and Allfrey, V. G. (1970): Selective synthesis of a nuclear acidic protein in liver cells stimulated by cortisol. *Nature,* 228:132–134.

271. Shorter, R. G., Moertel, C. G., Titus, J. L., and Reitemeier, R. J. (1964): Cell kinetics in the jejunum and rectum of man. *Am. J. Dig. Dis.,* 9:760–763.

272. Shorter, R. G., Spencer, R. J., and Hallenbeck, G. A. (1966): Kinetic studies of the epithelial cells of the rectal mucosa in normal subjects and patients with ulcerative colitis. *Gut,* 7:593–596.

273. Silen, W., Peloso, O., and Jaffe, B. F. (1966): Kinetics of intestinal epithelial proliferation: Effect of vagotomy. *Surgery,* 60:127–135.

274. Spencer, R. J., Huizenga, K. A., Hammer, C. S., and Shorter, R. G. (1969): Further studies of the kinetics of rectal epithelium in normal subjects and patients with ulcerative or granulomatous colitis. *Dis. Colon Rectum,* 12:406–408.

275. Stanley, M. D., Coalson, R. E., Grossman, M. I., et al. (1972): Influence of secretin and pentagastrin on acid secretion and parietal cell number in rats. *Gastroenterology,* 63:264–269.

276. Steel, G. G. (1968): Cell loss from experimental tumours. *Cell Tissue Kinet.,* 1:193–207.

277. Steel, G. G. (1973): Cytokinetics of neoplasia. In: *Cancer Medicine,* edited by J. F. Holland and E. Frie, pp. 125–140. Lea & Febiger, Philadelphia.

278. Steel, G. G., Adams, K., and Barrett, J. C. (1966): Analysis of the cell population kinetics of transplanted tumors of widely differing growth rate. *Br. J. Cancer,* 20:784–800.

279. Stellwagen, R., and Cole, R. (1969): Chromosomal proteins. *Annu. Rev. Biochem.,* 38:951–990.

280. Stemmermann, G. N., and Hayashi, T. (1968): Intestinal metaplasia of the gastric mucosa: A gross and microscopic study of its distribution in various disease states.

281. Stockdale, R. E., and Holtzer, H. (1961): DNA synthesis and myogenesis. *Exp. Cell Res.,* 24:508–520.

282. Stoecker, E. (1966): Proliferation in kidneys and liver. *Verh. Dtsch. Ges. Pathol.,* 50:53–74.

283. Swanson, V. L., and Thomassen, R. W. (1965): Pathology of the jejunal mucosa in tropical sprue. *Am. J. Pathol.,* 46:511–551.

284. Tanaka, J. (1968): Autoradiographic studies on the cell proliferation of the human gastric mucosa in supravital condition. *Acta. Pathol. Jpn.,* 18:307–318.

285. Taylor, E. W. (1963): Relation of protein synthesis to the division cycle in mammalian cell cultures. *J. Cell Biol.,* 19:1–18.

286. Taylor, J. H., Woods, P. S., and Hughes, W. L. (1957): The organization and duplication of chromosomes as revealed by autoradiographic studies using tritium labeled thymidine. *Proc. Natl. Acad. Sci. U.S.A.,* 43:122–128.

287. Temin, H. M. (1967): Control by factors in serum of multiplication of uninfected cells and cells infected and converted by avian sarcoma viruses. In: *Growth Regulating Substances for Animal Cells in Culture,* edited by V. Defendi and M. Stoker, pp. 103–116. Wistar Inst. Symp. Monograph No. 7, Philadelphia.

288. Temin, H. (1968): Carcinogenesis by avian sarcoma viruses. X. The decreased requirement for insulin-replaceable activity in serum for cell multiplication. *Int. J. Cancer,* 3:771–787.

289. Terz, J. J., Curatchet, H. P., and Lawrence, W. (1971): Analysis of the cell kinetics of human solid tumors. *Cancer,* 28:1100–1110.

290. Thake, D. C., Moon, H. W., and Lambert, G. (1973): Epithelial cell dynamics in transmissible gastroenteritis of neonatal pigs. *Vet. Pathol.,* 10:330–341.

291. Thrasher, J. D. (1967): Comparison of the cell cycle and cell migration in the intestinal epithelium of suckling and adult mice. *Experientia,* 23:1050–1051.

292. Tobey, R. A., Petersen, D. F., and Anderson, E. C. (1971): Biochemistry of G_2 and mitosis. In: *The Cell Cycle and Cancer,* edited by R. Baserga, pp. 309–353. Marcel Dekker, New York.

293. Tominaga, K. (1975): Distribution of parietal cells in the antral mucosa of human stomachs. *Gastroenterology,* 69:1201–1207.

294. Townsend, S. F. (1961): Regeneration of gastric mucosa in rats. *Am. J. Anat.,* 109:133–147.

295. Trier, J. S. (1962): Morphologic alterations induced by methotrexate in the mucosa of the human proximal intestine. I. Serial observations by light microscopy. *Gastroenterology,* 42:295–305.

296. Trier, J. S. (1962): Morphologic alterations induced by metho-trexate in the mucosa of the human proximal intestine. II. Electron microscopic observations. *Gastroenterology*, 43:407-424.

297. Trier, J. S., and Browning, T. H. (1966): Morphologic response of the mucosa of the human small intestine to x-ray exposure. *J. Clin. Invest.*, 45:194-204.

298. Trier, J. S., and Browning, T. H. (1970): Epithelial-cell renewal in cultured duodenal biopsies in celiac sprue. *N. Engl. J. Med.*, 283:1245-1250.

299. Trier, J. S., Lorenzsonn, V., and Groehler, K. (1967): Pattern of secretion of Paneth cells of the small intestine of mice. *Gastroenterology*, 53:240-249.

300. Troncale, F., Hertz, R., and Lipkin, M. (1971): Nucleic acid metabolism in proliferating and differentiating cells of man and neoplastic lesions of the colon. *Cancer Res.*, 31:463-467.

301. Troughton, W. E., and Trier, J. S. (1969): Paneth and goblet cell renewal in mouse duodenal crypts. *J. Cell Biol.*, 41:251-268.

302. Turkington, R. W. (1968): Hormone-induced synthesis of DNA by mammary gland in vitro. *Endocrinology*, 82:540-546.

303. Turkington, R. W., and Topper, Y. J. (1967): Androgen inhibition of mammary gland differentiation in vitro. *Endocrinology*, 80:329-336.

304. Tutton, P. J. M. (1973): Control of epithelial cell proliferation in the small intestinal crypt. *Cell Tissue Kinet.*, 6:211-216.

305. Tutton, P. J. M. (1974): The influence of serotonin on crypt cell proliferation in the jejunum of the rat. *J. Anat.*, 118:389.

306. Tutton, P. J. M. (1975): Neural stimulation of mitotic activity in the crypts of Lieberkuhn in rat jejunum. *Cell Tissue Kinet.*, 8:259-266.

307. Tutton, P. J. M., and Helme, R. D. (1974): The influence of adrenoreceptor activity on crypt cell proliferation in the rat jejunum. *Cell Tissue Kinet.*, 7:125-136.

308. Verbin, R. S., and Farber, E. (1967): Effect of cycloheximide on the cell cycle of the crypts of the small intestine in the rat. *J. Cell Biol.*, 35:649-658.

309. Vischer, E., and Chargaff, E. (1947): The separation and characterization of purines in minute amounts of nucleic acid hydrolysates. *J. Biol. Chem.*, 168:781-782.

310. Voorhees, J. J., Duell, E., and Kelsey, W. (1972): Dibutyl cyclic AMP inhibition of epidermal cell division. *Arch. Dermatol.*, 105:384-386.

311. Watson, J. D., and Crick, F. H. C. (1953): Genetic implications of the structure of deoxyribonucleic acid. *Nature*, 171:964-967.

312. Weiser, M. M. (1972): Membrane glycoprotein synthesis by intestine: An index of cell differentiation. *J. Clin. Invest.*, 51:101a-102a (abstr).

313. Weiss, S. B. (1960): Enzymatic incorporation of ribonucleoside triphosphates into the interpolynucleotide linkages of ribonucleic acid. *Proc. Natl. Acad. Sci. U.S.A.*, 46:1020-1030.

314. Welin, S., Youker, J., and Spratt, J. S. (1963): The rates and patterns of growth of 375 tumors of the large intestine and rectum observed serially by double contrast enema study (Malmo technique). *Am. J. Roentgenol.*, 90:673-687.

315. Weser, E., and Hernandez, M. H. (1971): Studies of small bowel adaptation after intestinal resection in the rat. *Gastroenterology*, 60:69-75.

316. Wessells, N. K. (1964): DNA synthesis, mitosis, and differentiation in pancreatic acinar cells in vitro. *J. Cell Biol.*, 20:415-433.

317. Whitfield, J. F., and MacManus, J. P. (1972): Calcium mediated effects of cyclic GMP on the stimulation of thymocyte proliferation by prostaglandin E_1. *Proc. Soc. Exp. Biol. Med.*, 139:818-824.

318. Whitfield, J. F., Rixon, R. H., MacManus, J. P., et al. (1973): Calcium, cyclic adenosine 3',5'-monophosphate, and the control of cell proliferation: A review. *In Vitro*, 8:257-278.

319. Wiendl, H. J., Schwabe, M., Becker, G., and Kowatsch, J. (1974): Feulgencytophotometric studies of gastric mucosal smears in malignant and benign diseases of the stomach. *Acta Cytol. (Baltimore)*, 18:222-230.

320. Willems, G. (1972): Cell renewal in the gastric mucosa. *Digestion*, 6:46-63.

321. Willems, G., Galand, P., Vansteenkiste, Y., et al. (1972): Cell population kinetics of zymogen and parietal cells in the stomach of mice. *Z. Zellforsch. Mikrosk. Anat.*, 134:505-518.

322. Willems, G., and Lehy, T. (1975): Radiographic and quantitative studies on parietal and peptic cell kinetics in the mouse. A selective effect of gastrin on parietal cell proliferation. *Gastroenterology*, 69:416-427.

323. Willems, G., Vansteenkiste, Y., and Limbosch, J. M. (1972): Stimulating effect of gastrin on cell proliferating kinetics in canine fundic mucosa. *Gastroenterology*, 62:583-589.

324. Willems, G., Vansteenkiste, Y., and Smets, P. H. (1971): Effects of ethanol on the cell proliferation kinetics in the fundic mucosa of dogs. *Am. J. Dig. Dis.*, 16:1057-1063.

325. Willems, G., Vansteenkiste, Y., and Smets, P. H. (1971): Effects of food ingestion on the cell proliferation kinetics in the canine fundic mucosa. *Gastroenterology*, 61:323-327.

326. Winawer, S. J., and Lipkin, M. (1969): Cell proliferation kinetics in the gastrointestinal tract of man. IV. Cell renewal in the intestinalized gastric mucosa. *J. Natl. Cancer Inst.*, 42:9-17.

327. Winborn, W. B., Seelig, L. L., Jr., Nakayama, H., et al. (1974): Hyperplasia of the gastric glands after small bowel resection in the rat. *Gastroenterology*, 66:384-395.

328. Wright, G. P. (1925): The relative duration of the various phases of mitosis in chick fibroblasts cultivated in vitro. *J. R. Microsc. Soc.*, 23:414-417.

329. Wright, N., Watson, A., Morley, A., Appleton, D., Marks, J., and Douglas, A. (1973): The cell cycle time in the flat (avillous) mucosa of the human small intestine. *Gut*, 14:603-606.

330. Wright, N., Watson, A., Morley, A., Appleton, D., and Marks, J. (1973): Cell kinetics in flat (avillous) mucosa of the human small intestine. *Gut*, 14:701-710.

331. Yeomans, N. D., St. John, D. J. B., and deBoer, W. G. R. M. (1973): Regeneration of gastric mucosa after aspirin-induced injury in the rat. *Am. J. Dig. Dis.*, 18:773-780.

332. Yeomans, N. D., and Trier, J. S. (1976): Epithelial cell proliferation and migration in the developing rat gastric mucosa. *Dev. Biol.*, 53:206-216.

333. Younger, L. R., King, J., and Steiner, D. F. (1966): Hepatic proliferative response to insulin in severe alloxan diabetes. *Cancer Res.*, 26:1408-1414.

334. Zagorulko, M. P., and Puzyrev, A. A. (1974): On proliferation of the epithelium of the duodenal mucosa in ulcerative disease. *Arkh. Patol.*, 36:(4)31-35.

335. Zufarov, K. A., Nurullaev, L. D., and Baibekov, I. M. (1973): Proliferation and migration of rat small intestinal epithelium during paratyphoid infection. *Biull. Eksp. Biol. Med.*, 75:79-82.

Physiology of the Gastrointestinal Tract, edited by
Leonard R. Johnson. Raven Press, New York © 1981.

Chapter 5

Regulation of Gastrointestinal Growth

Leonard R. Johnson

Classically the gastrointestinal system has been studied because of its digestive functions of motility, enzymatic digestion, secretion, and absorption. The purification of gastrin, secretin, and cholecystokinin in the early 1960s followed by the isolation of numerous other gastrointestinal peptides led to the realization that the gastrointestinal tract is the largest and perhaps most complex endocrine organ in the body. The hypothesis in 1969 that gastrin stimulated growth of oxyntic gland and duodenal mucosa (87) introduced the concept that gastrointestinal hormones regulate the growth of their target tissues in the same manner as had been demonstrated for the other endocrines. Gastrointestinal hormones are now known to interact with other endocrines in the regulation of growth of digestive tract mucosa and the exocrine pancreas (49). This knowledge has stimulated new approaches to and interpretations of experiments on intenstinal adaptation in response to surgery, diabetes, lactation, and feeding in general. The role of gastrointestinal hormones in the developmental changes which occur in young animals has also been in-

vestigated. This information has renewed interest in effects of other endocrines such as growth hormone, thyroxin, and the glucocorticoids on mucosal growth and their relationships to the gastrointestinal hormones. In addition, there is a large amount of recent evidence indicating that gastrointestinal secretions and specific nutrients influence mucosal growth. This chapter will attempt to correlate the information available in these fields of research, bring it up to date, and point out those areas and directions where, in the reviewer's opinion, emphasis should be placed in the future.

GROWTH PROPERTIES OF GASTROINTESTINAL MUCOSA

The mucosa of the gastrointestinal tract has one of the most rapid turnover rates of any tissue in the body. The functions of the various differentiated cells are dependent on the continuation of normal division by the proliferating cells deep within the mucosa. Normal proliferation occurs in undifferentiated precursor or stem cells located in the crypts of the small intestine and colon and in the mucous neck cells within the glands of the gastric mucosa. Proliferation and growth are balanced by cell loss through exfoliation of surface cells, so that under normal conditions cell populations are maintained at a steady state. Insufficient cell production or increased cell loss may result in ulceration or atrophy. Increased cell production or the prolonged life of certain cell types may result in hyperplasia. Due to the rapid turnover times of most of the cell populations, therefore, any alteration in the processes regulating growth is likely to produce functional changes.

In the oxyntic gland mucosa, [³H]thymidine is incorporated into DNA and cells divide in the middle third of the glands (126,138). Most newly produced cells migrate rapidly to the surface while differentiating into mucous cells. The migration time represents the time for replacement of the total cell population above the dividing zone and is about 3 days in the rat (31) and 4 to 6 days in the dog and human (126,194). Most studies agree that parietal cells are unable to divide (126,153, 189), and some newly formed cells slowly migrate down the gland to differentiate into acid-producing cells (189). Parietal cells in the mouse have been shown to survive for 90 days, which is also the time it takes for downward migration to the bottom of the glands (153). Observations indicate the zymogen cells can originate from undifferentiated cells after injury (106,134) but not in normal adult mucosa (189) where they are replaced by mitosis.

Since antral gastrin content varies considerably with feeding, fasting, and other events (117), the means and regulation of renewal of the G-cell population are important physiological questions. In the mouse analysis of labeling index curves during and after [³H]thymidine injection confirmed that the majority of G cells were renewed by mitosis of other G cells. Differentiation of G cells from other antral cells was not excluded, and the turnover time was estimated to be between 2 and 4 months (112). A recent abstract by Fugimoto et al. (56a) reports that most G cells in the hamster arise from a regenerative focus in the necks of the pyloric glands. G cells then migrate to the lower parts of the gland, and turnover time is 10 to 15 days. Whether the discrepancies between this report and the above one are due to a species difference or to inadequate methods remains to be determined. The mechanisms regulating the replication of G cells are unknown.

The mucosa of the small intestine is characterized by finger- or leaf-like extensions of the epithelial surface called villi. The villi are surrounded by the crypts of Lieberkuhn which contain the crypt base columnar cells believed to be the stem cell for the other epithelial cell types (23). Villi are tallest in the duodenum and shortest in the ileum, and they are surrounded by more crypts

in the doudenum (123). This is the so-called villus gradient of the small intestine. Following division of the stem cells the immature cells migrate out of the crypt and up the villus where they are extruded from the villus tip. This process is most rapid in the proximal gut and may occur within 2 days in the duodenum (11). As an individual cell migrates it matures into either a columnar cell, enteroendocrine cell, goblet cell, or Paneth cell (23).

The colonic surface is flat, lacking villous projections. Tubular crypts extend down toward the muscularis mucosae and contain columnar epithelial, mucous, Paneth, and enteroendocrine cells. Each of these differentiated cells is derived from a single stem cell, the vacoulated, crypt base columnar cell (23). Turnover time of the epithelial cells of the colonic mucosa is approximately 3 to 4 days (123).

It is also important to realize that the growth characteristics of the mucosa change with age. Thus hormone levels, receptor concentrations, and diet change dramatically from birth to adult. This is especially true in the rat, which goes through a definitive period of weaning during which important changes occur in the growth and function of the gastrointestinal mucosa.

GENERAL METHODS

In order to prove that an agent stimulates growth, one must demonstrate an increased number of cells in the target tissue following exposure to the agent. Increased DNA synthesis and tissue content of DNA are biochemical indicators of a trophic effect. Protein and RNA synthesis and content also increase during growth; however, these parameters can increase when cell numbers are not increasing. An increase in cell number is referred to as hyperplasia and is indicated biochemically by an increased DNA content. An increase in protein or RNA content respective to cell number, i. e., an increased volume: DNA ratio, is hypertrophy.

Ideally one must be able to demonstrate an increase in total DNA content of the organ to ensure that a measured increase in DNA synthesis is not being matched by an increase in cell turnover. This is not possible in short-term experiments, since it takes at least 48 hr after stimulation for DNA to accumulate sufficiently to show a statistically significant increase. The best approach has proven to be a combination of short- and long-term experiments, whereby different doses, tissues, and agents can be rapidly screened for trophic effects by measuring DNA synthesis. Once optimal conditions are established, a chronic study can be done to demonstrate a significant increase in total tissue DNA. In a long-term study a steady state has usually been reached and the incorporation of [³H]thymidine into DNA expressed per microgram DNA will be no different from control, although total organ [³H]thymidine incorporated may be increased, indicating an increase in proliferative pool size.

Autoradiographic techniques which measure the uptake of [³H]thymidine into nuclei are another means of assessing growth responses. Such data should always be combined with a measurement of actual mitoses, since autoradiography cannot distinguish between uptake of label and actual incorporation of label into DNA.

Measurements of DNA, RNA, and protein content are best expressed per whole tissue. This is easy when dealing with a discrete organ such as the pancreas or liver, but becomes more difficult when the boundaries of the tissue are vague as is the case for the oxyntic gland or duodenal mucosa. After some practice, one becomes fairly adept at visualizing the antral-fundic border and scraping off the oxyntic gland mucosa. Some investigators divide the small intestine into manageable segments after suspending it under constant tension. This technique incorrectly assumes that each intestine will stretch the same amount under a given tension. The error involved, however, is probably less than with any other method.

In order to demonstrate that a hormone physiologically regulates growth, one must demonstrate the effect with endogenous hormone. Usually one removes the endocrine gland which produces the hormone in question, observes the effect of the absence of the hormone, supplies the hormone exogenously, and observes a reversal of the effect caused by the absence of the gland. From the description of the normal growth of gastrointestinal mucosa in the previous section, it is obvious that the endocrine cells are scattered throughout the mucosa instead of occurring in isolated glands. This makes total surgical removal of a hormone source impossible.

Gastrin is the only gastrointestinal hormone whose endogenous levels can be effectively manipulated. Surgical removal of the rat antrum results in a decrease of serum gastrin levels to approximately 20% of normal (38,147). The remaining radioimmunoassayable gastrin is serum probably comes from the duodenum. Fasting rats for 48 hr lowers serum gastrin to 20% of normal and antral gastrin to about 50% of normal (117). Fasting for longer periods of time further reduces gastrin levels, but results of growth experiments are difficult to interpret because of the metabolic and endocrinologic changes produced by starvation. This problem has been circumvented by feeding rats parenterally, using the techniques of intravenous alimentation (170) or by feeding chemically defined liquid diets (174). Rats maintained for 7 to 10 days in positive nitrogen balance by intravenous alimentation increased body weight by 20% (89). In the same animals, antral gastrin decreased to 30% and serum gastrin to 15% of normal (96). Feeding a solution of glucose and amino acids for 7 days dropped gastrin levels to less than 20% of normal while still allowing the rats to gain weight (174). These two

techniques have proven extremely useful for providing well-nourished, gastrin-depleted animals for chronic studies involving the trophic actions of this hormone. Such models are critical, for just as it is almost impossible to demonstrate trophic effects of growth hormone in a nonhypophysectomized animal, it is extremely difficult to demonstrate similar effects of gastrin in animals with normal levels of the hormone.

In order to prove that the effect of a hormone is physiological, one must demonstrate that the action in question occurs in response to a dose of exogenous hormone which does not raise serum levels of the hormone above the levels encountered following normal endogenous release. Gastrin is the only gastrointestinal hormone for which there is a reliable radioimmunoassay in general use (127,199). This has made it difficult to ascertain the significance of the effects of cholecystokinin (CCK) and secretin on growth. The usual standard of comparing postprandial hormone levels with those produced by exogenous administration may be valid for digestive effects of gastrointestinal hormones but invalid for trophic effects. The continuing presence of hormone rather than a transient increase may be more important for producing responses with a long latency.

FACTORS AFFECTING GROWTH OF MUCOSA

Most of the factors affecting the growth of gastrointestinal mucosa are summarized in Fig. 1. In general there are two types of stimulation which result in growth: (a) nongastrointestinal hormones such as thyroxin (19,108) and growth hormone (6) have long been known to alter mucosal growth; (b) numerous other factors are brought into play by the ingestion and digestion of food. The importance of food was noted, for example, by Steiner et al. (171) who demonstrated in rats starved for 6 days that the small intestine lost 53% of

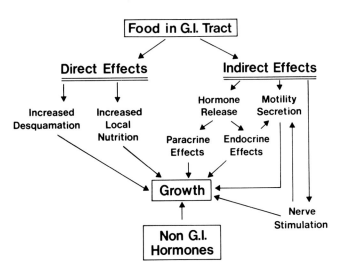

FIG. 1. Summary of factors influencing the growth of gastrointestinal mucosa.

its weight as opposed to only 32% for the whole body. They further found that the total intestinal cell population decreased and the RNA, protein, and water content of the individual cells was diminished compared to that in nongastrointestinal mucosal tissues.

The effects of food are divided into direct and indirect effects. Direct effects are further broken down into increased desquamation and local nutrition. In a number of tissues the mitotic rate is regulated through a negative feedback mechanism involving some type of chalone. These chalones, which ensure that lost cells are replaced by equal numbers of new cells, have been identified in epidermis (14), liver (182), and small intestine (179), plus numerous other tissues. Exfoliation of cells removes chalones and their negative influence on dividing cells. Thus the increased loss of cells following a meal is one possible explanation for the postprandial increase in mucosal cell renewal (62). Philpott (151) has shown that extracts from mature chick gastric mucosa decreased the number of cells entering the proliferative pool in stomachs from younger chicks. The inhibitory substance appeared to be protein in nature and was tissue specific. This type of mechanism may play an important role in regulating the proliferative response to damage. Willems et al. (193) observed that ethanol placed in the stomach results in superficial exfoliation which is followed 8 to 12 hr later by a stimulation of DNA synthesis and mitotic activity. Further work on the gastric chalone has not been reported, but it appears that purification of this substance is necessary before its role can be established.

On the other hand, local nutrition has received considerable attention from several groups of investigators as a possible explanation of the growth-promoting effects of food in the gut—especially in the case of intestinal adaptation in response to surgical resection. Interpretation of data in this field has been confused by use of the term "luminal nutrition." In 1974 Dowling (42) used it to mean nutrition derived by the absorbing enterocytes from absorbed foodstuffs. Riecken and Menge (155), however, defined it as "the presence of nutrient material in the intestinal lumen" and stated that "this does not imply that nutrients must be absorbed to exert their effect." The latter definition then is meant to include both direct and indirect effects. In a later paper Dowling's group (52) apparently agreed with Riecken and Menge but for some reason separated luminal nutrition from hormonal effects and the effects of pancreaticobiliary secretions. The term "local nutrition" avoids the imprecise connotations of "luminal" and conveys the notion of a direct effect on the mucosa rather than a systemic one. Therefore, during the remainder of this chapter "local nutrition" will be used to mean the nutritional effect of absorbed digestion products exerted directly on the absorbing cells before the nutrients are recirculated systemically.

Indirect effects of food include those produced by gastrointestinal hormones, increased motor and secretory activity, and nerve stimulation. Obviously these are interrelated since hormonal and nervous activities can both stimulate motility and secretion and nervous activity may release hormones. There are, however, direct effects of the gastrointestinal hormones on growth of the mucosa; and although not well studied, perhaps there are also direct effects of nervous stimulation on growth of the mucosa. The salivary gland is an excellent example of a tissue related to the digestive tract whose growth is regulated by nervous activity (164).

The effects of peptides can be further broken down into endocrine, paracrine, and neurotransmitter effects. A paracrine effect is one produced by a hormone on cells near its site of release which are reached by simple diffusion or via local circulation. Because of the dispersed nature of gut endocrine cells and the wide distribution of a single endocrine cell type within the mucosa, a number of gastrointestinal peptides are ideally suited to exert their effects as paracrines. The existence of such a paracrine effect, however, is difficult to demonstrate experimentally and remains to be proven. A number of peptides found in gut endocrine cells are also present in the nerves of the gastrointestinal tract. These include gastrin (180), vasoactive intestinal peptide (105), somatostatin (29, and enkephalin (122). Whether these peptides actually serve a transmitter function has not been determined. Vasoactive intestinal peptide, however, is released by vagal stimulation and is a candidate for the transmitter involved in the noncholinergic, nonadrenergic inhibitory system of the gut (50). The possibility that peptides which regulate growth can act as paracrines or neurotransmitters provides an explanation for the so-called direct effects of local nutrition.

GASTROINTESTINAL HORMONES

Historical

Presumptive evidence that gastrointestinal hormones affect the growth of their target tissues is provided by studies describing changes in human oxyntic gland mucosa following antrectomy or in the presence of increased gastrin levels. Lees and Grandjean (110) biopsied the gastric mucosal remnant in 33 healthy postantrectomy patients. Only one of these was considered normal while the rest had varying degrees of mucosal atrophy. Results from a similar study of 56 patients showed a significant decrease in the thickness of the parietal cell layer from 0.71 mm before antrectomy to 0.51 mm 12 months later (60). These results cannot be explained on the basis of disuse hypotrophy, for vagotomy which also decreases acid secretion about 60% does not cause mucosal atrophy (137). The opposite picture occurs in patients with hypergastrinemia from

Zollinger-Ellison syndrome (64). Gastric mucosal hyperplasia and an increased parietal cell count are characteristics of this disease (46). Clinically, therefore, the overproduction of gastrin is associated with gastrointestinal mucosal growth and the lack of the hormone with mucosal atrophy.

These observations could be explained if gastrin were a trophic hormone and led us to examine the effect of pentagastrin on protein synthesis (87). Rats were divided into three groups and injected with either saline, pentagastrin, or histamine. Doses of pentagastrin ranged from threshold to supramaximal for gastric acid secretion. The animals were killed 90 min after a single injection and homogenates of various tissues incubated with [^{14}C]leucine. A dose of pentagastrin, submaximal for acid secretion, caused a 60 to 100% stimulation of protein synthesis in oxyntic glandular mucosa and a 300% stimulation in duodenal mucosa (87). There was no stimulation of protein synthesis in either liver or skeletal muscle. Histamine had no effect on protein synthesis in any of the tissues examined. The stimulation of leucine incorporation was related to the dose of pentagastrin in a typical sigmoid manner. From this study we concluded that: (a) gastrin stimulates protein synthesis, (b) this effect is specific to certain tissues of the digestive tract, and (c) the effect is independent of secretory phenomena. In addition, we hypothesized that gastrin was a trophic hormone and regulated the growth of gastrointestinal tract mucosa (87).

The above conclusions have been supported by numerous studies, and gastrin has been shown to stimulate most of the metabolic responses associated with growth. In addition, secretin and CCK are now known to affect the growth of the exocrine pancreas, and secretin may interact with gastrin to regulate mucosal growth (84).

Effects of Exogenous Hormones

Gastrin

Parameters measured. Chronic *in vivo* administration of pharmacological amounts of pentagastrin causes oxyntic gland hyperplasia with increased mucosal height, volume, weight, and parietal cell mass (33). Crean et al. (33) attributed these results to either increased acid secretion or a direct effect of pentagastrin. Chronic administration of pentagastrin increased the secretory capacity due to the increased parietal cell mass (168). Treatment of rats with 3 daily injections of pentagastrin (250 μg/kg) for 2 weeks increased parietal cell counts from 34.0 to 54.6 million (168). Using autoradiography Willems and Lehy (191) found a significant increase in the production of new parietal cells following gastrin treatment in the mouse. The parietal cell population increased because of a stimulation in fundic stem cell DNA synthesis and shortened maturation time.

Gastrin apparently does not increase the number of chief cells in the gastric mucosa. In the experiments mentioned above in which Crean et al. (33) and Willems and Lehy (191) demonstrated that gastrin increased parietal cell numbers, there were no significant changes in peptic cell mass. These findings are supportive of the concept, mentioned earlier, that most peptic cells arise by mitosis of mature peptic cells and are not derived from stem cells. Thus it appears that gastrin acts directly on the stem or progenitor cells, resulting in increased numbers of stem, mucous, and parietal cells.

The biochemical processes regulated by trophic hormones include increased amino acid uptake, stimulation of protein, RNA, and DNA synthesis, and decreased protein catabolism. Collectively this reaction to a growth-stimulating substance is called the pleiotypic response. Stimulation of RNA, protein, and DNA syntheses have all been shown to occur with gastrin (84). In rats treated repeatedly with gastrin for at least 48 hr the increases in tissue content of protein and nucleic acids become significant (84).

As mentioned earlier, pentagastrin stimulates the *in vitro* incorporation of leucine into protein of gastric and duodenal mucosa (87). Synthetic human gastrin also caused a significant stimulation of *in vivo* protein synthesis in both duodenal and gastric mucosa (86). This study was the first to examine the trophic effects of a pure circulating form of gastrin.

Protein synthesized under the stimulation of pentagastrin appears to be confined to the gastric mucosal cells rather than secreted. Enochs and Johnson (48) injected rats with pentagastrin or saline and incubated pieces of oxyntic gland mucosa in tissue culture medium containing labeled amino acid. Over a period of time, labeled protein appeared in both mucosa and the medium. However, the amounts appearing in the medium were the same for both groups of rats whereas there was considerable stimulation of the synthesis of protein in the tissue (48). Sutton and Donaldson (173) supported this finding by demonstrating that the *in vitro* addition of pentagastrin to isolated gastric mucosa maintained by organ culture increased the overall incorporation of [^{14}C]leucine into gastric mucosal protein. Acetylcholine, cholecystokinin, secretin, and pentagastrin all stimulated the secretion of newly synthesized protein, but only pentagastrin increased synthesis of tissue protein (173).

Three injections of 250 μg/kg pentagastrin resulted in a significant stimulation of RNA synthesis in both duodenal and gastric mucosa (22). RNA synthesis was measured by following the incorporation of [^{14}C]orotic acid into RNA. Gastrin did not stimulate RNA synthesis in the liver. Pentagastrin prevents the decrease in RNA and DNA content of fundic and duodenal mucosa in antrectomized animals (88). Chronic administration of pentagastrin increases the total amount of pancreatic

RNA in both normal (135) and hypophysectomized rats (136). Studies of this effect have been restricted to the acinar cells. Duodenal and gastric RNA synthesis appears to peak 2 to 3 hr after a single injection of pentagastrin. The synthesis of all species of RNA is increased (48).

Numerous studies have documented the stimulatory effect of pentagastrin on DNA synthesis and DNA levels in the rat (48,90–92). Using autoradiography, Willems et al. (192) found stimulation of [³H]thymidine incorporation into canine gastric mucosa after a 4-hr infusion of porcine gastrin. Thymidine uptake was significantly increased 12 hr after gastrin infusion and peaked at 16 hr. Cell division began 20 hr after gastrin infusion. In the rat, DNA synthesis also peaks 16 hr following gastrin injection (48).

These effects of exogenous gastrin on parameters related to growth are well established. They are essentially identical to those which have been described for other trophic hormones such as growth hormone, androgens, and estrogens (82,178,195).

Tissue specificity. Gastrin appears to be a trophic hormone for the oxyntic gland mucosa and the mucosa of the entire small and large intestines. The trophic effects of exogenous gastrin on the gastric and duodenal mucosa have been described in the preceding section. The effects in other tissues are essentially identical. Using similar studies gastrin has also been shown to stimulate DNA synthesis and increase DNA, RNA, and protein content of ileal (85,91) and proximal large bowel mucosa (85,94). Gastrin does not appear to stimulate growth of gut smooth muscle (86). Figure 2 illustrates the DNA synthetic response to gastrin in mucosa from most regions of gastrointestinal tract plus skeletal muscle.

The most notable exceptions to the trophic action of gastrin are the mucosa of the antrum and esophagus (85). It is not surprising that gastrin stimulates the growth of the two tissues, oxyntic gland and duodenal mucosa, proximal and distal to the antrum without affecting the antrum itself. Regulation of antral growth by gastrin would be in opposition to the general concepts of endocrine physiology, for this tissue is the origin of most physiologically released gastrin. Thyroxin, cortisol, androgens, and estrogens regulate metabolism and growth in a number of tissues, but not in their glands of origin. The growth of the thyroid, adrenals, and sex glands is regulated by pituitary peptide hormones. Endocrine cells of the antrum proliferate during periods of chronic gastrin release. Antrocolic transposition results in significant increases in enterochromaffin cells (109,111) and gastrin cells (111). Lichtenberger et al. (120) have demonstrated that fasting reduced both antral and serum gastrin content. Both were increased by feeding. In general, stimulation of gastrin release results in higher levels of antral gastrin.

There is no evidence that hypergastrinemia of non-antral origin produces antral hypertrophy or G-cell hyperplasia. Marked antral hypoplasia has actually been reported in patients with Zollinger-Ellison syndrome (142). Chronic administration of pentagastrin restores the weights of the oxyntic gland and pancreas but not the antrum to normal in hypophysectomized rats (136). Casteleyn et al. (20) actually found that gastrin significantly decreased both labeling and mitotic indices in rat antral mucosa while increasing these parameters in oxyntic gland, duodenal, and jejunal mucosa. Since antral gastrin cells may proliferate from stem cells (56a), and since the relationship between antral stem cell kinetics and G-cell renewal has not been investigated, it is unknown whether gastrin or other factors regulate G-cell population. The regulation of G-cell population is an

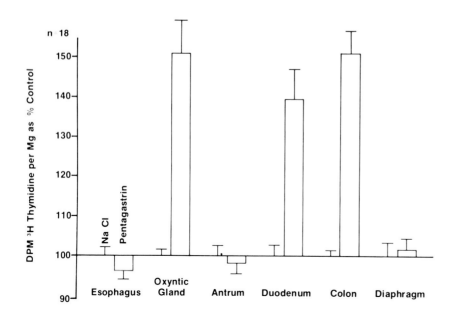

FIG. 2. Disintegration per minute (dpm) of [³H]thymidine incorporated into tissues from rats injected with saline or pentagastrin (250 μg/kg) expressed as a percentage of control (NaCl). Stimulation was significant (p < 0.001) for oxyntic gland, duodenal and colonic mucosa. Bars represent means and SEM of observations in 18 rats in each group. From Johnson (85).

unsolved and obviously important physiological problem with broad clinical implications.

There have been no trophic effects described for gastrin in any tissue outside the gastrointestinal tract proper except the pancreas. Both exogenous (129,135, 136) and endogenous (38) gastrin are strongly implicated in the regulation of the growth of the exocrine pancreas. This subject is treated elsewhere in this volume (see Chapter 36 by T. Solomon). Tissues outside of the gastrointestinal tract which have been examined for trophic effects of gastrin include liver (81,87,90, 136), skeletal muscle (85,87), kidney (96,136), spleen (96,136), and testes (96).

Responses in different species. As in the case of most fields of study involving acute biochemical experiments, the standard animal employed for the investigation of the trophic effects of gastrin has been the rat. Most of the experiments described in the preceding discussion have utilized this animal. Gastrin stimulates thymidine uptake and increases the mitotic index in the dog (192). Physiologic serum levels of gastrin also have been shown to stimulate DNA synthesis in the canine Heidenhain pouch as well as in the normally innervated stomach (158). In addition, gastrin stimulates thymidine uptake and cell division in the oxyntic gland mucosa of the mouse (191) and increases protein synthesis in rabbit mucosa maintained by organ culture (173). stimulates thymidine uptake and cell division in the oxyntic gland mucosa of the mouse (191) and increased

Most evidence of the trophic action of gastrin in man is indirect, stemming in large part from observations of mucosal hyperplasia in patients with hypergastrinemia (46,142) and atrophy in patients having undergone antrectomy (60,110). Olbe (146), however, was partially able to prevent the decrease in acid secretion in man following antrectomy by infusing pentagastrin continuously during the week after surgery. This finding indicates that exogenous gastrin prevents postantrectomy mucosal atrophy in man. Hansen et al. (70) found increased DNA synthesis in human oxyntic gland mucosa after high, but not low, doses of gastrin. This question, however, has not been approached with a carefully controlled and well-designed experiment utilizing a significant number of subjects.

Independence from secretion. Many experiments involving the trophic action of gastrin have included a group of histamine-injected animals to control for acid secretion. The results of these studies have been unanimous in that metabolic actions of gastrin were not duplicated by histamine in the species examined. These experiments have demonstrated gastrin stimulation of parietal cell hyperplasia (33), pancreatic hyperplasia (135), gastric and duodenal protein synthesis (87), gastric and duodenal RNA synthesis (22), DNA synthesis and growth of cultured duodenal cells (118), and gastric, duodenal, and ileal DNA synthesis (90,91).

The studies listed above were done on rats, and histamine is an extremely poor secretagogue in the rat compared to gastrin (83). Therefore, it can be argued that these experiments were not effectively controlled for the effects of acid secretion. For this reason, the study by Willems et al. (192) using the dog is especially significant. They infused either gastrin or histamine over a period of 4 hr in doses producing nearly identical acid outputs. Thymidine uptake into gastric mucosal cells and cell division were significantly stimulated in the animals receiving gastrin. There was no stimulation in any histamine-infused dog.

Further evidence that the trophic actions of gastrin are independent of secretory effects is provided by a study in which DNA synthesis in response to pentagastrin was studied in the presence of inhibitors of gastric acid secretion (91). Metiamide, a histamine receptor antagonist which also inhibits gastrin-stimulated acid secretion, was administered in combination with pentagastrin in a dose shown to block acid secretion almost completely. In this experiment pentagastrin alone caused a 40% stimulation of DNA synthesis in the oxyntic gland mucosa and an 80% increase in duodenal mucosa. These values were not significantly altered when metiamide was administered with pentagastrin.

From the foregoing discussion, it is also obvious that gastrin stimulates growth in numerous parts of the digestive tract which do not secrete acid. Other areas, such as the lower small intestinal mucosa, colonic mucosa, and the pancreas, are never exposed to acid. Yet doses of gastrin trophic for the mucosa of the oxyntic gland are trophic for these tissues as well. Secretin, which inhibits the trophic action of gastrin in the oxyntic gland area, is just as potent an inhibitor in small and large bowel mucosa. As one body of data these studies provide overwhelming evidence that the growth response to gastrin is unrelated to its secretory effects.

Evidence that gastrin acts directly. The best evidence that a hormone is acting directly on its target cells is the *in vitro* demonstration of its effects. Such a demonstration, of course, does not eliminate the possibility that a second messenger, such as one of the cyclic nucleotides, is involved in stimulating processes within the cell. It does, however, mean that the hormone is not causing the synthesis and/or release of a second agent which is transported by the blood to react with receptors in the target cells. Growth hormone and somatomedin offer the best example of this second type of process (35,36). Stimulation of sulfate uptake and protein synthesis in cartilage are widely recognized effects of growth hormone. These effects cannot be produced by adding growth hormone directly to cartilage *in vitro*. Plasma from normal rats added to cartilage from hypophysectomized rats, however, stimulates sulfate and amino acid incorporation (36). This "sulfation factor" contained in normal plasma has been identified as a peptide whose synthesis in the liver is dependent on growth hormone. This substance has been named somatomedin and is responsible for many, and perhaps most, of the effects of growth hormone (35).

There are several studies demonstrating trophic actions of gastrin *in vitro*. Miller et al. (139) found that pentagastrin at a concentration of 500 ng/ml maintained tissue cultures of rat and human oxyntic gland mucosa. Saline-treated cultures contained primarily fibroblasts whereas epithelial cells with junctional complexes predominated in the gastrin-inoculated flasks. At confluency, the mitotic activity of the pentagastrin-treated culture was more than twice that of controls. Gastrin-treated cultures contained twice the amount of protein when compared to control cultures started at the same time with identical inocula (139). Using organ cultures of oxyntic gland mucosa, Sutton and Donaldson (173) showed that although most secretagogues stimulated pepsinogen synthesis, only gastrin was capable of stimulating the synthesis of structural protein.

Lichtenberger et al. (118) examined the effects of pentagastrin on duodenal cells growing in tissue culture. After cultures of adult rat duodenal cells were established, the contents of half the flasks were exposed to pentagastrin once daily and half to saline. After 3 months, the pentagastrin-treated cultures contained approximately 90% epithelial cells and 10% fibroblasts, whereas the control cultures constituted an epithelial cell–fibroblast admixture of about 50% each. Epithelial cells appeared quite similar in structure to crypt cells, although a positive identification was not made. However, because gastrin-stimulated cultures of gastric mucosal cells also contained poorly differentiated cells, this evidence suggests that the trophic effect of gastrin is on generative cells in the mitotic locus and not on secretory cells. Pentagastrin-treated cultures had a faster doubling time, 19.5 hr compared with 31.5 hr for saline-treated controls. This was attributed in part to the greater percentage of cells in the proliferative population in the hormone-treated cultures, 73% in comparison to the controls, 36%. This latter measurement was arrived at by radioautographic determination of [³H]thymidine incorporation into DNA (Fig. 3).

The results of these *in vitro* studies employing organ and tissue culture techniques are proof that the trophic action of gastrin is due to a direct interaction of the hormone with receptors on its target cells, and not to a secondary factor released or synthesized by gastrin.

Molecular forms of gastrin and trophic activity. Most experiments involving the trophic effects of exogenous gastrin have utilized the synthetic analogue, pentagastrin. Gastrin was originally isolated by Gregory and Tracy (65) from porcine antral mucosa as the heptadecapeptide now referred to as G-17 or "little gastrin." Subsequently Yalow and Berson (200) found that the major circulating form of gastrin was a 34 amino acid peptide (G-34) which they named "big gastrin." Qualitatively the actions of pentagastrin, G-17, and G-34 in mammalian systems have proven to be identical although their potencies differ (183). The results of a study designed to compare the trophic activity of the circulating gastrins with that of pentagastrin were not unexpected (93). Those results were in general agreement with the structure-activity relationships of the gas-

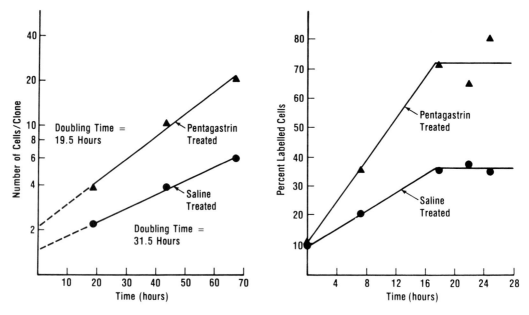

FIG. 3. Growth curves of duodenal cells in culture (*left panel*) show doubling times of pentagastrin- and saline-treated cells. Each point represents the mean number of cells per clone from 20 readings. *Right panel* shows percentage of cells in proliferative pools of pentagastrin- and saline-treated cultures. Each point represents the percentage of cells labeled with [³H]thymidine in a field of 1,000 cells. From Lichtenberger et al. (118).

trin molecules as determined for their stimulation of acid secretion. The maximal effects of G-34 II, G-17 I, G-17 II, and pentagastrin on DNA synthesis and DNA accumulation in duodenal and oxyntic gland mucosa were equal (Fig. 4). Peek stimulation occurred with 6.75 nmoles/kg G-34 II, 13.5nmoles/kg G-17 I and G-17 II, and 32.5nmoles/kg pentagastrin. From this study we concluded that the naturally occurring gastrins possess trophic activity, sulfation has no effect on trophic activity, and G-17 and G-34 are at least as effective in stimulating growth as they are in stimulating gastric acid secretion (93).

Doses required for trophic effect. In order for an effect of a hormone to be considered physiological, that effect should occur with an infusion of exogenous hormone which does not increase serum levels of the hormone above those which result after the release of the hormone by normal stimuli. Ryan et al. (158) tested whether exogenous gastrin, at a dose which increased serum gastrin levels the same amount as a meat meal, would stimulate DNA synthesis in dog oxyntic gland mucosa. After a 24-hr fast either saline, histamine (24 μg/kg-hr, or G-17 II (160 ng/kg-hr) was infused into conscious dogs for 4 hr. The doses of histamine and gastrin used elicited one-half maximal gastric acid secretion in the same dogs. At various times before, during, and after infusion mucosal biopsies were taken from both the vagally denervated pouches and the gastric remnant. Gastrin caused significant three- to five-fold increases in DNA synthesis 16 and 20 hr after the start of infusion when compared to zero time or to results with saline and histamine at the same time. Feeding a meat meal to the same dogs produced similar increases in DNA synthesis. Serum gastrin levels in response to gastrin infusion and the meat meal were not statistically different. The authors concluded that the trophic effect of gastrin was a physiological action of the hormone (158).

CCK

CCK is structurally and functionally related to gastrin. The active C-terminal tetrapeptide amide of gastrin is duplicated in CCK. The major structural difference which dictates whether a peptide of the CCK-gastrin family has a gastrin-like or CCK-like pattern of activity is the position of the tyrosyl residue and whether or not it is sulfated (98). Qualitatively the actions of gastrin and CCK are identical, but gastrin has high affinity for receptors stimulating acid secretion and low affinity for those involved in gallbladder contraction and pancreatic enzyme secretion. The opposite pattern prevails for peptides more closely related to CCK. Owing to the overlapping activity patterns and the tendency for CCK to have a higher affinity for tissues located more distally in the digestive tract, it seemed likely that CCK would have trophic influences on the pancreas and small intestine.

Most studies involving the trophic action of CCK have been conducted on the pancreas and are covered in Chapter 34 of these volumes together with the actions of all the gut hormones and pancreatic growth. The effects of CCK on growth of oxyntic gland and duodenal mucosa have been examined in only one published study (92). Low doses of CCK octapeptide (CCK-OP) causing a small but significant increase in pancreatic DNA synthesis had no stimulatory effect on mucosa of the oxyntic gland area or duodenum of the same animals. DNA concentration of the pancreas was also increased, indicating that the increase in synthesis was not matched by an increase in turnover. At higher doses of CCK-OP there was a slight increase in duodenal DNA synthesis and concentration which was of borderline statistical significance. Further increasing the dose of CCK-OP inhibited the trophic effect of pentagastrin in both the stomach and duodenum. We concluded that although

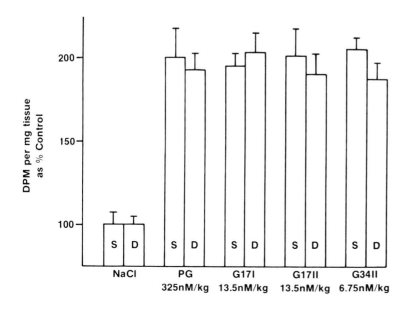

FIG. 4. Incorporation of [³H]thymidine into DNA of oxyntic gland (S) and duodenal (D) mucosa in response to maximally effective (as determined by dose-response curves) doses of pentagastrin (PG), G-17 I, G-17 II, and G-34 II. Means and SEs from 12 observations. From Johnson and Guthrie (93).

CCK is probably a physiologically important regulator of growth of the exocrine pancreas, it is unlikley that it exerts a trophic influence on either the stomach or duodenum (92).

Secretin

There have been relatively few studies involving the trophic action of secretin on the mucosa of the gastrointestinal tract. In general, secretin appears to inhibit the trophic actions of gastrin and to have no antitrophic activity of its own. In one study, rats having gastric cannulas were injected three times daily for 2 weeks with pentagastrin, secretin, pentagastrin plus secretin, or saline (168). Basal and maximal acid outputs were measured before, during, and after the injection period. Parietal cell mass was determined at the end of the study. Pentagastrin injection led to a 90% increase in maximal acid output. This increase failed to occur in the rats receiving secretin in addition to pentagastrin. The parietal cell population increased by 70% in the gastrin-injected rats. This too was prevented by secretin. The animals receiving only secretin had slightly lower secretory capacities and parietal cell counts than the saline-injected controls (168).

Secretin has been shown to inhibit the gastrin stimulation of DNA synthesis and accumulation in mucosa of the oxyntic gland area of the stomach, the duodenum (91), and the colon (94). The effects of secretin do not depend on its ability to inhibit gastrin-stimulated acid secretion, since metiamide, a potent inhibitor of acid secretion, had no significant effect on the trophic response to gastrin (91). Pansu et al. (148) found that secretin prevented the peaks in the labeling and mitotic indices in the circadian rhythm of rat jejunal mucosa. Pentagastrin, on the other hand, prevented the nadirs. These authors concluded that secretin and gastrin act as trophic factors for intestinal mucosa producing opposite effects on cell proliferation (148).

The remaining question is whether secretin has antitrophic activity of its own or whether it acts solely by inhibiting the growth-promoting effects of gastrin. Considering the profound inhibition of gastrin trophic activity caused by secretin, it is entirely possible that these antitrophic effects were due to the inhibition of endogenous gastrin. Because it is almost impossible to remove all sources of gastrin surgically, this point will best be settled by studying the metabolic effects of secretin on *in vitro* systems involving cell or organ culture.

The trophic effects of two additional members of the secretin family, vasoactive intestinal peptide (VIP) and glaucagon, have been examined in mucosa of the oxyntic gland and proximal colon (84). Like secretin, VIP had no effect on DNA synthesis when given by itself and inhibited the stimulation caused by gastrin. Glu-

cagon, however, stimulated DNA synthesis at several doses. The maximal effect of glucagon equalled about 50% of the increase caused by pentagastrin in the same experiments. Glucagon produced no inhibition of the trophic action of gastrin. There is no evidence supporting a physiological role for either VIP or glucagon in the regulation of mucosal growth.

Epidermal Growth Factor

Originally isolated by Cohen (27) from mouse submaxillary glands, epidermal growth factor (EGF) has been shown to stimulate epithelial cell proliferation in a number of tissue and organ culture systems from the human, mouse, and chicken (28). In 1972, Savage et al. (162) isolated and purified EGF showing that it was a polypeptide containing 53 amino acids.

Gregory (63) purified urogastrone in 1975 and noted that it closely resemebled EGF. Urogastrone also contains 53 amino acid residues and 37 of these are identical to those of EGF. Although it is likely that EGF and urogastrone are identical substances, it remains to be proven since their structures have not been determined in the same species.

Urogastrone was discovered following the observation that extracts of urine from pregnant women had a beneficial effect on experimental ulcers in dogs (161). Urogastrone was named for its ability to inhibit gastric acid secretion, and this action is shared by EGF (28). Also, urogastrone competes with EGF for receptor sites on cultured human fibroblasts (79). Human urogastrone also stimulates precocious eye opening in newborn mice in doses identical to EGF (79).

Feldman et al. (51) have shown that EGF stimulates ornithine decarboxylase activity in the stomach and duodenum of 8-day-old mice. Ornithine decarboxylase is a necessary enzyme in the synthesis of polyamines. Evidence exists relating polyamines to RNA synthesis and indicating that ornithine decarboxylase may actually activate RNA polymerase I (157). Thus the induction of ornithine decarboxylase activity has been used as an index of the trophic response.

Recently, Johnson and Guthrie (95) examined the trophic effects of EGF on gastrointestinal mucosa comparing them to those of pentagastrin. EGF was a potent stimulator of DNA synthesis in the oxyntic gland mucosa with maximal effects equal to those of pentagastrin. Unlike pentagastrin, EGF did not stimulate growth of duodenal and colonic mucosa. Neither peptide altered DNA synthesis in the skin. Secretin inhibited the trophic activity of pentagastrin but not EGF. Chronic administration (5 days) of EGF caused significant increases in oxyntic gland mucosal DNA, RNA, and protein content. EGF, therefore, is a potent stimulant of oxyntic gland mucosal growth in the rat. Whether this action is biologically significant depends on the demonstration that EGF is released into either the blood or gastric mucosa in amounts adequate to stimulate growth.

Endogenous Gastrin and Growth

Another criterion which must be satisfied before a particular action of an exogenously administered hormone can be proven to be physiological is that the effect in question can be produced by endogenous hormone. The lack of readily available and reproducible radioimmunoassays for secretin and CCK has made it impossible to correlate endogenous levels of these hormones with growth. There have been recent improvements in the secretin assay, but they have not yet been applied to studies involving growth of the mucosa. There are also no accepted methods for producing chronic alterations in serum secretin and CCK levels. On the other hand, endogenous levels of gastrin (as discussed earlier) can be altered chronically over a wide range of values and quantitated by standardized radioimmunoassays.

Growth of human oxyntic gland mucosa can be correlated with endogenous gastrin in cases of Zollinger-Ellison syndrome or partial gastric resection (as previously discussed in detail). Gastrin levels have been altered experimentally in animals by surgery or feeding experiments.

Antrectomy

In a recent study rats were either antrectomized to remove the primary source of gastrin or subjected to a sham operation (38). Three weeks later half the antrectomized rats were injected with pentagastrin (250 μg/kg) 4 times per day for 7 days. Antrectomy lowered serum gastrin levels to one-third normal. Serum gastrin levels in these three groups are shown in Fig. 5. Since pentagastrin is not recognized by the antibody used for the radioimmunoassay, and also because it is rapidly de-

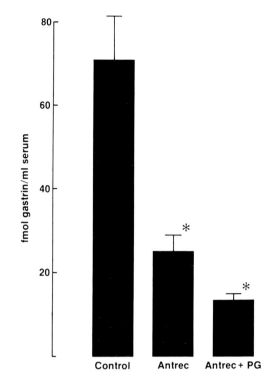

FIG. 5. Serum gastrin levels in control, antrectomized, and antrectomized rats treated with pentagastrin. Means and SEM of 23 observations in each group. *, $p < 0.001$ compared to control. From Dembinski and Johnson (38).

stroyed, the rats receiving pentagastrin also have low serum gastrin levels. Organ weight, DNA synthesis, and RNA and DNA content were significantly reduced in all tissues where gastrin is known to exert a trophic effect (pancreas and mucosa of the oxyntic gland area, duodenum, and colon), but not in the liver or the kidney. In each case pentagastrin treatment of antrectomized rats prevented the decreases. The data for RNA and DNA of colonic mucosa are shown in Fig. 6. These results indicate that endogenous gastrin has an important role in regulation of the growth of these tissues and sup-

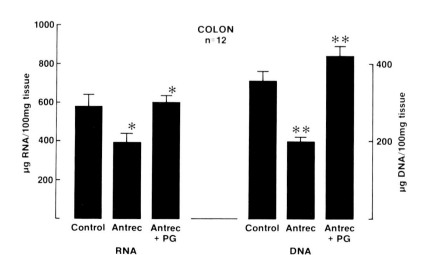

FIG. 6. Colonic DNA and RNA content of mucosa from rats described in Fig. 5 *, $p < 0.001$ compared to both control and antrectomy plus pentagastrin. From Dembinski and Johnson (38).

port previous studies involving duodenal and oxyntic gland mucosa in which serum gastrin was not measured (73,89,133).

In the studies by Martin et al. (133) and Helander (73) mentioned above, antrectomy caused decreases in peptic cell counts. In fact, 9 weeks after antrectomy peptic cell counts had decreased from 67 to 16 million (133). It has been previously mentioned that long-term administration of exogenous pentagastrin to normal, intact rats increases parietal but not peptic cell counts (33,191). This apparent discrepancy between the effects of exogenous and endogenous gastrin has several possible explanations. First, the sensitivities of the preparations are different. A normal, intact rat has sufficient circulating gastrin to maintain normal growth. Large doses of exogenous gastrin must be used to see a further effect, and the parietal cell mass may be increased more easily than the peptic cell mass. Second, maintenance of peptic cell mass may require a background presence of gastrin which is removed by antrectomy. Third, antrectomy could have resulted in gastritis which in turn, caused a loss of all cells. The question of whether gastrin regulates peptic cell growth could be answered by measuring peptic cell mass in control, antrectomized, and antrectomized animals treated chronically with gastrin.

Following antrectomy in the rat, the number and granularity of oxyntic gland endocrine-like cells also decrease (67). Hakanson et al. (67) found that the two main endocrine cell types, enterochromaffin-like cells and A-like cells, had fewer granules, smaller granules, and a lower concentration of granules in the cytoplasm following antrectomy. They interpreted their findings as indicating that gastrin had trophic effects on oxyntic gland endocrine cells as well as the secretory cells.

The role of endogenous gastrin in the growth of oxyntic gland mucosa was approached somewhat differently by Willems et al. (190). They first produced hypergastrinemia in dogs with Heidenhain pouches by removing the antrums from exposure to acid. Following this procedure, DNA synthesis, acid secretion, and the mitotic index increased significantly. Subsequent antrectomy resulted in a reduction of these parameters. In all cases, DNA synthesis was positively correlated with serum gastrin levels.

Gastric mucosal atrophy in humans following antrectomy is well documented (60,110). There have, however, been two studies designed to examine the role of endogenous gastrin on growth of the human stomach. Sipponen et al. (166) examined 41 patients who had undergone antrectomy 17 to 18 years earlier. Twenty-seven of these had atrophic gastritis and thirteen had a selective loss of parietal cells without gastritis or other inflammation. They concluded that these changes were due to the absence of the trophic effects of gastrin. Hansen et al. (69) measured *in vitro* [³H]thymidine in-

corporation into fundic mucosal biopsy samples from normal and antrectomized humans. DNA synthesis was accelerated after antrectomy, which they attributed to gastritis. This study, therefore, did little to elucidate the role of gastrin in human mucosal growth. It is obvious that because of problems in designing human studies, it will be extremely difficult to obtain definitive measurements of the trophic action of gastrointestinal hormones in man.

Feeding Studies

Evidence that the trophic actions of gastrin are physiologically significant comes from examining growth of the gastrointestinal tract after natural alteration of serum and antral gastrin levels. Gastrin levels change dramatically due to a number of developmental and physiological events. It is possible to exaggerate and prolong these changes without resorting to surgery.

Starvation is known to cause changes in small intestinal structure and function. Villus and crypt height in the rat are diminished after 3 to 6 days starvation (3, 128), and mucosal RNA, DNA, and protein content are markedly decreased after 3 to 6 days starvation (120, 171). These decreases are significantly greater than the loss of body weight. Over 3 days of starvation, rat antral gastrin levels dropped from 32 μg/g of wet weight to 5 μg/g of wet weight, and serum gastrin concentration decreased from 330 to 70 pg/ml (120). In these same animals, intestinal DNA, RNA, and protein content decreased significantly compared with body weight. Specific lactase and maltase activity increased. Animals injected with pentagastrin during the period of starvation showed significantly smaller changes than the starved saline-injected control rats (120).

Ingestion of a meal is followed by increases in DNA synthesis and in the mitotic index of canine fundic mucosa (193). This pattern can be reproduced by a 4-hr infusion of gastrin (192), suggesting that gastrin might be one of the factors responsible for postprandial cell renewal.

Although the studies mentioned above implicate decreased gastrin levels as part of the cause of the profound deleterious effects which short periods of starvation have on the gut, interpretation of these studies is made difficult by the inability to separate the metabolic changes associated with starvation from those caused purely by the absence of food from the gut. Our laboratory has used the intravenously alimented rat as a model to study gut structure and function in the well-nourished animal whose gastrointestinal tract has gone unexposed to food and the stimuli arising from its ingestion and presence. Several findings from these studies are of special significance. First, the parenterally fed animals often gained weight and always remained in positive nitrogen balance (21). Second, tissue to body weight ratios for oxyntic gland area, small intestine, and pancreas were significantly decreased in the parenterally fed animals, whereas the weights of other organs were unaffected (89,96). Third, specific and total activities of the different disaccharidase enzymes were only a fraction of those found in the orally fed controls (21, 96). Fourth, the parenterally fed animals were nearly depleted of antral gastrin (89,96). Fifth, these results could not be completely explained on the basis of food intake, dietary constituents, enzyme induction, or the absence of luminally derived nutrition in the parenterally fed animals.

In the latest of these studies, one group of parenterally nourished animals received a continuous infusion of 6.0 µg/kg-hr pentagastrin, a dose considerably less than the D_{50} for acid secretion in this species (96). The animals were killed approximately 2 weeks later and compared with parenterally fed rats which had received either histamine or nothing in addition to the intravenous diet. Serum as well as antral gastrin concentrations decreased significantly in all groups of parenterally fed animals. Weights of the oxyntic gland area, small intestine, and pancreas decreased significantly in all parenterally fed rats except those receiving gastrin. Gastrin completely prevented the decrease in disaccharidase activity normally associated with total parenteral nutrition. These data were interpreted to indicate that the oral ingestion of food and its presence in the gastrointestinal tract are necessary to maintain endogenous gastrin levels, and that the trophic action of endogenous gastrin is essential for the day-to-day maintenance of the structural and functional integrity of the gut (96).

Viewed as one body of evidence, the parallelism between serum and antral gastrin levels and growth of gastrointestinal tract tissue is striking. In each instance, decreased endogenous gastrin levels were associated with decreased growth, and the addition of exogenous gastrin was able to significantly increase growth towards normal levels. In the study involving parenterally fed animals the dose of gastrin infused was well below the limit considered to be physiological. Since the effects of exogenous gastrin in this study were dramatic (96), it may indicate that the continuing presence of a low level of the hormone is more effective in stimulating growth than periodic extreme fluctuations in hormone concentration. In summary, the results from studies of the effects of exogenous gastrin on mucosal growth and the correlation between endogenous gastrin levels and growth of the mucosa provide strong evidence that the trophic effect of gastrin is an important physiological action—as important as any action of the hormone.

Biochemical Mechanisms

The initial binding of a peptide hormone to its receptor begins a chain of events leading to the overt manifestation of hormone action. This process can be divided into the receptor-hormone interaction itself, transmission of that interaction to the synthetic processes of the cell, and, finally, the biochemical responses which result in the action in question. Knowledge of these processes for the gastrointestinal hormones lags far behind that of similar events related to other endocrines. These events have been best described in the digestive tract for the stimulation of pancreatic acinar cell secretion (*see* Chapter 33). The only similar studies on mucosal tissues and the only studies relating to growth have been with gastrin.

Receptors

A receptor is a macromolecule that specifically binds a hormone, forming a hormone-receptor complex. This binding is the recognition step which initiates cellular events eventually manifested as the physiological effects of the hormone. Biologically active labeled hormone and a standardized assay system are the first steps necessary for studying the interaction of a hormone with its receptor. In order to establish that the binding measurements obtained are a true reflection of hormone-receptor interaction in a pharmacological and a biological sense, five criteria must be satisfied. First, the receptor must have a finite binding capacity. Second, the binding reaction should have an affinity sufficiently high to be in accord with the tissue sensitivity to physiological levels of the hormone. Third, the receptor must bind the hormone specifically. Fourth, the receptor should be restricted to organs or tissues with a physiological sensitivity to the ligand. Fifth, a receptor-dependent hormonal response should be identified.

Takeuchi et al. (175) have recently reported the development of a standardized assay for measuring the binding of biologically active [^{125}I]15-leucine gastrin-17 to rat mucosal membranes and described some of the physical characteristics of the binding (176). The receptor and its interaction with gastrin satisfy the first four criteria listed above (175). The binding is saturable with a dissociation constant (K_D) of 4×10^{-10}M. This K_D compared favorably with serum gastrin levels in the rat which range from 2 to 4×10^{-10}M. The receptor is present in equal amounts in duodenal and oxyntic gland mucosa and absent from antral mucosa, spleen, kidney, and liver. The receptor binds G-17 and to a lesser extent cholecystokinin, cerulein, and pentagastrin. Secretin inhibits binding but does so in a noncompetitive fashion.

Whether this receptor is responsible for the trophic effect of gastrin is unknown. It is present in both duodenal and oxyntic gland mucosa whose growth is influenced by gastrin, and absent from antral mucosa, which is not affected. One characteristic of several trophic peptide hormones is that they regulate the numbers of their own receptors (58,152). Since hormone receptors turn over rapidly, the regulation of receptor concentration may play an important part in the overall endocrine regulation of physiological responses. In partial fulfillment of the criterion that hormone binding be associated with a biological response, the gastrin binding capacity has been shown to be related directly to serum gastrin levels (177). Decreasing serum gastrin levels by fasting, feeding liquid diets, or antrectomy caused significant decreases in receptor numbers. These decreases were prevented by treating the rats with exogenous pentagastrin. Vagotomy significantly increased both serum gastrin levels and the concentration of gastrin receptors. These data indicate that gastrin stimulates the production of its own receptor. The upregulation of the receptor was evident if binding capacity was expressed per milligram protein, per microgram DNA, or per amount of [^{125}I]cholergen specifically bound to the same membrane preparations.

Final proof that the receptor in question is responsible for the trophic action of gastrin awaits experiments correlating that binding with a trophic response *in vitro*. Nevertheless, it is likely that the trophic receptor present in cells which divide such as the mucous neck cells of the oxyntic gland mucosa is identical to the gastrin receptor present on differentiated cells which have arisen from the stem cell. The finding that the concentration of gastrin receptors is regulated and that regulation is at least in part due to gastrin introduces into gastrointestinal physiology the entire concept of hormone receptor regulation. This concept has many obvious ramifications in explaining end-organ response to hormones. The acid secretory dose-response curve to gastrin, for example, is shifted to the left in patients with duodenal ulcer disease. Whether this and other examples of incongruency between serum hormone levels and response can be explained by changes in receptor concentrations awaits further study.

Second Messengers

The second messengers involved in the trophic responses to gastrointestinal hormones have not been studied. This is obviously an area for future investigation. Chapter 34 of this volume contains a discussion of second messengers for the action of gastrointestinal hormones on the pancreas, the tissue for which most information is available.

Macromolecular Synthesis

The earliest response related to growth following the administration of gastrin is a significant increase in mRNA (48). Significant increases in mRNA occur 30 to 60 min after gastrin treatment. By 2 to 3 hr, all other species of RNA are also significantly increased (48). Majumdar and Goltermann (130) found a 100% increase in the number of gastric mucosal polysomes 1 hr after the injection of pentagastrin in fasted rats. This observation supports the finding of Enochs and Johnson (48) that stimulation of mRNA production is one of the earliest events associated with the trophic action of gastrin. Protein synthesis begins to increase 2 to 4 hr after gastrin injection and peaks at 6 hr (48). In organ cultures of gastric mucosa, protein synthesis was increased 7 hr after gastrin treatment (173). Inhibition of mRNA synthesis with actinomycin-D prevents the gastrin-induced stimulation of protein synthesis (48). Sixteen hours after gastrin injection DNA synthesis is maximally elevated in the gastric mucosa of both the rat (48) and dog (192). The mitotic index in canine gastric mucosa is increased five-fold at 20 and 24 hr (192). The time courses of the changes in protein and nucleic acid synthesis following gastrin injection are summarized in Fig. 7.

Majumdar and Goltermann (131) have provided evidence that chronic treatment with pentagastrin increases

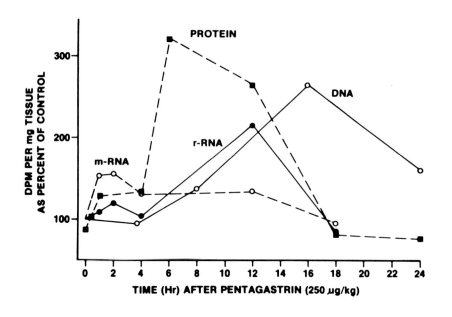

FIG. 7. Comparison of time sequences for the stimulation of macromolecular synthesis in the rat oxyntic gland mucosa following a single injection of pentagastrin (250 μg/kg) at 0 time. Results are expressed as percentages of data from saline-injected control animals killed at the same times. From Enochs and Johnson (48).

the translational ability of the ribosomes in addition to stimulating mRNA synthesis and polysome formation (transcription). Following chronic administration of the hormone the capacity of gastric mucosal ribosomes to synthesize both endogenous and exogenous mRNA-(poly(U))-directed protein in a cell-free system is stimulated, whereas after a single injection of gastrin only endogenous mRNA-directed protein synthesis is increased (130). Further evidence that chronic treatment with gastrin increased translational ability of the ribosomes was the observation that mRNA-free ribosomes had a greater capacity for polyphenylalanine synthesis than similar ribosomes from control animals (131).

This picture of the biochemical events following the injection of gastrin is consistent with the known mechanisms of action of other trophic hormones. Korner (102) has shown that hypophysectomized animals have a deficiency in the formation of polyribosomes which can be corrected by addition of polyuridine, indicating a decreased availability of mRNA. The addition of growth hormone resulted in an initial stimulation of mRNA followed by increases in all types of RNA and the stimulation of protein synthesis (103). Subsequent experiments indicated that growth hormone facilitated the formation of DNA-RNA polymerase complex and hence RNA synthesis (150).

The next step in elucidating the mechanism by which gastrin stimulates growth of gastrointestinal mucosa would be the *in vitro* correlation of receptor binding with one of the above-mentioned components of the pleiotypic response. Ideally one would then proceed to correlate binding and this response with the formation or uptake of a second messenger.

NONGASTROINTESTINAL HORMONES

Pituitary Hypophysectomy

General effects of the pituitary gland on growth are based on studies of hypophysectomized animals. The literature is replete with evidence that the pituitary is necessary to maintain the normal functional and structural development and integrity of the gastrointestinal tract (6,32,113,136).

Hypophysectomy leads to a marked decrease in gastric acid secretion in man, dog, rat, and cat (32). This decrease occurs rapidly with a 50% reduction in secretion 3 days after surgery in the rat. Under the same conditions pepsin output falls 90% within a week. These functional changes are accompanied by degranulation and involution of chief cells (6), involution of parietal cells, and decreased total activity of oxidative enzymes (6,8). In the rat, these decreases occur steadily over the first 12 days after hypophysectomy and then plateau (32).

In the pancreas, as in the stomach, total enzymatic activity is reduced by cellular atrophy, but the specific activities remain the same. Total pancreatic weight and RNA content are decreased (136).

Atrophic changes in the small intestine after hypophysectomy include decreased wet and dry weight, mitotic activity, villus height, and intestinal diameter (81, 183). Hypophysectomy also decreased the incorporation of thymidine and orotic acid into DNA and RNA of gut mucosa (114). The incorporation of amino acids into protein is also lowered, but the proportion of polysomes remains the same. Following hypophysectomy, however, the ability of polysomes to incorporate amino acids is impaired (114).

Despite the well-documented changes following hypophysectomy which are outlined above, there are numerous reports showing no change or opposite effects. These discrepancies have several sources which one should be aware of:

1. The completeness of hypophysectomy has not always been verified.

2. There are differences in response between species.

3. Hypophysectomy leads to a marked decrease in appetite, yet few studies have accounted for the difference in food intake. Pair feeding should be utilized to eliminate the effects of varied nutritional status, local nutrition, and gastrointestinal hormones on the metabolic and functional activity of the gastrointestinal tract. Pair feeding itself, however, creates a difficult problem. On the one hand, reduced appetite and food intake in the presence of reduced metabolic requirements affect gastrointestinal function in hypophysectomized animals. On the other hand, feeding intact animals the same diet as hypophysectomized animals induces in the former a state of semi-starvation with its incumbent and incompletely understood metabolic and hormonal effects.

4. The response to hypophysectomy and hormonal replacement may vary seasonally.

5. Proliferative activity in both the stomach and intestine follows a circadian rhythm. In rats, mitotic activity of the mucous neck cells of the gastric mucosa is greatest between 4 and 8 a.m. (24). In contrast, peak mitotic activity in the jejunum occurs around 11 p.m. (148). Hypophysectomy increased the mitotic rate of immature mucous cells while decreasing that of the mucous neck cells in the rat (24). Thus the time of day animals are killed may affect results differently in different tissues, and the effect seen may depend on the cell type.

6. Finally, and perhaps most importantly, the interpretation of studies involving hypophysectomy is difficult, since one is dealing with changes in many hormones as well as stress.

Of particular interest is the concept that hypophysectomy is associated with decreased release and tissue levels of gastrointestinal hormones. As early as 1952, Dorchester and Haist (40,41) reported that the secretin content of the small intestine was decreased 50% in hypophysectomized rats. It was not until 1973 that the relationship between the pituitary and gastrointestinal hormones was re-examined. Mayston and Barrowman (136) demonstrated that atrophic changes in the pancreas and duodenal mucosa of hypophysectomized rats could be prevented with pentagastrin. This finding led to the examination of gastrin levels in hypophysectomized rats. Hypophysectomy resulted in a 60% decrease of serum gastrin and an 80% decrease in antral gastrin content compared to normal, intact, pair-fed controls (47).

Interesting information regarding the role of the pituitary in gut growth has recently been provided by Lichtenberger and Bartke (115). Snell dwarf mice which have a hereditary deficiency of prolactin, growth hormone, and TSH were found to have only 30% of the antral gastrin concentration of their normal littermates. In addition, the duodenal mucosa of the mutants was thin, and there were significant reductions in the number of mitoses per crypt, crypt length, and villus height. Transplantation of a normal pituitary under the renal capsule significantly increased gastrin levels, mitoses, and the crypt length (115).

The identification of the pituitary hormone responsible for the maintenance of gastrin levels is not certain. Evidence discussed below indicates that growth hormone is involved. The relationships between gastrointestinal and pituitary and pituitary-dependent hormones have only just begun to be identified. This field promises to be one of the more interesting areas of gastrointestinal endocrinology in the future.

Growth Hormone

In view of its known function in promoting general body and tissue growth, there is a surprising paucity of information concerning the trophic activity of growth hormone on gastrointestinal tissues. In the few studies that are available, interpretation is made difficult by the fact that most animals were not pair fed. In some of the earlier studies, reviewed by Crean (32), it was suggested that growth hormone (GH), in combination with other anterior pituitary hormones, cortisone, and thyroxin was capable of reducing cellular atrophy in the stomach of hypophysectomized animals. This ability was dependent on almost immediate replacement therapy. If replacement was delayed beyond 2 weeks, cytological changes were inevitable although gastric secretion was restored.

Evidence of trophic activity following GH treatment is fairly conclusive and consistent. However, whether these are direct effects of GH or secondary effects of increased food intake, improved nutrition, or the food-

stimulated release of secondary hormones, such as gastrin, is difficult to determine. Sesso and Valeri (165) showed an increase in pancreatic weight as well as DNA and RNA content in GH-treated hypophysectomized rats. Leblond and Carriere (108) demonstrated that GH stimulated an increase in mitotic rate in the crypt cells of the duodenum in hypophysectomized or thyroidectomized rats. However, these rats were not pair fed.

The possibility that GH stimulates secondary gastrointestinal hormone release was first suggested by the experiments of Dorchester and Haist (41) in which weight and secretin content of atrophic small intestine of hypophysectomized rats were increased by multiple injections of GH, ACTH, or anterior pituitary extracts. Thyroid extracts had no effect on either intestinal weight or secretin content. An increase in secretin content was not stimulated in pair-fed intact rats except by anterior pituitary extracts. The fact that secretin content in hypophysectomized rats was increased to intact levels, but not greater, would suggest a permissive role for GH and ACTH. The purity of these hormonal preparations was questionable so that cross-contamination is a possibility. Whether the increase in secretin content was the result of a specific stimulus or of a general increase in protein synthesis and anabolic activity is not known. Since both GH and ACTH stimulate acid secretion, which in turn stimulates secretin release, it is also possible that increased secretin content was secondary to increased acid output. Acid secretion was not measured.

The work of Mayston and Barrowman (136) strongly suggests that pituitary hormones influence gastrin release. The fact that pentagastrin treatment prevents atrophy of the pancreas, duodenum, and gastric fundic mucosa in hypophysectomized rats implies that gastrin levels are low in the latter. Several other reports suggest that GH might stimulate gastrin release. Patients with acromegaly exhibit parietal cell hyperplasia and elevated maximal histamine response (68). Pearse and Bussolati (149) found increased antral G cell numbers and antral gastrin content in acromegalic patients. In order to explore this possibility, Enochs and Johnson (47) looked at serum and antral gastrin levels in pair-fed hypophysectomized and intact rats treated for 10 days with bovine GH. Growth hormone elevated both serum and antral gastrin concentrations only in hypophysectomized rats. It was ineffective at low doses (100 to 200 µg/ day) or after a single injection. Doses of 500 µg/day restored serum gastrin to intact levels and partially restored antral gastrin. Therefore the persistent presence of adequate levels of circulating GH may be permissive for the release and possibly for the synthesis of gastrin. Since antral gastrin, although elevated, remained significantly lower than in intact animals, it is probable that GH alone is not a sufficient stimulus for complete restoration of antral activity. It is quite likely that other pituitary hormones such as prolactin and ACTH, or corticosteroids, are also necessary. The decreased food intake of hypophysectomized animals may account in part for incomplete recovery of antral gastrin content. On the other hand, GH release-inhibiting hormone, somatostatin, which is present in large quantities in the stomach and pancreas as well as in the hypothalamus, has been shown to inhibit gastrin release.

Thus the evidence for a physiological role of GH in regulating growth of gastrointestinal tissues, although sparse, is consistent and convincing in light of its known anabolic effects on other tissues. However, this effect may, in part, be mediated by secondary factors such as improved nutrition and gastrin release.

The trophic effect of growth hormone on the gastric mucosa has been implicated as a possible mechanism for the protective effect growth hormone exerts against both stress (156) and steroid (181) induced gastric ulcers. Interestingly, gastrin, by virtue of its trophic effects, also protects against stress-induced ulcers (174). Almost all research into the mechanisms of ulcer formation has been directed toward the destructive factors (acid, pepsin, bile) acting on the gastric mucosa. It appears that those influences stimulating cell regeneration are also important and should be the subject of future studies in this field.

Thyroid Hormone

Thyroxin in physiological quantities exerts an anabolic effect leading to increased total body growth, as well as growth of most tissues. This anabolic effect derives from a general increase in metabolic rate including an increase in protein and RNA synthesis. The regulation of body growth depends on adequate amounts of both GH and thyroxin as evidenced by the development of dwarfism in cases of isolated GH or thyroid deficiency. The interdependence of these two hormones is also evident in the study of gastrointestinal growth. Rats thyroidectomized shortly after weaning fail to exhibit a normal increase in body weight or an increase in the number of cells and mitoses in the duodenal crypts (19, 108). Administration of thyroxin over an extended period of time resulted in body weight gain and restoration of crypt cell number and mitotic activity. Growth hormone led to similar but less pronounced increases. In hypophysectomized rats, thyroxin failed to increase the mitotic rate unless administered with GH, whereas GH alone was effective. Eartly and Leblond (45) suggested that at least part of the trophic action of thyroxin was secondary to increased endogenous release of GH. Unfortunately, effects of increased food intake were not ruled out. However, as shown by Levin (113), the effect of thyroxin is probably not entirely due to increased food consumption. Administration of 0.1% dinitrophenol in the diet of intact rats mimicked hyperphagic and temperature changes elicited by thyroxin. However, no increase in intestinal weight occured, whereas thyroxin or thyroid extract produced intestinal hypertrophy in intact rats.

The effects of thyroidectomy are apparently less pronounced in the stomach, where gastric secretion, but not mucosal growth, is decreased (32). In the pancreas of hypophysectomized rats, thyroxin leads to weight gain and an increase in RNA content and concentration, but no change in DNA content (165). Growth hormone led to similar increases, including an increase in DNA content. It was concluded that thyroxin could produce hypertrophy of the pancreas, but that hyperplasia depended on the presence of GH. The restoration of normal pancreatic proteolytic activity was dependent on the combined administration of GH, corticosterone, thyroxin, and insulin (7). It was found that thyroid extracts were completely ineffective in preventing the loss of secretin content of the small intestine (41).

ACTH and the Adrenals

An evaluation of the role of ACTH and the adrenocortical hormones on growth of the gastrointestinal tract is made difficult by the large number of contradictory reports in the literature. The effects of these hormones depend on dose, type of steroid, duration of treatment, and age of the animal being studied. Adrenal hormones have a well-established role in gut development, which will be covered in the next section. The current discussion will be restricted to effects in adult animals.

The effects of adrenalectomy and treatment with ACTH and adrenal cortical hormones have been extensively reviewed by Crean (32). Adrenalectomy leads to reduced secretory function in man and experimental animals. In the rat, this decrease is accompanied by marked involution of zymogen cells but not parietal cells. The rat appears to be remarkably resistant to the effects of adrenalectomy, since the parietal cell population and mucosal volume remain intact. In contrast, the cat and man exhibit various degrees of gastric and intestinal atrophy following adrenalectomy. However, these changes are much less marked than those produced by hypophysectomy. The atrophy also depends on whether or not the adrenalectomized animals are maintained on saline or tap water (113). Those given saline retain normal appetites and less atrophy results.

Studies of the effects of ACTH and adrenal steroids on gastric secretory function are contradictory and vary with duration of treatment. In general, acute studies have failed to show an increase in acid or pepsin secretion (32). More prolonged administration of these substances has been shown to increase acid content, volume, and pepsin secretion in rats and dogs (32,167). In man, Hitzelberger and Glass (78) noted an inconsistent increase in acid and volume, and a twofold increase in pepsin secretion after several weeks of steroid treatment. In one study, intravenous administration of ACTH increased acid secretion in the dog by 61% (59). Antral resection decreased this response, and antrectomy plus vagatomy completely abolished the effect. This study suggests that both the antrum and vagal innervation modify the effects of ACTH.

Recent studies indicate that glucocorticoids have a regulatory influence on gastrin production by the antrum, and therefore provide presumptive evidence that the effects of ACTH and glucocorticoids are in part mediated by gastrin as was suggested above. In the rat, hydrocortisone significantly increased antral gastrin levels within 90 min after injection of 16 or 32 mg/kg. Serum gastrin levels were unchanged (159). Adrenalectomy did not significantly alter either serum or antral gastrin. Hypophysectomy decreased both serum and antral gastrin to a small fraction of normal. Corticosterone completely prevented the decrease in antral gastrin and significantly increased serum gastrin levels in hypophysectomized rats (159). In the dog, chronic, exogenous high doses of adrenal cortical steroid resulted in a 137% increase in gastrin cell mass with an associated enhancement of meal-stimulated peak serum gastrin levels. Adrenalectomy reduced gastrin cell numbers by 50% without significantly changing serum gastrin levels (37). The data in both the rat and dog, therefore, suggest that the adrenals have their greatest effect on antral gastrin levels, perhaps directly increasing the number of gastrin cells, and that increases in serum gastrin levels may be the result of increased tissue content of the hormone.

One would assume, given the evidence that ACTH and adrenal steroids increase secretory function and gastrin release, that such treatment would result in increased parietal and chief cell populations as well as gastric mucosal hyperplasia. On the contrary, the vast majority of studies has shown that such treatment leads to a decrease in mucosal growth. Again, this effect appears to vary with dosage and length of treatment. Rasanen (154) studied changes in mitotic index in rat gastric and duodenal mucosa following ACTH, glucocorticoids, and stress. Multiple low doses of ACTH (2 IU for 4 days) caused a nonsignificant increase in the number of mitoses in the stomach and no change in the duodenum. On the other hand, a single large dose (15 IU) led to a significant 66% reduction in gastric mucosal mitoses but no change in the duodenum. Multiple injections of several glucocorticoids reduced mitoses in both gastric and duodenal mucosa with a greater decrease in the stomach and greatest inhibition with dexamethasone (highest potency steroid). Prolonged stress due to asbestos-induced peritonitis led to decreased mitoses in both stomach and duodenum. Stress plus low doses of ACTH further decreased mitoses in the stom-

ach but did not change the response in the duodenum. An acute stress (forced swimming) decreased gastric mitoses significantly by 80% but caused an insignificant decrease in the duodenum. Therefore, stress, ACTH, and glucocorticoids all decrease cell proliferation in the stomach and have much more moderate effects in the duodenum. The decrease in mucosal growth has been implicated in the increased incidence of peptic ulcer under various conditions of stress or steroid therapy (32, 167).

Summary

As the observant reader will have noticed, most of the papers cited in the preceding sections describing the effects of growth hormone, thyroxin, ACTH, and adrenal hormones on the growth of gastrointestinal mucosa were published in the fifties and sixties. There has been little recent interest in his area. A number of recent papers, however, have implicated growth hormone (47, 136) and adrenal hormones (37,159) in the regulation of tissue and serum gastrin levels and suggested that gastrin may in fact be responsible for some of the effects of these other hormones on the mucosa of the gut. Given the pituitary's function of directly or indirectly regulating the growth of most tissues, it is not unreasonable to suppose that its hormones also regulate the synthesis, release, and/or expression of the known trophic hormones of the digestive tract. These interrelationships should be thoroughly investigated in the future and may provide the answers to a number of important questions.

DEVELOPMENT

The structural and functional properties of the gut in the suckling animal undergo dramatic changes before adult patterns are developed. Most of these changes occur at or around the third week of postnatal life in the rat and the mouse. These changes have been reviewed in detail by Henning and Kretchmer (75). At this time, the diet changes from milk to solid food with high sucrose and maltose and low lactose content. Pinocytosis decreases, and the activities of gastric and pancreatic proteases and intestinal peptidases increase. Lactase activity decreases and is replaced by striking increases in sucrase, maltase, isomaltase, and pancreatic amylase. In addition to these functional changes there are structural changes and a rapid increase in the growth of the intestine. The rate of synthesis of protein, RNA, and DNA accelerates. This results in an increased mitotic index, increased crypt depth, and an enlargement of the gut (75).

A number of regulatory influences have been implicated in these changes, including glucocorticoids, dietary substrates, intestinal flora (which increase after weaning), and gastrin (75,116). The influence of these agents has been tested largely by injecting or introducing them at various times prior to weaning and by prolonging weaning. There is copious evidence that maturation and enzymatic function are dependent on the adrenal steroids. Injection of cortisol into 9-day-old rats led to premature cessation of pinocytosis in the distal small intestine (25). This change occurred in the differentiated function of new cells migrating up from the crypts, but not in mature cells already on the villi. Early induction and stabilization of pepsinogen activity in the gastric mucosa also follows injection of either ACTH or hydrocortisone (57). Glucocorticoids are also necessary to the development of pancreatic enzymes (39,160). The dramatic drop in lactase and rise in sucrase and maltase, which normally occur during the third postnatal week, can be precociously elicited by cortisone injections between days 4 and 18 (75,101,140).

The relative importance of cortisol and dietary constituents on intestinal development was investigated by Lebenthal et al. (107). Feeding 9-day-old rats a diet rich in sucrose via gastrostomies led to premature induction of α-glucosidase activities and an increase in mitotic index and depth of intestinal crypts. Adrenalectomy, however, prevented induction of these changes by sucrose. Neither does premature weaning halt pinocytosis (75). Therefore, dietary change in this stage of development is incapable, by itself, of producing development. However, if cortisone and sucrose are given to 9-day-old adrenalectomized rats, the increases in sucrase and maltase activities, as well as crypt proliferation, are synergistic (107). In adult animals, neither cortisol nor adrenalectomy affects these enzyme activities.

Ferguson et al. (54) suggested that the major factor in intestinal development is the innate capability of the genome, which is independent of, but can be modulated by, external stimuli such as cortisol. In support of this theory, these authors demonstrated that isografts of mouse fetal intestine, implanted in host kidneys, underwent normal developmental changes. Lactase and sucrase activities of both isograft and intact intestines exhibited immature patterns at day 11 and mature activities after day 14. A bolus injection of cortisone into both host and control animals at day 10 resulted in premature enzyme changes in both isografts and intact intestine.

The evidence discussed above leaves little doubt that the functional differentiation of the gastrointestinal tract depends in part on adrenal steroids. The role of these steroids in structural maturation of the gut has been less thoroughly investigated. During the third week of development, the rates of protein and nucleic acid synthesis in the intestinal mucosa increase. The ratio of protein/DNA does not change following weaning, indicating parallel increases in both fractions. The RNA-DNA ratio, however, increases two- to threefold (100). When rats were injected over a period of 4 days with

cortisone beginning between days 11 and 18, the ratio of RNA/DNA increased in a dose-dependent manner. Cortisone had no effect on this ratio in adult rats. Similar increases in crypt size and mitotic rate in response to cortisol have already been mentioned (76,107). This would suggest that both structural and functional changes at the time of weaning are cortisol dependent. However, similar structural increases have been attributed to gastrin. Lichtenberger and Johnson (116) prevented rats from weaning and compared enzyme and growth changes with those in weaned controls. Prevention of weaning slowed the rate of increase in RNA, DNA, and protein content as compared to that in weaned controls. It also prevented lactase activity from decreasing to normal weaned levels, but it had no effect on the normal development of maltase and alkaline phosphatase activities. Maintenance of high lactase may have been due to prolongation of a milk diet. Since cortisol levels presumably increase normally in rats prevented from weaning (food intake has not been shown to alter steroid secretion), the developmental changes in maltase and phosphatase activities were cortisol but not substrate dependent. However, changes in lactase activity and growth did not proceed normally.

Chronic injections of pentagastrin into rats prevented from weaning led to nearly parallel increases in both DNA and protein content and a greater increase in RNA; protein and RNA levels were similar to those of weaned animals. These changes resulted in an increase in the RNA/DNA ratio similar to that reported by Koldovsky and Sunshine (101) following cortisone. Pentagastrin had no effect on enzyme activities. Antral gastrin levels are normally very low until about day 18, when they rise dramatically. However, in 24-day-old rats that were prevented from weaning, antral gastrin remained low, implicating the role of the switch to solid food in the elevation of gastrin levels.

As a result of the gastrin study in weaning animals (116), it was hypothesized that gastrin does not affect the development of disaccharidase patterns; that since both cortisol and gastrin elicited similar increases in parameters related to growth and since cortisol levels develop independently of food intake, the effects of cortisol on growth may depend on gastrin; and that injection of cortisol prior to weaning may stimulate a premature release of gastrin accounting for the trophic effects of cortisol in these animals. Serum gastrin levels in newborn rats had not been measured, and it was assumed incorrectly that since antral levels of the hormone were low, serum levels were also low. Several recent findings have shed considerable light on the relationships among cortisol, gastrin, and growth. First, serum gastrin levels are quite high in newborn puppies (132) and rats (K. Takeuchi, W. Peitsch, and L. R. Johnson, *unpublished*). Second, the pH of the gastric contents is high in both species (no doubt accounting for high serum gastrin levels, since there would be no acid inhibition of gastrin release). Third, exogenous gastrin injection fails to elicit a secretory response in either newborn rats or dogs and fails to stimulate DNA synthesis in the oxyntic gland mucosa of preweaning rats. Fourth, there is no gastrin receptor present in the oxyntic gland mucosa of newborn rats until weaning (K. Takeuchi, W. Peitsch, and L. R. Johnson, *unpublished*). Fifth, response to exogenous pentagastrin occurs at about the same time the gastrin receptor appears. Sixth, there is a large increase in free serum corticosterone 2 days prior to weaning in the rat, which lasts for about 10 days (74). Seventh, injection of corticosterone on day 7 results in the premature appearance of the gastrin receptor on day 9 and the ability of the rats to secrete acid in response to exogenous gastrin (K. Takeuchi, W. Peitsch, and L. R. Johnson, *unpublished*).

The above findings indicate that corticosterone is responsible for the initial induction of synthesis of the gastrin receptor. Full development of the gastrin receptor to adult levels may depend on food intake and subsequent gastrin release, since it has been shown that gastrin upregulates its own receptor (117). Once normal levels of gastrin receptor have been attained, the growth of the mucosa may become gastrin dependent. These hypotheses offer explanations for the lack of an effect of cortisol on growth if injected after weaning has taken place (100). They also explain why the prevention of weaning decreases but does not totally prevent growth of the mucosa (116).

Obviously many more studies must be completed to fully understand the relationships among cortisol, gastrin, and development. However, knowledge of gastrin receptor levels sheds considerable light on these questions and offers a new approach to understanding the development of the gastrointestinal tract.

ADAPTATION

Adaptation is best defined for our purposes as a modification in an organism to better suit a change in its environment. In connection with the growth of the gastrointestinal tract, this word is used to describe the increase in mucosal mass which occurs in response to some types of surgery which decrease the amount or alter the position of absorbing mucosa. The increased growth of mucosa in lactating females is also often thought of as adaptation.

Surgical Studies

Five basic types of surgical alterations have been devised to test the three major mechanisms hypothesized to account for gastrointestinal mucosal growth. Antrectomy has been performed to examine the effects of endogenous gastrin removal. This has been fully cov-

ered in a previous section and will be dealt with here only as it applies to adaptation. Transplantation of the duodenal papilla to the ileum exposes distal gut mucosa to increased amounts of pancreatic and biliary secretions. Ileojejunal transposition exposes a segment of former ileum to increased amounts of gut contents while decreasing the exposure of a segment of jejunum. Resection of a portion of intestine exposes the distal bowel to increased amounts of both secretions and nutrients. Intestinal bypass and formation of a Thiry-Vella fistula removes a loop of bowel from continuity and exposure to luminal factors while preserving the influence of systemic factors.

Papilla Transplantation

The major appeal of the pancreaticobiliary secretion and local nutrition hypotheses is that they are gradient based. That is, the proximal bowel would normally be exposed to the highest concentrations of both nutrients and secretions, and any effects they might exert would be expected to decrease distally. These mechanisms could, therefore, explain the presence of the intestinal villus height and crypt depth gradient (123), the atrophy of proximal bowel removed from continuity as a Thiry-Vella loop (61), the observation that transposition of proximal and distal segments results in hyperplasia of the former distal segment and hypoplasia of the former proximal segment (4,66), and the often reproduced finding that resection of a segment of proximal bowel leads to hyperplasia of the remaining distal intestinal mucosa (186).

Altmann and Leblond (4) identified what they termed "villus enlarging factors" which were presumed to be secreted by the stomach or duodenum. In the same paper they obtained evidence that secretions emanating from the duodenal papilla also contained "enlarging factors." Therefore, in a second study Altmann (2) transplanted a small segment of duodenum containing the papilla to the lower ileum. Within a month the villus size index increased significantly on either side of the transplanted papilla. In fact, the lengths of the ileal villi near the papilla approached those of the duodenum (2). It was concluded that a villus enlarging factor reached the intestine through the duodenal papilla and that pancreatic secretions appeared to play a major role. Data from this same paper, however, are a strong argument against a trophic influence for pancreatic and biliary secretions. Following transplantation of the papilla to the ileum, the size of proximal gut villi, now removed from the influence of these secretions, did not decrease in the slightest (2).

In a recent study, Weser et al. (186) found that transplantation of the duodenal papilla to the ileum resulted in ileal hyperplasia, and a subsequent 60% increase in the weight of the entire small bowel. The authors attributed these effects to trophic substances within bile and pancreatic juice. This study failed to ask several important questions. First, why should the weight of the entire small bowel increase 60%? If the secretions are a physiologically important mechanism for maintaining and regulating growth, certainly the proximal bowel should have undergone hypoplasia after removal of the papilla. Second, how much of the induced "growth" of the ileum was an inflammatory response to bile and pancreatic juice?

In general, progress in this field has been slow since Altmann's original observations. Work in this area has been almost totally descriptive. The time has come to isolate the mysterious "enlarging factors" present in bile and pancreatic juice and define the biochemical mechanisms under their control which result in growth of the mucosa.

Ileojejunal Transposition

As originally described by Altmann and Leblond (4), transposition of ileal and jejunal segments results in decreased villus size of the transposed jejunal segment and increased villus size of the transposed ileal segment. This general finding has been supported by others (66). These studies do not shed light on the mechanism involved since they do not differentiate between effects of local nutrition and secretions. They do, however, implicate a gradient oriented mechanism.

Resection and Bypass

The most widely used model for studying intestinal adaptation and growth of mucosa following changes in exposure of mucosa to luminal contents is partial (usually proximal) intestinal resection or bypass. Following the resection of one part of the small intestine in many species including man, the remaining intestinal mucosa undergoes both structural (12,55,124,144) and functional (15,43,143,184,187) changes, including small bowel dilation, villus enlargement, epithelial cell hyperplasia, increased cell migration rate, and increased absorptive capacity per length of intestine.

Direct evidence that the presence of foodstuffs (luminal contents and/or their ingestion) is necessary for the development of postresectional hyperplasia was recently provided by Feldman et al. (52). They examined the adaptational response in two groups of jejunectomized dogs. One group was fed totally by the intravenous route and the other group was pair-fed by mouth. There was no evidence of either functional or structural adaptation in the parenterally nourished animals, whereas those fed orally exhibited intestinal hyperplasia, increased gut enzyme activities, and an increased ability to absorb glucose. These studies, however, do not pro-

vide evidence regarding the mechanism(s) involved in the response. Intravenous feeding has been shown to decrease pancreatic secretion (97) and gastrin levels (89) as well as removing the effects of local nutrition.

Although most investigators suggest that alterations in local nutrition account for some or all of the hyperplasia following resection, it is obvious that other mechanisms must also be in operation. In 1914, Stassoff (169) described gastric hypersecretion following partial resection of the intestine. This observation has been confirmed more recently in humans (56), dogs (104, 188), and rats (18). Winborn et al. (197) have demonstrated dramatic hyperplasia of gastric epithelial cells in the rat following either distal or proximal small bowel resection. Distal small bowel resection causes hyperplasia of the proximal small bowel mucosa (145), and removal of the colon results in hyperplasia of the ileum (198). It is obvious that none of these findings can be accounted for by a gradient-oriented mechanism.

Hanson et al. (71) described hypoplasia in Thiry-Vella loops of both jejunal and ileal origin. Following 60% resection of the intestine in continuity, however, hyperplasia occurred not only in the residual intestine but in the bypassed loops of both jejunum and ileum. Cell counts of villus and crypt columns were increased along with tritiated thymidine uptake per crypt. This is direct evidence that the systemic mechanism responsible for some of the response to partial intestinal resection stimulates growth of gut mucosa as well as gastric mucosa.

All of the above results of resection could be explained if serum gastrin levels were elevated after resection. It is, therefore, not surprising that marked hypergastrinemia in the fasting and fed states was observed by Straus et al. (172) in four patients with short bowel syndrome. Normal gastrin levels were found in a patient with jejunoileal bypass. Subsequent studies have confirmed the presence of normal serum gastrin levels in patients with intestinal bypass (30). In the dog intestinal resection causes marked hypergastrinemia (188). Bowen et al. (13) recently studied the relationship between gastrin levels and gastric mucosal growth in both resected and bypassed rats. Serum and antral gastrin levels were significantly elevated in the resected but not the bypassed group. Similarly, the weight of the oxyntic gland area of the stomach was increased in animals with intestinal resection. Oxyntic gland weights of the bypassed group were comparable to those of controls. A recent report indicates that the gastrin response to a meal in patients who have undergone bypass is elevated significantly compared to preoperative levels. Thus the effect of bypass surgery on human serum gastrin levels appears to be controversial and may depend on whether basal or stimulated levels are measured (5).

As one body of evidence, these data strongly implicate gastrin as being responsible for the trophic effects of intestinal resection on the stomach. They further demonstrate the existence of a humoral mechanism which is responsible for some of the effects of resection on the adaptation of the small bowel.

The existence of a humoral mechanism which stimulates growth of the mucosa following resection has been tested directly by experiments with parabiotic rats. Loran and Carbone (125) linked rats with cutaneous parabiosis and found intestinal hyperplasia in the unoperated animal following intestinal resection in the other. A recent study employing vascular parabiosis has demonstrated that both transsection and resection of the intestine of one rat result in hyperplasia of the mucosa of the paired animal (196).

Although the hormone responsible for the humoral component of intestinal adaptation in response to resection has not been identified, several lines of evidence indicate that gastrin is not solely responsible. In one study rats were divided into two groups: one fed totally by vein and one intragastrically (44). One week after surgery, the animals were killed and the incontinuity bowel and the bypassed bowel were examined. The animals fed by vein showed decreased weight and reduced DNA and protein content of bypassed bowel and segments of jejunum and ileum left in continuity. Since the bypassed gut was already removed from the effects of luminal contents, the fact that it was significantly smaller in the animals fed by vein was interpreted to mean that the luminal contents in the intragastrically fed animals released a trophic hormone. The authors found that serum gastrin levels were twice as high in the animals fed by stomach tube (103 pg/ml) compared to the parenterally fed group (52 pg/ml). However, because of the extreme variation in their assay, the difference were not significant. They, therefore, concluded that gastrin was not the trophic hormone involved (44). Due to the scatter of their radioimmunoassay data, it is obvious that this conclusion is unwarranted. Nevertheless, it is probably correct. Oscarson et al. (147) have shown that intestinal hyperplasia in response to resection was not decreased by antrectomy. In similar studies, we have found that following resection in antrectomized animals the adaptational response of the distal small intestine is left intact but the hyperplasia which normally occurs in the mucosa of oxyntic gland, duodenum, and colon is lost (A. B. Dembinski and L. R. Johnson, *unpublished*). Morin and Ling (141) reported that rats fed parenterally failed to develop mucosal hyperplasia of the distal small intestine, duodenum, or oxyntic gland following proximal gut resection. Another group treated identically but infused continuously with pentagastrin developed hyperplasia of the duodenal and oxyntic gland mucosa but not that of the distal gut. These authors concluded that gastrin was necessary for the postresectional response of the stomach and duodenum but not the remainder of the small intestine.

Mechanisms

This section on gastrointestinal mucosal adaptation in response to surgery is best summarized by examining the mechanisms proposed to explain the results. There are basically four such mechanisms. Gastrin, a humoral factor other than gastrin, local nutrition, and pancreatic and biliary secretions. The first two of these are well established although the identity of the humoral agent(s) other than gastrin is unknown. Gastrin appears to account for the adaptational response of the oxyntic gland and duodenal mucosa, but not the distal intestinal mucosa. Some but not all of the growth of distal gut mucosa following resection is stimulated by another humoral agent(s). The role of pancreatic and biliary secretions must be questioned since removal of these secretions to the distal gut does not result in hypoplasia of the proximal mucosa normally exposed to them (2, 186). No growth factors have been isolated from these secretions, nor have the biochemical mechanisms been elucidated which would account for their effects. The concept of local nutrition, however, remains popular (185) and deserves closer examination.

Whether local nutrients stimulate gut growth has been tested by infusing various substances into Thiry-Vella loops. Although some of the data from these studies are contradictory, they do provide further insight into possible mechanisms. Liquid elemental diets have been reported to cause hyperplasia (80) of bypassed mucosa and to have no effect (99)—not reversing the hypoplasia produced by bypass. Clarke (26) has approached this problem by infusing isotonic solutions of specific substances into surgically prepared sacs of upper small intestine. Infusion of galactose, α-methylglucoside, and NaCl stimulated cell production to the same extent as glucose. This observation cannot be explained by the increased local nutrition theory, since neither galactose, α-methylglucoside, nor Na^+ is metabolized significantly by the mucosa. However, they are all actively transported, as is glucose, and Clarke (26) has suggested that this is evidence that functional work load influences the growth of gut mucosa. This concept was further supported in that mannose, although metabolized, did not stimulate cell production. The active component of mannose absorption is so slight that it is negligible (9). These findings indicate that active absorptive or secretory work requires the replacement of cells; irrespective of the nutrient value of the absorbed material. This idea is a rational explanation for most of the mucosal growth responses which cannot be explained by hormones. This so-called functional demand theory is all the more attractive in that it has been applied to many other tissues (77), and it is unlikely that the growth of gut mucosa is regulated by a completely different mechanism from those (hormones, growth factors, functional demand) known to regulate the growth of other parts of the body.

Nevertheless, epithelial cells of the small intestine are capable of incorporating orally administered amino acids into protein (1,77), and it has been suggested that luminally derived amino acids might be important in the nutrition of the small intestinal mucosa during protein deprivation (77). If one compares the protein distribution of orally administered amino acids with parenterally administered ones, the patterns are quite different (1). After intravenous amino acid administration, proteins from cells of the crypts and villus-crypt junctions are most heavily labeled. After intraluminal administration protein from cells near the villus tips is most heavily labeled. In other words, mature, nondividing enterocytes near the villus tips incorporate luminal amino acids into protein. The cells responsible for growth, the crypt cells, are supplied from the bloodstream. This should be considered as strong evidence against the local nutrition concept.

The GI mucosa is the largest endocrine organ in the body. Hormone- and peptide-containing cells are scattered throughout the mucosa from the stomach to, and including, the colon. Theoretically, these hormones could influence the metabolism and function of mucosal cells without appearing in the general circulation. The paracrine effects of these hormones are unknown and have not been studied. Released by luminal contents, these growth factors could easily satisfy the criterion of a gradient-oriented mechanism which some deem necessary to explain a portion of the data. Without changing any of our concepts about the regulation of cell growth, the paracrine action of these peptides explains the concept of local nutrition.

Lactation

Lactation is associated with hyperplasia and hypertrophy of gastrointestinal mucosa in numerous species. The weight and nitrogen content of the lactating rat's stomach and intestine increase progressively from the time the pups are born until they are weaned (53). Proliferation of intestinal epithelial cells increases, resulting in elongation of the crypts and villi (16,72). The number of parietal and chief cells in the oxyntic gland mucosa increases dramatically during lactation (34), correlating with the increased acid secretory capacity of the stomach (121). The mechanism which stimulates gut growth during lactation is unknown. A number of possibilities, hyperphagia, gastrin, prolactin, or another hormone, have been suggested.

Hyperphagia is definitely associated with lactation (53,54,119) and has been the most commonly invoked mechanism to explain the growth which occurs. Campbell and Fell (17) restricted the diets of lactating rats to those of virgin controls and found no increases in mucosal growth. Lichtenberger and Trier (119) demonstrated that mucosal growth during lactation was correlated more strongly with food intake than with either antral or serum gastrin levels. On the other hand, Harding and Cairnie (72) found mucosal hyperplasia of the intestines of lactating rats placed on restricted diets, although the changes were not equal to those in animals fed *ad libitum*. Crean and Rumsey (34) reported that changes in food intake did not parallel the mucosal growth response of the stomach and suggested that other factors were involved.

Due to the well-known relationship between food intake and gastrin levels (89,96,117), several investigators have examined the possibility that gastrin mediates the growth changes in lactating animals. Lichtenberger and Trier (119) have examined this relationship and found that both serum and antral levels of gastrin are elevated. In a definitive experiment, however, hyperplasia of duodenal mucosa in lactating rats occurred to the same extent in antrectomized animals as it did in sham-operated lactating controls (119). This study rules out the possibility that gastrin is a major factor in intestinal hyperplasia during lactation. Whether it is responsible for some of the changes in the gastric mucosa is unknown.

The mechanism of lactation-induced hyperplasia remains unclear. Prolactin has been shown not to stimulate hyperplasia of the intestine to any great extent in Snell dwarf mice, which have a hereditary deficiency of prolactin, growth hormone, and TSH (115). Whether prolactin is effective in the presence of normal growth hormone levels has not been investigated. The observation that the weight and DNA content of the rat pancreas increase significantly during lactation and then decrease after weaning (10) implies a hormonal mechanism, since the pancreas does not come into contact with food. The identity of this hormone should be the object of future experiments.

FUTURE DIRECTIONS

Throughout this chapter I have tried to reach conclusions regarding the mechanisms influencing the growth of gastrointestinal mucosa under a variety of conditions. Attempts have been made to indicate those areas of investigation which seem to offer the best possibilities for providing answers to unsolved questions. This final section briefly comments on the significance of the trophic action of gastrin and summarizes what appear to be the important areas of future research.

The establishment of gastrin as a physiologically significant regulator of the growth of the gastrointestinal tract mucosa has had many implications. These include the interactions of nongastrointestinal trophic hormones with gastrin, the changes which occur during development, lactation, and surgically induced adaptation. It seems likely that the most important action of gastrin is its trophic one. Secretion and motility are regulated by nerves and direct stimulation as well as by hormones. Absorption is largely unregulated. These processes occur adequately in the absence of hormones. The maintenance of the structural and functional integrity of the mucosa is necessary for life; gastric secretion *per se* is not. It, therefore, seems possible that the trophic action of gastrin, rather than its digestive function, is responsible for its evolution and persistence in the phylogeny of species.

The clinical significance of the trophic action of gastrin is obvious in the Zollinger-Ellison syndrome and following antrectomy in man. The demonstration that endogenous and exogenous gastrin prevents stress ulcer through its trophic action (174) suggests that this hormone is important in preventing damage to the mucosa which might be caused by a variety of agents. The question of whether gastrointestinal hormones are important factors in the growth of mucosal tumors remains unexplored.

One area that has not been dealt with and which has important ramifications for all the actions of gastrointestinal hormones is the regulation of the synthesis and release of this group of peptides. There is little information available concerning the steps in gastrointestinal hormone synthesis. These will have to be elucidated before the biochemical controls of the pathways can be defined. Hopefully investigators will apply the techniques now available from other fields to this area. As indicated previously, it is now known that growth hormone and adrenal glucocorticoids influence gastrin levels. The whole area of pituitary-gastrointestinal peptide interactions promises to be a fruitful one for research in the near future. This is especially true since the realization that many gastrointestinal peptides are located in nerves and the brain. On the other hand, somatostatin is present in large amounts in the gastrointestinal tract and may regulate hormone release through a paracrine action. Interactions between gut hormones and other endocrines may prove to be important in explaining developmental changes in the digestive tract as well as those during adaptation to surgery and lactation.

The concept of paracrine action is especially attractive to gastrointestinal physiology since many peptides are located in endocrine cells dispersed over wide areas of the digestive tract mucosa. Local release of growth factors may play an important role in the trophic response to local stimuli provided by food ingestion and secretions. The method of proving the existence of a paracrine effect, however, has not been found, but this problem is certainly an important one worth solving.

The finding that the levels of the gastrin receptor in oxyntic gland mucosa are regulated by both gastrin itself and corticosterone introduces the concept of hormone receptor regulation to gastrointestinal physiology. This area, as well as the many others mentioned, promises to have great significance for understanding the regulation of mucosal growth.

REFERENCES

1. Alpers, D. H. (1972): Protein synthesis in intestinal mucosa: The effect of route of administration of precursor amino acids. *J. Clin. Invest.*, 51:167–173.
2. Altmann, G. G. (1971): Influence of bile and pancreatic secretions on the size of the intestinal villi in the rat. *Am. J. Anat.*, 132:167–178, 1971.
3. Altmann, G. G. (1972): Influence of starvation and refeeding on mucosal size and epithelial renewal in the rat small intestine. *Am. J. Anat.*, 133:391–400.
4. Altmann, G. G., and Leblond, C. P. (1970): Factors influencing villus size in the small intestine of adult rats as revealed by transposition of intestinal segments. *Am. J. Anat.*, 127:15–36.
5. Atkinson, R. L., Dahms, W. T., Bray, G. A., Lemmi, C., and Schwartz, A. A. (1979): Gastrin secretion after weight loss by dieting and intestinal bypass surgery. *Gastroenterology*, 77:696–699.
6. Baker, B. L., and Abrams, G. D. (1954): Effect of hypophysectomy on the cytology of the fundic glands of the stomach and on the secretion of pepsin. *Am. J. Physiol.*, 177:409–412.
7. Baker, B. L., Clapp, H. W., Annable, C. R., and Dewey, M. M. (1961): Elevation of proteolytic activity in the pancreas of hypophysectomized rats by hormonal therapy. *Proc. Soc. Exp. Biol. Med.*, 108:238–242.
8. Baker, B. L., and Clark R. H. (1961): Influence of hypophysectomy on oxidative enzymes and size of parietal cells in gastric mucosa. *Proc. Soc. Exp. Biol. Med.*, 106:65–67.
9. Barnett, J. E. C., Ralph, A., and Munday, K. A. (1970): Structural requirements for active intestinal transport. *Biochem. J.*, 118:843–850.
10. Barrowman, J. A., and Mayston, P. D. (1973): Pancreatic secretion in lactating rats. *J. Physiol. Lond.*, 229:41P–42P.
11. Bertalanfly, F. D., and Nagy, K. P. (1961): Mitotic activity and renewal of the epithelial cells of human duodenum. *Acta Anat., (Basel)*, 45:362–370.
12. Booth, C. C., Evans, K. T., Meuzies, T., and Street, D. F. (1959): Intestinal hypertrophy following partial resection of the small bowel in the rat. *Br. J. Surg.*, 46:403–410.
13. Bowen, J. C., Paddack, G. L., Bush, J. C., Wilson, R. J., and Johnson, L. R. (1978): Diverse gastric responses to small intestinal resection and bypass in rats. *Surgery*, 83:402–405.
14. Bullough, W. S. (1972): The control of epidermal thickness. *Br. J. Dermatol.*, 87:347–394.
15. Bury, K. D. (1972): Carbohydrate digestion and absorption after massive resection of the small intestine. *Surg. Gynecol. Obstet.*, 135:177–187.
16. Cairnie, A. B., and Bentley, R. E. (1967): Cell proliferation studies in the intestinal epithelium of the rat: hyperplasia during lactation. *Exp. Cell Res.*, 46:428–440.
17. Campbell, A. M., and Fell, B. F. (1964): Gastrointestinal hypertrophy in the lactating rat and its relation to food intake. *J. Physiol. Lond.*, 170:90–97.
18. Cardis, D. T., Roberts, M., and Smith, G. (1969): The effect of small bowel resection on gastric acid secretion in the rat. *Surgery*, 65:292–297.
19. Carriere, R. M. (1967): The influence of thyroid and testicular hormones on the epithelium of the crypts of Lieberkuhn in the rat's intestine. *Anat. Rec.*, 156:423–429.
20. Casteleyn, P. P., Dubrasquet, M., and Willems, G. (1977): Opposite effects of gastrin on cell proliferation in the antrum and other parts of the upper-gastrointestinal tract in the rat. *Am. J. Dig. Dis.*, 22:798–804.
21. Castro, G. A., Copeland, E. M., Dudrick, S. J., and Johnson, L. R. (1975): Intestinal disaccharidase and peroxidase activity in parenterally nourished rats. *J. Nutr.*, 105:776–781.
22. Chandler, A. M. and Johnson, L. R. (1972): Pentagastrin stimulated incorporation of [14C] orotic acid into RNA of gastric and duodenal mucosa. *Proc. Soc. Exp. Biol. Med.*, 141:110–113.
23. Cheng, H., and Leblond, C. F. (1974): Origin differentiation and renewal of the four main epithelial cell types in the mouse small intestine. V. Unitarian theory of the origin of the four epithelial cell types. *Am. J. Anat.*, 141:537–562.

24. Clark, R. H., and Baker, B. L. (1963): Effect of hypophysectomy on mitotic proliferation in gastric epithelium. *Am. J. Physiol.,* 204:1018-1022.

25. Clark, S. L. (1971): The effects of cortisol and BUDR on cellular differentiation in the small intestine in suckling rats. Am. J. Anat., 132:319-338.

26. Clarke, R. M. (1977): 'Luminal nutrition' versus 'functional work-load' as controllers of mucosal morphology and epithelial replacement in the rat small intestine. *Digestion,* 15:411-424.

27. Cohen, S. (1962): Isolation of a mouse submaxillary gland protein accelerating incisor eruption and eyelid opening in the newborn animal. *J. Biol. Chem.,* 237:1155-1162.

28. Cohen, S., and Taylor, J. M. (1974): Epidermal growth factor: Chemical and biological characterization. *Recent. Prog. Horm. Res.,* 30:533-550.

29. Costa, M., Patel, J. B., Furness, J. B., and Arimura, A. (1977): Evidence that some intrinsic neurons of the intestine contain somatostatin. *Neurosci. Lett.,* 6:215.

30. Coutsoftides, T., Baranowski, J., and Himal, H. S. (1976): Gastric acid and serum gastrin secretion before and after by-pass of the small intestine for morbid obesity. *Surg. Gynecol. Obstet.,* 142:521-523.

31. Creamer, B., Shorter, R. G., and Barnforth, J. (1961): The turnover and shedding of epithelial cells. I. The turnover in the gastrointestinal tract. *Gut,* 2:110-118.

32. Crean, G. P. (1963): The endocrine system and the stomach. *Vitam. Horm.,* 21:215-280.

33. Crean, G. P., Marshall, M. W., and Rumsey, R. D. E. (1969): Parietal cell hyperplasia induced by the administration of pentagastrin (ICI 50, 123) to rats. *Gastroenterology,* 57:147-156.

34. Crean, G. P., and Rumsey, R. D. E. (1971): Hyperplasia of the gastric mucosa during pregnancy and lactation in the rat. *J. Physiol. (Lond.),* 215:181-197.

35. Daughaday, W. H. (1974): The adenohypophysis. In: *Textbook of Endocrinology,* edited by R. H. Williams, pp. 31-79. W. B. Saunders Co., Philadelphia.

36. Daughaday, W. H., and Garland, J. T. (1972): The sulfation factor hypothesis: Recent observations. In: *Growth and Growth Hormone,* edited by A. Pecile and E. E. Muller, pp. 168-179. Excerpta Medica, Amsterdam.

37. Delaney, J. P., Michel, H. M., Bonsack, M. E., Eisenberg, M. M., and Dunn, D. H. (1979): Adrenal corticosteroids cause gastrin cell hyperplasia. *Gastroenterology,* 76:913-916.

38. Dembinski, A. B., and Johnson, L. R. (1979): Growth of pancreas and gastrointestinal mucosa in antrectomized and gastrin-treated rats. *Endocrinology,* 105:769-773.

39. Deschodt-Lanckman, M., Robberecht, P., Camus, J., Baya, C., and Christophe, J. (1974): Hormonal and dietary adaptation of rat pancreatic hydrolases before and after weaning. *Am. J. Physiol.,* 226:39-44.

40. Dorchester, J. E. C., and Haist, R. E. (1952): The secretin content of the intestine in normal and hypophysectomized rats. *J. Physiol.,* 118:188-195.

41. Dorchester, J. E. C., and Haist, R. E. (1952): The effect of anterior pituitary extracts, desiccated thyroid, growth-hormone preparations, and ACTH on the extractable secretin of the intestines of hypophysectomized and intact rats. *J. Physiol.,* 119:266-273.

42. Dowling, R. H. (1974): The influence of luminal nutrition on intestinal adaptation after small bowel resection and by-pass. In: *Intestinal Adaptation,* edited by R. H. Dowling and E. O. Rieken, pp. 35-45. F. K. Schattauer Verlag, Stuttgart.

43. Dowling, R. H., and Booth, C. C. (1967): Structural and functional changes following small bowel resection in the rat. *Clin. Sci.,* 32:139-149.

44. Dworkin, L. D., Levine, G. M., Farber, N. J., and Spector, M. H. (1976): Small intestinal mass of the rat is partially determined by indirect effects of intraluminal nutrition. *Gastroenterology,* 71:626-630.

45. Eartly, H., and Leblond, C. P. (1954): Identification of the effects of thyroxine mediated by the hypophysis. *Endocrinology,* 54:249-271.

46. Ellison, E. H., and Wilson, S. D. (1967): Further observations on factors influencing the symptomatology manifest by patients with Zollinger-Ellison syndrome. In: *Gastric Secretion,* edited by T. K. Shnitka, J. A. L. Gilbert, and R. C. Harrison, pp. 363-369. Pergamon, New York.

47. Enochs, M. R., and Johnson, L. R. (1976): Effect of hypophysectomy and growth hormone on serum and antral gastrin levels in the rat. *Gastroenterology,* 70:727-732.

48. Enochs, M. R., and Johnson, L. R. (1977): Changes in protein and nucleic acid synthesis in rat gastric mucosa after pentagastrin. *Am. J. Physiol.,* 232:E223-E228.

49. Enochs, M. R., and Johnson, L. R. (1977): Hormonal regulation of the growth of gastrointestinal tract; biochemical and physiological aspects. In: *Progress in Gastroenterology, Vol. III,* edited by G. B. Jerzy Glass, pp. 3-28. Grune & Stratton, New York.

50. Fahrenkrug, J., Schaffalitzky de Muckadell, O. B., and Holst, J. J. (1978): Nervous release of VIP. In: *Gut Hormones,* edited by S. R. Bloom, pp. 488-491. Churchill Livingstone, Edinburgh.

51. Feldman, E. J., Aures, D., and Grossman, M. I. (1978): Epidermal growth factor stimulates ornithine decarboxylase activity in the digestive tract of the mouse. *Proc. Soc. Exp. Biol. Med.,* 159:400-402.

52. Feldman, E. J., Dowling, R. H., McNaughton, J., and Peters, T. J. (1976): Effects of oral versus intravenous nutrition on intestinal adaptation after small bowel resection in the dog. *Gastroenterology,* 70:712-719.

53. Fell, B. F., Smith, K. A., and Campbell, R. M. (1963): Hypertrophic and hyperplastic changes in the alimentary canal of the lactating rat. *J. Pathol. Bacteriol.,* 85:179-188.

54. Ferguson, A., Gerskowitch, V. P., and Russell, R. I. (1973): Pre- and postweaning disaccharidase patterns in isografts of fetal mouse intestine. *Gastroenterology,* 64:292-297.

55. Flint, J. M. (1912): The effect of extensive resection of the small intestine. *Johns Hopkins Med. J.,* 23:127-144.

56. Frederick, P. L., Sizer, J. S., and Osborne, M. P. (1965): Relation of massive bowel resection to gastrin secretion. *N. Engl. J. Med.,* 272:509-514.

56a. Fugimoto, S., Kawai, K., Hattori, T., and Fujita, S. (1979): Tritiated thymidine autoradiographic study on origin and renewal of gastrin cells in pyloric area of hamsters. *Gastroenterology,* 76:1136.

57. Furichata, C., Kawachi, T., Sagimura, T. (1972): Premature induction of pepsinogen in developing rat gastric mucosa by hormones. *Biochem. Biophys. Res. Commun.,* 47:705-711.

58. Gavin, J. R., Roth, J., Neville, D. M., Jr., Demeytes, P., and Buell, D. N. (1974): Insulin-dependent regulation of insulin receptor concentrations: A direct demonstration in cell culture. *Proc. Natl. Acad Sci. U.S.A.,* 71:84-91.

59. Gerity, P. J., Camilleri, J. A., and Hayes, M. A. (1954): Mechanism for potentiation of gastrin secretion by ACTH. *Surg. Forum,* 5:285-287.

60. Gjurldsen, S. T., Myren, J., and Fretheim, B. (1968): Alterations of gastric mucosa following a graded partial gastrectomy. *Scand. J. Gastroenterol.,* 3:465-470.

61. Gleeson, M. H., Cullen, J., and Dowling, R. H. (1972): Intestinal structure and function after small bowel by-pass in the rat. *Clin. Sci.,* 43:731-742.

62. Grant, R., Grossman, M. I., and Ivy, A. C. (1953): Histological changes in gastric mucosa during digestion and their relationship to mucosal growth. *Gastroenterology,* 25:218-231.

63. Gregory, H. (1975): Isolation and structure of urogastrone and its relationship to epidermal growth factor. *Nature,* 257:325-327.

64. Gregory, R. A., Grossman, M. I., Tracy, H. J., and Bentley, P. H. (1967): Nature of the gastric secretagogue in Zollinger-Ellison tumors. *Lancet,* 2:543-544.

65. Gregory, R. A., and Tracy, H. J. (1964): The constitution and properties of two gastrins extracted from hog antral mucosa. I. The isolation of two gastrins from hog antral mucosa. *Gut,* 5:103-114.

66. Gronqvist, B., Engstrom, B., and Grimelius, L. (1975): Morphological studies of the rat small intestine after jejunoileal transposition. *Acta Chir. Scand.,* 141:208-217.

67. Hakanson, R., Larsson, L.-I., Liedberg, G., Oscarson, J., Sundler, F., and Vang, J. (1976): Effects of antrectomy and portacaval shunting on the histamine-storing endocrine-like cells in oxyntic mucosa of rat stomach. *J. Physiol.,* 259:785-800.

68. Hall, W. (1971): The parietal cell mass: Growth hormone relationship in man. *Am. J. Dig. Dis.,* 16:139–143.
69. Hansen, O. H., Larsen, J. K., and Svendsen, L. B. (1978): Changes in gastric mucosal cell proliferation after antrectomy or vagotomy in man. *Scand. J. Gastroenterol.,* 13:947–952.
70. Hansen, O. H., Pedersen, T., Larsen, J. K., and Rehfeld, J. F. (1976): Effect of gastrin on gastric mucosal cell proliferation in man. *Gut,* 17:536–541.
71. Hanson, W. R., Rijke, R. P. C., Plaisier, H. M., Van Ewik, W., and Osborne, J. W. (1977): The effect of intestinal resection on Thiry-Vella fistulae of jejunal and ileal origin in the rat: evidence for a systemic control mechanism of cell renewal. *Cell Tissue Kinet.,* 10:543–555.
72. Harding, J. D., and Cairnie, A. B. (1975): Changes in intestinal cell kinetics in the small intestine of lactating mice. *Cell Tissue Kinet.,* 8:135–144.
73. Helander, H. F. (1978): Quantitative ultrastructural studies on rat gastric zymogen cells under different physiological and experimental conditions. *Cell Tissue Res.,* 189:287–303.
74. Henning, S. J. (1978): Plasma concentrations of total and free corticosterone during development in the rat. *Am. J. Physiol.,* 235:E451–E456.
75. Henning, S. J., and Kretchmer, N. (1973): Development of intestinal function in mammals. *Enzyme,* 15:3–23.
76. Herbst, J. J., and Sunshine, P. (1969): Postnatal development of the small intestine of the rat. Changes in morphology at weaning. *Pediatr. Res.,* 3:27–33.
77. Hirschfield, J. S., and Kern, F. (1969): Protein starvation and the small intestine. III. Incorporation of orally and intraperitoneally administered 1-leucine 4,5-^{3}H into intestinal protein of protein-deprived rats. *J. Clin. Invest.,* 48:1224–1229.
78. Hitzelberger, A. L., and Glass, G. B. J. (1962): Effects of corticosteroids in human beings on the secretion of large molecular substances of gastric juice. *J. Lab. Clin. Med.,* 59:575–587
79. Hollenberg, M. D., and Gregory, H. (1976): Human urogastrone and mouse epidermal growth factor share a common receptor. *Life Sci.,* 20:267–274.
80. Jacobs, L. R., Taylor, B. R., and Dowling, R. H. (1975): Effect of luminal nutrition on the intestinal adaptation following Thiry-Vella by-pass in the dog. *Clin. Sci. Mol. Med.,* 49:26 (abstr.).
81. Jacobson, E. D., and Magnani, T. J. (1964): Some effects of hypophysectomy on gastrointestinal function and structure. *Gut,* 5:473–479.
82. Jensen, E. V., and DeSombre, E. R. (1972): Estrogen and progestins. In: *Biochemical Actions of Hormones, Vol. III,* edited by G. Litwack, pp. 215–256. Academic Press, New York.
83. Johnson, L. R. (1971): The control of gastric secretion: No room for histamine? *Gastroenterology,* 61:106–118.
84. Johnson, L. R. (1976): The trophic action of gastrointestinal hormones. *Gastroenterology,* 70:278–288.
85. Johnson, L. R. (1977): New aspects of the trophic action of gastrointestinal hormones. *Gastroenterology,* 72:788–792.
86. Johnson, L. R., Aures, D., and Hakanson, R. (1969): Effect of gastrin on the *in vivo* incorporation of [^{14}C] leucine into protein of the digestive tract. *Proc. Soc. Exp. Biol. Med.,* 132:996–998.
87. Johnson, L. R., Aures, D., and Yuen, L. (1969): Pentagastrin-induced stimulation of protein synthesis in the gastrointestinal tract. *Am. J. Physiol.,* 217:251–254.
88. Johnson, L. R., and Chandler, A. M. (1973): RNA and DNA of gastric and duodenal mucosa in antrectomized and gastrin-treated rats. *Am. J. Physiol.,* 224:937–940.
89. Johnson, L. R., Copeland, E. M., Dudrick, S. J., Lichtenberger, L. M., and Castro, G. A. (1975): Structural and hormonal alterations in the gastrointestinal tract of parenterally fed rats. *Gastroenterology,* 68:1177–1183.
90. Johnson, L. R., and Guthrie, P. D. (1974): Mucosal DNA synthesis: A short term index of the trophic action of gastrin. *Gastroenterology,* 67:553–559.
91. Johnson, L. R., and Guthrie, P. D. (1974): Secretin inhibition of gastrin-stimulated deoxyribonucleic acid synthesis. *Gastroenterology,* 67:601–606.
92. Johnson, L. R., and Guthrie, P. D. (1976): Effect of cholecystokinin and 16,16-dimethyl prostaglandin E$_2$ on RNA and DNA of gastric and duodenal mucosa. *Gastroenterology,* 70:59–65.
93. Johnson, L. R., and Guthrie, P. D. (1976): Stimulation of DNA synthesis by big and little gastrin (G-34 and G-17). *Gastroenterology,* 71:599–602.
94. Johnson, L. R., and Guthrie, P. D. (1978): Effect of secretin on colonic DNA synthesis. *Proc. Soc. Exp. Biol. Med.,* 158:521–523.
95. Johnson, L. R., and Guthrie, P. D. (1980): Stimulation of rat oxyntic gland mucosal growth by epidermal growth factor. *Am. J. Physiol.,* 238:G45–G49.
96. Johnson, L. R., Lichtenberger, L. M., Copeland, E. M., Dudrick, S. J., and Castro, G. A. (1975): Action of gastrin on gastrointestinal structure and function. *Gastroenterology,* 68:1184–1192.
97. Johnson, L. R., Schanbacher, L. M., Dudrick, S. J., and Copeland, E. M. (1977): Effect of long-term parenteral feeding on pancreatic secretion and serum secretin. *Am. J. Physiol.,* 233:E524–E529.
98. Johnson, L. R., Stening, G. F., and Grossman, M. I. (1970): The effect of sulfation on the gastrointestinal actions of caerulein. *Gastroenterology,* 58:208–216.
99. Keren, D. F., Elliot, H. L., Brown, G. D., and Yardley, J. H. (1975): Atrophy of villi with hypertrophy and hyperplasia of Paneth cells in isolated (Thiry-Vella) ileal loops in rabbits. *Gastroenterology,* 68:83–93.
100. Koldovsky, O., Herbst, J. J., Barke, J., and Sunshine, P. (1970): RNA and DNA in intestinal mucosa during development of normal and cortisone-treated rats. *Growth,* 34:359–367.
101. Koldovsky, O., and Sunshine, P. (1970): Effect of cortisone on the developmental pattern of the neutral and the acid b-galactosidase of the small intestine in the rat. *Biochem. J.,* 117:467–471.
102. Korner, A. (1963): Growth hormone control of messenger RNA synthesis. *Biochem. Biophys. Res. Commun.,* 13:386–389.
103. Korner, A. (1964): Regulation of the rate of synthesis of messenger RNA by growth hormone. *Biochem. J.,* 92:449–456.
104. Landor, J. H., and Baker, W. K. (1964): Gastric hypersecretion produced by massive small bowel resection in dogs. *J. Surg. Res.,* 4:518–522.
105. Larsson, L.-I., Fahrenkrug, J., Schattalitzky de Muckadell, O., Sundler, F., and Hakanson, R. (1976): Localization of vasoactive intestinal peptide (VIP) to central and peripheral neurons. *Proc. Natl. Acad. Sci. USA,* 73:3197–3200.
106. Lawson, H. H. (1970): The origin of chief and parietal cells in regenerating gastric mucosa. *Br. J. Surg.,* 57:139–141.
107. Lebenthal, E., Sunshine, P., and Kretchner, N. (1972): Effect of carbohydrate and corticosteroids on activity of α-glucosides in intestine of the infant rat. *J. Clin. Invest.,* 51:1244–1250.
108. Leblond, C. P., and Carriere, R. M. (1955): The effect of growth hormone and thyroxine on the mitotic rate of the intestinal mucosa of the rat. *Endocrinology,* 56:261–266.
109. Lechago, J., and Benscome, S. A. (1973): The encodrine cells of the upper gut mucosa in dogs with transplantation of the pyloric antrum to the colon. *Z. Zellforsch. Mikrosk. Anat.,* 146:237–242.
110. Lees, F., and Grandjean, L. C. (1968): The gastric and jejunal mucosae in healthy patients with partial gastrectomy. *Arch. Intern. Med.,* 101:9437–9451.
111. Lehy, T., Voillemot, N., Dubrasquet, M., and Dufougeray, F. (1975): Gastrin cell hyperplasia in rats with chronic antral stimulation. *Gastroenterology,* 68:71–82.
112. Lehy, T., and Willems, G. (1976): Population kinetics of antral gastrin cells in the mouse. *Gastroenterology,* 71:614–619.
113. Levin, R. J. (1969): The effects of hormones on the absorptive, metabolic, and digestive functions of the small intestine. *J. Endocrinol.,* 45:315–348.
114. Leviton, R., and Havivi, E. (1970): Effect of hypophysectomy on amino acid, thymidine, and orotic acid incorporation into the mucosa of the small bowel. *Can. J. Biochem.,* 48:828–830.
115. Lichtenberger, L. M., and Bartke, A. (1979): Pituitary-induced alterations in gastrin levels and gastrointestinal growth in normal and genetically dwarf mice. *Proc. Soc. Exp. Biol. Med.,* 161:289–294.
116. Lichtenberger, L. M., and Johnson, L. R. (1974): Gastrin in the ontogenic development of the small intestine. *Am. J. Physiol.,* 227:390–395.

117. Lichtenberger, L. M., Lechago, J., and Johnson, L. R. (1975): Depression of antral and serum gastrin concentration by food deprivation in the rat. *Gastroenterology,* 68:1473-1479.
118. Lichtenberger, L. M., Miller, L. R., Erwin, D. N., and Johnson, L. R. (1973): The effect of pentagastrin on adult duodenal cells in culture. *Gastroenterology,* 65:242-251.
119. Lichtenberger, L. M., and Trier, J. S. (1979): Changes in gastrin levels, food intake, and duodenal mucosal growth during lactation. *Am. J. Physiol.,* 237:E98-E105.
120. Lichtenberger, L. M., Welsh, J. D., and Johnson, L. R. (1975): Relationship between the changes in gastrin levels and intestinal properties in the starved rat. *Am. J. Dig. Dis.,* 21:33-38.
121. Lilja, B., and Svensson, S. E. (1967): Gastric secretion during pregnancy and lactation in the rat. *J. Physiol. (Lond.),* 190:261-272.
122. Linnoila, I., DiAugustine, R. P., Miller, R., Chang, I., and Cuatracasas, P. (1978): Distribution of [Met^5]-[Leu^5]- enkephalin in the gastrointestinal tract. *Fed. Proc.,* 37:666.
123. Lipkin, M., Sherlock, P., and Bell, B (1963): Cell proliferation kinetics in the gastrointestinal tract of man. II. Cell renewal in stomach, ileum, colon, and rectum. *Gastroenterology,* 45:721-729.
124. Loran, M. R., and Althausen, T. L. (1960): Cellular proliferation of intestinal epithelia of the rat two months after partial resection of the ileum. *J. Biophys. Biochem. Cytol.,* 7:667-671.
125. Loran, M. R., and Carbone, J. V. (1968): The humoral effect of intestinal resection on cellular proliferation and maturation in parabiotic rats. In: *Gastrointestinal Radiation Injury,* edited by M. F. Sullivan, pp. 127-141. Excerpta Medica Foundation, Amsterdam.
126. McDonald, C., Trier, J. S., and Everett, B. 1964): Cell proliferation and migration in the stomach, duodenum and rectum of man. *Gastroenterology,* 46:405-417.
127. McGuigan, J. E., and Trudeau, W. L. (1968): Immunochemical measurement of elevated levels of gastrin in the serum of patients with pancreatic tumors of the Zollinger-Ellison variety. *N. Engl. J. Med.,* 278:1308-1313.
128. McNeil, L. K., and Hamilton, J. R. (1971): The effect of fasting on disaccharidase activity in the rat small intestine. *Pediatrics,* 47:65-72.
129. Mainz, D. L., Black, O., and Webster, P. D. (1973): Hormonal control of pancreatic growth. *J. Clin. Invest.,* 52:2300-2304.
130. Majumdar, A. P. N., and Goltermann, N. (1977): Effects of fasting and pentagastrin on protein synthesis by isolated gastric mucosal ribosomes in a cell-free system. *Gastroenterology,* 73:1060-1064.
131. Majumdar, A. P. N., and Goltermann, N. (1978): Chronic administration of pentagastrin: Effect on gastric mucosal protein synthesis in rats. *Mol. Cell. Endocrinol.,* 11:137-143.
132. Malloy, M. H., Morriss, F. H., Denson, S. E., Weisbrodt, N. W., Lichtenberger, L. M., and Adcock, E. W., III (1979): Neonatal gastric motility in dogs: Maturation and response to pentagastrin. *Am. J. Physiol.,* 236:E562-E566.
133. Martin, F., Macleod, I. B., and Sircus, W. (1970): Effects of antrectomy on the fundic mucosa of the rat. *Gastroenterology,* 59:437-444.
134. Matsuyama, M., and Suzuki, H. (1970): Differentiation of immature mucosal cells into parietal, argyrophil and chief cells in stomach grafts. *Science,* 169:385-387.
135. Mayston, P. D., and Barrowman, J. A. (1971): The influence of chronic administration of pentagastrin on the rat pancreas. *Q. J. Exp. Physiol.,* 56:113-122.
136. Mayston, P. D., and Barrowman, J. A. (1973): The influence of chronic administration of pentagastrin on the pancreas in hypophysectomized rats. *Gastroenterology,* 64:391-399.
137. Melrose, A. G., Russell, R. I., and Dick, A. (1964): Gastric mucosal structure and function after vagotomy. *Gut,* 5:546-549.
138. Messier, B. (1960): Radioautographic evidence for the renewal of the mucous cells in the gastric mucosa of the rat. *Anat. Rec.,* 136:242-247.
139. Miller, L. R., Jacobson, E. D., and Johnson, L. R. (1973): Effect of pentagastrin on gastric mucosal cells grown in tissue culture. *Gastroenterology,* 64:254-267.
140. Moog, F., Denes, A. W., and Powell, P. M. (1973): Disaccharidases in the small intestine of the mouse: Normal development and influence of cortisone, actinomycin D, and cycloheximide. *Dev. Biol.,* 35:143-159.
141. Morin, C. L., and Ling, V. (1978): Effect of pentagastrin on the rat small intestine after resection. *Gastroenterology,* 75:224-229.
142. Neuberger, P., Lewin, M., and Bonfils, S. (1972): Parietal and chief cell populations in four cases of the Zollinger-Ellison syndrome. *Gastroenterology,* 63:937-942.
143. Nygaard, K. (1966): Resection of the small intestine in rats. I. Nutritional status and adaptation of fat and protein absorption. *Acta Chir. Scand.,* 132:731-742.
144. Nygaard, K. (1967): Resection of the small intestine in rats. III. Morphological changes in the intestinal tract. *Acta Chir. Scand.,* 133:233-248.
145. Nygaard, K. (1974): Small bowel resection and by-pass. In: *Intestinal Adaptation,* edited by R. H. Dowling and E. O. Rieken, pp. 47-59. F. K. Schattauer Verlag, Stuttgart.
146. Olbe, L. (1974): Differences between human and animal gastric acid secretion. In: *Syllabus for AGA Postgraduate Course on Peptide Ulcer Disease. (Unpublished)* San Francisco.
147. Oscarson, J. E. A., Veen, H. F., Williamson, R. C. N., Ross, J. S., and Malt, R. A. (1977): Compensatory postresectional hyperplasia and starvation atrophy in small bowel: Dissociation from endogenous gastrin levels. *Gastroenterolgy,* 72:890-895.
148. Pansu, D., Berard, A., Dechelette, M. A., and Lambert, R. (1974): Influence of secretin and pentagastrin on the circadian rhythm of cell proliferation in the intestinal mucosa of rats. *Digestion,* 11:266-274.
149. Pearse, A. G. C., and Bussolati, G. (1970): Immunofluoresence studies of the distribution of gastrin cells in different clinical states. *Gut,* 11:646-648.
150. Pegg, A. E., and Korner, A. (1965): Growth hormone action on rat liver RNA polymerase. *Nature,* 205:904-905.
151. Philpott, G. W. (1971): Tissue-specific inhibition of cell proliferation in embryonic stomach epithelium *in vitro. Gastroenterology,* 61:25-34.
152. Posner, B. I., Kelly, P. A., and Friesen, H. G., (1975): Prolactin receptors in rat liver: Possible induction by prolactin. *Science,* 188:57-59.
153. Ragins, H., Wincze, F., and Liu, S. M. (1968): The origin of gastric parietal cells in the mouse. *Anat. Rec.,* 162:99-110.
154. Rasanen, T. (1963): Fluctuations in the mitotic frequency of the glandular stomach and intestine of the rat under the influence of ACTH, glucocorticoids, stress and heparin. *Acta Physiol. Scand.,* 58:211-220.
155. Riecken, E. O., and Menge, H. (1977): Nutritive effects of food constituents on the structure and function of the intestine. *Acta Hepatogastroenterol. (Stuttg.),* 24:388-399.
156. Robert, A., Phillips, J. P., and Nezamis, J. E. (1966): Gastric secretion and ulcer formation after hypophysectomy and administration of somatotrophic hormone. *Am. J. Dig. Dis.,* 11:546-552.
157. Russell, D. H., Byus, C. V., and Manen, C. A. (1976): Proposed model of major sequential biochemical events of a trophic response. *Life Sci., 19:1297-1306.*
158. Ryan, G. P., Copeland, E. M., and Johnson, L. R. (1978): Effects of gastrin on vagal denervation on DNA synthesis in canine fundic mucosa. *Am. J. Physiol.,* 235:E32-E36.
159. Sander, L. D., Enochs, M. R., and Johnson, L. R. (1978): Effects of ACTH and the adrenals on serum and antral gastrin levels in the rat. *Proc. Soc. Exp. Biol. Med.,* 158:609-613.
160. Sanders, T. G., and Rutter, W. J. (1970): The developmental regulation of amylolytic and proteolytic enzymes in the embryonic rat pancreas. *J. Biol. Chem.,* 249:3500-3509.
161. Sandweiss, D. J., Saltzstein, H. C., and Farbman, A. (1938): The prevention or healing of experimental peptic ulcer in Mann-Williamson dogs with the anterior pituitary-like hormone (Antuitrin-S). *Am. J. Dig. Dis.,* 5:24-30.
162. Savage, C. R., Jr., Inagami, T., and Cohen, S. (1972): The primary structure of epidermal growth factor. *J. Biol. Chem.,* 247:7612-7621.
163. Schapiro, H., Wruble, L. D., and Britt, L. G. (1970): The effect of hypophysectomy on the gastric intestinal tract. A review of the literature. *Am. J. Dig. Dis.,* 15:1019-1030.

164. Schneyer, C. A., and Hall, H. D. (1970): Autonomic regulation of postnatal changes in cell number and size of rat parotid. *Am. J. Physiol.,* 219:1268–1272.

165. Sesso, A., and Valeri, V. (1958): Nucleic acid patterns in the pancreas of hypophysectomized rats after administration of growth hormone and of thyroxine. *Exp. Cell Res.,* 14:201–203.

166. Sipponen, P., Hakkiluoto, A., Kalima, T. V., and Siurala, M. (1976): Selective loss of parietal cells in the gastric remnant following antral resection. *Scand. J. Gastroenterol.,* 11:813–816.

167. Spiro, H. N., and Milles, S. S. (1960): Clinical and physiological implications of the steroid-induced peptic ulcer. *N. Engl. J. Med.,* 263:285–294.

168. Stanley, M. D., Coalson, R. E., Grossman, M. I., and Johnson, L. R. (1972): Influence of secretin and pentagastrin on acid secretion and parietal cell number in rats. *Gastroenterology,* 63:264–269.

169. Stassoff, B. (1914): Experimentelle untersachungen uberdie kompeusatorischen vorange ker darmresektionen. *Beitr. Klin. Chir.,* 89:527–533.

170. Steiger, E., Vars, H. M., and Dudrick, S. J. (1972): A technique for long term intravenous feeding in unrestrained rats. *Arch. Surg.,* 104:330–332.

171. Steiner, M., Boughes, H. R., Freedman, L. S., and Gray, S. J. (1968): Effect of starvation on the tissue composition of the small intestine in the rat. *Am. J. Physiol.,* 215:75–77.

172. Straus, E., Gerson, C. D., and Yalow, R. S. (1974): Hypersecretion of gastrin associated with the short bowel syndrome. *Gastroenterology,* 66:175–180.

173. Sutton, D. R., and Donaldson, R. M. (1975): Synthesis and secretion of protein and pepsinogen by rabbit gastric mucosa in organ culture. *Gastroenterology,* 69:166–174.

174. Takeuchi, K., and Johnson, L. R. (1979): Pentagastrin protects against stress ulceration in rats. *Gastroenterology,* 76:327–334.

175. Takeuchi, K., Speir, G. R., and Johnson, L. R. (1979): Mucosal gastrin receptor. I. Assay standardization and fulfillment of receptor criteria. *Am. J. Physiol.,* 237:E284–E294.

176. Takeuchi, K., Speir, G. R., and Johnson, L. R. (1979): Mucosal gastrin receptor. II. Physical characteristics of binding. *Am. J. Physiol.,* 237:E295–E300.

177. Takeuchi, K., Speir, G. R., and Johnson, L. R. (1980): Mucosal gastrin receptor. III. Regulation by gastrin. *Am. J. Physiol.,* 238:G135–G140.

178. Tomkins, G. M., and Gelehrter, T. D. (1972): The present status of genetic regulation by hormones. In: *Biochemical Actions of Hormones, Vol. II,* edited by G. Litwack, pp. 1–20. Academic Press, New York.

179. Tutton, P. J. M. (1973): Control of epithelial cell proliferation in the small intestinal crypt. *Cell Tissue Kinet.,* 6:211–216.

180. Uvnas-Wallensten, K., Rehfeld, J. F., Larsson, L.-I., and Uvnas, B. (1977): Heptadecapeptide gastrin in the vagal nerve. *Proc. Natl. Acad. Sci. USA,* 74:5707–5710.

181. Vanamee, P., Winawer, S. J., Sherlock, P., Sonenberg, M., and Lipkin, M. (1970): Decreased incidence of restraint-stress induced gastric erosions in rats treated with bovine growth hormone. *Proc. Soc. Exp. Biol. Med.,* 135:259–263.

182. Verly, W. G., Deschamps, V., Pushpathadam, J., and Desrosiers, M. (1971): The hepatic chalone. Assay method for the hormone and purification of the rabbit liver chalone. *Can. J. Biochem.,* 49:1376–1383.

183. Walsh, J. H., and Grossman, M. I. (1975): Gastrin. *N. Engl. J. Med.,* 292:1324–1332, 1377–1384.

184. Weinstein, D. L., Shoemaker, C. P., and Hersh, T. (1969): Enhanced intestinal absorption after small bowel resection in man. *Arch. Surg.,* 99:560–562.

185. Weser, E. (1978): Role of gastrin in intestinal adaptation after small bowel resection. *Gastroenterology,* 75:323–324.

186. Weser, E., Heller, R., and Tawil, T. (1977): Stimulation of mucosal growth in the rat ileum by bile and pancreatic secretions after jejunal resection. *Gastroenterology,* 73:524–529.

187. Weser, E., and Hernandez, M. H. (1971): Small bowel adaptation after intestinal resection in the rat. *Gastroenterology,* 60:69–75.

188. Wickbom, G., Landor, J. H., Bushkin, F. L., and McGuigan, J. E. (1975): Changes in canine gastric acid output and serum gastrin levels following massive small intestinal resection. *Gastroenterology,* 69:448–452.

189. Willems, G., Galand, P., and Vansteenkiste, Y. (1972): Cell population kinetics of zymogen and parietal cells in the stomachs of mice. *Z. Zellforsch, Mikrosk. Anat.,* 134:505–518.

190. Willems, G., Gepts, W., and Bremer, A. (1977): Endogenous hypergastrinemia and cell proliferation in the fundic mucosa of the dog. *Am. J. Dig. Dis.,* 22:419–423.

191. Willems, G., and Lehy, T. (1975): Radioautographic and quantitative studies on parietal and peptic cell kinetics in the mouse. *Gastroenterology,* 69:416–426.

192. Willems, G., Vansteenkiste, Y., and Limbosch, J. M. (1972): Stimulating effect of gastrin on cell proliferation kinetics in canine fundic mucosa. *Gastroenterology,* 62:323–327.

193. Willems, G., Vansteenkiste, Y., and Smets, P. L. (1971): Effects of ethanol on the cell proliferation kinetics in the fundic mucosa of dogs. *Am. J. Dig. Dis.,* 15:1057–1064.

194. Willems, G., Vansteenkiste, Y., and Verbeustel, S. (1971): Autoradiographic study of cell renewal in fundic mucosa of fasting dogs. *Acta Anat. (Basel),* 80:23–32.

195. Williams-Ashman, H. G., and Reddi, A. M. (1972): Androgenic regulation of tissue growth and function. In: *Biochemical Actions of Hormones, Vol. II,* edited by G. Litwack, pp. 257–294. Academic Press, New York.

196. Williamson, R. C. N., Buchholtz, T. W., and Malt, R. A. (1978): Humoral stimulation of cell proliferation in small bowel after transection and resection in rats. *Gastroenterology,* 75:249–254.

197. Winborn, W. B., Seelig, L. L., Jr., Nakayama, H., and Weser, E. (1974): Hyperplasia of gastric glands after small bowel resection in the rat. *Gastroenterology,* 66:384–395.

198. Wright, H. K., Poskitt, T., and Cleveland, J. C. (1969): The effect of total colectomy on morphology and absorptive capacity of the ileum in the rat. *J. Surg. Res.,* 9:301–304.

199. Yalow, R. S., and Berson, S. A. (1970): Radioimmunoassay of gastrin. *Gastroenterology,* 58:11–14.

200. Yalow, R. S., and Berson, S. A. (1970): Size and charge distinctions between endogenous human plasma gastrin in peripheral blood and heptadecapeptide gastrins. *Gastroenterology,* 58:609–615.

Physiology of the Gastrointestinal Tract, edited by
Leonard R. Johnson. Raven Press, New York © 1981.

Chapter 6

Structure of Muscles and Nerves in the Gastrointestinal Tract

Giorgio Gabella

Analysis of the motor activity of the alimentary tract is founded on interpretation of the structure of the musculature and its nerves. The muscle coat is a conspicuous and tough component of the wall of the gastrointestinal tract. It is a continuous structure made of smooth muscle and extending from the upper part of the esophagus to the anal canal. The continuity is not disrupted by the presence of largely expanded segments, such as stomach and cecum, or by the opening of other canals, such as the hepatopancreatic duct into the duodenum. At the connections between segments rearrangement of the musculature occurs, sometimes forming an easily recognizable sphincter; sphincterial properties, however, more often reside in physiological and pharmacological characteristics of the musculature of certain portions of the tract, which are based on fine structural features of the innervation.

The intestinal muscle cells are relatively small (they are about two-thirds the volume of a hepatocyte), and of paramount importance are the structures at their surface that establish junctions between adjacent cells. These junctions are essential to produce mechanical cooperativity and communication between the cells. Special problems arise from several facts: there are no Z lines providing an easily recognized attachment site for the myofilaments; there are no proper tendons; there is a low myosin content by comparison with skeletal muscles but an ability to generate an equal amount of force; and there is the ability to shorten to as little as one-quarter the resting length, and to maintain contractions for long periods with little fatiguing. Smooth muscles can work partly against each other, or against a hydrostatic pressure within the lumen, but have a more complex relation with each other than that between agonist and antagonist skeletal muscles.

The intestines are richly supplied with nerves; in particular, they possess intramural ganglionated plexuses. These constitute the most peripheral nervous relays and are farther from the central nervous system than any other ganglia. They are situated at the end of sympathetic and parasympathetic (efferent) pathways, and they constitute the metasympathetic system or more appropriately the enteric nervous system.

The plexuses are readily accessible and may constitute a useful and interesting model for neurobiological studies. Yet they are so closely associated with the effectors themselves, both muscular and secretory, that they present special problems to physiological and pharmacological investigations. The number of neurons present within the gastrointestinal wall is enormous. They are connected to the sympathetic ganglia and to the central nervous system by means of a relatively small number of afferent and efferent fibers, but most of their spontaneous and reflex activities are little affected by decentralization—the basic mechanism of coordinated transport in the small intestine survives an extrinsic denervation of the gut. There is little evidence of hierarchical organization among intramural neurons.

FINE STRUCTURE OF SMOOTH MUSCLE CELLS

Visceral muscle cells are uninucleated and spindle shaped. At rest they measure 500 to 700 μm in length, but in isotonic contraction they can shorten to less than one-quarter of their resting length. Their volume is about 3500 μm^3 (106,219). The cell volume increases during postnatal development, but it does not change later in life. There are only small differences in muscle cell volume between animal species (Fig. 1), and cell size is not correlated with body size.

Because of their minute volume, visceral smooth muscle cells have a high surface-to-volume ratio (Fig. 2). The surface of one cell (not including the caveolae) amounts to slightly more than 5,000 μm^2 (106,219) and there is about 1.5 μm^2 of cell surface for every cubic micrometer of cell volume (106). The amount of cell surface (cell membrane) available for exchanges with the extracellular space is considerable, approximately 1 m^2/g tissue. Several structural specializations are present at the cell surface, and they include cell-to-cell junctions and junctions between a cell and the surrounding connective tissue stroma (see p. 205). Visceral muscle cells are invested by a basal lamina, except in the few areas of close cell-to-cell apposition such as the nexuses (p. 205).

The cell membrane has flask-shaped invaginations or caveolae over most of its surface (Fig. 3). Caveolae measure about 70 nm across and 120 nm in length, and their long axis is orthogonal to the cell surface. They are not penetrated by the basal lamina and open into the intercellular space through a narrow neck. Caveolae may occur singly at the cell surface but they are usually arranged in rows that run parallel to the long axis of the cell. Several rows are present on the profile of a cell in transverse section, and they alternate with parts of the membrane occupied by dense bands (this page) (222, 237,254,317) (Fig. 3). There are 20 to 30 caveolae per square micrometer of cell surface and a total of about 170,000 caveolae per cell (106). They increase the amount of cell membrane present at the cell surface by 50 to 70% (106,133). More than one-third of the plasma membrane at the cell surface forms caveolae, whereas

the rest of it forms the cell surface proper. Both the number of caveolae and the diameter of their necks are unaffected by shortening or stretching of the muscle cells (113). An interesting feature revealed by freeze-fracture is that intramembrane particles are abundant in the cell membrane immediately adjacent to the necks of the caveolae (113,317), whereas they are rare in the membrane of the caveolae themselves (113,253).

Caveolae of smooth muscle cells are accessible to extracellular space tracers such as ferritin, colloidal lanthanum, and peroxidase, but they show no micropinocytotic activity (69). In view of their constant occurrence and distribution, the caveolae can be regarded as organelles of smooth muscle cells, although their role remains unknown. Caveolae are also found in cardiac and skeletal muscles, in endothelial cells, and in some epithelial cells, but in each cell type they have some unique structural features and they probably serve different roles.

In the areas of the cell surface which are not occupied by caveolae, electron-dense material adheres to the inner side of the cell membrane and constitutes the so-called dense bands (or dense patches) (Fig. 3). These are about 0.2 to 0.4 μm in width and extend for 1 to 2 μm or more along the cell length; they are about 30 to 100 nm thick. Thin (actin) filaments and intermediate filaments penetrate into the dense bands (46,106,242) (Fig. 4A). Filaments are thus cemented to the cell membrane by means of a dense band, but they do not seem to reach or penetrate the membrane itself.

Dense bands are distributed all over the cell surface. In the middle portions of a cell—for example, at the level of the nucleus—30 to 50% of the cell profile can be occupied by dense bands and the percentage can be greater toward the tapering ends of the cell. On the average, between one-half and one-third of the cell surface (depending on the type of muscle) is occupied by dense bands (106). The majority of dense bands are apposed to microfibrils of the extracellular space. The possibility of a mechanical link between the two is discussed elsewhere. A dense band may match a similar structure in an adjacent cell, forming an intermediate junction (p. 205). The dense bands are undoubtedly points of attachment of the thin filaments to the cell membrane. It is characteristic of smooth muscle cells that this attachment is not confined to the ends of the cell but is widely spread over the entire cell surface. The protein alpha-actinin (which is also a structural component of Z lines of skeletal muscle fibers) has been localized by immunohistochemistry in the dense bands and the dense bodies of smooth muscle cells (275). Both this observation and the distribution of myofilaments support the notion, first discussed by Pease and Molinari (242), that dense bands and dense bodies are the equivalent of Z disks. Intermediate filaments (p. 204) probably connect some or most of the dense bands

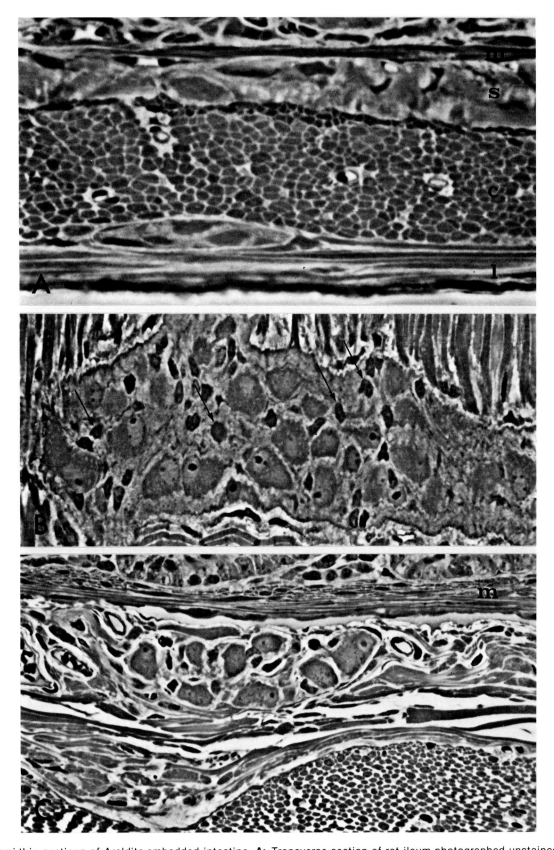

FIG. 1. Semi-thin sections of Araldite-embedded intestine. **A:** Transverse section of rat ileum photographed unstained in phase contrast. The mucosa is at top, the serosa at the bottom. m, muscularis mucosae; s, submucosa; c, circular muscle layer; l, longitudinal muscle layer. Between the two muscle layers is a ganglion of the myenteric plexus. At the innermost part of the circular muscle, note a thin layer of small and dark muscle cells (*arrow*). Magnification: 670 ×. **B:** Tangential section of muscle coat of guinea pig ileum, showing a large ganglion of the myenteric plexus. The circular muscle is at the bottom and the longitudinal muscle at top. Between the ganglion neurons are many glial cells (a few are arrowed), in which mainly the dark nuclei are visible. Magnification: 670 ×. **C:** Transverse section of sheep ileum. At bottom is part of the circular musculature, at top, the mucosa; m, muscularis mucosae with muscle cells running circularly (*upper part*) and cells running longitudinally (*bottom part*). In the submucosa surrounded by blood vessels and bundles of collagen, is a ganglion of the submucosal plexus, showing eight neurons and several glial cells. Magnification: 680 ×.

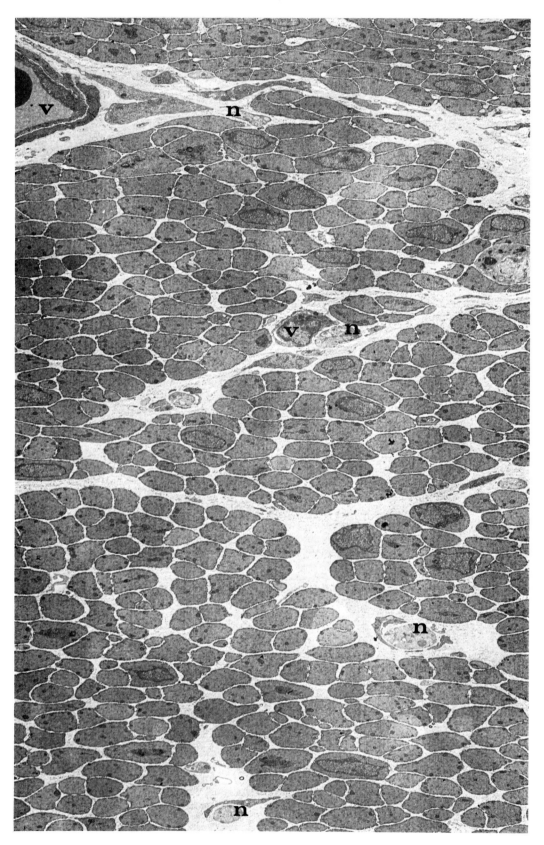

FIG. 2. Transverse section of the circular muscle layer of guinea pig proximal colon. Blood vessels (v) and intramuscular nerves (n) are scattered among the muscle cells. Note the variability in size of the muscle cell profiles. Magnification: 3,300 ×.

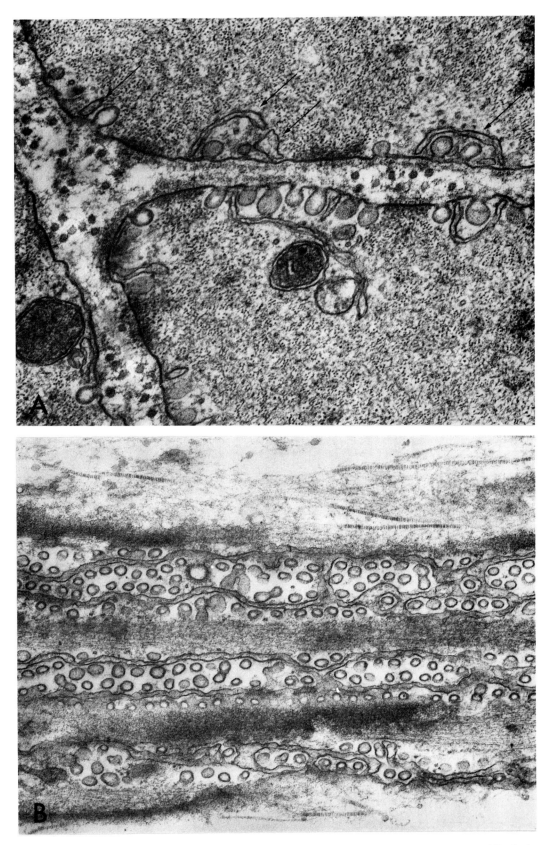

FIG. 3. A: Circular muscle layer of guinea pig ileum. Three muscle cells transversely sectioned show several flask-shaped caveolae closely associated with sarcoplasmic reticulum (*arrows*). The areas of the membrane free of caveolae are occupied by dense bands. The cells are coated by a basal lamina which appears thicker at the level of the dense bands. Collagen fibrils transversely sectioned are present in the intercellular space. Magnification: 67,000 ×. **B:** Longitudinal section of the guinea pig taenia coli. The cell membrane of a muscle cell is tangentially cut and shows caveolae (which are cross-sectioned and appear as isolated vesicles) associated with tubules of sarcoplasmic reticulum. Between the rows of caveolae, some dense bands are seen *en face*. At top, the basal lamina is included in the section and it appears associated with cross-banded collagen fibrils. This arrangement suggests a structural link between myofilaments, dense bands, cell membrane, basal lamina, and collagen fibrils. Magnification: 45,500 ×.

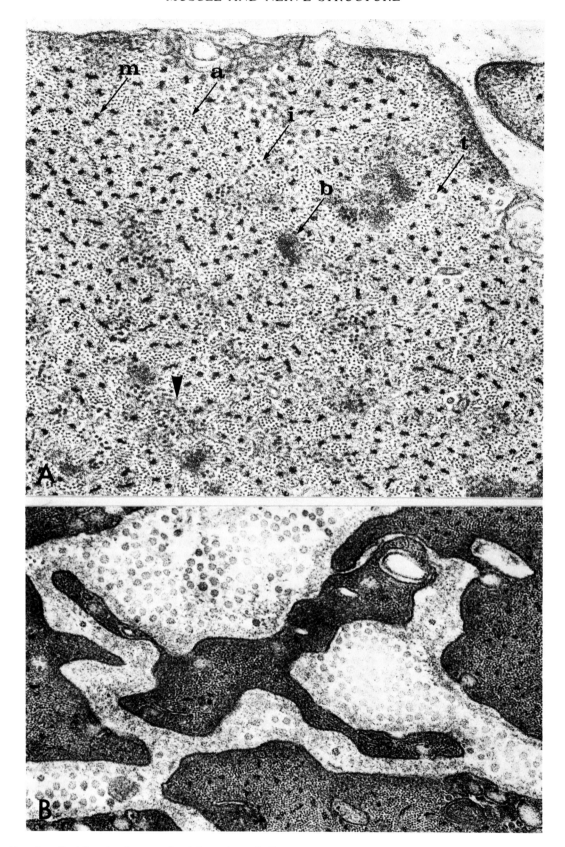

FIG. 4. A: Muscle cell of the circular muscle of the guinea pig ileum in transverse section, showing details of the filaments. a, bundles of thin (or actin) filaments; m, thick (or myosin) filaments; i, intermediate (or 10-nm) filaments; b, dense body. Note that in areas not occupied by myofilaments (for example, at the *arrowhead*), there are groups of intermediate filaments and other materials, including filaments, not readily identified. At top right, the cell membrane has a dense band. There are several microtubules (t). Magnification: 95,000 ×. B: Transverse section of guinea pig taenia coli. A cell profile of complex shape corresponds to the end part of a muscle cell. Note the thick basal lamina which seems to anchor the laminar processes to the adjacent muscle cells and to the numerous collagen fibrils. Magnification: 66,000 ×.

to the dense bodies situated more deeply in the sarcoplasm. In isotonically contracted muscle cells, most of the dense bands are retracted and the areas of the membrane-bearing caveolae are pushed outward.

Numerous microtubules are consistently found in smooth muscle cells (Fig. 4A). Other organelles include centrioles (often found on one side of the nucleus), a Golgi apparatus (in the regions of sarcoplasm near the nuclear poles), lysosomes, and sarcoplasmic reticulum (Fig. 3A). In developing muscle cells rough sarcoplasmic reticulum predominates, whereas in adult muscle cells cisternae of smooth reticulum are far more abundant. Some cisternae lie near the nucleus and among the filaments, but most of the reticulum is situated near the cell surface (Fig. 3). Large cisternae of smooth sarcoplasmic reticulum can be found immediately beneath and parallel to the cell membrane: the gap between the two structures is only about 10 nm, and regularly spaced electron densities have been observed in it (69). This arrangement is comparable to the "peripheral coupling" observed in cardiac muscle (87,298). Other parts of the reticulum may form a trough partly enclosing the caveolae or a network of tubules lying among the caveolae. Most of the sacs of reticulum have at least a small area where they lie close to the cell membrane. The total volume occupied by sarcoplasmic reticulum is in the region of 2% of the cell volume (69,218,252). The granular and some of the smooth sarcoplasmic reticulum are probably involved in synthetic processes (turnover of membranes, of filaments, and of collagen and other intercellular materials). The smooth sarcoplasmic reticulum is probably a major intracellular compartment for calcium sequestration and release. During activation of a smooth muscle, the influx of calcium from the extracellular space plays a greater role than in striated muscles; there are, however, also intracellular stores of calcium in smooth muscles, although they are not as well understood as in skeletal fibers. Histochemical studies on calcium localization in smooth muscles have indicated that the sarcoplasmic reticulum is the main site for calcium storage and release (66,149,186,251,324). Fast calcium uptake is also found in purified microsomal fractions obtained from smooth muscles (92,255). Recently by electron probe analysis on vascular smooth muscle cells calcium has been localized in the sarcoplasmic reticulum (295).

Mitochondria are found mainly near the cell surface or in the proximity of the nuclear poles. Elongated, parallel to the myofilaments, and usually with a dense matrix and intramitochondrial granules, they are closely associated with sacs and tubules of sarcoplasmic reticulum (106). An association between mitochondria and caveolae has also been reported (135,213,291,297). The volume occupied by mitochondria varies between 5 and 9%, depending on the type of intestinal muscle (112). Mitochondria of smooth muscle cells can take up and accumulate divalent cations, including calcium (293,294). Several authors have suggested that mitochondria participate in the regulation of calcium concentration in the sarcoplasm (11,297,315), although in this respect, at least in taenia coli, the role of the sarcoplasmic reticulum appears more important (255). It has recently been shown by electron probe analysis that smooth muscle mitochondria (in blood vessels) can be massively loaded with calcium in damaged cells but play no major role in regulating sarcoplasmic calcium concentration during physiological contraction (296).

Filaments

Actin and myosin can be extracted from smooth muscles, and the two prominent populations of thin and thick filaments are regarded as actin and myosin filaments. At least one other type of filament is clearly identified in smooth muscle cells, the intermediate or 10 nm filaments (Fig. 4A). In general, the structure and distribution of filaments in smooth muscle cells are less well understood than in striated muscles.

The thin filaments measure about 7 nm in diameter, they are readily preserved in most preparations (after glutaraldehyde fixation), they are often arranged in regular bundles, but their length has not been determined. Estimates of the ratio of thin to thick filaments in visceral muscles are about 12:1 (25,148,227), but there are probably variations between different smooth muscles. In some preparations, the thin filaments are arranged in rosettes around the much less numerous thick filaments, but this is often not the case. Thin filaments can be seen to penetrate into the amorphous material of the dense bands associated with the cell membrane and of the dense bodies (7,46,242).

The thick filaments are considerably more difficult to preserve, and their appearance in electron micrographs varies widely with the preparation procedure used. They have an irregular profile in transverse section, measure 15 to 17 nm in diameter, and have tapered ends (7). In vascular muscle cells, they measure 2.2 μm in length (7). Thick filaments isolated from the guinea pig taenia coli by gentle homogenization are mostly less than 3 μm in length, but long filaments up to 8 μm or more are also found; some of the thick filaments aggregate side by side and in such a way that the cross-bridge repeat is always in register (283). Much shorter values for the length of the myosin filaments in visceral muscles are quoted by other authors (228).

Cross-bridges in smooth muscle myosin filaments are not so readily demonstrated as in skeletal muscles, but they probably have a helical arrangement along the filament (289,292). X-ray diffraction studies have shown a 14.4 nm meridional reflection in smooth muscles, which is considered to arise from the myosin filaments and to represent the axial periodicity of myosin heads (and therefore cross-bridges) (211,279). A bare area in the middle portion of smooth muscle myosin filaments has not been demonstrated (289). Some authors, however, have reported the presence of a bare area in myosin filaments (188,228), whereas others have concluded that the definitive absence of a bare area in visceral muscle myosin filaments indicates that the arrangement of myosin molecules is different from that found in skeletal fiber myosin filaments (283,287) (see below). *In vitro,* myosin molecules obtained from smooth muscle appear identical to those from striated muscle (82). However, it is not known how myosin molecules are assembled in the thick filaments of smooth muscles. Thick filaments can be reassembled *in vitro,* and recently it has been shown that smooth muscle myosin is assembled not only in short bipolar filaments, similar to those obtained from skeletal muscle myosin (171), but also in filaments with two faces along their entire length, and the myosin heads are oriented in opposite directions in each face (57). *In vivo* the myosin filaments of striated fibers have myosin heads with the same orientation in each half of the filament. This may be the case also in smooth muscle myosin, but according to Sobieszek (287), who has put forward the best known model of the molecular packing in the myosin filaments of smooth muscle, the filaments are made of bipolar building units, most likely an antiparallel myosin dimer (two myosin molecules linked tail-to-tail with an overlap of about 60 nm and a twist of 180°). On the basis of optical diffraction analysis, Sobieszek (287) has proposed that such dimers are arranged on a six-stranded helix of 72 nm repeats. The absence of a central bare zone (286,288), the finding that the terminal portions of *in vitro* myosin filaments are devoid of projections (or cross-bridges) (bare edges) (287), and the occurrence of a 14.4 nm continuous repeat are all accounted for by this model (151,287).

Although the composition of actins isolated from a variety of smooth and striated muscles is similar (reviewed in 145), the composition of myosin is less uniform. Antibodies against smooth muscle myosin do not react with skeletal muscle myosin (138), and there are also chemical differences between myosins from various smooth muscles or from different species (250). The high ratio of thin filaments to thick filaments, especially when compared with skeletal muscle fibers where the ratio is 2:1, roughly corresponds to a ratio of actin to myosin that is several times higher than that found in skeletal muscles, the difference being accounted for by a low concentration of myosin in smooth muscle (223,311). Since the amount of tension developed by a striated muscle is related to the number of cross-bridges acting in parallel (170), it is of considerable interest to find that visceral and vascular smooth muscles can generate a tension per unit transverse sectional area that is as large as that of skeletal muscles (107,223).

The third type of filament found in smooth muscle cells is the intermediate filament or 100-A° or 10-nm filament (on account of its approximate diameter). These filaments are present in all smooth muscle cells, but their numbers vary considerably even within the same population of cells. They may be bundled to form a core in the central part of the cell (46) or may occur individually or in small groups among the myofilaments or in association with dense bodies and dense bands (259,292,294) (Fig. 4A). Intermediate filaments are abundant in developing and cultured smooth muscle cells (39,312) and in pathological conditions such as response to injury (294) or experimental hypertrophy (108). In transverse section the intermediate filaments have a clear-cut profile, often with a clear area in the center (259,285,312). They are formed by four filamentous subunits of 3.5 nm diameter (285). Intermediate filaments can be seen associated with the amorphous material of dense patches (46) and to encircle some of the dense bodies (7), probably forming a mechanical link with them. It has been suggested that intermediate filaments form inside smooth muscle cells a supporting framework, similar to the cytoskeleton that intermediate filaments form in obliquely striated muscles of invertebrates (266).

Intermediate filaments identical in appearance to those described in smooth muscle cells are found in developing skeletal muscle fibers (177), in cardiac muscle cells (256), and in several nonmuscle cells (178). Among the last are fibroblasts, endothelial cells, epithelial keratin cells (in which the 10-nm filaments are called tonofilaments), glial cells (gliofilaments) (see Fig. 18), and neurons (neurofilaments). The term *desmin filaments* has been proposed for the intermediate filaments of muscle cells (166,205), the term *vimentin filaments* for the intermediate filaments found in mesenchymal cells and some of their derivatives (93,172). Keratins are a complex family of proteins, and their filaments differ substantially in composition and substructure from other intermediate filaments (29,303). The major constituents of the other intermediate filaments are proteins of 55,000 to 58,000 daltons. There is similarity in the composition of these proteins between different cell types [particularly similar are smooth muscle intermediate filaments and neurofilaments (65,284)], but there are important immunological differences, and a complex classification of biochemical types of intermediate filaments is emerging (17,204).

The arrangement of filaments in smooth muscle cells is poorly known. Their spatial distribution is probably more difficult to preserve for microscopy and also less regular and less uniform than in striated fibers. Thin filaments can be arranged in rosettes around thick filaments (7,292), but they also occur in compact bundles of 20 or more filaments. Thin filaments penetrate into the amorphous and electron-dense material of dense bodies and dense bands (242,292). Some regularity in the arrangement of thick filaments has been observed in vascular muscle cells studied in serial sections, and these groups of filaments (3 to 5 thick filaments and the associated thin filaments) could constitute a sort of mini-sarcomere (7). A full comparition of the myofilaments into proper sarcomeres has also been proposed (282). In visceral smooth muscles myofilaments are arranged parallel to the cell long axis or form a small angle with it (265). They probably remain almost parallel even during intense shortening of the muscle (109). It has, however, been suggested that in isotonically contracted cells the bundles of filaments become rearranged and run obliquely across the cell, forming an angle of 30° to 50° with the cell axis (88,91,283).

JUNCTIONS BETWEEN MUSCLE CELLS: ELECTRICAL AND MECHANICAL COUPLING

Important features of smooth muscles are cell-to-cell junctions involving specializations of the cell membrane and the adjacent structures (reviewed in refs. 146 and 109).

An area of the cell membrane receiving attachment of myofilaments (dense band) can be matched by a similar area in an adjacent cell, and they form a symmetrical, usually elongated junction known as the intermediate junction (Fig. 5A). The cleft between the membranes is 30 to 40 nm and is occupied by an ill-defined band of electron-dense material that often shows a periodicity and is in continuity with the basal laminae of the two cells. Other structural details of these junctions, including the relation of the dense material with the myofilaments, are identical to those found in the single dense bands. The latter could be regarded as hemi-junctions linking the contractile apparatus to the collagen and elastic framework of the muscle. The intermediate junctions seem to provide direct mechanical links between muscle cells. Their structure suggests that they transmit force from a bundle of myofilaments in a cell to a bundle in the neighboring one. These junctions are different from desmosomes, mainly in that there is no multilayered material in the intercellular gap and there are no groups of large intramembrane particles (in freeze-fractured preparations).

Other junctions which are similar but somewhat distinct from those described above are smaller in size and spot-like and display a symmetric condensation of electron-dense material that is not associated with myofilaments (Fig. 5A). The intercellular gap is of uniform width and measures 15 to 20 nm. The significance of these junctions is not clear. They sometimes occur between a smooth muscle cell and a nerve ending.

Another well-known junction found in a number of smooth muscles is the gap junction or nexus (Fig. 5B). This is a disk- or oval-shaped area of the cell membrane, closely apposed to an identical area in an adjacent cell. The intercellular gap is reduced to a space 2 to 3 nm wide that is bridged by subunits regularly arranged and probably containing the channels for the direct, private exchange of ions and certain molecules between the two cells (reviewed in 131,246 and 302). The narrow intercellular gap can be penetrated by extracellular electron-dense tracers, such as colloidal lanthanum, which give it the appearance of a thin, dark line separating the two membranes. In a flat view of the junction (the junction has a total thickness of about 20 nm and can therefore be fully included in a microtonic section for an *en face* view), the regularly arranged discontinuities within the gaps, due to subunits bridging the two membranes, become apparent as areas not filled by the tracer (reviewed in 246 and 302). In the area of the nexus the interior of the membrane, as visualized by freeze-fracture, shows a highly characteristic clustering of intramembrane particles on the P-face (Fig. 6A). On the E-face, there is a set of shallow dimples (intramembrane pits) closely matching in number and distribution the particles of the P-face, and an identical pattern is found in the adjacent membrane (Fig. 6B). Gap junctions have been studied more extensively and are better characterized in certain epithelial tissues (such as the liver, gastric mucosa, and lens) than in smooth muscles. Each intermembrane particle is thought to represent the fractured aspect of an intercellular channel which spans the thickness of the two membranes and the narrow intercellular gap, and allows transit of certain ions and small molecules. The result of this communication is an electrical or metabolic coupling between the cells. The possibility of interruption of the communication (uncoupling) (for example, by an increase of the intracellular concentration of calcium or by a decrease of the pH) is well documented, and there have been suggestions as to the structural changes that cause the uncoupling (244,245,314). The gap junctions of smooth muscle are considered to conform to the characteristics found in these junctions in other tissues (95,114,121) and to provide electrical coupling between the muscle cells (9).

Gap junctions appear in freeze-fracture preparations as patches of intramembrane particles 8 to 10 nm in diameter (Fig. 6A). In the circular muscle of the guinea pig ileum, the area of a nexus ranges between 0.01 and 0.15 μm^2, and the packing density of intramembrane particles is about 7,000 μm^{-2}. In this muscle each cell has about 250 nexuses, and all together the nexuses of one cell occupy about 0.22% of the cell surface (114).

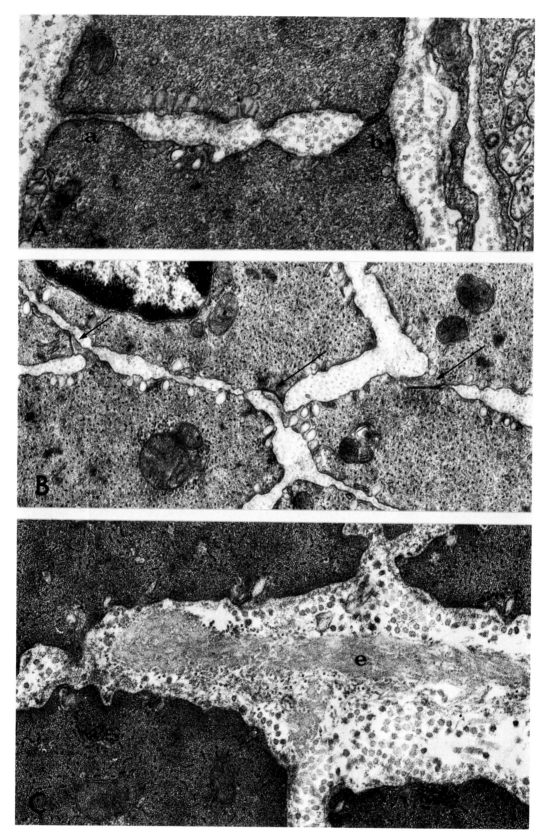

FIG. 5. A. Transverse section of an intestinal muscle. The two muscle cells are linked by intermediate junctions of two different types. The one at left (a) is broader, with an intercellular gap of approximately 30 nm, which is occupied by a band of electron-dense material. The junction is basically formed by two dense bands matching each other in adjacent cells and receiving insertion of thin filaments. The junction at right (b) is smaller, has an intercellular gap of about 15 nm, and shows prominent electron-dense material associated with the cell membrane. The laminar process of an interstitial cell and a nerve are present at far right. **B:** Circular muscle of rat ileum. Three gap junctions between muscle cells (*arrows*). Magnification: 25,000 ×. **C:** Transverse section of guinea pig taenia coli. An elastic fiber (e) closely associated with the basal lamina of two muscle cells. As is often the case in intestinal muscles, the elastic fiber runs at right angle to the long axis of the muscle cells. Magnification: 52,000 ×.

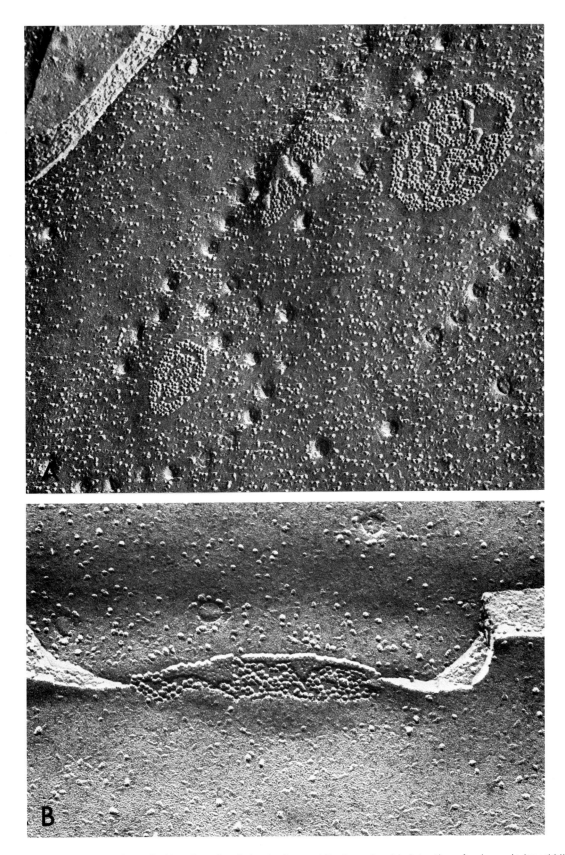

FIG. 6. Freeze-fracture preparations. **A:** Muscle cells of circular layer of the hypertrophic intestine of guinea pig (see 111). The fracture plane exposes the P-face of the cell membrane. There are three large clusters of intramembrane particles which are identified as gap junctions or nexuses. In addition to numerous dispersed intramembrane particles, the membrane shows crater-like structures which are caveolae fractured at the level of their necks. Modified from Gabella (111). Magnification: 92,000 ×. **B:** Circular layer of guinea pig ileum. Two muscle cells of which the P-face (*top*) and the E-face (*bottom*) are exposed. A gap junction occurs between the two cells and is exposed partly on the P-face (where it appears as a conglomeration of particles) and partly on the E-face (where it appears as a conglomeration of pits). The whitish streak on either side of the gap junction is the intercellular space. Magnification: 84,000 ×.

For some time after the original observations on the presence of nexuses in smooth muscles were reported (70,71), these junctions were considered to be a consistent feature of all smooth muscles. More recent studies, particularly by freeze-fracture, have shown that this is not the case. There are muscles, such as the longitudinal muscle of the ileum or of the vas deferens of the guinea pig, that have good cable properties (and their cells are therefore electrically coupled) but are devoid of nexuses. In taenia coli gap junctions are small and few in number (95) or extremely rare (113). Gap junctions are abundant in the circular muscle of the guinea pig ileum and even more abundant in that of the duodenum; they are, however, not found in the adjacent longitudinal musculature and are virtually absent in the rectum (115). Similarly, in the small intestine of the dog, nexuses are abundant in the circular muscle but absent in the longitudinal muscle (147), and in the stomach they are found in the circular musculature of the antrum but are absent in both muscle layers of the fundus (63). The failure to identify nexuses in muscles with good cable properties suggests that in some muscles electrical coupling can be obtained by means other than gap junctions. In the small intestine of the cat gap junctions are seen in both muscle layers (310), but in freeze-fracture preparations those of the longitudinal musculature are much fewer in number and smaller in size than those of the circular layer (110). During experimentally induced hypertrophy of the small intestine, the percentage surface of the circular muscle cells which is occupied by gap junctions more than doubles (111) and a similar increase is observed in another smooth muscle, the vas deferens of the rat, upon denervation (319). Treatment of a smooth muscle *in vitro* with metabolic inhibitors leads to reduction or disappearance of the gap junctions, whereas treatment with a hypertonic solution hardly changes their number (63).

Occasional gap junctions are found between a muscle cell and an interstitial cell: in the avian intestine (175), in the guinea pig taenia coli (106), and in the small intestine of the dog (63), the mouse (323), and the cat (310). In the last case, it has been suggested that gap junctions between smooth muscle and interstitial cells, albeit infrequent, can provide coupling between the longitudinal and the circular musculature. (Junctions between nerve endings and muscle cells are described on p. 219.)

ARRANGEMENT OF CELLS IN A SMOOTH MUSCLE

Smooth muscle cells in the muscle coats are densely packed. There are about 180,000 cells/mm³ (106). The cells are separated by spaces measuring only a few tens

of nanometers, mainly occupied by collagen fibrils, and by a few larger spaces occupied by nerves, capillaries, interstitial cells and intramuscular septa of connective tissue (Fig. 2). The volume of the intercellular space—as estimated from electron micrographs analyzed morphometrically—varies between 10% and 30% (109). Somewhat larger estimates are obtained with the use of tracers (such as inulin, co-EDTA, or polyethylene glycol), and there is therefore some uncertainty as to the actual extent of the extracellular space *in vivo* (27,134,304).

Muscle cells lie approximately parallel to each other, usually forming sheet-like layers or coats. In the intestine the two layers are superimposed, and their cells run at right angles (orthogonal) to each other—circular and longitudinal musculature, the former often being subdivided into two components. In the cecum and in parts of the colon (to an extent which varies between species) the longitudinal musculature is extremely attenuated except in three regions around the circumference of the organs, where it forms thick cords (the taeniae). In the stomach, the arrangement of the musculature is more complex, and in some areas there are three layers; the muscle cells in one layer are still orthogonal or near by orthogonal to those of the adjacent layer. Exchange of muscle cells between adjacent layers is rare, but it has been reported in the cat intestine (40) and in the guinea pig taenia coli (106).

In the small intestine, the innermost part of the circular layer is made of special muscle cells which are much smaller and more electron dense than those of the bulk of the circular layer (Fig. 1A) (104,209,280,307). Between the two components run a large number of nerve fibers with abundant varicosities (104,280,307), and it has been suggested that some of these are sensory fibers working in conjunction with the small muscle cells in the manner of a stretch receptor (104).

The muscle cells within a layer are subdivided into groups by laminar intramuscular septa, which span the full thickness of the layer. The septa are parallel to the muscle cells and extend only for a few hundred microns; they are then replaced by other septa in different positions. Thus the muscle is not subdivided into clear-cut bundles by the occurrence of septa, but all groups of muscle cells are continuous with each other. In cord-like muscles, such as the taeniae, septa are prominent but of short length and again the muscle is not subdivided into identifiable bundles (106), although electrophysiologically the effector unit of visceral smooth muscles is not a single cell but a muscle cell bundle (18). The occurrence of muscle bundles is clear in other muscles such as the circular musculature of the cecum and colon, but here again they always divide or merge with other bundles. A perimysium is not present in intestinal muscles.

During isotonic contraction the individual muscle

cells shorten approximately by the same amount as the whole muscle. The surface of the cell, which is fairly smooth in the cell at rest, becomes highly corrugated, being thrown into prominent folds (Fig. 7). Many of the folds, and the grooves which separate them, are obliquely arranged with respect to the cell long axis and may interdigitate with some of the grooves and folds of neighboring cells. The intramuscular septa of isotonically contracted muscles remain parallel to the long axis of the muscle. The muscle cells, however, at least in the guinea pig taenia coli, seem to undergo some torsion when they shorten maximally and their long axes deviate somewhat from the axis of the muscle.

Abundant collagen fibrils are present within visceral smooth muscles. Characteristically they measure 30 to 35 nm in diameter (whereas those of the submucosa and serosa measure about 50 nm) and display a transverse banding with a repeat of about 65 nm. They are grouped in bundles to form the collagen fibers of intramuscular septa or occur individually around the muscle cells. The collagen content of a visceral smooth muscle is 3 to 4 times larger than that of a skeletal muscle, and this observation has led to the suggestion that in a smooth muscle, which is devoid of tendons, the abundant collagen constitutes a kind of intramuscular tendon (109). The septa, for example, would bear the tension produced by a group of muscle cells and would transmit it longitudinally to other groups of muscle cells. Collagen fibrils probably play a major role in the transmission of force along a smooth muscle. Some morphological evidence suggests a link between the cell membrane, covered by a basal lamina, and adjacent collagen fibrils, mainly by means of microfibrils. These connections are more evident at the level of the dense bands, an observation suggesting the propagation of force generated by the myofilaments to the collagen framework of the muscle. Microfibrils connecting the specialized cell membrane and the collagen fibrils have also been demonstrated in cardiac and skeletal muscles (144) and in vascular smooth muscle cells (268,289). Since the dense bands are distributed over the entire length of a smooth muscle cell, most of the cell surface (and not only the two ends of the cell) is involved in this process. However, the biochemistry and the structural details of these junctions between the contractile apparatus (via the dense bands) and the stroma are poorly understood. They include not only junctions with collagen fibrils but also a small number of junctions with elastic fibers (Fig. 5C). In some smooth muscles—for example, the taenia coli—the end portions of many muscle cells acquire an elaborate profile with laminar projections (Fig. 4B), and there are complex apparatuses linking two muscle cells end-to-end (Fig. 8) (109). The significance of these structures is probably to enhance cell-to-cell and cell-to-stroma linkage.

The gastrointestinal tract contains smooth muscle also in the wall of its vessels and in the muscularis mucosae, situated at the boundary between the mucosa and submucosa. The muscularis mucosae is very thin (usually not more than 2 to 5 cells thick) in the small intestine (Fig. 1A and B): it is formed by muscle cells running longitudinally, or by two layers, one longitudinal, the other (on the mucosal side) circular. The muscularis mucosae is more prominent in the esophagus, particularly near the gastroesophageal junction, and in the large intestine, particularly toward the terminal part of the rectum; the longitudinal component always predominates. The muscularis mucosae is made of smooth muscle cells, whose fine structure has been investigated by Lane and Rhodin (198).

Commonly found within the intestinal musculature are the interstitial cells. These cells have attracted considerable attention after Cajal (37) suggested that they were modified sympathetic neurons relaying motor nerve endings to smooth muscle cells. Like neurons they can be stained with intravital methylene blue and silver impregnation (307). In the electron microscope, however, these cells show no similarity to nerve cells, but rather have many structural features in common with fibroblasts (110,264,307) (see Fig. 11). The cytoplasm is rich in cisternae of smooth and rough endoplasmic reticulum, with a content of medium electron density. A basal lamina is usually absent [it has, however, been observed in interstitial cells of the small intestine of the mouse (323) and lovebird (175)]. Interstitial cells are intensely positive for nonspecific cholinesterase (142,190), are often associated with intramuscular nerves or spread over the surface of a ganglion, and have a characteristic stellate shape with long processes. The latter can reach out toward a number of muscle cells and with them they occasionally form gap junctions (see p. 208). Some interstitial cell processes reach within 20 nm of a vesicle-containing nerve ending, and the proposal that these may be synaptic contacts has been put forward (140,164).

In the light of the ultrastructural evidence, Cajal's hypothesis appears untenable, although some authors (175) accept that interstitial cells may transmit stimuli from nerve endings to smooth muscle cells. It has also been suggested that interstitial cells are undifferentiated or immature smooth muscle cells (323), and that they may provide electrical coupling (in the cat small intestine) between circular and longitudinal muscle cells (310). As already suggested by Dogiel (74), interstitial cells are probably modified fibroblasts, but their functional role within a muscle remains to be elucidated.

Other cells found within smooth muscle are macrophages [recognized by their phagocytotic activity (307)], mast cells (45), and myoblast-like cells (323). The intramuscular blood vessels are mainly capillaries.

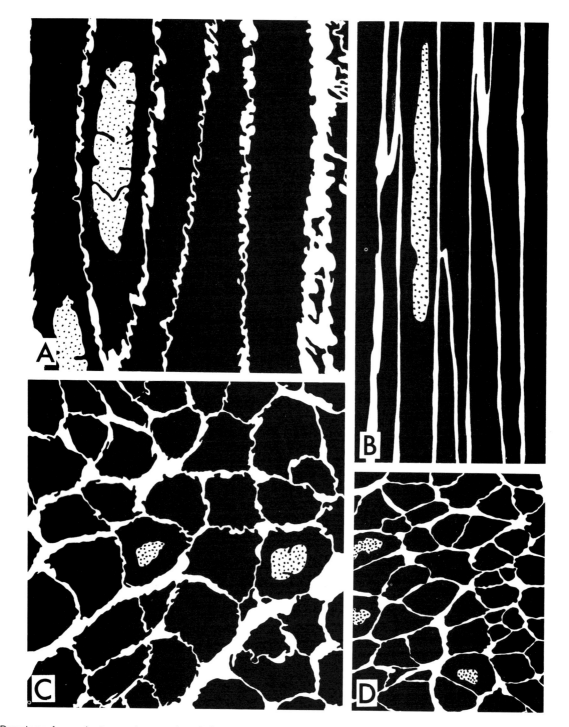

FIG. 7. Drawings from electron micrographs of the guinea pig taenia coli. **A:** Strip isotonically contracted against 1 g load in longitudinal section. **B:** Strip relaxed and stretched, in longitudinal section. **C:** Transverse section of an isotonically contracted strip. **D:** Transverse section of a stretched strip. Note that with isotonic contraction, the muscle cells markedly fatten and their profiles become highly corrugated. Changes occur also in the length and the shape of the nuclei (*dotted areas*). Magnification: **A** and **B**, 4,600 ×; **C** and **D**, 3,100 ×.

EXTRINSIC AND INTRINSIC INNERVATION OF THE ALIMENTARY TRACT: SOURCE AND DISTRIBUTION OF EXTRINSIC NERVES

The chief components of the nervous apparatus controlling the motility of the gut are the intramural plex-

uses. From these plexuses motor fibers emerge to innervate the muscle cells, and afferent fibers penetrate into the plexuses projecting back from the muscle to the ganglia. In addition to entirely intrinsic neurons (whose axons constitute the great majority of the nerve fibers within the gut), the gastrointestinal wall contains nerve fibers of extrinsic origin. These reach the gut via the

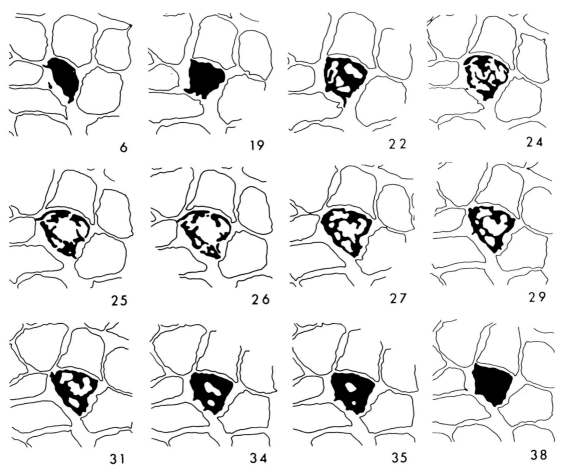

FIG. 8. Guinea pig taenia coli. Drawings of smooth muscle cell profiles from transverse serial sections. The level along the series is indicated by the number below each section, which is the distance in microns from the beginning of the series. Two muscle cells, whose full profile is seen in the first and the last drawing, are shaded; they join each other end-to-end by means of elaborate laminar and finger-like processes.

vagus nerve, the mesenteric nerves, and the pelvic nerves.

The largest components of the vagus nerve are afferent fibers issued by neurons of the nodose and jugular ganglia. In the cervical portion of the nerve in the cat, the fibers that degenerate after intracranial vagotomy (i.e., vagotomy above the ganglia) represent only 20 to 25% of the total; however, in the abdominal vagus 90% of the fibers survive this operation and can therefore be considered to originate from the vagal ganglia; whereas the fibers that do degenerate are probably efferent fibers issued by neurons in the medulla (2,84). These efferent fibers are preganglionic parasympathetic fibers. In the vagus nerves of the rabbit and cat they are mainly unmyelinated; they often begin as thinly myelinated fibers and lose their sheath along their course. In small animal species, such as the rat, rabbit, and cat, myelinated fibers in the abdominal vagus amount to less than 1% of the total number of fibers. However, in humans and sheep this portion of the nerve contains thousands of myelinated fibers (173,272).

The vagus nerve may contain a small number of adrenergic fibers originating from the superior cervical ganglion (207,224) and probably also from the stellate ganglion (4). Afferent and efferent fibers (of the latter there is probably more than one type, as evidenced by pharmacological studies) cannot be distinguished morphologically.

There is abundant evidence on the influence of vagal fibers on secretion and motility, but the projection of these fibers in the stomach and intestine is not well understood. The evidence at hand is chiefly based on silver impregnation studies (185,273,274), and suffers therefore from the difficulty of tracking degenerating autonomic axons, particularly within the viscera.

The mesenteric nerves emerge from the prevertebral (also paraaortic or preaortic) ganglia: the celiac, superior, and inferior mesenteric ganglia. They lie in the mesentery and are satellites of the large arteries for the stomach and intestines. Each artery is accompanied by 3 to 6 small nerves (paravascular nerves) that run at some distance from its adventitia. The adventitia in its turn is richly supplied with adrenergic fibers that mainly provide motor control of the vascular musculature (perivascular nerve fibers). The bulk of the fibers in mesenteric nerves are efferent fibers originating from neurons of the prevertebral ganglia. They are sympathetic, postganglionic, adrenergic fibers. The vast majority are unmyelinated.

The prevertebral ganglia are made up of neurons fairly uniform in size (67), slightly larger than those of the sympathetic chain (94), multipolar, and with long and complex dendrites. By fluorescence microscopy these neurons are identified as adrenergic and they are the source of the adrenergic supply to the gut (199,229). An indication of the relative extent of the prevertebral ganglia is given by the following nerve cell counts in the mouse (189): superior cervical ganglion, 14,500 neurons; stellate ganglion, 19,000; cardiac ganglion, 11,000; celiac ganglion, 25,000; superior mesenteric ganglion, 25,000. The inferior mesenteric ganglion is usually by far the smallest of the three prevertebral ganglia.

The ganglion neurons receive numerous synaptic endings mainly on their dendrites, less often on the cell bodies (80,307). There are also specialized junctions between axons (possible axoaxonic synapses) and dendrodendritic junctions (81). Many synaptic endings are from preganglionic fibers originating from the neurons in the intermediolateral column approximately from the levels between T-4 and L-3 or L-4 (in humans) (216). The fibers first travel in the ventral roots, then in the white rami communicantes; they pass without interruption through the ganglia of the sympathetic chain from which they emerge to form the conspicuous thoracic splanchnic nerves and the much smaller lumbar splanchnic nerves. These fibers are cholinergic and, after extensive branching, synapse on the adrenergic ganglion neurons. Whereas in the ganglia of the sympathetic chain virtually the entire synaptic input is contributed by the preganglionic fibers, in the prevertebral ganglia there are also synaptic endings from neurons situated in adjacent ganglia (e.g., synaptic connections from the celiac ganglion to the inferior mesenteric ganglion and vice versa). These fibers, whose occurrence has been shown by intracellular recording from ganglion neurons (58,194), are presumably adrenergic; they probably correspond to the fibers seen by fluorescence microscopy forming prominent pericellular nests around some ganglion neurons (143,229). Moreover, the prevertebral ganglia receive a synaptic input from neurons situated within the walls of the viscera. The pioneering work of Kuntz (195,196) on intramural afferent neurons whose axons project on neurons of the prevertebral ganglia has been confirmed by intracellular recording studies (58,59,194). These afferent neurons have not been identified morphologically or electrophysiologically, but those located in the gallbladder or in the colon of the guinea pig are known to respond to distension of the wall (mechanoreceptors) (see p. 234). An electrophysio-

logical study of the celic ganglion of the guinea pig has shown a high degree of convergence of different inputs on individual ganglion neurons (193).

A large proportion of neurons in the prevertebral ganglia (about 60% in the guinea pig) contain the peptide somatostatin (see p. 230) (156). These neurons are adrenergic (as shown by a positive reaction with antiserum for dopamine-beta-hydroxylase) and contain norepinephrine; they are thus an example of neurons in which two substances active in nerve transmission are stored in the same cell. In addition, the prevertebral ganglia contain substance P-immunoreactive fibers (perhaps originating from the dorsal root ganglia and reaching the wall of the gut (158), fibers with gastrin/cholecystokinin-like immunoreactivity (203), fibers with VIP immunoreactivity (157), and fibers with enkephalin immunoreactivity (278). The prevertebral ganglia also contain a certain number of small, intensely fluorescent cells (SIF cells, or chromaffin cells) (see an exhaustive review in 308).

A third source of extrinsic fibers to the alimentary tract is the pelvic plexus. This is a laminar ganglionated plexus situated on either side of the rectum (200,220). From the ganglia originate numerous small nerves which reach the urogenital organs and the aboral part of the alimentary tract. Cholinergic neurons are present in these ganglia, which receive synapses from parasympathetic, preganglionic, cholinergic fibers originating from the sacral portion of the spinal cord. Other neurons in these ganglia are adrenergic and there are also a number of lumbar sympathetic fibers (197). Therefore, in many species at the pelvic level the sympathetic and parasympathetic pathways cannot be clearly separated and some functional interaction may take place between the two. But in the colon of the rabbit, for example, the sympathetic and the parasympathetic fibers reach the organ via separate nerves, the lumbar colonic nerves and the pelvic nerves, respectively (119). The preganglionic parasympathetic fibers to the colon (of the cat) are unmyelinated and conduct at a velocity of only 0.5 to 1.4 m/sec (68).

DISTRIBUTION OF INTRAMURAL PLEXUSES

The two ganglionated plexuses are situated in the submucosa (submucosal or Meissner's plexus) and between the layers of the muscle coat (myenteric or Auerbach's plexus). The two plexuses are coextensive with the smooth musculature, from the esophagus to the anal canal, and they extend without discontinuities through the various portions of the alimentary tract. The plexuses can be visualized as mesh-like laminar structures, i.e., wide and thin ganglia spread over a surface and joined to each other by connecting strands (Fig. 9). Small nerves emerge from the plexuses and connect the two or provide nerve endings to the layers of the wall.

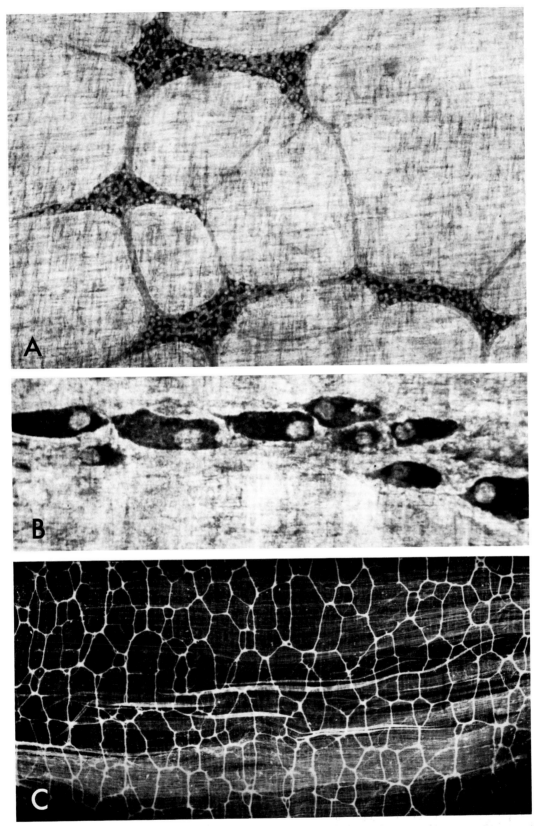

FIG. 9. A: Myenteric plexus of guinea pig rectum stained *in toto* with a histochemical method for DPN diaphorase. The stretch preparation includes the longitudinal musculature which appears in the background. Three large ganglia are packed with neurons and are linked by connecting strands. From Gabella (105). Magnification: 133 ×. **B:** Nerve ganglion cells of the myenteric plexus stained as in **A**. Magnification: approximately 800 ×. **C:** Myenteric plexus of rabbit ileum, lying over the longitudinal musculature. The tissue was incubated for the histochemical detection of acetylcholinesterase (thiocholine method). The print was obtained by placing the microscope slide directly in the enlarger and producing a reverse (or negative) image on photographic paper. Magnification 8.4 ×.

The mesh formed by the ganglia and the connecting strands has a regular, although not quite geometrical, pattern, which is characteristic of each segment of the alimentary tract and to some extent also of the animal species. Whether these patterns have any significance and whether they bear any relation to the functional properties of the organ are unknown. As a manifestation of order, they represent a challenging problem of morphogenesis and intercellular organization.

The number of neurons in each ganglion of the myenteric plexus varies from 50 or more to only a few. In some species, e.g., the rat, the ganglia are not well individualized and appear more as lines of neurons arranged circumferentially. In the colon of the guinea pig the ganglia are so large that they tend to merge with each other without a clear-cut separation (110,176) (Fig. 10C). Occasionally, neurons are not grouped in a ganglion but occur isolated within a connecting strand. In the small intestine there is little difference in the appearance of the plexus near the attachment of the mesentery and at the antimesenterial border (Figs. 10A and B) (although ganglion neurons are reported to be smaller near the mesenterial border); however, in the stomach Auerbach's ganglia are large and numerous near the lesser curvature and are sparse or absent near the greater curvature. In the colon of the guinea pig Auerbach's plexus is extremely thick in the proximity of the peritoneal attachment and becomes progressively more wide-meshed toward the opposite border (Fig. 10C).

The number of neurons in the myenteric plexus amounts to several thousand per square centimeter of serosal surface. Representative figures (per square centimeter) from the guinea pig are as follows: cardia, 3,500; duodenum, 10,000; ileum, 7,500; cecum between taeniae, 4,500; cecum beneath taeniae, 12,000; colon, 15,000 to 19,000; rectum, 18,000 (176). The number of neurons per unit surface is somewhat related to the thickness of the adjacent musculature, as exemplified by the greater density of neurons beneath the taeniae of the cecum as compared with the rest of the cecum. Similar figures have been obtained for other species (110), but with increase in body size the ganglia become more sparse and the number of neurons per unit surface is smaller. The small intestine of the rat contains about 1.85×10^6 neurons in the myenteric plexus (102), whereas in the cat the figure for both plexuses together is around 6×10^6 (271).

In the submucosal plexus of the guinea pig and rat ileum and colon, the neurons are about half as numerous as in the myenteric plexus (105,234), whereas they are 2 to 3 times more numerous in the cat ileum (271). In certain species (e.g., pig, cat, sheep) some authors distinguish in the submucosal plexus a Henle's plexus, situated near the inner aspect of the circular musculature, and a Meissner's plexus, situated near the muscularis mucosae (141,300).

GENERAL STRUCTURE OF INTRAMURAL GANGLIA

Broadly speaking, there are two cell types in intramural ganglia, nerve cells and glial cells, and they are associated with a neuropil formed by neuronal processes (some of extrinsic origin, and other issued by intrinsic neurons) and glial processes (Fig. 11). The ganglia are compact structures, very much reminiscent of the general architecture of the central nervous system, usually with no penetration of connective tissue (Figs. 11 and 12). Each ganglion and connecting strand is surrounded by a basal lamina and collagen fibrils, but these—for example, in the adult guinea pig—do not penetrate inside the plexus. Small bundles or septa of collagen are occasionally found within enteric ganglia of other animal species (cat, sheep).

The intramural ganglia are therefore basically different from the sympathetic and parasympathetic ganglia, in which generally each neuron with its short processes and the incoming synapses constitutes a unit wrapped by satellite cells and surrounded by a basal lamina and collagen fibrils. All the neurons of an intramural ganglion are surrounded by a common basal lamina and they are separated from each other by glial cells (Fig. 11). The anatomical separation between neurons is certainly much less than in other autonomic ganglia. During development, large areas of direct apposition between the neuronal perikarya are often encountered; in the adult, only a thin glial laminar process may intervene between adjacent neurons, and limited areas of direct apposition between perikarya may persist. In this connection it should be mentioned that the contraction and relaxation of the muscle layers alter considerably the shape and thickness of the ganglia. The effect on the fine structure of the ganglia has not been studied, but the mechanical activity of the adjacent muscles undoubtedly produces changes in shape of ganglionic neuronal and glial cells. The latter cells, being so rich in slender laminar processes, probably facilitate a certain topographical rearrangement within the ganglion without alteration of the crucial intercellular contacts.

A unique feature of the enteric plexuses (the myenteric plexus in particular) is that large areas of the surface of the perikaryon and the larger dendrites lie at the surface of the ganglion in direct contact with the basal lamina (Figs. 11 and 19). The neuronal surface is thus directly exposed to the extracellular space at large and to the connective tissue (103). In the cytoplasm of the neurons a band of microfilamentous material is

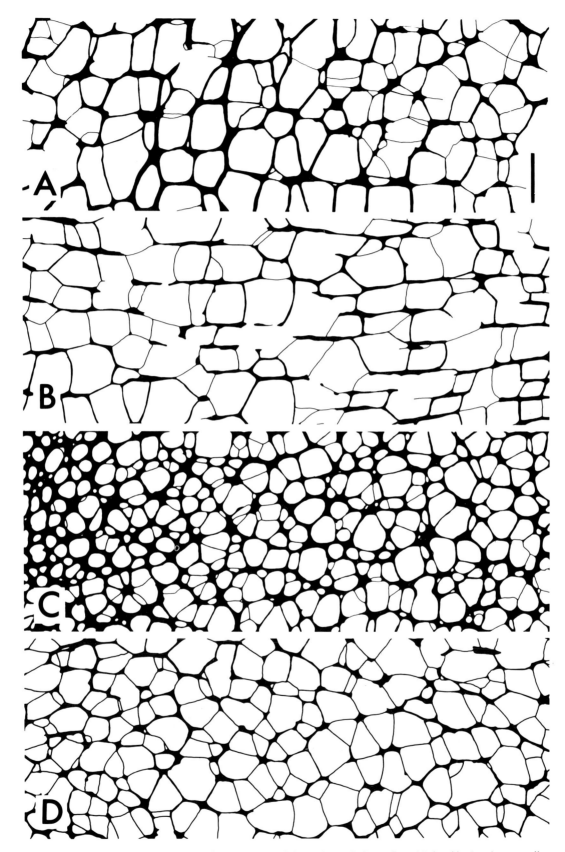

FIG. 10. Drawings of the myenteric plexus from different parts of the guinea pig intestine obtained by tracing ganglia and connecting meshes from photographic montages of stretch preparations such as that illustrated in Fig. 9A. **A:** Duodenum, **B:** Ileum, **C:** Proximal colon, **D:** Rectum. In each preparation, the left side is near the peritoneal attachment, and the longitudinal axis of the intestine runs vertically. Note that in the proximal colon, the ganglia are more closely packed near the peritoneal attachment than elsewhere. In the ileum, the ganglia are markedly elongated in the direction of the circular musculature. From Gabella (110). Magnification: 8 ×.

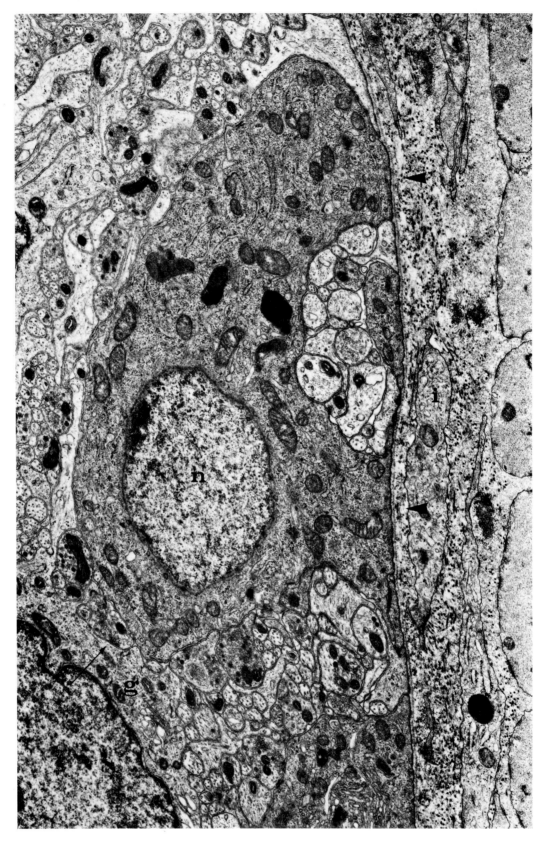

FIG. 11. Ganglion of the myenteric plexus of guinea pig ileum with part of the adjacent circular musculature (*far right*). In the center is a ganglion neuron with its nucleus (n); in the perikaryon, there are mainly mitochondria, ribosomes, lysosomes, and rough endoplasmic reticulum. Parts of the neuronal membrane reach the surface of the ganglion and are directly covered by the basal lamina (*arrowheads*). g, glial cell; i, process of an interstitial cell. Note the densely packed neuropil formed by dendrites, axons, and glial processes. There are several axosomatic synapses and a neuroglial junction (*arrow*). Magnification: 16,000 × .

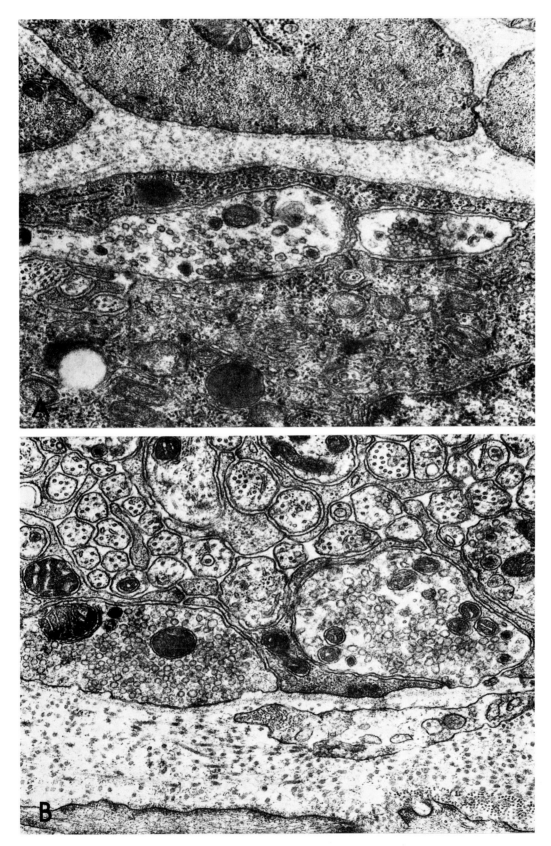

FIG. 12. A: Two varicosities containing mainly small agranular vesicles make synaptic contacts with the perikaryon of a ganglion neuron. At top are muscle cells of the circular layer. Magnification: 36,000 ×. **B:** Two varicosities at the surface of the ganglion, separated by a glial process. The two varicosities are probably of different types since they differ in the size and appearance of their vesicles and their mitochondria. At bottom is a muscle cell of the longitudinal layer. Magnification: 36,000 ×.

often found associated with these areas of the plasma membrane (see Fig. 19).

Small blood vessels can lie near ganglia of the myenteric plexus (without penetrating into them, with very rare exceptions), but in several species (sheep, rat, and guinea pig) there seems to be no special vascular architecture in connection with the ganglia (103). However, in the intestine of the pig and the cat, capillaries are very numerous in the proximity of the ganglia and form characteristic periganglionic networks (179,301).

Neurons, glial cells, and their processes are closely packed together within the ganglia. An apparent space of only about 20 nm is present between the membrane of adjacent structures. There are some doubts as to the real amount of this space [a similar problem, as to the extent of the extracellular space, is encountered in the central nervous system (56)], but with most preparative techniques there is hardly any space in addition to the thin gap of 20 nm between adjacent processes. Glial cells in particular are moulded so as to "fill in" the spaces remaining between neuronal processes, which are usually rounder. The spaces between processes are easily reached by a systemically injected tracer (such as horseradish peroxidase) (36,181).

Outside the ganglia and the large interconnecting strands lie interstitial cells which are flattened and have long laminar processes (Fig. 11). The intervening space contains the basal lamina of the ganglion, microfibrils, and a few collagen fibrils. There are, however, occasional areas of more intimate contact (with a gap of only about 20 nm) between a cellular element at the ganglion surface and an interstitial cell or a smooth muscle cell. The interstitial cells may form a continuous sheath all around a ganglion, but it is more common, particularly in small ganglia, to find only a partial covering: in this case large areas of the ganglion directly face smooth muscle cells (Fig. 12). The interstitial cells do not appear to provide a proper sheath or a "capsule" to the ganglia of the myenteric plexus, and their presence around the connecting meshes (or around the submucosal ganglia) is even more irregular (110). Other authors describe (in the same ganglia) a supporting cell sheath which fully surrounds the plexus and acts as a barrier to the penetration of certain substances, such as albumin, into the plexus (122).

It has been claimed that there is a blood-myenteric plexus barrier to small protein molecules, analogous to the blood-brain barrier. The main evidence put forward to support this notion is the absence of fenestrations in the capillaries of the muscularis externa (122). The issue of the accessibility of the ganglia to blood-borne substances is obviously of considerable interest, not least in the analysis of the effects of injected drugs, and deserves further investigation.

TYPES OF NEURONS

The vast population of intramural nerve ganglion cells represents a heterogeneous set of neurons. Most other autonomic ganglia are considerably simpler in the sense that they are made of a fairly uniform population of neurons that differ in the projection of their long axons but are organized in a rather uniform and simpler fashion. In terms of size, the enteric neurons are distributed over an extremely wide range, roughly from the size of cerebellar granule cells to that of Purkinje cells (110). The histograms of neuron sizes vary in different parts of the alimentary tract. In the myenteric plexus of the rat, small neurons are more abundant in the small intestine than in the stomach or the large intestine. The largest percentage of large neurons is found in the cecum, where the range of sizes is also wider than in other parts of the gut (102). In some species the ganglion cells of the submucous plexus are smaller and less heterogeneous in size than those of the myenteric plexus (89,141,234).

Elaborate classifications of the enteric neurons have been produced on the basis of silver impregnation and methylene blue studies. The best known of them is that of Dogiel (74), who described three types of methylene blue stained neurons according to the number, extent, and branching characteristics of the neuronal processes. Dogiel's classification has been modified or used in different ways by many authors (reviewed in 274). Some have expressed doubts on the existence of clear-cut morphological types (e.g., 185), and there are also reservations on the reliability of silver impregnation methods. Other classifications based on silver impregnation have been put forward, by among others, Hill (150), Botar et al. (26), and Rintoul (261). Some investigators have distinguished argentophile and argentophobe neurons (163); multipolar, bipolar, and unipolar neurons (274); or separate classes of neurons on the basis of the size of the perikaryon (89).

In the myenteric plexus of the cat the neurons range in size between 15,000 and 60,000 μm^3, and they have been grouped into three distinct categories: small, medium, and large cells (89). The majority (83%) of the neurons in the submucosal plexus of the cat small intestine are unipolar or bipolar, and their processes can be traced into the mucosa, an observation suggesting that they are afferent neurons (89; see also 30). The remaining neurons are multipolar and are considered to provide the motor innervation to the muscularis mucosae (89).

In investigations which have begun only recently, tracers such as horseradish peroxidase, Procion Yellow, and Lucifer Yellow have been injected in the myenteric neurons, and it has become possible to study the morphology of enteric ganglion cells in a highly selected way

(154,226). These studies have revived the interest in the search for cell types based on the morphology of the processes, but for the moment little correlation has been found between electrophysiological properties and neuronal morphology (154); these studies have, however, confirmed the extraordinary structural complexity and variability of the enteric neurons. Classifications of the enteric neurons based on their electrophysiological properties have been proposed (see Chapter 1), but the structural features of the various efferent neurons and the mechanosensitive neurons have not yet been worked out.

NEURONAL PROCESSES, NERVE ENDINGS, AND SYNAPSES

Intramural ganglia have a neuropil of remarkable complexity, rich in dendrites and axons. The description that follows is a tentative one since only a limited number of studies have been published and there are no three-dimensional reconstructions from serial section studies.

Nerve endings occur as expansions along an axon (and this part of the axon is by definition its terminal portion); the *endings* are, therefore, usually not the true anatomical ending of a fiber but varicosities along its length. The occurrence of varicosities is well documented in the case of adrenergic fibers, since they are readily seen in fluorescence microscopy (Fig. 13). However, it seems that most other types of axons in the gastrointestinal tract are also varicose. The distribution of varicosities (along adrenergic axons) is fairly regular in those axons running intramuscularly or within a connecting mesh of either plexus. These varicosities measure about 1 to 2 μm in diameter and are spaced with the frequency of about 250 to 300/mm (62,214,230), but often much less. Indirect estimations carried out in the iris and the hind leg of rats indicate that an adrenergic neuron has a total of about 26,000 varicosities on the terminal portions of its axons (61). The varicosities of an adrenergic neuron together contain more than 100 times more norepinephrine than the corresponding cell body (61,120). There are, unfortunately, no equivalent data for the adrenergic fibers supplying the gut. The extent of arborization of these fibers and the number of their varicosities must be substantial considering the numerical ratio between intramural ganglion neurons and prevertebral ganglion neurons (see p. 212). But whether the arborization of the other types of fibers (nonadrenergic) is equally large is doubtful. The significance of a structural pattern with varicosities, as opposed to one with nerve endings only at the terminal points of the arborization, has not been clarified. One of the effects of this pattern is to obtain a much larger number of functional endings for a given length of the axonal arborization than would be possible with endings located only at the ends of the axonal branches.

Adrenergic varicosities present within the ganglia of the plexuses are less uniform in size and distribution than those found elsewhere in the intestinal wall, and the individual fibers are hard to follow in the fluorescence microscope (Fig. 9). Little is known about the varicose patterns in other nerve types of the gut, but it seems that the varicosities along a fiber are rather variable in terms of size, spacing, and shape. There are also differences in the packing densities of vesicles within varicosities and probably in the amount of transmitter stored.

The intervaricose portions of an axon are of narrow diameter (some axons are less than 0.2 μm in diameter); they usually contain microtubules, and occasionally a synaptic vesicle, a mitochondrion, neurofilaments, and some endoplasmic reticulum. The microtubules penetrate into the varicosity and some are occasionally seen to proceed without interruption to the next intervaricose segment. Some microtubules appear to end within a varicosity, but it is not clear whether they are in any way anchored to the plasma membrane. Mitochondria are often found in the varicosities, but the most common components are the so-called synaptic vesicles. These are characterized by their size, shape, electron density, and distribution, and constitute the basis (albeit an uncertain one) for the classification and identification of nerve endings in the electron microscope. Morphological classifications of nerve endings in the gut have been put forward by several investigators. The work is still in an early phase and is limited to few species and to few portions of the gut, and many doubts still exist on the type of endings present and their significance. More investigations and some discussion on the types of neurotransmitter involved are presented in the section Neurotransmitters: Morphological Studies.

In the myenteric plexus of humans, rhesus monkeys, and guinea pigs, three types of nerve profiles have been described (14). One type is characterized by numerous agranular vesicles, 35 to 60 nm in diameter, and a few large (80 to 110 nm) vesicles with a granule of medium electron density. These varicosities, some of which synapse on ganglion neurons, are interpreted as cholinergic. A second type of ending contains vesicles 50 to 90 nm in diameter, with an intensely osmiophilic granule, mixed with an equal number of agranular vesicles and a few large (90 to 130 nm) granular vesicles. These endings are never found to form synaptic contacts and are interpreted as adrenergic since they degenerate after 6-hydroxydopamine treatment and the electron density of their granules is enhanced by 5-hydroxydopamine treatment. Endings of the third and most common type contain, in addition to a few agranular vesicles, vesicles 85 to 160 nm in diameter with a large granule of medium electron density and not clearly separated from the vesi-

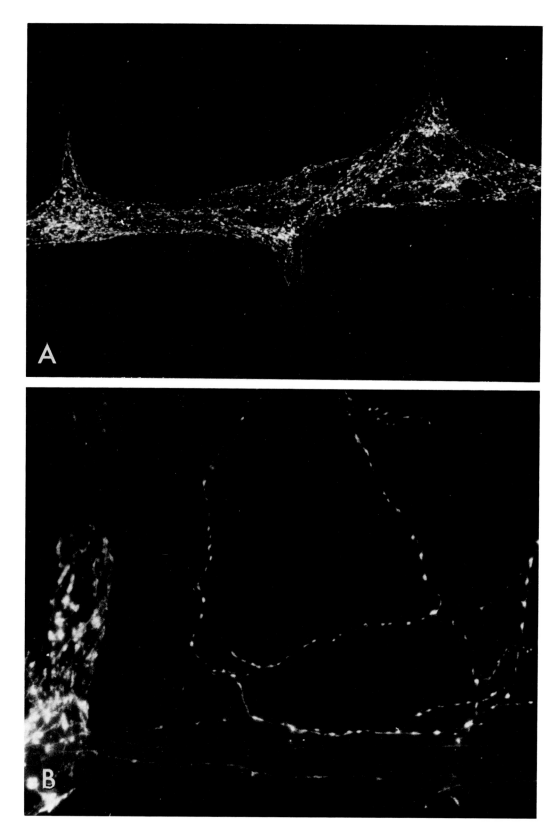

FIG. 13. Fluorescence microscopy for catecholamines (formaldehyde method). Myenteric plexus of the guinea pig. **A:** A large ganglion and its connecting strands. The fluorescent axons are varicose and form an intricate mesh around ganglion neurons (these appear as dark areas since they do not contain catecholamines). Magnification: approximately 250 ×. **B:** At right is a ganglion with many fluorescent varicosities (adrenergic endings). Also, fluorescent fibers running outside the ganglion and the connecting strands clearly display their beaded structure. The fluorescent varicosities vary in size and spacing, and many of those in the ganglion are larger than those outside. Magnification: approximately 600 ×

cle membrane. These nerve profiles are labeled p-type varicosities, where p stands for polypeptide. Endings rich in large granular vesicles ("neurosecretory type") had already been noted in the nerves of the gut (137,307).

In the guinea pig ileum many nerve endings synapse on the soma or dendrites of myenteric ganglion neurons, and several types have been tentatively identified (103). The prominence of synaptic specializations is variable. In some endings there are conspicuous presynaptic dense projections, around which vesicles are clustered, extending for most of the area of contact with the postsynaptic element; the latter show thickening of the membrane. Other endings display a much less obvious junctional specialization, confined to an area of only a few tenths of a micron in diameter. Some endings are packed with small agranular vesicles 40 to 60 nm in diameter (Fig. 12A). These endings are interpreted as cholinergic, and like other cholinergic endings a nerve profile may contain one or two large granular vesicles, in addition to mitochondria and isolated cisternae of endoplasmic reticulum. There are also several endings in which the agranular vesicles predominate (particularly in the proximity of the prejunctional membrane), but there are also a substantial number of large granular vesicles. These endings too may be cholinergic, but the content and the significance of their large granular vesicles are not clear (p. 224).

Some synaptic nerve profiles are characterized by granular vesicles 90 to 140 nm in diameter having a dense core of variable appearance and occasional discontinuities in their membrane (Fig. 14A). These endings, which are common in the small intestine of the guinea pig, rabbit, and cat, and are (at least in the guinea pig) of intrinsic origin, are probably similar to the p-type profiles described above (14), and their vesicles were labeled heterogeneous granular vesicles (HGV) because of their morphological variety (103). Characteristically, in the region near the presynaptic membrane, where junctional specializations are visible, one finds almost exclusively small agranular vesicles (Fig. 14A); granular vesicles are generally not observed closer than 200 nm to the presynaptic membrane.

Another type of synaptic nerve profile (which, like the previous two, is found in both the myenteric and the submucosal plexus) contains mainly small granular vesicles (Fig. 15A and B); their cores are electron dense and can be eccentrically located. These endings may synapse on cell bodies or on dendrites or on spines from either, and have been interpreted as adrenergic (103). Other authors have disputed this view and regard these endings as "not noradrenergic" (100). Some of the small granular vesicle-containing endings in the myenteric plexus of the guinea pig may not be adrenergic (136). The three types of endings described above can converge on a single neuron (see Fig. 17) (103), and most neurons seem to receive synapses from more than one kind of nerve end-

ing. Another type of synaptic nerve profile contains large granular vesicles 90 to 150 nm in diameter with an intensely electron-dense core, separated from the membrane by a clear halo (Fig. 14B); the region immediately adjacent to the presynaptic membrane often contains only small agranular vesicles (103). A small number of endings contain mainly flat agranular vesicles, together with mitochondria and endoplasmic reticulum, and synapse on ganglion cell bodies of the myenteric plexus (103). It has recently been suggested that these are adrenergic nerve endings (100).

Some of the nerve endings described above are situated at the surface of ganglia of the myenteric plexus, and part of their membrane is directly covered by the basal lamina (Fig. 12B). Endings containing chiefly agranular vesicles and endings with flat vesicles are often found in this position. The occasional presence of dense projections and clustering of vesicles in the axonal membrane contacting the basal lamina may indicate release of transmitters in the spaces around the ganglion, and there is also the possibility that some of these endings are sensory. Nerve endings with vesicles loaded with 5-hydroxydopamine (105) or tritiated norepinephrine (110) or stained with potassium permanganate (215) (therefore presumably adrenergic, see p. 225) are also found in this location; they should probably be of those containing flat vesicles in conventional preparations. Varicosities of cholinergic and adrenergic types lying in contact with each other, and both at the surface of the ganglion (in the myenteric plexus of the rabbit) have been described by Manber and Gershon (215), who interpret them as axoaxonic synapses. Numerous nerve endings form specialized junctions with glial cells, which are described on p. 230.

In a more elaborate classification, eight or more morphological types of endings are identified in the myenteric plexus of the guinea pig (44). It is possible that each type represents a different type of neuron and that perhaps the variety of vesicles reflects the occurrence of a conspicuous number of neurotransmitters. Other authors have advanced a more skeptical view and have suggested that there is no structural distinction in the gut of vertebrates between axons that are cholinergic and axons that are nonadrenergic inhibitory (64).

Campbell and Gibbins (38) have investigated the ultrastructure of the nonadrenergic, noncholinergic inhibitory nerves, which are a major component of the intrinsic innervation of the gut (see p. 224). On the basis of their studies on the anococcygeus muscle (218) and on other organs, including the gut, they conclude that the p-type nerve profiles (14) can be subdivided into two groups: (a) the small p-type endings, with small clear vesicles and large granular vesicles ranging from 90 to 120 nm in diameter, which the authors identify as the noncholinergic nonadrenergic inhibitory (purinergic) nerves; and (b) the large p-type endings, with large gran-

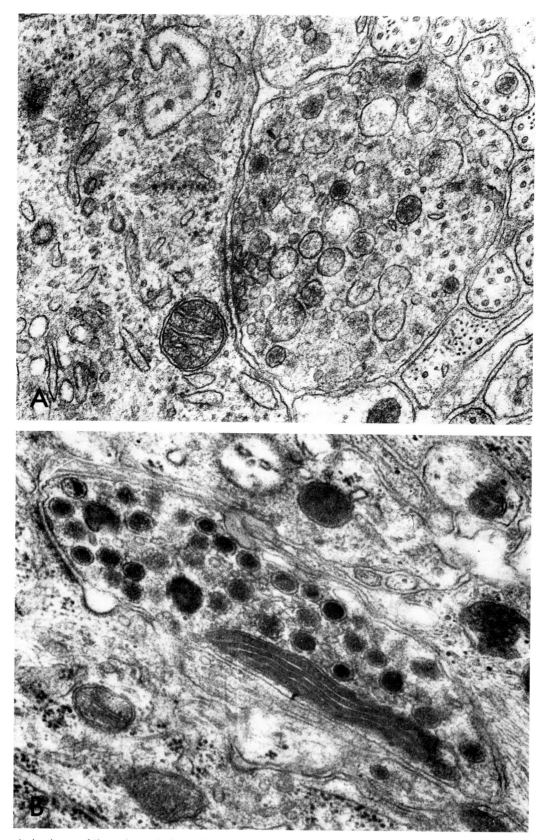

FIG. 14. Myenteric plexus of the guinea pig ileum. **A:** Varicosity forming an axosomatic synapse and containing a heterogeneous population of vesicles. The vesicles vary in size and in the density of their granules. Microtubules are present at right part of the varicosity. Note that in the immediately presynaptic area there are only small agranular vesicles. Magnification: 68,000 ×. **B:** Varicosity containing mainly large granular vesicles with synapses on the perikaryon of a ganglion neuron. Magnification: 60,000 ×.

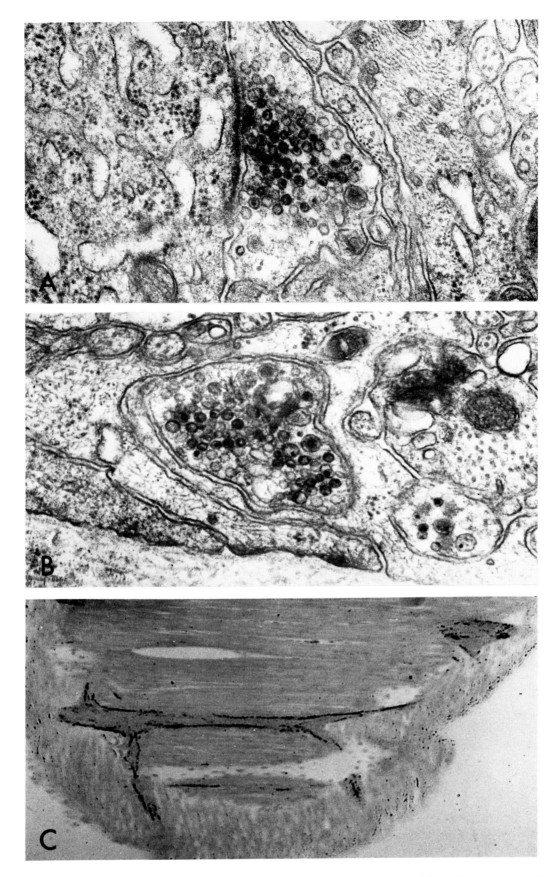

FIG. 15. A: Myenteric plexus of guinea pig jejunum. Varicosity packed with small granular vesicles with synapses on the perikaryon of a ganglion neuron. Magnification: 41,000 ×. **B:** Same preparation as in **A** showing a similar nerve ending wrapped by a glial process. Magnification: 41,000 ×. **C:** Autoradiograph of guinea pig ileum after incubation in tritiated norepinephrine. Silver grains (indicating sites of uptake of norepinephrine) are found mainly over the ganglia of the myenteric plexus, whereas there are only few grains in the muscle layers. Note that the grains are mainly at the edges (therefore at the surface) of the ganglia. From Gabella (110). Magnification: 125 ×.

ular vesicles ranging from 140 to 200 nm in diameter, containing as unknown transmitter (38).

The identification and classification of nerve endings on the basis of vesicle type have dominated the ultrastructural studies of the intramural plexuses. It should not be forgotten, however, that the enteric ganglia offer many other morphological questions which need to be pursued — for example, the synaptic specializations, the emergence of cell processes from the cell bodies, and the type and arrangement of processes. On these points, as on many other, there are only a few observations. The emergence of the axon has not been identified with certainty in any intramural neuron. The axon probably originates not from the cell body but rather from one of the large and irregular expansions of the perikarya. The extent of the synaptic specializations is variable, and it is not clear how this aspect correlates with the morphological types of endings and with the type of neurotransmitter. And it is not known how many of the myriad nerve endings found in a ganglion have no synaptic specialization. The structure of the cell processes and their shape and arborization appear in the electron microscope more elaborate than silver impregnation suggested (and this will become even clearer when three-dimensional reconstructions of whole neurons are carried out).

NEUROTRANSMITTERS: MORPHOLOGICAL STUDIES

Pharmacological studies clearly indicate that several neurotransmitters are released from intramural nerves of the gut. In addition to norepinephrine and acetylcholine, other substances which may play the role of neurotransmitters in the gut include serotonin (5-hydroxytryptamine 5-HT), adenosine triphosphate (ATP), and several peptides, such as substance P, vasoactive intestinal peptide (VIP), somatostatin, and enkephalin. Morphological studies can provide only supportive evidence as to the identification of a neurotransmitter, but their contribution can be valuable in view of the complexity and variety of neuronal types present in the gut. Histochemical and electron microscope techniques have chiefly been applied to this problem.

Acetylcholine

Many neurons of the myenteric plexus and the submucous plexus are intensely positive for the acetylcholinesterase reaction (141, 307), and they may therefore be cholinergic neurons. The results are, however, uncertain since there is a wide range of intensities within a population of ganglion cells, there is considerable variability among species, there are doubts about the specificity of the methods used, and a positive reaction for acetylcholinesterase is not invariably indicative of a cho-

linergic neuron. Moreover, the resoltion of the method (which has been used only at the light microscopic level) does not allow one to identify nerve endings. The distribution of cholinergic nerve endings has thus not been worked out; that their number must be considerable is indicated by the extraordinarily large amount of acetylcholine stored and released by the myenteric plexus (72, 318).

By electron microscopy cholinergic endings are recognized as varicosities containing small agranular vesicles: apart from an occasional large granular vesicle, the vesicles are of uniform type (about 50 nm in diameter), and in size and appearance they resemble those found in identified cholinergic endings such as those of the sphincter pupillae or in striated muscles. Nerve endings of this type occur within the intestinal muscles (where they may form neuromuscular contacts, see p. 232) and within the plexuses: here they are found either lying at the surface of a ganglion, directly beneath the basal lamina, or synapsing on cell bodies or dendrites. When synaptic specializations are present in a nerve profile, they are usually prominent. However, only a minority of the endings within the intramural ganglia display this "typical" cholinergic appearance, and it is therefore probable that other morphological types of endings should be considered cholinergic (see p. 221). Conversely, some of the endings containing agranular vesicles may ergic, as has been suggested for some tryptaminergic neurons in the central nervous system (239).

Catecholamines

The main sympathetic input to the gut comes from fibers releasing norepinephrine. They are postganglionic fibers of the prevertebral ganglia (see p. 212); there may also be a few fibers originating from the thoracolumbar chain. In the rat and the dog, adrenergic fibers from the cervical sympathetic ganglia reach the gastrointestinal tract via the vagus nerve (4,235). The stellate ganglion provides adrenergic fibers to the gastroesophageal junction in the dog and cat (132). The distribution of adrenergic fibers within the intestinal wall has been established by the Falck and Hillarp method for localization of catecholamines in fluorescence microscopy (Figs. 13A and B). There are numerous adrenergic endings in the myenteric and submucous ganglia, and in the connecting strands (Fig. 13A) there are a few intramuscular and periglandular varicose fibers, and there are several fibers associated with blood vessels (which are numerous in the submucosa). Apart from a few exceptions (see p. 225), there are no adrenergic cell bodies in the wall of the gut (Fig. 13A) and all the adrenergic fibers present are of extrinsic origin. After excision of the prevertebral ganglia or severance of their efferent nerves, all fluorescent fibers disappear from the affected part of the gut and the neuronal catecholamine content falls virtually to zero. There is, however, a short period in embryonic life (between days 12 and 18 in the rat) during which neurons in the esophagus and stomach (and to lesser extent in the cranial part of the intestine) display catecholamine fluorescence and tyrosine hydroxylase (the rate-limiting enzyme in catecholamine biosynthesis) activity (42). In the rat and guinea pig stomach, a few neurons of the myenteric plexus are immunoreactive for dopamine-beta-hydroxylase (the enzyme catalyzing the conversion of dopamine into norepinephrine) (277), although catecholamine-containing neurons are not found there.

Exceptions to the absence of adrenergic neurons within the gut wall are found in the chicken gizzard (21), the guinea pig colon (49,52,97), and the large intestine of the lizard (258). In the myenteric plexus of the guinea pig colon, about 1% of the neurons contain a histochemically detectable amount of catecholamines (97). Extrinsic denervation of this part of the gut produces a fall of only 40% of the neuronal catecholamine content, the remaining amount representing, therefore, the content due to intrinsic adrenergic ganglion cells (117). Isolated adrenergic neurons are occasionally found also in the myenteric plexus of the guinea pig rectum (98).

The transmitter in adrenergic nerves in the mammalian gut is norepinephrine (3): the fibers also contain traces of dopamine, the intermediate precursor of norepinephrine. In the teleost gut the adrenergic transmitters are serotonin (5-HT) and dopamine (12,316), whereas epinephrine is the predominant catecholamine in the amphibian gut (86,258). The number of adrenergic fibers running within the musculature is usually small (the features of the neuromuscular junctions are described on p. 232). In the small intestine they are usually found in the innermost part of the circular muscle (281) near a layer of special muscle cells (p. 208). Adrenergic fibers usually are absent from the longitudinal muscle of the ileum, but they are found in the taenia coli and in the longitudinal muscle of the rectum. By contrast, intramuscular adrenergic fibers are numerous at certain junctions between segments of the alimentary tract. The musculature of the gastroesophageal junction is richly supplied with adrenergic fibers (116), in sharp contrast with the musculature of the stomach; a similar arrangement, however, has not been found in the rat (130), cat, or monkey (15). In the lower esophageal sphincter of the cat and dog, the motor control is provided by adrenergic fibers, which originate from the stellate ganglion (8,132).

A particularly rich supply of adrenergic fibers is found in the internal anal sphincter of the cat (165) and guinea pig (54), and probably humans (13). This is the densest adrenergic innervation found in the alimentary tract; most of the fibers originate from the superior mesenteric ganglion, but some are issued by ganglion neurons of the sacral sympathetic chain (50). Adrenergic fibers are plentiful in the sphincter of Oddi of guinea pigs and rabbits (221).

The distribution of adrenergic fibers in the myenteric plexus is clearly seen in stretch preparations of the longitudinal musculature with the plexus attached. The fluorescent nerve endings are numerous. They form fairly regular varicose fibers in the connecting strands of the plexus, whereas in the ganglia their arrangement is more irregular and individual adrenergic axons are difficult to recognize. They occasionally form basket-like structures suggesting the presence of nets of adrenergic fibers around certain ganglion neurons. The distribution of adrenergic fibers, as seen in fluorescence microscopy, appears rather uniform in the myenteric ganglia of the various parts of the gut (54). This observation is confirmed by quantitative fluorimetric studies of the guinea pig, which show that the norepinephrine content in the myenteric plexus (and longitudinal muscle) of the various segments of the gut between stomach and rectum varies little (with the exception of the colon, where the higher norepinephrine content is accounted for by the presence of intrinsic adrenergic neurons, see this page) (187). In the guinea pig ileum about one-sixth of the neuronal catecholamine content of the wall is in the myenteric plexus. The other five-sixths is accounted for by adrenergic fibers inside the musculature, in the submucous plexus, around the glands of the mucosa, and, above all, around blood vessels of the submucosa (105).

In the electron microscope adrenergic endings can be identified as nerve profiles with a predominance of granular vesicles, 40 to 60 nm in diameter. Granularity can be enhanced by using "false transmitters" (such as 5-hydroxydopamine), which are specifically taken up by adrenergic endings (Fig. 16). In general, preservation of dense cores in adrenergic vesicles, particularly within the intramural plexuses, is somewhat erratic, even with a consistent preparative technique. Fixation methods involving the use of dichromate salts or permanganate give a better yield of small granular vesicles, although the general preservation of the tissue is less good than with glutaraldehyde. The increase in granularity following treatment of the gut with 5-hydroxydopamine is noticeable in the perivascular and intramuscular adrenergic endings and in those of the submucous plexus, but it is usually less good in those of the myenteric plexus. The ultrastructural identification of adrenergic endings is, therefore, not always easy. When the dense cores are not preserved, an adrenergic ending may look rather similar to a cholinergic one. On the other hand, the presence of a minute dense core in synaptic vesicles may arise as an effect of fixation [for example, the high calcium content of the fixative (249)], and there are dense-cored vesicles containing transmitters other than catecholamines. Moreover, in some regions of the gut (e.g., the colon of the guinea pig) there are adrenergic

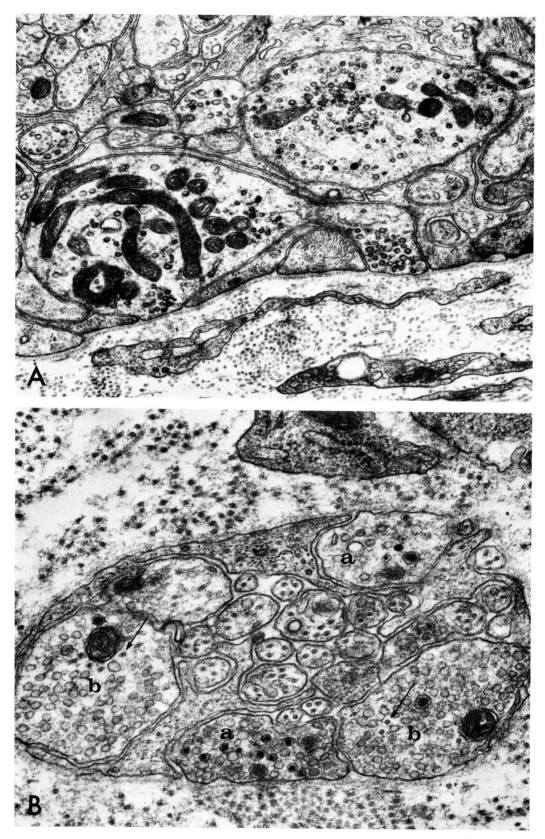

FIG. 16. A: Myenteric plexus of guinea pig cecum after incubation with 5-hydroxydopamine. The false transmitter has been taken up by some nerve varicosities and has enhanced the electron density of their small granular vesicles. One of these profiles (identified as adrenergic) reaches the surface of the ganglion and is partly in contact with its basal lamina; it is particularly rich in mitochondria. Magnification: 25,500 ×. **B:** Proximal colon of guinea pig treated with several injections of 5-hydroxydopamine. An intramuscular nerve shows several axons, most of which are 0.15 to 0.40 μm in diameter and contain mainly microtubules; they are probably intervaricose portions of axons. Of the axons containing synaptic vesicles (varicosities), two have small granular vesicles (whose granularity is probably enhanced by the false transmitter) and are identified as adrenergic (a). Two other larger varicosities (b) are packed with small agranular vesicles and are probably cholinergic; both varicosities also contain a number of microtubules (*arrows*). Magnification: 49,000 ×.

endings containing vesicles which are of medium size and less electron dense than the small granular vesicles (14,103).

In the guinea pig ileum some adrenergic endings synapse on neuronal cell bodies (Fig. 15A) and on large dendrites (details of synaptic junctions are described on p. 219); these varicosities are somewhat larger than intramuscular adrenergic endings (103). In permanganate-fixed ganglia less than 1% of the total number of varicosities is of the adrenergic type, and they are mainly located near the surface of the ganglia (215). Also, the endings which take up exogenous (tritiated) norepinephrine are situated mainly at the surface of the myenteric ganglia (110,215) (Fig. 15C), whereas they are usually well inside the ganglia in the submucous plexus (110). Taxi and Droz (309) found tritiated norepinephrine localized in nerve endings synapsing on dendrites in both intramural plexuses of the rat intestine. Nerve endings containing small granular vesicles (some synapsing on ganglion neurons) appeared in degeneration after injection of 6-hydroxydopamine (chemical sympathectomy) in the cat myenteric plexus (90). A close apposition between cholinergic and adrenergic nerve endings has been described in the myenteric plexus of the guinea pig ileum and has been interpreted as an axoaxonic synapse (215). One important effect of sympathetic stimulation or of exogenously applied norepinephrine is to inhibit the release of acetylcholine from cholinergic endings of the plexus (191,240). Norepinephrine has, however, no effect on the membrane potential of the ganglion neurons (152,226). Intestinal relaxation by sympathetic stimulation is achieved without changes in electrical activity of the myenteric plexus (306). The complexity of the responses to adrenergic stimulation is clearly shown by experiments on the rabbit colon [where the sympathetic and parasympathetic pathways to the intestinal wall run in separate nerves (119)], in which the inhibitory effects are obtained through adrenergic receptors on the muscle cells and on the ganglion neurons (129).

Serotonin

Gershon and collaborators (123,125,126) have proposed that serotonin (5-hydroxytryptamine) is a neurotransmitter used by a population of neurons (serotoninergic neurons) in the enteric ganglia. [The intestinal wall contains also large amounts of 5-HT stored in chromaffin cells (16)]. The amount of neuronal 5-HT must be small and at very low concentration since it is not detected by fluorescence microscopy (3). Evidence of the occurrence of serotoninergic neurons in the gut is based on fluorescence microscopy and uptake studies after pharmacological treatments (126,263). Moreover, some intramural neurons can be stained immunohistochemically for tryptophan hydroxylase (the enzyme catalyzing the first step in the synthesis of 5-HT from tryptophan) (124). Electrophysiological studies on the myenteric plexus of the guinea pig suggest a role of 5-HT in the production of excitatory postsynaptic potentials (322), as well as a presynaptic inhibition of acetylcholine release (231). Studies on developing gut (269) and on organ cultures (75,76) confirm the existence in the mammalian myenteric plexus of intrinsic neurons able to synthesize and take up serotonin.

Purines

The intestine contains a vast population of inhibitory neurons which are nonadrenergic and noncholinergic (19,31,33,34,217). Strong inhibitory responses are elicited by transmural stimulation, and they are not affected by sympathectomy (96) or adrenolytic drugs; moreover, this inhibition has been demonstrated in the anal sphincter of the cat (118), which is contracted by catecholamines. Intramural inhibitory nerves can be demonstrated in the developing fetal rabbit before the appearance of adrenergic nerves (127).

Nonadrenergic noncholinergic inhibitory nerves are present in several other organs (see a review in 32). Their endings have been identified, after excluding the cholinergic and the adrenergic endings, as endings mainly displaying large vesicles, 80 to 200 nm in diameter, with an electron-dense granule separated from the vesicle membrane by an electron-lucent halo (large opaque vesicles) (262). The identification of these endings in the gut may be more difficult than in other organs in view of the presence of still more numerous types of nerves. No less than nine morphological different types of neurons have been described in the myenteric plexus of the guinea pig (44), although other authors have more conservative estimates (14,103,323). Campbell and Gibbins (38) have recently suggested that these inhibitory nerves in the gut are a subcategory of the p-type nerve endings (the small p-type endings, with large granular vesicles measuring 90 to 120 nm in diameter) (see p. 221).

Evidence that the inhibitory transmitter of these intramural neurons may be adenosine triphosphate or a related purine has been put forward by Burnstock and collaborators (35). A fluorescence histochemical staining with the antimalarial drug quinacrine has been developed (236), and it has been suggested that it may stain ATP stores. In the mammalian myenteric plexus 10 to 16% of the neurons stain intensely with this method and they may represent intrinsic inhibitory neurons rich in ATP (60).

Peptides

A number of biologically active peptides have been known for some time to be present in the intestinal wall. These "intestinal hormones" have been mainly local-

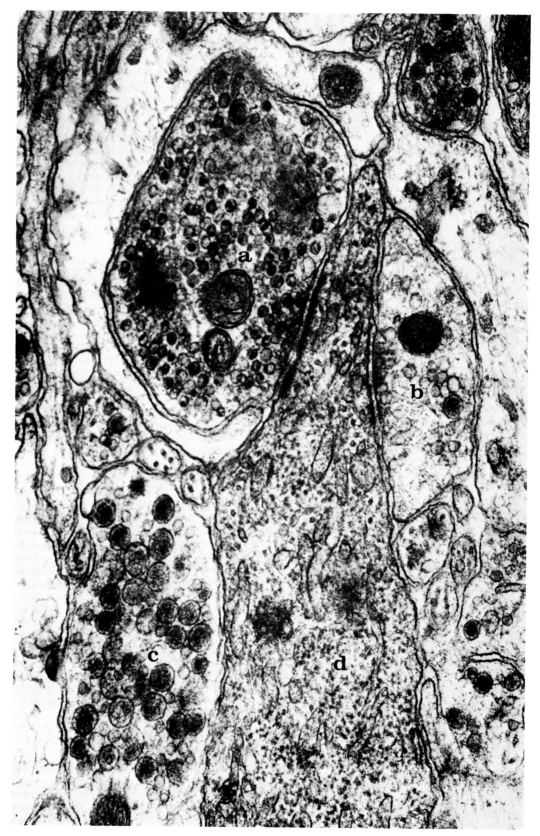

FIG. 17. Myenteric plexus of guinea pig ileum. A large dendrite (d) receives synapses from three different nerve endings: one varicosity (a) contains mainly small granular vesicles, another (b) has small agranular vesicles, and the third (c) contains mainly large granular vesicles. From Gabella (112). Magnification: 38,000 ×.

ized in enterochromaffin cells. Recently, thanks to more sensitive and specific immunofluorescence techniques, biologically active peptides have also been localized in neuronal elements of the gut. The list of these peptides includes vasoactive intestinal peptide, substance P, enkephalins, somatostatins, gastrins, cholecystokinin, neurotensin, and bombesin, and more will probably be added. Peptide-containing neurons are present in sympathetic ganglia (see p. 212), in dorsal root ganglia, and in various regions of the central nervous system (reviewed in 161). Peptides are widely distributed in neuronal elements of the gut. Extensive studies have recently been published (e.g., 277) with detailed mapping of various immunofluorescent structures. The concentration of peptides within neurons is much higher in nerve fibers than in cell bodies. Positive cell bodies are usually not readily detectable unless organs are treated *in vivo* with drugs such as vinblastine or colchicine: by impairing axonal transport, these drugs increase in the cell body the concentration of various substances including catecholamines (155) and peptides (10,162). A limited number of experiments have been carried out to see whether more than one peptide may be present in the same neuron. The evidence suggests that in the enteric neurons each of the known peptides is localized in a separate population of neurons (277). However, it is likely that peptides coexist with the transmitter acetylcholine in some ganglion neurons in the gut (see p. 221), as they do in other autonomic ganglia (212). Somatostatin is localized in adrenergic neurons of the prevertebral ganglia (156) (see p. 212), enkephalin in neurons of the cervical ganglion (278), and substance P in 5-HT-containing neurons of the brainstem (239).

Substance P

Substance P is a chemical originally extracted from the intestine and the brain (83) and characterized as an undecapeptide (41). The high content of substance P in sensory ganglia and dorsal roots (162,238) is in agreement with the suggestion that this peptide is involved in transmission in afferent fibers (208). Substance P is present in nerve cell bodies and fibers of the myenteric and submucosal plexuses, and in nerve fibers in the circular muscle, around the glands of the mucosa, and around blood vessels (225,241,277,305). In the guinea pig ileum about 11% of the neurons in the submucosal plexus contain histochemically detectable amounts of substance P, and about 3.5% in the myenteric plexus (48, 100); the fibers containing this peptide are mainly of intrinsic origin (276). In tissue culture studies on the guinea pig ileum, substance P containing neurons were found only in the myenteric plexus, whereas their nerve endings occurred mainly in the submucosal plexus (184).

VIP

Vasoactive intestinal peptide is composed of 28 aminoacids and has been isolated in large amounts from the intestine (270). VIP-immunoreactive nerve cell bodies are found in both enteric plexuses (201,202), but there are large quantitative differences between various parts of the gut (277). In the guinea pig ileum about 42% of the ganglion cells are positive in the submucosal plexus and about 2.5% in the myenteric plexus; their axons project only in the anal direction (51). In the guinea pig cecum (as studied in tissue culture) VIP-positive neurons are found only in the submucosal plexus while their endings are mainly in the myenteric plexus (184). VIP-immunoreactive axons are found in the circular muscle, around blood vessels, and in the mucosa; they are abundant in the longitudinal musculature of the stomach in the rat and guinea pig (277). Particularly rich in VIP-containing fibers is the musculature of the gastroesophageal junction, the pylorus, and the sphincter of Oddi (and also the junction of uterus and urethra with the bladder) (5). Dose-related inhibitory effects of VIP on sphincteric muscles have been reported in the opossum abdominal esophagus (257) and in the cat pylorus (77). Electrical or reflex (by distension of the upper esophagus) stimulation of intrinsic inhibitory neurons of the cat stomach is accompanied by release of VIP (85), and the gastric relaxation is mimicked by intraarterial infusion of VIP (78). Some VIP-containing fibers originating in intramural ganglia project to prevertebral ganglia (160).

Enkephalins

Enkephalins are pentapeptides which have high affinity for opiate receptors (167,169) and are present in large amounts in certain areas of the brain and in the gastrointestinal tract (168). Some effects of these substances have been extensively investigated, in particular inhibition of the release of acetylcholine from the myenteric plexus (reviewed in 192) and hyperpolarization and inhibition of firing of myenteric neurons of the guinea pig ileum (232, 233). Enkephalin-containing cell bodies are found mainly in the myenteric plexus (6,79,210,276,277); they are absent in the submucosal plexus (with the exception of duodenum and colon of the rat and cecum of the guinea pig) (277). About one-quarter of the myenteric neurons of the guinea pig ileum contain detectable amounts of enkephalins (100). There are enkephalin-positive fibers within the myenteric plexus and in the circular muscle layer, but they are rare in the submucosa and mucosa (277). Enkephalin-like immunoreactivity has been observed in the myenteric plexus of the human gut (248).

Somatostatin

Somatostatin is a 14-amino acid peptide originally isolated from the hypothalamus (28). It has been localized by immunofluorescence in varicose fibers of the myenteric and submucosal plexuses (55,159) and in some nerve cell bodies; the latter are less numerous than those which stain for substance P, VIP, or enkephalins (277). In the guinea pig ileum, about 5% of the neurons stain for somatostatin in the myenteric plexus, and about 17% in the submucosal plexus (53). Since somatostatin-containing nerve fibers are found mainly within the plexuses, it has been suggested that this peptide may be localized in interneurons (55). The pharmacological effects of somatostatin—inhibition of release of acetylcholine (43,139) and depression of firing of myenteric neurons (321)—also seem to be mainly at the level of the plexuses. Somatostatin-containing neurons of the myenteric plexus in the guinea pig ileum have axons projecting in the anal direction for 8 to 12 mm (53).

Other Peptides, Amino Acids, and Derivatives

Other peptides which have recently been localized by immunofluorescence in neuronal structures of the gastrointestinal tract include gastrin and cholecystokinin (203), bombesin (24, 73), and angiotensin (101). The dipeptide homocarnosine has been detected by paper chromatography in tissue culture of the myenteric plexus of the newly born guinea pig cecum. (183). There is no definite evidence that amino acids, such as glycine or glutamate, can be neurotransmitters in the gut. However, 4-aminobutyrate (gamma-aminobutyrate or GABA), a decarboxylation derivative of glutamate, is specifically taken up by some neurons of the myenteric plexus can be synthesized there from glutamate (183). These results support the suggestions that in the gastrointestinal tract GABA may serve as a neurotransmitter (153).

GLIAL CELLS

Glial cells are readily indentified in the intramural ganglia on the basis of their shape, position, and ultrastructural features (103). They are smaller and more numerous than ganglion neurons (in the myenteric plexus of the guinea pig ileum they outnumber nerve cells by 2 to 1) (Fig. 1B). In the connecting meshes of the plexuses, apart from the rare occurrence of neuronal perikarya, all the cells are glial cells.

Some of the glial cells are closely related to neuronal perikarya which they cover with long laminar extensions of their cell bodies (Fig. 11). This glial covering is, however, incomplete in the areas where the neuronal membrane is directly "exposed" at the ganglion surface. The glial covering is not found at the sites of the synapses or at the numerous sites where nerve processes lie directly over the perikaryal surface. A glial covering is also missing where two perikarya are in direct membrane-to-membrane contact; these contacts are found only ocasionally in ganglia of adult animals, whereas they are common during development.

Some glial cells have processes that extend tens of microns away from the cell body and are mainly related to nerve processes. The glial processes expand between axons and dendrites, occupying the angular space among them (Fig. 12). Some nerve processes are fully surrounded by a glial expansion (Fig. 18A), but more often the wrapping is only partial (Fig. 14A) and neuronal processes lying in direct membrane-to-membrane contact with each other are common. It is not clear whether there are different types of glial cells within the enteric ganglia, since the glial cells associated with neuronal perikarya can also have prominent expansions between nerve processes. Myelin sheaths are not found (there are rare exceptions in the stomach and rectum).

The enteric glial cells are rich in gliofilaments, which are arranged in sheafs and bundles extending into the glial processes (Fig. 18). Mitochondria, microtubules, ribosomes, and rough endoplasmic reticulum are well represented (45,103). The gliofilaments have conspicuous attachments at the cytoplasmic aspect of the membrane in that part of the process in contact with the basal lamina (Fig. 18B) (103). There are numerous symmetrical cell-to-cell junctions of the puncta adherens type between glial cells or between a glial cell and a neuron. Gap junctions are only rarely found on glial cells. A very common type of specialized junction (found in the myenteric and submucosal plexus of several mammalian species) occurs between vesicle-containing axons and glial cell bodies or glial processes (Figs. 11 and 18A) (103,105). These nerve varicosities contain vesicles, usually of the lucent type, which are clustered in a focal area around a dense projection similar to those found in synapses. The glial membrane that is abutted by this nerve ending does not show, however, structural specializations. The significance of these axoglial junctions is completely obscure.

The glial cells of the connecting strands are usually situated at the center of the strand and have radially arranged processes extending up to the surface. A single glial cell can be associated with several hundred axons.

The glial cells found in the enteric ganglia are structurally different from the Schwann cells of peripheral nerves (including those found in the intestinal wall (p. 232) and from the satellite cells supporting the neurons of sympathetic ganglia. They are referred to as enteric glial cells, and they may constitute a special type of glial cell. Their morphology and their relation to neurons are certainly more reminiscent of astrocytes of the central nervous system than of other glial cells of the peripheral

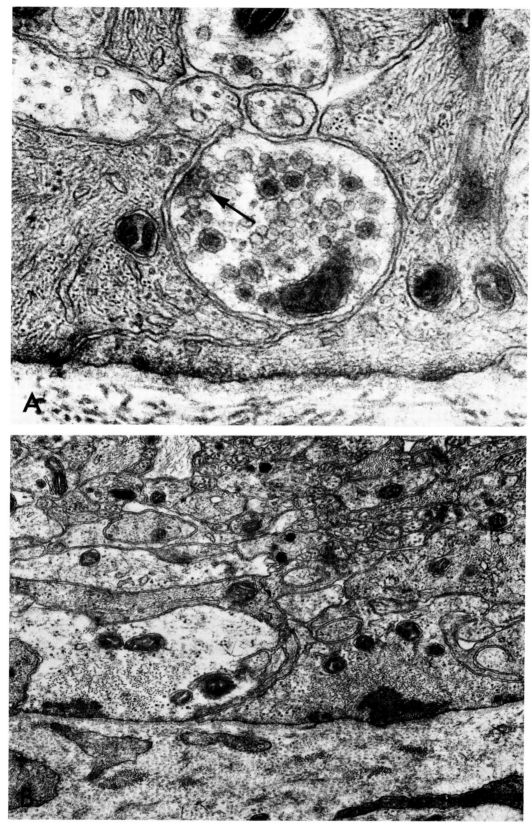

FIG. 18. A: Myenteric plexus of the rabbit ileum. A vesicle-containing nerve profile abuts on a glial process. Clustering of vesicles and membrane specialization are visible (*arrow*). Magnification: 66,500 ×. **B:** Myenteric plexus of guinea pig ileum. Two glial processes with numerous gliofilaments reach the surface of the ganglion and lie beneath its basal lamina. Note the conspicuous electron-dense material associated with the cell membrane and into which the gliofilaments penetrate. Mitochondria and microtubules are also present in the glial processes. Collagen fibrils, elastic fibers, and processes of interstitial cells are visible outside the ganglion. Magnification: 26,000 ×.

nervous system. In recent immunohistochemical study of these cells it has been found that the enteric glial cells (unlike the glial cells of other peripheral ganglia) are rich in glial fibrillary acid protein, a protein associated with gliofilaments and previously detected only in the astrocytes of the central nervous system (182).

INNERVATION OF THE VARIOUS PARTS OF THE INTESTINAL WALL

From a morphological point of view, the presence of nerve fibers within a tissue or part of an organ constitutes *innervation*. Physiological studies are needed to establish whether coexistence of nerves and muscle tissue represents a functional relation between the two and what sort of interaction the encounter between a nerve fiber and a muscle cell achieves. Morphologically, the significance of the innervation of a tissue or an organ can be assessed only if a quantitative analysis of several parameters is available, such as number of nerves, types of nerve fibers, distance between nerves and effectors, and branching pattern of nerve fibers. The nerve fibers which innervate the various layers of the intestinal wall are postganglionic and are unmyelinated. Since only a small percentage of endings degenerate after extrinsic denervation of the gut, the large majority of nerve fibers are of intrinsic origin.

Muscle Coat

Generally the longitudinal musculature of the small intestine is poorly innervated. No nerve fibers are usually found in the longitudinal muscle of the ileum and jejunum of the rat and guinea pig (but a small number of cholinergic and adrenergic axons run in the slightly thicker longitudinal musculature of the duodenum). Neurotransmitters probably reach the longitudinal musculature from the numerous nerve endings situated at the surface of the myenteric ganglia (Fig. 12B). In addition, small nerve bundles can be present between the myenteric plexus and longitudinal muscle cells, usually with some close neuromuscular contacts (Fig. 19). In species of larger body size, such as the rabbit and cat, the ileal longitudinal musculature is thicker and contains small intramuscular nerve bundles (307,310). In the taenia coli adrenergic and cholinergic axons are readily detectable with histochemical methods (1). There are also varicosities mainly containing large opaque vesicles which are interpreted as endings of the intrinsic inhibitory fibers (32). It was reported some years ago that in the guinea pig taenia coli the muscle cells near the serosal surface have an extensive intrinsic inhibitory innervation, but a sparse cholinergic and adrenergic innervation, and also that at intervals of about 1 mm there

is a marked decrease in the number of small nerve bundles (20). The density of innervation of the longitudinal musculature increases in the rectum and becomes particularly rich in the proximity of the anal canal (reviewed in 99).

The circular musculature of the small intestine contains several intramuscular nerve bundles. There are hundreds of axons per square millimeter of transverse sectional area, but it has not been established how many of these are in transit between the two plexuses and how many constitute functional innervation. In the ileum the terminal axons (the axons with vesicle-containing varicosities) are not uniformly distributed throughout the circular layer: they are preferentially found in small bundles at the same level as the myenteric plexus, i.e., in the gap between circular and longitudinal musculature, and near the submucosal border of the circular muscle, in the proximity of a layer of small and dense muscle cells (see p. 208) (Fig. 1A). The great majority of axons are grouped into bundles with supporting Schwann cells. Large and medium-sized intramuscular nerves are often accompanied by interstitial cells (see p. 209). Even the axons which are more intimately associated with muscle cells are often part of a small bundle and are accompanied by thin cytoplasmic processes from Schwann cells. Individual axons are encountered only rarely; although they are by no means absent, they seem much less numerous than in other smooth muscles such as the spincter pupillae or the vas deferens.

Intramuscular axons tend to run parallel to the smooth muscle cells. They are varicose, and the varicosities are regarded as the sites where neurotransmitters are released. It is still uncertain what the conduction velocity of impulses is in the varicose portion of an axon and how many varicosities (if not all) are activated to release neurotransmitter for each impulse traveling along an axon. There is also some uncertainty as to what constitutes a neuromuscular contact (or junction) in the intestinal muscles. The characteristic specializations of the cell membrane visualized by freeze-fracture in the end plates of skeletal fibers are not found in the smooth muscle cells lying close to a nerve ending.

The varicosities usually contain numerous synaptic vesicles but show few of the specializations associated with synaptic junctions. Dense projections are often absent in the varicosities, and when they are present they are small and few in number. The vesicles may be clustered close to some area of the membrane of the varicosity, but more often they show no association with the plasma membrane. Another parameter which seems to vary markedly even within the same axon is the distance between varicosity and muscle cell. Some varicosities are nowhere near a muscle cell but lie fully embedded in collagen fibrils or surrounded by interstitial cell processes. Most commonly a varicosity is separated from a muscle cell by a gap measuring from 40 to over 100 nm. This is generally considered the type

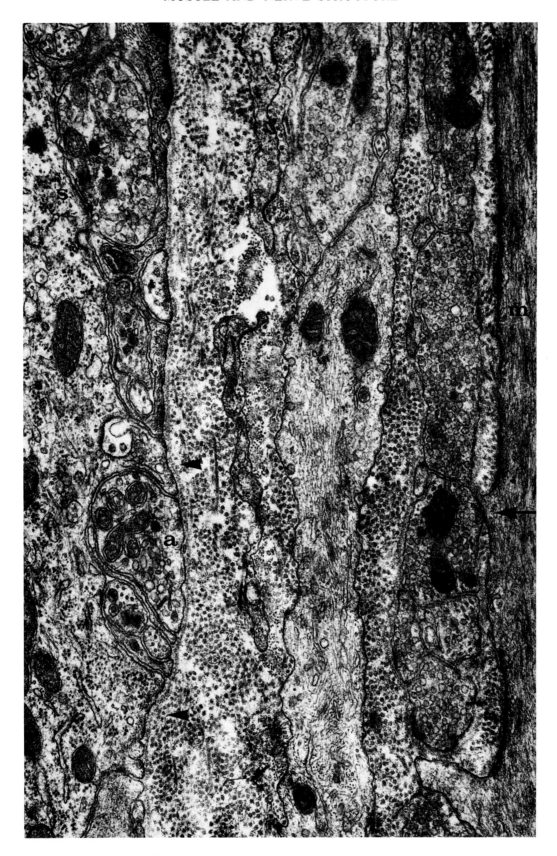

FIG. 19. Myenteric plexus of guinea pig ileum. The micrograph includes a muscle cell of the longitudinal layer (*m*). Several varicosities packed with small agranular vesicles are situated between the myenteric ganglion and the longitudinal musculature. In one area (*arrow*), a close neuromuscular contact is formed. Within the ganglion, a neuron is visible, receiving a synapse (s) and reaching the surface of the ganglion (*arrowheads*). Another varicosity is situated at the surface of the ganglion (a). From Gabella (112). Magnification: 35,000 ×.

of neuromuscular junction characteristic of intestinal muscles (260,274,307), as opposed, for example, to that of the muscles of the iris or the vas deferens. In the latter examples the neuromuscular gaps are more uniform in width and mostly measure about 20 nm. However, on closer examination, also in the intestine there are neuromuscular contacts whose gap is reduced to about 20 nm. Endings identified as cholinergic and adrenergic have been found in this relation to muscle cells (110).

Muscles of Sphincters

The innervation of the musculature is particularly dense at the level of most sphincters. A rich adrenergic innervation is found in the internal anal sphincter (p. 225) and in other sphincters. Nerve fibers containing the peptide VIP are numerous in the musculature of the gastroesophageal junction and the pylorus and in the sphincter of Oddi (5) (p. 225). Detailed ultrastructural studies of the innervation of the sphincteric musculature in the alimentary canal have not been published.

Muscularis Mucosae

Several small nerve bundles pierce the muscularis mucosae and penetrate into the mucosa. It is, however, not clear how many of the axons establish functional relations with the muscle cells. The relative importance of neuronal and myogenic control mechanisms on the muscularis mucosae remains to be established.

Blood vessels

A rich adrenergic supply (originating from the sympathetic ganglia) is seen by fluorescence microscopy around the blood vessels of the gut wall, particularly around the arteries (reviewed in 99). These adrenergic nerve endings are clearly recognized by electron microscopy, and they are accompanied by a small number of nerve fibers of different morphology. By immunohistochemistry it has recently been shown that nerve fibers containing neuropeptides are closely associated with blood vessels of the submucosa (277). Physiologically, vasodilator fibers have been found in intestinal blood vessels, originating from neurons of the intramural ganglia (22,23). Biber (22) has suggested that intestinal blood flow is regulated by fibers originating from the prevertebral ganglia and by fibers of local origin.

THE PROBLEM OF AFFERENT FIBERS

Afferent mechanisms play an important part in the activity of the gastrointestinal tract. They are at work in all the reflex and coordinated activities of the gut, and afferent impulses can reach the central nervous system (sensory mechanisms). However, there is little convincing anatomical evidence on the structures involved in afferent mechanisms. The intestinal wall is endowed with chemoreceptors and mechanoreceptors, but these have not yet been identified morphologically. Chemoreceptors are situated in the mucosa, a part of the wall which is particularly rich in nerve fibers. However, encapsulated nerve endings and sensory receptors are not found by electron microscopy. By silver impregnation methods some nerve fibers are seen forming complex arborizations in the mucosa and are interpreted as afferent fibers (299). Mechanoreceptors are mainly situated in the muscle coat and are stimulated by distension of the wall and by active contraction of the muscle. The physiological characteristics of these receptors, as can be studied by recording from nerve fibers in the vagus and the mesenteric nerves, have often been reviewed (174,206,320).

The structures in the gut wall in which mechanical stimuli are transformed into nervous impulses have not been identified. They may be "free" nerve endings within the circular muscle coat, or they can be some of the numerous nerve endings associated with the small and dense muscle cells at the innermost aspect of the circular muscle coat (Fig. 1A), or some of the endings within the myenteric plexus, particularly those situated at the surface of the ganglia.

Some afferent fibers originate from intramural neurons, so that a great deal of reflex activity persists after extrinsic denervation of a segment of intestine. These neurons have been investigated electrophysiologically (see Chapter 1, *this volume*), but they are not yet identified in the electron microscope. Afferent fibers of extrinsic origin (mainly from the vagal ganglia and from dorsal root ganglia) are also present in the gastrointestinal tract. They travel within the vagus and the splanchnic nerves, and transmit to the brainstem and the spinal cord.

In the enteric ganglia, there are also neurons (as yet unidentified) which project an axon centripetally to the prevertebral ganglia, where the axon synapses on ganglion neurons (195,196) (see p. 212). These axons are activated by distension of the intestinal wall, and their activity can be detected by intracellular recording from the prevertebral ganglion cells (58,59). After partial resection of the small intestine, degenerating nerve endings have been seen in the celiac ganglion of the cat (313). In the mesenteric nerves of the rabbit as many as 30% of the axons remain intact distal to a surgical division of the nerves and therefore originate from intramural neurons (267).

It seems that there are at least three levels for the reflex activity of the gut. One is entirely intrinsic with afferent and efferent fibers probably relaying in the enteric ganglia. Another involves connections between afferent and efferent pathways in the prevertebral ganglia, and the third one involves connections in the spinal cord and the medulla.

References

1. Åberg, G., and Eränkö, O. (1967): Localization of noradrenaline and acetylcholinesterase in the taenia of the guinea-pig caecum. *Acta Physiol. Scand.,* 69:383-384.

2. Agostoni, E., Chinnock, J. E., Daly, M. D. B., and Murray, J. G. (1975): Functional and histological studies of the vagus nerve and its branches to the heart, lungs and abdominal viscera in the cat. *J. Physiol. (Lond.),* 135:182-205.

3. Ahlman, H., and Enerbäck, L. (1974): A cytofluorimetric study of the myenteric plexus of the guinea pig. *Z. Zellforsch.,* 153:248-259.

4. Ahlman, B. H., Lundberg, J. M., Dahlström, A., Larsson, I., Pettersson, G., Kewenter, J., and Nyhus, L. M. (1978): Evidence for innervation of the small intestine from cervical sympathetic ganglia. *J. Surg. Res.,* 24:142-149.

5. Alumets, J., Fahrenkrug, J., Håkanson, R., Schaffalitzky de Muckadell, O., Sundler, F., and Uddman, R. (1979): A rich VIP nerve supply is characteristic of sphincters. *Nature (Lond.),* 280:155-156.

6. Alumets, J., Håkanson, R., Sundler, F., and Chang, K.-J. (1978): Leu-enkephalin-like material in nerves and enterochromaffin cells in the gut. *Histochemistry,* 56:187-196.

7. Ashton, F. T., Somlyo, A. V., and Somlyo, A. P. (1975): The contractile apparatus of vascular smooth muscle: intermediate high voltage stereo electron microscopy. *J. Mol. Biol.,* 98:17-29.

8. Baisset, A., and Montastruc, R. (1956): Contribution expérimentale à l'étude de l'innervation sympathique du cardia chez le chien. *C.R. Soc. Biol.,* 150:2003-2007.

9. Barr, L., Berger, W., and Dewey, M. M. (1968): Electrical transmission of the nexus between smooth muscle cells. *J. Gen. Physiol.,* 51:347-369.

10. Barry, J., Dubois, M. P., and Poulain, P. (1973): LRF producing cells of the mammalian hypothalamus. A fluorescent antibody study. *Z. Zellforsch.,* 146:351-366.

11. Batra, S. C. (1973): Effect of some estrogens and progesterone on calcium release by myometrial mitochondria. *Biochem. Pharmacol.,* 22:803-809.

12. Baumgarten, H. G. (1967): Vorkommen und Verteilung adrenerger Nervenfasern im Darm der Scheie. *Z. Zellforsch.,* 76:248-259.

13. Baumgarten, H. G. (1967): Über die Verteilung von Catecholaminen in Darm des Menschen. *Z. Zellforsch.,* 83:133-146.

14. Baumgarten, H. G., Holstein, A.-F., and Owman, Ch. (1970): Auerbach's plexus of mammals and man: electron microscopic identification of three different types of neuronal processes in myenteric ganglia of the large intestine from rhesus monkeys, guinea-pigs and man. *Z. Zellforsch.,* 106:376-397.

15. Baumgarten, H. G., and Lange, W. (1969): Adrenergic innervation of the oesophagus in the cat (*Felix domestica*) and rhesus monkey (*Macacus rhesus*). *Z. Zellforsch.,* 95:529-545.

16. Benditt, E. P., and Wong, R. L. (1957): On the concentration of 5-hydroxytryptamine in mammalian enterochromaffin cells and its release by reserpine. *J. Exp. Med.,* 105:509-520.

17. Bennett, G. S., Fellini, S. A., Croop, J. M., Otto, J. J., Bryan, J., and Holtzer, H. (1978): Differences among 100 Å filament subunits from different cell types. *Proc. Natl. Acad. Sci. U.S.A.,* 75:4364-4368.

18. Bennett, M. R. (1972): *Autonomic Neuromuscular Transmission.* Cambridge University Press, London.

19. Bennett, M. R., Burnstock, G., and Holman, M. E. (1966): Transmission from intramural inhibitory nerves in the smooth muscle of the guinea-pig taenia coli. *J. Physiol. (Lond.),* 182:541-558.

20. Bennett, M. R., and Rogers, D. C. (1967): A study of the innervation of the taenia coli. *J. Cell Biol.,* 33:573-596.

21. Bennett, T., Malmfors, T., and Cobb, J.L.S. (1973): Fluorescence histochemical observations on catecholamine-containing cell bodies in Auerbach's plexus. *Z. Zellforsch.,* 139:69-81.

22. Biber, B. (1973): Vasodilator mechanisms in the small intestine. *Acta Physiol. Scand. [Suppl. 40].*

23. Biber, B., Fara, J., and Lundgren, O. (1973): Intestinal vasodilation in response to transmural electrical field stimulation. *Acta Physiol. Scand.,* 87:277-282.

24. Bloom, S. R., Ghatei, M. A., Wharton, J. W., Polak, J. M., and Brown, M. M. R. (1979): Distribution of bombesin in human alimentary tract. *Gastroenterology,* 76:1103.

25. Bois, R. M. (1973): The organization of the contractile apparatus of vertebrate smooth muscle. *Anat. Rec.,* 177:61-78.

26. Bótar, J., Battancs, L., and Becker, A. (1942): Die Nervenzellen des Dünndarms. *Anat. Anz.,* 93:138-149.

27. Brading, A. F., and Jones, A. W. (1969): Distribution and kinetics of CoEDTA in smooth muscle, and its use as an extracellular marker. *J. Physiol. (Lond.),* 200:387-402.

28. Brazeau, P., Vale, W., Burgus, R., Ling, N., Butcher, M., Rivier, J., and Guillemin, R. (1973): Hypothalamic polypeptide that inhibits the secretion of immunoreactive pituitary growth hormone. *Science,* 179:77-79.

29. Brysk, M. M., Gray, R. H., and Bernstein, I. A. (1977): Tonofilament protein from newborn rat epidermis. *J. Biol. Chem.,* 252:2127-2133.

30. Bülbring, E., Lin, R. C. Y., and Schofield, G. C. (1958): An investigation of the peristaltic reflex in relation to anatomical observations. *Q. J. Exp. Physiol.,* 43:26-37.

31. Bülbring, E., and Tomita, T. (1966): Evidence supporting the assumption that the 'inhibitory potential' in the taenia coli of the guinea-pig is a post-synaptic potential due to nerve stimulation. *J. Physiol. (Lond.),* 185:24-25P.

32. Burnstock, G. (1975): Comparative studies of purinergic nerves. *J. Exp. Zool.,* 194:103-134.

33. Burnstock, G., Campbell, G., Bennett, M., and Holman, M. E. (1963): Inhibition of the smooth muscle of the taenia coli. *Nature (Lond.),* 200:581-582.

34. Burnstock, G., Campbell, G., Bennett, M., and Holman, M. E. (1964): Are there intrinsic inhibitory nerves which are distinct from sympathetic nerves? *Int. J. Neuropharmacol,* 3:163-166.

35. Burnstock, G., Campbell, G., Satchell, D., and Smythe, A. (1970): Evidence that adenosine triphosphate or a related nucleotide is the transmitter substance released by nonadrenergic inhibitory nerves in the gut. *Br. J. Pharmacol.,* 40:668-688.

36. Bursztajn, S., and Gershon, M. D. (1977): Discrimination between nicotinic receptors in vertebrate ganglia and skeletal muscle by alpha-bungarotoxin and cobra venoms. *J. Physiol. (Lond.),* 269:17-31.

37. Cajal, S. R. (1893): Sur les ganglions et le plexus nerveux de l'intestin. *C.R. Soc. Biol. (Paris),* 5:217-223.

38. Campbell, G., and Gibbins, I. L. (1979): Nonadrenergic, noncholinergic transmission in the autonomic nervous system: Purinergic nerves. In: *Trends in Autonomic Pharmacology, Vol. 1,* edited by S. Kalsner, pp. 103-144. Urban & Schwarzenberg, Baltimore and Munich.

39. Campbell, G. R., Chamley-Campbell, J., Gröschel-Stewart, U., Small, J. V., and Anderson, P. (1979): Antibody staining of 10-nm (100-Å) filaments in cultured smooth, cardiac, and skeletal muscle cells. *J. Cell Sci.,* 37:303-322.

40. Carey, E. J. (1921): Studies on the structure and function of the small intestine. *Anat. Rec.,* 21:189-215.

41. Chang, M. M., Leeman, S. E., and Niall, H. D. (1971): Aminoacid sequence of substance P. *Nature [New Biol.],* 232:86-87.

42. Cochard, P., Goldstein, M., and Black, I. B. (1978): Ontogenetic appearance and disappearance of tyrosine hydroxylase and catecholamine biosynthesis in the rat embryo. *Proc. Natl. Acad. Sci. U.S.A.,* 75:2986-2990.

43. Cohen, M. L., Rosing, E., Wiley, K. S., and Slater, I. H. (1978): Somatostatin inhibits adrenergic and cholinergic neurotransmission in smooth muscle. *Life Sci.,* 23:1659-1664.

44. Cook, R. D., and Burnstock, G. (1976): The ultrastructure of Auerbach's plexus in the guinea-pig. I. Neuronal elements. *J. Neurocytol.,* 5:171-194.

45. Cook, R. D., and Burnstock, G. (1976): The ultrastructure of Auerbach's plexus in the guinea-pig. II. Non-neuronal elements. *J. Neurocytol.,* 5:195-206.

46. Cooke, P. (1976): A filamentous cytoskeleton in vertebrate smooth muscle fibers. *J. Cell Biol.,* 68:539–556.

47. Cooke, P. H. (1976): A filamentous cytoskeleton in vertebrate smooth muscle fibers. *J. Cell Biol.,* 68:539–556.

48. Costa, M., Cuello, A. C., Furness, J. B., and Franco, R. (1980): Distribution of enteric neurons showing immunoreactivity for substance P in the guinea-pig ileum. *Neuroscience,* 5:323–331.

49. Costa, M., and Furness, J. B. (1971): Storage, uptake and synthesis of catecholamines in the intrinsic adrenergic neurons in the proximal colon of the guinea-pig. *Z. Zellforsch.,* 120:364–385.

50. Costa, M., and Furness, J. B. (1973): The origins of the adrenergic fibre which innervate the internal anal sphincter, the rectum, and other tissues of the pelvic region in the guinea-pig. *Z. Anat. EntwGesch.,* 140:129–142.

51. Costa, M., Furness, J. B., Buffa, R., and Said, S. I. (1980): Distribution of enteric nerve cell bodies and axons showing immunoreactivity for vasoactive intestinal polypeptide in the guinea-pig intestine. *Neuroscience,* 5:587–596.

52. Costa, M., Furness, J. B., and Gabella, G. (1971): Catecholamine-containing nerve cells in the mammalian myenteric plexus. *Histochemie,* 25:103–106.

53. Costa, M., Furness, J. B., Llewellyn-Smith, I. J., Davies, B., and Oliver, J. (1980): An immunohistochemical study of the projections of somatostatin-containing neurons in the guinea-pig intestine. *Neuroscience,* 5:841–852.

54. Costa, M., and Gabella, G. (1971): Adrenergic innervation of the alimentary canal. *Z. Zellforsch.,* 122:357–377.

55. Costa, M., Patel, Y., Furness, J. B., and Arimura, A. (1977): Evidence that some intrinsic neurons of the intestine contain somatostatin. *Neurosci. Lett.,* 6:215–222.

56. Cragg, B. (1979): Overcoming the failure of electronmicroscopy to preserve the brain's extracellular space. *Trends Neurosci.,* 2: 159–161.

57. Craig, R., and Megerman, J. (1977): Assembly of smooth muscle myosin into side-polar filaments. *J. Cell Biol.,* 75:990–996.

58. Crowcroft, P. J., Holman, M. E., and Szurszewski, J. H. (1971): Excitatory input from the distal colon to the inferior mesenteric ganglion of the guinea-pig. *J. Physiol. (Lond.),* 219:443–461.

59. Crowcroft, P. J., and Szurszewski, J. H. (1971): A study of the inferior mesenteric and pelvic ganglia of guinea-pig with intracellular electrodes. *J. Physiol. (Lond.),* 219:421–441.

60. Crowe, R. (1980): *(personal communication).*

61. Dahlström, A. (1971): Axoplasmic transport (with particular respect to adrenergic neurons). *Philos. Trans. R. Soc. Lond. [Biol.],* 261:325–358.

62. Dahlström, A., and Häggendal, J. (1966): Some quantitative studies of the noradrenaline content in the cell bodies and terminals of a sympathetic adrenergic neuron system. *Acta Physiol. Scand.,* 67:271–277.

63. Daniel, E. E., Daniel, V. P., Duchon, G., Garfield, R. E., Nichols, M., Malhotra, S. K., and Oki, M. (1976): Is the nexus necessary for cell-to-cell coupling of smooth muscle? *J. Membr. Biol.,* 28:207–239.

64. Daniel, E. E., Taylor, G. S., Daniel, V. P., and Holman, M. E. (1977): Can nonadrenergic inhibitory varicosities be identified structurally? *Can. J. Physiol. Pharmacol.,* 55:243–250.

65. Davison, P. F., Hong, B. S., and Cooke, P. (1977): Classes of distinguishable 10 nm cytoplasmic filaments. *Exp. Cell Res.,* 109:471–474.

66. Debbas, G., Hoffman, L., Landon, E. J., and Hurwitz, L. (1975): Electron microscopic localization of calcium in vascular smooth muscle. *Anat. Rec.,* 182:447–472.

67. De Castro, F. (1932): Sympathetic ganglia: normal and pathological. In: *Cytology and Cellular Pathology of the Nervous System, Vol. 1,* edited by W. Penfield, pp. 319–379. Paul B. Hoeber, New York.

68. De Groat, W. C., and Krier, J. (1975): Preganglionic C-fibres: a major component of the sacral autonomic outflow to the colon of the cat. *Pflügers Arch.,* 359:171–176.

69. Devine, C. E., Somlyo, A. V., and Somlyo, A. P. (1972): Sarcoplasmic reticulum and excitation-contraction coupling in mammalian smooth muscle. *J. Cell Biol.,* 52:690–718.

70. Dewey, M. M., and Barr, L. (1962): Intercellular connection between smooth muscle cells: the nexus. *Science,* 127:670–672.

71. Dewey, M. M., and Barr, L. (1964): A study of the structure and distribution of the nexus. *J. Cell Biol.,* 23:553–583.

72. Dikshit, B. B. (1938): Acetylcholine formation by tissues. *Q. J. Exp. Physiol.,* 28:243–251.

73. Dockray, G. J., Vaillant, C., and Walsh, J. H. (1979): The neuronal origin of bombesin-like immunoreactivity in the rat gastrointestinal tract. *Neuroscience,* 4:1561–1568.

74. Dogiel, A. S. (1899): Ueber den Bau der Ganglien in den Geflechten des Darms und der Gallenblase des Menschen und der Saügetiere. *Arch. Anat. Physiol. Anat.,* :130–158.

75. Dreyfus, C. F., Bornstein, M. B., and Gershon, M. D. (1977): Synthesis of serotonin by neurons of the myenteric plexus in situ and in organotypic tissue culture. *Brain Res.,* 128:125–139.

76. Dreyfus, C. F., Sherman, D. L., and Gershon, M. D. (1977): Uptake of serotonin by intrinsic neurons of the myenteric plexus grown in organotypic tissue culture. *Brain Res.,* 128:109–123.

77. Edin, R., Lundberg, J. M., Ahlman, H., Kewenter, J., Dahlström, A., Fahrenkrug, J., and Hökfelt, T. (1979): On the VIPergic innervation of the feline pylorus. *Acta Physiol. Scand.,* 107:185–187.

78. Eklund, S., Jodal, M., Lundgren, O., and Sjöquist, A. (1979): Effects of Vasoactive intestinal polypeptide on blood flow motility and fluid transport in the gastrointestinal tract of the cat. *Acta Physiol. Scand.,* 105:461–468.

79. Elde, R., Hökfelt, T., Johansson, O., and Terenius, L. (1976): Immunohistochemical studies using antibodies to leucine-enkephalin: initial observations on the nervous system of the rat. *Neuroscience,* 1:349–351.

80. Elfvin, L.-G. (1971): Ultrastructural studies on the synaptology of the inferior mesenteric ganglion of the cat. I. Observations on cell surface of the postganglionic perikaya. *J. Ultrastructr. Res.,* 37:411–425.

81. Elfvin, L.-G. (1971): Ultrastructural studies on the synaptology of the inferior mesenteric ganglion of the cat. II. Specialized serial neuronal contacts between preganglionic end fibers. *J. Ultrastructr. Res.,* 37:426–431.

82. Elliott, A., Offer, G., and Burridge, K. (1976): Electron microscopy of myosin molecules from muscle and non-muscle sources. *Proc. R. Soc. Lond. [Biol.],* 193:45–53.

83. Euler, U. S. von, and Gaddum, J. H. (1931): An unidentified depressor substance in certain tissue extracts. *J. Physiol. (Lond.),* 72:74–87.

84. Evans, D. H. L., and Murray, J. G. (1954): Histological and functional studies on the fibre composition of the vagus nerve of the rabbit. *J. Anat.,* 88:320–337.

85. Fahrenkrug, J., Haglund, U., Jodal, M., Lundgren, O., Olbe, L., and Schaffalitzky de Muckadell, O. B. (1978): Nervous release of vasoactive intestinal polypeptide in the gastrointestinal tract of cats: possible physiological implications. *J. Physiol. (Lond.),* 284:291–305.

86. Falck, B., Häggendal, J., and Owman, Ch. (1963): The localization of adrenaline in adrenergic nerves of the frog. *Q. J. Exp. Physiol.,* 48:253–257.

87. Fawcett, D. W., and McNutt, N. S. (1969): The ultrastructure of the cat myocardium. I. Ventricular papillary muscle. *J. Cell Biol.,* 42:1–45.

88. Fay, F. S., and Delise, C. M. (1973): Contraction of isolated smooth muscle cells. Structural changes. *Proc. Natl. Acad. Sci. U.S.A.,* 70:641–645.

89. Féher, E., and Vajda, J. (1972): Cell types in the nerve plexus of the small intestine. *Acta Morphol. Acad. Sci. Hung.,* 20:13–25.

90. Féher, E., and Vajda, J. (1976): Selective sympathetic denervation induced by a 6-hydroxy-dopamine in the small intestine. *Acta Morphol. Acad. Sci. Hung.,* 24:121–128.

91. Fisher, B. A., and Bagby, R. M. (1977): Reorientation of myofilaments during contraction of a vertebrate smooth muscle. *Am. J. Physiol.,* 232:C5–C14.

92. Ford, G. D., and Hess, M. L. (1975): Calcium-accumulating properties of subcellular fractions of bovine vascular smooth muscle. *Circ. Res.,* 37:580–587.

93. Franke, W. W., Schmid, E., Osborn, M., and Weber, K. (1978): Different intermediate-sized filaments distinguished by immunofluorescence microscopy. *Proc. Natl. Acad. Sci. U.S.A.,* 75:5034–5038.

94. Fredricsson, B., and Sjöquist, F. (1962): A cytomorphological study of cholinesterase in sympathetic ganglia of the cat. *Acta Morphol. Neerl. Scand.,* 5:140-166.

95. Fry, G. N., Devine, C. E., and Burnstock, G. (1977): Freeze-fracture studies of nexuses between smooth muscle cells. *J. Cell Biol.,* 72:26-34.

96. Furness, J. B. (1969): An electrophysiological study of the innervation of the smooth muscle of the colon. *J. Physiol. (Lond.),* 205:549-562.

97. Furness, J. B., and Costa, M. (1971): Morphology and distribution of intrinsic adrenergic neurons in the proximal colon of the guinea-pig. *Z. Zellforsch.,* 120:346-363.

98. Furness, J. B., and Costa, M. (1973): The ramifications of adrenergic nerve terminals in the rectum, anal sphincter and anal accessory muscles of the guinea-pig. *Z. Anat. EntwGesch.,* 140:109-128.

99. Furness, J. B., and Costa, M. (1974): The adrenegic innervation of the gastrointestinal tract. *Ergebn. Physiol.,* 69:1-51.

100. Furness, J. B., and Costa, M. (1980): Types of nerves in the enteric nervous system. *Neuroscience,* 5:1-20.

101. Fuxe, K., Hökfelt, T., Said, S. I., and Mutt, V. (1977): Vasoactive intestinal polypeptide and the nervous system. Immunohistochemical evidence for localization in central and peripheral neurons, particularly intra-cortical neurons of the cerebral cortex. *Neurosci. Lett.,* 5:241-246.

102. Gabella, G. (1971): Neuron size and number in the myenteric plexus of the newborn and adult rat. *J. Anat.,* 109:81-95.

103. Gabella, G. (1972): Fine structure of the myenteric plexus in the guinea-pig ileum. *J. Anat.,* 111:69-97.

104. Gabella, G. (1974): Special muscle cells and their innervation in the mammalian small intestine. *Cell Tissue Res.,* 153:63-77.

105. Gabella, G. (1976): *Structure of the Autonomic Nervous System.* Chapman & Hall, London.

106. Gabella, G. (1976): Quantitative morphological study of smooth muscle cells of the guinea-pig taenia coli. *Cell Tissue Res.,* 170:161-186.

107. Gabella, G. (1976): The force generated by a visceral smooth muscle. *J. Physiol. (Lond.),* 263:199-213.

108. Gabella, G. (1979): Hypertrophic smooth muscle. IV. Myofilaments, intermediate filaments and some mechanical properties. *Cell Tissue Res.,* 201:277-288.

109. Gabella, G. (1979): Smooth muscle cell junctions and structural aspects of contraction. *Br. Med. Bull.,* 35:213-218.

110. Gabella, G. (1979): Innervation of the gastrointestinal tract. *Int. Rev. Cytol.,* 59:129-193.

111. Gabella, G. (1979): Hypertrophic smooth muscle. III. Increase in number and size of gap junctions. *Cell Tissue Res.,* 201:236-276.

112. Gabella, G. (1980): Structure of smooth muscle. In: *Smooth Muscle: An Assessment of Current Knowledge,* edited by E. Bülbring, A. F. Brading, A. W. Jones, and T. Tomita, pp. 1-46. Edward Arnold, London.

113. Gabella, G., and Blundell, D. (1978): Effect of stretch and contraction on caveolae of smooth muscle cells. *Cell Tissue Res.,* 190:255-271.

114. Gabella, G., and Blundell, D. (1979): Nexuses between the smooth muscle cells of the guinea-pig ileum. *J. Cell Biol.* 82:239-247.

115. Gabella, G., and Blundell, D. (1981): Distribution of gap junctions in the musculature of the guinea-pig intestine. (In preparation).

116. Gabella, G., and Costa, M. (1967): Le fibre adrenergiche nel canale alimentare. *Giorn. Accad. Med. (Torino),* 130:199-221.

117. Gabella, G., and Juorio, A. V. (1975): Effect of extrinsic denervation on endogenous noradrenaline and (^{3}H) noradrenaline uptake in the guinea-pig colon. *J. Neurochem.,* 25:631-634.

118. Garrett, J. R., and Howard, E. R. (1975): Neural control of the internal anal sphincter of cats after chemical sympathectomy with 6-hydroxydopamine. *J. Physiol. (Lond.),* 247:25-27P.

119. Garry, R. C., and Gillespie, J. S. (1954): An *in vitro* preparation of the distal colon of the rabbit with orthosympathetic and parasympathetic innervation. *J. Physiol. (Lond.),* 123:60-61P.

120. Geffen, L. B., and Livett, B. G. (1971): Synaptic vesicles in sympathetic neurons. *Physiol. Rev.,* 51:98-157.

121. Geisweid, G., and Wermbter, G. (1974): Die Feinstruktur des Nexus zwischen glatten Muskelzellen der Taenia coli in Gefrierätzbild. *Cytobiologie,* 9:121-130.

122. Gerhon, M. D., and Bursztajn, S. (1978): Properties of the enteric nervous system: limitation of access of intravascular macromolecules to the myenteric plexus and muscularis externa. *J. Comp. Neurol.,* 180:467-487.

123. Gershon, M. D., Drakontides, A. B., and Ross, L. L. (1965): Serotonin: Synthesis and release from the myentric plexus of the mouse intestine. *Science,* 149:197-199.

124. Gershon, M. D., Dreyfus, C. F., Pickel, V. M., Joh, T. H., and Reis, D. J. (1977): Serotonergic neurons in the peripheral nervous system: identification in gut by immunohistochemical localization of tryptophan hydroxylase. *Proc. Natl. Acad. Sci. U.S.A.,* 74:3086-3089.

125. Gershon, M. D., Dreyfus, C. F., and Rothman, T. P. (1979): The mammalian enteric nervous system: a third autonomic division. In: *Trends in Autonomic Pharmacology, Vol. 1,* edited by S. Kalsner, pp. 59-101. Urban & Schwarzenberg, Baltimore and Munich.

126. Gershon, M. D., Robinson, R. G., and Ross, L. L. (1976): Serotonin accumulation in the guinea-pig myenteric plexus: ion dependence, structure-activity relationship and the effect of drugs. *J. Pharmacol. Exp. Ther.,* 198:548-561.

127. Gershon, M. D., and Thompson, E. (1973): The maturation of neuromuscular function in a multiply innervated structure: development of the longitudinal smooth muscle of the foetal mammalian gut and its cholinergic excitatory, adrenergic inhibitory innervation. *J. Physiol. (Lond.),* 234:257-277.

128. Gibbins, I. L., and Haller, C. J. (1979): Ultrastructural identification of non-adrenergic non-cholinergic nerves in the rat anococcygeous muscle. *Cell Tissue Res.,* 200:257-271.

129. Gillespie, J. S., and Khoyi, M. A. (1977): The site and receptors responsible for the inhibition by sympathetic nerves of intestinal smooth muscle and its parasympathetic motor nerves. *J. Physiol. (Lond.),* 267:767-789.

130. Gillespie, J. S., and Maxwell, J. S. (1971): Adrenergic innervation of the sphincteric and nonsphincteric smooth muscle in the rat intestine. *J. Histochem. Cytochem.,* 19:676-681.

131. Gilula, N. B. (1978): Structure of intercellular junctions. In: *Intercellular Junctions and Synapses,* edited by J. Feldman, N. B. Gilula, and J. D. Pitts, pp. 1-22. Chapman & Hall, London.

132. Gonella, J., Niel, J. P., and Roman, C. (1979): Sympathetic control of lower oesophageal sphincter motility in the cat. *J. Physiol. (Lond.),* 287:177-190.

133. Goodford, P. J. (1970): Ion movements in smooth muscle. In: *Membranes and Ion Transport,* edited by E. Bittar, pp. 33-74. John Wiley & Sons, New York.

134. Goodford, P. J., and Hermansen, K. (1961): Sodium and potassium movements in the unstriated muscle of the guinea-pig taenia coli. *J. Physiol. (Lond.),* 158:426-448.

135. Goodford, P. J., and Wolowyk, M. W. (1972): Localization of cation interactions in the smooth muscle of the guinea-pig taenia coli. *J. Physiol. (Lond.),* 224:521-535.

136. Gordon-Weeks, P. R., and Hobbs, M. J. (1979): A non-adrenergic nerve ending containing small granular vesicles in the guinea-pig gut. *Neurosci. Lett.,* 12:81-86.

137. Grillo, M. A., and Palay, S. L. (1962): Granule-containing vesicles in the autonomic nervous system. Fifth International Conference on Electron Microscopy, Philadelphia, Vol. 2, p. 6.

138. Gröschel-Stewart, U. (1971): Comparative studies of human smooth and striated muscle myosins. *Biochim. Biophys. Acta,* 229:322-334.

139. Guillemin, R. (1976): Somatostatin inhibits the release of acetylcholine induced electrically in the myenteric plexus. *Endocrinology,* 99:1653-1654.

140. Güldner, F.-H., Wolff, J. R., and Keyselingk, D. G. (1972): Fibroblasts as a part of the contractile system in duodenal villi of rat. *Z. Zellforsch.,* 135:349-360.

141. Gunn, M. (1968): Histological observations of the myenteric and sub-mucous plexuses of mammals. *J. Anat.,* 102:223-239.

142. Gunn, M. (1971): Cholinergic mechanisms in the gastrointestinal tract. *J. Neurovisc. Rel.,* 32:224-240.

143. Hamberger, B., Norberg, K. A., and Ungerstedt, U. (1975):

Adrenergic synaptic terminals in autonomic ganglia. *Acta Physiol. Scand.*, 64:285–286.

144. Hanak, H., and Böck, P. (1971): Die Feinstruktur der Muskel-Sehnenverbindung von Skelett- und Herzmuskel. *J. Ultrastructr. Res.*, 36:68–85.

145. Hartshorne, D. J., and Gorecka, A. (1980): Biochemistry of the contractile proteins of smooth muscle. In: *Handbook of Physiology, Section 2, Vol. II*, pp. 93–120. American Physiological Society, Washington, D.C.

146. Henderson, R. M. (1975): Cell-to-cell contacts. In: *Methods in Pharmacology, Vol. 3*, edited by E. E. Daniel and D. M. Paton, pp. 47–77. Plenum, New York.

147. Henderson, R. M., Duchon, G., and Daniel, E. E. (1971): Cell contacts in duodenal smooth muscle layers. *Am. J. Physiol.*, 221:564–574.

148. Heumann, H.-G. (1969): Gibt es in glatten Vertebratenmuskeln dicke Filamente? Elektronenmikroskopische Untersuchungen an der Darmmuskulatur der Hausmaus. *Zool. Anz. Verh. Zool. Ges.*, 33:416–424.

149. Heumann, H.-G. (1976): The subcellular localization of calcium in vertebrate smooth muscle: calcium-containing and calcium-accumulating structures in muscle cells of mouse intestine. *Cell Tissue Res.*, 169:221–231.

150. Hill, C. J. (1927): A contribution to our knowledge of the enteric plexuses. *Philos. Trans. R. Soc. Lond. [Biol.]*, 215:355–387.

151. Hinssen, H., D'Haese, J., Small, J. V., Sobieszek, A. (1978): Mode of filament assembly of myosin from muscle and nonmuscle cells. *J. Ultrastruct. Res.*, 64:282–302.

152. Hirst, G. D. S., and McKirdy, H. C. (1974): A nervous mechanism for descending inhibition in guinea-pig small intestine. *J. Physiol. (Lond.)*, 228:129–143.

153. Hobbiger, F. (1958): Effects of α-aminobutyric acid on the isolated mammalian ileum. *J. Physiol. (Lond.)*, 142:147–164.

154. Hodgkiss, J. P., and Lees, G. M. (1978): Correlated electrophysiological and morphological characteristics of myenteric plexus neurones. *J. Physiol. (Lond.)*, 285:19–20P.

155. Hökfelt T., and Dahlström, A. (1971): Effects of two mitosis inhibitors (colchicine and vinblastine) on the distribution and axonal transport of noradrenaline storage particles, studied by fluorescence and electron microscopy. *Z. Zellforsch.*, 119:460–482.

156. Hökfelt, T., Elfvin, L.-G., Elde, R., Schultzberg, M., Goldstein, M., and Luft, R. (1977): Occurrence of somatostatin-like immunoreactivity in some peripheral noradrenergic neurons. *Proc. Natl. Acad. Sci. U.S.A.*, 74:3587–3591.

157. Hökfelt, T., Elfvin, L.-G., Schultzberg, M., Fuxe, K., Said, S. I., Mutt, V., and Goldstein, M. (1977): Immunohistochemical evidence of vasoactive intestinal polypeptide-containing neurons and nerve fibers in sympathetic ganglia. *Neuroscience*, 2:885–896.

158. Hökfelt, T., Elfvin, L.-G., Schultzberg, M., Goldstein, M., and Nilsson, G. (1977): On the occurrence of substance P-containing fibers in sympathetic ganglia: immunohistological evidence. *Brain Res.*, 132:29–41.

159. Hökfelt, T., Johansson, O., Efendić, S., Luft, R., and Arimura, A. (1975): Are there somatostatin-containing nerves in the rat gut? Immunohistochemical evidence for a new type of peripheral nerve. *Experientia*, 31:852–854.

160. Hökfelt, T., Johansson, O., Ljungdahl, Å., Lundberg, J. M., Schultzberg, M., Terenius, L., Goldstein, M., Elde, R., Steinbusch, H., and Verhofstad, A. (1978): Histochemistry of transmitter interactions. Neuronal coupling and coexistence of putative transmitters. *Adv. Pharmacol. Ther.*, 2:131–143.

161. Hökfelt, T., Johansson, O., Ljungdahl, Å., Lundberg, J. M., and Schultzberg, M. (1980): Peptidergic neurons. *Nature (Lond.)*, 284:515–521.

162. Hökfelt, T., Kellerth, J.-O., Nilsson, G., and Pernow, B. (1975): Experimental immunohistochemical studies on the localization and distribution of substance P in cat primary sensory neurons. *Brain Res.*, 100:235–252.

163. Honjin, R., Izumi, S., and Osugi, H. (1959): The distribution and morphology of argentophile and argentophobe nerve cells in the myenteric plexus of the digestive tube of the mouse: a quantitative study. *J. Comp. Neurol.*, 111:291–319.

164. Honjin, R., Takahashi, A., and Tasaki, Y. (1975): Electron microscopic studies of nerve endings in the mucous membrane of the human intestine. *Okajimas Folia Anat. Jpn.*, 40:409–427.

165. Howard, E. R., and Garrett, J. R. (1973): The intrinsic myenteric innervation of the hind-gut and accessory muscles of defecation in the cat. *Z. Zellforsch.*, 136:31–44.

166. Hubbard, B. D., and Lazarides, E. (1979): Copurification of actin and desmin from chicken smooth muscle and their copolymerization in vitro to intermediate filaments. *J. Cell Biol.*, 80:166–182.

167. Hughes, J. (1975): Isolation of an endogenous compound from the brain with pharmacological properties similar to morphine. *Brain Res.*, 88:295–308.

168. Hughes, J., Kosterlitz, H. W., and Smith, T. W. (1977): The distribution of methionine-enkephalin and leucine-enkephalin in the brain and peripheral tissues. *Br. J. Pharmacol.*, 61:639–647.

169. Hughes, J., Smith, T. W., Kosterlitz, H. W., Fothergill, L. H., Morgan, B. A., and Morris, H. R. (1975): Identification of two related pentapeptides from the brain with potent opiate agonist activity. *Nature (Lond.)*, 258:577–579.

170. Huxley, A. F. (1973): Muscular contraction. *J. Physiol. (Lond.)*, 243:1–43.

171. Huxley, H. E. (1963): Electron microscopic studies on the structure and synthetic protein filaments from striated muscle. *J. Mol. Biol.*, 7:281–308.

172. Hynes, R. O., and Destree, A. T. (1978): 10 nm filaments in normal and transformed cells. *Cell*, 13:151–163.

173. Iggo, A. (1956): Central nervous control of gastric movements in sheep and goats. *J. Physiol. (Lond.)*, 131:248–256.

174. Iggo, A. (1966): Physiology of visceral afferent systems. *Acta Neuroveg. (Wien)*, 28:121–134.

175. Imaizumi, M., and Hama, K. (1969): An electron microscopic study of the interstitial cells of the gizzard in lovebirds (*Uroloncha domestica*). *Z. Zellforsch.*, 97:351–357.

176. Irwin, D. A. (1931): The anatomy of Auerbach's plexus. *Am. J. Anat.*, 49:141–166.

177. Ishikawa, H., Bischoff, R., and Holtzer, H. (1968): Mitosis and intermediate-sized filaments in developing skeletal muscle. *J. Cell Biol.*, 38:538–555.

178. Ishikawa, H., Bischoff, R., and Holtzer, H. (1969): Formation of arrowhead complexes with heavy meromyosin in a variety of cell types. *J. Cell Biol.*, 43:312–328.

179. Iwanow, J. F., and Radostina, T. N. (1937): Über die Blutversorgung der intramuralen Nervengeflechte des Darms. *Anat. Anz.*, 84:354–360.

180. Jacobowitz, D. (1967): Histochemical studies of the relationship of chromaffin cells and adrenergic nerve fibers to the cardiac ganglia of several species. *J. Pharmacol. Exp. Ther.*, 158:227–240.

181. Jacobs, J. M. (1977): Penetration of systemically injected horseradish peroxidase into ganglia and nerves of the autonomic nervous system. *J. Neurocytol.*, 6:607–618.

182. Jessen, K. R., and Mirsky, R. (1980): Glial cells in the enteric nervous system contain glial fibrillary acidic protein. *Nature*, 286:736–737.

183. Jessen, K. R., Mirsky, R., Dennison, M. E., and Burnstock, G. (1979): GABA may be a neurotransmitter in the vertebrate peripheral nervous system. *Nature (Lond.)*, 281:71–74.

184. Jessen, K. R., Polak, J. M., Van Noorden, S., Bloom, S. R., and Burnstock, G. (1980): Peptide-containing neurones connect the two ganglionated plexuses of the enteric nervous system. *Nature (Lond.)*, 283:391–393.

185. Johnson, S. E. (1925): Experimental degeneration of the extrinsic nerves of the small intestine in relation to the structure of the myenteric plexus. *J. Comp. Neurol.*, 38:299–314.

186. Jonas, L., and Zelch, U. (1974): The subcellular calcium distribution in the smooth muscle cells of the pig coronary artery. *Exp. Cell Res.*, 89:352–358.

187. Juorio, A. V., and Gabella, G. (1974): Noradrenaline in the guinea pig alimentary canal: regional distribution and sensitivity to denervation and reserpine. *J. Neurochem.*, 22:851–858.

188. Kaminer, B. (1969): Synthetic myosin filaments from vertebrate smooth muscle. *J. Mol. Biol.*, 39:257–274.

189. Klingman, G. I., and Klingman, J. D. (1967): Catecholamines in peripheral tissues of mice and cell counts of sympathetic ganglia after the prenatal and postnatal administration of nerve growth factor antiserum. *Int. J. Neuropharmacol.*, 6:501–508.

190. Koelle, G. B. (1951): The elimination of enzymatic diffusion artifacts in the histochemical localization of cholinesterases and a survey of their cellular distributions. *J. Pharmacol. Exp. Ther.*, 103:153–171.

191. Kosterlitz, H. W., Lydon, R. J., and Watt, A. J. (1970): The effects of adrenaline, noradrenaline and isoprenaline on inhibitory α- and β-adrenoceptors in the longitudinal muscle of the guinea-pig ileum. *Br. J. Pharmacol. Chemother.*, 39:398–413.

192. Kosterlitz, H. W., and Waterfield, A. A. (1975): In vitro models in the study of structure activity relationships of narcotic analgesics. *Annu. Rev. Pharmacol.*, 15:29–47.

193. Kreulen, D. L., and Szurszewski, J. H. (1979): Nerve pathways in celiac plexus of the guinea-pig. *Am. J. Physiol.*, 237: E90–E92.

194. Kreulen, D. L., and Szurszewski, J. H. (1979): Reflex pathways in the abdominal prevertebral ganglia: evidence for a colocolonic inhibitory reflex. *J. Physiol. (Lond.)*, 295:21–32.

195. Kuntz, A. (1938): The structural organization of the celiac ganglia. *J. Comp. Neurol.*, 69:1–12.

196. Kuntz, A. (1940): The structural organization of the inferior mesenteric ganglia. *J. Comp. Neurol.*, 72:371–382.

197. Kuntz, A., and Moseley, R. L. (1936): An experimental analysis of the pelvic autonomic ganglia in the cat. *J. Comp. Neurol.*, 64:63–75.

198. Lane, B. P., and Rhodin, J. A. G. (1964): Fine structure of the lamina muscularis mucosae. *J. Ultrastruct. Res.*, 10:489–497.

199. Langley, J. N. (1921): *The Autonomic Nervous System.* Cambridge University Press, London.

200. Langley, J. N., and Anderson, H. K. (1896): The innervation of the pelvic and adjoining viscera. V. Position of the nerve cells on the course of the efferent nerve fibres. *J. Physiol. (Lond.)*, 19:131–139.

201. Larsson, L.-I. (1977): Ultrastructural localization of a new neuronal peptide (VIP). *Histochemistry*, 54:173–176.

202. Larsson, L.-I., Fahrenkrug, J., Schaffalitzky de Muckadell, O., Sundler, F., Håkanson, R., and Rehfeld, J. F. (1976): Localization of vasoactive intestinal polypeptide (VIP) to central and peripheral neurons. *Proc. Natl. Acad. Sci. U.S.A.*, 73: 3197–3200.

203. Larsson, L.-I., and Rehfeld, J. (1979): Localization and molecular heterogeneity of cholecystokinin in the central and peripheral nervous system. *Brain Res.*, 165:201–218.

204. Lazarides, E. (1980): Intermediate filaments as mechanical integrators of cellular space. *Nature (Lond.)*, 283:249–256.

205. Lazarides, E., and Hubbard, B. D. (1976): Immunological characterization of the subunit of the 100 Å filaments from muscle cells. *Proc. Natl. Acad. Sci. U.S.A.*, 73:4344–4348.

206. Leek, B. F. (1972): Abdominal visceral receptors. In: *Handbook of Sensory Physiology, Vol. III, 1,* edited by E. Neil, pp. 113–160. Springer, Berlin.

207. Leidberg, G., Nielseu, U. C., Owman, C., and Sjöberg, N.-O. (1973): Adrenergic contribution to the abdominal vagus nerve in the cat. *Scand. J. Gastroenterol.*, 8:177.

208. Lembeck, F. (1953): Zur Frage der zentralen Übertragung afferenter Impulse. III. Das Vorkommen und die Bedeutung der Substanz P in den dorsalen Wurzeln des Rückenmarks. *Naunyn Schmiedeberg's Arch. Pharmacol.*, 219:197–213.

209. Li, P. (1937): Neve Beobachtungen über die struktur der Zirkulämuskels im Dünndarm bei Wirbeltieren. *Z. Anat. Entwickl.*, 107:212–222.

210. Linnoila, R. I., Diagustine, R. P., Miller, R. J., Chang, K. J., and Cuatrecasas, P. (1978): An immunohistological and radio-immunological study of the distribution of met[5]- and leu[5]-enkephalin in the gastrointestinal tract. *Neuroscience*, 3:1187–1196.

211. Lowy, J., Poulsen, F. R., and Vibert, P. J. (1970): Myosin filaments in vertebrate smooth muscle. *Nature (Lond.)*, 225:1053–1054.

212. Lundberg, J. M., Hökfelt, T., Schultzberg, M., Uvnäs-Wallenstein, K., Köhler, C., and Said, S. I. (1979): Occurrence of vasoactive intestinal polypeptide (VIP)-like immunoreactivity in certain cholinergic neurons of the cat: evidence from combined immunohistochemistry and acetylcholinesterase staining. *Neuroscience*, 4:1539–1559.

213. Makita, T., and Kiwaki, S. (1978): Connection of microtubules, caveolae, mitochondria and sarcoplasmic reticulum in the taenia coli of guinea-pigs. *Arch. Histol. Jpn.*, 41:167–176.

214. Malmfors, T. (1965): Studies on adrenergic nerves. The use of rat and mouse iris for direct observations on their physiology and pharmacology at cellular and subcellular levels. *Acta Physiol. Scand. [Suppl.]*, 248:1–93.

215. Manber, L., and Gershon, M. D. (1979): A reciprocal adrenergic-cholinergic axoaxonic synapse in the mammalian gut. *Am. J. Physiol.* 236:E738–E745.

216. Massazza, A. (1923): La citoarchitettonica del midollo spinale umano. *Arch. Anat. Histol. Embryol.*, 2:1–56.

217. Martinson, J., and Muren. A. (1963): Excitatory and inhibitory effects of vagus stimulation on gastric motility in the cat. *Acta Physiol. Scand.*, 57:309–316.

218. McGuffee, L. J., and Bagby, R. M. (1976): Ultrastructure, calcium accumulation, and contractile response in smooth muscle. *Am. J. Physiol.*, 230:1217–1224.

219. Merrillees, N. C. R. (1968): The nervous environment of individual smooth muscle cells of the guinea-pig vas deferens. *J. Cell Biol.*, 37:794–817.

220. Mitchell, G. A. G. (1953): *Anatomy of the Autonomic Nervous System.* Churchill Livingstone, Edinburgh.

221. Mori, J., Azuma, H., and Fujiwara, M. (1971): Adrenergic innervation and receptors in the sphincter of Oddi. *Eur. J. Pharmacol.*, 14:365–373.

222. Muggli, R., and Baumgartner, H. R. (1972): Pattern of membrane invaginations at the surface of smooth muscle cells of rabbit arteries. *Experientia*, 28:1212–1214.

223. Murphy, R. A., Herlihy, J. T., and Megerman, J. (1974): Force-generating capacity and contractile protein content of arterial smooth muscle. *J. Gen. Physiol.*, 64:691–701.

224. Muryobayashi, T., Mori, J., Fujiwara, M., and Shimamoto, K. (1968): Fluorescence histochemical demonstration of adrenergic nerve fibers in the vagus nerve of cats and dogs. *Jpn. J. Pharmacol.*, 18:285–293.

225. Nilsson, G., Larsson, L.-I., Brodin, E., Pernow, P., and Sundler, F. (1975): Localization of substance P-like immunoreactivity in mouse gut. *Histochem.*, 43:97–99.

226. Nishi, S., and North, R. A. (1973) : Intracellular recording from the myenteric plexus of the guinea-pig ileum. *J. Physiol. (Lond.)*, 231:471–491.

227. Nonomura, Y. (1976): Fine structure of myofilaments in chicken gizzard smooth muscle. In: *Recent Progress in Electron Microscopy of Cells and Tissues,* edited by E. Yamada, V. Mizuhira, K. Kurosumi, and T. Nagano, pp. 40–48. Georg Thieme, Stuttgart.

228. Nonomura, Y., and Ebashi, S. (1980): Calcium regulatory mechanism in vertebrate smooth muscle. *Biomed. Res.*, 1:1–14.

229. Norberg, K.-A. (1967): Transmitter histochemistry of the sympathetic adrenergic nervous system. *Brain Res.*, 5:125–170.

230. Norberg, K.-A., and Hamberger, B. (1964): The sympathetic adrenergic neuron. *Acta Physiol. Scand. [Suppl.]*, 238:1–42.

231. North, R. A., Henderson, G., Katayama, Y., and Johnson, S. M. (1980): Electrophysiological evidence for presynaptic inhibition of acetylcholine release by 5-hydroxytryptamine in the enteric nervous system. *Neuroscience*, 5:581–586.

232. North, R. A., Katayama, Y., and Williams, J. T. (1979): On the mechanism and site of action of enkephalin on single myenteric neurons. *Brain Res.*, 165:67–77.

233. North, R. A., and Williams, J. T. (1976): Enkephalin inhibits firing of myenteric neurones. *Nature (Lond.)*, 264:460–461.

234. Ohkubo, K. (1936): Studies on the intrinsic nervous system of the digestive tract. I. The submucous plexus of guinea-pig. *Jpn. J. Med. Sci. Anta.*, 6:1–20.

235. Ohsumi, K., Tsunekawa, K., and Fujiwara, M. (1974): Fluorescence histochemical studies on adrenergic nerve fibres in the vagus nerve of rat. In: *Amine Fluorescence Histochemistry,* edited by M. Fujiwara and C. Tanaka, pp. 000. Igaku Shoin Ltd., Tokyo.

236. Olson, L., Ålund, M., and Norberg, K. A. (1976): Fluorescence microscopical demonstration of a population of gastrointestinal nerve fibres with a selective affinity for quinacrine. *Cell Tissue Res.*, 171:407–423.

237. Orci, L., and Perrelet, A. (1973): Membrane-associated particles: increase at sites of pinocytosis demonstrated by freeze-etching. *Science,* 181:868–869.

238. Otsuka, M., Konishi, S., and Takahashi, T. (1972): *Proc. Jpn. Acad.,* 48:342–346.

239. Palay, S. L., and Chan-Palay, V. (1975): A guide to the synaptic analysis of the neuropil. *Cold Spring Harbor Symp. Quant. Biol.,* 40:1–16.

240. Paton, V. D. M., and Vizi, E. S. (1969): The inhibitory action of noradrenaline and adrenaline on acetylcholine output by guinea pig ileum longitudinal muscle strip. *Br. J. Pharmacol. Chemother.,* 35:10–28.

241. Pearse, A. G. E., and Polak, J. M. (1975): Immunocytochemical localization of substance P in mammalian gut. *Histochem.,* 41: 373–375.

242. Pease, D. C., and Molinari, S. (1960): Electron microscopy of muscular arteries; pial vessels of the cat and monkey. *J. Ultrastruct. Res.,* 3:447–468.

243. Pelletier, G., and Leclerc, R. (1979): Localization of Leu-enkephalin in dense core vesicles of axon terminals. *Neurosci. Lett.,* 12:159–163.

244. Peracchia, C. (1977): Gap junctions. Structural change after uncoupling procedures. *J. Cell Biol.,* 72:628–641.

245. Peracchia, C. (1978): Calcium effects on gap junction structure and cell coupling. *Nature (Lond.),* 271:669–671.

246. Peracchia, C. (1980): Structural correlates of gap junction permeation. *Int. Rev. Cytol.,* 66:81–146.

247. Pickel, V. M., Joh, T. H., Reis, D. J., Leeman, S. E., and Miller, R. J. (1979): Electron microscopic localization of substance P and enkephalin in axon terminals related to dendrites of catecholaminergic neurons. *Brain Res.,* 160:387–400.

248. Polak, J. M., Bloom, S. R., Sullivan, S. N., Facer, P., and Pearse, A. G. E. (1977): Enkephalin-like immunoreactivity in the human gastrointestinal tract. *Lancet,* 1:972–974.

249. Politoff, A. L., Rose, S., and Pappas, G. D. (1974): The calcium binding sites of synaptic vesicles of the frog neuromuscular junctions. *J. Cell Biol.,* 61:818–823.

250. Pollard, T. D., and Weihing, R. R. (1974): Actin and myosin and cell movement. *CRC Crit. Rev. Biochem.,* 2:1–65.

251. Popescu, L. M., and Diculescu, I. (1975): Calcium in smooth muscle sarcoplasmic reticulum *in situ. J. Cell Biol.,* 67:911–918.

252. Popescu, L. M., Diculescu, I., Zelek, U., and Ionescu, N. (1974): Ultrastructural distribution of calcium in smooth muscle cells of guinea-pig taenia coli. *Cell Tissue Res.,* 154:357–378.

253. Prescott, L., and Brightman, M. W. (1976): The sarcolemma of *Aplysia* smooth muscle in freeze-fracture preparations. *Tissue Cell,* 8:158–241.

254. Prosser, C. L., Burnstock, G., and Kahn, J. (1960): Conduction in smooth muscle: comparative structural properties. *Am. J. Physiol.,* 199:545–552.

255. Raeymaekers, L., Wuytack, F., Batra, S., and Casteels, R. (1977): A comparative study of the calcium accumulation by mitochondria and microsomes isolated from the smooth muscle of the guinea-pig taenia coli. *Pflügers Arch.,* 368:217–223.

256. Rash, J. E., Biesele, J. J., and Grey, G. O. (1970): Three classes of filaments in cardiac differentiation. *J. Ultrastructr. Res.,* 33:408–435.

257. Rattan, S., Said, S. I., and Goyal, R. K. (1977): Effect of vasoactive intestinal polypeptide (VIP) on the lower esophageal sphincter pressure (LESP). *Proc. Soc. Exp. Biol. Med.,* 155:40–43.

258. Read, J. B., and Burnstock, G. (1968): Comparative histochemical studies of adrenergic nerves in the enteric plexuses of vertebrate large intestine. *Comp. Biochem. Physiol.,* 27:505–517.

259. Rice, R. V., Moses, J. A., McManus, G. M., Brady, A. C., and Blasik, L. M. (1970): The organization of contractile filaments in a mammalian smooth muscle. *J. Cell Biol.,* 47:183–197.

260. Richardson, K. C. (1958): Electron microscopic observations on Auerbach's plexus in the rabbit with special reference to the problem of smooth muscle innervation. *Am. J. Anat.,* 103:99–136.

261. Rintoul, J. R. (1960): Comparative morphology of the enteric nerve plexuses. M. D. Thesis, University of St. Andrews, St. Andrews, Fife, Scotland.

262. Robinson, P. M., McLean, J. R., and Burnstock, F. (1971): Ultrastructural identification of non-adrenergic inhibitory nerve fibers. *J. Pharmacol. Exp. Ther.,* 179:149–160.

263. Robinson, R. G., and Gershon, M. D. (1971): Synthesis and uptake of 5-hydroxytryptamine by the myenteric plexus of the guinea-pig ileum: a histochemical study. *J. Pharmacol. Exp. Ther.,* 178:311–324.

264. Rogers, D. C., and Burnstock, G. (1966): The interstitial cell and its place in the concept of the autonomic ground plexus. *J. Comp. Neurol.,* 126:255–284.

265. Rosenbluth, J. (1965): Smooth muscle: an ultrastructural basis for the dynamics of its contraction. *Science,* 184:1337–1339.

266. Rosenbluth, J. (1967): Obliquely striated muscle. III. Contraction mechanism of *Ascaris* body muscle. *J. Cell Biol.,* 34:15–33.

267. Ross, J. G. (1957): On the presence of centripetal fibres in the superior mesenteric nerves of the rabbit. *J. Anat.,* 92:189–197.

268. Ross, R., and Klebanoff, S. J. (1971): The smooth muscle cell. I. In vivo synthesis of connective tissue proteins. *J. Cell Biol.,* 50:159–171.

269. Rothman, T. P., Ross, L. L., and Gershon, M. D. (1976): Separately developing axonal uptake of 5-hydroxytryptamine and norepinephrine in the fetal ileum of the rabbit. *Brain Res.,* 115:437–456.

270. Said, S. I., and Mutt, V. (1970): Polypeptide with broad biological activity. Isolation from small intestine. *Science,* 169:1217–1218.

271. Sauer, M. E., and Rumble, C. T. (1946): The number of nerve cells in the myenteric and submucous plexuses of the small intestine of the cat. *Anat. Rec.,* 96:373–381.

272. Schnitzlein, H. N., Rowe, L. C., and Hoffman, H. H. (1958): The myelinated compound of the vagus nerves in man. *Anat. Rec.,* 131:649–667.

273. Schofield, G. C. (1962): Experimental studies on the myenteric plexus in mammals. *J. Comp. Neurol.,* 119:159–184.

274. Schofield, G. C. (1968): Anatomy of muscular and neural tissues in the alimentary canal. In: *Handbook of Physiology, Section 6, Vol. IV,* pp. 1579–1627. American Physiological Society, Washington, D.C.

275. Schollmeyer, J. E., Furcht, L. T., Goll, D. E., Robson, R. M., and Stromer, M. H. (1976): Localization of contractile proteins in smooth muscle cells and in normal and transformed fibroblasts. In: *Cell Motility,* edited by R. Goldman, T. Pollard, and J. Rosenbaum, pp. 361–388. Cold Spring Harbor Laboratory, Cold Spring Harbor, N.Y.

276. Schultzberg, M., Dreyfus, C. F., Gershon, M. D., Hökfelt, T., Elde, R., Nilsson, G., Said, S., and Goldstein, M. (1978): VIP; enkephalin- substance P-, and somatostatin-like immunoreactivity in neurons intrinsic to the intestine: immunohistochemical evidence from organotypic tissue cultures. *Brain Res.,* 155:239–248.

277. Schultzberg, M., Hökfelt, T., Nilsson, G., Terenius, L., Rehfeld, J. F., Brown, M., Elde, R., Goldstein, M., and Said, S. (1980): Distribution of peptide- and catecholamine-containing neurons in the gastro-intestinal tract of rat and guinea-pig: immunohistochemical studies with antisera to substance P, vasoactive intestinal polypeptide, enkephalins, somatostatin, gastrin/cholecystokinin, neurotensin and dopamine-β-hydroxylase. *Neuroscience,* 5:689–744.

278. Schultzberg, M., Hökfelt, T., Terenius, L., Elfvin, L.-G., Lundberg, J. M., Brandt, J., Elde, R. P., and Goldstein, M. (1979): Enkephalin immunoreactive nerve fibres and cell bodies in sympathetic ganglia of the guinea-pig and rat. *Neuroscience,* 4:249–270.

279. Shoenberg, C. F., and Haselgrove, J. C. (1974): Filaments and ribbons in vertebrate smooth muscle. *Nature (Lond.),* 249: 152–154.

280. Silva, D. G. (1971): The fine structure and innervation of the inner circular muscle layer of the cat. *Anat. Rec.,* 169:428 (abstr.).

281. Silva, D. G., Ross, G., and Osborne, L. W. (1971): Adrenergic innervation of the ileum of the cat. *Am. J. Physiol.,* 220: 347–352.

282. Small, J. V. (1974): Contractile units in vertebrate smooth muscle cells. *Nature (Lond.),* 249:325–327.

283. Small, J. V. (1977): Studies on isolated smooth muscle cells: the contractile apparatus. *J. Cell Sci.,* 24:327–349.

284. Small, J. V., and Sobieszek, A. (1977): Studies on the function and composition of the 10 nm (100 Å) filaments of vertebrate smooth muscle. *J. Cell Sci.,* 23:243-268.

285. Small, J. V., and Squire, J. M. (1972): Structural basis of contraction in vertebrate smooth muscle. *J. Mol. Biol.,* 67:117-149.

286. Sobieszek, A. (1972): Cross bridges on self-assembled smooth muscle myosin filaments. *J. Mol. Biol.,* 70:741-744.

287. Sobieszek, A. (1977): Vertebrate smooth muscle myosin. Enzymatic and structural properties. In: *The Biochemistry of Smooth Muscle,* edited by N. L. Stephens, pp. 413-443. University Park Press, Baltimore.

288. Sobieszek, A., and Small, J. V. (1972): Filaments from purified smooth muscle myosin. *Cold Spring Harbor Symp. Quant. Biol.,* 37:109-112.

289. Somlyo, A. V. (1980): Ultrastructure of vascular smooth muscle. In: *Handbook of Physiology, Section 2, Vol. II,* pp. 33-67. American Physiological Society, Washington, D.C.

290. Somlyo, A. V., Ashton, F. T., Lemanski, L., Vallieres, J., and Somlyo, A. P. (1977): Filament organization and dense bodies in vertebrate smooth muscle. In: *Biochemistry of Smooth Muscle,* edited by N. L. Stephens, pp. 445-471. University Park Press, Baltimore.

291. Somlyo, A. P., Devine, C. E., Somlyo, A. V., and North, S. R. (1971): Sarcoplasmic reticulum and the temperature-dependent contraction of smooth muscle in calcium-free solutions. *J. Cell Biol.,* 51:722-741.

292. Somlyo, A. P., Devine, C. E., Somlyo, A. V., and Rice, R. V. (1973): Filament organization in vertebrate smooth muscle. *Philos. Trans. R. Soc. Lond. [Biol.],* 265:223-229.

293. Somlyo, A. V., and Somlyo, A. P. (1971): Strontium accumulation by sarcoplasmic reticulum and mitochondria in vascular smooth muscle. *Science,* 174:955-958.

294. Somlyo, A. P., and Somlyo, A. V. (1975): Ultrastructure of smooth muscle. In: *Methods in Pharmacology,* edited by E. E. Daniel and D. M. Paton, pp. 3-43. Plenum, New York.

295. Somlyo, A. P., Somlyo, A. V., Ashton, F. T., and Valliéres, J. (1976): Vertebrate smooth muscle: ultrastructure and function. In: *Cell Motility,* edited by R. Goldman, T. Pollard, and J. Rosenbaum, pp. 165-183. Cold Spring Harbor Laboratory, Cold Spring Harbor, N.Y.

296. Somlyo, A. P., Somlyo, A. V., and Shuman, H. (1979): Electron probe analysis of vascular smooth muscle. *J. Cell Biol.,* 81:316-335.

297. Somlyo, A. P., Somlyo, A. V., Devine, C. E., Peters, P. D., and Hall, T. A. (1974): Electron microscopy and electron probe analysis of mitochondrial calcium accumulation in smooth muscle. *J. Cell Biol.,* 61:723-742.

298. Sommer, J. R., and Johnson, E. A. (1968): Cardiac muscle. A comparative study of Purkinje fibers and ventricular fibers. *J. Cell Biol.,* 36:497-526.

299. Stach, W. (1976): Afferente Nervenendigungen im Dünndarm und Magen. Licht- und electronenmikropische Untersuchungen. *Z. Mikrosk. Anat. Forsch.,* 90:790-800.

300. Stach, W. (1977): Neuronstruktur und -architektur im Plexus submucosus externus (Schabadasch) des Duodenums. *Verh. Anat. Ges.,* 71:867-871.

301. Stach, W. (1978): Die Gefässversorgung des Plexus myentericus (Auerbach) in Dünndarm von Schwein und Katze. *Acta Anat. (Basel),* 100:161-169.

302. Staehelin, L. A. (1974): Structure and function of intercellular junctions. *Int. Rev. Cytol.,* 39:191-283.

303. Steinert, P. M., Idler, W. W., and Zimmerman, S. B. (1976): Self-assembly of bovine epidermal keratin filaments *in vitro. J. Mol. Biol.,* 108:547-567.

304. Stephens, N. L., Mitchell, R. W., and Kroeger, E. A. (1977): Smooth muscle biochemistry and hypoxia. In: *The Biochemistry of Smooth Muscle,* edited by N. L. Stephens, pp. 679-701. University Park Press, Baltimore.

305. Sundler, F., Håkanson, R., Larsson, L. I., Brodin, E., and Nilsson, G. (1977): Substance P in the gut: an immunochemical and immunohistochemical study of its distribution and development. In: *Substance P,* edited by U.S. von Euler and B. Pernow, pp. 59-65. Raven Press, New York.

306. Takayanagi, I., Sato, T., and Takari, K. (1977): Effects of sympathetic nerve stimulation on electrical activity of Auerbach's plexus and intestinal smooth muscle tone. *J. Pharm. Pharmacol.,* 29:376-377.

307. Taxi, J. (1965): Contribution a l'étude des connexions des neurones moteurs du systéme nerveux autonome. *Ann. Sci. Nat. Zool.,* 7:413-674.

308. Taxi, J. (1979): The chromaffin and chromaffin-like cells in the autonomic nervous system. *Int. Rev. Cytol.,* 57:283-343.

309. Taxi, J., and Droz, B. (1969): Radioautographic study of the accumulation of some biogenic amines in the autonomic nervous system. In: *Cellular Dynamics of the Neurons,* edited by S. H. Barondes, pp. 175-190. Academic Press, New York.

310. Taylor, A. B., Kreulen, D., and Prosser, C. L. (1977): Electron microscopy of the connective tissue between longitudinal and circular muscle of the small intestine of cat. *Am. J. Anat.,* 150:427-442.

311. Tregear, R. T., and Squire, J. M. (1973): Myosin content and filament structure in smooth and striated muscle. *J. Mol. Biol.,* 77:279-290.

312. Uehara, Y., Campbell, G. R., and Burnstock, G. (1971): Cytoplasmic filaments in developing and adult vertebrate smooth muscle. *J. Cell Biol.,* 50:484-497.

313. Ungváry, Gy., and Léránth, Cs. (1970): Termination in the prevertebral abdominal sympathetic ganglia of axons arising from the local (terminal) vegetative plexus of visceral organs. *Z. Zellforsch.,* 110:185-191.

314. Unwin, P. N. T., and Zampighi, G. (1980): Structure of the junction between communicating cells. *Nature (Lond.),* 283:545-549.

315. Valliéres, J., Scarpa, A., and Somlyo, A. P. (1975): Subcellular fractions of smooth muscle. Isolation, substrate utilization and Ca^{2+} transport by main pulmonary artery and mesenteric vein mitochondria. *Arch. Biochem. Biophys.,* 170:659-669.

316. Watson, A. H. D. (1979): Fluorescent histochemistry of the teleost gut: evidence for the presence of serotonergic neurones. *Cell Tissue Res.,* 197:155-164.

317. Wells, G. S., and Wolowyk, M. K. (1971): Freeze-etch observations on membrane structure in the smooth muscle of guinea-pig taenia coli. *J. Physiol. (Lond.),* 218:11-13P.

318. Welsh, J. H., and Hyde, J. E. (1944): Acetylcholine content of the myenteric plexus and resistance to anoxia. *Proc. Soc. Exp. Biol. Med.,* 55:256-257.

319. Westfall, D. P., Lee, T. J.-F., and Stitzel, R. E. (1975): Morphological and biochemical changes in supersensitive smooth muscle. *Fed. Proc.,* 34:1985-1989.

320. Widdicombe, J. G. (1974): Enteroceptors. In: *The Peripheral Nervous System,* edited by J. I. Hubbard, pp. 455-485. Plenum, New York.

321. Williams, J. T., and North, R. A. (1978): Inhibition of firing of myenteric neurons by somatostatin. *Brain Res.,* 155:165-168.

322. Wood, J. D., and Mayer, C. J. (1979): Serotonergic activation of tonic-type enteric neurons in guinea pig small bowel. *J. Neurophysiol.,* 42:582-593.

323. Yamamoto, M. (1977): Electron microscopic studies on the innervation of the smooth muscle and the interstitial cell of cajal in the small intestine of the mouse and bat. *Arch. Histol. Jpn.,* 40:171-201.

324. Zelch, U., Jonas, L., and Wiegershausen, B. (1972): Ultrahistochemischer Nachweiss von Calcium in glatten Muskelzellen der Arteria coronaria sinistra des Schweins. *Acta Histochem. (Jena),* 44:180-182.

Physiology of the Gastrointestinal Tract, edited by
Leonard R. Johnson. Raven Press, New York © 1981.

Chapter 7

Biochemistry of the Contractile Process in Smooth Muscle

David J. Hartshorne

The aim of this chapter is to outline the basic biochemistry of the contractile process. Not enough data are available to restrict the discussion to visceral muscle, and information obtained from several different smooth muscles will be considered. Although there are obviously some differences between different muscle tissues, this generalization is justified since in terms of the biochemistry of the contractile proteins there appears to be a reasonable degree of uniformity. Frequently, especially in the earlier phases of smooth muscle biochemistry, there was a tendency to use skeletal muscle as a model since this system is better understood. It is often useful to use a comparative approach, and in many instances I have tried to indicate the major biochemical differences that exist between the two muscle types.

It is established for all muscle types that an increase in the intracellular concentration of Ca^{2+} initiates contraction. The major emphasis of this review will be concerned with the effects of Ca^{2+} on the contractile apparatus. This will involve a prior description of the properties of the contractile proteins. A brief discussion on the sarcoplasmic reticulum will also be presented. However, the mechanism and initial consequences of excitation are beyond the scope of this review, and the reader is referred to other chapters in this volume. Another feature that is dealt with in only a cursory fashion is smooth muscle ultrastructure, and here reviews by Somlyo (184) and Gabella, Chapter 6, *(this volume)* offer more detailed presentations.

CONTROL OF INTRACELLULAR Ca^{2+} CONCENTRATION—ROLE OF THE SARCOPLASMIC RETICULUM

Following excitation, the concentration of intracellular Ca^{2+} rises to between 1 and 10 μM which then promotes contraction. The structures that are primarily responsible for the regulation of the Ca^{2+} level within the cell are the sarcoplasmic reticulum and the plasma membrane. It is thought that the action potential probably represents some influx of Ca^{2+} (15), and the question that remains to be answered for each smooth muscle is how much of the activating Ca^{2+} enters during the action potential and how much is released from intracellular sites, primarily the sarcoplasmic reticulum. To evaluate this requires a knowledge of the extent of Ca^{2+} binding to the total available intracellular sites, e.g., calmodulin and myosin, and this is not known with any accuracy. However, the concensus of opinion is that many smooth muscles contain a sarcoplasmic reticulum which functions in an analogous manner to that in skeletal muscle, i.e., it acts as an intracellular Ca^{2+} sink. It has been shown (184) that the volume of sarcoplasmic reticulum varies in different smooth muscles and that this is correlated to the contractile response in Ca^{2+}-free media (102). The larger volume of sarcoplasmic reticulum was found in the more tonic smooth muscles, e.g., rabbit main pulmonary artery, and the smaller volume was observed in some phasic muscle, e.g., taenia coli. It was pointed out, however, that the volume of sarcoplasmic reticulum may also be a reflection of other functions associated with this organelle, such as synthesis of extracellular proteins. In this context, it should be mentioned that the smooth and rough portions of the reticulum are continuous (184).

Several studies have been undertaken to determine by electron microscopy the localization of Ca^{2+} in smooth muscle. Sr^{2+} (used as a Ca^{2+} analogue) was detected in mitochondria and sarcoplasmic reticulum of vascular smooth muscle by electron microscopy and electron probe analysis (186,187). In other studies, Ca^{2+} was localized in the sarcoplasmic reticulum of mouse intestinal muscle (84); in mitochondria, sarcoplasmic reticulum, and at the plasma membrane of thoracic aorta (39); and at the plasma membrane and sarcoplasmic reticulum of guinea pig taenia coli (195). Thus there is considerable evidence to indicate that the sarcoplasmic reticulum of smooth muscle can accumulate Ca^{2+} and thereby act as a Ca^{2+} sink as it does in skeletal muscle. There is also evidence that mitochondria accumulate various cations and thus could be involved in the regulation of the intracellular Ca^{2+} concentration. However, this seems unlikely for the following reasons: the K_m for respiratory-driven Ca^{2+} uptake is quite high (17 μM) relative to the concentrations of Ca^{2+} expected to induce contraction, and it was found (188) that following a K^+ contracture there was no evidence of mitochondrial Ca^{2+} sequestration. It seems likely therefore that the observed uptake of cations by mitochondria was artifactual and was probably the result of cell damage (188).

The sarcoplasmic reticulum is located centrally within the cell and is also frequently found immediately beneath the plasma membrane where the gap between the two membranes (10 to 12 nm) is transversed by electron-opaque connections. It is thought that this surface coupling, which is similar in appearance to the junctional sarcoplasmic reticulum of cardiac and skeletal muscle, might be involved in the release of Ca^{2+} from the sarcoplasmic reticulum following an action potential (184). In many instances, the sarcoplasmic reticulum is also in close association with surface vesicles (see Fig. 2) or caveolae (65) and often forms a fenestrated network surrounding the vesicles (184). The caveolae are flask-shaped invaginations of the cell membrane (see Fig. 2) between 50 and 80 nm in diameter and are found in several cell types in addition to smooth muscle. There is evidence that they are not randomly distributed in smooth muscle but tend toward a longitudinal orientation (184). The caveolae appear to be analogous to the T-tubule system of striated muscle cells (59), although presumably they would not be required to serve an identical function since the smooth muscle cell is relatively small and the rapid transmission of the depolarization wave does not present a problem.

The isolation of a membrane fraction representative of the sarcoplasmic reticulum has been attempted by several investigators (see review 15). In general, these studies are hampered by the difficulty in preparing homogeneous membrane fractions; but it is clear that a microsomal fraction can be obtained which demonstrates ATP-dependent Ca^{2+} uptake. It was calculated for the membranous fraction obtained from bovine vascular smooth muscle that this had the capability or capacity to act as both a sink and a source for the activating Ca^{2+} (60). Thus the evidence in support of a functional sarcoplasmic reticulum in smooth muscle is supported by both morphological and biochemical studies.

The mechanism of Ca^{2+} release from the sarcoplasmic reticulum is not established for either the smooth muscle or skeletal muscle system. In smooth muscle, it is possible that Ca^{2+} entering during the action potential releases Ca^{2+} from the sarcoplasmic reticulum (15). It has also been suggested that Ca^{2+} is released from intracellular sites following excitation with acetylcholine, norepinephrine, and angiotensin (15). These agents are capable of initiating contraction in the absence of external Ca^{2+} or in the presence of La^{3+}, which is thought to block transmembrane Ca^{2+} transport.

Many of the details concerning the functioning of the sarcoplasmic reticulum are obviously missing, but it is reasonable at this stage to assume that the sarcoplasmic reticulum serves to control, at least partially, the level of Ca^{2+} in the cell which is available to the contractile proteins. Once the concentration of Ca^{2+} increases above a threshold level, the contractile system is activated, and this will be discussed in more detail in subsequent sections. It is interesting that in isolated toad stomach smooth muscle cells, the increase in intracellular concentration of Ca^{2+} following stimulation precedes by a wide margin the development of tension (56). This suggests that Ca^{2+} release is relatively rapid and that the rate-limiting step for contraction is probably associated with the contractile apparatus.

CONTRACTILE APPARATUS

The protein components of the cell that respond to the increase of Ca^{2+} and utilize the chemical energy of ATP to produce shortening and/or the development of tension are termed collectively the contractile apparatus. This includes the major contractile proteins—myosin, actin, and tropomyosin—and also the proteins that are involved in the Ca^{2+}—dependent regulation of contractile activity. For the sake of convenience and hopefully clarity, the following more detailed discussion of the contractile apparatus of smooth muscle will be considered under several categories.

Content of Contractile Proteins

This section deals primarily with the amount of myosin, actin, and tropomyosin in smooth muscle. These values are necessary as a basis for the correlation of some of the data derived from biochemical and physiological studies, plus they are useful from a practical point of view when attempting to isolate or localize the various contractile proteins. It has been known for many years since the pioneering studies of Csapo (31) and Needham and Cawkwell (146) that smooth muscles contain actomyosin, and the general impression from these and other studies was that the content of actomyosin was less than that in skeletal muscle. A qualitative difference was also observed as it was found that smooth muscle actomyosin could be extracted at low ionic strength (95,112), in contrast to the requirement of high ionic strength for skeletal and cardiac muscle. This led to the term "tonoactomyosin" (72,114) to imply a different type of actomyosin that was thought to be involved in tonic contractions (113). The existence of a specialized form of actomyosin is no longer accepted (160), and the reason for the solubility of the actomyosin at low ionic strength is not fully understood. It seems to be a general property and has been shown for many different smooth muscles. A factor that could be involved is the high content of actin that exists in all smooth muscles.

The advent of sodium dodecylsulfate (SDS) electrophoresis has greatly facilitated the analytical determinations, and to a large extent the figures that are accepted today are derived using this technique. Shown in Table 1 are the cellular contents of myosin, actin, and tropomyosin for several smooth muscles. For comparative purposes representative values for these proteins in skeletal muscle are approximately: myosin 62, actin 22, tropomyosin 5, each given as mg/g cell weight. It is clear from Table 1 that the amount of myosin in smooth muscle is considerably lower than in skeletal muscle, and the amount of actin in smooth muscle tends to be higher. However, it was found that smooth muscle can be divided roughly into two groups, one group being arterial, which contains more actin than the second group, nonarterial (25). It appears that arterial smooth muscle develops more force than most other smooth muscles, and it is possible that this could be due, in part, to the higher actin content (140). If these values are expressed as molar ratios (the assumed molecular weights are 470,000, 42,000, and 68,000 daltons for myosin, actin, and tropomyosin, respectively) relative to myosin, for the arterial myosin there are approximately 28 molecules of actin and 5 molecules of tropomyosin for each myosin molecule, and for the nonarterial muscles the values are 16:3:1, respectively. When compared to the molar ratios obtained from skel-

TABLE 1. *Cellular myosin content, actin/myosin weight ratios and actin/tropomyosin weight ratios of various porcine smooth muscles*

| | Cellular protein contents | | | Weight ratios | |
Tissue	Myosin[a]	Actin (mg/g cell wet wt)	Tropomyosin	Actin/myosin	Actin/tropomyosin
Arterial					
Carotid	19.8 ± 3.3	48.5 ± 6.1	13.5 ± 1.8	2.6 ± 0.3	3.5 ± 0.2
Aorta (thoracic)	18.3 ± 1.2	40.9 ± 3.6	12.5 ± 1.9	2.3 ± 0.3	3.7 ± 0.6
Coronary (left anterior descending)	20.6 ± 3.4	60.6 ± 11.9	16.0 ± 2.6	2.9 ± 0.1	3.4 ± 0.3
Nonarterial					
Esophagus	22.1 ± 4.9	30.4 ± 5.4	7.7 ± 1.4	1.5 ± 0.1	4.2 ± 0.3
Trachea	16.7 ± 2.5	25.1 ± 4.4	7.2 ± 1.2	1.5 ± 0.1	3.5 ± 0.2
Intestine					
Circular	19.4 ± 1.5	29.0 ± 4.4	7.8 ± 1.2	1.6 ± 0.2	3.8 ± 0.3
Longitudinal	16.8 ± 2.2	29.2 ± 2.8	7.4 ± 0.9	1.7 ± 0.1	4.0 ± 0.2
Uterus	22.5 ± 2.7	23.9 ± 2.9	8.1 ± 2.0	1.1 ± 0.1	3.5 ± 0.5
Means					
Arterial	19.6 ± 0.7	50.0 ± 4.7	14.0 ± 1.2	2.6 ± 0.2	3.5 ± 0.1
Nonarterial	19.5 ± 1.3	27.5 ± 1.8[b]	7.7 ± 0.6[b]	1.5 ± 0.1[b]	3.8 ± 0.1

[a]Calculated by multiplying the myosin heavy chain estimates by 1.9 to correct for light chain weights.
[b]Significantly different ($p < 0.05$) from the mean of arterial tissues.
Table taken from Cohen and Murphy (25).

etal muscle—4 actins: 0.6 tropomyosin: 1 myosin—it is obvious that a considerable excess of actin exists in smooth muscle. If it is assumed that the density of the smooth muscle is unity, then the concentrations of myosin, actin, and tropomyosin for arterial and non-arterial muscles are approximately: 0.04 mM, 1.2mM, 0.2mM and 0.04 mM, 0.66 mM and 0.11 mM, respectively. The corresponding concentrations of myosin, actin, and tropomyosin in skeletal muscle are approximately: 0.13 mM, 0.5 mM, and 0.07 mM, respectively. In general, the higher content of actin relative to myosin in smooth muscle is reflected by the number of thin (actin) and thick (myosin) filaments (see section Intracellular Filaments).

The figures presented in Table 1 can also be applied to clarify the situation with respect to tropomyosin. The concentration of tropomyosin in smooth muscle is higher than in skeletal muscle, and this has been known for many years; however, tropomyosin plus actin should be considered. The molar ratio of actin to tropomyosin for both skeletal and smooth muscle is between 6–7 to 1. It has been established from many studies with the skeletal muscle system that this is the stoichiometry found in thin filaments, and it is reasonable to assume that all of the tropomyosin in smooth muscle is bound to F-actin and is localized with the thin filaments. There is no justification, therefore, to regard the tropomyosin content of smooth muscle as anomalously high, and the high concentration of tropomyosin is merely a consequence of the higher actin content. It was suggested (181) that tropomyosin forms the core of thick filaments, and based on this discussion this is unlikely.

The proteins myosin, actin, and tropomyosin form the major constituents of the contractile apparatus, but there are minor components necessary for the normal functioning of the actomyosin system, particularly those involved in the regulatory mechanism, and these should be included in the above tabulation. However, a complete itemization is not available and the concentration of only one additional protein, calmodulin (see section on Regulation) has been calculated. It was found (69) that the amount of calmodulin in rabbit uterus represented 0.42% of the total protein. Assuming that the total protein contributes 15% of the wet weight of the cell, the content of calmodulin would be 0.63 mg/g wet weight, and using the same assumptions as above and a molecular weight of 17,000 daltons, the concentration would be approximately 0.037 mM. It is known, however, that calmodulin is implicated in many enzymic mechanisms (24), and only a fraction of the total calmodulin would be expected to be associated with the contractile apparatus.

Properties of the Contractile Proteins

Most of the following discussion will be concerned with the proteins myosin, actin, and tropomyosin.

These three proteins constitute the bulk of the contractile apparatus, but other proteins are required for normal functioning. These are the regulatory components which will be dealt with in a separate section (Regulation). For a more comprehensive treatment than is presented here, see Hartshorne and Gorecka (76). Many of the properties of the major contractile proteins together with some properties of other muscle components for smooth and skeletal muscle are summarized in Table 2. It is hoped that this table will be useful for comparative purposes and will also serve as a rapid source of reference.

Myosin

Physical properties. In general, the techniques which were developed for the isolation of skeletal muscle myosin are not adequate for the isolation of homogeneous myosin from smooth muscle sources. The most common problem is the removal of actin, since the actomyosin of smooth muscle is more resistant to dissociation. However, methods have been developed, some adapted from the skeletal muscle procedures, and myosin has been isolated from a wide variety of smooth muscles (76). The physical parameters of smooth muscle myosin are quite similar to those of skeletal and cardiac muscle myosins, although clearly the different myosins associated with each muscle type are quite distinct. These distinctions are apparent with respect to the amino acid compositions (143), ATPase characteristics (see later), subunit composition (see later), and several other features [reviewed by Murphy and Megerman (143)].

The molecular weight of the myosin molecule is about 470,000 daltons. The molecule is composed of two large identical subunits of about 200,000 daltons each, and four smaller subunits: two of about 17,000 daltons each and two of about 20,000 daltons. The two large subunits interact to form an extensive region of a coiled-coil α-helix which directs the molecule into a rod-like shape. At the N-terminal region of the molecule the coiled-coil interaction is changed into a more globular conformation, and it is here that the smaller subunits, the myosin light chains, are associated. This is also the part of the molecule that possesses the enzymatic and actin-binding sites. This is depicted diagrammatically in Fig. 1. Part of the α-helical portion of the myosin molecule, the "tail" region, interacts with others to form the body of the thick filament. The globular head regions of the molecules protrude from the thick filament and constitute the cross-bridges, which are the sites for ATP hydrolysis and tension development. For skeletal muscle myosin it is thought that the cross-bridges originate at a more flexible part of the α-helical region, and this is often referred to as the hinge region. Whether or not a similar situation exists with smooth muscle myosin is not known, although in this context it is interesting that

TABLE 2. *Summary of the contractile apparatus of smooth and skeletal muscles*

	Smooth muscle		Skeletal muscle
Myosin			
Location	Thick filaments		Thick filaments
Subunits	200,000 (2)	Heavy chains	200,000(2)
	200,000 (2) ⎱	Lights chains	⎰ 18,000 (2)
	17,000 (2) ⎰		⎱ 25,000 (2) or 16,000 (2)
Concentration			
mg/g cell	20		62
Approx. molarity	0.04		0.13
Ca^{2+}-ATPase activity	∼60 (low ionic strength)		∼800 (no increase at high ionic strength)
(nmoles P_i/min/mg myosin)	∼250 (high ionic strength)		
Mg^{2+}-ATPase activity	∼2		∼2
(nmoles P_i/min/mg myosin)	Activation by actin requires additional factors		Activation by actin to ∼850; no additional factors required
Actin			
Location	Thin filaments		Thin filaments
Molecular weight	42,000		42,000
Concentration			
mg/g cell	50 (arterial): 28 (nonarterial)		22
Approx. molarity	1.2	0.7	0.5
Isoelectric variant	γ		α
Tropomyosin			
Location	Thin filaments		Thin filaments
Subunits	33,000 (2)		33,000 (2)
	Precise M.W. not established		α and β isomers
	Isomeric forms not established		
Regulatory system	Myosin light chain kinase plus Myosin light chain phosphatase Myosin-linked or leiotonin A and C Actin-linked		Troponin plus tropomyosin on thin filaments
Other components			
α-Actinin: subunits	100,000 (2)		100,000 (2)
Location	Dense bodies		Z-lines

Frederiksen (64) found that aorta myosin is less flexible than its skeletal counterpart, and thus may not possess an easily recognized hinge region.

The head region of the molecule contains the ATPase sites, and in this general area the myosin light chains are located. The exact function of the light chains is not known, although they are implicated in some way in the normal functioning of myosin since their removal results in a complete loss of ATPase activity. For smooth muscle myosin and also for myosins from several non-muscle sources, the larger of the two light chains are involved in the Ca^{2+}-dependent regulation of activity, and this will be discussed in more detail in the Regulation section of these volumes. If one compares myosins from several muscle and non-muscle sources, it is evident that the light chain composition is, to a degree, characteristic of the muscle type. In myosin from white skeletal muscle three classes of light chains are seen, with molecular weights of 16,000, 18,000, and 25,000 (207). Each myosin contains two of the 18,000 light chains, and two of either of the other two classes (121, 208). Myosins from slow (red) skeletal and cardiac muscle contain predominantly two classes of light chains, of approximately 20,000 and 27,000 M.W. (122). The myosins of smooth muscle and nonmuscle sources contain two light chains of 20,000 M.W. and two light chains of 17,000 M.W. (43,107,117,135,158,179,180, 204,214). Recently it was found that several of the heavy chain components of skeletal muscle myosin are heterogeneous (38,89,161), although this has not been ob-

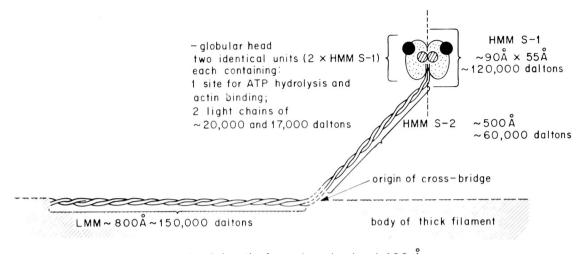

FIG. 1. Diagrammatic representation of the myosin molecule. The coiled-coil α-helical portion of the molecule is depicted as a rope-like structure. At the origin of the cross-bridge, i.e., at one end of the heavy meromyosin subfragment 2 (HMM S-2) molecule, it is not known whether the α-helical structure is retained *(dashed line)*. The position of the 4 light chains is arbitrary, although it is known that they are located in the globular head region, which is composed essentially of two heavy meromyosin subfragment 1 (HMM S-1) molecules. The body of the thick filament is formed from the aggregation of the tail region of the myosin molecules, i.e., light meromyosin (LMM). Figure taken from Hartshorne and Gorecka (76).

served for smooth muscle myosin. The immunochemical distinction between skeletal and smooth muscle myosins has been known for several years (76). It is clear, therefore, that myosin exists in several isoenzymic forms, although the subunit composition (i.e., two heavy chains and 2 × 2 light chains) and overall geometry of each myosin type are similar.

Proteolytic fragments. Much of our knowledge about the geometry and functioning of the myosin molecule was derived from studies using controlled proteolytic degradation. Myosin can be hydrolyzed with trypsin into two major fragments representing the tail portion of the molecule and the head portion of the molecule. These are referred to as light meromyosin (LMM) and heavy meromyosin (HMM), respectively. This cleavage is shown in Fig. 1. The site of cleavage into the LMM and HMM portions approximates a division of the myosin molecule into that region which is involved in the formation of the body of the thick filament (LMM) and that part of the molecule which forms the cross-bridge (HMM). The cross-bridge originates at what is frequently called the hinge region, and although there is little chemical evidence to support this nomenclature, it is interesting that molecules of skeletal muscle myosin examined by electron microscopy frequently showed a sharp bend at a site which is consistent with the expected LMM-HMM cleavage site (52). At low ionic strength, LMM is insoluble and aggregates to form paracrystalline arrays, HMM on the other hand is soluble and retains the biological proportion of the parent molecule. By using different conditions of proteolysis, it is possible to ob-

tain other fragments. Papain (126) or α-chymotrypsin (208) is frequently used to generate smaller enzymatically active molecules which are called heavy meromyosin subfragment 1 (HMM S-1). Each myosin head (or HMM) contains two molecules of HMM S-1, and these correspond to the two actin-binding and two ATPase sites that the myosin molecule possesses. Again this dissection is depicted diagrammatically in Fig. 1. The advantage of these various fragments lies not only in their contribution to the molecular geometry of myosin, but also because they are more suitable for use in various kinetic analyses due to their solubility at low ionic strength.

The above pattern of proteolysis was demonstrated using skeletal muscle myosin, and it is now evident that a similar pattern is obtained from smooth muscle myosin. Some differences in the products have been observed (see review 76), although probably the most significant consideration in the production of these proteolytic fragments from smooth muscle myosin is associated with the lability to proteolysis of the 20,000 light chain. As will be evident from the subsequent discussion (section on Regulation), this component is intimately involved in the regulatory mechanism, and it is difficult to preserve full regulation of ATPase activity following proteolysis of the myosin. For example, HMM from chicken gizzard myosin retained only about 60% of the parent myosin properties (148,164), and in HMM S-1 the 20,000 light chain was completely lost (107,182).

Myosin aggregation—filament formation. Myosin aggregates at low ionic strength to form structures which can be quite similar to the *in situ* thick filament structure. This was discovered initially for skeletal muscle myosin (93) and later demonstrated using smooth muscle myosin (74,104,168,169). However, the shape and size of the artificial filaments were extremely variable and depended on many of the experimental parameters (e.g., ionic strength, pH, concentration of myosin). Thus it was difficult to assign any one filament type as an *in vivo* model. More recently longer filaments have been observed which do not show a central bare zone, and these have been used as models for various modes of myosin assembly. Sobieszek (179) suggested that the building unit of the filaments was an antiparallel myosin dimer with an overlay of about 600Å, and the tails of the myosin molecules twisted around each other by a total of 180°; a six-stranded helix gave the best fit to his data. The same basic structure was more recently shown for several types of myosin (86), and it was suggested that the structural organization of thick filaments from smooth muscle and nonmuscle myosins was distinct from that observed with skeletal muscle myosin. In this model adjacent rows of cross-bridges have opposite polarities. It should be pointed out, however, that to date thick filaments in nonmuscle cells have not been unequivocally demonstrated. Wachsberger and Pepe (204) found that as the ionic strength of a rabbit uterine myosin solution was reduced, short tapered bipolar filaments with a central bare zone were formed. In the presence of 5 to 10 mM Mg^{2+}, these short filaments aggregated by end-to-end overlap of the tapered ends to form longer filaments (0.7 to 1.2 μm) with the obliteration of the bare zone region. Two filament types, either bipolar or nonpolar, were observed with chicken gizzard myosin by Suzuki et al. (196), and it was suggested that the formation of one or the other type of filament depended on the speed of dilution of the myosin solution. Similarly, the short bipolar filaments were observed by Craig and Megerman (29), and in addition a longer side-polar filament was also found. In the latter type, the cross-bridges on one side of the filament had opposite polarity to those on the other side of the filament. This aggregate did not show a helical arrangement of the myosin molecules and resulted rather in a rectangular profile where the cross-bridges were found only on two opposite faces. The advantage of this geometry is that it would allow interaction with actin along the entire filament length and could accommodate the wide range of shortening of which smooth muscle is capable. In skeletal muscle an additional component of the thick filament, C protein (30,130,154), is known to affect the structure of the filament (111,154). Since smooth muscle does not contain C protein (204), this is unlikely to be a contributing complication. It is clear from this discussion that the assembly mode of myosin giving rise to the *in vivo* filaments is not established and must be clarified in the future.

ATPase activity. It is generally true that the ATPase activities of smooth muscle myosin are lower than those of skeletal muscle myosin. The characteristics of the ATPase activities are also different, and each myosin type shows a general pattern of behavior characteristic of the muscle type. Three different ATPase activities are usually measured. These are Ca^{2+}-ATPase activity, where Ca^{2+} and ATP are approximately equimolar and thus Ca^{2+}-ATP is the substrate; K^+-EDTA ATPase activity, where divalent cations are removed with EDTA and K^+ acts as the counterion to ATP; and Mg^{2+}-ATPase activity, where Mg^{2+} and ATP are in the same concentration range and Mg^{2+}-ATP is the substrate. The latter is the only activity of physiological relevance. However, the other activities are useful to characterize the myosin and they also indicate the differences between skeletal and smooth muscle myosin. The K^+-EDTA ATPase activity is about 30% of the fast skeletal muscle myosin value, but otherwise its properties (effect of actin, SH modification, etc.) are similar. The Ca^{2+}-ATPase activity is quite different, and shows a marked activation on increasing the ionic strength. This effect was first noted several years ago for uterine actomyosin (146), and subsequently it was shown that an activation of Ca^{2+}-ATPase activity also occurred on tryptic digestion or the addition of various denaturing agents to gizzard myosin (11). More recently, it was found that the Ca^{2+}-ATPase activity of rabbit stomach myosin reached its optimum value at approximately 0.3 M KCl (105). This behavior is not a characteristic of skeletal muscle myosin although it does appear to be common with nonmuscle myosins [as an example, myosin from fibroblasts is activated by KCl (214)]. Another difference observed with the Ca^{2+}-ATPase activity is that smooth muscle myosin does not show the classic activation (165) of activity associated with the modification of the sulfhydryl 1 residue (203,211). Other characteristics of the Ca^{2+}-ATPase activity are discussed elsewhere (76).

The Mg^{2+}-ATPase activity of smooth muscle myosin, in the absence of contaminating proteins, is similar to that of skeletal muscle myosin and is in the order of 2 nmoles P_i liberated/min/mg myosin. Both myosin types show a similar, but unusual, pH profile in that maximum activity is observed at acidic (approximately 5) and alkaline (approximately 10) pH values (43). This obviously has no physiological relevance, but it is useful in clarifying earlier reports that smooth muscle actomyosin showed maximum activity at nonphysiological pH values (13,15,138,139), which apparently were due to myosin alone rather than to the actin-activated ATPase activity. In fact, the pH optimum for the activation of Mg^{2+}-ATPase activity by actin is close to neutrality (43), as is the pH optimum for tension development in glycerinated fibers (132). The most significant difference in the Mg^{2+}-ATPase activity of smooth muscle and striated muscle myosins is found in the effect of actin. The Mg^{2+}-ATPase activity of striated muscle myosin is activated over 100-fold on the addition of actin. With smooth muscle myosin the activation by actin is much less (11,43,211), and if the myosin and actin are pure, the activation is negligible. In contrast, the Mg^{2+}-ATPase activity of actomyosin extracted as a complex from the muscle, i.e., in an impure form, is much higher. Originally this discrepancy was thought to be due to the denaturation of myosin during the isolation procedures, but it is now accepted that the activation of smooth muscle myosin by actin requires additional factors and these proteins constitute the regulatory components of the actomyosin complex (see section on Regulation).

At this point, it is convenient to discuss the Mg^{2+}-ATPase activity of actomyosin with the understanding that the enzyme from smooth muscle sources contains components in addition to actin and myosin. In general, the Mg^{2+}-ATPase activity of skeletal muscle actomyosin (0.5 to 1.0 μmoles P_i liberated/min/mg actomyosin) is higher than that of smooth muscle actomyosin. Values for the latter are extremely variable and range between 10 and 300 nmoles P_i liberated/min/mg actomyosin (35,43,135,162,178,182,183,189). The majority of reports, however, favor values toward the lower end of this range. At the present time, there is no adequate explanation to account for this wide range of activities, although it is known that alterations in the assay conditions [e.g., Mg^{2+} and protein concentration, ionic strength (76)] influence the activity. The amount of the regulatory proteins, i.e., activating components, that a given actomyosin contains is also a potential variable, and the extent of phosphorylation of the myosin molecule (see section on Regulation) is an important consideration. In addition, the kinetics of the ATP hydrolysis by actomyosin is complex and often shows a rapid initial phase followed by a slower rate of hydrolysis.

In view of this uncertainty about the specific activity of the isolated smooth muscle actomyosin, it is relevant to ask what range of values might be derived from physiological measurements. It is established that for each cross-bridge cycle (attachment to and detachment from actin) one molecule of ATP is hydrolyzed. Further, it is accepted that the specific Mg^{2+}-ATPase activity of actomyosin reflects the potential cross-bridge cycling rate. It was calculated (134) for arterial muscle at 37°C that the cross-bridge cycling rate is of the order of 1 sec^{-1} (at least an order of magnitude slower than most skeletal muscles). This corresponds to an ATPase activity of about 37 nmoles P_i/min/mg myosin at 37°C, and assuming a Q_{10} of 3 (43), an activity at 25°C of about 10 nmoles P_i/min/mg myosin can be estimated. This value is subject to many ambiguities but lends some confidence to the correlation of the biochemical and physiological data.

It is customary in muscle biochemistry to use actomyosin as a model for the contractile apparatus. One illustration of this in terms of the ATPase activity has already been noted. Another widely used example is the investigations of the Ca^{2+}-dependent regulatory mechanisms. It is established that an increase in the intracellular Ca^{2+} concentration initiates contraction and that Mg^{2+}-ATP is the fuel for this process. Thus the *in vitro* analogue to this situation is actomyosin in which the Mg^{2+}-ATPase activity is regulated by alterations of the Ca^{2+} concentration over a range of approximately 10^{-5} (active) to 10^{-7} (inactive). Historically, meeting this requirement proved elusive, and it was not until 1970 that Sparrow et al. (189) described a Ca^{2+}-sensitive actomyosin isolated from arterial muscle. Since this time several groups have isolated Ca^{2+}-sensitive actomyosins from a variety of smooth muscles (see review 76), and in general these have been useful in furthering our understanding of the regulatory mechanism. The assay that is used to estimate Ca^{2+} sensitivity is usually to measure the Mg^{2+}-ATPase activity in the presence of Ca^{2+} and in the presence of a Ca^{2+} chelating agent, commonly, 2,2'-ethylenedioxybis [ethyliminodi (acetic acid)], abbreviated EGTA, to achieve a low ($<10^{-7}$ M) Ca^{2+} concentration. Under the latter condition the Mg^{2+}-ATPase activity of Ca^{2+}-sensitive actomyosin is reduced, and the extent of the inhibition is a measure of the Ca^{2+} sensitivity. As the activation of the Mg^{2+}-ATPase activity occurs only in the presence of Ca^{2+}, the requirements for the Ca^{2+}-dependent regulation are established. Some actomyosin preparations do not show any Ca^{2+} dependency, and this is often due to membrane contaminants or proteolytic degradation of the regulatory components (45,77) or myosin. Ca^{2+}-sensitive actomyosin from smooth muscle does not contain subunits similar to those of skeletal muscle troponin (19,43,180) as judged by electrophoretic techniques.

Actin

Of the three major proteins of the contractile apparatus, actin from a wide variety of sources shows the least variation. The molecular weight of G-actin, 42,000, as derived from the amino acid sequence of skeletal muscle actin (26,53), is constant as is the ability of G-actin to polymerize to F-actin, which is assembled into a double-stranded helical array. F-actin forms the basis of all thin filaments. Other common features of actin include the ability of F-actin to activate the Mg^{2+}-ATPase activity of skeletal muscle myosin; the binding of one molecule of nucleotide—either ADP in F-actin or ATP in G-actin (54)—per G-actin molecule; and the ability of F-actin to bind tropomyosin. These constant features (see review 76) are found in actins isolated from both muscle and nonmuscle sources. However, it has recently been discovered by isoelectric focusing techniques that slight differences are apparent and three variants of actin have been identified. These are referred to as α, β, and γ (159,209). The most acidic form, α, is characteristic of skeletal and cardiac muscle actin, cytoplasmic actin (i.e., nonmuscle actin) contained the β and γ forms and smooth muscle actin co-migrated with the γ form (159,201). The difference in isoelectric points between the skeletal muscle (α) and smooth muscle (γ) actins seems to be restricted to a few amino acids at the N-terminus (200,216), and the rest of the sequence is similar. For the β and γ forms, a substitution of three N-terminal aspartic acid residues (β) for three glutamic acid residues (γ) accounts for the distinction in their isoelectric points (200). Recently it was suggested that γ actin binds Mg ADP more strongly than β actin (7). However, these distinctions are relatively minor, and in their biological properties skeletal muscle and smooth muscle actins are very similar. The majority of investigators are of the opinion that skeletal and smooth muscle actin can be used interchangeably, i.e., in hybrid systems with myosin. An exception to this generalization is the work of Ebashi and collaborators (49,50) who found a specific requirement for smooth muscle actin in their studies on the regulatory mechanism in smooth muscle. Another distinction between the α and γ forms of actin was reported by Suzuki et al. (197) who found that the inclusion of Ca^{2+} during the preparative procedure altered the properties of actin isolated from chicken gizzard.

Tropomyosin

It has been known for several years that tropomyosin is a component of smooth muscle (see review 76). With respect to their gross physical properties, tropomyosins from all muscle sources are similar. The molecule is asymmetric or rod-like, with dimensions of approximately 42×2 nm. It is composed of two similar subunits arranged in register in a coiled-coil configuration, and the secondary structure is almost entirely α-helical. At low ionic strength, tropomyosin forms an end-to-end polymer which is disrupted by increasing the ionic strength. It is assumed that on the thin filaments the tropomyosin exists as the polymeric form and one strand of tropomyosin molecules is associated with each of the two actin strands (144). The stoichiometry of the tropomyosin interaction with actin is approximately one tropomyosin per seven actins, and this ratio is maintained in hybrid systems where the actin and tropomyosin are isolated from different muscle sources. The affinity of the tropomyosin binding to actin is enhanced in the presence of troponin (44), and since it is thought that troponin is not present in smooth muscle it would be expected that tropomyosin is more easily dissociated from the thin filaments of smooth muscle as compared to those of skeletal muscle. This affords an explanation for the relatively common observation that tropomyosin

is extracted from smooth muscle under a variety of different solvent conditions.

A few years ago it was found that contrary to earlier opinions, the tropomyosin subunits were not all identical and to a limited degree, the tropomyosin subunit composition was characteristic of the muscle type. This was discovered initially in rabbit psoas muscle where two subunits, α and β, were identified (33). The relative amounts of each differed and α was present in greater amounts (33,103). In slow (red) skeletal muscle (34,111) and in fetal muscle (5) the proportion of β is increased, whereas in rabbit and avian cardiac muscle only α is found (32,34,125). The β subunit is also found in the larger mammalian hearts (116,149). It is suggested that in muscles where both subunits exist only the $\alpha\alpha$- and $\alpha\beta$-dimers are formed (51,194,210), i.e., the $\beta\beta$-dimer is not found. Despite the difference in the electrophoretic mobility of the α and β subunits (33), it was found recently that both contain the same number of amino acids, 284, and thus have a similar molecular weight of approximately 33,000 (125,193). The complete sequence of both α (192,193) and β tropomyosin (125) has been determined and found to differ in 39 amino acid substitutions. To date there is no clear indication of any marked functional differences between the two (116). Both show periodic distributions of amino acids which are thought to reflect a repeat of the actin binding sites (125,150,191,193).

The tropomyosin of smooth muscle has not been as extensively characterized as that of skeletal muscle. It is known, however, that different subunits can be detected, for example, the tropomyosin of chicken gizzard shows two components of approximately equal proportions (19,34,43). The faster of the two gizzard tropomyosin subunits has a mobility on SDS polyacrylamide electrophoresis similar to that of the skeletal muscle β-tropomyosin, although it is not chemically equivalent (34). The subunit molecular weights for the two gizzard tropomyosin components have not been established. In view of the finding that the α and β components of skeletal muscle tropomyosin have similar sizes and yet different electrophoretic mobilities, the apparent molecular weights based on SDS polyacrylamide electrophoresis of 36,000 and 39,000 for the gizzard subunits must be confirmed by alternate techniques. Strasburg and Greaser (194) found that the gizzard tropomyosin is a homodimer, either $2 \times 36,000$ or $2 \times 39,000$, and the heterodimer is not formed. Tropomyosin has been identified in other smooth muscles—rabbit and pig uterus (34), hog carotid artery (142), and calf aorta (58)—and found to consist predominantly of a single subunit species. It has been known for some time that the tropomyosins of skeletal and smooth muscles are immunochemically distinct (34). It was also suggested that each tropomyosin subunit has a specific antigenic site in addition to sites which are common to each tropomyosin subunit (80).

The function of tropomyosin in smooth muscle is not fully understood. It is known that tropomyosin can activate the Mg^{2+}-ATPase activity of phosphorylated myosin (see section on Regulation) plus actin (77,183), and it appears therefore that the actin-tropomyosin complex serves as a better activator of the myosin ATPase activity than actin alone. Activation was optimal at the expected tropomyosin:actin molar stoichiometry of about 1:5 (77). In this sense the function of tropomyosin can be regarded as secondary to that of the regulatory system. In striated muscle tropomyosin functions with troponin as a regulatory complex, and it is interesting that although troponin is absent from smooth muscle, its tropomyosin still retains a troponin binding site (49,76,190) and is able to function in the skeletal muscle system. Thus there is a consensus of opinion that tropomyosin, like actin, is capable of functioning in a variety of hybrid systems, and this reflects the conservation on the tropomyosin molecule of several basic properties, i.e., binding to actin and to troponin. An exception to the universal role of tropomyosin is apparent from the work of Ebashi and colleagues (49), who found a requirement for smooth muscle tropomyosin in their studies on the regulatory mechanism of smooth muscle.

Intracellular Filaments

The accepted model to account for length changes in skeletal muscle is based on the sliding filament theory. It was found independently by A. F. Huxley and Niedergerke (92) and H. E. Huxley and Hanson (94) that the shortening of striated muscle was the result of a relative sliding between two sets of filaments. These filament types are the thick (myosin-containing) and thin (actin-containing) filaments. During any length change, the length of the two filament types does not alter and the change in the muscle length is achieved by varying the degree of filament overlap. This model is a fundamental component of any treatment of the contractile process in skeletal muscle, and as such, a similar situation was sought in smooth muscle. However, a double-filament array in smooth muscle was not demonstrated until several years after its discovery in skeletal muscle. Thin filaments were numerous and were observed in many types of smooth muscle, but the existence of thick filaments was not established until the late sixties (40,106, 147). It appears that the thick filaments of smooth muscle are more labile than their skeletal muscle counterparts, and, to a large extent, the demonstration of thick filaments in smooth muscle requires more refined fixation techniques (see review 184). However, it is now accepted that the thick and thin filament array does exist in smooth muscle and thick filaments have been ob-

served in many types of smooth muscle. This is an important conclusion since it suggests that the fundamental mechanism of contraction is similar in both the skeletal and smooth muscle systems. In the sliding filament model, tension is generated as a consequence of the interaction of the myosin cross-bridges with actin and the associated hydrolysis of ATP. In the relaxed muscle, the interaction between the two filament types is prevented, and the sites of tension development are not formed. An increase in the intracellular concentration of Ca^{2+} initiates contraction, and this occurs by promoting the cross-bridge actin interaction. In the simplest concept, it is the function of the regulatory components of the contractile apparatus to recognize the Ca^{2+} transients within the cell and to translate these to result in either an increase or decrease in the extent of cross-bridge contacts with actin.

The thin filaments (5 to 8 nm diameter) in smooth muscle are numerous and appear similar to skeletal muscle thin filaments (73,93). The backbone of the filament is organized in a two-stranded helical array with an axial repeat of 36 to 38 nm. The F-actin, which consists of two linear polymers of G-actin monomer repeat, is about 5.5 nm. The length of the thin filaments in smooth muscle has not been determined, although it is assumed that they are at least as long as the skeletal muscle thin filaments (approximately 1 μm). The only other major protein component of the smooth muscle thin filament is tropomyosin, and this is found at a stoichiometry of about 1 tropomyosin molecule for each 6 or 7 actin molecules. Troponin is not found in smooth muscle thin filaments (42,182), and this is the major difference between the smooth and striated muscle filaments. It is interesting that despite the absence of troponin, X-ray diffraction data indicate that the position of tropomyosin on smooth muscle thin filaments is altered on activation of the muscle (151,202). In striated muscle, the movement of tropomyosin from a blocking to a nonblocking position, corresponding to the relaxed and contracted states, respectively, has been suggested as a critical component of the regulatory mechanism (see review 76). However, regulation in striated muscle requires the participation of troponin, which is thought to direct and stabilize the tropomyosin positions. Thus the significance of the tropomyosin movement in smooth muscles is not understood, although it may reflect some interactions of the myosin cross-bridges with the actin filaments.

One end of the thin filament appears to be associated with amorphous structures, called dense bodies. These are found attached to the plasma membrane and also within the cytoplasm. Although it is not conclusive, it is likely that both forms of the dense bodies are analogous to the Z-lines of striated muscle (see review 184) and probably serve to anchor the thin filaments. In support of this, α-actinin, which is known to be a component of Z-lines, has been localized in the dense bodies (163). Another type of filament also appears to be associated with the dense bodies. These are the 100 Å or intermediate filaments which are found not only in smooth muscles but in many other eukaryotic cells (115). The function of these filaments is not established, although it is clear that they do not participate directly in the contractile process. Perhaps their function is associated with the finding that they form a cytoskeletal network (8,27,28,177), which could aid in the distribution of tension throughout the cell.

Thick filaments are now an accepted component of the ultrastructure of the smooth muscle cell. They have been seen in a wide variety of smooth muscles (see review 184), and together with the thin filaments they are assumed to constitute a sliding filament model to account for length changes in smooth muscle. Yet despite their recent popularity, several features about them are not established. One of these is the length of the thick filaments. Ashton et al. (8), using intermediate high-voltage stereo electron microscopy, determined a length of 2.2 μm for the thick filaments in rabbit portal anterior mesenteric vein, which is considerably longer than the filaments of rabbit skeletal muscle (93). Longer filaments up to 8 μm were reported in homogenates of taenia coli (174), although it is not clear whether or not these represented aggregates of smaller filaments. The 2.2 μm filaments (8) were found to have tapered ends which is consistent with a packing of the myosin molecules in a manner similar to that in skeletal muscle. However, a central bare zone, which is predicted from this mode of assembly, has not been unequivocally demonstrated for smooth muscle thick filaments. This is an important point as it reflects the arrangement of the cross-bridges on the thick filament. Cross-bridges have been observed on smooth muscle thick filaments (8,40, 185), and although a helical arrangement is consistent with the observations (see review 184), this is not firmly established. The distribution of thick filaments within the smooth muscle cell is obviously not as regular as in skeletal muscle, although there is some indication that a longitudinal ordering of filaments occurred in vascular tissue (8), and it was suggested that these approximate a mini-sarcomere (Fig. 3). The results obtained with fluorescent antibodies to myosin also suggest some regularity in the arrangement of myosin (9,23,71).

One of the most striking features about the ultrastructure of the smooth muscle cell is the large number of actin filaments relative to the number of thick filaments (Figs. 2 and 3). This is consistent with the concentration of actin and myosin within the smooth muscle cell, as discussed above. In rabbit skeletal muscle, there are about two thin filaments to one thick filament. This ratio for smooth muscle is much higher, and filament counts by several investigators all indicate an excess of actin filaments: 10–14:1 (83) and 12:1 (14) for intestinal muscle and between 12:1 and 15:1 (40,185) for vascular muscle. As shown earlier, the content of actin in vascular muscle is higher than in nonvascular muscle, and assuming that the lengths of the filaments in both muscle groups are the same, one would expect somewhat higher actin:myosin filament ratios for the vascular tissues (140). The actin:myosin filament counts are higher in smooth compared to skeletal muscle partly because the actin content is higher but, more significantly, because the myosin content is lower. This is interesting because it was shown that smooth muscle can generate a tension approximately equal to that of skeletal muscle (142), and it is known that the force developed by a muscle is proportional to the number of cross-bridges acting in parallel (91), which in turn is proportional to the concentration of myosin. Thus the low content of myosin must be compensated for in some way, and several suggestions have been put forward, including the longer thick filaments in smooth compared to skeletal muscle, the higher content of actin in smooth muscle, and possibly different cross-bridge kinetics for the smooth muscle system. These and other possibilities are discussed by Somlyo (184) and Murphy (140).

Many of the features that have been discussed are apparent from the electron micrographs presented in Figs. 2 and 3. A longitudinal section of vascular smooth muscle is shown in Fig. 2. The excess of thin filaments compared to thick filaments is clearly illustrated. The caveolae and some elements of the sarcoplasmic reticulum are also visible. In Fig. 3, the same vascular muscle tissue was chemically skinned using the detergent saponin, fixed, and a longitudinal section taken. This treatment destroys much of the membrane structure but allows a much clearer visualization of the three filament types. The thick filaments are surrounded by thin filaments thus resembling a "mini-sarcomore." The 100 Å filaments appear to be closely associated with the dense bodies from which the thin filaments also originate.

Regulation of the Contractile Apparatus

The changes in the intracellular concentration of Ca^{2+} result in either contraction, at higher Ca^{2+} levels, or relaxation, at lower Ca^{2+} levels. As discussed previously, the level of Ca^{2+} is controlled in part by the sarcoplasmic reticulum, and the subject of this section is to examine those components of the contractile apparatus which recognize the Ca^{2+} fluctuations and can then modify the system to result in either contraction or relaxation.

Requirements for Regulation

The best understood regulatory system is that of skeletal muscle, where the complex of troponin and tro-

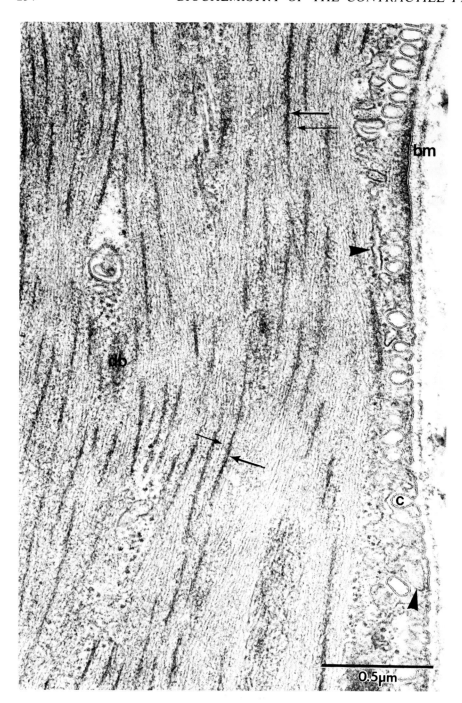

FIG. 2. Longitudinal section from the rabbit portal anterior mesenteric vein illustrating thick myosin filaments *(large arrows)* surrounded with adjacent parallel actin filaments *(small arrows).* Dense bodies, db; sarcoplasmic reticulum, *arrowheads;* dense basement membrane, bm; and caveolae, c. Figure supplied by Dr. A. V. Somlyo, University of Pennsylvania.

pomyosin located on the thin filament regulates contractile activity. Following the historical precedent (46), smooth muscle was accordingly analyzed for troponin-like components. Several groups reported success (20, 45,98,99,167,190). However, more recent investigations have found that troponin-like proteins are not present in Ca^{2+}-sensitive actomyosin (19,43,180) nor on smooth muscle thin filaments (43,182), and the current consensus of opinion is that troponin as it exists in skeletal muscle is not found in smooth muscle. Progress in understanding the regulatory mechanism of vertebrate smooth muscle was facilitated by results obtained with invertebrate muscle. Szent-Györgyi and his colleagues

discovered that in molluscan muscle regulation was associated with the myosin molecule (108,118) and was a function of the myosin light chains (109,198). A simple and elegant test was devised to distinguish between actin-linked and myosin-linked muscles (118,119), and using this procedure Bremel (18) found that in chicken gizzard actomyosin the control system was also associated with the myosin molecule. However, this discovery raised a puzzling feature since it was known that as the smooth muscle myosin was purified its activation by actin decreased (11,43,211), in contrast to the molluscan and vertebrate skeletal muscle systems. It became apparent that an additional factor was required for acti-

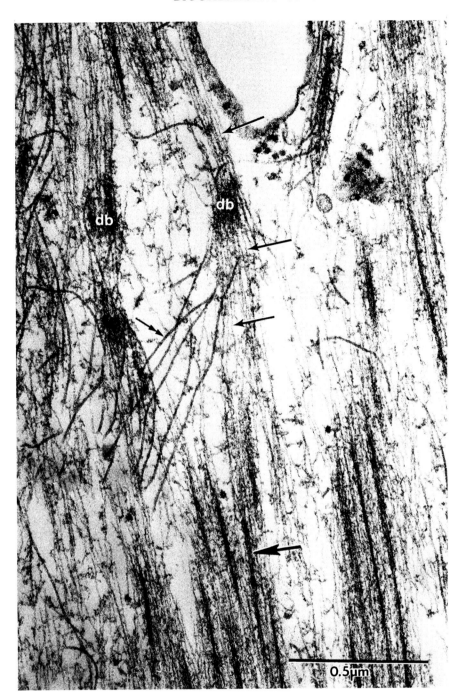

FIG. 3. Longitudinal section from a saponin-skinned portal anterior mesenteric vein smooth muscle cell. Tannic acid used during fixation. Some of the soluble cytoplasmic proteins have washed out of the cell allowing better visualization of the thin actin filaments *(small arrows)* running into the dense bodies (db). Intermediate or 100 Å filaments *(double arrowhead)* are associated with the dense bodies. Some of the actin filaments can be traced from the dense bodies to myosin filaments *(large arrowhead)* forming a "mini-sarcomere." Figure supplied by Dr. A. V. Somlyo, University of Pennsylvania.

vation, and that this was lost during the purification procedures. Further, it was clear that the activation of the Mg^{2+}-ATPase activity of smooth muscle myosin by actin occurred only in the presence of Ca^{2+} (in the μM range). This type of regulation is distinct from that seen in many invertebrates where a mixture of pure myosin and actin is adequate for a regulated and active actomyosin. However, even though additional components are necessary, it is still myosin-linked since it is proposed that activation is achieved by a modification of myosin. The existence of a myosin-linked regulatory mechanism in chicken gizzard has been confirmed (19, 75,97,182) and extended to actomyosins from other

smooth muscles (16,63,135,199). It should be noted that even though myosin-linked regulation in smooth muscle is accepted by most investigators, it is not unanimously accepted (50).

The basic requirements for regulation in smooth muscle are, however, accepted universally. These are that the Mg^{2+}-ATPase activity of actomyosin is activated in the presence of Ca^{2+}, at those Ca^{2+} concentrations necessary to initiate contraction, and that in the absence of Ca^{2+} no activation is achieved. The basic concept for this mechanism is quite different from that existing in striated muscle where regulation is achieved by inhibiting an active state in the absence of Ca^{2+}, and this is the function of troponin. The mechanism in smooth muscle operates by activating a dormant state in the presence of Ca^{2+}. This basic difference has been stressed repeatedly by Ebashi and co-workers (48–50). The controversies that exist are in the nature of the activating factor and whether it is myosin- or actin-linked.

Three possibilities have been suggested as the regulatory components in smooth muscle: (a) that a troponin-like system is operative, (b) that activation of actomyosin is mediated by the phosphorylation of the 20,000 light chains of the myosin molecule, and (c) that activation of actomyosin is achieved by a system termed leiotonin. The first suggestion, however, is not likely. From the above discussion it is apparent that the function of "classic" troponin is to inhibit, rather than activate, ATPase activity. Further, it is established that proteins corresponding to the troponin subunits, I and T, are not present in smooth muscle actomyosin preparations. Thus if a "troponin-like" principle is operative in smooth muscle, it would be expected to serve an inhibitory control function which is secondary to the activating regulatory system. This possibility cannot be eliminated, but it is unlikely to be effected by a protein similar to skeletal muscle troponin. The remaining two possibilities, leiotonin and phosphorylation, form the basis of the current controversy and will be considered below.

Phosphorylation of Myosin as a Regulatory Mechanism

This theory of regulation in smooth muscle is the most widely accepted. It was reported initially by Sobieszek (179) and Bremel et al. (19), who found that chicken gizzard myosin and actomyosin were phosphorylated on the 20,000 light chains of myosin and that this event occurred at a similar concentration of Ca^{2+} as that necessary for the activation of ATPase activity. One mole of phosphate was found per mole of light chain. It was suggested as a result of this work that the actin-myosin interaction in smooth muscle is regulated via the phosphorylation of the myosin molecule. Since

the original observations, several groups have demonstrated a phosphorylation of smooth muscle myosin (4, 12,22,41,61,67,90,96,97,178,179,183), and, in general, these reports can be summarized to state what is believed to be the key facts of the phosphorylation theory: (a) the two 20,000 light chains of the myosin molecule can be phosphorylated by a specific enzyme, the myosin light chain kinase (MLCK); (b) phosphorylation occurs only in the presence of Ca^{2+} and at Ca^{2+} concentrations similar to those required to initiate contraction; (c) phosphorylation is a prerequisite for the activation by actin of the Mg^{2+}-ATPase activity of smooth muscle myosin; and (d) an additional enzyme is required to deactivate the contractile apparatus, and this is a myosin light-chain phosphatase which removes the phosphate groups from the myosin light chains.

There is considerable evidence to support each of the above contentions, and if the validity of each is accepted, then a cyclic scheme to summarize the role of myosin phosphorylation in the regulation of smooth muscle actomyosin can be formulated and this is presented in Fig. 4. Several distinct phases can be identified within this scheme. Myosin is phosphorylated by the MLCK in the presence of Ca^{2+}, and this initiates the cross-bridge interactions with actin. One can regard this as the activation phase. In the presence of actin, the phosphorylated myosin will undergo repetitive cycles of ATP hydrolysis, corresponding to the cross-bridge cycling, and this phase will continue as long as Ca^{2+} is present. Tentatively this can be correlated to steady-state tension development. When Ca^{2+} is removed the MLCK is rendered inactive and the phosphatase removes the phosphate groups from the light chains. The net result of this is that the actin and myosin dissociate (the cross-bridge interactions are prevented) and relaxation occurs.

Several features of this scheme should be considered in more detail, and these are numerically identified in Fig. 4.

Composition of the myosin light chain kinase. One of the original objectives in our laboratory was to isolate the kinase from smooth muscle with the idea that

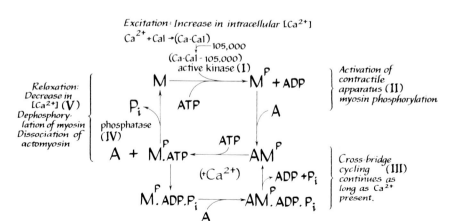

FIG. 4. Schematic representation of the role of phosphorylation and dephosphorylation in smooth muscle. Each phase of the cycle, I–V, is discussed in the text. Abbreviations used: M, M^P, dephosphorylated and phosphorylated myosin, respectively; P_i, inorganic phosphate; A, actin.

a clearer understanding of the regulatory mechanism would be available only when each one of the components in the actomyosin system was adequately characterized. It was found during these studies that the MLCK from chicken gizzard was composed of two distinct proteins (35) and both were required for MLCK activity. The molecular weights of these are approximately 105,000 and 17,000. The two subunits were purified and it was found (37) that the smaller component was identical to calmodulin (which was previously called modulator protein, calcium-dependent regulator protein, and phosphodiesterase activator protein; see review 24). It was known from many other studies that calmodulin binds Ca^{2+} and it directs the Ca^{2+} dependence of several enzyme systems (24,206). Thus by analogy with these previous results it is suggested that calmodulin is the Ca^{2+} receptor of the MLCK, and its position in the regulatory mechanism of smooth muscle is equivalent to that served by troponin C in striated muscle. On excitation of the muscle the intracellular Ca^{2+} concentration increases, Ca^{2+} is bound to calmodulin, and the Ca^{2+}-calmodulin complex interacts with the larger subunit to form the active myosin light chain kinase. The stoichiometry of the calmodulin kinase complex is 1:1 (78). Subsequently, these findings were confirmed by Adelstein and co-workers (3) using turkey gizzard smooth muscle, although the larger component of the kinase was reported to be 125,000 M.W.

At about the same time that our work on the gizzard MLCK was reported, other investigators found that the MLCK from skeletal muscle was also composed of two subunits, one of which was calmodulin (205,212). The larger subunit, however, was smaller and has a molecular weight of about 80,000 (213). A similar molecular weight was reported earlier by Pires and Perry (156), although the requirement for calmodulin was not realized at this time and was confirmed in a later report (145). The function of MLCK in skeletal muscle is not known. It phosphorylates two of the myosin light chains, referred to as the DTNB [5,5'-dithiobis-(2-nitrobenzoic acid)] light chains, P-light chains (62), or regulatory light chains (100), but this modification does not markedly affect the actin-activated Mg^{2+}-ATPase activity of skeletal or cardiac muscle myosin as it does with smooth muscle myosin. Recently other systems have been studied, and calmodulin-dependent myosin light chain kinases have been identified in blood platelets (36,79), brain (36), and fibroblasts (215).

Some of the properties of the gizzard kinase have been reported. The K_m of the kinase for ATP is about 65 μM (78); the V_{max} for phosphorylation of the isolated myosin light chains is between 5 and 15 μmoles P transferred/min mg^{-1} kinase at 25°C (3,78), although with intact myosin as the substrate the rate of phosphorylation might be slower (133). The Q_{10} for the enzyme is close to 2, and optimal activity is found in the neutral pH range (133). It is well known that maximum ATPase

activity or tension development in smooth muscle requires Mg^{2+} concentrations in excess of the ATP concentration (57,76,162). It was found that the MLCK does not show a requirement for free Mg^{2+} (78), and therefore the unusual Mg^{2+} dependency of the smooth muscle actomyosin probably is a reflection of the myosin molecule itself. When the effect of cAMP and cGMP was assayed using purified preparations of actomyosin or MLCK, no marked alteration of activity was observed (137,173,205). However, Adelstein and colleagues (3) found that the larger subunit of the MLCK was phosphorylated by the cAMP-dependent kinase, and this phosphorylation resulted in a decrease of the MLCK activity. Subsequently in assays carried out with actomyosin preparations which contained (either intrinsic or added) cAMP-dependent kinase, an inhibition of ATPase activity (137,173) and myosin light chain phosphorylation (173) was observed. It was proposed (3) that an increase in cAMP concentration might function physiologically not only by lowering the intracellular concentration of available Ca^{2+} but also by modifying the contractile apparatus directly and thereby regulating smooth muscle contraction.

Calmodulin is similar in its physical properties to troponin C. Both are acidic proteins, bind Ca^{2+}, have similar molecular weights (although calmodulin is slightly smaller—16,700 as compared to about 18,200), and have some sequence homologies (24). Calmodulin will also function with skeletal muscle troponin I in the regulation of skeletal muscle actomyosin (6), although troponin C will not activate the myosin light chain kinase (37). The similarity of the two proteins led to the report of a troponin C-like component from smooth muscle (82), and it was suggested that the identification of this protein reflected the presence of an actin-linked regulatory system. It is now accepted that the protein isolated was in fact calmodulin (68,81), and troponin C is not present in smooth muscle. This does not eliminate the existence of a thin-filament-based regulatory system, but in view of the multiple functions of calmodulin, its presence is not by itself sufficient to suggest actin-linked regulation in smooth muscle.

In summary, it may be proposed that the enzyme responsible for the activation of the contractile apparatus (initiation of contraction) is the MLCK, which consists of two distinct protein components. The smaller component is the Ca^{2+} receptor and the regulatory moiety of the enzyme and is identical with calmodulin. The larger kinase subunit provides the active site for the phosphotransferase activity but is inactive in the absence of calmodulin. This mode of regulation is distinct from the cAMP-dependent protein kinase, where the dissociated catalytic subunit is active and the complex with the cAMP-binding subunit is inactive.

Activation phase. If the phosphorylation theory is accepted then it is mandatory that the phosphorylation of myosin precedes the contractile response. In a biochemical sense this can be rephrased to state that phosphorylation is essential for the Mg^{2+}-ATPase activity of actomyosin. In general, the bulk of the experimental evidence supports this contention. Sobieszek (179) suggested that phosphorylation of the myosin molecule regulates *in vivo* the actin-myosin interaction, and in studies using the purified MLCK (35) we found that the increase of Mg^{2+}-ATPase activity of actomyosin paralleled the extent of myosin phosphorylation. However, the exact relationship between myosin phosphorylation and specific Mg^{2+}-ATPase activity of actomyosin has not been established. It is not known, for example, if one phosphate group per myosin molecule (i.e., where one of the two 20,000 light chains is phosphorylated) results in an "active" molecule, or if phosphorylation of both sites is required. In this context it is not known whether or not there exists a cooperative response between the two myosin heads, or active sites. These and other relationships must be clarified before the details of the activation phase can be fully appreciated.

One of the obvious points to investigate is the rate at which activation can be achieved. Since phosphorylation is proposed as a prerequisite for the subsequent cross-bridge cycling, it is pertinent to ask whether or not the phosphorylation rate can be rate limiting to tension development. As mentioned previously (section on myosin ATPase activity) the published values for the Mg^{2+}-ATPase activity of smooth muscle actomyosin are variable, but if a value of 100 nmoles P_i liberated/ min/mg myosin at 25°C is chosen as a representative value, this gives a turnover number of about 0.8 sec^{-1}. Assuming that the ATPase rate is indicative of the cross-bridge cycling rate, this would mean that the myosin-actin interactions occur at a frequency of slightly faster than once per second. In order for the phosphorylation of myosin to be limiting, this would require a MLCK rate of about (or less than) this frequency. If one assumes a value of 10 μmoles/min/mg kinase for the V_{max} of the MLCK (see previous section), a turnover number of about 18 sec^{-1} is obtained. This suggests that the contraction speed as indicated by the specific ATPase activity of the actomyosin is at least an order of magnitude slower than the phosphorylation of myosin. On this basis, then, it would be predicted that the activation of myosin is not a rate-limiting step in the initiation of contraction. However, the kinase rates were measured using isolated myosin light chains as the substrate, and preliminary evidence (133) indicates that when myosin is used as the substrate the phosphorylation rates might be slower. Other factors could also affect the kinase activity *in situ,* and therefore the above conclusion can be regarded as only tentative.

Steady-state cycling rate. Once the myosin is phosphorylated, it can enter into repetitive cycles of ATP hydrolysis which will continue as long as Ca^{2+} is present. One difficulty associated with the analysis of this phase is the nonlinear kinetics frequently observed with smooth muscle actomyosin. The time course of ATP hydrolysis often shows a rapid initial phase followed by a slower rate. The finding of Murphy and colleagues (141) that in pig carotid a high initial velocity of shortening corresponded to a rapid phosphorylation of myosin and that subsequently both rates declined suggests that the biphasic or nonlinear response is also found in intact tissue. The factors that influence the time course of ATP hydrolysis are not known, and this is one of the intriguing problems that must be resolved in the future.

When viewed conservatively, probably the only statement that can be made at this time is that phosphorylation appears to be a prerequisite for the actin activation of the Mg^{2+}-ATPase activity of myosin, and it is generally found that the level of phosphorylation is proportional to the ATPase activity. Obviously the highest ATPase activity is expected when the myosin molecule is fully phosphorylated, i.e., 2 moles phosphate per mole myosin. Different extents of phosphorylation is probably the major contributor to the wide range of ATPase values that have been reported. Why the phosphorylation of the light chains should affect the active sites of myosin which are located on the heavy chains is not known, but some theories can be considered. One suggestion is that the state of aggregation of the myosin molecules is related to ATPase activity, with the aggregated myosin showing higher activity (196). The effect of phosphorylation is to stabilize the filamentous state of myosin in the presence of ATP, which would disperse the nonphosphorylated myosin aggregates. The disadvantage of this theory is that it requires the absence of thick filaments in relaxed muscle and their assembly following the phosphorylation of myosin. Although there is still some controversy on this point, most available evidence indicates that thick filaments are present in both the relaxed and contracted states. Another possibility is that phosphorylation alters the inhibition by ATP of the myosin active site. In this hypothesis ATP at millimolar concentrations inhibits the Mg^{2+}-ATPase activity of unphosphorylated actomyosin, and the event of phosphorylation shifts the range of inhibitory ATP to higher concentrations which are not encountered under physiological conditions, thus effectively allowing the actin activation of the myosin ATPase activity. At the present time, however, this mechanism is purely speculative: the molecular events that occur as a consequence of phosphorylation are not established and must be regarded as one of the priorities for future research.

Myosin light chain phosphatase. This enzyme has not been isolated from smooth muscle, although a myosin light chain phosphatase from skeletal muscle has been characterized (131) and shown to have a molecular weight of about 70,000. The presence of phosphatase activity, however, has been detected in several smooth muscle preparations (4,22,96) and some of its properties are known. Removal of the light chain phosphate groups can occur in the absence of Ca^{2+}, and this is consistent with the role of the phosphatase in the relaxation phase. In general, the phosphatase rate is much lower than the kinase rate, and in the presence of phosphatase, kinase, and Ca^{2+} a net phosphorylation of myosin is usually achieved. Thus even though it is thought that the phosphatase is active in both the presence and absence of Ca^{2+}, its influence on the contractile mechanism is obvious only when the kinase is deactivated by the removal of Ca^{2+}. It is not known whether the phosphatase is subject to regulation in the intact cell, although the *in vitro* evidence has not revealed any regulatory processes. Calmodulin does not affect the phosphatase activity.

It was suggested (61) that in smooth muscle, the amount of phosphatase relative to the myosin content is higher than in skeletal muscle. Thus if one assumes a similar level of kinase activity, it would be expected that the average level of myosin phosphorylation is lower in smooth than in skeletal muscle.

Role of Ca^{2+} in the relaxation phase. The role of Ca^{2+} in contraction is relatively simple: it is thought to bind to calmodulin and activate the MLCK. However, the mechanism that promotes relaxation or the removal of Ca^{2+} is not as well accepted. The confusion stems from the observation that some invertebrate myosins are regulated by the binding of Ca^{2+} to the myosin light chains (198) and are inhibited when these Ca^{2+} sites are not occupied. It is known also that smooth muscle myosin binds Ca^{2+} (19,182). The possibility arose that a similar mechanism might operate in smooth muscle, and thus the relative importance of the removal of phosphate groups and the removal of Ca^{2+} from the light chains was questioned. The simplest mechanism to account for relaxation is that the reduced intracellular Ca^{2+} concentration inactivates the kinase and allows the phosphatase to dephosphorylate the myosin. In this situation, the important point is whether or not the myosin is phosphorylated, and it does not take into account the interaction of Ca^{2+} with the myosin light chains. The second possibility is that the Ca^{2+}-light chain interaction is dominant and the removal of Ca^{2+} from the light chain sites inhibits ATPase activity irrespective of the state of phosphorylation. The former view was favored by Small and Sobieszek (175,176) and Ikebe et al. (96) and the latter by Chacko et al. (22). In order to decide between the two possibilities, the actin-activated Mg^{2+}-ATPase activity of phosphorylated myosin should be assayed in the presence and absence of Ca^{2+}. Although the concept is extremely simple, its practical application was not as straightforward, and the major difficulty stemmed from the presence of contaminating kinase and/or phosphatase. Thus the approach that we took toward solving the problem (166) was to design exper-

iments in which the effects of the above contaminants might be reduced. One example was to use adenosine 5'-0 (3-thiotriphosphate), abbreviated by ATPγS. (These experiments are discussed because they constitute one line of evidence in support of the phosphorylation theory of regulation.) ATPγS serves as a substrate for the MLCK, and a thiophosphate group is transferred to the 20,000 light chain. The thiophosphorylated light chain, however, is a poor substrate for the phosphatase (66,70, 131). The net result is that the myosin is "frozen" in the phosphorylated state and may be assayed without the complications associated with contamination by phosphatase. The experimental observations were that as the extent of thiophosphorylation increased, the degree of Ca^{2+}-sensitivity decreased with the ATPase activity of the actomyosin in the absence of Ca^{2+} becoming equal to that shown in the presence of Ca^{2+}, i.e., the myosin was locked into an active and unregulated state. Thus the conclusion from these experiments is that phosphorylated myosin is active regardless of whether or not Ca^{2+} is present and does not support the idea that an additional regulatory function is associated with the binding of Ca^{2+} to myosin. Recently the effects of ATPγS were tested using mechanically disrupted chicken gizzard fibers (88) and functionally skinned rabbit ileum strips (21), and it was found that the thiophosphorylation resulted in the loss of Ca^{2+} control and the generation of an active state. Thus the consensus of opinion at this time is that a direct myosin control system, such as found in the invertebrates, is not present in smooth muscle (for discussion see 166). It should be pointed out, however, that the minority opinion of Chacko et al. (22) was developed using vas deferens. This tissue has not been analyzed by other investigators and might represent an exception to the general pattern of relaxation in smooth muscle.

Evidence to support the phosphorylation theory. The initial evidence to suggest a regulatory function for myosin phosphorylation was that the actin-activated ATPase activity of smooth muscle myosin was increased as the extent of phosphorylation increased. This is still generally accepted. The relationship between the activation of ATPase activity and phosphorylation is maintained when purified kinase components are used (35), and this reduces the possibility that the activation is due to the presence of contaminants in the protein preparations. The activation of ATPase activity as a result of myosin phosphorylation is not unique to smooth muscle and is also found with several nonmuscle systems (1,2). In skeletal and cardiac muscle phosphorylation of myosin is also observed (10,62,155–157), but in these systems a marked activation of ATPase activity is not found and the function of myosin phosphorylation in striated muscle is not clear.

In studies concerning intact muscle preparations it was shown that contraction is associated with the phosphorylation of the 20,000 light chain of myosin (12,

101), and similar results were obtained using various types of skinned fibers (88,110). The correlation of tension development and increase in phosphorylation is certainly consistent with the hypothesis that the phosphorylation of myosin serves a regulatory function, but it is not by itself conclusive. It is known that Ca^{2+} both activates the MLCK and induces tension development, and the concomitant occurrence of both processes could be fortuitous. Thus what is required is to correlate in a more direct manner the event of phosphorylation (or dephosphorylation) with another parameter, e.g., ATPase activity or tension development. The use of ATPγS as a substrate for the MLCK achieves this purpose. As discussed previously this compound supports the thiophosphorylation of the myosin light chains, but the resultant product is resistant to the action of the phosphatase and the myosin becomes locked into the phosphorylated state. In *in vitro* assays it was found (166) that increasing extents of thiophosphorylation was accompanied by a decrease in the Ca^{2+} sensitivity of the actomyosin. The loss of Ca^{2+} regulation following preincubation with ATPγS was also found with mechanically disrupted chicken gizzard fibers (88) and functionally skinned rabbit ileum strips (21). The major advantage associated with the use of ATPγS is that it caused an alteration in the actomyosin characteristics, and this perturbation was reflected in, and correlated with, two independent assays (i.e., Ca^{2+} sensitivity and ATPase activity, and Ca^{2+} sensitivity and tension development). A similar situation is achieved by monitoring the effects of various phenothiazine derivatives. It was shown by Levin and Weiss (120) that trifluoperazine binds with a high affinity to calmodulin and prevents the activation of phosphodiesterase activity. It is established that the MLCK requires calmodulin for activity (37), and it was shown that various pharmaceutical agents that interact with calmodulin inhibited the Ca^{2+}-dependent phosphorylation of chicken gizzard myosin (85) and in functionally skinned rabbit ileum and pulmonary artery strips induced relaxation by inactivating the kinase and allowing the dephosphorylation of the myosin (110). Specific inhibition of the MLCK by the phenothiazine derivatives coupled with subsequent relaxation of the muscle strips provides strong evidence in support of the phosphorylation theory.

Additional supportive evidence comes from the use of proteolytically degraded kinases. Brief proteolysis of an impure kinase preparation resulted in the loss of Ca^{2+} sensitivity and the subsequent activation of the Mg^{2+}-ATPase of actomyosin and the phosphorylation of myosin, both in the absence of Ca^{2+} (77). These results, as with the ATPγS experiments, clearly correlate the events of ATPase activation with the phosphorylation of myosin. One approach which is not particularly useful in this context is the correlation of tension development or ATPase activation and phosphorylation of myosin as a function of the Ca^{2+} concentration. It was shown earlier that the activation of actomyosin ATPase activity and the degree of myosin phosphorylation exhibited a similar requirement for Ca^{2+} (4,41, 179). However, these experiments cannot eliminate the possibility that an additional mechanism of activation exists with a Ca^{2+} requirement similar to that of the MLCK.

Leitonin System

The major controversy concerning the regulatory process in smooth muscle is to identify the mechanism that activates the Mg^{2+}-ATPase activity of actomyosin in the presence of Ca^{2+}. The most popular theory is that the phosphorylation of myosin is implicated, although an alternate system has been proposed by Ebashi and his colleagues and termed leiotonin (47,129). The two theories are similar in that each causes an activation of the actomyosin activity in the presence of Ca^{2+}, but they differ in many other respects. The major distinction is that the activation of ATPase activity by leiotonin is thought to be achieved without an accompanying phosphorylation of myosin (128). The leitonin is located on the thin filament where it is functional at relatively high molar ratios of actin to leiotonin, of the order of 100:1 (47). Recent evidence to support the actin-linked nature of leiotonin was obtained by Mikawa (127), who found that cross-linking of smooth muscle thin filaments by glutaraldehyde in the presence or absence of Ca^{2+} resulted in an actin filament frozen in either the activated or inhibited state, respectively. This would argue in favor of a control system which operates via the modification of actin rather than myosin. The leiotonin system also shows a preference for smooth muscle actin and tropomyosin (50) as compared to the skeletal muscle proteins, and this preference is not observed with the phosphorylation mechanism. Originally it was felt that leiotonin was composed of a single protein of molecular weight about 80,000 (47,87), although more recently it was resolved into two components of molecular weights 80,000 and 18,000, and termed leiotonin A and leiotonin C, respectively (129). The latter is an acidic protein which is similar to, but not identical with, calmodulin.

The mechanism of action of leiotonin is not known. It is felt that since such small amounts of leiotonin are required for regulation, its role could not be structural in the sense that the skeletal muscle troponin and tropomyosin components are. Probably its mechanism of action involves an enzymic function, although there is no evidence to support this. Clearly before the relative merits of the leiotonin and the phosphorylation systems can be evaluated, much more information must be obtained.

Summary of the Regulatory Mechanism

It is known that the contractile activity in smooth muscle is regulated by changes in the intracellular concentration of Ca^{2+}. The system that is responsible for the control by Ca^{2+} is different from that found in skeletal muscle (i.e., troponin and tropomyosin) and functions by the activation of a dormant state when the Ca^{2+} concentration is increased. The controversy that exists is centered on identification of the activating principle. The most popular theory is that the state of phosphorylation of the myosin molecule governs the ATPase activity of its complex with actin. A myosin light chain kinase phosphorylates the two 20,000 light chains of myosin and allows activation by actin. This process occurs only in the presence of Ca^{2+} ($> 10^{-6}$ M) and is thought to initiate the contraction of the smooth muscle. As long as the Ca^{2+} concentration remains above that required for activation, the phosphorylated myosin will undergo repeated cycles of actin-mediated ATP hydrolysis, corresponding to the cross-bridge cycles. When the Ca^{2+} concentration is reduced below threshold, the kinase is inactivated and a second enzyme, a myosin light chain phosphatase, removes the phosphate groups from the myosin light chains and returns the myosin molecule to its dormant state. This results in relaxation. An alternative system has been proposed as the regulatory mechanism in smooth muscle, termed leiotonin. It is thought that the leiotonin system does not involve the phosphorylation of myosin and is located on the thin filaments. Its mechanism of action is not known. At the present time the significance of the two distinct theories of regulation has not been resolved. It is possible of course that both mechanisms operate, either within one cell or in different cells, and one system could supplement the other. However, this is pure conjecture and much more data are required before any evaluation can be attempted.

Mechanism of Contraction

This section is intended as a summary of some of the previous discussions. A few key points are abstracted and, in some instances, extended or extrapolated based on our knowledge of the skeletal muscle theory of contraction. The idea is to try to provide a best guess for what is assumed to be the contractile mechanism in smooth muscle. Some aspects of the mechanism remain to be elucidated, and where these are obvious they will be indicated.

The initial assumption is that length changes in smooth muscle occur as a result of varying degrees of overlap of the thick and thin filaments, i.e., the sliding filament mechanism. There is no direct evidence to conclude this, largely because of the lack of a well-ordered filament array in smooth muscle (for further discussion see 55 and 140), but the available data are consistent with this hypothesis. The next assumption is that tension is generated as a consequence of the cyclic cross-bridge–actin interaction, which is associated with the hydrolysis of ATP. Cross-bridges have been observed on smooth muscle thick filaments by electron microscopy (see section on Intracellular Filaments), and low-angle X-ray diffraction data have shown a 14.4 nm meridional reflection (123,124,170) characteristic of cross-bridges projecting from the thick filament with this repeat. A further requirement for the sliding filament theory is that the tension generated by the cross-bridge interactions can be extended or transmitted throughout the cell. In skeletal muscle, the continuous sarcomere structure and thereby the function of the Z-lines in joining adjacent I bands fulfills this requirement. In smooth muscle, it appears that the requirement is also satisfied since the dense body structures are thought to be analogous to Z-lines and interact with the thin filaments, in some instances providing a connection with the plasma membrane. The 100 Å filaments may also serve a passive role in force generation since these are thought to be associated with the dense bodies. Thus the qualitative pattern of the contractile elements in smooth and skeletal muscle has certain similarities which are easily adaptable into a sliding filament mechanism. Some of the unknowns in the smooth muscle system include the way in which the myosin molecules pack to form the thick filament, the lengths of both the thick and thin filaments, and the stoichiometry and spatial relationships between the thick filaments and interacting thin filaments.

Little is known about the kinetics of ATP hydrolysis by smooth muscle actomyosin (i.e., the cross-bridge cycle), and the working hypothesis is that the kinetic scheme is qualitatively similar to that established for the skeletal muscle system. In its simplest form this scheme is presented in Fig. 5. The myosin cross-bridge is dissociated from actin by binding ATP. In the detached state the ATP is hydrolyzed to form ADP and inorganic phosphate, which remain bound to the active site. As a result of hydrolysis, the conformation of the myosin head is altered to assume an "activated" state. This interacts with actin, which accelerates the release of the products of hydrolysis, and the myosin returns to its "ground" state. The latter constitutes the power stroke for contraction. ATP then binds to the vacated myosin active sites and the cross-bridge is dissociated from actin. A point to emphasize is that hydrolysis of ATP occurs with the dissociated cross-bridges (or in *in vitro* assays with myosin alone) and that rapid turnover of ATP molecules will occur only by facilitating release of the hydrolysis products and this is the role of actin. The role of Ca^{2+} in this process is to regulate the cross-bridge–actin interactions. In relaxed muscle the cross-bridges are dissociated and are frozen in the myosin-

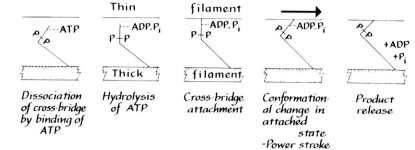

FIG. 5. Schematic representation of the cross-bridge cycle and associated hydrolysis of ATP. The myosin in this scheme is phosphorylated. Only one of the two active sites of myosin is depicted. The reaction sequence shown corresponds to one cycle of the steady-state cycling rate (III) which is discussed earlier.

products complex, only a slow release of ADP and P_i occurs, and this reflects the Mg^{2+}-ATPase of myosin alone.

Details of an equivalent cycle for smooth muscle are not established, and only a few of the steps have been investigated. It has been suggested (126a,136) that the overall pathways for smooth and skeletal muscle are similar, and Marston and Taylor (126a) found that two of the kinetic steps were markedly slower in smooth muscle. One was associated with the hydrolysis of ATP to form the myosin-products complex, and the other reflected a conformational change occurring with the actomyosin-products complex prior to a relatively rapid release of products. The latter was proposed as the rate-limiting step of ATP hydrolysis at 25 °C (as it probably is in the skeletal muscle system). The significance of this finding is that in smooth muscle one would therefore expect the presence of a relatively long-lived attached complex (cross-bridges to actin), and this might help to explain not only the slow maximum speed of contraction but also the high holding economy characteristic of smooth muscle. One criticism of these studies is that they were performed using the myosin fragment, heavy meromyosin subfragment-1, which does not contain its native complement of the 20,000 light chain, and its ATPase activity is not sensitive to changes in the Ca^{2+} concentration. Thus the conclusions mentioned above should be accepted only when they are confirmed using preparations that more closely reflect the properties of the parent myosin molecule. In other studies (199), it was found that the rate of formation of the myosin-products complex for Mg^{2+}-ATP was about the same for arterial and skeletal muscle myosins, and this was apparent also from the work of Marston and Taylor (126a). In summary, the correlation of the known slow rate of smooth muscle contraction with the available kinetic data suggests that the rate-limiting step for contraction is associated with a slow process occurring in the attached cross-bridge state. Some of the events occurring in the detached state are probably also slower for smooth muscle compared to skeletal muscle [e.g., the binding of ATP to myosin (136)], but these are not adequate to account for the observed low rate of Mg^{2+}-ATP hydrolysis by smooth muscle actomyosin.

A note of caution should be added. The previous discussions were based on the assumption that a single rate-limiting event was operative. However, in the smooth muscle literature, there are several indications to suggest that more complex kinetic pathways occur. For example, it was found (171,172) that in taenia coli at intermediate Ca^{2+} levels there was a resistance to stretch which disappeared at lower Ca^{2+} concentrations. This was interpreted to indicate noncycling cross-bridge attachments, i.e., analogous to rigor bonds. Murphy and his collaborators (141) found in pig carotid strips that an initial high rate of shortening velocity was correlated to a rapid phosphorylation of myosin but that after the rapid initial phases both decreased markedly although tension remained relatively constant. In our laboratory we have found that the kinetics of myosin phosphorylation and Mg^{2+}-activated ATPase activity of actomyosin are not linear, and both show a rapid initial phase followed by a slower phase. These examples illustrate that the contractile behavior of smooth muscle does not follow a simple pattern, and it is therefore possible that different kinetic steps are rate limiting at different stages of the contraction sequence. This is relevant in view of the well-known observation (152,153) that smooth muscle can maintain tension in relatively low ATP usage, and it is important to establish the details of the cross-bridge kinetics that will adapt to both the phasic and tonic responses.

ACKNOWLEDGMENT

The author is supported by Grant HL 23615 from the National Institutes of Health.

REFERENCES

1. Adelstein, R. S. (1978): Myosin phosphorylation, cell motility and smooth muscle contraction. *Trends Biochem. Sci.,* 3:27–30.
2. Adelstein, R. S., and Conti, M. A. (1975): Phosphorylation of platelet myosin increases actin-activated myosin ATPase activity. *Nature,* 256:597–598.
3. Adelstein, R. S., Conti, M. A., Hathaway, D. R., and Klee, C. B. (1978): Phosphorylation of smooth muscle myosin light chain kinase by the catalytic subunit of adenosine 3':5'-monophosphate-dependent protein kinase. *J. Biol. Chem.,* 253:8347–8350.
4. Aksoy, M. O., Williams, D., Sharkey, E. M., and Hartshorne, D. J. (1976): A relationship between Ca^{2+} sensitivity and phosphorylation of gizzard actomyosin. *Biochem. Biophys. Res. Commun.,* 69:35–41.

5. Amphlett, G. W., Syska, H., and Perry, S. V. (1976): The polymorphic forms of tropomyosin and troponin I in developing rabbit skeletal muscle. *FEBS Lett.,* 63:22–26.

6. Amphlett, G. W., Vanaman, T. C., and Perry, S. V. (1976): Effect of the troponin C-like protein from bovine brain (brain modulator protein) on the Mg^{2+}-stimulated ATPase of skeletal muscle actomyosin. *FEBS Lett.,* 72:163–168.

7. Anderson, N. L. (1979): The β and γ cytoplasmic actins are differentially thermostabilized by Mg ADP; γ actin binds Mg ADP more strongly. *Biochem. Biophys. Res. Commun.,* 89:486–490.

8. Ashton, F. T., Somlyo, A. V., and Somlyo, A. P. (1975): The contractile apparatus of vascular smooth muscle: intermediate high voltage stereo electron microscopy. *J. Mol. Biol.,* 98:17–29.

9. Bagby, R. M., and Pepe, F. A. (1977): Striations in antimyosin-stained isolated adult smooth muscle cells. *Fed. Proc.,* 36:602.

10. Bárány, M., and Bárány, K. (1980): Phosphorylation of the myofibrillar proteins. *Ann. Rev. Physiol.,* 42:275–292.

11. Barany, M., Barány, K., Gaetjens, E., and Bailin, G. (1966): Chicken gizzard myosin. *Arch. Biochem. Biophys.,* 113:205–221.

12. Barron, J. T., Bárány, M., and Bárány, K. (1979): Phosphorylation of the 20,000-dalton light chain of myosin of intact arterial smooth muscle in rest and in contraction. *J. Biol. Chem.,* 254:4954–4956.

13. Bohr, D. F., Filo, R. S., and Guth, K. F. (1962): Contractile protein in vascular smooth muscle. *Physiol. Rev. [Suppl. 5],* 42:98–112.

14. Bois, R. M. (1973): The organization of the contractile apparatus of vertebrate smooth muscle. *Anat. Rec.,* 117:61–78.

15. Bolton, T. B. (1979): Mechanisms of action of transmitters and other substances on smooth muscle. *Physiol. Rev.,* 59:606–718.

16. Borejdo, J., and Oplatka, A. (1976): Evidence for myosin-linked regulation in guinea pig taenia coli muscle. *Pfluegers Arch. Eur. J. Physiol.,* 366:177–184.

17. Bose, R., and Stephens, N. L. (1977): Mechanism of action of hypoxia in smooth muscle. Role of contractile proteins. In: *The Biochemistry of Smooth Muscle,* edited by N. L. Stephens, pp. 499–512. University Park Press, Baltimore.

18. Bremel, R. D. (1974): Myosin linked calcium regulation in vertebrate smooth muscle. *Nature,* 252:405–407.

19. Bremel, R. D., Sobieszek, A., and Small, J. V. (1977): Regulation of actin-myosin interaction in vertebrate smooth muscle. In: *The Biochemistry of Smooth Muscle,* edited by N. L. Stephens, pp. 533–549. University Park Press, Baltimore.

20. Carsten, M. E. (1971): Uterine smooth muscle: troponin. *Arch. Biochem. Biophys.,* 147:353–357.

21. Cassidy, P. S., Hoar, P. E., and Kerrick, W. G. L. (1979): Irreversible thiophosphorylation and activation of tension in functionally skinned rabbit ileum strips by [^{35}S] ATPγS. *J. Biol. Chem.,* 254:11148–11153.

22. Chacko, S., Conti, M. A., and Adelstein, R. S. (1977): Effect of phosphorylation of smooth muscle myosin on actin activation and Ca^{2+} regulation. *Proc. Natl. Acad. Sci. U.S.A.,* 74:129–133.

23. Chamley, J. H., Campbell, G. R., McConnell, J. D., and Groeschel-Stewart, U. (1977): Comparison of vascular smooth muscle cells from adult human, monkey and rabbit in primary culture and in subculture. *Cell Tissue Res.,* 177:503–522.

24. Cheung, W. Y. (1980): Calmodulin plays a pivotal role in cellular regulation. *Science,* 207:19–27.

25. Cohen, D. M., and Murphy, R. A. (1978): Differences in cellular contractile protein contents among porcine smooth muscles: evidence for variation in the contractile system. *J. Gen. Physiol.,* 72:369–380.

26. Collins, J. H., and Elzinga, M. (1975): The primary structure of actin from rabbit skeletal muscle. *J. Biol. Chem.,* 250:5915–5920.

27. Cooke, P. A. (1976): A filamentous cytoskeleton in vertebrate smooth muscle fibers. *J. Cell Biol.,* 68:539–556.

28. Cooke, P. H., and Fay, F. S. (1972): Correlation between fiber length, ultrastructure, and the length-tension relationship of mammalian smooth muscle. *J. Cell Biol.,* 52:105–116.

29. Craig, R., and Megerman, J. (1977): Assembly of smooth muscle myosin into side-polar filaments. *J. Cell Biol.,* 75:990–996.

30. Craig, R., and Offer, G. (1976): The location of C-protein in rabbit skeletal muscle. *Proc. R. Soc. Lond. [Biol.],* 192:451–461.

31. Csapo, W. (1948): Actomyosin content of the uterus. *Nature,* 162:218–219.

32. Cummins, P. (1979): The homology of the α-chains of cardiac and skeletal rabbit tropomyosin. *J. Mol. Cell. Cardiol.,* 11:109–114.

33. Cummins, P., and Perry, S. V. (1973): The subunits and biological activity of polymorphic forms of tropomyosin. *Biochem. J.,* 133:765–777.

34. Cummins, P., and Perry, S. V. (1974): Chemical and immunochemical characteristics of tropomyosins from striated and smooth muscle. *Biochem. J.,* 141:43–49.

35. Dabrowska, R., Aromatorio, D., Sherry, J. M. F., and Hartshorne, D. J. (1977): Composition of the myosin light chain kinase from chicken gizzard. *Biochem. Biophys. Res. Commun.,* 78:1263–1272.

36. Dabrowska, R., and Hartshorne, D. J. (1978): A Ca^{2+}- and modulator-dependent myosin light chain kinase from non-muscle cells. *Biochem. Biophys. Res. Commun.,* 85:1352–1359.

37. Dabrowska, R., Sherry, J. M. F., Aromatoria, D. K., and Hartshorne, D. J. (1978): Modulator protein as a component of the myosin light chain kinase from chicken gizzard. *Biochemistry,* 17:253–258.

38. d'Albis, A., Pantaloni, C., and Bechet, J.-J. (1979): An electrophoretic study of native myosin isozymes and of their subunit content. *Eur. J. Biochem.,* 99:261–271.

39. Debbas, G., Hoffman, L., Landon, E. J., and Hurwitz, L. (1975): Electron microscopic localization of calcium in vascular smooth muscle. *Anat. Rec.,* 182:447–471.

40. Devine, C. E., and Somlyo, A. P. (1971): Thick filaments in vascular smooth muscle. *J. Cell Biol.,* 49:636–649.

41. DiSalvo, J., Gruenstein, E., and Silver, P. (1978): Ca^{2+} dependent phosphorylation of bovine aortic actomyosin. *Proc. Soc. Exp. Biol. Med.,* 158:410–414.

42. Driska, S. P. (1976): Calcium control of smooth muscle contractile proteins. Ph. D. thesis, Carnegie-Mellon University, Pittsburgh.

43. Driska, S., and Hartshorne, D. J. (1975): The contractile proteins of smooth muscle. Properties and components of a Ca^{2+}-sensitive actomyosin from chicken gizzard. *Arch. Biochem. Biophys.,* 167:203–212.

44. Eaton, B. L., Kominz, D. R., and Eisenberg, E. (1975): Correlation between the inhibition of the acto-heavy meromyosin ATPase and the binding of tropomyosin to F-actin: effects of Mg^{2+}, KCl, troponin I, and troponin C. *Biochemistry,* 14:2718–2725.

45. Ebashi, S., Iwakura, H., Nakajima, H., Nakamura, R., and Ooi, Y. (1966): New structural proteins from dog heart and chicken gizzard. *Biochem. Z.,* 345:201–211.

46. Ebashi, S., Kodama, A., and Ebashi, F. (1968): Troponin I. Preparation and physiological function. *J. Biochem. (Tokyo),* 64:465–477.

47. Ebashi, S., Mikawa, T., Hirata, M., Toyo-oka, T., and Nonomura, Y. (1977): Regulatory proteins of smooth muscle. In: *Excitation-Contraction Coupling in Smooth Muscle,* edited by R. Casteels, T. Godfraind, and J. C. Rüegg, pp. 325–334. Elsevier/North-Holland Biomedical Press, Amsterdam.

48. Ebashi, S., Nonomura, Y., Kitazawa, T., and Toyo-oka, T. (1975): Troponin in tissues other than skeletal muscle. In: *Calcium Transport in Contraction and Secretion,* edited by E. Carofoli, F. Clementi, W. Drabikowski, and A. Margreth, pp. 405–414. North-Holland, Amsterdam.

49. Ebashi, S., Nonomura, Y., Toyo-oka, T., and Katayama, E. (1976): Regulation of muscle contraction by the calcium-troponin-tropomyosin system. In: *Calcium in Biological Systems,* edited by C. J. Duncan, pp. 349–360. Cambridge University Press, London.

50. Ebashi, S., Toyo-oka, T., and Nonumura, Y. (1975): Gizzard troponin. *J. Biochem. (Tokyo),* 78:859–861.

51. Eisenberg, E., and Kielley, W. W. (1974): Troponin-tropomyosin complex. Column chromatographic separation and activity of the three active troponin components with and without tropomyosin present. *J. Biol. Chem.,* 249:4742–4748.

52. Elliott, A., and Offer, G. (1978): Shape and flexibility of the myosin molecule. *J. Mol. Biol.,* 123:505–519.

53. Elzinga, M., Collins, J. H., Kuehl, W. M., and Adelstein, R. S. (1973): Complete amino-acid sequence of actin of rabbit skeletal muscle. *Proc. Natl. Acad. Sci. U.S.A.,* 70:2687–2691.

54. Engel, J., Fasold, H., Hulla, F. W., Waechter, F., and Wegner, A. (1977): The polymerization reaction of muscle actin. *Mol. Cell. Biochem.,* 18:3–13.

55. Fay, F. S., Rees, D. D., and Warshaw, D. M. (1980): Contractile mechanism of smooth muscle. In: *Membrane Structure and Function,* edited by E. Bittar. John Wiley and Sons, New York *(in press).*

56. Fay, F. S., Shlevin, H. H., Granger, W. C., Jr., and Taylor, S. R. (1979): Aequorin luminescence during activation of single isolated smooth muscle cells. *Nature,* 280:506–508.

57. Filo, R. S., Bohr, D. F., and Ruegg, J. C. (1965): Glycerinated skeletal and smooth muscle: Calcium and magnesium dependence. *Science,* 147:1581–1583.

58. Fine, R. E., and Blitz, A. L. (1975): A chemical comparison of tropomyosins from muscle and non-muscle tissues. *J. Mol. Biol.,* 95:447–454.

59. Forbes, M. S., Rennels, M. L., and Nelson, E. (1979): Caveolar systems and sarcoplasmic reticulum in coronary smooth muscle cells of the mouse. *J. Ultrastruct. Res.,* 67:325–339.

60. Ford, G. D., and Hess, M. L. (1975): Calcium-accumulating properties of subcellular fractions of bovine vascular smooth muscle. *Circ. Res.,* 37:580–587.

61. Frearson, N., Focant, B. W. W., and Perry, S. V. (1976): Phosphorylation of a light chain component of myosin from smooth muscle. *FEBS Lett.,* 63:27–32.

62. Frearson, N., and Perry, S. V. (1975): Phosphorylation of the light-chain components of myosin from cardiac and red skeletal muscles. *Biochem. J.,* 151:99–107.

63. Frederiksen, D. W. (1976): Myosin-mediated Ca^{++}-regulation of actomyosin-adenosinetriphosphatase from porcine aorta. *Proc. Natl. Acad. Sci. U.S.A.,* 73:2706–2710.

64. Frederiksen, D. W. (1979): Physical properties of myosin from aortic smooth muscle. *Biochemistry,* 18:1651–1656.

65. Gabella, G. (1971): Caveolae intracellulares and sarcoplasmic reticulum in smooth muscle. *J. Cell Sci.,* 8:601–609.

66. Gergely, P., Vereb, G., and Bot, G. (1976): Thiophosphate-activated phosphorylase kinase as a probe in the regulation of phosphorylase phosphatase. *Biochim. Biophys. Acta,* 429:809–816.

67. Gorecka, A., Aksoy, M. O., and Hartshorne, D. J. (1976): The effect of phosphorylation of gizzard myosin on actin activation. *Biochem. Biophys. Res. Commun.,* 71:325–331.

68. Grand, R. J. A., and Perry, S. V. (1978): The amino acid sequence of the troponin C-like protein (modulator protein) from bovine uterus. *FEBS Lett.,* 92:137–142.

69. Grand, R. J. A., Perry, S. V., and Weeks, R. A. (1979): Troponin C-like proteins (calmodulins) from mammalian smooth muscle and other tissues. *Biochem. J.,* 177:521–529.

70. Gratecos, D., and Fischer, E. H. (1974): Adenosine 5′-o(3-thiotriphosphate) in the control of phosphorylase activity. *Biochem. Biophys. Res. Commun.,* 58:960–967.

71. Groeschel-Stewart, U., Chamley, J. H., Campbell, G. R., and Burnstock, G. (1975): Changes in myosin distribution in dedifferentiating and redifferentiating smooth muscle cells in tissue culture. *Cell Tissue Res.,* 165:13–22.

72. Hamoir, G., and Laszt, L. (1962): Tonomyosin of arterial muscle. *Nature,* 193:682–684.

73. Hanson, J., and Lowy, J. (1963): The structure of F-actin and of actin filaments isolated from muscle. *J. Mol. Biol.,* 6:46–60.

74. Hanson, J., and Lowy, J. (1964): The problem of the location of myosin in vertebrate smooth muscle (discussion). *Proc. R. Soc. Lond. [Biol.],* 160:523–524.

75. Hartshorne, D. J., Abrams, L., Aksoy, M. O., Dabrowska, R. Driska, S., and Sharkey, E. M. (1977): Molecular basis for the regulation of smooth muscle actomyosin. In: *The Biochemistry of Smooth Muscle,* edited by N. L. Stephens, pp. 513–532. University Park Press, Baltimore.

76. Hartshorne, D. J., and Gorecka, A. (1980): The biochemistry of the contractile proteins of smooth muscle. In: *Handbook of Physiology, Section 2. The Cardiovascular System, Vol. II. Vascular Smooth Muscle,* edited by D. F. Bohr, A. P. Somlyo, and H. V. Sparks, pp. 93–120. American Physiology Society, Bethesda, Md.

77. Hartshorne, D. J., Gorecka, A., and Aksoy, M. O. (1977): Aspects of the regulatory mechanism in smooth muscle. In: *Excitation-Contraction Coupling in Smooth Muscle,* edited by R. Casteels, T. Godfraind, and J. C. Rüegg, pp. 377–384. Elsevier/North-Holland Biomedical Press, Amsterdam.

78. Hartshorne, D. J., Siemankowski, R. F., and Aksoy, M. O. (1980): Ca regulation in smooth muscle and phosphorylation: Some properties of the myosin light chain kinase. In: *Regulatory Mechanism of Muscle Contraction,* edited by S. Ebashi, K. Maruyama, and M. Endo, pp. 287–301. Japan Soc. Promotion of Sci. and Fujihara Found. of Sci., Tokyo.

79. Hathaway, D. R., and Adelstein, R. S. (1979): Human platelet myosin light chain kinase requires the calcium-binding protein calmodulin for activity. *Proc. Natl. Acad. Sci. U.S.A.,* 76:1653–1657.

80. Hayashi, J., Ishimoda, T., and Hirabayashi, T. (1977): On the heterogeneity and organ specificity of chicken tropomyosins. *J. Biochem. (Tokyo),* 81:1487–1495.

81. Head, J. F., Mader, S., and Kaminer, B. (1977): Troponin-C-like modulator protein from vertebrate smooth muscle. In: *Calcium Binding Proteins and Calcium Function,* edited by R. H. Wasserman, R. A. Corradino, E. Carafoli, R. H. Kretsinger, D. H. MacLennan, and F. L. Siegel, pp. 275–277. Elsevier/North-Holland Publishing Co., Amsterdam.

82. Head, J. F., Weeks, R. A., and Perry, S. V. (1977): Affinity-chromatographic isolation and some properties of troponin C from different muscle types. *Biochem. J.,* 161:465–471.

83. Heumann, H.-G. (1969): Gibt es in glatten Vertebraten muskeln dicke Filamente? Elektronenmikroskopische Untersuchungen an der Darm-muskulature der Hausmaus. *Zool Anz. [Suppl. BD] Verh. Zool. Ges.,* 33:416–424.

84. Heumann, H.-G. (1976): The subcellular localization of calcium in vertebrate smooth muscle: Calcium-containing and calcium-accumulating structures in muscle cells of mouse intestine. *Cell Tissue Res.,* 169:221–231.

85. Hidaka, H., Naka, M., and Yamaki, T. (1979): Effect of novel specific myosin light chain kinase inhibitors on Ca^{2+}-activated Mg^{2+}-ATPase of chicken gizzard actomyosin. *Biochem. Biophys. Res. Commun.,* 90:694–699.

86. Hinssen, H., D'Haese, J., Small, J. V., and Sobieszek, A. (1978): Mode of filament assembly of myosins from muscle and nonmuscle cells. *J. Ultrastruct. Res.,* 64:282–302.

87. Hirata, M., Mikawa, T., Nonomura, Y., and Ebashi, S. (1977): Ca^{2+} regulation in vascular smooth muscle. *J. Biochem. (Tokyo),* 82:1793–1796.

88. Hoar, P. E., Kerrick, W. G. L., and Cassidy, P. S. (1979): Chicken gizzard: Relation between calcium-activated phosphorylation and contraction. *Science,* 204:503–506.

89. Hoh, J. F. Y., and Yeoh, G. P. S. (1979): Rabbit skeletal myosin isoenzymes from fetal, fast-twitch and slow-twitch muscles. *Nature,* 280:321–323.

90. Huszar, G., and Bailey, P. (1979): Relationship between actin-myosin interaction and myosin light chain phosphorylation in human placental smooth muscle. *Am. J. Obstet. Gynecol.,* 135:718–726.

91. Huxley, A. F. (1957): Muscle structure and theories of contraction. *Prog. Biophys. Mol. Biol.,* 7:257–318.

92. Huxley, A. F., and Niedergerke, R. (1954): Structural changes in muscle during contraction. *Nature,* 173:971–973.

93. Huxley, H. E. (1963): Electron microscope studies on the structure of natural and synthetic protein filaments from striated muscle. *J. Mol. Biol.,* 7:281–308.

94. Huxley, H. E., and Hanson, J. (1954): Changes in the cross-striations of muscle during contraction and stretch and their structural interpretation. *Nature,* 173:973–976.

95. Huys, J. (1963): Données nouvelles sur l'actomyosine d'uterus human gravide. *Bull. Soc. R. Belge Gynecol. Obstet.,* 33:429–443.

96. Ikebe, M., Aiba, T., Onishi, H., and Watanabe, S. (1978): Calcium sensitivity of contractile proteins from chicken gizzard muscle. *J. Biochem. (Tokyo),* 83:1643–1655.

97. Ikebe, M., Onishi, H., and Watanabe, S. (1977): Phosphorylation and dephosphorylation of a light chain of the chicken gizzard myosin molecule. *J. Biochem. (Tokyo)*, 82:299–302.

98. Ito, N., and Hotta, K. (1976): Regulatory protein of bovine tracheal smooth muscle. *J. Biochem. (Tokyo)*, 80:401–403.

99. Ito, N., Takagi, T., and Hotta, K. (1976): Regulatory protein of vascular smooth muscle. *J. Biochem. (Tokyo)*, 80:899–901.

100. Jakes, R., Northrop, F., and Kendrick-Jones, J. (1976): Calcium binding regions of myosin 'regulatory' light chains. *FEBS Lett.*, 70:229–234.

101. Janis, R. A., and Gualteri, R. T. (1978): Contraction of intact smooth muscle is associated with the phosphorylation of a 20,000 dalton protein. *Physiologist*, 21:59.

102. Johansson, B., and Somlyo, A. P. (1980): Electrophysiology and excitation-contraction coupling. In: *Handbook of Physiology, Section 2. The Cardiovascular System, Vol. II. Vascular Smooth Muscle*, edited by D. F. Bohr, A. P. Somlyo, and H. V. Sparks, pp. 301–323. American Physiology Society, Bethesda, Md.

103. Johnson, L. S. (1974): Non-identical tropomyosin subunits in rat skeletal muscle. *Biochim. Biophys. Acta*, 371:219–225.

104. Kaminer, B. (1969): Synthetic myosin filaments from vertebrate smooth muscle. *J. Mol. Biol.*, 39:257–264.

105. Katoh, N., and Kubo, S. (1977): Purification and some properties of rabbit stomach myosin. *J. Biochem. (Tokyo)*, 81:1497–1503.

106. Kelley, R. E., and Rice, R. V. (1968): Localization of myosin filaments in smooth muscle. *J. Cell Biol.*, 37:105–116.

107. Kendrick-Jones, J. (1973): The subunit structure of gizzard myosin. *Philos. Trans. R. Soc. Lond. [Biol.]*, 265:183–189.

108. Kendrick-Jones, J., Lehman, W., and Szent-Györgyi, A. G. (1970): Regulation in molluscan moscles. *J. Mol. Biol.*, 54:313–326.

109. Kendrick-Jones, J., Szentkiralyi, E. M., and Szent-Györgyi, A. G. (1976): Regulatory light chains in myosins. *J. Mol. Biol.*, 104:747–775.

110. Kerrick, W. G. L., Hoar, P. E., and Cassidy, P. S. (1980): Ca^{2+}-activated tension: The role of myosin light chain phosphorylation. *Fed. Proc.*, 39:1558–1563.

111. Koretz, J. F. (1979): Effects of C-protein on synthetic myosin filament structure. *Biophys. J.*, 27:433–446.

112. Laszt, L. (1961): Properties of vessel muscle proteins extracted with water or salt solutions of low ionic strength. *Nature*, 189:230.

113. Laszt, L. (1964): Was ist Gefässtonus? Untersuchunger über die Beziehungen Zwischen Gefässmuskelkon, traktion und-volumen änderung. *Angiologica*, 1:346–356.

114. Laszt, L., and Hamoir, G. (1961): Etude par electrophorèse et ultracentrifugation de la composition protéinique de la conche musculaire des carotides de bovidé. *Biochim. Biophys. Acta*, 50:430–449.

115. Lazarides, E. (1980): Intermediate filaments as mechanical integrators of cellular space. *Nature*, 283:249–256.

116. Leger, J., Bouveret, P., Schwartz, K., and Swynghedauw, B. (1976): A comparative study of skeletal and cardiac tropomyosin. Subunits, thiol group content and biological activities. *Pfluegers Arch.*, 362:271–277.

117. Leger, J. J., and Focant, B. (1973): Low molecular weight components of cow smooth muscle myosins: Characterization and comparison with those of striated muscle. *Biochim. Biophys. Acta*, 328:166–172.

118. Lehman, W., Kendrick-Jones, J., and Szent-Györgyi, A. G. (1972): Myosin-linked regulatory systems: comparative studies. *Cold Spring Harbor Symp. Quant. Biol.*, 37:319–330.

119. Lehman, W., and Szent-Györgyi, A. G. (1975): Regulation of muscular contraction. Distribution of actin control and myosin control in the animal kingdom. *J. Gen. Physiol.*, 66:1–30.

120. Levin, R. M., and Weiss, B. (1977): Binding of trifluoperazine to the calcium-dependent activator of cyclic nucleotide phosphodiesterase. *Mol. Pharmacol.*, 13:690–697.

121. Lowey, S., Benfield, P. A., Silberstein, L., and Lang, L. M. (1979): Distribution of light chains in fast skeletal myosin. *Nature*, 282:522–524.

122. Lowey, S., and Risby, D. (1971): Light chains from fast and slow muscle myosins. *Nature*, 234:81–85.

123. Lowy, J., Poulsen, F. R., and Vibert, P. J. (1970): Myosin filaments in vertebrate smooth muscle. *Nature*, 225:1053–1054.

124. Lowy, J., Vibert, P. J., Haselgrove, J. C., and Poulsen, F. R. (1973): The structure of the myosin elements in vertebrate smooth muscles. *Philos. Trans. R. Soc. Lond. [Biol.]*, 265:191–196.

125. Mak, A. S., Lewis, W. G., and Smillie, L. B. (1979): Amino acid sequences of rabbit skeletal β- and cardiac tropomyosins. *FEBS Lett.*, 105:232–234.

126. Margossian, S. S., and Lowey, S. (1973): Substructure of the myosin molecule. III. Preparation of single-headed derivatives of myosin. *J. Mol. Biol.*, 74:301–311.

126a. Marston, S. B., and Taylor, E. W. (1978): Mechanism of myosin and actomyosin ATPase in chicken gizzard smooth muscle. *FEBS Lett.*, 86:167–170.

127. Mikawa, T. (1979): Freezing of the calcium-regulated structures of gizzard thin filaments by glutaraldehyde. *J. Biochem. (Tokyo)*, 85:879–881.

128. Mikawa, T., Nonomura, Y., and Ebashi, S. (1977): Does phosphorylation of myosin light chain have direct relation to regulation in smooth muscle? *J. Biochem. (Tokyo)*, 82:1789–1791.

129. Mikawa, T., Nonomura, Y., Hirata, M., Ebashi, S., and Kakiuchi, S. (1978): Involvement of an acidic protein in regulation of smooth muscle contraction by the tropomyosin-leiotonin system. *J. Biochem. (Tokyo)*, 84:1633–1636.

130. Moos, C., Offer, G., Starr, R., and Bennett, P. (1975): Interaction of C-protein with myosin, myosin rod and light meromyosin. *J. Mol. Biol.*, 97:1–9.

131. Morgan, M., Perry, S. V., and Ottaway, J. (1976): Myosin light-chain phosphatase. *Biochem. J.*, 157:687–697.

132. Mrwa, U., Achtig, I., and Rüegg, J. C. (1974): Influences of calcium concentration and pH on the tension development and ATPase activity of the arterial actomyosin contractile system. *Blood Vessels*, 11:277–286.

133. Mrwa, U., and Hartshorne, D. J. (1980): Phosphorylation of smooth muscle myosin and myosin light chains. *Fed. Proc.* 39:1564–1568.

134. Mrwa, U., Paul, R. J., Kreye, V. A. W., and Rüegg, J. C. (1975): The contractile mechanism of vascular smooth muscle. *INSERM*, 50:319–326.

135. Mrwa, U., and Rüegg, J. C. (1975): Myosin-linked calcium regulation in vascular smooth muscle. *FEBS Lett.*, 60:81–84.

136. Mrwa, U., and Trentham, D. (1975): Transient kinetic studies of the Mg^{2+}-dependent arterial myosin and actomyosin adenosine triphosphatases isolated from porcine carotids. *Hoppe-Seylers Z. Physiol. Chem.*, 356:255.

137. Mrwa, U., Troschka, M., and Rüegg, J. C. (1979): Cyclic AMP-dependent inhibition of smooth muscle actomyosin. *FEBS Lett.*, 107:371–374.

138. Murphy, R. A. (1969): Contractile proteins of vascular smooth muscle: Effects of hydrogen and alkali metal cations on actomyosin adenosine triphosphatase activity. *Microvasc. Res.*, 1:344–353.

139. Murphy, R. A. (1971): Arterial actomyosin: Effects of pH and temperature on solubility and ATPase activity. *Am. J. Physiol.*, 220:1494–1500.

140. Murphy, R. A. (1979): Filament organization and contractile function in vertebrate smooth muscle. *Annu. Rev. Physiol.*, 41:737–748.

141. Murphy, R. A., Aksoy, M. O., and Dillon, P. F. (1980): Regulation in vascular smooth muscle: Ca^{2+}-dependent myosin light chain phosphorylation mediates cross-bridge cycling rates. *Fed. Proc.*, 39:1817.

142. Murphy, R. A., Herlihy, J. T., and Megerman, J. (1974): Force-generating capacity and contractile protein content of arterial smooth muscle. *J. Gen. Physiol.*, 64:691–705.

143. Murphy, R. A., and Megerman, J. (1977): Protein interactions in the contractile system of vertebrate smooth muscle. In: *The Biochemistry of Smooth Muscle*, edited by N. L. Stephens, pp. 473–498. University Park Press, Baltimore.

144. Murray, J. M., and Weber, A. (1974): The cooperative action of muscle proteins. *Sci. Am.*, 230:58–71.

145. Nairn, A. C., and Perry, S. V. (1979): Calmodulin and myosin light-chain kinase of rabbit fast skeletal muscle. *Biochem. J.*, 179:89–97.

146. Needham, D. M., and Cawkwell, J. M. (1956): Some properties of the actomyosin-like protein of the uterus. *Biochem J.*, 63:337–344.

147. Nonomura, Y. (1968): Myofilaments in smooth muscle of guinea pig's taenia coli. *J. Cell Biol.*, 39:741–745.

148. Onishi, H., and Watanabe, S. (1979): Chicken gizzard heavy meromyosin that retains the two light-chain components, including a phosphorylatable one. *J. Biochem. (Tokyo)*, 85:457–472.

149. Ookubo, N., Ueno, H., and Ooi, T. (1975): Similarities and differences of the α and β components of tropomyosin. *J. Biochem. (Tokyo)*, 78:739–747.

150. Parry, D. A. D. (1975): Analysis of the primary sequence of α-tropomyosin from rabbit skeletal muscle. *J. Mol. Biol.*, 98:519–535.

151. Parry, D. A. D., and Squire, J. M. (1973): Structural role of tropomyosin in muscle regulation: Analysis of the x-ray diffraction patterns from relaxed and contracting muscles. *J. Mol. Biol.*, 75:33–55.

152. Paul, R. J., Glück, E., and Rüegg, J. C. (1976): Cross-bridge ATP utilization in arterial smooth muscle. *Pfluegers Arch.*, 361:297–299.

153. Paul, R. J., and Rüegg, J. C. (1976): Biochemistry of vascular smooth muscle: Energy metabolism and the proteins of the contractile apparatus. In: *Microcirculation*, edited by B. M. Altura and G. Kaley, pp. 41–82. University Park Press, Baltimore.

154. Pepe, F. A., and Drucker, B. (1975): The myosin filament. III. C-protein. *J. Mol. Biol.*, 99:609–617.

155. Perrie, W. T., Smillie, L. B., and Perry, S. V. (1973): A phosphorylated light-chain component of myosin from skeletal muscle. *Biochem. J.*, 135:151–164.

156. Pires, E. M. V., and Perry, S. V. (1977): Purification and properties of myosin light-chain kinase from fast skeletal muscle. *Biochem. J.*, 167:137–146.

157. Pires, E., Perry, S. V., and Thomas, M. A. W. (1974): Myosin light chain kinase, a new enzyme from striated muscle. *FEBS Lett.*, 41:292–296.

158. Pollard, T. D., and Weihing, R. R. (1974): Actin and myosin and cell movement. *CRC Crit. Rev. Biochem.*, 2:1–65.

159. Rubenstein, P. A., and Spudich, J. A. (1977): Actin microheterogeneity in chick embryo fibroblasts. *Proc. Natl. Acad. Sci. U.S.A.*, 74:120–123.

160. Rüegg, J. C., Strassner, E., and Schirmer, R. H. (1965): Extraktion und Reinigung von Arterien-Actomyosin, Actin, und Extraglobulin. *Biochem. Z.*, 343:70–85.

161. Rushbrook, J. I., and Stracher, A. (1979): Comparison of adult, embryonic, and dystrophic myosin heavy chains from chicken muscle by sodium dodecyl sulfate/polyacrylamide gel electrophoresis and peptide mapping. *Proc. Natl. Acad. Sci. U.S.A.*, 76:4331–4334.

162. Russell, W. E. (1973): Insolubilization and activation of arterial actomyosin by bivalent cations. *Eur. J. Biochem.*, 33:459–466.

163. Schollmeyer, J. E., Furcht, L. T., Goll, D. E., Robson, R. M., and Stromer, M. H. (1976): Localization of contractile proteins in smooth muscle cells and in normal and transformed fibroblasts. In: *Cell Motility, Vol. 3, book A*, edited by R. Goldman, T. Pollard, and J. Rosenbaum, pp. 361–388. Cold Spring Harbor Labs., Cold Spring Harbor, N.Y.

164. Seidel, J. C. (1978): Chymotryptic heavy meromyosin from gizzard myosin: A proteolytic fragment with the regulatory properties of the intact myosin. *Biochem. Biophys. Res. Commun.*, 85:107–113.

165. Sekine, T., Barnett, L. M., and Kielley, W. W. (1962): The active site of myosin adenosine triphosphatase. I. Localization of one of the sulfhydryl groups. *J. Biol. Chem.*, 237:2769–2772.

166. Sherry, J. M. F., Gorecka, A., Aksoy, M. O., Dabrowska, R., and Hartshorne, D. J. (1978): Roles of calcium and phosphorylation in the regulation of the activity of gizzard myosin. *Biochemistry*, 17:4411–4418.

167. Shibata, N., Yamagami, T., Yoneda, S., Akagami, H., Takeuchi, K., Tanaka, K., and Okamura, Y. (1973): Identification of myosin A, actin and native tropomyosin constitution of arterial contractile protein (myosin B) and their characteristics. *Jpn. Circ. J.*, 37:229–252.

168. Shoenberg, C. F. (1965): Contractile proteins of vertebrate smooth muscle. *Nature*, 206:526–527.

169. Shoenberg, C. F. (1969): An electron microscope study of the influence of divalent ions on myosin filament formation in chicken gizzard extracts and homogenates. *Tissue Cell*, 1:83–96.

170. Shoenberg, C. F., and Haselgrove, J. C. (1974): Filaments and ribbons in vertebrate smooth muscle. *Nature*, 249:152–154.

171. Siegman, M. J., Butler, T. M., Mooers, S. U., and Davies, R. E. (1976): Calcium-dependent resistance to stretch and stress relaxation in resting smooth muscles. *Am. J. Physiol.*, 231:1501–1508.

172. Siegman, M. J., Butler, T. M., Mooers, S. U., and Davies, R. E. (1976): Cross-bridge attachment, resistance to stretch, and viscoelasticity in resting mammalian smooth muscle. *Science*, 191:383–385.

173. Silver, P. J., and DiSalvo, J. (1979): Adenosine $3':5'$-monophosphate-mediated inhibition of myosin light chain phosphorylation in bovine aortic actomyosin. *J. Biol. Chem.*, 254:9951–9954.

174. Small, J. V. (1977): Studies on isolated smooth muscle cells: The contractile apparatus. *J. Cell Sci.*, 24:327–349.

175. Small, J. V., and Sobieszek, A. (1977): Myosin phosphorylation and Ca-regulation in vertebrate smooth muscle. In: *Excitation-Contraction Coupling in Smooth Muscle*, edited by R. Casteels, T. Godfraind, and J. C. Rüegg, pp. 385–393. Elsevier/North-Holland Biomedical Press, Amsterdam.

176. Small, J. V., and Sobieszek, A. (1977): Ca-regulation of mammalian smooth muscle actomyosin via a kinase-phosphatase-dependent phosphorylation and dephosphorylation of the 20,000-M_r light chain of myosin. *Eur. J. Biochem.*, 76:521–530.

177. Small, J. V., and Sobieszek, A. (1977): Studies on the function and composition of the 10-nm (100 Å) filaments of vertebrate smooth muscle. *J. Cell Sci.* 23:243–268.

178. Sobieszek, A. (1977): Ca-linked phosphorylation of a light chain of vertebrate smooth-muscle myosin. *Eur. J. Biochem.*, 73:477–483.

179. Sobieszek, A. (1977): Vertebrate smooth muscle myosin. Enzymatic and structural properties. In: *The Biochemistry of Smooth Muscle*, edited by N. L. Stephens, pp. 413–443. University Park Press, Baltimore.

180. Sobieszek, A., and Bremel, R. D. (1975): Preparation and properties of vertebrate smooth-muscle myofibrils and actomyosin. *Eur. J. Biochem.*, 55:49–60.

181. Sobieszek, A., and Small, J. V. (1973): The assembly of ribbon-shaped structures in low ionic strength extracts obtained from vertebrate smooth muscle. *Philos. Trans. R. Soc. Lond. [Biol.]*, 265:203–212.

182. Sobieszek, A., and Small, J. V. (1976): Myosin-linked calcium regulation in vertebrate smooth muscle. *J. Mol. Biol.*, 102:75–92.

183. Sobieszek, A., and Small, J. V. (1977): Regulation of the actin-myosin interaction in vertebrate smooth muscle: Activation via a myosin light-chain kinase and the effect of tropomyosin. *J. Mol. Biol.*, 112:559–576.

184. Somlyo, A. V. (1980): Ultrastructure of vascular smooth muscle. In: *Handbook of Physiology, Section 2. The Cardiovascular System, Vol. II. Vascular Smooth Muscle*, edited by D. F. Bohr, A. P. Somlyo, and H. V. Sparks, pp. 33–67. American Physiology Society, Bethesda, Md.

185. Somlyo, A. P., Devine, C. E., Somlyo, A. V., and Rice, R. V. (1973): Filament organization in vertebrate smooth muscle. *Philos. Trans. R. Soc. Lond. [Biol.]*, 265:223–229.

186. Somlyo, A. V., and Somlyo, A. P. (1971): Strontium accumulation by sarcoplasmic reticulum and mitochondria in vascular smooth muscle. *Science*, 174:955–958.

187. Somlyo, A. P., Somlyo, A. V., Devine, C. E., Peters, P. D., and Hall, T. A. (1974): Electron microscopy and electron probe analysis of mitochondrial cation accumulation in smooth muscle. *J. Cell Biol.*, 61:723–742.

188. Somlyo, A. P., Somlyo, A. V., and Shuman, H. (1979): Electron probe analysis of vascular smooth muscle. Composition of mitochondria, nuclei, and cytoplasm. *J. Cell Biol.*, 81:316–335.

189. Sparrow, M. P., Maxwell, L. C., Rüegg, J. C., and Bohr, D. F. (1970): Preparation and properties of a calcium ion-sensitive actomyosin from arteries. *Am. J. Physiol.*, 219:1366–1372.

190. Sparrow, M. P., and van Bockxmeer, F. M. (1972): Arterial tropomyosin and a relaxing protein fraction from vascular smooth muscle. Comparison with skeletal tropomyosin and troponin. *J. Biochem. (Tokyo),* 72:1075–1080.

191. Stewart, M., and McLachlan, A. D. (1975): Fourteen actin-binding sites on tropomyosin? *Nature,* 257:331–333.

192. Stone, D., and Smillie, L. V. (1978): The amino acid sequence of rabbit skeletal α-tropomyosin. The NH$_2$-terminal half and complete sequence. *J. Biol. Chem.,* 253:1137–1148.

193. Stone, D., Sodek, J., Johnson, P., and Smillie, L. B. (1974): Tropomyosin: correlation of amino acid sequence and structure. *FEBS Lett.,* 31:125–136.

194. Strasburg, G. M., and Greaser, M. L. (1976): The native subunit pattern of tropomyosin. *FEBS Lett.,* 72:11–14.

195. Sugi, H., and Daimon, T. (1977): Translocation of intracellularly stored calcium during the contraction-relaxation cycle in guinea pig taenia coli. *Nature,* 269:436–438.

196. Suzuki, H., Onishi, H., Takahashi, K., and Watanabe, S. (1978): Structure and function of chicken gizzard myosin. *J. Biochem. (Tokyo),* 84:1529–1542.

197. Suzuki, K., Yamaguchi, M., and Sekine, T. (1978): Two forms of chicken gizzard F-actin depending on preparation with or without added calcium. *J. Biochem. (Tokyo),* 83:869–878.

198. Szent-Györgyi, A. G., Szentkiralyi, E. M., and Kendrick-Jones, J. (1973): The light chains of scallop myosin as regulatory subunits. *J. Mol. Biol.,* 74:179–203.

199. Takeuchi, K., and Tonomura, Y. (1977): Kinetic and regulatory properties of myosin adenosinetriphosphatase purified from arterial smooth muscle. *J. Biochem. (Tokyo),* 82:813–833.

200. Vandekerckhove, J., and Weber, K. (1978): Actin amino-acid sequences. Comparison of actins from calf thymus, bovine brain, and SV 40-transformed mouse 3T3 cells with rabbit skeletal muscle actin. *Eur. J. Biochem.,* 90:451–462.

201. Vandekerckhove, J., and Weber, K. (1978): Mammalian cytoplasmic actins are the products of at least two genes and differ in primary structure in at least 25 identified positions from skeletal muscle actins. *Proc. Natl. Acad. Sci. U.S.A.,* 75:1106–1110.

202. Vibert, P. J., Haselgrove, J. C., Lowy, J., and Poulsen, F. R. (1972): Structural changes in actin-containing filaments of muscle. *J. Mol. Biol.,* 71:757–767.

203. Wachsberger, P., and Kaldor, G. (1971): Studies on uterine myosin A and actomyosin. *Arch. Biochem. Biophys.* 143:127–137.

204. Wachsberger, P. R., and Pepe, F. A. (1974): Purification of uterine myosin and synthetic filament formation. *J. Mol. Biol.,* 88:385–391.

205. Waisman, D. M., Singh, T. J., and Wang, J. H. (1978): The modulator-dependent protein kinase. A multifunctional protein kinase activatable by the Ca^{2+}-dependent modulator protein of the cyclic nucleotide system. *J. Biol. Chem.,* 253:3387–3390.

206. Wang, J. H. (1977): Calcium-regulated protein modulator in cyclic nucleotide systems. In: *Cyclic, 3', 5'-Nucleotides: Mechanisms of Action,* edited by H. Cramer and J. Schultz, pp. 37–56. John Wiley and Sons, Lond.

207. Weeds, A. G., and Lowey, S. (1971): Substructure of the myosin molecule. II. The light chains of myosin. *J. Mol. Biol.,* 61:701–725.

208. Weeds, A. G., and Taylor, R. S. (1975): Separation of subfragment-1 isoenzymes from rabbit skeletal muscle myosin. *Nature,* 257:54–56.

209. Whalen, R. G., Butler-Browne, G. S., and Gros, F. (1976): Protein synthesis and actin heterogeneity in calf muscle cells in culture. *Proc. Natl. Acad. Sci. U.S.A.,* 73:2018–2022.

210. Yamaguchi, M., Greaser, M. L., and Cassens, R. G. (1974): Interactions of troponin subunits with different forms of tropomyosin. *J. Ultrastruct. Res.,* 48:33–58.

211. Yamaguchi, M., Miyazawa, Y., and Sekine, T. (1970): Preparation and properties of smooth muscle myosin from horse esophagus. *Biochim. Biophys. Acta,* 216:411–421.

212. Yazawa, M., Kuwayama, H., and Yagi, K. (1978): Modulator protein as a Ca^{2+}-dependent activator of rabbit skeletal myosin light-chain kinase. Purification and characterization. *J. Biochem. (Tokyo),* 84:1253–1258.

213. Yazawa, M., and Yagi, K. (1978): Purification of modulator-deficient myosin light-chain kinase by modulator protein-Sepharose affinity chromatography. *J. Biochem. (Tokyo),* 84:1259–1265.

214. Yerna, M.-J., Aksoy, M. O., Hartshorne, D. J., and Goldman, R. D. (1978): BHK 21 myosin: Isolation, biochemical characterization and intracellular localization. *J. Cell Sci.,* 31:411–429.

215. Yerna, M.-J., Dabrowska, R., Hartshorne, D. J., and Goldman, R. D. (1979): Calcium-sensitive regulation of actin-myosin interactions in baby hamster kidney (BHK-21) cells. *Proc. Natl. Acad. Sci. U.S.A.,* 76:184–188.

216. Zechel, K. (1979): Localization of the charge differences in the actins of rabbit skeletal muscle and chicken gizzard by two-dimensional gel electrophoretic analysis of tryptic fragments. *Hoppe-Seyler's Z. Physiol. Chem.,* 360:777–782.

Physiology of the Gastrointestinal Tract, edited by
Leonard R. Johnson. Raven Press, New York © 1981.

Chapter 8

Smooth Muscle: Mechanochemical Energy Conversion Relations Between Metabolism and Contractility

Richard J. Paul

This chapter focuses on the role of smooth muscle as the ultimate effector of gastrointestinal motility. Although smooth muscle has other notable talents, as, for example, the ability to synthesize elastin and collagen fibers, its primary function is the conversion of chemical to mechanical energy. In generating force, shortening, or performing mechanical work, muscle is unusual among mechanical devices in that it effects the direct conversion of chemical energy into a mechanical output. Its efficiency and wide range of operating specifications surpass those of most man-made devices.

Our knowledge of smooth muscle, although not as detailed as that of skeletal muscle, is now coming of age. Skeletal muscle properties are no longer needed as models for smooth muscle, but can be used in a true comparative sense to illustrate differences that may ultimately lead to the understanding of molecular mechanisms. Smooth muscle generally operates at lower contraction speeds in lower power output ranges and is much more economical than its skeletal muscle counterpart. Smooth and skeletal muscle also both utilize ATP as their immediate source of chemical energy, but here again one finds considerable differences in the strategies of metabolic synthesis involved. As both smooth and skeletal muscle contractile systems are composed of similar actin and myosin components, the mechanisms underlying these differences are of considerable interest among muscle physiologists.

The first step to understanding any mechanochemical process, whether one deals more comfortably with the language of chemical input and mechanical output or with that of metabolism and contractility, is to characterize both ends of the energy conversion. I have chosen to begin with the output or mechanics as it will better serve to orient one to smooth muscle studies. This is followed by a consideration of the energy metabolism of smooth muscle. With this information, the next stage is to develop a picture of the relation between mechanics and energetics. While primarily dealing at the cellular level, I will attempt to pull together what is known about these processes working toward the reductionist goal of explaining smooth muscle mechanochemistry in terms of molecular mechanisms while also trying to relate the relations between metabolism and contractility to their role in the context of the whole organism.

I have approached this review from a didactic rather than a pedagogic point of view. My point of view may be made clearer in light of the following analogy. For astronomers, the Copernican view of the universe is generally regarded as the more correct model than the Ptolemeic. The Copernican system can well account for the erratic behavior of a few exceptional heavenly bodies. However, in navigation the Ptolemeic view of an earth-centered universe produces a much simpler method of finding one's path through the darkness. When possible, I have opted for simple descriptive models to navigate through the current body of smooth muscle knowledge, fully aware that more complex hypotheses will eventually be needed to describe the intricacies of smooth muscle behavior. In keeping with a didactic approach, the references cited are illustrative and not intended to be exhaustive.

I would like to apologize to many researchers whose work was not cited, and emphasize that the references were chosen only as samples from a rapidly growing literature. I have freely borrowed from recent reviews and would like to acknowledge these sources for additional references. For skeletal muscle mechanics, Simmons and Jewell (122); for smooth muscle mechanics, Murphy (95), Johansson (70), and Peterson (109); for smooth muscle mechanochemistry, Paul and Peterson (106) and Paul (103); for smooth muscle in general, Stephens (125).

I would further like to emphasize that smooth muscle is not a homogeneous entity. Differences between smooth muscles can be as great as those between smooth and skeletal muscle. However, I am forced for brevity and didactic reasons to generalize about smooth muscle, presuming a degree of homogeneity that may not exist. This may be somewhat counterbalanced by my personal idiosyncrasy of stressing what is not known with certainty over the generally accepted. Hopefully with this in mind, one can better grasp the overview that I am attempting to present.

MECHANICS—SMOOTH MUSCLE OUTPUT

The most striking characteristic of muscle tissue is its ability to shorten and generate force. Measurement of these mechanical parameters is deceptively simple; interpretation of mechanical data, however, is not as straightforward. As with most physiological problems, questions can be formulated at subcellular, cellular, tissue, and organ levels, and it is quite exceptional that any single experimental design can successfully provide information at several levels. Unfortunately, much ambiguity arises in the literature on smooth muscle mechanics when extrapolating to cellular and subcellular mechanisms on the basis of mechanical experiments on strips of tissue cut from smooth muscle containing organs. As our knowledge of cellular level properties is primarily based on such evidence, I will point out some of the hazards in the interpretation of these results.

Interpretation of Mechanical Data

Cellular Orientation, Content, and Type

A prerequisite for cellular level interpretation is a knowledge of the orientation of the smooth muscle cells. This is of particular importance in whole tissue studies in which results are often complicated by mul-

tiple cellular orientations. One must be aware of both longitudinal and circumferential cell layers, for example, in esophagogastric preparations. One also must bear in mind that cell orientation may be altered by changes in tissue length, a particular pitfall encountered when helically cut preparations are used. Although useful information can be obtained from *in vitro* strips studies, extrapolation to cellular properties requires precise knowledge of cell orientation.

Along with orientation, cellular content plays an important role in analysis of whole tissue mechanical studies. Comparison of the force-generating capacities between tissues at the level of cellular components requires knowledge of the cellular content as well as orientation. Although this fact appears obvious, in practice this is not often achieved. In general, histological evidence on each preparation is laborious to obtain; minimally, force should be normalized to tissue cross-sectional area to provide a first-order basis for comparison. As our knowledge of smooth muscle increases in sophistication, the types of cells present may become of increasing importance in interpretation of mechanical data. At the present time, little information on the homogeniety of smooth muscle cells within a particular cell layer is available. Differences in the mechanical properties and agonist sensitivity of smooth muscle from circumferential and longitudinal layers of various smooth muscles are summarized by Vanhoutte (137). This opens the possibility that within a single layer, different smooth muscle types, analogous to different skeletal muscle fiber types, may exist. Although consideration of these factors may at first appear to add unnecessary complexity to interpretation of smooth muscle mechanics, future progress in relating the mechanical behavior at tissue and organ levels to cellular properties will depend on experiments designed in view of these potential complexities.

Mechanical State

The factors thus far discussed in relation to interpretation of mechanical data have all related to anatomical or histological properties of the tissue preparation under investigation. These structural factors are not particular to smooth muscle studies and are equally applicable to muscle mechanics in general. The functional definition and measurement of smooth muscle activity, however, has plagued interpretation of mechanical data to a far greater extent than its counterpart in skeletal muscle studies. Skeletal muscle activity has a clearly measurable resting state, characterized by negligible contractile activity, against which various levels of muscle activity can be referenced. Many smooth muscles, on the other hand, always appear to have some level of activity, and assessment of the true "resting state" has proven to be a considerable stumbling block in interpreting mechanical studies. With the advantage of hindsight, we can define muscular activity in terms of molecular events as the level of actomyosin interaction. Muscle activity in the smooth muscle literature goes by various names: tonus, tone, contractility, and active state, among the most frequently used. Although we are currently in a better position to define smooth muscle activity, measurement of a reference or resting state is still as formidable a problem with many smooth muscle preparations as it was for physiologists at the earlier part of this century (14,100). This is of particular significance in studies of intestinal smooth muscle where spontaneous rhythmic activity may be superimposed on a constant level of tone. Attempts to achieve a reference state of reduced muscle activity have included inhibition of activity by cooling (46) or the use of metabolic poisons (22). However, it has been reported (57,113) that anoxia and substrate removal have differential effects on the tonic and phasic components of whole tissue activity. This evidence also raises the possibility of different smooth muscle types and suggests further caution in assessing the measurements of the reference state. In the absence of readily obtainable basal state activity, experiments are often designed to measure changes in muscle activity in response to a given intervention either as a change in muscle length under a fixed load or as a change in isometric force at a fixed reference length. Although both protocols can yield useful information, the latter is generally easier to interpret. Because of the effects of passive tension and the relation between force and length, changes in muscle length are not linearly related to muscle activity. Thus shortening does not produce a measure of activity as easily as changes in isometric force; this is of particular importance in understanding metabolic studies [see Paul (102) and below]. Although listing these reservations about interpretations of mechanical data at this point runs the risk of setting into nihilistic a tone, the goal is to set a reasonably critical attitude to the broad generalizations I will make about smooth muscle that a review of this nature requires.

Statics

Isometric Contraction

Measurement of force at fixed overall tissue length can provide considerable information about muscle properties. The most striking feature of smooth muscle is the variety of responses encountered. In the unstimulated state, one observes a range of responses from spontaneous, maintained levels of isometric force or rhythmic contractions, to, as with many tissues, no apparent activity. Even greater variability is seen in response to agonists. To understand the basis for this behavior, one would have to do tissue-by-tissue analysis.

Most evidence suggests that these phenomena have little to do with mechanics *per se*, but instead relate to variability in excitation and excitation-contraction coupling in smooth muscle. These latter topics are considered elsewhere in this volume, and, although important, only tend to complicate mechanical studies. Of interest in the context of this review is the time course and estimation of the maximum force-generating capacity. Both parameters are important to the understanding of function at both cellular and organ levels. Table 1 gives these parameters for various smooth muscles studied. The major determinants of isometric force are tissue length (discussed in detail in the next section) and level of activation of actomyosin interaction. Although the optimum length can be determined with relative ease, the time course and maximization of activation are difficult to assess. As time course studies depend on techniques and parameters more suitably dealt with after consideration of transient steady-state behavior, its discussion will be deferred for the moment. Experimental conditions leading to maximum or at least constant levels of actomyosin interaction, essential to straightforward interpretation of mechanical data at the molecular level, are often difficult to obtain with certainty. Depolarization of the muscle membrane by electrical stimulation or altering the external K^+ concentration does not generally produce the maximum isometric force in smooth muscle. Agonists such as carbachol, epinephrine, or histamine often elicit much larger forces.

The concentration of intracellular Ca^{2+} is the major determinant of actomyosin activity and hence isometric force in smooth muscle (37). However, most vertebrate smooth muscle studied shows a myosin-linked regulatory mechanism with the possibility that this may coexist with a thin-filament regulatory mechanism as well. This allows for multiple sites for control, and in particular for modulation of the Ca^{2+} sensitivity itself, for example, by phosphorylation of the light chain kinase (3). Thus the variety of responses cannot be uniquely ascribed to differential effects of agonist on Ca^{2+} concentration.

In practice, one has little recourse in attempting to maximize isometric force in intact tissue preparations other than utilizing a variety of agonists or combinations of agonists and optimizing the response. The relation of this value to the maximum tissue capacity is a matter of one's bias. Preparations in which the sarcolemma has been removed or made permeable by various "skinning" procedures would appear to be one experimental way to approach the question of maximum force-generating capacity, as controlled levels of Ca^{2+} may be easily adjusted. Up to this point, such preparations generally develop less isometric force under supposedly optimum Ca^{2+} concentrations. This may be due to impairment by the skinning procedure of the intercellular connections (see below) related to force

TABLE 1. *Isometric force characteristics*

Muscle type	Temp. °C	Stimulus	Maximum isometric tension P_0 mN/mm^2	Time to $\frac{1}{2}$ max force $t_{1/2}$ (sec)	Reference
Skeletal muscle					
Frog	10	Tetanic	345	0.1	Hodgkin and Horowicz (62)
Semitendinosus	20	100 mMK$^+$	363	0.5	Hodgkin and Horowicz (62)
Frog sartorius	0	Tetanic	250	0.2	Kushmerick (78)
Cat calf muscles	In vivo	Nerve stim.	127	—	Helander and Thulen (52)
Mouse soleus	24.5	Tetanic	100	0.1	Edwards et al. (34)
Crayfish extensor Carpopoditi	18–24	173 mMK$^+$	759	0.3	Zacher and Zacharova (145)
Vascular smooth muscle					
Bovine mesenteric artery	37	Epinephrine	206	150	Lundholm and Mohme-Lundholm (83)
Bovine mesenteric vein	37	Epinephrine	73	30	Paul and Peterson (105)
Hog carotid artery (media)	37	30 mMK$^+$	223	70	Seidel and Murphy (120)
Hog carotid artery (media)	37	Histamine	87	30	Glück and Paul (43)
Rat mesenteric artery	37	155 mMK$^+$	74	1.5	Halpern et al. (48)
Visceral smooth muscle					
Taenia coli, guinea pig	37	Carbachol	417	7	Gabella (41)
Taenia coli, guinea pig	37	Electrical field	260	4	Lowy and Mulvany (80)
Taenia coli, guinea pig	37	K$^+$	178	1	Åberg and Axelsson (2)
Taenia coli, rabbit	22	Electrical field	87	2.5	Gordon and Siegman (46)
Cat duodenum	30	Electrical field	73	1.5	Meiss (87)
Rabbit mesotubarium	25	Electrical field	25	0.3	Meiss (88)
Rabbit uterus	27	Electrical field	13	2	Czapo and Goodall (28)
Dog trachaelis	37	Electrical field	108	3	Stephens and Niekerk (129)
Invertebrate smooth muscle					
Mytilus, ABRM	20	Phasic	700	30	Baguet and Gillis (11)
	20	Tonic	350	30	Baguet and Gillis (12)

transmission in the tissue or of the regulatory system itself. These points are purely speculative, and further discussion is beyond the scope of this review. The values given in Table 1 should be viewed, then, as only the best operational definitions of maximum force-generating ability.

The values of maximal isometric force in Table 1 show considerable variability, not unanticipated in light of the above discussion. One can conclude, however, that smooth muscle is capable of generating at least as much force as skeletal muscle. This is an important bit of evidence to be reconciled in the molecular mechanism of smooth muscle force production, for smooth muscle contains only between 1/10 to 1/5 of the myosin contained in skeletal muscle (51,96,132). For a thorough investigation of this point, one is referred to the work of Murphy (95) and Gabella (41). A basis for large force-generating capacity relative to myosin content in smooth muscle has been proposed on both structural and functional grounds.

When normalized to cellular content, guinea pig taenia coli is reported to generate 734 mN/mm^2(41). Gabella (41) suggests that these large forces may be due to the intercellular structures in the tissue through which the individual cells transfer force. He presents evidence

for structures in smooth muscle analogous to the intramuscular tendons of pennate skeletal muscle types. In this type of structural arrangement, one has effectively more cells exerting their forces in parallel, and hence a larger apparent force per cross-sectional area.

At the subcellular level, long sarcomeres relative to skeletal muscle could also provide a structural basis for more parallel force-generating units, i.e., the myosin cross-bridges, and larger force per cellular cross-sectional area. Although evidence on the effective sarcomere length in smooth muscle is scanty, the length of smooth muscle thick filaments is not dramatically larger than that of their skeletal muscle counterparts (9). Thus an intracellular structural basis appears unlikely to be a predominant factor for the large force-generating capacities of smooth muscle cells as estimated from whole tissue measurements. The contribution of effective sarcomere length will be reconsidered in terms of the economy of smooth muscle tension maintenance (below); a comprehensive account of the effect of such structural factors is presented by Rüegg (117).

The relatively large forces generated by vascular smooth muscle, on the other hand, cannot be explained in terms of pennate-like transmission of cellular forces. Driska and Murphy (33) present evidence indicating that force transmission in arterial tissue behaves as though the smooth muscle cells were in series. An important implication of this work is that in this tissue cellular mechanical properties can be inferred from whole tissue studies which would not be as straightforward for other possible arrangements.

The recent work of Fay and co-workers (35,36) on the mechanical properties of isolated smooth muscle cells from the toad (*Bufo marinus*) stomach has shed considerable light on the question of the force-generating capacity at the cellular level. Fay has reported maximum isometric focus for single cells to be on the order of 260 mN/mm^2, although considerable variability in this parameter was seen. Thus the large forces seen in certain tissues can be accounted for solely in terms of cellular properties, without invoking intercellular structural factors.

The values presented in Table 1 can also be used to estimate physiological properties at the organ level. For example, one can estimate a "safety factor," in terms of the whole organ's capacity to react to loads. This requires accurate knowledge of organ geometries and the assumptions and approximations inherent in material stress analysis (31,112). Fortunately, many smooth muscle lined organs have tubular geometries and reasonable estimates can be made; for example, the force per cross-sectional area required by a vessel to contract against a given blood pressure can be readily estimated (102). These estimated forces when compared to forces developed by isolated vascular strips indicate that there is a considerable safety factor for all sizes of vessels studied.

Isometric Force–Tissue Length Relation

The relation between the isometric force capacity and tissue length has been intensively studied in smooth muscle. Similar studies on skeletal muscle (44) have provided the basis for the accepted sliding filament model of muscle contraction as well as defining the physiological range of length over which muscle tissue can effectively operate.

Interpretation of force-length relations at any level of cellular organization is subject to all the reservations previously discussed and, with the addition of a new variable, even more caution. In particular, mechanical interpretations of data presume that cell orientation and the level of activation are not functions of length. In cardiac muscle, for example, changes in muscle activity with tissue length are a major determinant of the force-length relation (67).

When smooth muscle force-length behavior has been characterized, the protocols and terminology have largely evolved from skeletal muscle experimentation. The relation between force and length is measured under unstimulated conditions, generating the "passive" length-

tension characteristics. This measurement is repeated under conditions designed to ensure maximum and constant activation, and as this measurement also contains the passive length-tension characteristics, the relation generated is called the total force-length relation. Operationally, the passive force-length relation is subtracted from the total force-length relation, generating the active force-length relation, so-called because it is designed to reflect the behavior of the active muscle elements, presumably the change in actomyosin interaction with length. These ideal characteristics are shown in Fig. 1, curves fit to data from bovine mesenteric vein (105). The model inherent to this analysis is often referred to as a Maxwell or Hill model. Other models based on series and parallel combinations of active and passive elements have been proposed, such as the Voigt model in which a parallel combination of an active and passive element is connected in series to another passive element. Although it is unrealistic to expect that any simple model could provide a complete description of the mechanics of these complicated structures, two parallel elements not only appear to be sufficient to explain the mechanical behavior, but also there is some evidence to indicate that it may be the correct model (32,93). Identification of the exact tissue structures corresponding to these parallel elements, however, cannot as yet be made with complete certainty. Of particular relevance are the recent reports of Bagby and Fisher (10), Fay et al. (36), and Mulvany and Warshaw (94). These studies on isolated cells or on a preparation in which the cells can be visualized allow for clearer separation between cellular and extracellular components of the force-length relation.

Passive tension in smooth muscle arises primarily from extracellular connective tissue, consisting mainly of collagen and elastin. The force-extension characteristics of this parallel passive element can be adequately described as an exponential spring; force $= Ae^{k\Delta l/l_o}$, where A and k are constants and $\Delta l/l_o$ the relative change in length. Although important physiologically as a major stress-bearing component, this element does not play a role in regulation and control of function. Changes in parallel passive element characteristics with age or myopathy, however, can play an important role in organ function [for example, see Dobrin (31)]. The major focus of interest in force-length studies has centered on the active isometric force-length characteristics, because of its importance both in describing organ function and in providing information on the mechanism of smooth muscle contractility. Representative active force-length relations for representative visceral and vascular smooth muscles are presented in Fig. 2. The active force-length curves are similar in form to those obtained from skeletal muscle; however, one must be cautious in assuming that this similarity can extend to the underlying structural basis. In skeletal muscle, sarcomere length can be

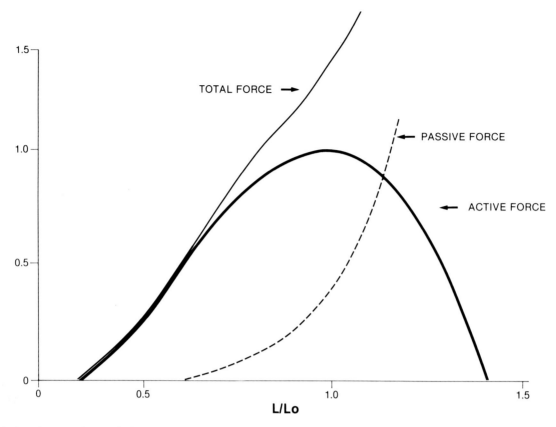

FIG. 1. Relations between isometric force and muscle length. Characteristics of bovine mesenteric vein adapted from Paul and Peterson (105). *Ordinate:* isometric force normalized to the maximum active isometric force. *Abscissa:* tissue length normalized to the length at which maximum active isometric force is measured. Passive force represents the characteristic measured in an unstimulated tissue. Total force represents the characteristic measured in a maximally stimulated tissue. Active force, ascribable to the active contractile elements, is the difference between total and passive force characteristics.

accurately measured and used as a true reference length. Smooth muscle unfortunately does not have readily identifiable structural features comparable to sarcomeres, and use of the optimum length for isometric force generation, l_o, as a reference length—although operationally useful—is not as precise.

Mulvany and Warshaw (94) have shown a proportionality between cell length and tissue length. The distribution of values was, however, quite broad and they further noted that the activation produced a substantial rearrangement of cells. It is thus quite probable that not all cells are at the same point on their force-length curves at a given tissue length. Whole tissue force-length curves must be viewed then as an average of individual smooth muscle cells properties. In view of this, and because of the different sizes of smooth muscle cells in vascular and visceral tissue, there is a surprising degree of similarity in the tissue force-length relations given in Fig. 2. Smooth muscle appears to have a slightly larger working range than skeletal muscle. Under maximum activation, skeletal muscle can shorten to 0.5 l_o (116), whereas smooth muscle can maximally contract at least to 0.3 to 0.4 l_o. Certain visceral muscles, canine bronchus (126), rabbit bladder (135), rabbit mesotubarium

(89), and isolated toad stomach cells (10,35) have been reported to shorten to as small as 0.2 l_o, although changes in cell orientation in whole tissues and uncertainty in assessment of a comparable l_o in isolated cells may reduce the significance of this value.

The descending limb of the force-length curve, of significance to tests of sliding filament theories, has proven to be a region of severe experimental difficulty in smooth muscle studies. In addition to the presence of large passive tensions, the irreversibility of measurements in this range (94,111) has complicated measurement of active isometric force. Fay (35) has found that use of isolated cells, in which passive tension was small at lengths up to 3 times the resting cell length, could overcome some of the experimental problems inherent in whole tissue studies. The length at which no force could be generated on the descending limb of the force-length curve in these single cells was longer than that estimated from whole tissue studies ($\sim$1.8 l_o). Whether this is a property of these large single cells or a tissue property of all smooth muscles but masked by cellular inhomogeneity cannot be determined. These lengths, however, are not significantly different from the lengths in skeletal muscle at which thin and thick filaments

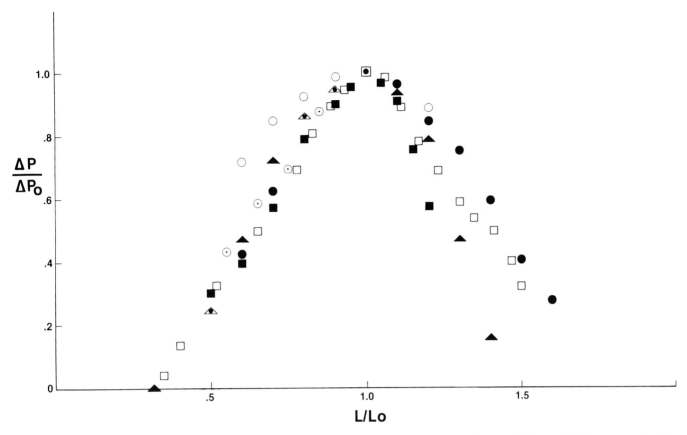

FIG. 2. Active force-length characteristic of various vascular and visceral smooth muscles. *Ordinate:* active isometric force normalized to the maximum isometric force. *Abscissa:* tissue length normalized to the length at which maximum active isometric force is generated. *Filled symbols* represent vascular smooth muscle: ●, rat mesenteric arterioles (94); ■, porcine carotid artery (58); ▲, bovine mesenteric vein (105). *Open symbols* represent visceral smooth muscle: ○, guinea pig taenia coil (80); □, cat intestinal muscle (87); △, rabbit taenia coli (45).

reach a nonoverlap configuration. Although the evidence is not as convincing as that for skeletal muscle, the active force-length curves measured in smooth muscle are most simply interpreted in terms of a sliding filament model analogous to that generally accepted for smooth muscle. A model of a sliding filament mechanism constructed to fit the less organized filament structure of smooth muscle is shown in Fig. 3.

Steady-State Relations Between Force and Velocity

Although much information has been derived from isometric measurements, studies under conditions in which muscle is allowed to contract are inherently more interesting physiologically. As for the isometric studies, the easiest conditions to study are those in which steady values of force and velocities are obtained, in which case transients, particularly those related to activation, can be ignored. However, because muscle length, and hence filament overlap, are continuously changing during contraction, a true steady state cannot be achieved. In skeletal muscle studies, this problem has been approached with a certain degree of success by extrapolating the measured values of force and velocity to the

initial study values. This procedure has been generally adopted for smooth muscle studies, although its application is considerably more arbitrary. In smooth muscle studies, assignment of initial study values is far less certain than for skeletal muscle. In fact, most records of smooth muscle velocity or force do not show a clearly defined steady period, and in general, some fixed time after the contraction is arbitrarily chosen for the measurement of force and velocity.

Three types of conditions for measurement of force-velocity characteristics have generally been used. The first is the classic afterloaded isotonic contraction in, which a muscle, whose length is initially determined by a preload, is constrained such that it cannot lengthen but can freely shorten isotonically when the force it develops is equal to the afterload placed on it. A second is the isometric release method in which a muscle is released from an isometric contraction to a fixed load against which it shortens. The third, less often reported, involves measurement of force when the muscle is constrained to contract at a fixed velocity. The force-velocity characteristic of skeletal muscle is reported to be independent of the experimental conditions used to generate the relation (61,68). For smooth muscle, however,

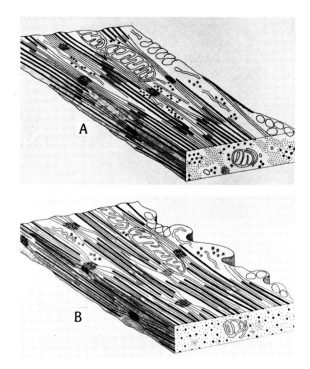

FIG. 3. Schematic diagrams of section of smooth muscle cell in relaxed (**A**) and contracted (**B**) state. In the relaxed muscle (**A**), the thick filaments are grouped together, separate from the thin filaments. The thin filaments are connected to the dense bodies. During contraction (**B**), the thin filaments slide and interdigitate between the thick filaments, and the thin and thick filaments form a more regular pattern. The contraction of the filament units is transferred to the cell membrane, where dense bodies are present. At long cell lengths, the average interaction between thick and thin filaments would be reduced, presumably accounting for the decline in isometric force at long tissue lengths as shown in Figs. 1 and 2. Adapted from Heumann (59).

the situation appears more complex. Peterson (108) reported that the characteristics of force-velocity relations were different when measured by afterload or isometric release conditions and attributed the differences in part to differences in initial contractile element length, inherent under afterload or isometric release conditions. Hellstrand and Johansson (55) also reported that the force-velocity characteristic of rat portal vein was dependent on whether afterload or isometric conditions were used. Their results were opposite to those of Peterson (108), with afterloaded contraction speeds being slower than that found under a similar load under isometric release conditions. This they attributed to incomplete activation under afterloaded conditions. In addition, interpretation of smooth muscle force-velocity data is further complicated by differences reported to be dependent on the mode of stimulation. For example, in vascular tissue K^+-depolarization can elicit larger isometric forces than electrical stimulation; shortening velocities, however, are greater at low loads with electrically stimulated tissue strips (95). Similar stimulus dependence of force-velocity characteristics has been reported (49,55).

Hill's (60) hyperbolic relation between force and velocity is the most common mathematical treatment of smooth muscle data, although these can be adequately described by many mathematical formulations. Data are fit to the formula $(P + a)(V + b) = b(P_o + a)$, where P is the developed force, V is the shortening velocity, P_o is the isometric force, and a and b are constants. Values of these Hill parameters for representative smooth muscles are given in Table 2. Because of the identity $a/P_o = b/V_{max}$, aP_o and V_{max} are sufficient to define the Hill equation which is shown graphically in Fig. 5. The parameters listed are descriptive of the active contractile elements in the muscle as experiments were generally performed at lengths at which passive elements could be neglected and also because contribu-

TABLE 2. *Force-velocity characteristics*

	a/P_0	$V_{max}(l_o/s)$	Reference	Notes[a]
Skeletal				
Frog sartorius	0.26	1.29	Hill (62)	0°C
Rat gracilis anticus		7	Bahler et al. (13)	17.5°C
Vascular smooth muscle				
Carotid media, hog	0.18	0.12	Herlihy and Murphy (58)	Isometric release
Mesenteric vein, calf	0.5	0.0175	Peterson (108)	Afterload
	0.1	0.0073	Peterson (108)	Isometric release
Mesenteric arteriole, rat	0.23	0.133	Mulvany (93)	Isometric release
	0.25	0.068		27°C " "
Portal vein, rat	0.73	0.74	Hellstrand and Johansson (55)	Isometric release Spontaneous contraction
Visceral smooth muscle				
Taenia coli, rabbit	0.331	0.031	Gordon and Siegman (45)	23°C
Taenia coli, guinea pig	0.18	0.1	Lowy and Mulvany (80)	23°C
Taenia coli, guinea pig	0.17	0.3	Mashima and Handa (85)	
Duodenal, circular, cat	0.24	0.094	Meiss (87)	30°C
Trachaelis, dog	0.23	0.3	Stephens (124)	

[a]Data obtained at 37°C unless otherwise noted.

tion of any elements in series with the active elements (see below) would be constant under these steady-state conditions. The a/P_o characteristic of the Hill equation shows a high degree of uniformity for all muscle types, with the exception of the portal vein (Table 2) which is potentially related to measurements made during a spontaneous, non-steady-state contraction, and it appears to be relatively insensitive to temperature. V_{max}, on the other hand, varies considerably with muscle type and temperature. Most mammalian smooth muscles appear to have maximum shortening capacities between 0.1 and 0.3 l_o/s at 37°C.

Although useful in describing the physiologically important relation between force and shortening velocity in a self-consistent manner, the Hill equation has proven somewhat of an enigma in terms of its underlying mechanism. In skeletal muscle studies, there have been numerous attempts to explain the molecular mechanism, particularly in relation to the parameters measured in muscle energetics (61,141). However, no hypothesis appears to be even close to acceptance in explaining the relation between force and velocity in contrast to the nearly universal acceptance of a sliding filament model to explain the relation between force and length.

For the case of smooth muscle, force-velocity data can be treated in a similar manner as in skeletal muscle studies; however, the degree of analogy is even less good than in the case of force-length comparisons. The Hill-type behavior of the force-velocity relation in smooth muscle, which for the present can be viewed only as an empirical fit, is useful in predicting such behavior at tissue levels although it may not reflect the same mechanisms as are found in skeletal muscle.

Studies of Mechanical Transients

A two-element model consisting of a passive element in parallel with a contractile element obeying Hill's force-velocity equation can adequately describe static and steady-state mechanical properties of muscle. This model cannot, however, account for responses to rapid changes in load or length. In 1938 Hill (60) proposed that the addition of an elastic element in series with the active contractile component could more accurately model muscle mechanical behavior, including rapid transients. This model element, known as the "series elastic element" (S.E.), was viewed as a passive element, and though much stiffer, showed similar exponential spring characteristics as the passive parallel element (P.E.) (68). In studies of whole muscle, the tendons could be readily identified with making a contribution to the S.E. and directed attention to other passive elements in series with the contractile elements. On the whole, inclusion of this element enables non-steady-state behavior of whole muscles, for example, the de-

velopment of force during an isometric tetanus, to be adequately portrayed. Adoption of this model has further allowed for a phenomenological description of the time course of an active state of the contractile elements. By various experimental procedures, the effects of the series component can be separated from the contractile component such that the time course of the maximum force-bearing capacity of the contractile component could be estimated. Although considerably slower than the time course of the active state for skeletal muscle (84), the active state of smooth muscle shows an analogous time course (46,69,87).

Within the last decade, there has been a tremendous resurgence of interest in the S.E. component, as it has been shown that part of the series elasticity can be related to active elements, and in particular to mechanics at the cross-bridge level itself (66). This change in viewing the S.E. component was brought about by various technical improvements (increased resolution of measuring apparatus and improved ability to impose rapid mechanical transients), and in particular to development of preparations and techniques in which extracellular series compliance and its effects could be reduced to a minimum.

The series elastic component is usually referred to in terms of its extension, $\Delta l/l_o$, when it is bearing a load equal to the maximum isometric force, P_o. Earlier measurements of this S.E. extension in whole skeletal muscle were on the order of 3 to 5% (68), whereas recent measurements on single skeletal fibers place the value at less than 1%. This latter value is critical as it translates to an extension of about 10 nm per half-sarcomere, the fundamental working unit of muscle (38). This value is compatible with the dimensions of the extension attributed to the head region of the myosin molecule, and suggests that the S.E. behavior may in part be related to contractile element function at the level of the myosin cross-bridge itself. This finding has precipitated intensive investigation into the behavior of mechanical transients in the hope of uncovering the molecular basis of contraction.

Two types of experiments have been generally used to investigate the properties of the series elastic component. One type involves measurement of force transients after imposition of rapid step changes in length, whereas the other relates to length transients following rapid step changes in force. These are illustrated in Fig. 4. Rapid changes are essential, for one needs to assume that the responses can be distinguished from the steady-state behavior of the contractile elements. The imposition of mechanical changes in times less than 1 msec, which creates considerable technical difficulty, is essential for skeletal muscle studies. At least four separate phases in the response of skeletal muscle to rapid changes in force or length have been observed, and several theories of cross-bridge mechanics have been put forth (1,25,38).

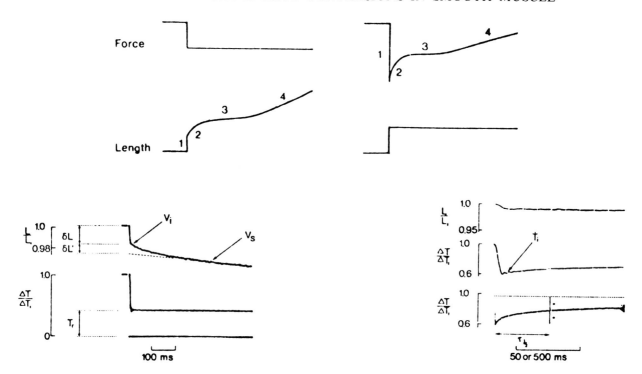

FIG. 4. Upper panel: Schematic drawing of mechanical transients as described in frog skeletal muscle (65). *Left panel* "velocity (or isotonic) transient." *Right panel* "force transient." Shortening is indicated as an upward deflection of the length record. In the model proposed by Huxley and Simmons (65, 66), phase 1 is attributed to elastic recoil in attached cross-bridges, phase 2 (1–2 msec at 0°C) to a viscoelastic relaxation in attached bridges, phase 3 (5–20 msec) to adjustment of the rates of attachment and detachment of bridges after the step, with change in detachment rate coming to an end first. Phase 4 represents shortening, or tension redevelopment, respectively, with attachment as the predominant process. After Hellstrand (54). **Lower panel:** Mechanical transients in rat arterioles at 37°C, from Mulvany (93). Shortening in this study is indicated by a downward deflection in the length record. *Left side:* Isotonic release recorded with oscilloscope showing imposed load change (*center trace*) and resulting displacement change (*top trace*). The *bottom trace* shows the resting tension before activation. *Right side:* Isometric release recorded with oscilloscope by using two different time bases: bar is 50 msec for upper two traces and 500 msec for bottom trace. Top trace shows imposed internal circumference change, *lower two traces* the wall tension response. The dashed line above the bottom trace shows the wall tension 10 sec after the release.

Treatment of the S.E. component of smooth muscle has predictably followed the lead of skeletal muscle physiology. In older literature, addition of an S.E. element was phenomenologically adequate to explain transient behavior. However, the S.E. extension of smooth muscle was considerably larger than its skeletal muscle counterpart, being in the range of 10 to 20% [see Murphy (95)]. In recent experiments, improved techniques appear to have also affected reduction in smooth muscle S.E. extension measurements, although the best estimates are substantially greater (3 to 7%) than can be attributed to cross-bridge properties. This is not unreasonable in light of smooth muscle structure where force must be transmitted via series connections between cells. This factor complicates interpretation of smooth muscle transient responses in terms of cross-bridge mechanics. This problem has been carefully investigated for various smooth muscle preparations by Hellstrand and Johansson (56), Meiss (89), Peterson (109), and Mulvany (93). Although their results vary somewhat, they do not report transient responses in smooth muscle to show the distinct four phases observed in skeletal muscle, although two different stages are clearly discernible. All groups report certain features, notably temperature de-

pendence, which suggests some involvement of cross-bridge mechanics in the observed responses to transient changes in force or length. Current interest focuses on the measurement of instantaneous stiffness, potentially a measure of the number of active cross-bridges, as a function of tissue during a contraction-relaxation cycle. At present, no one method has given a clear indication of separating extracellular from cross-bridge contributions to S.E. behavior. However, mechanical studies at this level will not doubt provide information on the molecular mechanisms underlying contractility in smooth muscle.

Time Course for Development of Isometric Force

The time course for development of isometric force differs widely between muscle types as well as between different muscles within a particular type. This can be seen by comparing the values for the time required to develop one-half of the maximum isometric tension listed in Table 1. Many factors bear on the determination of this time course, and can be roughly divided into those involving activation and those pertaining to the intrinsic mechanical properties of the tissue. The former include such factors as the time course of development of excitation in response to an agonist and the spread of excitation across and between cells. These factors are treated elsewhere in this volume. The mechanical factors have been developed with the model given in Fig. 5 as the conceptual framework (61). Influencing the rate of tension development in this model are (a) the active state, defined in terms of the ability of the contractile component to bear tension; (b) the series elastic component characteristics; and (c) the intrinsic contractile velocity. In the current molecular view of smooth muscle contraction, the time course of the active state would be related to the activation of the actomyosin ATPase through the phosphorylation of the myosin light chains mediated by a Ca^{2+}-sensitive kinase. The determination of the active state from mechanical parameters (26) is dependent for its interpretation on the two-element model. As the current view of skeletal muscle places the elasticity within the contractile element, that is, in the cross-bridges themselves, thus the interpretation of these mechanically defined ''active states'' is not straightforward (71). As mentioned above, mechanically defined active states for smooth muscle (46,69) have been measured, and although subject to reservation, are potentially closer to reflecting actomyosin interaction as smooth muscle behavior is better approximated by the two-element model. The extent of the series elasticity, in effect the amount of slack that is needed to be taken up before contractile element force becomes total force, and the speed at which this can be done, i.e., contractile element shortening speed, are

major factors which can be experimentally separated from active state considerations by measuring the time course following a large change in length from a previously maximally activated isometric contraction. Risking a generalization, it appears that the intrinsic shortening speed is probably the major factor for the range of differences in the time course of tension development shown in Table 1.

Summary of Mechanical Properties of Smooth Muscle

The observations on the mechanical properties discussed can be summarized in the model presented in Fig. 5. Although always a simplification, this model can adequately describe the behavior of smooth muscle under a variety of conditions. The parallel elastic element is a passive structure, and such elastic structures can be readily identified in smooth muscle containing tissues. The contractile component obeys force-length and force-velocity relations analogous to those measured in skeletal muscle. This behavior most likely reflects the geometry and interaction of thick and thin, myosin and actin containing filaments of smooth muscle. The series elastic component is necessary to accommodate transient behavior. The structures responsible are less readily identified and are likely to be a combination of cross-bridge and intercellular force-transmitting connections. Although this model is phenomenologically adequate in terms of describing mechanical responses, the molecular basis of these responses is as yet poorly understood.

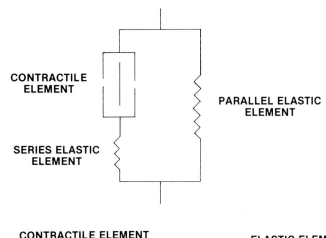

CONTRACTILE ELEMENT

SERIES ELASTIC ELEMENT

PARALLEL ELASTIC ELEMENT

CONTRACTILE ELEMENT ACTIVE MECHAN O CHEMICAL ENERGY CONVERTER

ELASTIC ELEMENTS PASSIVE ELEMENTS

FIG. 5. Model for the mechanical properties of smooth muscle. *Upper schematic:* Mechanical analogue based on steady-state and transient mechanical responses of smooth muscle. *Lower graphs* schematically show the relations between force, length, and velocity for the model elements.

CHEMICAL ENERGY—SMOOTH MUSCLE INPUT

Smooth muscle, like all muscle machines, is a mechanochemical engine. The ability to generate force, shorten, and produce mechanical work is directly dependent on the input of chemical free energy. Adenosine triphosphate (ATP) hydrolysis, catalyzed by myosin, is the immediate driving reaction coupled to mechanical output. Although the actomyosin ATPase is a major component of ATP utilization in active muscle, it is not the only energy-dependent contractile process. Excitation and the coupling of excitation to contraction involve energy-dependent processes, as, for example, ion pumps involved in Ca^{2+} translocation and in response to altered Na^+ and K^+ gradients. The sources, stores, and coordination of ATP synthesis will be considered in relation to contractile ATP utilization. I should like to reemphasize that there are considerable differences among smooth muscles. In a recent review restricted to vascular smooth muscle, I have treated this in considerable detail. It is impossible in this review to treat all smooth muscle types as exhaustively. Using this base, I have attempted to expand the scope in this chapter to treat most smooth muscle types, fully aware of the necessary shortcomings of the generalization involved.

Energy Sources: ATP Synthesis in Smooth Muscle

The biochemical pathways for ATP synthesis in smooth muscle appear to be similar to those of skeletal muscle, which has served as the experimental system for much of our understanding of energy metabolism. Although not as extensively characterized as their skeletal muscle counterparts, the enzymes of the Embden-Meyerhof pathway, the tricarboxylic acid cycle, and the respiratory chain have been identified in smooth muscle (63,72,142,146). The *in vivo* operation of these pathways can be indirectly inferred from (a) the ability of fatty acids, tricarboxylic acid cycle intermediates and glucose to restore contractility in substrate-depleted tissue strips, (39,40,113); and (b) the effects of specific metabolic inhibitors (47,115).

Although the biochemical pathways for synthesis of ATP from any of the potential substrates are present in smooth muscle, it is impossible to generalize about the energy source(s) under physiological conditions. In fact, the evidence is often contradictory. Respiratory quotients (RQ) based on gas-exchange experiments in the presence of glucose (73,75,140) strongly indicate that carbohydrate is the predominant substrate oxidized. However, studies using isotopically labeled glucose indicate that only a small fraction of the glucose carbon is found as CO_2 (90,92,99), most of the label appearing as lactate. Glucose uptake is appreciable in smooth muscle and has been shown to follow Michaelis-Menten kinetics (7). There is evidence suggesting that membrane transport is the rate-limiting step for glucose metabolism; however, as compared to skeletal muscle, smooth muscle is relatively insensitive to insulin (6,15). Glucose uptake has been reported to be both greater (7,73) as well as less than that which could be accounted for in terms of respiration and glycolysis. The role of glycogen is equally confusing.

The activity of glycogen phosphorylase appears to be related to contractile activity (30,97) as well as to agonists promoting relaxation via stimulation of β-adrenergic receptors (5); the evidence for the opposite has also been presented (18). The stimulation of glycogenolysis was found, however, not to be consistently related to smooth muscle contraction (83). A balance of carbohydrate utilization in terms of glycolysis, glycogenolysis, and respiration has not been reported for smooth muscle.

The lack of carbon balance in smooth muscle suggests that other substrates, presumably endogenous fatty acids, play a considerable role in smooth muscle energy metabolism. This is supported by the inability to exhaust tissue glycogen stores in the absence of glucose (57,82,131). Evidence for the role of fatty acids in smooth muscle metabolism is scanty. β-Hydroxybutyrate is reported to be equally as effective as glucose in terms of supporting contractile and electrical activity (17) as well as respiration (19). Even less is known about amino acid catabolism in smooth muscle, although amino acids can be degraded (91) and maintain respiration in rat aorta (16).

In summary, the substrate utilization pattern of smooth muscle *in situ* is not known with certainty. Glucose uptake is appreciable; however, there is conflicting evidence on the nature of the substrate for oxidative metabolism. Although this lack of knowledge is formidable, consideration of overall steady-state metabolic rates in terms of respiration and glycolysis (see Energy Utilization, below) can produce a more coherent pattern of ATP synthesis in smooth muscle.

Energy Sources

Short Term

The immediate source of chemical energy is the ATP molecule. Included in the immediate energy sources are other so-called high-energy compounds or phosphagens linked to ATP synthesis by rapid chemical reactions. The Lohmann reaction, involving the transfer of a phosphoryl group from phosphocreatine (PCr) to ADP, is an example of these sources. The presence of myokinase, which catalyzes the formation of ATP from two ADP molecules in smooth muscle, suggests that this reaction should be included in the immediate phosphagen pool as well.

In general, smooth muscle has very low phosphagen reserves in comparison to skeletal muscle (20,102). In terms of ATP content, the range reported for smooth muscle, 2 to 3 μmol/g blot, is not substantially below the range of 3 to 5 μmol/g blot reported for skeletal muscle; these differences are likely to be due to the lower cellular content of smooth muscle tissue. The major difference in the smooth and skeletal muscle phosphagen pool is ascribable to the significant difference in phosphocreatine content. The phosphocreatine content of skeletal muscle is on the order of 30 μmol/g blot and forms such an effective buffer against changes in ATP content that ATP changes in skeletal muscle cannot be observed during contraction. The phosphocreatine content of smooth muscle is on the same order of magnitude as the ATP content. In this respect, smooth muscle is more similar to other cell types than to skeletal muscle. This low phosphagen pool in smooth muscle makes this tissue dependent on continuous ATP synthesis and its coordination with metabolic demands in the absence of ongoing ATP synthesis.

Long Term

Endogenous substrates available for the maintenance of cellular ATP include the usual complement of carbohydrates, lipids, and proteins. Quantifying the relative importance of each source to smooth muscle is somewhat arbitrary in view of the lack of information of the nature of the preferred substrate under physiological conditions. The role of glycogen because of its importance as an energy store in skeletal muscle has received considerable attention. The glycogen content of smooth muscle is in a range of 1 to 10 μmol/g (81,102), considerably less than the average concentration of about 75 μmol/g found in skeletal muscle. In the absence of exogenous glucose, the amount of glycogen in smooth muscle would provide ATP for at least 15 min and up to several hours at basal levels of utilization, and for about one-half that time under conditions of maximum contractile activity. This time, calculated on the basis of glycogen content, agrees roughly with the duration of time before isometric force begins to decline in the absence of exogenous substrate. The role of glycogen as a preferred energy source is complicated by the above-mentioned fact that glycogen is difficult to deplete from smooth muscle and is not totally exhausted even when the tissues cannot support contractile function after prolonged periods without external substrate. Furthermore, external glucose is reported to inhibit glycogenolysis (81,121), and lactate, the major end-product of carbohydrate catabolism in smooth muscle, appears to arise almost entirely from glucose. Exogenous glucose would seem to be the most likely candidate as a preferred energy source. This is, however, contra-

dicted by a fair amount of data indicating that little glucose is converted to CO_2 in studies employing isotopically labeled glucose. Add to this rather confusing picture the fact that glycogen phosphorylase activity, the apparently controlling step of glycogenolysis, is well coordinated with contractility (30,97). Although the evidence is far from complete, glycolysis appears not to be correlated with glycogenolysis, suggesting some form of compartmentalization of carbohydrate catabolism in smooth muscle. Other stores such as fatty acids and proteins are not as easy to quantify in ATP units. Fatty acids under physiological conditions form a large store; however, they appear not to affect glucose utilization (50).

In sum, the phosphagen pool of smooth muscle is considerably lower than that of skeletal muscle, principally due to lower levels of phosphocreatine. Maintenance of ATP thus requires continuous and well-regulated synthesis. Sources and substrate stores for ATP synthesis are quite ubiquitous in smooth muscle. The preferred substrate (if any) under physiological conditions is not know with certainty.

Energy Utilization

Although the exact nature of the substrate utilization pattern is uncertain, one can quantify the rate of chemical energy utilization with a fair degree of precision.

Energy utilization is expressed in units of moles of ATP, which, as the main intermediary in many energy transfer processes, not only is more relevant to the biochemistry than the usual heat equivalent units of calorimetry but also has theoretical advantages (86). Direct measurement of ATP breakdown is complicated by the resynthesis of ATP by intermediary metabolism. Straightforward application of the techniques employed to measure ATP breakdown in skeletal muscle poses severe problems. In this methodology, resynthesis is blocked by metabolic poisons (N_2, iodoacetate), and changes in the phosphagen pool are estimated using freeze clamping techniques to stop phosphagen breakdown at various points in time. The low phosphagen pool of smooth muscle coupled with the relatively high rates of ATP utilization at physiological temperatures makes interpretation of results using metabolic inhibitors difficult. This disadvantage can be turned around, however, by the use of intermediary metabolism itself to estimate ATP utilization.

For smooth muscle, as for most other cell types, the through-put of ATP plays a much larger role than the ATP concentration in energy utilization considerations. Using oxygen consumption and lactate production to measure the rates of intermediary metabolism, one can calculate cellular ATP synthesis. Under steady-state conditions, for example, basal metabolism, the ATP content is constant, thus ATP synthesis is equal to its utilization, and rates of intermediary metabolism can be directly related to ATP utilization. The attainment of steady states in smooth muscle is supported by both direct measurement of ATP content and indirect measurements, i.e., the constancy of the rates of intermediary metabolism. Thus measures of intermediary metabolism as oxygen consumption and lactate production in smooth muscle provide a reasonable guide to the tissue's ATP utilization. Because of uncertainty in the substrate for oxidative metabolism, the absolute values are subject to error, although at most by about 20% by conservative estimates (102). The ATP utilization of various muscles based on measurements of intermediary metabolism are presented in Table 3. As can be seen in Table 3, lactate production in smooth muscle is of approximately the same magnitude on a molar basis as oxygen consumption. The relative phosphorylation efficiency of oxidative metabolism is such, however, that most ATP is provided by oxidation. For example, if the rate of O_2 consumption (J_{O_2}) were equal to the rate of lactate production (J_{lac}), 85% of the total rate of ATP synthesis (J_{ATP}) would be attributable to oxidative phosphorylation. Nevertheless, these high rates of lactate production are peculiar to smooth muscle and few other cell types (76). Potential mechanisms underlying this unusual aerobic glycolysis are discussed below (Relations Between Smooth Muscle Metabolism and Contractility). Another difference between smooth and skeletal muscle that is apparent from Table 3 is that the maximum J_{ATP} in smooth muscle is far less than that in skeletal, even at similar levels of maintained force. This economy of operation of smooth muscle has been recognized as one of its characteristic features for many years (14). The question of economy will be treated below. At the risk of redundancy, the data in Table 3 point

out the phosphagen pool being small compared to ATP utilization over time periods relevant to smooth muscle considerations. For example, bovine mesenteric vein takes about 10 min to reach the peak of an isometric contraction, whereas its preformed phosphagen pool could supply the required ATP for only 1 ½ min.

RELATIONS BETWEEN SMOOTH MUSCLE INPUT AND OUTPUT

Relations Between Smooth Muscle Metabolism and Contractility

Smooth muscle metabolism, like all cells under physiological conditions, is acceptor limited; that is, ADP is required for both oxidative and glycolytic metabolism. Thus if metabolism is stimulated, one seeks to identify the ATPase that is providing the ADP underlying the observed increase in metabolism. As can be seen from Table 3, the ATP utilization of smooth muscle increases between two- and threefold under maximum stimulation. Under controlled isometric conditions, this increase in metabolism is correlated with increases in active isometric force. In earlier times, there was a fair bit of controversy on this point [see Paul (102) for historical review], and much confusion in the literature concerning smooth metabolism has arisen because measurements made on smooth muscle rings, strips, or slices left the mechanical condition, a major determinant of metabolism, uncontrolled. In recent years, the evidence supporting the linear relation between force and metabolism has been extended to many smooth muscles including airways (128), visceral (19,118), vascular (43,53,107), and invertebrate (11). It is possible that the increase in metabolism with force is not pre-

TABLE 3. *Energy utilization parameters of muscle*

Tissue	$\sim$P[a] content μmol/g	unstimulated μmol/(g·min)			maximum stimulated			Reference
		J_{O_2}	J_{lac}	J_{ATP}	J_{O_2}	J_{lac}	J_{ATP}	
Rat portal vein	3.3	0.39	0.38	3.0	1.2	—	7.7	Hellstrand (53) Hellstrand et al. (57)
Rabbit aorta	0.6	0.10	0.11	0.78	0.14	0.25	1.2	Needleman and Blehm (98) Paul (*unpublished*)
Hog carotid artery	0.7	0.069	0.11	0.58	0.13	0.26	1.2	Glück and Paul (43) Van Harn et al. (136)
Bovine mesenteric vein	1.5	0.069	0.17	0.65	0.12	0.29	1.1	Peterson and Paul (110)
Guinea pig taenia coli	6	0.28	0.16	2.0	0.50	0.84	4.3	Casteels and Wuytack (24) Wuytack and Casteels (143)
Dog trachealis	2.4	0.75	0.12	5.0	1.3	—	8.3	Stephens and Skoog (128) Stephens et al. (127)
Rat myometrium	1.6	0.28	0.28	2.1	0.33	0.45	2.7	Kroeger (77); Walaas and Walaas (138)
Skeletal Dog semitendinosus	15–30[b]	0.2	—	1.25	7.8	—	50	Stainsby and Barclay (123)

[a]ATP + PCr except for hog carotid artery, for which ATP only is given.
[b]Range reported for skeletal muscle.

dominantly due to actomyosin ATPase and the correlation is not causal but related through a third variable such as the increase in intracellular Ca^{2+} accompanying contraction (133). Two lines of evidence suggest this possibility is unlikely.

Smooth muscle actomyosin ATPase measured in homogenates of purified actomyosin is in good agreement with the increase in metabolism associated with active isometric force (104,119). Furthermore, when isometric force is altered by changing muscle length only, keeping the stimulation constant, the metabolic rate is found to parallel the changes in active isometric force (53,105). Approximately 80% of the increase in J_{O_2} observed at the tissue length at which maximum isometric force is developed is not present at lengths at which no force is developed. The change in isometric force with muscle length at constant stimulus levels is likely to be attributable solely to variations in actomyosin ATPase due to changes in the effective overlap of thick and thin filaments. Thus the tension-dependent metabolism observed under these conditions is likely to be causally related to the actomyosin ATPase. These relations are shown schematically in Fig. 6.

As oxidative phosphorylation provides the bulk of smooth muscle ATP synthesis, the relation between metabolism and force primarily depends on correlation between J_{O_2} and force. The relation of aerobic glycolysis to contractility is of interest, for although it does not serve as a major ATP source, this pathway accounts for most of the glucose utilized by smooth muscle. The observed glycolysis in smooth muscle under fully oxygenated conditions is unusual and this "defect" in the Pasteur effect (76) is found in relatively few other cell types, such as tumor (114) and retinal cells. The mechanisms underlying aerobic glycolysis have been the topic of speculation for some time (79), and trivial explanations such as hypoxic zones, paucity of mitochondria, or anomalies of *in vitro* conditions do not appear to be likely mechanisms (102). There is a growing body of evidence, although far from conclusive, that glycolysis is preferentially coupled to the energy requirements of the Na-K pump. Based on similarities in the response of electrical and mechanical parameters to glucose removal or Li^+ substitution for Na^+, a coupling between glycolysis and some Na^+-dependent process was suggested (131). Differential effects of substrate depletion and anoxia (4,74) support the concept of compartmentalization of metabolism according to function. However, it appears that in uterine smooth muscle, both aerobic and glycolytic processes can support Na-K pumping (115). Recent data from porcine coronary arteries (103) indicate that if Na-K transport processes are inhibited by ouabain or by removal of K^+ or Na^+, lactate production is also inhibited. Ouabain, moreover, increases isometric force in these vessels which is correlated with an increase in J_{O_2} concomitant with the decrease in J_{lac}. Ouabain also has little effect on J_{O_2} in taenia coli (134). Readmission of K^+ to tissues incubated in K^+-free medium stimulates aerobic glycolysis in the porcine vessels and taenia coli (24), presumably due to stimulation of Na-K transport. The evidence supports the concept of metabolic compartmentalization but not of an absolute

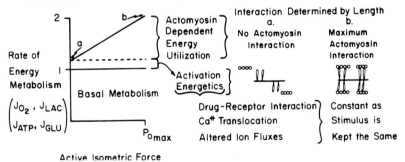

A. Maximal Activation at Various Muscle Lengths

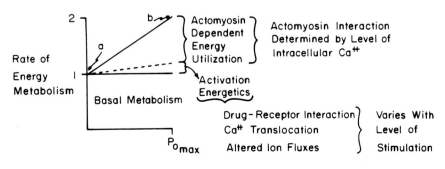

B. Fixed Muscle Length at Various Degrees of Activation

FIG. 6 Determinants of vascular smooth muscle energy metabolism under isometric conditions. **A:** Top line represents total metabolic rate as a function of active isometric force, measured under conditions of maximal stimulation at various muscle lengths. Metabolic rates are given in terms of ATP utilization in arbitrary units. The ordinate, however, could be expressed in terms of the rates of oxygen consumption, lactate production, or glucose consumption, as these metabolic parameters show a similar dependence on isometric force. Changes in isometric force are assumed to reflect change in number of available actomyosin interaction sites. Solid horizontal line represents basal metabolism measured in the absence of stimulation. Distance between solid and broken horizontal line represents requirements of activation processes. **B:** Top line represents total metabolic rate as a function of active isometric force measured under conditions of fixed muscle length with graded contractions produced at various levels of activation. Difference in slopes of relation between metabolism and force under the different conditions (a, b) can be attributed to different levels of activation at the same force. Broken line represents metabolism associated with activation processes.

kind. It can be best distinguished when output is altered. Changes in force or Na-K transport appear to preferentially affect J_{o_2} and J_{lac}, respectively. However, force in some tissues can be supported by glycolytically generated ATP under anaerobic conditions and Na-K transport can be supported by oxidative processes in the absence of glucose. The data support a functional rather than structural compartmentalization such that membrane processes as Na-K pumping use glucose from external sources and membrane-bound glycolytic enzymes, whereas the ATP required for actomyosin interaction is provided by localized mitochondria. This area is open to many exciting questions concerning biochemical regulation of metabolism. For example, how can glycolysis be inhibited while oxidative phosphorylation is stimulated as is found in the presence of ouabain? Although much needs to be done, the possibility of utilizing J_{o_2} as an index of actomyosin interaction and J_{lac} as a measure of Na-K pumping is intriguing.

Muscle Energetics

Muscle energetics is a name given to the field of investigation which attempts to quantify the relation between the chemical input, the role of ATP hydrolysis, and the mechanical output under various loading conditions. These data provide information at two important levels. On the one hand, they can be analyzed to provide information on the kinetics of actomyosin ATPase in the intact, structured muscle. This is becoming of increased importance as many of the recent advances in our understanding of muscle contraction at the molecular level have been derived from biochemical studies of isolated muscle proteins (130). This effect of imposition of the three-dimensional structure of the intact tissue on kinetic parameters is not known and is an exciting arena for biophysical correlation of structure and function. A further interest in studies of energetics is that measurements of input-output parameters can provide information enabling thermodynamic limits on muscle performance to be determined. These limits can be used to provide unique criteria to evaluate kinetic models of contraction.

Muscle energetics is currently undergoing a revival of interest, generated by data which conflict with the evidence used to formulate the classic picture developed by A.V. Hill and his school (61). The cornerstone of the classic theories was the use of measurements of muscle heat production to estimate ATP turnover. Recent experiments [see Curtin and Woledge (27) and Homsher and Kean (64)], however, indicate that the assumed proportionality between heat production and phosphagen breakdown is not valid. Furthermore, comparison of ATP breakdown during contraction to oxidative resynthesis of ATP (78,101) suggests that a large fraction of the ATP breakdown occurs after mechanical relaxation. Thus, for better or worse, the consideration of smooth muscle energetics cannot fall back on a reference frame generated from skeletal muscle studies.

The most striking feature of smooth muscle energetics is the economical cost in metabolic terms of maintaining isometric force. The tension cost, i.e., the rate of ATP utilization per unit isometric force, of various muscles is presented in Table 4. Smooth muscle can maintain isometric forces of similar or greater magnitude than skeletal muscle at tension costs of up to several hundredfold less. The underlying mechanisms have been considered in detail (102,117), and both structural and biochemical factors play a role. Structural considerations show that muscles with long effective sarcomere lengths have more cross-bridges in parallel. Assuming equal force per ATP breakdown per cross-bridge, muscles with long sarcomeres would have a lower tension cost than muscles with short sarcomeres. Long sarcomere structured muscles would also be associated with a slower velocity of contraction for a given cross-bridge speed, which is also a characteristic of smooth muscle. Such structural considerations play a larger role in invertebrate smooth muscle which may have sarcomeres 10 times larger than skeletal muscle. Mammalian smooth muscle, however, does not appear to have myofilaments or sarcomeres (9) that are dramatically longer than skeletal muscle, and it is unlikely that more than a factor of 5 in tension cost can be attributed to structure. The major determinant of the lower tension cost in smooth muscle appears to be biochemical. The low tension cost and contraction velocity is correlated with a lower actomyosin ATPase. The actomyosin ATPase of hog carotid artery is about 100-fold less than that of skeletal muscle. In view of current theories of cross-bridge interaction

TABLE 4. *Tension cost of various muscles*

Muscle	Temp °C	Tension cost μmol ATP/min·g wet weight mN/mm²	Tension cost[a] comparison at equivalent temperature	Reference
Mouse soleus	24.5	930	2,920	Edwards et al. (34)
Rat portal vein	37	116	120	Hellstrand (53)
Guinea pig taenia coli	37	25	25	Saito et al. (118)
Dog trachaelis	37	11	11	Stephens and Skoog (128)
Hog carotid artery	37	6	6	Paul et al. (104)
Mytilas ABRM (tonic)	20	0.4	2	Baguet and Gillis (12)

[a]Calculations based on a Q_{10} for ATP turnover of 2.5.

(130), a low ATPase could allow for a longer time of attachment of actin to myosin during a cross-bridge cycle, with a resulting lower tension cost. Although attractive, this hypothesis requires more detailed information on the kinetics of actomyosin interaction in smooth muscle before definitive statements on the mechanism of the low tension cost of smooth muscle can be made.

Of critical interest to theories of muscle energetics is the measurement of the ATP turnover under conditions in which the muscle is producing work. The turnover rate at maximum contraction velocity (unloaded contraction) is also important in distinguishing between theories of muscle contraction (23). It is somewhat surprising that these critical parameters are not known with certainty for skeletal muscle. Under conditions of maximum work production, the rate of ATP breakdown is greater in skeletal muscle by up to threefold over the isometric rate (42). Similar studies on taenia coli (21) also show that the ATP breakdown increases by as much as 2.7 times over the isometric rate when actively shortening as loads less than isometric. In vascular tissue, on the other hand, the rate of ATP estimated from measurements of O_2 consumption is not significantly different from the isometric rate when allowed to contract against a load (53) or in isovelocity contractions (106). Whether this difference is related to difference in technique or tissue is not known, and like many other questions concerning smooth muscle, its resolution requires more experiments. In summary, other than the low cost of maintaining tension, our knowledge of smooth muscle energetics is limited. In lieu of answers, perhaps it is better to summarize questions. Is the low tension cost matched by efficiency under work performing conditions? What is the ATP cost of shortening under zero loads, i.e., the efficacy of shortening? How do the structure and mechanical constraints imposed by the intact tissue modulate the actomyosin ATPase? The answers to these questions will allow meaningful discussion of smooth muscle energetics to begin.

Coordination of Metabolism and Contractility

The details of the mechanisms matching ATP synthesis to its utilization are beyond the scope of both this chapter and indeed the available evidence. However, some general patterns can be discerned although they should be viewed with caution. Smooth muscle mitochondria, like their skeletal muscle counterparts, are limited by the ADP concentration. In the presence of adequate substrate, they will effectively rephosphorylate any ADP available. This is useful as mitochondrial ATP output is automatically coordinated with the ADP produced by various cellular ATPases, in this case predominantly the ADP resulting from actomyosin ATPase activity.

Although the evidence is not as solid, glycolysis is also probably regulated by ADP through its effects on the presumably rate-limiting enzyme phosphofructokinase. In seeking coordinating mechanisms, one can thus shift one's attention to steps that control the mobilization of substrate. It is well documented that the level of intracellular Ca^{2+} is the predominant factor regulating actomyosin interaction and hence contractility in smooth muscle (139). It is thus not unreasonable to suspect Ca^{2+} concentration as a possible factor in the control of substrate entry. This is supported by the fact that glycogen phosphorylase in smooth muscle, a rate-limiting enzyme in glycogenolysis, is activated by intracellular Ca^{2+} (29, 97). As indicated above, however, the carbohydrate source for the large component of aerobic glycolysis appears to be exogenous glucose. Membrane transport appears to be the rate-limiting step for glycolysis in the smooth muscle of rabbit colon and bovine mesenteric arteries (8); however, again one cannot generalize as this apparently does not hold for rabbit aorta (144). Intracellular Ca^{2+} has been shown to regulate glucose transport in skeletal and cardiac muscle, and this mechanism also appears to be valid for rat detrusor smooth muscle. Thus calcium could play a major role in coordination of carbohydrate catabolism with contractility. There are many other potential modulating substances, cyclic nucleotides, for example; however, their role in coordination of metabolism with contractility is less clear. As outlined above, the exact nature of the substrates oxidized by smooth muscle is open to question, and their regulation is thus even less clear. Again, one is left with directions for further research rather than answers.

SMOOTH MUSCLE MECHANOCHEMISTRY

Review of the available mechanical and chemical evidence on smooth muscle indicates that a model based on sliding filaments and cyclic interaction between actin and myosin, i.e., a cross-bridge cycle, is adequate to explain smooth muscle mechanochemistry. Any model must be able to explain the physiological adaptations peculiar to smooth muscle, particularly the low tension cost and show contractile velocities. Current evidence favors these properties residing on the molecular level, in terms of modification of the actomyosin ATPase. On the physiological level, this molecular adaptation allows circulatory regulation by vascular smooth muscle to occur at minimal metabolic cost. For example, a vasculature lined with skeletal muscle would require twice the basal metabolism of the whole organism solely for maintenance of vessel diameter against blood pressure (102). The low maintenance cost of muscle is less relevant to visceral physiology as shortening rather than force maintenance appears to be the predominant mode of operation of its muscle coat. Although potentially even less efficient than skeletal muscle under shortening conditions, smooth muscle is adapted to operate under much lower input and output power requirements.

Thus, to the organism, smooth muscle is essential to match the required motility. Again, one will probably find the underlying mechanisms to involve the specialized actomyosin ATPase. Our knowledge of smooth muscle mechanochemistry has developed to the point of pushing such physiologically relevant questions as tension cost and efficiency to the molecular level—a region where much needs to be done.

ACKNOWLEDGMENT

This work is in part supported by American Heart Association Grant #78-1080, National Institutes of Health.

REFERENCES

1. Abbott, R. H., and Steiger, G. J. (1977): Temperature and amplitude dependence of tension transients in glycerinated skeletal and insect fibrillar muscle. *J. Physiol.*, 266:13–42.
2. Aberg, A. K. G., and Axelsson, J. (1965): Some mechanical aspects of an intestinal smooth muscle. *Acta Physiol. Scand.*, 64:15–27.
3. Adelstein, R. S. (1978): Myosin phosphorylation, cell motility and smooth muscle contraction. *Trends Biochem. Sci.*, 3:27–29.
4. Altura, B. M., and Altura, B. T. (1970): Differential effects of substrate depletion on drug-induced contraction of rabbit aorta. *Am. J. Physiol.*, 219:1698–1705.
5. Andersson, R., and Mohme-Lundholm, E. (1970): Metabolic actions in intestinal smooth muscle associated with relaxation mediated by adrenergic α- and β-receptors. *Acta Physiol. Scand.*, 79:244–261.
6. Arnqvist, H. J. (1972): Characteristics of monosaccharide permeability in arterial tissue and intestinal smooth muscle; Effect of insulin. *Acta Physiol. Scand.*, 85:217–227.
7. Arnqvist, H. J. (1973): Effects of increasing glucose concentrations on the glucose metabolism in arterial tissue and intestinal smooth muscle. *Acta Physiol. Scand.*, 88:481–490.
8. Arnqvist, H. J. (1977): Glucose transport and metabolism in smooth muscle. Action of insulin and diabetes. In: *The Biochemistry of Smooth Muscle*, edited by N. L. Stephens, University Park Press, Baltimore, pp. 127–158.
9. Ashton, F. T., Somlyo, A. V., and Somlyo, A. P. (1975): The contractile apparatus of vascular smooth muscle: Intermediate high voltage stereo electron microscopy. *J. Mol. Biol.*, 98:17–29.
10. Bagby, R. M., and Fisher, B. A. (1973): Graded contractions in muscle strips and single cells from Bufo marinus stomach. *Am. J. Physiol.*, 255:105–109.
11. Baguet, F., and Gillis, J. M. (1967): The respiration of the anterior byssus retractor muscle of *Mytilus edulis* (ABRM) after a phasic contraction. *J. Physiol. (Lond.)*, 188:67–82.
12. Baguet, F., and Gillis, J. M. (1968): Energy cost of tonic contraction in a lamellibranch catch muscle. *J. Physiol. (Lond.)*, 198:127–143.
13. Bahler, A. S., Fales, J. T., and Zieler, K. L. (1968): The dynamic properties of mammalian skeletal muscle. *J. Gen. Physiol.*, 51:369–384.
14. Bethe, A. (1911): Die Dauerverkurzung der Muskeln. *Pfleugers Arch.*, 142:291–336.
15. Bihler, I., Sawh, P. C., and Elbrink, J. (1977): Membrane transport of sugars in smooth muscle: Its relationship to carbohydrate metabolism and its regulation by physiological and pharmacological factors. In: *The Biochemistry of Smooth Muscle*, edited by N. L. Stephens, pp. 113–126. University Park Press, Baltimore.
16. Briggs, F. N., Chernick, S., and Chaikoff, I. L. (1949): The metabolism of arterial tissue. I. Respiration of rat thoracic aorta. *J. Biol. Chem.*, 179:103–111.
17. Bueding, E., Bülbring, E., Gercken, G., Hawkins, J. T., and Kuriyama, H. (1967): The effects of adrenaline on the adenosinetriphosphate and creatine phosphate content of intestinal smooth muscle. *J. Physiol.*, 193:187–212.
18. Bueding, E., Bülbring, E., Gercken, G., and Kuriyama, H. (1962): Lack of activation of phosphorylase by adrenaline during its physiological action on smooth muscle. *Nature*, 196:944.
19. Bülbring, E., and Golenhofen, K. (1967): Oxygen consumption by the isolated smooth muscle of guinea pig taenia coli. *J. Physiol.*, 923:212–224.
20. Bütler, T. M., and Davies, R. E. (1980): High energy phosphate metabolism of smooth muscle. In: *Handbook of Physiology, Section on Circulation II*, edited by D. F. Bohr, A. P. Somlyo, and H. V. Sparks, pp. 237–252. American Physiological Society, Bethesda, Md.
21. Butler, T. M., Siegman, M. J., and Mooers, S. U. (1979): Mammalian smooth muscle: Economical but inefficient. *Biophys. J.*, 25:269a.
22. Butler, T. M., Siegman, M. J., Mooers, S. U., and Davies, R. E. (1978): Chemical energetics of single isometric tetani in mammalian smooth muscle. *Am. J. Physiol.*, 235(1):L1–L7.
23. Caplan, S. R. (1968): Autonomic energy conversion. II. An approach to the energetics of muscular contraction. *Biophys. J.*, 8:1167–1193.
24. Casteels, R., and Wuytack, F. (1975): Aerobic and anaerobic metabolism in smooth muscle cells of taenia coli in relation to active ion transport. *J. Physiol.*, 250:203–220.
25. Civian, M. M., and Podolsky, R. J. (1966): Contraction kinetics of striated muscle fibres following quick changes in load. *J. Physiol.*, 184:512–534.
26. Close, R. I. (1972): Dynamic properties of mammalian skeletal muscles. *Physiol. Rev.*, 52:129–197.
27. Curtin, N. A., and Woledge, R. C. (1978): Energy changes and muscular contraction. *Physiol. Rev.*, 58:690–761.
28. Czapo, A., and Goodall, M. (1954): Excitability, length-tension relation and kinetics of uterine muscle contraction in relation to hormonal status. *J. Physiol.*, 126:384–395.
29. Diamond, J. (1973): Phosphorylase, calcium, and cyclic AMP in smooth muscle contraction. *Am. J. Physiol.*, 225:930–937.
30. Diamond, J., and Brody, T. M. (1966): Relationship between smooth muscle contraction and phosphorylase activation. *J. Pharmacol. Exp. Ther.*, 152:212–220.
31. Dobrin, P. B. (1978): Mechanical properties of arteries. *Physiol. Rev.*, 58:397–460.
32. Dobrin, P., and Canfield, T. (1977): Identification of smooth muscle series elastic component in intact carotid artery. *Am. J. Physiol.*, 232:H122–H131.
33. Driska, S. P., and Murphy, R. A. (1978): Estimate of cellular force generation in an arterial smooth muscle with a high actin:myosin ratio. *Blood Vessels*, 15:26–32.
34. Edwards, R. H. T., Hill, D. K., and Jones, D. A. (1975): Metabolic changes associated with slowing of relaxation in fatigued mouse muscle. *J. Physiol. (Lond.)*, 251:287–301.
35. Fay, F. S. (1975): Isometric contractile properties of single isolated smooth muscle cells. *Nature*, 265:553–556.
36. Fay, F. S., Cooke, P. H., and Canaday, P. G. (1976): Contractile properties of isolated smooth muscle cells. In: *Physiology of Smooth Muscles*, edited by E. Bülbring and M. F. Shuba, pp. 249–264. Raven Press, New York.
37. Filo, R. S., Bohr, D. F., and Rüegg, J. C. (1965): Glycerinated skeletal and smooth muscle, calcium and magnesium dependence. *Science*, 147:1581–1583.
38. Ford, L. E., Huxley, A. F., and Simmons, R. M. (1977): Tension responses to sudden length change in stimulated frog muscle fibers near slack length. *J. Physiol.*, 269:441–515.
39. Furchgott, R. F. (1966): Metabolic factors that influence contractility of vascular smooth muscle. *Bull. N.Y. Acad. Med.*, 42:996–1006.
40. Furchgott, R. F., and Wales, M. R. (1952): Utilization of compounds of Krebs cycle for contraction energy by rabbit intestinal smooth muscle. *Am. J. Physiol.*, 169:326–336.
41. Gabella, G. (1976): The force generaged by a visceral smooth muscle. *J. Physiol.*, 263:199–213.
42. Gilbert, C., Kretzschmar, K. M., and Wilkie, D. R. (1972): Heat work and phosphocreatine splitting during muscular contraction. *Symp. Quant. Biol.*, 37:613–618.

43. Glück, E., and Paul, R. J. (1977): The aerobic metabolism of porcine carotid artery and its relationship to isometric force: Energy cost of isometric contraction. *Pfluegers Arch.,* 370:9–18.

44. Gordon, A. M., Huxley, A. F., and Julian, F. J. (1966): The variation in isometric tension with sarcomere length in vertebrate muscle fibers. *J. Physiol. (Lond.),* 184:170–192.

45. Gordon, A. R., and Siegman, M. J. (1971): Mechanical properties of smooth muscle. I. Length-tension and force-velocity relations. *Am. J. Physiol.,* 221:1243–1249.

46. Gordon, A. R., and Siegman, M. J. (1971): Mechanical properties of smooth muscle. II. Active state. *Am. J. Physiol.,* 221:1250–1254.

47. Greenberg, S., Wilson, W. R., and Long, J. P. (1973): Effect of metabolic inhibitors on mesenteric arterial smooth muscle. *Arch. Int. Pharmacodyn. Ther.,* 206:214–227, 1973.

48. Halpern, H., Mulvany, M. J., and Warshaw, D. M. (1978): Mechanical properties of smooth muscle cells in the walls of arterial resistance vessels. *J. Physiol.,* 275:85–101.

49. Hardung, V., and Laszt, L. (1966): Die Beziehung zwischen Last und Verkürzunggeschwindigheit beim Gefässmuskel. *Angiologica,* 3:100–113.

50. Hashimoto, S., and Dayton, S. (1977): Fatty acid metabolism of normal aortic tissue and its alterations induced by atherosclerosis. In: *The Biochemistry of Smooth Muscle,* edited by N. L. Stephens, pp. 219–240. University Park Press, Baltimore.

51. Helander, E. (1957): On quantitative muscle protein determination. *Acta Physiol. Scand. [Suppl. 141],* 41.

52. Helander, E., and Thulin, C.-A. (1962): Isometric tension and the myofilamental cross-section area in striated muscle. *Am. J. Physiol.,* 202:824–826.

53. Hellstrand, P. (1977): Oxygen consumption and lactate production of the rat portal vein in relation to its contractile activity. *Acta Physiol. Scand.,* 100:91–106.

54. Hellstrand, P. (1979): Mechanical and metabolic properties related to contraction in smooth muscle. *Acta Physiol. Scand. [Suppl.],* 464:1–54.

55. Hellstrand, P., and Johansson, B. (1975): The force-velocity relation in phasic contractions of venous smooth muscle. *Acta Physiol. Scand.,* 93:157–166.

56. Hellstrand, P., and Johansson, B. (1979): Analysis of the length response to a force step in smooth muscle from a rabbit urinary bladder. *Acta Physiol. Scand.,* 106:221–238.

57. Hellstrand, P., Johansson, B., and Norberg, K. (1977): Mechanical, electrical and biochemical effects of hypoxia and substrate removal on spontaneously active vascular smooth muscle. *Acta Physiol. Scand.,* 100:69–83.

58. Herlihy, J. T., and Murphy, R. A. (1974): Force-velocity and series elastic characteristics of smooth muscle of the hog carotid artery. *Circ. Res.,* 34:461–466.

59. Heumann, H.-G. (1973): Smooth muscle: Contraction hypothesis based on the arrangement of actin and myosin filaments in different states of contraction. *Philos. Trans. R. Soc. Lond. [Biol.],* 265:213–218.

60. Hill, A. V. (1938): The heat of shortening and the dynamic constants of muscle. *Proc. Roy. Soc. Lond. [Biol.],* 126:136–195.

61. Hill, A. V. (1965): *Trails and Trials in Physiology,* pp. 1–374. Edward Arnold, London.

62. Hodgkin, A. L., and Horowicz, P. (1960): Potassium contractures of single muscle fibers. *J. Physiol.,* 153:386–403.

63. Hollmann, S. (1949): Über die anaerobe Glykolyse in der Uterusmuskulatur. *Z. Physiol. Chem.,* 284:89.

64. Homsher, E., and Kean, C. J. (1978): Skeletal muscle energetics and metabolism. *Annu. Rev. Physiol.,* 40:90–131.

65. Huxley, A. F. (1974): Review lecture: muscular contraction. *J. Physiol.,* 243:1–43.

66. Huxley, A. F., and Simmons, R. M. (1971): Proposed mechanism for force generation in striated muscle. *Nature,* 233:533–538.

67. Jewell, B. R. (1977): A reexamination of the influence of muscle length on myocardial performance. *Circulation,* 40:221–230.

68. Jewell, B. R., and Wilkie, D. R. (1958): An analysis of the mechanical components in frog's striated muscle. *J. Physiol.,* 143:575–540.

69. Johansson, B. (1973): Active state in the smooth muscle of the rat portal vein in relation to electrical activity and isometric force. *Circ. Res.,* 32:246–258.

70. Johansson, B. (1978): Vascular smooth muscle biophysics. In: *Microcirculation, Vol. II,* edited by G. Kaley and B. M. Altura, pp. 83–118. University Park Press, Baltimore.

71. Julian, F. J., and Moss, R. L. (1976): The concept of active state in striated muscle. *Circ. Res.,* 38:53–59.

72. Kirk, J. E. (1969): *Enzymes of the Arterial Wall.* Academic Press, New York.

73. Kirk, J. E., Effersoe, P. G., and Chiang, S. P. (1954): The rate of respiration and glycolysis by human and dog aortic tissue. *J. Gerontol.,* 9:10–35.

74. Knull, H. R., and Bose, D. (1975): Reversibility of mechanical and biochemical changes in smooth muscle due to anoxia and substrate depletion. *Am. J. Physiol.,* 229:329–333.

75. Kosan, R. L., and Burton, A. C. (1966): Oxygen consumption of arterial smooth muscle as a function of active tone and passive stretch. *Circ. Res.,* 18:79–88.

76. Krebs, H. A. (1972): The Pasteur effect and the relations between respiration and fermentation. *Essays Biochem.,* 8:1–34.

77. Kroeger, E. A. (1976): Effect of ionic environment on oxygen uptake and lactate production of myometrium. *Am. J. Physiol.,* 230:158–162.

78. Kushmerick, M. J. (1977): Energy balance in muscle contraction: A biochemical approach. *Curr. Top. Bioenerg.,* 6:1–37.

79. Lehninger, A. L. (1969): The metabolism of the arterial wall. In: *The Arterial Wall,* edited by A. I. Lansing, pp. 220–246. Bailliere, Tindall and Cox, London.

80. Lowy, J., and Mulvany, M. J. (1973): Mechanical properties of guinea pig taenia coli muscles. *Acta Physiol. Scand.,* 88:123–136.

81. Lundholm, L., Andersson, R. G., Arnqvist, H. J., and Mohme-Lundholm, E. (1977): Glycolysis and glycogenolysis in smooth muscle. In: *The Biochemistry of Smooth Muscle,* edited by N. L. Stephens, pp. 159–207. University Park Press, Baltimore.

82. Lundholm, L., and Mohme-Lundholm, E. (1960): The carbohydrate metabolism and tone of smooth muscle. *Acta Pharmacol. Toxicol.,* 16:374–388.

83. Lundholm, L., and Mohme-Lundholm, E. (1963): Contraction and glycogenolysis of smooth muscle. *Acta Physiol. Scand.,* 56:125–129.

84. MacPherson, L., and Wilkie, D. R. (1954): The duration of the active state in a muscle twitch. *J. Physiol.,* 124:292–299.

85. Mashima, H., and Handa, M. (1969): The force-velocity relation and the dynamic constants of the guinea pig taenia coli. *J. Physiol. Soc. Jpn.,* 31:565–566.

86. McGilvery, R. W. (1970): *Biochemistry: A Functional Approach,* p. 520. W. B. Saunders Co., Philadelphia.

87. Meiss, R. A. (1971): Some mechanical properties of cat intestinal muscle. *Am. J. Physiol.,* 220:2000–2007.

88. Meiss, R. A. (1975): Graded activation in rabbit mesotubarium smooth muscle. *Am. J. Physiol.,* 229:455–465.

89. Meiss, R. A. (1978): Dynamic stiffness of rabbit mesotubarium smooth muscle: Effect of isometric length. *Am. J. Physiol.,* 234:C14–C26.

90. Morrison, A. D., Berwick, L., Orci, L., and Winegrad, A. I. (1976): Morphology and metabolism of an aortic intima-media preparation in which an intact endothelium is preserved. *J. Clin. Invest.,* 57:650–660.

91. Morrison, E. S., Scott, R. F., Frick, J., and Kroms, M. (1976): Oxidation of amino acids by swine aorta. *Fed. Proc.,* 35:449 (abst.).

92. Morrison, E. S., Scott, R. F., Kroms, M., and Frick, J. (1972): Glucose degradation in normal and atherosclerotic aortic intima-media. *Atherosclerosis,* 16:175–184.

93. Mulvany, M. (1979): The undamped and damped series elastic components of a vascular smooth muscle. *Biophys. J.,* 26:401–414.

94. Mulvany, M., and Warshaw, D. M. (1979): The active tension-length curve of vascular smooth muscle related to its cellular components. *J. Gen. Physiol.,* 74:84–104.

95. Murphy, R. A. (1976): Contractile system function in mammalian smooth muscle. *Blood Vessels,* 13:1–23.

96. Murphy, R. A., Herlihy, J. T., and Megerman, J. (1974): Force-generating capacity and contractile protein content of arterial smooth muscle. *J. Gen. Physiol.,* 64:691–705.

97. Namm, D. H. (1971): The activation of glycogen phosphorylase in arterial smooth muscle. *J. Pharmacol. Exp. Ther.*, 178:299-310.

98. Needleman, P. H., and Blehm, D. (1970): Effect of epinephrine and potassium chloride contraction and energy intermediates in rabbit thoracic aorta strips. *Life Sci.*, 9:1181-1189.

99. Newmark, M. Z., Malfer, C.D., and Wiese, C. D. (1972): Regulation of arterial metabolism. I. The effects of age and hormonal status upon the utilization of glucose *in vitro* by rat aorta. *Biochim. Biophys. Acta.*, 261:9-20.

100. Parnas, J. (1910): Energetik glatter Muskeln. *Pfluegers Arch.*, 134:441-495.

101. Paul, R. J. (1980): Physical and biochemical energy balance during an isometric tetanus and steady state recovery in frog sartorius at 0°C. *J. Physiol. (in press)*.

102. Paul, R. J. (1980): The chemical energetics of vascular smooth muscle. Intermediary metabolism and its relation to contractility. In: *Handbook of Physiology, Section on Circulation II*, edited by D. F. Bohr, A. P. Somlyo, and H. V. Sparks, pp. 201-236. American Physiological Society, Bethesda, Md.

103. Paul, R. J., Bauer, M., and Pease, W. (1979): Vascular smooth muscle: Aerobic glycolysis linked to Na-K transport processes. *Science*, 206:1414-1416.

104. Paul, R. J., Glück, E., and Rüegg, J. C. (1976): Cross-bridge ATP utilization in arterial smooth muscle. *Pfluegers Arch.*, 361:297-299.

105. Paul, R. J., and Peterson, J. W. (1975): Relation between length, isometric force, and O_2 consumption rate in vascular smooth muscle. *Am. J. Physiol.*, 228:915-922.

106. Paul, R. J., and Peterson, J. W. (1977): The mechanochemistry of smooth muscle. In: *The Biochemistry of Smooth Muscle*, edited by N. L. Stephens, pp. 15-39. University Park Press, Baltimore.

107. Paul, R. J., Peterson, J. W., and Caplan, S. R. (1973): Oxygen consumption rate in vascular smooth muscle: Relation to isometric tension. *Biochim. Biophys. Acta*, 305:474-480.

108. Peterson, J. W. (1974): Rates of metabolism and mechanical activity in vascular smooth muscle, Ph.D. thesis. Harvard University, Cambridge, Mass.

109. Peterson, J. W. (1978): Relation of stiffness, energy metabolism and isometric tension in a vascular smooth muscle. In: *Mechanism of Vasodilation*, edited by P. M. Vanhoutte and I. Leusen, pp. 79-88. S. Karger, Basel.

110. Peterson, J. W., and Paul, R. J. (1974): Aerobic glycolysis in vascular smooth muscle: Relation to isometric tension. *Biochim. Biophys. Acta*, 357:167-176.

111. Peterson, J. W., and Paul, R. J. (1974): Effects of initial length and active shortening on vascular smooth muscle contractility. *Am. J. Physiol.*, 227:1019-1024.

112. Peterson, L. H. (1962): Properties and behavior of living vascular wall. *Physiol. Rev. [Suppl. 5]*, 42:309-327.

113. Pfaffman, M., Urakawa, N., and Holland, W. C. (1965): Role of metabolism in K^+-induced tension changes in guinea pig taenia coli. *Am. J. Physiol.*, 208:1203-1205.

114. Racker, E. (1976): Why do tumor cells have high aerobic glycolysis? *J. Cell. Physiol.*, 89:697-700.

115. Rangachari, P. K., Paton, D. M., and Daniel, E. E. (1972): Aerobic and glycolytic support of sodium pumping and contraction in rat myometrium. *Am. J. Physiol.*, 223(5):1009-1015.

116. Rüdel, R., and Taylor, S. R. (1971): Striated muscle fibres: facilitation of contraction at short lengths by caffeine. *Science*, 172:387-388.

117. Rüegg, J. C. (1971): Smooth muscle tone. *Physiol. Rev.*, 51:201-248.

118. Saito, Y., Sakai, Y., Ikeda, M., and Urakawa, N. (1968): Oxygen consumption during potassium induced contracture in guinea pig taenia coli. *Jpn. J. Pharmacol.*, 18:321-331.

119. Seidel, C. L., Bauer, H., and Paul, R. J. (1979): Metabolism of relaxed and contracted rat aorta. *Fed. Proc.*, 38(3):12450.

120. Seidel, C. L., and Murphy, R. A. (1976): Stress relaxation in hog carotid artery as related to contractile activity. *Blood Vessels*, 13:78-91.

121. Südhof, H. (1950): Über den Kohlenhydraststoffwechsel der Arterienwand. *Pfluegers Arch.*, 252:551-565.

122. Simmons, R. M., and Jewell, B. R. (1974): Mechanics and

models of muscular contraction. In: *Recent Advances in Physiology, No. 9*, edited by R. J. Linden, pp. 87-147. Churchill Livingstone, Edinburgh.

123. Stainsby, W. N., and Barclay, J. K. (1971): Relation of load, rest length, work and shortening to oxygen uptake by *in situ* dog semitendinosus. *Am. J. Physiol.*, 221:1238-1242.

124. Stephens, N. L. (1973): Effect of hypoxia on contractile and series elastic components of smooth muscle. *Am. J. Physiol.*, 224:318-321.

125. Stephens, N. L. (ed.) (1977): *Smooth Muscle Biochemistry*. University Park Press, Baltimore.

126. Stephens, N. L., Meyers, J. L., and Cherniack, J. L. (1968): Oxygen, carbon dioxide, H^+ ion, and bronchial length-tension relationships. *J. Appl. Physiol.*, 25:376-383.

127. Stephens, N. L., Mitchell, R. H., and Kroeger, E. A. (1977): Smooth muscle biochemistry and hypoxia. In: *Smooth Muscle Biochemistry*, edited by N.L. Stephens, pp. 679-702. University Park Press, Baltimore.

128. Stephens, N. L., and Skoog, C. M. (1974): Tracheal smooth muscle and rate of oxygen uptake. *Am. J. Physiol.*, 226:1462-1467.

129. Stephens, N. L., and Van Niekerk, W. (1977): Isometric and isotonic contractions in airways smooth muscle. *Can. J. Physiol. Pharmacol.*, 55:833-838.

130. Taylor, E. W. (1979): Mechanism of actomyosin ATPase and the problem of muscle contraction. *CRC Crit. Rev. Biochem.*, 6:103-164.

131. Timms, A. R. (1964): The coupling of electrical and mechanical activities in intestinal smooth muscle in relation to metabolism. *Trans. N.Y. Acad. Sci.*, [II], 26:902-913.

132. Tregear, R. T., and Squire, J. M. (1973): Myosin content and filament structure in smooth and striated muscle. *J. Mol. Biol.*, 77:279-290.

133. Urakawa, N., Ikeda, N., Saito, Y., and Sakai, Y. (1968): Effects of calcium depletion on oxygen consumption in guinea pig taenia coli. *Jpn. J. Pharmacol.*, 18:500-508.

134. Urakawa, N., Ikeda, M., Saito, Y., and Sakai, Y. (1969): Effects of factors inhibiting tension development on oxygen consumption of guinea pig taenia coli in high K medium. *Jpn. J. Pharmacol.*, 19:578-586.

135. Uvelius, B. (1976): Isometric and isotonic length-tension relations and variations in cell length in longitudinal smooth muscle from rabbit urinary bladder. *Acta Physiol. Scand.*, 97:1-72.

136. Van Harn, G. L., Rubio, R., and Berne, R. M. (1977): Formation of adenosine nucleotide derivatives in isolated hog carotid artery strips. *Am. J. Physiol.*, 233(2):H299-H304.

137. Vanhoutte, P. M. (1978): Heterogeneity in vascular smooth muscle. In: *Microcirculation*, Vol. II, edited by G. Kaley and B. M. Altura, pp. 181-309. University Park Press, Balitmore.

138. Walass, O., and Walass, F. (1960): The content of adenosine-triphosphate in uterine muscle of rats and rabbits. *Acta Physiol. Scand.*, 21:1.

139. Weiss, G. (1977): Calcium and contractility in vascular smooth muscle. In: *Advances in General and Cellular Pharmacology, Vol. II*, edited by T. Narahashi and C. P. Bianchi, p. 71. Plenum Press, New York.

140. Wertheimer, H. E., and Ben-Tor, V. (1960): Age and hormonal influences on aortic tissue metabolism. *Arch. Kreislaufforsch.*, 33:25-33.

141. Woledge, R. C. (1971): Heat production and chemical change in muscle. *Prog. Biophys. Mol. Biol.*, 22:37-74.

142. Wrogemann, K., and Stephens, N. L. (1977): Oxidative phosphorylation in smooth muscle. In: *The Biochemistry of Smooth Muscle*, edited by N. L. Stephens, pp. 41-50. University Park Press, Baltimore.

143. Wuytack, F., and Casteels, R. (1972): The energy-rich phosphates in smooth muscle of the guinea pig taenia coli during metabolic depletion. *Arch. Int. Physiol. Biochim.*, 80:829-830.

144. Yalcin, S., and Winegrad, A. I. (1963): Defect in glucose metabolism in aortic tissue from alloxan diabetic rabbits. *Am. J. Physiol.*, 205:1253-1259.

145. Zachar, J., and Zacharová, D. (1966): Potassium contractures in single muscle fibres of the crayfish. *J. Physiol.*, 186:596-616.

146. Zemplenyi, T. (1968): *Enzyme Biochemistry of the Arterial Wall*. Lloyd-Luke, London.

Physiology of the Gastrointestinal Tract, edited by
Leonard R. Johnson, Raven Press, New York © 1981.

Chapter 9

Extrinsic Control of Digestive Tract Motility

C. Roman and J. Gonella

The extrinsic control of gastrointestinal motility differs in importance among the organs. In this respect, the extrinsic nerves closely control both ends of the alimentary canal (the cervical esophagus and the external anal sphincter) since the muscular coat of these areas is striated muscle that is paralyzed after denervation. The rest of the digestive tract having smooth muscle coats possesses the ability to function fairly normally in the absence of extrinsic nerves. This functional autonomy is partly due to intrinsic reflexes mediated through intramural nervous ganglia. The role of the extrinsic nerves is mainly to "modulate" the intrinsic reflexes and to achieve the integration of activity in widely separated regions of the alimentary canal. In fact, there

are several degrees in the autonomy of the digestive smooth muscle effector. Thus motility in the stomach and colon is more dependent on extrinsic nerve activity than it is in the small intestine. Since marked structural and functional differences exist among various regions of the gastrointestinal tract, the esophagus, the stomach, the small intestine, and the large intestine will be treated separately.

EXTRINSIC CONTROL OF ESOPHAGUS

The esophagus may be regarded as a tube extending from pharynx to stomach and serving to transport material between these two organs. At rest (i.e., between swallows and regurgitations), sphincter mechanisms at either end of the tube prevent easy access of air from above and gastric content from below. For purposes of clarity, the control of the tubular esophagus (or esophageal body) and that of the sphincter areas will be dealt with separately, after a review of some general features of esophageal innervation.

Anatomical and Histological Data About the Esophageal Innervation

Vagal Innervation

The motor innervation of the esophagus is supplied by the vagus nerves (Fig. 1). Classically, the cervical esophagus is innervated by the recurrent laryngeal nerves and the rest of the tube by branches from the thoracic vagal trunks (157). Still Hwang et al. (153) have demonstrated that the cervical portion of the esophagus, at least its upper end, receives its innervation either from the pharyngoesophageal nerve (e.g., dog, cat, rabbit) or from the external branch of the superior laryngeal nerve (e.g., monkey, guinea pig, rat). The pharyngoesophageal nerve (leaving the vagus nerve above the superior laryngeal nerve) also supplies the cervical esophagus of sheep (89,275). In humans, nerves of similar anatomic distribution have not been described (152).

A myenteric plexus of Auerbach lies between the longitudinal and circular muscle layers of esophagus. These intramural neurons are generally considered as relay neurons between the vagal fibers and the smooth muscle cells (201). But a myenteric plexus does also exist in the striated muscle coat, i.e., in the proximal part of the human esophagus and throughout the esophagus of various species whose esophageal muscle coat is composed entirely of striated muscle (2,157,164,217). The function

of this intramural plexus within the striated muscle esophagus remains obscure since many histological studies have suggested that the efferent vagal fibers did not synapse on cells of the myenteric plexus but ended directly on the striated muscle cells at neuromuscular junctions similar to those of skeletal muscle fibers elsewhere (2,102,132,161,287).

The vagus nerves also contain sensory fibers originating from the esophagus. These fibers have their cell bodies in the nodose ganglion. As indicated by various experiments using section, stimulation, and recording (see below), the sensitive fibers from the upper cervical esophagus of dog, rat, cat, and sheep join the vagus high in the neck through the superior laryngeal nerve (7,151,226,275,277). Those innervating the rest of the esophagus join the vagus within the thorax either through the recurrent laryngeal nerves (lower cervical and upper thoracic esophagus) or through esophageal branches of the vagus (lower thoracic esophagus). Histological works have shown the existence of many sensory endings in the mucosa, submucosa, and muscular layers (2,161,162,308,334). These endings are generally simple, free endings. But a few encapsulated structures resembling neuromuscular spindles have also been described in the striated muscle esophagus of humans (308) and various animals (162). Most of these various endings likely belong to vagal sensory fibers, although solid support of such a contention is lacking.

Sympathetic Innervation

The esophagus seems to receive an abundant sympathetic innervation, but the origin and course of these fibers remain unclear. As for their termination within the esophageal wall, more precise information has been obtained, with the Falk and Hillarps histofluorescence technique by Baumgarten and Lange (16), according to

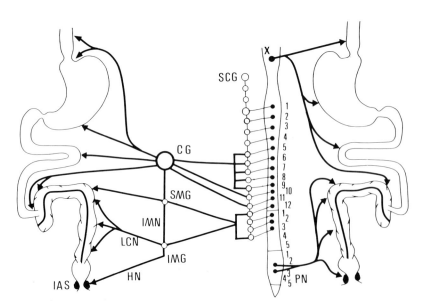

FIG. 1. Schema of the extrinsic efferent innervation of the gut. The sympathetic innervation is represented on the left of the figure, the parasympathetic on the right. This representation is a synthesis of various data and may present variations according to different species. SCG, superior cervical ganglion; CG, celiac ganglion; SMG, superior mesenteric ganglion; IMG, inferior mesenteric ganglion; IMN, intermesenteric nerve; LCN, lumbar colonic nerves; HN, hypogastric nerves; X, vagus dorsal motor nucleus and vagus nerve; PN, pelvic nerves; IAS, internal anal sphincter.

whom the sympathetic fibers which enter the cat and rhesus monkey esophagus not only supply the vessels but also mainly innervate ganglia of the myenteric plexus and the muscularis mucosae. Only a few fibers are confined to the muscular layers of the distal esophagus (smooth muscle). Surprisingly, densely innervated myenteric ganglia are also observed in the upper and middle portion of the esophagus even though the muscular wall is exclusively or mainly composed of striated muscle. As for the lower esophageal sphincter, the sympathetic innervation is similar to that of the adjacent nonsphincter area, with a dense innervation of the ganglia and few fibers to the musculature.

Extrinsic Control of Esophageal Body

The esophageal transport of material in the aboral direction is due to a propagated contraction generally recognized as peristalsis (56,138,157). According to its method of elicitation, esophageal peristalsis was divided by Meltzer (229,230) into primary and secondary types: primary peristalsis is initiated by swallowing; secondary peristalsis is independent of swallowing and starts in the esophagus in response to a local stimulus. Such a local stimulus can be provided either by a bolus of food that remains stuck in the gullet, or by a rubber balloon suddenly inflated.

The esophageal muscular coat is composed entirely of striated muscle in some species (e.g, dog, sheep), but in others (opossum, cat, monkey, humans) striated muscle is found in the cervical and smooth muscle in the distal thoracic esophagus (138,157). The importance of the extrinsic control of the two kinds of muscle being different, the striated and smooth muscle esophagus will be considered separately (except for data about the sensory fiber activity).

Striated Muscle Esophagus

Effects of extrinsic nerve stimulation. Stimulation of *vagal efferent fibers* by a single shock or train of pulses triggers, after a short latency, a twitch or a tetanus which are typical of striated muscle responses. If the stimulation is delivered on the cervical vagus below the nodose ganglion, the response observed in most mammals is restricted to the middle and lower esophagus, because the upper esophagus receives its motor fibers either from the pharyngoesophageal nerve or from the external branch of the superior laryngeal nerve (see above).

It has been possible to calculate the conduction velocity of the vagal efferent fibers by varying the site of nerve stimulation while using EMG recording techniques. Data obtained in sheep indicate values ranging between 15 and 30 m/sec for fibers controlling the cervical esophagus and between 40 and 60 m/sec for fibers controlling the thoracic esophagus (39).

The motor effects of vagal stimulation on the striated muscle esophagus are suppressed by neuromuscular blocking agents such as curare or succinylcholine (15, 86,157,275,324). This indicates that they are cholinergic in nature. In contrast, atropine has no effect (157,324).

Distension of the esophagus is probably one of the most physiological ways to stimulate the *vagal afferent fibers*. Such a stimulus induces a reflex contraction of the gullet, a secondary peristalsis. This response is present throughout the length of the esophagus, but the threshold for its initiation is higher in the cervical portion than in the thoracic one (151,157,275).

Reflex esophageal contractions may also be elicited by electrical stimulation of the central end of one vagus cut in the neck, the other one remaining intact. This was first established by Chauveau (46) in horse and later by Meltzer and Auer (231) in dog. Similar experiments have been more recently resumed by Roman and Car (277) who stimulated sheep afferent vagal fibers at different levels. An interesting feature emerging from these last data is that the area concerned with the reflex contraction is more restricted than the one innervated by the whole stimulated afferent fibers. For example, the cervical vagus carries the afferent fibers innervating the whole esophagus except the upper cervical portion, but stimulation of the central end of this nerve triggers only the contraction of the lower cervical esophagus (and not that of the thoracic portion). This fact may be explained by an inhibition exerted by sensitive fibers of the proximal parts of the gullet on the activity usually triggered by fibers of distal parts. This inhibition is of the same nature as that induced by a natural stimulation of afferent fibers, i.e, by a balloon distension. Indeed, distension of a limited portion of the esophagus inhibits contractile activity (either primary or secondary) distal to the distended area (151,275).

Effects of extrinsic fiber section. Many investigators did not find any change in various animals in esophageal function following section or stimulation of the different possible components of the *sympathetic supply* to the esophagus (27,131,157). In humans, extensive sympathectomy also failed to alter esophageal motility (157). Knight (193) reported somewhat different results in cat, but his findings have not been duplicated by others.

Bilateral *vagotomy* is followed by a paralysis of the striated muscle esophagus (44,131,142,157). When the section is performed below the nodose ganglion, the cervical esophagus in the dog and many other animals is not affected. But this part of the gullet is also paralyzed if the pharyngoesophageal nerves or the external branch of the superior laryngeal nerves are severed.

The observations concerning the thoracic esophagus after low cervical vagotomy do not allow one to distinguish between the role of afferent and efferent fibers since both are severed by the operation. However, a distinction is possible for the cervical esophagus because in many animals the afferent and efferent pathways are separated (different branches of the vagus). Section of afferent fibers (superior laryngeal nerves) in dog and sheep abolishes the secondary peristalsis of the cervical esophagus while the primary peristalsis over this region is retained (151,275).

Recording of extrinsic nerve activity. After microdissection of the superior laryngeal nerve in the anesthetized rat, Andrew (7) recorded the activity of *vagal sensory fibers* innervating the upper part of the cervical esophagus. At rest, these fibers fired spontaneously at a low frequency (4 to 15 spikes/sec). They were strongly excited (frequency up to 200 or 300 spikes/sec) by the presence of a bolus in the cervical esophagus or by the passage of a peristaltic wave through the ending zone.

The activity of vagal sensory fibers has also been successfully recorded by implanting microelectrodes in the nodose ganglion of anesthetized cats (226,228) or sheep (98). From these accurate studies, it appears that sensory fibers are in the majority myelinated fibers belonging to the B type. They originate from mechanoreceptors which in cat are distributed throughout the esophagus although they are more concentrated in two areas: at the beginning of the thoracic esophagus and at the lower esophageal sphincter. Most of the mechanoreceptors are slowly adapting receptors (Fig. 2), probably located within the muscular layer and activated by slight passive distension or contraction of the esophagus (either spontaneous or vagally induced contractions). In addition, there are a few rapidly adapting receptors, very likely located in the serosa, and exhibiting an on-off discharge only during strong displacements and distensions of esophagus (Fig. 3).

In addition to these mechanoreceptors, chemosensitive vagal endings have also been reported in the cat esophagus (135). These chemoreceptors, mainly located in the distal esophagus, are sensitive to acid or alkaline solutions.

After microdissection of the superior laryngeal nerve in anesthetized rats, Andrew (7) recorded the swallowing discharge of a few *vagal motor fibers* controlling the upper cervical esophagus. Following Andrew's pioneer work, more extensive studies have been performed in conscious sheep and monkey by Roman (274,275,280)

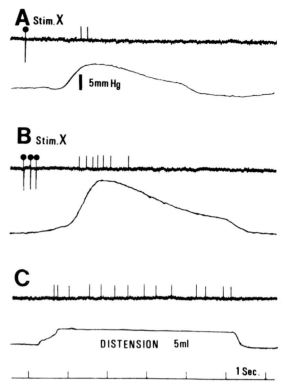

FIG. 2. Discharge of a vagal muscular receptor located in the lower part of the thoracic esophagus. The recording was made in anesthetized cat by means of a glass extracellular microelectrode inserted in the nodose ganglion of the vagus. **A**: Response to a moderate contraction produced by a single stimulation of the contralateral vagal nerve (Stim. X). **B**: Response to a stronger contraction elicited by stimulations of the contralateral vagal nerve. **C**: Response to esophageal distension. From MEI (*unpublished*).

by means of a nerve suture technique. In these animals, the central end of the left vagus had been sutured to the peripheral end of the left spinal accessory nerve. When reinnervation was effective, the activity of motor units of the sternocleidomastoideus and trapezius muscles indicated vagal motor fiber activity. Using electromyographic techniques for unit detection (by a Bronk needle) in the unanesthetized sheep or monkey, it was thus possible to study the discharge of the vagal fibers that previously supplied the esophagus (Fig. 4). The main results emerging from these experiments may be summarized as follows:

1. The vagal motor fibers have no spontaneous discharge at rest. This means that there is no tonic con-

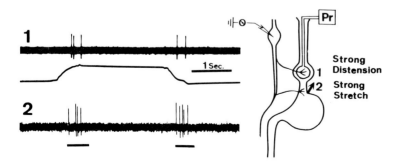

FIG. 3. Activity of vagal nonmuscular receptors located in the lower part of the esophagus. Recording as for Fig. 2. **1**: This receptor was activated by a strong distension of the esophagus. Pr, pressure transducer. **2**: This receptor responded to stretching (*bars*) of the lower esophageal sphincter. From MEI (*unpublished data*).

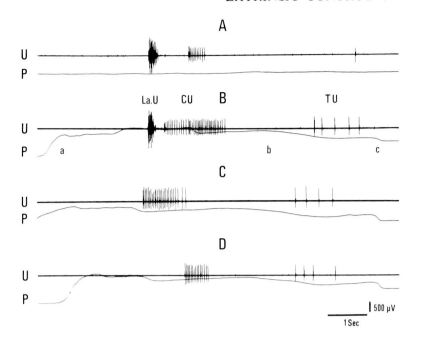

FIG. 4. Discharge of esophageal motor fibers during primary and secondary peristalsis in baboon. All the recordings of this figure were obtained using a nerve suture technique *(see text)*. *Upper trace:* discharge of 3 different vagal efferent fibers which originally supplied the larynx (La.U), the cervical esophagus (CU), and the distal thoracic esophagus (TU). *Lower trace:* pressure variations recorded by an intraesophageal balloon propelled by the peristaltic wave. a, balloon, inflation; b, passage through the narrow area of the beginning of the thoracic esophagus; c, balloon entering the stomach. **A:** Reference swallowing induced by injection of a small amount of water in the back of the mouth; the balloon is empty. **B:** Deglutition of a bolus (balloon inflated with 10 ml air). **C** and **D:** Secondary peristalsis with a bolus of same size as in **B**. Note the difference in the discharge pattern of vagal fibers supplying the striated (CU) and the smooth muscle esophagus (TU); see also the increased discharge of both kinds of fibers during the deglutition of a bolus (comparison between **A** and **B** recordings). From Roman and Tieffenbach (280).

traction of the esophagus, a conclusion in keeping with data obtained by direct EMG recording of esophageal muscle activity (9,139,243). They fire with a burst of spikes only during esophageal peristalsis, either primary or secondary. Their discharge frequency is fairly high and typical of a striated muscle command (mean frequency between 15 and 30 spikes/sec; instantaneous frequency between 20 and 70 spikes/sec).

2. During peristalsis, the various vagal motor fibers controlling the different portions of the esophagus discharge in succession (Fig. 4).

3. During primary peristalsis, the vagal motor discharges are reinforced by stimulation of afferent fibers from the esophagus: deglutition of a bolus elicits a more powerful discharge than that occurring during a "dry" swallow (Fig. 4).

4. During secondary peristalsis, the activity of the vagal motor fibers is usually weaker than that exhibited during primary peristalsis (Fig. 4).

5. Firing of vagal motor fibers is inhibited during the buccopharyngeal stage of deglutition or after distension of an esophageal portion above their innervation area. This inhibition has a central origin (see below); its effects have also been observed directly on esophageal motility either by manometric (157) or by EMG techniques (139,166).

Central mechanisms responsible for esophageal peristalsis. The organization of esophageal motility takes place within the swallowing center, which in fact is responsible for all the phenomena observed during deglutition, i.e., the buccopharyngeal component and esophageal peristalsis.

A large body of evidence resulting from the destruction of various nervous structures or sections of the brainstem at different levels (see references in 87) in-

dicates that the circuits necessary to the swallowing motor performance are contained within the rhombencephalon (medulla and pons). The rhombencephalic *swallowing center,* or more exactly the two half centers (left and right), may be divided into three stages or subsystems (87,175,275): afferent (inputs), efferent (outputs, i.e., motoneurons), and organizing stages (internuncial system).

The sensory fibers responsible for elicitation of swallowing have been demonstrated by nerve stimulation in the superior laryngeal branch of the vagus, the vagus itself, the glossopharyngeus, and the maxillary branch of the trigeminal nerve (87). At the central level, the afferents from these nerves converge in two systems: the solitary tract and the descending trigeminal tract (Fig. 5). It seems that lastly the swallowing fibers of the trigeminal tract also enter the solitary system (87). Finally, the solitary tract represents the central afferent system for swallowing. Its stimulation elicits deglutition as readily as excitation of peripheral nerves (40). Involvement of the central afferent system may also account for swallowing triggered by stimulation of the floor of the fourth ventricle (233).

The motoneurons involved in swallowing and esophageal motility (striated muscle) lie in the trigeminal, facial, and hypoglossal nuclei and nucleus ambiguus (87). Since Marinesco and Parhon (220), the nucleus ambiguus is generally agreed on as the vagal nucleus responsible for the innervation of striated muscles controlled by the vagus. Motoneurons of this nucleus innervate indeed the pharynx, larynx, and esophagus (87). Histological studies of muscle representation within the nucleus have provided evidence that esophageal motoneurons are concentrated in the rostral portion (87). This point has been fully confirmed by electrical stim-

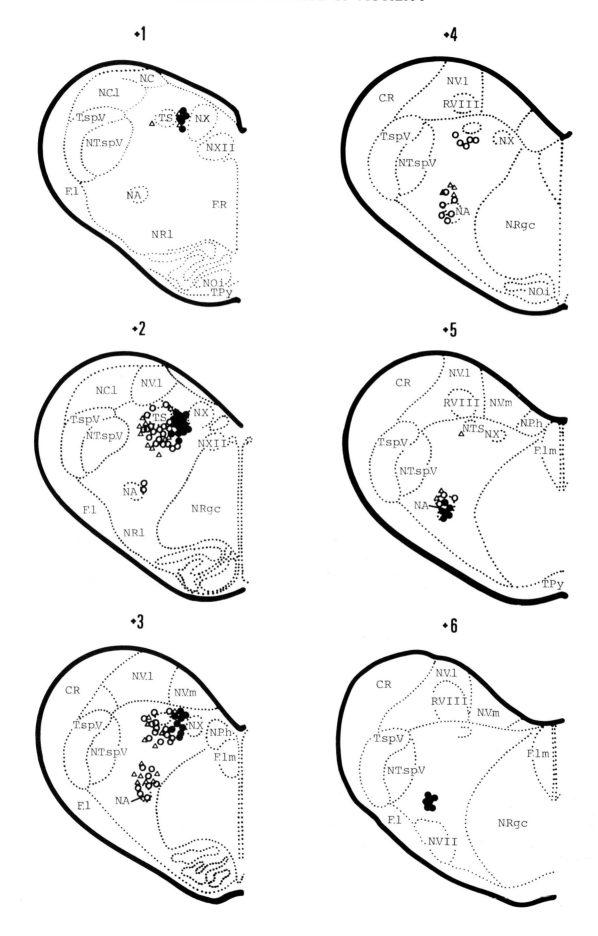

ulation of the medulla either in rabbit (205) or sheep (276). In addition, microelectrode recordings in the nucleus ambiguus have revealed the swallowing discharge of motoneurons occurring during either the buccopharyngeal (175,310) or the esophageal stage of deglutition (178) (Fig. 5). It was noticed that motor innervation of the smooth muscle esophagus is probably provided by the dorsal motor nucleus of the vagus instead of by the nucleus ambiguus. Such a statement is supported by histological data (220). In addition, after lesions of the vagal dorsal motor nucleus in cat, the motility of the distal esophagus (smooth muscle) is markedly impaired (143). Lastly, when horseradish peroxidase is injected into the last centimeters of the cat esophagus, labeled cell bodies are observed in the dorsal motor nucleus of the vagus (253), although some are also seen in the nucleus ambiguus.

The organizing stage consists of an internuncial system that programs the successive excitation of motoneurons, thereby organizing the whole motor sequence of deglutition. These programming interneurons are obviously placed between the afferents and the motoneurons, but their exact location remains disputed. Doty et al. (88) have reported that lesions of the reticular substance between the posterior pole of the facial nucleus and the rostral pole of the inferior olive, 1 to 3 mm dorsal to these structures and about 1.5 mm off the midline, suppressed swallowing induced by superior laryngeal nerve stimulation. According to Doty et al. (88), the destroyed area would correspond to the organizing stage of the swallowing center. Subsequent experiments based on stimulation of the medulla failed to confirm this interpretation (40,275). In addition, microelectrode soundings indicated that the medullary neurons exhibiting a swallowing activity, except the motoneurons, were located in the solitary tract nucleus (STN) and the underlying reticular substance, a few millimeters (2 to 4) in front of the obex (175,177,252, 310) (Fig. 5).

These STN or reticular neurons present either a phasic discharge only when swallowing occurs or a spontaneous activity that is altered during deglutition (increased or inhibited). Depending on the temporal relationship of their activity with the mylohyoideus contraction (onset of deglutition), the phasic swallowing neurons have been classified into three categories by Jean (175,177): "early" neurons firing before or during the buccopharyngeal stage, and "late" and "very late" neurons discharging during the esophageal stage (Fig. 6). Apart from their swallowing activity, these neurons

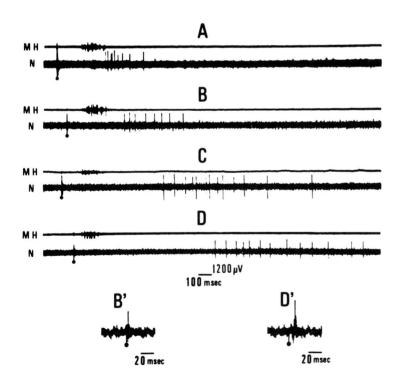

FIG. 6. Activity of late and very late swallowing interneurons. Anesthetized sheep. In all recordings: *upper trace,* mylohyoideus EMG (MH) indicating the onset of swallowing; *lower trace,* discharge of the mudullary swallowing interneuron (N). Dots indicate the stimulation artifacts. In all four recordings (A-D), the beginnings of the MH contraction have been alignated. **A-D:** "Swallowing activity" of late (**A** and **B**) and very late (**C** and **D**) interneurons during swallowing induced by SLN stimulation (single shock). **B′:** "Initial activity" of the late interneuron shown in **B**; stimulation of SLN by single shock. **D′:** "Initial activity" of the very late interneuron shown in **D**; stimulation of the cervical vagus by single shock. From Jean (175).

FIG. 5. Localization of swallowing neurons in sheep. Each map represents a hemi-medulla. The numbers indicate (in mm) the transverse sections rostral to the obex (+ 1 = 1 mm rostral to the obex, etc.). *open circles:* early neurons; *closed circles:* late and very late neurons; *triangles;* neurons with spontaneous activity. CR, corpus restiformis; F.l fasciculus lateralis; F.l.m, fasciculus longitudinalis medialis; F.R., formatio reticularis; N.A., nucleus ambiguus; N.C., nucleus cuneatus; N.C.l., nucleus cuneatus lateralis (von Monakov); N.O.i., nucleus olivaris inferior; N.P.h., nucleus praepositus hypoglossi; N.R.gc., nucleus reticularis gigantocellularis; N.R.l., nucleus reticularis lateralis; N.T.S., nucleus tractus solitarius; N.T.sp.V., nucleus tr. spinalis n. trigemini; N.V.l., nucleus vestibularis lateralis; N.V.m., nucleus vestibularis medialis; N.VII, nucleus n. facialis; N.X, nucleus dorsalis n. vagi; N.XII, nucleus n. hypoglossi; R.VIII, radices descendentes n. vestibuli; T.Py., tractus pyramidalis; T.S., tractus solitarius; T.sp.V., tractus spinalis n. trigemini; From Jean (175,177).

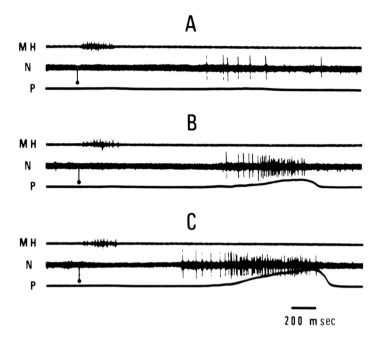

FIG. 7. Effect of a slight esophageal distension upon the swallowing activity of a late interneuron. Anesthetized sheep. In all recordings: *upper trace*, mylohyoideus EMG (MH); *middle trace*, discharge of the medullary interneuron (N); *lower trace*, recording of the intraesophageal pressure (P). The three recordings (**A–C**) were obtained during swallowing induced by SLN stimulation (*dots*). The balloon is deflated in **A**, inflated with 5 ml air in **B**, and with 10 ml in **C**. Note the large increase of swallowing activity in **B** and particularly in **C**. From Jean (175).

may also exhibit a short-latency activation on electrical stimulation of afferent fibers lying in either the superior laryngeal nerve (early and late neurons) or the cervical vagus nerve (very late neurons). The late and very late neurons are activated by localized distensions of the proximal or distal esophagus, respectively (Fig. 7). Taking into account these reflex activations and the fact that STN is usually regarded as a relay nucleus for the vagal sensory fibers, it might be argued that the swallowing discharge of STN neurons actually corresponds to a feedback phenomenon, a reflex activity due to afferent fiber activation during deglutition. However, this interpretation does not seem correct, since Jean (175, 177) observed that the swallowing activity of the STN or reticular neurons in response to superior laryngeal nerve stimulation was not markedly altered after curarization of the animal (Fig. 8). Hence it appears that these neurons are truly interneurons which take part in the programming of the motor sequence of deglutition.

This conclusion is further supported by the effects resulting from STN lesions: After electrical coagulation, either extensive (177) or restricted (176), deglutitions elicited by superior laryngeal nerve stimulation disappear either totally or only in part (suppression of the esophageal stage). All the preceding results point out that an important portion of the swallowing center lies in the STN, which is not simply a relay nucleus for afferent information but also and chiefly an integrative area subserving the organization of motor performances, in this case, that of deglutition.

Neurophysiological mechanisms are involved in the programming of esophageal peristalsis. Current concepts about the nervous mechanisms of esophageal peristalsis in particular, and deglutition in general, have been deeply influenced by pioneer works of Mosso (246) and Meltzer (229). From these fundamental works, especially those of Meltzer, emerged the concept of central programming of deglutition. This old established

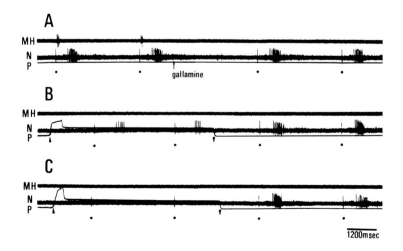

FIG. 8. Inhibition of the discharge of a very late interneuron by distension of a proximal esophageal region. Anesthetized sheep. **A**: Swallowing activity of a very late interneuron (N) corresponding to the beginning of the thoracic esophagus during several deglutitions (SLN stimulation at the dots) before and after curarization (gallamine). The intraesophageal balloon (P) located at the level of the cervical esophagus is deflated. Note that after curarization the mylohyoideus EMG (MH) disappears, while the swallowing activity of the interneuron persists. **B**: First the balloon is inflated with 10 ml air (*arrow*); the swallowing activity of the interneuron is then weaker and delayed. After balloon deflation (*arrow*) the swallowing activity returns to normal (end of tracing). **C**: The distension is stronger (20 ml air). The neuronal discharge is absent as long as the balloon is inflated. From Jean, (175).

concept has regained at the present time a renewal of interest in neurophysiology. Meltzer described the mechanism of primary peristalsis as follows:

> The first afferent impulse which is conveyed from the periphery to the centre of deglutition and which causes the coordinated contraction of the mylohyoid, pharyngeal and laryngeal group of muscles, travels further within the centre through several groups of ganglia, sends down successively along its route efferent impulses to the several divisions of the esophagus including the cardia and causes hereby their successive contraction without the aid of new afferent stimuli.

In other words, the motor sequence of deglutition would depend on a central mechanism (connections between neurons) which, after starting, could run its entire course without any new afferent support. This opinion was based on a fact already noticed by Mosso (246), that, in dog, primary peristalsis could jump a gap produced by esophageal transsection. According to Meltzer, the mechanism of secondary peristalsis, quite different from that of primary peristalsis, would consist of a succession of reflexes originating in esophageal receptors sequentially stimulated by a moving bolus. In support of this difference, Meltzer argued that in dog, secondary peristalsis, unlike primary, cannot jump a gap produced by esophageal transsection (229,230).

More recent studies of the effects of esophageal transsection have confirmed the theory of the central programming of primary peristalsis in the striated muscle esophagus (44,131). In addition, microelectrode recordings have shown that, in sheep, the swallowing discharge of medullary neurons (either motoneurons or interneurons) persisted after curarization of the animals (175,177,178) (Fig. 8). This means that the swallowing program triggered by superior laryngeal nerve stimulation can run its full course within the center even if muscles are paralyzed (striated muscle) so that no bolus is transported. Actually, these results do not mean that afferents from esophagus have no role under physiological circumstances. They only indicate that in the absence of afferent input the central program is able to organize the motor sequence of peristalsis, at least in sheep. It is possible that, according to the species, the central program deprived of afferent reinforcement becomes subliminal for motoneuronal activity. This might be the case in dog, since Longhi and Jordan (212) have observed in this animal that deviation of the swallowed bolus from the esophagus by means of an esophageal cannula or through an esophagostomy eliminated all peristaltic activity below the level of bolus deviation. These last data have been fully confirmed by Janssens and co-workers (137,166,169) who showed that deviation of the swallowed bolus at the cervical level eliminated all peristaltic activity in the thoracic esophagus. However, accurate studies performed on several species

led Janssens (166) to assume that the necessity of an intraluminal bolus for the progression of primary peristalsis in the striated muscle esophagus is valid only for the cervical esophagus of dog, since esophageal transsection and bolus deviation at the thoracic level in dog and at any level in rabbit, opossum, and rhesus monkey does not eliminate primary peristalsis in the esophageal segment below the level of deviation. Janssens (166) concluded that the regulation of primary peristalsis in the canine esophagus is the exception rather than the rule, a statement which casts serious doubt on the use of the canine esophagus as an adequate model for the study of esophageal physiology.

Even if an afferent feedback is not necessary for primary peristalsis, under normal circumstances when a bolus is swallowed esophageal receptors are stimulated (see above, recording of vagal sensory fiber activity). This afferent stimulation increases the discharge of the various esophageal motoneurons (see recordings of vagal motor fiber activity). A similar facilitation is observed at the level of the interneurons that program the motor sequence of peristalsis (175,177) (Fig. 7). Thus the central program may function in the absence of afferent support, but under normal circumstances, this program is permanently modified by esophageal afferents that adjust the force and progression velocity of the peristaltic contraction according to the esophageal content.

Concerning secondary peristalsis, various investigators (63,101,151,168,302) have brought evidence that its central mechanism should not be very different from that of primary peristalsis. The motoneurons and interneurons involved in both cases are the same (175,177, 274,275). During primary peristalsis, however, the central chain of neurons which programs deglutition is excited from its beginning, whereas during secondary peristalsis the excitation starts at the level of one or another link of the chain. According to Roman (275) and Jean (177), an effect of this difference would be that, in sheep at least, excitation of the central organizing system is weaker during secondary than during primary peristalsis. Then, if this central excitation was not permanently reinforced by afferent feedback during secondary peristalsis, it would not proceed to the end of the central neuronal chain, contrary to what is observed during primary peristalsis.

The central mechanism responsible for the successive excitation of interneurons during deglutition is not yet understood. However, it may be assumed that it is probably different from a simple transmission of excitation between neurons. In this connection, attention must be paid to the inhibitory phenomena that have already been mentioned about activity of motor neurons (see above recording of vagal motor fibers' activity). Inhibition is also observed at the level of interneurons, within the central system, subserving the programming of deglutition. Indeed, Jean (175,177) has shown that in sheep all the esophageal interneurons were strongly inhibited during the buccopharyngeal stage of deglutition. In addition, the interneurons controlling a distal esophageal segment were also inhibited when interneurons controlling more proximal segments were called into play (Fig. 8). Jean (177) put forward arguments supporting the assumption that the successive activation of the swallowing interneurons might result, at least in part, from a succession of postinhibitory rebounds. From a conceptual point of view, it is noteworthy that Jean's hypothesis provides a mechanism of programming (series of postinhibitory rebounds) rather similar to those already demonstrated in the nervous system of invertebrates, for example, that subserving the food intake behavior in decapod crustacea (296).

Reflex and cortical triggering of the swallowing center. These points will not be dealt with in detail since they are not directly related to the nervous control of esophageal motility.

Swallowing can be reflexly elicited by stimulation of specific areas of palate, pharynx, and epiglottis, which are innervated by the maxillary branch of trigeminal nerve, the glossopharyngeal nerve, and the superior laryngeal nerve (SLN) (87). However, when these nerves are electrically stimulated, only stimulation of the SLN is really effective in causing swallowing in all the species tested. Stimulation of the SLN, even with a single pulse, elicits the swallowing discharge of all the swallowing center neurons and, in addition, a short-latency activation of neurons controlling the muscles of pharynx, larynx, and the beginning of the esophagus (175,177). These short-latency activations are the neurophysiological support of "elementary reflexes" often mentioned in the literature (87).

Stimulation of the glossopharyngeal nerve and maxillary branch of the trigeminal nerve gives rise to unclear and controversial results (87,91,138,304). More recent studies in sheep (50) have shown that glossopharyngeal nerve stimulation produced a facilitation of medullary interneurons controlling the buccopharyngeal stage of deglutition (early interneurons). This facilitation was usually unable to trigger swallowing but sufficient to inhibit a primary or secondary peristalsis already in progress. This inhibition had been noticed a century ago by Kronecker and Meltzer (199), who claimed that the glossopharyngeal nerve was a specific inhibitor nerve for peristalsis, especially responsible for the inhibition of esophageal motility during the buccopharyngeal stage of deglutition. Obviously, this interpretation was not correct since the inhibition observed by these authors likely expressed an intrinsic property of the swallowing center, i.e., suppression of the activity of late and very late interneurons when the early ones were called into play.

Concerning the maxillary branch of the trigeminal nerve, recent data also obtained in sheep have indicated that its stimulation had no effect on the activity of medullary swallowing neurons and so was unable to trigger swallowing (51).

Cortical and subcortical controls also influence swallowing. Early reports (87) mention the possibility of inducing swallowing by stimulation of the cerebral cortex. More recently, this point has been fully confirmed by Sumi (311) in rabbits and by Car (37) in sheep. The effective area which lies in the frontal cortex projects onto the swallowing zone of the medullary STN through a polysynaptic pathway (38). For swallowing to be elicited, the cortical area must be stimulated by a train of shocks. Stimulation by single pulses produces only a weak discharge of the early interneurons of the STN and of some motoneurons of the nucleus ambiguus (179). These results indicate that the swallowing area can closely control the activity of medullary neurons involved in the buccopharyngeal stage of deglutition.

In addition to its control by the cortical area, deglutition can be elicited or facilitated by stimulation of various subcortical structures including the internal capsule, subthalamus, amygdala, hypothalamus, substantia nigra, and mesencephalic reticular formation (38,91). Some of these structures certainly belong to the corticobulbar swallowing pathway.

Smooth Muscle Esophagus

Effects of severing the extrinsic nerves: the "autonomous" peristalsis. In contrast to the striated muscle esophagus, the smooth muscle portion of esophagus is not paralyzed by bilateral vagotomy (24,27,35,81,187, 279,326). Indeed, the smooth muscle esophagus remains able to exhibit peristaltic contractions in response to liquid injection or balloon distension. Similar responses can be observed *in vitro* on the isolated organ (49), indicating that the responses observed after vagotomy alone were not due to a possible involvement of the sympathetic nervous system. In this connection, it may be recalled that according to Burgess et al. (27) the sympathectomy alone performed *in vivo* does not change the function of the feline smooth muscle esophagus.

The peristalsis occurring in the smooth muscle esophagus deprived of its extrinsic innervation was termed "tertiary peristalsis" by Cannon (35) and Jurica (187). This term had two advantages; first, it has a physiological meaning in that it denotes a peristalsis which, contrary to the primary and secondary types, is independent of the extrinsic innervation; second, from a historical point of view, it is in lineal descent from the two previous terms (primary and secondary) proposed by Meltzer. Unfortunately, the term is now confusing since clinicians use it to describe nonpropulsive contractions occurring in elderly patients. Thus, to be as clear as possible, the adjective "autonomous" will be employed in the place of "tertiary" in the following text.

Effects of efferent fiber stimulation. Available data concern only the effects of vagal stimulation. With pressure or suction electrodes on the cat smooth muscle esophagus during *in vivo* or *in vitro* experiments, it is possible to record two kinds of EMG responses induced by stimulation of vagal efferent fibers with single shocks or short pulse trains.

Excitatory responses (Fig. 9) consist of excitatory junction potentials (EJPs), slow depolarizations which may give rise to a burst of spikes inducing a contraction of the muscle (79,81,126,323). EJPs are recorded from the two muscle layers, the circular EJPs having a higher threshold than the longitudinal ones (126). These excitatory responses are suppressed by atropine or hexamethonium. This indicates that the excitatory pathway is entirely cholinergic, composed of cholinergic preganglionic fibers exciting cholinergic intramural neurons that in turn activate smooth muscle.

Inhibitory responses (Fig. 10) consist of inhibitory junction potentials (IJPs) corresponding to slow hyperpolarizations of smooth muscle fibers that are often followed by a transient depolarization that may initiate spikes (postinhibitory rebounds). IJPs are more easily recorded on the circular muscle (79,126) and after atropine treatment (126). They are not affected by antiad-

renergic drugs but they are suppressed by hexamethonium (126). In view of the preceding results, IJPs might result from stimulation of cholinergic preganglionic fibers that excite intramural inhibitory neurons whose mediator is neither epinephrine nor acetylcholine. These could be the "purinergic" nerves described by Burnstock (28,29). As already known for other parts of the digestive tract (184,223), it is likely that preganglionic vagal fibers leading to inhibition have a smaller diameter, a higher excitation threshold, and a lower conduction velocity than those leading to excitation (126).

When long trains of pulses are delivered to the distal cut end of one vagus, two kinds of responses can be elicited from the circular muscle: the "on-response" during stimulation and the "off-response" after the end of stimulation. These two sorts of responses have been observed either in cat (86,323) or in opossum (84).

The off-responses appear to be resistant to atropine (84,86). Thus they might correspond to a passive rebound phenomenon associated with membrane depolarization after active hyperpolarization due to stimulation of the vagal fibers synapsing with the nonadrenergic noncholinergic intramural inhibitory neurons (see above). Some investigators (84,86,323) have found that the off-responses were not propagated. Mukhopadhyay and

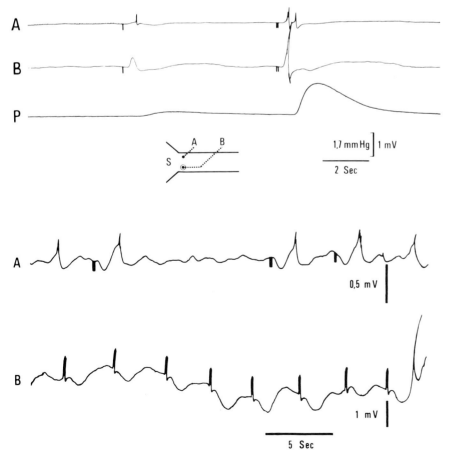

FIG. 9. Excitatory vagal responses recorded *in vitro* on longitudinal and circular muscle of the cat LES. **A** and **B**: EMG; monopolar records with pressure electrodes; RC amplification (time constant 0.1 sec). Recording **A**, on longitudinal muscle; **B**, on circular muscle (window through the longitudinal layer). **P**: Intramural pressure; DC amplification. The first vagal stimulation (single pulse, 1 msec, 15 V) evokes an EJP which initiates a spike on the longitudinal muscle and only an EJP of high amplitude on circular muscle. The second stimulation (2 pulses, 30 Hz, 1 msec, 15 V) evokes EJPs initiating two small spikes on longitudinal muscle and one large spike on circular muscle. Circular muscle contraction leads to a high intraluminal pressure increase. From Gonella et al. (126).

FIG. 10. Inhibitory vagal responses recorded *in vitro* in the presence of atropine on longitudinal and circular muscle of the cat LES. In **A** and **B**, EMG recorded from 2 different animals; monopolar records; RC amplification. **A**: Electrode on longitudinal muscle (R-C = 0.1 sec). **B**: Electrode on circular muscle (window through longitudinal muscle; R-C = 2.5 sec). Stimulation of the vagus with brief trains (5 pulses at 30 Hz, 1 msec, 18 V). IJPs are observed on both muscle layers. In **A**, each IJP is followed by a rebound depolarization with one or several spikes superimposed. In **B**, the rebound occurs at the end of the series of stimuli. From Gonella et al. (126).

Weisbrodt (247) reported otherwise, but they used short trains of pulses which according to Dodds et al. (84) did not allow differentiation between on and off-responses.

The on-responses are suppressed by atropine (84,86). Therefore, they result from excitation of the vagal excitatory (cholinergic) pathway. According to Tieffenbach and Roman (323), the on-responses observed in cat distal esophagus were more-or-less simultaneous. However, Dodds et al. (86) observed in the same species that the on-contractions generally had a latency gradient simulating peristalsis, although the tracings they showed were not fully convincing in that respect. In opossum, Dodds et al. (84) recorded also on-responses which propagated with a velocity very similar to that of peristalsis. However, the aspect of the response was greatly dependent on the stimulation parameters since high stimulus frequency and long pulse widths tended to make the contractions more simultaneous.

Finally, vagal stimulation is an artificial method for the nervous control study because it calls into play at the same time a great number of preganglionic fibers synapsing with excitatory or inhibitory intramural neurons of various esophageal regions. When, in addition, stimulation is performed with a long train of pulses (at a frequency likely different from that of the spontaneous discharge), complex summation and occlusion phenomena must take place within the plexuses. This makes the interpretation of stimulating effects still less clear, since nearly nothing is known about the esophageal myenteric circuitry. Taking into account these nonphysiological conditions plus the possible depressant action of anesthesia on myenteric circuits (*in vivo* experiments), it would be surprising to produce something resembling the normal working of the esophagus.

Possible roles of the vagal extrinsic innervation in the motility of the smooth muscle esophagus. The existence of an autonomous peristalsis in the smooth muscle portion of the esophagus raises several questions. What may be the role of the vagal fibers supplying this region? Is there any central programming of peristalsis during deglutition? One might speculate that, in opossum, cat, monkey, and human, the proximal esophagus (striated muscle) is under central control, whereas peristalsis of the distal esophagus (smooth muscle) would only depend on a peripheral mechanism (myenteric neurons) triggered by arrival of the bolus in this area. This assumption does not fit in with several experimental data. First, there is an extrinsic vagal supply whose stimulation induces excitatory and inhibitory effects, even with single-pulse stimulation, which underlines the powerful influence exerted by the vagal fibers on esophageal smooth muscle. On the other hand, various experiments strongly suggest the existence of an extrinsic command during deglutition. For instance, deviation of the swallowed bolus at the level of cervical esophagus in opossums or rhesus monkeys does not eliminate the primary

peristalsis in the thoracic esophagus (166,167). In other words, the smooth muscle esophagus does not need the presence of an intraluminal bolus for the progression of primary peristalsis. An identical conclusion can be drawn from curarization experiments. In baboons, primary peristalsis of the smooth muscle esophagus, occurring during swallowing induced by SLN stimulation, is still elicited after curarization of the animal to paralyze the oropharynx and cervical esophagus (323). Since no bolus can reach the thoracic esophagus after curarization, the persistent contractions of the smooth muscle must be due to central orders. Similar observations have also been made by Janssens (166) on three human beings having severe cerebral trauma but a preserved function of the swallowing center and who needed curarization because of the artificial respiration. In addition, Ryan et al. (286) have observed in the anesthetized opossum that bilateral vagal cooling or vagotomy decreased significantly the primary peristalsis occurring in the smooth muscle segment of esophagus in response to a pharyngeal stimulation.

Using a nerve suture technique previously described (see above), Roman and Tieffenbach (280) recorded in the conscious monkey the spontaneous discharge of vagal efferent fibers controlling the smooth muscle esophagus. These fibers fired in succession during either primary or secondary peristalsis (Fig. 4). Their discharge was weak with only a few spikes at a frequency lower than 5 spikes/sec. According to Roman and Tieffenbach, the main effect of these discharges would be to facilitate the intramural neurons which are by themselves able to organize esophageal motility. In other words, the vagal fibers whose activity was recorded would belong to the vagal excitatory pathway that is called into play during primary or secondary peristalsis. As already mentioned, the vagal excitatory effects on smooth muscle are blocked by atropine. Thus the primary peristalsis should also be suppressed under atropine. This seems to be true in cat (86) but not in opossum or humans (85,190,247). In humans, intravenous injection of anticholinergic drugs is followed by disturbances of esophageal motility resembling those of diffuse spasm or presbyesophagus (139).

Nerve stimulation experiments have also indicated the existence of vagal preganglionic fibers that act to inhibit esophageal motility (vagal inhibitory pathway). At present, it is possible only to speculate about the physiological role of such fibers. They might be involved in the deglutitive inhibition of esophageal peristalsis. In monkey and humans, EMG studies have shown that the distal progression of primary peristalsis in the thoracic esophagus could be stopped by a second swallow (138, 139,166). It is possible that this inhibition results, at least in part, from an active inhibition of esophageal smooth muscle, for suppression of vagal excitatory discharges alone should not impede the progression of an autonomous peristalsis initiated by the arrival of the swallowed bolus in the distal esophagus. On the other hand, it is known that inhibition induced by nonadrenergic noncholinergic intramural neurons is followed by a rebound excitation, a contraction of the smooth muscle. In opossum smooth muscle strips electrically stimulated, Weisbrodt and Christensen (330) observed that the time interval between the end of stimulus and the onset of postinhibitory rebound was longer for strips taken from more distally located esophageal segments. This observation led Weisbrodt and Christensen (330) to propose that primary peristalsis in smooth muscle esophagus could simply result from a rebound excitation. According to these authors:

> After a swallow the responsible nerves (presumably the nonadrenergic inhibitory nerves) to the entire smooth muscle segment are excited simultaneously. This causes the circular muscle to be inhibited. Since all of the muscle except the distal esophageal sphincter is already maximally inhibited, relaxation occurs only at the distal esophageal sphincter. Upon recovery from this inhibition, the muscle at all levels demonstrates a rebound contraction. Because of the gradient in latency of this contraction, this response appears as a peristaltic sweep down the esophagus.

This attractive hypothesis is not fully satisfactory because it provides no role for the excitatory vagal pathway which still does exist. In addition, during their recording experiments, Roman and Tieffenbach (280) did not observe the simultaneous excitation of the vagal fibers as predicted in the proposal of Weisbrodt and Christensen. Anyway, it remains that rebound contractions do exist and that they very likely take part in peristalsis organization even if they are coupled with other phenomena.

Extrinsic Control of Sphincters

Upper Esophageal Sphincter

EMG evidence of an active closure. The closing and opening mechanisms of the upper esophageal sphincter are still controversial. Since many investigators had been unable to record a tonic EMG activity of the muscles surrounding the pharyngoesophageal junction (especially the cricopharyngeus), Doty (87) concluded that "the pharyngoesophageal junction must normally be closed only by passive elasticity of surrounding tissues, that active closure is readily induced by a variety of reflexes serving to contract the cricopharyngeus and that during swallowing the orifice is opened passively by hyoid and laryngeal movements while all contraction of cricopharyngeus is initially forestalled by the swallowing center exerting a powerful inhibition on cricopharyngeal motoneurons." Subsequent EMG studies performed either in humans using intraluminal probes (139,243) or in sheep and dog having chronic implanted electrodes (41,138,166) have shown that at rest there is a more or less permanent tonic activity of the cricopharyngeal muscle. In the dog, this activity is minimal when the animal is very quiet. But the slightest excitation gives rise to a continuous spiking activity more or less modulated by respiration. In humans, the tonic resting discharge is usually more intense probably because of a reflex excitation due to the intraluminal recording device. With a swallow, the continuous spiking activity is immediately and completely inhibited while intraluminal pressure falls. This inhibition is followed by an intense burst of spikes which corresponds to the deglutitive contraction of the pharyngoesophageal sphincter (peak of intraluminal pressure). Then, the EMG activity and the intraluminal pressure return to their resting level.

Central control during swallowing. The behavior of the striated muscle of the pharyngoesophageal sphincter is necessarily the direct consequence of motor fiber discharge. Indeed, Andrew (7) demonstrated that the vagal motor fibers supplying the upper sphincter had a spontaneous discharge that was inhibited during the buccopharyngeal stage of deglutition and then resumed at a transient raised level. This inhibition of the tonic discharge once more expresses one main feature of the swallowing center organization, the inhibition of activity in aboral segments when more oral segments are called into play.

Reflex control. In sheep and dog, the tonic EMG activity of the upper sphincter is reinforced when the proximal cervical esophagus is slightly distended either by inflation of a balloon (41) or by injection of water in it (166,168). In humans, similar effects have been observed by recording the intrasphincteric pressure during intraesophageal infusion of water and NaCl or HCl solutions at various concentrations (117). Infusion with each solution increased the sphincter resting pressure (volume response). The increase was greater for HCl infusion than for other solutions, indicating a selective response to acid.

All these reflex responses are probably due to excitation of vagal afferents from the esophagus since electrical stimulation of these afferents in sheep readily elicits reflex contractions of the cricopharyngeus (277).

Lower Esophageal Sphincter

Effects of extrinsic nerve section or pharmacological blockade on lower esophageal sphincter (LES) function. During experiments *in vitro* on the terminal esophagus of the guinea pig and kitten (216) or dog (321), it was demonstrated that some resting tone persisted in the LES totally deprived of its extrinsic innervation. In addition, Mann et al. (216) showed that transient distension of the esophageal body produced a sphincter relaxation immediately followed by a phasic contraction that closed the gastroesophageal junction. Thus the sphincter function is preserved at least in part after extrinsic denervation. Then, what is changed by comparison with the normal animal? What are the net effects of vagal or sympathetic sections? Many investigators have attempted to answer these questions. For a detailed bibliography from before 1958, the reader is referred to the review of Ingelfinger (157); only works since 1958 will be individually cited in the following text.

The results of *vagotomy* can be summarized as follows: (a) it produces difficulty or impossibility for LES to relax during swallowing, which constitutes in sum an experimental achalasia (24,27,44,142,157), data that have been more recently confirmed by vagal cooling experiments (58,286); (b) it increases resting tone, to create a "spasm" that may be a permanent, transient, or even late occurrence (27,157,272); (c) it does not alter resting tone (58,157); (d) it decreases resting tone (44, 131,142,157,181).

In addition, the closer to the diaphragm the vagotomy is performed, the less pronounced is the effect on LES (45,58). On the other hand, relaxation induced by esophageal distension is also suppressed in those species such as dog having striated muscle throughout the esophagus (338). But this is not true for species having smooth muscle in the distal esophagus (58,216) because in that case there is an intramural nervous mechanism which provides descending inhibition like that described for intestine (17,144).

Concerning the effects of atropine, the results are less variable than those for vagotomy since most of the data indicate some fall of the resting tone (181,208,264,305). This is not surprising because, as indicated below, the vagus nerve likely exerts a double control on LES, both excitatory and inhibitory. Now, atropine only blocks the vagal excitatory pathway while vagotomy also suppresses the inhibitory one.

With *sympathetic nerve section* or pharmacological blockade, the results are also conflicting. After various sympathetic denervations, very often no clear change of the sphincter resting tone has been observed, but sometimes a slight decrease has been reported (157). More recent studies in the opossum have shown that adrenergic denervation by 6-hydroxydopamine resulted in decreased basal pressure (83) and that phentolamine, an adrenergic alpha-receptor antagonist, prevented the transient sphincter hypertension caused by vagotomy (272). On the other hand, sphincter relaxation during swallowing was unaffected by sympathectomy (83).

In sum, the control exerted on LES tone by the adrenergic supply, if there is any, appears to be mainly excitatory. This fact has been confirmed by nerve stimulation experiments (see below).

Effects of efferent nerve stimulation and of cholinergic and sympathetic agonists and antagonists. Liter-

ature before 1958 (157) indicates that repetitive stimulation of the distal cut end of the cervical *vagus* in various animals (dog, rabbit, cat) produces conflicting results: either a sphincter contraction or a relaxation often followed by a contraction after the end of the stimulation. It is also reported that the type of response might depend on the stimulation parameters or on the initial state of sphincter tone.

Subsequent works have somewhat clarified the problem. Thus it is established that vagal stimulation in cat and opossum relaxes the LES (52,79,126,272). EMG recordings show that relaxation follows from a hyperpolarization of the circular muscle (79,126) (Fig. 10). When stimulation is performed with long trains of pulses, the hyperpolarization is permanent; but when single pulses or short trains of pulses are used, the hyperpolarization consists of brief inhibitory junction potentials. Usually these inhibitory responses are followed by a rebound excitation, a membrane depolarization that gives rise to spikes thereby inducing a muscle contraction (Fig. 10). All these data easily explain an early and often reported observation (157) according to which vagal stimulation produced a sequence of both responses, a sphincter relaxation followed by a contraction.

In opossum, it seems that vagal stimulation induces only inhibitory effects, i.e., sphincter relaxation (272). But in cat, excitatory responses are also elicited in both muscular layers (126). With single-pulse stimulation, the excitatory responses consist of brief muscle depolarizations or excitatory junction potentials that may give rise to spike potentials triggering muscle contraction (Fig. 9). EJPs are suppressed either by atropine or by hexamethonium, indicating that these responses are due to stimulation of preganglionic cholinergic fibers that excite intramural postganglionic neurons: their mediator, responsible for muscle excitation, is also acetylcholine.

As for inhibitory responses, they would involve preganglionic fibers synapsing with intramural postganglionic neurons whose mediator is neither acetylcholine nor epinephrine (126,129). These intramural inhibitory neurons very likely correspond to the so-called purinergic neurons (28,29).

Sympathetic nerves have also been studied. Epinephrine and norepinephrine cause contraction of the LES of various animals *in vivo* and *in vitro* (47,48,127,130, 157). These motor effects involve alpha-adrenergic receptors since they are also produced by phenylephrine (83) and blocked by phentolamine or ergotamine (83, 127). The LES is also said to possess beta-adrenergic receptors whose stimulation leads to inhibition of resting tone in opossum (83) and in humans (339).

According to many investigators, electrical stimulation of the various components of the sympathetic supply has no effect on LES motility; for others, however, a contraction resembling a "spasm" can be obtained (157). Recent experimental data in cats are in keeping

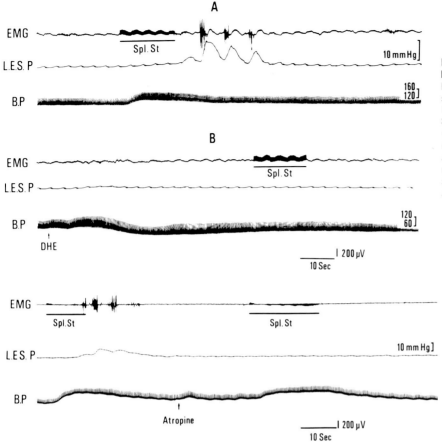

FIG. 11. Motor response of the cat LES evoked by splanchnic nerve stimulation *in vivo.* EMG, bipolar recording made with extracellular pressure electrodes (RC = 0.06 sec); LESP, intraluminal pressure; BP, arterial blood pressure; Spl. St, splanchnic nerve stimulation (30 Hz, 0.5 msec, 16 V). **A** and **B** recordings were made on the same animal. **A,** control; **B,** after dihydroergotamine (DHE) injection (1 mg/kg) at the arrow. Note in **B** the suppression of the LES response. From Gonella et al. (127).

FIG. 12. Effect of atropine on LES response evoked by splanchnic nerve stimulation *in vivo.* EMG, bipolar recording (RC = 0.06 sec); LESP, endoluminal pressure; BP, arterial blood pressure; Spl.St, splanchnic nerve stimulation (30 Hz, 0.5 msec, 16 V). Note that after atropine (0.1 mg/kg) the rise in blood pressure is still present while the LES response is abolished. From Gonella et al. (127).

with this last conclusion (127,278). From these data, the following points emerge. Sympathetic fibers supplying the cat LES come from the stellate ganglion or run along the splanchnic nerve. Repetitive stimulation of these fibers induces, with a long latency (5 to 8 sec), a sustained or rhythmic contraction of the sphincter that is suppressed by adrenergic alpha antagonists (phentolamine, dihydroergotamine) and greatly reduced by atropine (Figs. 11 and 12). This surprising effect of atropine suggests that norepinephrine released by sympathetic endings might act chiefly (but not exclusively) on the myenteric cholinergic neurons to release acethycholine which in turn excites sphincter muscle. The existence of a cholinergic link in the sympathetic control of LES is further supported by recent findings (128) showing a

release of labeled acethycholine by LES muscular strips under the action of norepinephrine.

Recording of efferent fiber activity. Available data concern only the vagal fibers whose activity has been studied in conscious dog using a nerve suture technique (236,238). It must be recalled that the muscular coat of the dog esophagus is entirely striated except for the LES area, where a band of circularly disposed smooth muscle becomes visible within the striated coat. Vagal fibers that might control the LES smooth muscle have a spontaneous discharge that is altered during swallowing. Two types of patterns can be distinguished (Fig. 13). For some fibers, the spontaneous firing rate (between 1.5 and 4.5 spikes/sec) is suddenly enhanced just after the buccopharyngeal stage of swallowing (from 12 to 16

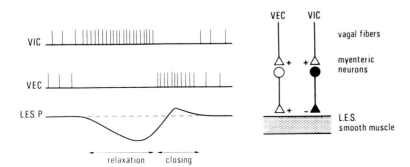

FIG. 13. Diagrammatic representation of the vagal control of LES (cardia). VEC, vagal excitatory fiber of the cardia; VIC, vagal inhibitory fiber of the cardia; LESP, endoluminal pressure recorded in the LES during esophageal peristalsis. The two types of fibers exhibit a spontaneous tonic discharge. During esophageal peristalsis (either primary or secondary), the firing of VIC fibers is increased while LES relaxes; this sustained activity is interrupted at the end of peristalsis, i.e., when LES closes again. The behavior of VEC fibers is exactly the opposite: cessation of discharge during LES relaxation and transient activation during sphincter closing. From Miolan and Roman (238).

spikes/sec). This discharge stops abruptly just before the end of esophageal peristalsis and starts again 2 or 3 sec later at a low frequency (from 1.5 to 4.5 spikes/sec). Other fibers which also have a low discharge frequency (from 1 to 3 spikes/sec) stop firing soon after the onset of swallowing and remain silent until the end of esophageal peristalsis. At this time, i.e., when the bolus enters the stomach, the discharge resumes with a transient increased frequency (from 5 to 9 spikes/sec).

According to Miolan and Roman (236,238) the former fibers, termed vagal inhibitory fibers of cardia (VIC), are preganglionic fibers that probably activate intramural inhibitory neurons, whereas the latter, called vagal excitatory fibers of cardia (VEC), are preganglionic fibers which very likely synapse with intramural excitatory neurons. It must be emphasized that both types of fibers have a spontaneous resting discharge, and that esophageal distension can alter this activity in the same way as swallowing (increased discharge for VIC fibers, decreased discharge for VEC fibers).

Possible roles of extrinsic fibers. Since the two types of *vagal fibers* (VEC, VIC) have a spontaneous resting discharge, it is difficult to predict the effect of the global vagal output on the LES tone. As mentioned above, vagotomy leads to conflicting results which do not allow firm conclusions. Moreover, the respective importance of excitatory and inhibitory pathways may differ from one species to another. Nevertheless, vagal activity may participate in maintenance of resting tone since atropine usually reduces the intraluminal pressure. This effect of atropine has generally been interpreted as indicating blockade of vagal cholinergic influences. But, as shown by Gonella et al. (127), atropine also antagonizes the motor effects of the sympathetic system on LES.

Although it is difficult to assess the role of vagal fibers in the maintenance of resting tone, it is clear that these fibers are involved in the changes of sphincter tone occurring during swallowing, after esophageal distension, or during gastric contractions.

The LES opening during swallowing or after esophageal distension very likely depends on an increased discharge of VIC fibers and on an inhibition of VEC fibers, at least in dog (Fig. 13). The closure observed afterward results from an opposite change in the two discharge types: The cessation of VIC fiber discharge must be followed by a rebound excitation that is probably reinforced by the transient acceleration of VEC fiber discharge (Fig. 13).

On the other hand, several investigators (42,52,80, 209,236) have reported an increase of LES tone occurring with increased gastric pressure due to gastric contractions. This response, obviously designed to prevent gastroesophageal reflux, appears to be a reflex effect mediated mainly by the vagus nerves since it is reduced or even abolished by vagotomy (80). In this connection, Miolan and Roman (238) have reported that the dis-

charge of VIC fibers was decreased when the intragastric pressure increased. At the same time, the activity of VEC fibers is enhanced (J. P. Miolan, *unpublished*). Afferents for such a reflex are probably sensory fibers from the stomach that are carried by the vagus nerves (see below). As for the efferent pathway, aside from the vagal fibers already mentioned, a possible involvement of the sympathetic supply of LES cannot be ruled out.

Data concerning the possible role of the *sympathetic supply* of LES are scarce. In anesthetized opossums, Di Marino and Cohen (83) observed that after pharmacological blockade of adrenergic nerves, the resting tone of LES was reduced by about 22%, but that relaxation during swallowing was not changed. However, these results obtained under anesthesia may not reflect the actual part taken by adrenergic fibers, especially in the maintenance of normal resting tone. Sympathetic fibers might also participate in reflex increase of the sphincter closure in response to various stimuli. In this connection, Rattan and Goyal (272) showed in the opossum that a reflex increase of LES pressure followed stimulation of the central cut end of one vagus (stimulation of sensitive fibers) even if the other vagus was severed. This reflex response was antagonized by phentolamine as well as by atropine, which can be easily interpreted taking into account what is known about the mechanism of action of sympathetic fibers on LES (see above).

EXTRINSIC CONTROL OF THE STOMACH

General Survey of Gastric Innervation

Efferent Innervation

The stomach, like the rest of the digestive tract, is innervated by the parasympathetic and sympathetic divisions of the autonomic nervous system (337) (Fig. 1). The parasympathetic supply corresponds to the vagus nerves whose efferent preganglionic fibers synapse with neurons of the gastric intrinsic plexuses. Postganglionic fibers from these plexuses innervate the smooth muscle and secretory cells. The cell bodies of vagal preganglionic neurons are classically located in the medulla within the dorsal motor nucleus of the vagus (119,220, 240,241). A recent histological study in the cat using the horseradish peroxidase technique has confirmed this localization (335). It showed, in addition, that a few cell bodies lie outside the dorsal motor nucleus, especially in the solitary tract nucleus.

The sympathetic supply to the stomach comes mainly from the 6th to 9th thoracic segments of the spinal cord, which contain the cell bodies of the preganglionic neurons. The cell bodies of the postganglionic neurons that supply the stomach and duodenum are located mostly in the celiac ganglion. The postganglionic fibers pass from the celiac ganglion to the stomach and duodenum along the branches of the celiac artery. Since the postganglionic fibers are adrenergic, the distribution of their terminals within the gastric wall can be visualized by fluorescence histochemical method. The main feature emerging from histofluorescence data is that most of the terminals supply the intramural ganglia and blood vessels, but that few fibers innervate the muscular coats or the muscularis mucosae (108).

Sensory Innervation

Vagal fibers. Two sorts of gastric vagal receptors have been described: stretch receptors and chemoreceptors. Stretch receptors presumably located within the muscular coat are activated by passive distension of the stomach (154,155,226,259) and also by contractions of the walls (154,155,226) (Fig. 14). Most of these receptors are found in the antrum, but some of them lie in proximal stomach near the LES. According to Takeshima (316), antral receptors respond to distension and peristalsis whereas those of the cardiac portion are activated only by changes in gastric volume. Chemoreceptors correspond to mucosal endings. Actually, they are rapidly adapting mechanoreceptors which act also as slowly adapting chemoreceptors (53,70,156); they respond to balloon distension of stomach by an on-off discharge. Their chemosensitivity is limited to acid or alkali in the cat (70,156) but it seems rather unspecific in the rat, since in this animal the same nerve ending can be excited by several of the following stimuli: organic and inorganic acids, water, alcohol, hypertonic saline, NaOH, NH_4Cl, $CuSO_4$, casein hydrolysate, mustard powder, and cayenne pepper (53).

Splanchnic fibers. According to Ranieri et al. (271), splanchnic mechanosensitive endings, especially those of the antrum and distal body, are present in the gastric wall. They are activated by spontaneous or vagally induced contractions and also by distension or compression of the stomach. Most of them exhibit a slowly adapting discharge, except for a few on-off receptors. The cell bodies of these sensitive fibers lie in spinal dorsal root ganglia between T-7 and T-11.

Effects of Severing the Extrinsic Nerves

Vagotomy

McSwiney (215), who surveyed the data available in 1931, concluded that section of both vagus nerves resulted in decreased tone, dilatation of stomach, weakened peristalsis, and delayed emptying. However, subsequent works have shown that gastric tone instead of being lowered was in fact increased after vagotomy. More precisely, vagotomy impairs the reservoir function of stomach. The adaptive relaxation of the proximal stomach in response to a gastric distension is no longer observed, and so the intragastric pressure of the distended stomach is higher than normal (43,165,170,222, 332). On the other hand, the gastric relaxation observed during swallowing or after esophageal distension (receptive relaxation) is also suppressed by vagotomy (36, 165,170). Proximal gastric vagotomy which only denervates the fundus and body is as effective as truncal vagotomy in producing these alterations of the gastric reservoir function (332).

Concerning gastric emptying, all investigators agree that truncal vagotomy slows the emptying of solids (60,

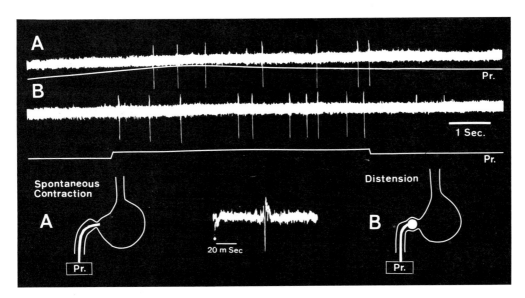

FIG. 14. Activity of a vagal muscular receptor located in the pyloric area. Recording as for Fig. 2. **A:** Response to a spontaneous contraction of antrum. **B:** Response to a distension. The conduction velocity for the corresponding fiber was determined by electrical stimulation of the ipsilateral vagal nerve. The circle indicates the stimulation artifact. Conduction velocity = 0.9 m/sec. (From Mei, *unpublished data*).

158,215,224,332) and, in contrast, increases that of liquids (60,224,332). The proximal gastric vagotomy also results in an increased emptying of liquids (23,332) but does not affect emptying of solids (60,158,332). These data indicate that the emptying of liquids depends to a great extent on the proximal stomach which adjusts intragastric pressure by its tension variations, while emptying of solids is chiefly under the control of the distal stomach. Since proximal gastric vagotomy effectively decreases the secretion of HCl and pepsin by the stomach while preserving a normal antral motility, this surgical intervention is now currently undertaken in man as an operative treatment for duodenal ulcer.

Delayed emptying of solids after truncal vagotomy or total gastric vagotomy very likely results from a decreased force of antral peristalsis (215,332) and not from a possible spasm of the pylorus since this sphincter has been shown to be patulous and open following vagotomy (215,268).

Regarding the gastric EMG, obvious disturbances can be observed during the few days immediately following a transthoracic vagotomy. The normal EMG activity of the canine or human distal stomach (lower body and antrum) consists of two successive potentials (Fig. 15). The initial potential or electrical control activity, ECA (67), is a rhythmic depolarization or upstroke potential (95) that is always present and that constitutes the basic electrical rhythm (BER). The initial potential is usually followed by a second potential or electrical response activity, ERA (67), which, on microelectrode recordings, consists of a plateau with superimposed oscillations or true spike potentials depending on the region

examined (95). Muscle contraction occurs only when the second potential achieves a critical amplitude and duration (Fig. 15). When the EMG is recorded with chronically implanted electrodes and R-C amplification, the plateau potential is not observed and then the ERA corresponds only to oscillations or spike potentials. Immediately after vagotomy, the antral electrical activity shows periods of total disorganization with groups of slow potentials, ECAs, exhibiting various amplitudes, frequencies, and configurations (191,234,262). At the same time the prevagotomy pattern of the BER is preserved in the gastric body so that the ECAs of the antrum and body are no longer synchronized (262). The abnormal antral ECAs are not followed by ERAs, and so they do not trigger muscular contractions. Usually the normal pattern of the antral BER is restored within a week, although some dogs continue to have occasional periods of disorganized rhythm for several months after vagotomy (191,262). After restoration of the normal antral BER, perturbations similar to those observed in the early postvagotomy period can be provoked by i.v. injection of atropine (262). Hence, EMG disturbance ensuing from vagotomy very likely expresses a decrease in the cholinergic tone, which is then able to recover, probably due to an adaptive function of intraparietal cholinergic structures.

Sympathectomy

Data about sympathectomy are less numerous than those concerning vagotomy. However, it is generally stated that section of splanchnic nerves results in accel-

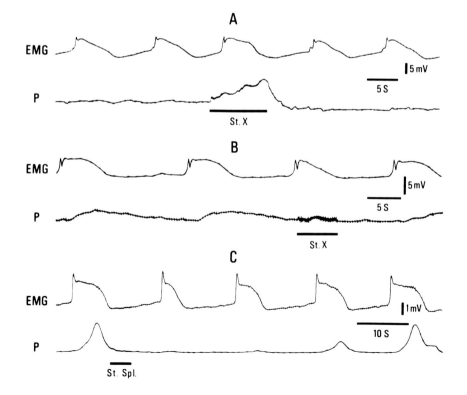

FIG. 15. Effects of vagal and splanchnic stimulations on dog gastric EMG. In vivo experiments: dogs anesthetized with pentobarbital. EMG, monopolar records made with a suction electrode; R-C amplification in **A** (time constant = 5 sec) and D-C amplification in **B** and **C**. P: Intraluminal pressure recorded by a balloon located in the distal antrum. **A**: In the absence of atropine, stimulation of the vagus (St. X; 10 V, 2 msec, 10 Hz) causes a gastric contraction and increases the amplitude and duration of the gastric complex action potential. **B**: In the presence of atropine, vagal stimulation (St. X) with identical parameters decreases the amplitude and duration of the plateau potential (inhibitory effect also recorded on the pressure tracing). **C**: Other animal nonatropinized; stimulation of splanchnic nerve (St. Spl.; 5 V, 0.5 msec, 30 Hz) results in gastric motility inhibition which is obvious on both EMG and pressure tracings. From Miolan and Roman (235).

erated gastric emptying, probably because of an increased tone and a more powerful peristalsis (6,194, 215). It is also agreed that splanchnic section has less disturbing effects on the stomach than vagotomy, and that animals have a more normal stomach if the splanchnics are cut after vagotomy.

Stimulation of Efferent Extrinsic Fibers

Strong statements can be found to the effect that stimulation of either vagus or splanchnic nerves produces both excitatory and inhibitory effects on gastric motility. The question has been successively reviewed by McSwiney (215), Thomas and Baldwin (318), and Kosterlitz (194). Analysis of historical and modern literature up to 1968 will not be reviewed in detail. The reader wishing such details should consult these reviews.

Vagal Efferent Fibers

The vagus nerves carry two kinds of preganglionic fibers, fibers whose stimulation leads to excitatory effects, and others whose stimulation leads to inhibitory effects. The former have a lower excitation threshold (hence a larger diameter) than the latter (221–223).

Excitatory effects. When recorded by manometry, the excitatory effects consist first of an increase in gastric tone that may chiefly reflect contraction of the proximal stomach, the fundus and body (215,223,263). At the antral level, vagal stimulation can trigger peristaltic contractions in the rat isolated stomach (10) and in the anesthetized opossum as well (288).

When the EMG of the distal stomach is recorded, the vagal excitatory effects are revealed by the occurrence or the facilitation of the ERAs in those species such as dog or pig that present complex gastric action potentials. Depending on the recording technique, an increase in the amplitude and duration of the plateau potential (235) (Fig. 15) or in the occurrence of spikes has been observed after each ECA (195,196,288). Sarna and Daniel (288) have also reported that intense vagal stimulation could cause premature control potentials, as could localized intraarterial injections of acetylcholine (66). In addition, Daniel and Sarna (68) have shown that there is a segmental distribution of the excitatory vagal fibers that reach the stomach through various branches of the two nerves of Latarjet.

The EMG of the guinea pig stomach differs from that of the canine stomach since it does not exhibit complex action potentials, but only true spike potentials occurring more or less continuously or grouped in bursts, especially at the antral level. Vagal excitatory responses recorded by intracellular microelectrodes from isolated guinea pig stomach (20) consist of EJPs, either pure or with superimposed spikes. These EJPs follow within 200 msec each vagal pulse and last about 400 to 500

msec. Then, vagal excitatory responses of guinea pig stomach resemble very much those of the cat smooth muscle esophagus (see above).

The consensus is that neuroeffector transmission from the excitatory vagal pathway is cholinergic and that consequently it is blocked by atropine or hyoscine (20,194,235,288).

The contraction induced by vagal stimulation is also abolished or at least markedly reduced by drugs such as hexamethonium that antagonize ganglionic transmission (194,196,288). Thus the excitatory vagal path appears to be composed of preganglionic cholinergic fibers synapsing with myenteric cholinergic neurons that excite smooth muscle.

Inhibitory effects. These are easily observed after atropine has been used to block the vagal excitatory effects. The inhibitory effects correspond to a relaxation of the gastric wall, especially evident in the proximal stomach (fundus and body) and well recorded by manometric techniques (32,221–223). On electrical recordings from the body of the guinea pig stomach, vagal inhibitory responses consist of IJPs, hyperpolarizations lasting 1,000 to 1,800 msec, following each stimulus pulse with a short latency (200 to 300 msec). When a train of pulses (20 Hz) is used, hyperpolarization is maintained but a rebound excitation, a train of spikes, occurs after the cessation of stimulation (20). EMG recording of antral activity in anesthetized dog has shown that vagal inhibition also affects the antrum, but the inhibition is not like that observed in the guinea pig stomach, since there is a decrease in amplitude and duration of the plateau of the complex action potential (235) (Fig. 15).

Vagal inhibitory effects were interpreted as being adrenergic in nature. Indeed, a large body of evidence indicates that the vagus of various species carries adrenergic fibers originating chiefly from the superior cervical and the stellate ganglia (207,213,249).

It is now widely accepted, however, that the vagal inhibitory responses differ from those induced by sympathetic stimulation or catecholamine injection. The vagal responses are generally stronger, develop more rapidly, and are obtained at a lower stimulation frequency than adrenergic responses (32,222). Furthermore, they are not blocked by such anti-adrenergic drugs as guanethidine, bretylium, or alpha- and beta-adrenergic antagonists (20,32,222). They are present in isolated stomachs of animals treated with reserpine in concentrations sufficient to deplete tissue stores of norepinephrine (136). The ability of ganglion blocking agents to greatly reduce the vagal inhibitory responses suggests the presence of cholinergic (nicotinic) synapses between extrinsic vagal fibers and nonadrenergic inhibitory intramural neurons (20,26,263). These inhibitory intramural neurons are very likely identical to those identified elsewhere in the digestive tract (28,29).

Sympathetic Efferent Fibers

Both inhibition and facilitation of gastric motility have been described in response to splanchnic nerve stimulation (194,215,318). The chief and the best known effect is the inhibitory one.

Relaxant responses. These correspond to a decreased tone of the proximal stomach and to a weakened peristalsis of the antrum (Fig. 15). These effects are adrenergic in nature since they are blocked by guanethidine (20,222) or by bretylium (32). In addition, when sympathetic stimulation is performed at the preganglionic level, the splanchnic nerve, the inhibitory effects are also abolished by the ganglion blocking agents, hexamethonium, nicotine, either applied to ganglia, the celiac and superior mesenteric, or injected intravenously (251,298).

It is now widely accepted that adrenergic nerves may reduce gastric motility by acting at two different sites, the myenteric neurons and the muscle itself. The action on myenteric neurons is strongly supported by the anatomical observation that adrenergic fibers ramify extensively in Auerbach's plexus (108). Also, experimental data gathered by Jansson and co-workers (170,172,174) indicate that the more powerful the cholinergic tone, representing activity of myenteric neurons, the stronger the splanchnic inhibition of the stomach. Thus the sympathetic inhibition is prompt and pronounced, even for weak stimulation frequencies when the two vagus nerves are intact. After acute vagotomy or atropine injection, the inhibitory responses are much weaker and retarded, and require higher stimulation frequencies.

Nevertheless, a direct action of adrenergic fibers on smooth muscle does exist. From histological data based on the fluorescence histochemical method, it can be stated that there is some adrenergic innervation of muscular coats (108). In addition, nerve stimulation *in vivo* indicates that some sympathetic inhibition remains under atropine (170). *In vitro,* sympathetic relaxation of muscular strips taken from guinea pig stomach does not appear to be changed under hyoscine or atropine (20, 118). Intracellular recording of the activity from guinea pig stomach muscle strips (20) showed that sympathetic stimulation at 10 to 20 Hz caused a hyperpolarization of the cell membrane and subsequently a rebound excitation. Beani et al. (20) did not mention whether such hyperpolarizations were also obtained in the presence of atropine. It seems likely that they are not due to a decreased activity of intramural cholinergic neurons, since it was observed on other strips that atropine *per se* did not change the resting membrane potential of muscular cells. In dog stomach *in vivo,* Miolan and Roman (235) showed that splanchnic stimulation at 30 Hz reduced the amplitude and duration of the plateau of the complex action potential (Fig. 15). *In vitro,* El Sharkawy and Szurszewski (96) observed similar modification of the complex action potential of the dog

stomach under the action of norepinephrine. According to El Sharkawy and Szurszewski (96), norepinephrine could act directly on smooth muscle since the gastric action potential is not altered by atropine or tetrodotoxin. However, it is quite possible that a part of the inhibitory responses observed *in vivo* by Miolan and Roman (235) results from an action on myenteric ganglion cells, because the most obvious inhibitory effects were observed when gastric peristalsis was powerful, therefore when the cholinergic tone was great.

As for the receptors involved in the effects of norepinephrine released from sympathetic nerves in mammalian gastrointestinal tissues, it has been suggested that inhibition of the acetylcholine release from intramural cholinergic neurons is mediated by alpha-adrenergic receptors, whereas direct muscle inhibition is chiefly achieved through beta receptors (108,122,327). Still, alpha receptors are also present in muscle and they mediate either excitation or inhibition, depending on the organ and the species. Also, another current concept is that norepinephrine acts directly on smooth muscle during sympathetic stimulation mainly from an overflow of transmitter from nerves supplying myenteric ganglia (108). This would explain why higher rates of stimulation are needed to produce inhibition in the absence of cholinergic tone, when inhibition of the myenteric ganglia has practically no effect.

Motor responses. According to McSwiney (215) and co-workers, motor effects can be elicited by stimulation of the splanchnic nerves or the periarterial nerves running to the stomach. The same authors reported that high-frequency stimulation led to inhibition, whereas low-frequency stimuli favored contraction of the body and fundus in particular. Splanchnic motor responses have been more recently confirmed by Semba and Hiraoka (298), Jansson (170), Nakazato et al. (251), and Semba and Mizonishi (300). These motor responses, or part of them, are suppressed by atropine. Therefore, they very likely result from cholinergic fiber stimulation. According to Semba and Hiraoka (298), the splanchnic cholinergic fibers would leave the spinal cord by the dorsal roots of rachidian nerves. Such cholinergic fibers emerging from the spinal cord in the dorsal roots of the spinal nerves have been extensively described in amphibians (34).

However, Nakazato et al. (251) have reported that in the atropinized dog, stimulation of splanchnic or periarterial nerves was still able to produce gastric contractions. A similar motor effect was also obtained by close intra-arterial injection of norepinephrine. In this connection, early observations of Muren (248) must be recalled. Muren noticed that injection of epinephrine or norepinephrine (2 μg/kg i.v.) in the dog produced gastric inhibition when the two vagus nerves were intact, i.e., when the gastric tone was important. The response was reversed to excitation when gastric tone was decreased by such means as vagus nerves section, deep anesthesia, or atropine injection. A similar inversion of epinephrine effects in the presence of atropine had also been reported by McSwiney (215) and co-workers in rabbit. These true sympathetic motor effects are very likely mediated by alpha-adrenergic receptors localized on smooth muscle, because, in the atropinized dog, they are blocked by phenoxybenzamine to be replaced by a relaxation that is, in turn, antagonized by beta receptor antagonists such as pronethalol (251). Moreover, the existence of gastric motor effects mediated by alpha-adrenergic receptors is attested by several reports concerning two other animal species, guinea pig (133,256) and rabbit (134).

In summary, it seems clear that motor effects can be induced by splanchnic stimulation. They result from involvement of muscarinic or alpha-adrenergic receptors. No information is available about their physiological significance.

Possible Roles of Extrinsic Innervation

Receptive Relaxation and Related Phenomena

The term receptive relaxation was proposed by Cannon and Lieb (36) to designate the relaxation that affects chiefly the fundus and the body during swallowing. As already mentioned by Cannon and Lieb (36), receptive relaxation is suppressed by vagotomy and hence it results from an extrinsic reflex. The fact that a vagal inhibitory pathway is the efferent link of this reflex has been demonstrated by extensive studies of Martinson and co-workers (3,165,170,222). The same investigators have also shown that similar gastric relaxation occurred in several different circumstances. Thus, apart from swallowing, another effective stimulus is provided by esophageal distension which usually must stimulate secondary peristalsis (170). Proximal stomach relaxation is also induced by distension of the whole stomach or by distension restricted to the antrum or even by close intraarterial injection of acetylcholine, which increases antral motility (3). Thus it seems reasonable to assume that slowly adapting antral stretch receptors activated either by distension or by forceful contractions are responsible for such relaxation of the corpus-fundus area. In additon to the vagally mediated reflex relaxation, antral distension can also elicit a sympathetic gastrogastric inhibitory reflex with both afferent and efferent links conveyed by the splanchnic nerves; the efferent adrenergic link of the reflex acts essentially by inhibiting the excitatory cholinergic neurons in the gastric walls (3). Lastly, gastric relaxation has also been produced artificially by electrical stimulation of fibers in the vagus nerve originating from various receptors located in the esophagus, stomach, and probably intestine (3,170,255). The physiological significance of all these reflex relaxations is that they

would prevent the gastric pressure from becoming too high during and after food ingestion, during the strong antral contractions of the emptying period. In addition, vagally mediated relaxations of the stomach are also observed during vomiting. (3). They correspond to a sort of receptive relaxation, since during vomiting the stomach is usually filled with ingesta returning from the upper intestine.

The discharge pattern of vagal efferent (preganglionic) fibers thought to be involved in the corpus-fundus relaxation has been studied in the dog by Miolan and Roman (237) using a nerve suture technique (Fig. 16). These vagal fibers fired spontaneously at low frequency (from 0 to 3 spikes/sec). During the proximal stomach relaxation, as caused by swallowing, esophageal distension, and strong antral contractions, two opposite patterns were observed: for many fibers, the discharge frequency was increased to 10 to 40 spikes/sec; for others, the firing was decreased or abolished (Fig. 16). From these results, Miolan and Roman (237) concluded that the proximal stomach relaxation resulted from a decreased activity of vagal preganglionic fibers synapsing with excitatory myenteric neurons, but also and chiefly from an activation of preganglionic fibers synapsing with inhibitory myenteric neurons. In the following text, these fibers will be termed the vagal excitatory fibers of the fundus (VEF) and the vagal inhibitory fibers of the fundus (VIF), respectively.

Gastric Motility During Fasting and Fed States

Motility patterns. By recording the EMG simultaneously at multiple sites along the small bowel of fasted conscious dogs, Szurszewski (312) noticed a caudad moving band of large-amplitude spike potentials (the activity front) sweeping in recurring cycles every 90 to 180 min along the entire small bowel. Later, Code and Marlett (55) demonstrated that the activity front is part of a complex (the migrating myoelectric complex, MMC) starting in the stomach. According to their description, the myoelectric complex is composed of four distinct phases that recur regularly at each point of detection. As far as the gastric antrum is concerned, these four phases can be described as follows. Phase 1 is characterized by the absence of spike potentials or ERA. Only ECA, pacesetter potentials, are recorded. This means that there is no mechanical activity. Persistent but random spike potential activity marks the onset of phase 2. During this phase, spike potentials increase in incidence and intensity. Phase 3 is characterized by the sudden onset and continuous occurrence of bursts of large action potentials with every ECA. During this period, strong rhythmic contractions are recorded. The end of this phase is nearly as sudden as its beginning. During phase 4, there is a rapid decrease in incidence and intensity of spike potentials and a return to phase 1 within a few minutes.

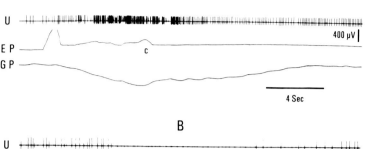

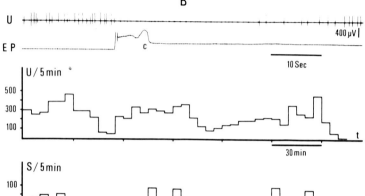

FIG. 16. Discharge pattern of vagal efferent fibers probably supplying the fundus in conscious dog. U, activity of vagal efferent fiber recorded using a nerve suture technique; U/5 min, number of vagal impulses per 5 min as a function of time; S/5 min, number of gastric spike potentials (antral EMG) per 5 min as a function of time. EP, esophageal pressure recorded by a free moving balloon propelled by a secondary peristaltic contracton. The last wave of the tracing (C) is recorded when the balloon enters the stomach. GP, gastric pressure recorded by an inflated balloon (100 ml air) located in the proximal stomach. A: During a secondary peristalsis the proximal stomach relaxes (receptive relaxation). At the same time, the vagal fiber is strongly excited (VIF type = vagal inhibitory fiber of fundus). B: Tracings during the receptive relaxation induced by a secondary peristalsis; this other type of vagal fiber is inhibited (VEF type = vagal excitatory fiber of fundus). Diagrams: on fasted dog, the discharge of the VEF fiber exhibits cyclic variations parallel with the MMCs recorded on gastric antrum. From Miolan (unpublished).

Recent data (160) confirming early reports have shown that the fundus and body of the stomach also contract in association with the antrum during the MMC.

After feeding, the antrum electric activity mainly consists of bursts of large spike potentials of long duration following every ECA. This intense contractile activity lasting several hours is responsible for the gastric emptying. The behavior of the proximal stomach during the postprandial period is not well known. However, it is generally stated that this region plays the role of a pressure regulator. So if intragastric pressure increases too much during the forceful antral contractions, the fundus and body relax, and, on the contrary, when intragastric pressure falls because of emptying, the fundus and body contract in order to maintain a certain load to the antral pump.

Controls. Concerning the control of MMCs, numerous data point out the importance of humoral factors, particularly of motilin, in the initiation or at least the regulation of the interdigestive motor activity (159,265, 322,333). It is widely accepted that the extrinsic nerves are of minor importance since vagal and splanchnic section do not suppress the MMCs (219,284,285,331). However, one cannot take for granted that section is the best experimental approach to get reliable information about the actual role of the extrinsic nerves. In this connection, it is noteworthy that atropine suppresses the MMCs, which indicates the prominent part taken by the cholinergic intramural nerves in interdigestive motor phenomena. It would be very surprising, too, if the activity of cholinergic intramural neurons during MMC should be controlled only by hormonal factors and not by extrinsic fibers at all.

Indeed, Miolan and Roman (239) have shown that the spontaneous discharge of vagal preganglionic fibers fluctuated with the various phases of the MMC occurring in the gastric antrum (Fig. 17): mean frequencies

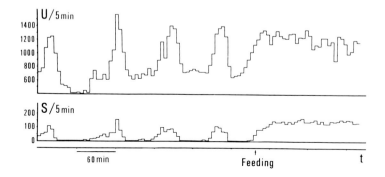

FIG. 17. Discharge pattern of a vagal efferent fiber probably supplying the antrum (VEA type = vagal excitatory fiber of antrum) during fasting and feeding in conscious dog. U/5 min, number of vagal impulses per 5 min as a function of time; recording made using a nerve suture technique; S/5 min, number of gastric spike potentials per 5 min as a function of time; recording made with electrodes chronically implanted in the antrum walls. In fasted dog, there are cyclic variations of vagal discharge with parallel variations in gastric motility (MMCs). Feeding increases both vagal discharge and gastric motility. From Miolan and Roman (239).

of about 0.1 to 1.5 spikes/sec during phase 1; 1.5 to 5 spikes/sec in phase 3; intermediate values for phases 2 and 4. These fibers were thought to supply the gastric antrum for the following reasons: (a) the discharge frequency was closely related to the spontaneous motility of the antrum; (b) firing was practically unaffected by receptive relaxation of stomach; (c) discharge was facilitated by a gastric distension which increased antral motility and relaxed the proximal stomach.

Taking into account that their discharge increased each time the gastric motility was enhanced, one could assess that these fibers belonged to the vagal excitatory pathway. Thus they will be termed VEA (vagal excitatory fibers of the antrum) in the rest of the text. More recent data (J.P. Miolan and C. Roman, *unpublished*) have revealed that vagal fibers controlling the proximal stomach, both VEF and VIF, were also concerned in the MMCs: the discharge of VEF fibers increased during phase 3 (Fig. 16), while that of VIF fibers decreased. After feeding, the discharge pattern of VEF and VIF fibers is not known. As for the VEA fibers, their discharge frequency increased as much as during phase 3 of a MMC (Fig. 17). This sustained activity, which started as soon as the food was offered, lasted several hours. If the food was only shown but not given afterward, the vagal hyperactivity lasted only a few minutes.

As to the physiological significance of the changes in vagal activity, two interpretations may be proposed. First, these changes represent the extrinsic inputs that cause gastric motor events. Second, vagal firing changes do not program the gastric motor events but provide an additional mechanism that facilitates the functioning of the intramural network responsible for motor programming. In support of the second hypothesis and against the first one, it should be noted that in dogs, the MMCs and the postprandial hypermotility are both still observed after bilateral vagotomy and bilateral splanchnicotomy. But it may be inferred that after extrinsic denervation, there is a recovery of function due to adaptive phenomena within intramural nervous circuits, so that the stomach is soon able to exhibit approximately normal motility. This does not mean that under normal physiological circumstances, the extrinsic circuits, the vagal ones in particular, do not have an important effect on the organization of gastric motor patterns. In support of such a role are recent findings of Diamant et al. (82) on conscious dogs whose vagosympathetic trunks were cooled in the neck. Blockade of nerve conduction resulted in abolition of the feeding pattern, whereas on release of vagal blockade the feeding pattern was reestablished. This provided, so far, the best evidence that vagal activity is of primary importance for gastric motor activity during the postprandial period. The same conclusion might also apply to the interdigestive period, to the MMCs, since the discharge of VEA fibers, for instance, is not different during phase 3 of the MMCs and after feeding (Fig. 17). But additional

data are obviously needed. In particular, it would be useful to know the effect of vagal cooling on MMCs.

Another important question concerning the vagal firing changes during MMCs or after feeding is that of their origin. One possibility is a reflex origin, changes resulting from stimulation of gastric stretch receptors that are known to be responsive to distension and to contraction of the stomach (see above). This interpretation seems plausible for changes observed after feeding. In this connection, Davison and Grundy (71) have shown that in anesthetized rats the discharge of single vagal efferent fibers was markedly altered (excitation or inhibition) by gastric inflation, gastric contractions, or compression of the stomach. According to these investigators, the opposite changes of vagal discharges would correspond to a reciprocal reflex control of antagonist excitatory and inhibitory vagal pathways. Thus it is likely that during the postprandial period, vagovagal gastrogastric reflexes play a prominent role, in addition to local reflexes which can substitute for them if necessary. However, it is difficult to assume that during MMCs the vagal firing changes also result from feedback phenomena (stimulation of gastric receptors by hypermotility), since, under atropine which suppresses motor expression of MMCs, identical changes of vagal discharges are observed (J. P. Miolan, *unpublished*).

Since Pavlov's demonstration of a cephalic phase of gastric secretion, it has been several times suggested that sight, smell, and taste of food could stimulate gastric motility. Some early observations are in keeping with this suggestion (318). The finding of Miolan and Roman (239) showing that the discharge of VEA fibers is enhanced as soon as food is offered also strongly supports the hypothesis of a cephalic phase of gastric motility. However, other data (318) have suggested otherwise by showing a decreased gastric motility at the sight or smell of food. These conflicting results may be ascribed to the gastric receptive relaxation or to the cephalic phase of acid secretion and the subsequent reflex gastric inhibition triggered by arrival of acid in the upper intestine (see below). Thus it is possible that, depending on experimental conditions, the cephalic facilitation of gastric motility may be overridden by inhibitory influences.

Enterogastric Reflex and Gastric Emptying

Appropriate chemical or mechanical stimulation of the mucosa of the upper intestine produces an inhibition of gastric peristalsis and hence a slowing of gastric emptying. This has been called the "enterogastric inhibitory reflex" by Thomas et al. (320).

Many stimuli have been found to initiate this reflex, e.g., mineral acids, fats and fatty acids, hypertonic solutions of various substances (salt, glucose, etc.), duodenal distension, and, more recently, duodenal thermal stimulation.

Response to acids. Slowing of gastric emptying by mineral acids (in particular, hydrochloric acid) has long been known (148,317). Extensive studies of the effect have been done by Hunt and Knox (148–150), who have clarified many aspects of acid effectiveness, namely, the influence of concentration, molecular weight, and pH. Judging from the effects of restricted intestinal perfusions, acid receptors appear to be located in the first 5 cm of the duodenum and in the jejunum (60–62). Electrophysiological studies have indicated that vagal sensory fibers could be activated by acid perfusion of the proximal intestine (8,53,70,260,261). These vagal receptors are probably mucosal endings that function both as rapidly adapting mechanoreceptors and as slowly adapting chemoreceptors.

As to the reflex circuits involved in acid inhibition of gastric motility, there are different opinions about the importance of vagal pathways. According to Thomas et al. (320) and Quigley and Meschan (270), the acid reflex in dog was abolished or at least greatly diminished by vagotomy. This result has been confirmed by Roze et al. (283) in pig. Schapiro and Woodward (293), however, reported that only celiac ganglionectomy was able to suppress acid-induced gastric inhibition in the dog. Thus the reflex circuit would consist of afferent fibers arising in the upper small intestine and synapsing with cell bodies of efferent adrenergic neurons lying in the celiac ganglion. Such connections have been demonstrated by recent electrophysiological work (198). It is quite possible that several different reflex mechanisms interact together. The fact that a sympathetic circuit is involved in the acid reflex has been confirmed by Cooke and Clark (62). In addition, Miolan (*unpublished*) has recently observed that the discharge of the vagal efferent fibers that control the dog stomach was modified when hydrochloric acid was introduced into the duodenum (Fig. 18). The activity of the excitatory fibers, both VEA and VEF, was decreased while that of inhibitory fibers (VIF) was enhanced.

Response to fat and fatty acids. The slowing of gastric emptying by fat and fatty acids is also well documented (60,148). The receptors responsible for this effect are more sensitive to fatty acids than to triglycerides. They appear to be located mainly in the jejunum, at least in dog (61); there is no available information about their electrophysiological properties. Moreover, the mechanism of fat inhibition is still a controversial subject. Since the observations of Farrel and Ivy (99), indicating that introduction of fats into the duodenum inhibited the motility of a transplanted fundic pouch, it is generally believed that a hormone, enterogastrone, is involved in the mediation of this inhibitory effect. However, according to Hunt and Knox (148), fat inhibition has a short latency and persists only for 1 or 2 min after withdrawal of stimulus; this makes a hormonal mechanism hardly credible. In addition, it has

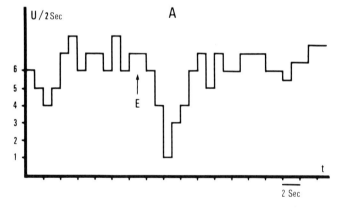

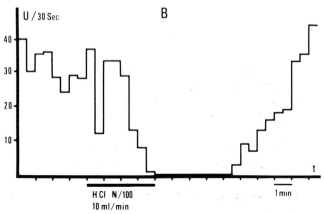

FIG. 18. Effect of mechanical or acid stimulation of duodenum upon the discharge of vagal efferent fibers probably supplying the antrum (VEA type). Conscious dog, recording of vagal activity made using a nerve suture technique. U/2 sec, U/30 sec, number of vagal impulses per 2 and 30 sec, respectively, as a function of time. **A**: A small balloon (2 ml air) initially located in the distal antrum is propelled into the duodenum by antral contractions. Soon after entering (E; *arrow*), the VEA fiber discharge is inhibited. This inhibition is of short duration because the balloon is driven away by intestinal contractions. **B**: Duodenal infusion with hydrochloric acid (intraluminal catheter) produces a pronounced and long-lasting inhibition of vagal discharge. From Miolan (*unpublished*).

been reported that vagotomy either reduced the slowing of gastric emptying by fats in man (328) or suppressed fat-induced gastric inhibition in dog (191) and pig (283).

Response to osmotic factors. In order to explain the fact that various hypertonic solutions can produce a slowing of gastric emptying, it has been postulated that osmoreceptors were present in intestinal walls (60,148). Such receptors seem localized to the duodenum in man (148,225) and to jejunum in dog (61). Nevertheless, electrophysiological evidence of the existence of specific receptors responding to the osmotic pressure *per se* is still lacking. Vagal intestinal receptors described by Clarke and Davison (53) in the rat were excited not only by hypertonic saline but also by water; also, they did not respond to hypertonic glucose. In contrast, the vagal glucoreceptors reported by Mei (227) responded only to glucose and various carbohydrates. Their discharge frequency increased when sugar concentration (and therefore osmolarity) was raised. But substances other than carbohydrates, e.g., NaCl, KCl of the same osmolarity, were ineffective; this indicated that the osmotic pressure *per se* was not directly related to the receptor activation. It is quite possible that activation of such vagal glucoreceptors instead of "true" osmoreceptors may account for the slowing of gastric emptying by sugar solutions. In this connection, it is significant that vagotomy in pig abolishes the inhibition of gastric motility induced by intestinal infusion of glucose (283).

Response to Intestinal Distension. Several studies have shown that duodenal distension, either by balloon inflation or as a consequence of gastric evacuation, exerts an inhibitory influence on the mechanical activity of the stomach (267,269,320). A similar effect can be observed on the electrical activity of the gastric musculature (69). Electrophysiological investigations have revealed the existence of many mechanoreceptors connected with vagal or splanchnic sensory fibers. The vagal mechanoreceptors are either stretch receptors located within the muscular layers or mucosal endings that are responsive to both chemical and mechanical stimuli (53,70,155,226,260,261). As for splanchnic mechanoreceptors, those described so far respond only to distension or to contraction of the intestine, thus resembling very much the vagal stretch receptors (271).

The inhibition of gastric motility in response to duodenal distension very likely involves a reflex mechanism mediated by extrinsic nerves, since it is not affected by the transsection of gastroduodenal junction, whereas it is markedly altered by vagotomy or by pharmacological blockade of the sympathetic system (69). The existence of a vagal reflex is further supported by the finding of Miolan and Roman (239) showing that the discharge of vagal excitatory fibers supplying the dog antrum (VEA type) was inhibited by duodenal distension (Fig. 18). On the other hand, it is well known that intestinal distension is able to elicit a sympathetic inhibition of gastric

motility that is part of the intestino-gastrointestinal sympathetic reflex (see below and 108). In contrast to what is generally believed, this reflex is not necessarily an unphysiological one, since it can be evoked for moderate intestinal distension that is probably in the physiological range (174).

Response to thermal stimuli. Recently, El Ouazzani and Mei (94) described vagal thermoreceptors in the walls of antrum and duodenum in cat. These receptors discharged with an optimum frequency when either warm (46° to 49°C) or cold (12° to 10°C) solutions were infused into the gastroduodenal area. They did not respond to mechanical stimuli, compression, and distension of the gut, or to chemical excitation (glucose, or acid solutions). Thus they must be considered to be true thermoreceptors responding specifically to temperature variations. By means of EMG recording, El Ouazzani and Mei (94) have observed that both cold and warm stimulation of the duodenum, stimuli able to elicit the optimum discharge of thermoreceptors, induced an inhibition of antral activity. This inhibition persisted after bilateral splanchnicotomy but disappeared after bilateral vagotomy. Thus it is likely that, in addition to the other enterogastric reflexes, duodenal thermal stimulation also elicits a reflex inhibition of gastric motility thereby providing an additional mechanism for the regulation of gastric emptying.

Pain Reflexes

It is well known that distension or mucosal irritation of one part of the gastrointestinal tract can inhibit the movements of other parts, including the stomach (108). Such gastric inhibition induced by distension of the intestine has been repeatedly reported (170,172,174). The efferent link of the reflex involves sympathetic adrenergic fibers that act mainly on the intramural cholinergic ganglion cells. Generally speaking, the sympathetic inhibitory reflexes are considered to be noxious because they are elicited by overdistension of the intestine. But it is now established that they are also induced by moderate distension of the gut (172,174). Thus they certainly may take a part in the normal regulation of gastrointestinal flow rate. Gastric motility can also be inhibited by noxious cutaneous stimuli (289,318) or by stimulation of somatic nerves (12,171). Most of these inhibitory reflexes induced from skin or somatic nerves involve a sympathetic efferent pathway (289).

Central Nervous Structures Involved in the Regulation of Gastric Motility

The existence of a cephalic influence on gastric motility is suggested by the association between disturbances of gastrointestinal motility and disturbed emotional states. Many authors after Cannon and Carlson (*see* 318) have reported that excitement, anxiety, and fear often caused inhibition of gastric motility. Accelerated gastric emptying and increase of motility have also been observed. All these effects demonstrate that cerebral influences are able to modify the usual gastric responses to food, suggesting a control exerted by higher centers on lower structures involved in the regulation of gastric function.

Our present knowledge of the role of the central nervous system in gastric motility is based on the effects of stimulation or destruction of various structures in anesthetized animals. In addition to the depressant action of anesthesia on the nervous system and the stomach itself, it is now well accepted that stimulation or destruction of nervous structures is a coarse method that allows only a rough estimate of the possible importance of these structures. By no means can they give precise information about the actual control exerted under physiological conditions. Only recording experiments performed in conscious animals could solve the problem. In the absence of such an approach, this section will consist mainly of a catalogue of the effects elicited by stimulation. This constitutes the first stage of knowledge that should lead to a more accurate study of the physiological involvement of the concerned areas.

Telencephalon

Sigmoid area. According to Eliasson (92), a facilitation of gastric motility was elicited in the cat by stimulating the anterior sigmoid area, whereas an inhibition was obtained from the posterior sigmoid area. Others saw (141,309) only inhibitory effects produced by stimulation of the whole area. These inhibitory effects disappeared after high spinal section, indicating that they were mediated by sympathetic efferents (141). In this connection, Eliasson (92) mentioned that inhibitory effects were only partly reduced while excitatory effects were suppressed by vagotomy.

Olfactory area. Eliasson (92) observed strong gastric contractions in the cat and increased peristalsis after stimulation of the olfactory bulb, tract, and tubercule and of the pyriform and prepyriform cortex. These effects appeared to be mediated by way of the splanchnic nerves and to be cholinergic in nature. In contrast, Ström and Uvnäs (309) reported, also in cat, that stimulation of the olfactory tract caused a marked inhibition of gastric tone.

Orbital area. Most of the investigators agree that stimulation of the orbital cortex leads to an inhibition of gastric tone and peristalsis. This has been observed in the cat (14,92,141), dog (12,13), and monkey (14, 188). However, some excitatory effects have also been reported in monkey (188) and in dog (12). All of these effects, both excitatory and inhibitory, are abolished by vagotomy (13,92,188).

Limbic area. Stimulation of the anterior cingulate cortex is usually followed by an inhibition of antral motility in dog (13), monkey (188), and cat (92). Conversely, the destruction of the same region results in an increase of the antropyloric motility (12). However, Eliasson (92) reported that, in addition to the antral inhibition, limbic stimulation could also produce contractions of the body. Both excitatory (body) and inhibitory (antrum) effects were suppressed by vagotomy.

Parietal area. From the anterior portion of the lateral and suprasylvian gyrus, Eliasson (92) was able to elicit excitatory effects on the body of the cat stomach. These effects were abolished by vagotomy and atropine.

Basal ganglia. Ström and Uvnäs (309) observed facilitation of the cat gastric motility from stimulating various basal structures, the putamen, the pallidum, the caudate nucleus, and the claustrum. Eliasson (92), however, obtained excitatory responses of the body only from stimulation of the pallidum.

Diencephalon

Thalamus. According to Eliasson (93), excitatory effects consisting of an increase of gastric tone and/or an augmentation of gastric movements were obtained in cat on stimulation of the reticular nucleus, the anterior part of the nucleus ventralis and lateral nucleus, the pulvinar, the entopeduncular nucleus, and the zona incerta. Inhibitory effects (decreased tone and inhibition of peristalsis) were elicited on stimulation of the posterolateral and posteromedial parts of the ventral nucleus and the anteromedial nucleus. All these effects were abolished after bilateral vagotomy or atropinization.

Hypothalamus. Literature previous to 1968 (318) indicates that both excitatory and inhibitory gastric responses can be elicited by stimulation of the hypothalamus. Eliasson (93) stated that "these effects could not be attributed to any special nuclei or fiber tracts." Particular attention, however, has been paid to the lateral hypothalamus from which effects have been more often obtained, particularly inhibitory ones. Folkow and Rubinstein (104) suggested that stimulation of the feeding area induced gastric relaxations of vagal origin, which could correspond to an anticipatory response of the stomach to food intake. But subsequent experiments of Lisander (210) have not confirmed this point: Gastric inhibition mediated through the vagal inhibitory pathway (inhibition present under atropine and after spinal cord section) was obtained from points scattered in the hypothalamus but not particularly concentrated in the feeding area.

Stimulation of the defense area located just below the feeding area also produces inhibitory effects (104,170, 173) that are due in part to a reduction of the vagal cholinergic excitatory tone (210), and in part to an increase in sympathetic discharge (76,170,173). These inhibitory sympathetic effects are more readily triggered by stimulation of the posterior part of the defense area, whereas from the anterior part a reduction of the sympathetic discharges to the stomach is more often obtained (76).

In the sympathetic inhibitory area behind the preceding ones, stimulation leads to a general reduction of the sympathetic tone resulting in a decrease of the blood pressure and heart rate, and to an increase of gastric tone (76). These results are generally in agreement with those of earlier workers (see 318) who found increases of motility from stimulation of the tuberal nucleus and supraoptic area and decreases from more posterior regions of hypothalamus.

Mesencephalon and Pons

Eliasson (93) obtained excitatory effects on stimulation of the superior colliculi, the area around the fasciculus longitudinalis, the ventrolateral parts of tegmentum, and reticular substance of pons. Inhibitory effects were elicited from the central and dorsal parts of tegmentum and reticular substance of pons, the medial lemniscus, and the area around the fasciculus longitudinalis.

Similar results were obtained by Hesser and Perret (141) who showed, in addition, that in animals with cervical cord transsected at C-5 level, predominantly augmentative effects were obtained from all the regions and especially from the central tegmentum and medial reticular substance (inhibitory areas in control animals). On the other hand, in vagotomized animals, only sparse inhibitory responses were elicited, probably because the effects of sympathetic activation are more difficult to show after suppression of the vagal excitatory tone.

Medulla

Stimulation of this structure produces powerful gastric effects. This is not surprising since the medulla contains the sensory and motor nuclei of the vagus and the fibers which carry the influences of higher centers either to the motor nuclei of the vagus or to the sympathetic cells. Both excitatory and inhibitory responses have been elicited from practically all the medullary regions, but preferably from the reticular substance, the region of the solitary tract, of the dorsal motor nucleus of vagus (DMNV), and the medial longitudinal fascicle (299).

Concerning the response elicited from the DMNV, it seems clear that part of the excitatory and inhibitory effects results from stimulation of the two kinds of vagal neurons corresponding to the excitatory and inhibitory vagal pathways, respectively. Indeed, these responses persist after spinalization, but they are suppressed by vagotomy or intravenous injection of hexamethonium (299). The excitatory responses are antagonized by atropine. Recently, Semba and Mizonishi (300) reported that DMNV stimulation could produce atropine-resistant excitatory responses that had a very long latency (more than 20 sec after the onset of stimulation). These responses were also obtained by stimulation of the cervical vagus. These responses very likely corresponded to postinhibitory rebounds, although the authors mentioned that inhibition preceding excitation was not always recorded. But this inhibition was probably difficult to demonstrate because the gastric motility was certainly markedly depressed in the anesthetized and atropinized preparations used by Semba and Mizonishi (300).

By stimulating the DMNV in vagotomized dogs, Semba et al. (299) have also obtained gastric excitatory responses that were suppressed either by atropine or by section of splanchnic nerves. Thus these responses were attributed to splanchnic cholinergic fibers. The splanchnic motor area of the DMNV was localized behind the vagal motor area (301). Nothing is known about the significance of this medullary splanchnic area. For example, it is not known whether these neurons are efferent neurons sending their axon directly to the splanchnic nerves or whether they are interneurons synapsing with spinal efferent neurons.

Excitatory and inhibitory responses mediated through the vagus nerves are also obtained by stimulation of structures around the DMNV, especially the solitary tract and the solitary tract nucleus (STN). These responses are probably indirect reflex responses. It is well known, indeed, that the solitary tract is a sensory structure collecting afferent fibers from various cranial nerves, in particular from the vagus nerve. These afferent fibers leave the solitary tract at various levels to synapse with cells of the STN. The axons of STN neurons end mainly on cells of the underlying reticular substance. No direct (monosynaptic) connections have been described between the STN and the DMNV. Therefore, the responses obtained from stimulation of the STN or from the dorsal reticular formation could represent an indirect (transsynaptic) activation of neurons of the DMNV. Some of these effects might also correspond to a direct activation of vagal preganglionic neurons, since a recent study using the horseradish peroxidase technique has revealed the presence of vagal cell bodies outside the DMNV and more precisely in the STN (335).

Excitatory responses mediated through the splanchnic nerves have also been elicited from structures around the DMNV, including the STN and the dorsal reticular formation (299). Here again, these responses might be indirect and relayed, for instance, by the splanchnic area of the DMNV; there is no experimental information in support of this suggestion.

As for the effects elicited from the medial longitudinal fascicle, the most plausible explanation could be that they correspond to stimulation of fibers conveying influences from higher centers. A similar explanation probably applies to the responses observed by Eliasson (93) to stimulation of the ventrolateral reticular formation.

Spinal Cord

Semba et al. (297) have reported that both inhibitory and excitatory effects could be obtained by stimulation of the dog thoracic cord.

Inhibition was observed on stimulation of the ventral horn of the gray matter, the intermediolateral and the intermediomedial nuclei. Excitatory responses were elicited from the dorsal nucleus, intermediolateral nucleus, dorsal column, and dorsal funiculus. The two types of responses were not affected by spinal transsections above and below the stimulated area. Semba et al. (297) gave no precise information about the rostrocaudal extent of the responsive area. They mentioned that inhibitory responses persisted after section of the dorsal spinal roots, whereas the excitatory ones were not affected by severing the ventral roots. According to these investigators, the inhibitory effects would correspond to stimulation of splanchnic fibers arising from ventral spinal roots, whereas excitatory responses would result from stimulation of splanchnic fibers running along the dorsal roots to leave the spinal cord. This interpretation is fully in agreement with Semba's previous results (298, 301). However, Jefferson et al. (180) have reported, in dogs under pentobarbital sodium (Nembutal), contractions of the stomach from stimuli applied to the spinal cord caudal to T-3, and to the intact ventral and dorsal roots from T-4 to L-2, and to the splanchnic nerves. These contractions were not abolished by removal of the stellate and celiac ganglia. These results seem to indicate that both ventral and dorsal thoracic roots carry motor fibers to the stomach and that these fibers apparently reach the stomach partly through the splanchnic nerves and partly through unknown pathways.

EXTRINSIC CONTROL OF INTESTINAL MOTILITY: SMALL AND LARGE INTESTINE

The extrinsic innervation of the small and large intestines, like that of esophagus and stomach, is achieved through parasympathetic and sympathetic nerves (Fig. 1). These extrinsic nerves are composed of afferent and efferent axons that connect the intestines to the central nervous system. Connecting pathways are generally well documented, but the localization of centers, and their functional role, remain controversial and unclear. Sympathetic nerves are inhibitory, except for those to sphincters, whereas parasympathetic nerves contain two distinct nerve fiber populations, one excitatory and the other inhibitory.

Organization of Extrinsic Nerve Pathways

Vagus Nerve

The vagus contains afferent and efferent axons that innervate the small intestine throughout its length (Fig. 1). Afferent neurons' cell bodies are located in the nodose ganglion, whereas those of efferent ones are situated in the vagus dorsal motor nucleus. Recent data obtained in the cat with horseradish peroxidase (HRP) retrograde transport technique (292), provide more precision concerning the localization of nerve cell bodies innervating the small intestine. Preganglionic neurons to the duodenum are located throughout the rostrocaudal extent of vagus dorsal motor nucleus, with a greater density at the level of the obex, where the ependymal canal widens to form the fourth ventricle. After HRP injection in the ileum wall, labeled neurons were mainly encountered in the dorsal motor nucleus rostral part. In addition, a few labeled neurons to the duodenum were found in the caudal part of the solitary tract nucleus, a region close to the dorsal motor nucleus (292).

It is generally accepted that, in man, vagal axons innervate the ascending and transverse colon, although their exact distribution remains unknown (325). In animals, the origin of parasympathetic colonic innervation, as well as the colon size and function, vary among species. The rabbit proximal colon is innervated by the vagus (184), whereas the distal colon receives its parasympathetic outflow from the pelvic nerves. In the cat, labeled neurons are observed in the vagus dorsal motor nucleus after HRP injection in the descending colon and upper rectum wall (292), but they seem to be less numerous than those innervating the small intestine.

Sacral Parasympathetic Nerves

In humans, the rectum and descending colon are innervated by the pelvic nerves issuing from S-2 to S-4 spinal roots and connecting to the pelvic plexus (325, 337). In rabbit, cat, and dog, the colon, rectum, and anal sphincter innervation has been extensively studied by Langley and Anderson (203,204). Recent studies indicate that after HRP injection in rectum and anal sphincters (internal and external), preganglionic labeled neurons are localized within three sacral cord nuclei. The first nucleus, composed of small neurons, is located in the gray matter intermediolateral part (with some neurons near the ependymal canal). It extends from S-2 to Cx-1 spinal roots, but most of the cell bodies are situated between S-2 and S-3. The second nucleus, consisting of relatively large neurons, is located in the ventromedial part of the ventral horn. The third nucleus, composed of very few large neurons, is located in the midventral part of the ventral horn (214). Cell bodies of the afferent axons are located in the corresponding spinal dorsal root ganglia. It must be pointed out that all the afferent axons do not run in dorsal spinal roots. Several findings (54,57) indicate that afferent axons innervating the rectum run in the sacral ventral roots. It will be necessary to take these data into account in physiological studies concerning the extrinsic nervous control of the large intestine.

Sympathetic Supply

The sympathetic efferent pathway consists of two distinct neurons: a cholinergic preganglionic neuron located in the mediolateral gray matter, and a noradrenergic postganglionic neuron located in peripheral extramural ganglia, either in paravertebral ganglia of the sympathetic chain or in prevertebral (previsceral) ganglia (celiac, superior mesenteric, inferior mesenteric ganglia). Although variations among species and individuals are frequent, the small intestine is mainly innervated by preganglionic axons issuing from T-9 to T-10 spinal roots running in the splanchnic nerves and synapsing in celiac and superior mesenteric ganglia (Fig. 1). The proximal part of the duodenum is innervated by axons having their cell bodies within the celiac ganglia and reaching the intestine in nerve bundles running along branches of the celiac artery (337). The ileum, jejunum, and the distal part of the duodenum receive their innervation from cell bodies located in the superior mesenteric ganglion. Their axons reach the effector in nerve satellites of the superior mesenteric artery (337). An indeterminate part of this last population innervates also the ascending and transverse colon.

Only noradrenergic nerve endings are present in the intestinal wall, except for the guinea pig colon in which intramural noradrenergic cell bodies have been described (33). It must be also pointed out that cholinergic postganglionic axons are also present in sympathetic nerves (28,30).

Effects of Stimulation and Section of Extrinsic Nerves

Small Intestine

Stimulation and section of vagus nerves. In acute animals, stimulation of the distal cut end of one vagus with a single shock has no effect. Stimulation with trains of pulses (Fig. 19) at a frequency around 10 Hz generally induces a contraction or enhances preexisting contractions. This excitation, which affects both muscle coats (17,19,106,123,250), is suppressed by atropine (106, 250). In the presence of atropine, vagal stimulation inhibits preexisting contractions. This inhibition is followed by a period of hypermotility (106), a consequence of a postinhibitory rebound. The parasympathetic innervation of the small intestine is quite similar to that described for the esophagus and stomach: the vagus nerves contain two distinct populations of preganglionic efferent axons, one connected with intramural cholinergic excitatory neurons, the other with intramural nonadrenergic noncholinergic inhibitory neurons. On the basis of various arguments, Burnstock (29) has proposed that these inhibitory neurons should be called purinergic neurons. This term will be subsequently used in the text.

In fact, the response to vagal stimulation consists very often of a mixture of both excitation and inhibition. Moreover, with manometric recording, inhibition is clearly observed only when "spontaneous contractions" are present. In nonspontaneously active intestine, the postinhibitory rebound excitation has often been inter-

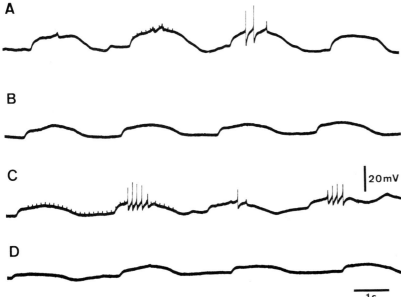

FIG. 19. Intracellular recordings from the longitudinal smooth muscle layer of rabbit duodenum. Traces **A–D** have been obtained during the same experiment; **B**, **C** and **D** are continuous recordings from the same cell. In **A** and **C**, right vagus stimulation, with two train pulses of different duration, indicated by the small-sized artifacts appearing in **A** on the second ECA and in **C** on the two first ones. The responses to vagal stimulation consists of spike potentials—also called electrical response activity (ERA)—superimposed on the 3rd ECA in **A** and on the 2nd, 3rd, and 4th one in **C**. Notice the absence of close relationship between nerve stimulation and smooth muscle cell response. From Gonella (123).

20mV

1 s.

preted as a pure excitatory effect (see 31,32). That is the case for the interpretation of the vagal effects proposed by Bayliss and Starling (17). These authors used atropine to prevent artifactual contraction or relaxation due to anemia from bradycardia. They concluded that vagal stimulation resulted in an inhibition followed by an excitation, the latter being unaltered by atropine, but permanently abolished by nicotine. Interpreted in the light of modern concepts, the findings of Bayliss and Starling show that the vagal inhibitory pathway is cholinergic.

Another matter of confusion came from the fact that vagal stimulation in the thorax and especially below the diaphragm could induce inhibition which was partially antagonized by adrenergic antagonists (see 192). The interpretation of these data was that inhibition was not parasympathetic but sympathetic in nature, and due either to the presence of adrenergic axons in the vagus or to the diffusion of stimulation to sympathetic nerves. It is now established that noradrenergic axons do exist in the vagus nerves but their participation in control of small intestine motility is not certain. As to the hypothesis of stimulus diffusion, it is only partly true (106). Also, inhibition by vagal stimulation in the neck, in the presence of atropine, has been clearly shown by Nakayama (250), although the interpretation he proposed at that time was not the one that is generally accepted now.

No marked difference has been noted between stimulation of both vagus nerves in excitatory or inhibitory effects (19,192). Optimal stimulation frequency ranges between 8 and 10 Hz (192); higher frequencies, around 20 Hz, are needed to obtain inhibition. In acute animals, section of the two vagus nerves in the neck or in the thorax does not produce any marked effect although a transient decrease of jejunal and ileal motility is noticed (19,192). It can be concluded that, at least in acute anesthetized animals, a vagal excitatory tone is virtually absent, but this is probably not the case in awake animals (238).

It is necessary to keep in mind that as far as upper small intestine segments are concerned, especially the duodenum, inhibition of motility induced by vagal stimulation may be the result of two different mechanisms. Inhibition may be due either to stimulation of a direct vagal inhibitory pathway to the duodenum or to activation of antral motility. Daniel (65) has shown in dogs that stimulation of the nerves of Latarjet, which induces antral contractions, simultaneously inhibits duodenal motility. This inhibition may be due to the activation of intramural inhibitory purinergic neurons running inside the gut wall from antrum to duodenum (65). This alternate activation of antrum and duodenum presumably is part of a regulatory mechanism that coordinates motility of the antrum and duodenum during gastric emptying (5,317,319). Electromyographic studies show that, in the duodenum, ERA is present only on those

control potentials that coincide with antral contractions (5,11,21,234). In fact, this last mechanism is presumably only partly intrinsic in origin, since in the early stages after vagotomy a deficient antroduodenal coordination is currently observed (234). This deficiency may account for gastric emptying disturbances following vagotomy. Dogs can recover from this dysfunction about 1 month after truncal vagotomy (4) probably because of adaptation of the intramural plexuses.

Stimulation and section of the sympathetic nerves. It has been known since the second half of the last century that stimulation of efferent splanchnic nerves leaving the spinal cord by thoracic and lumbar roots inhibits small intestine motility. However, various authors also described excitation (for references see 17,108). Also, the inhibitory mechanism itself was disputed. Some authors considered inhibition to be a direct effect, and others thought it was the consequence of anemia due to vasoconstriction. Bayliss and Starling (19) observed, in acute experiments on rabbits, cats, and dogs, an inhibition of small intestine motility in response to splanchnic nerve stimulation, followed by an excitation at the end of the stimulus. They postulated that this excitation (described by several authors) could correspond to a misinterpretation of a postinhibitory activation. They ruled out the possibility of secondary circulatory effects during splanchnic nerve stimulation by demonstrating that the inhibition of small intestine movements could be produced by mesenteric nerves stimulation "several minutes after the small intestine has been cut out of the body."

Thirty years later, Finkleman (100) showed that low concentrations of epinephrine mimic the inhibitory effect induced in isolated organs by mesenteric nerve stimulation. It was later established that mesenteric nerve stimulation releases mainly norepinephrine (97); this result has been confirmed by several authors using biochemical methods (108). It is now well documented that the small intestine sympathetic innervation is noradrenergic and inhibitory.

Splanchnic nerve section, in contrast to vagus section, is followed, in acute experiments, by a marked increase in intestinal motility (17). After administration of such sympatholytic drug as guanethidine or ergotamine, vagus nerve stimulation evokes strong contractions throughout the small intestine, whereas in the absence of such drugs vagal stimulation elicits weak responses in the duodenum and little or no response in the ileum (192). These results suggest that sympathetic nerves exert tonic inhibitory influences on the small intestine that are presumably stronger in distal segments than in proximal ones. From these data, Kewenter (192) proposed that sympathetic inhibitory tone blocks transmission in intramural excitatory nerve pathways. This interpretation is supported by numerous morphological findings that show the presence of a dense noradrenergic innervation around intramural ganglia, especially those of the myenteric plexus (163,164,254).

There is still a question about the site of action of norepinephrine released by sympathetic nerve stimulation. A current concept, based on pharmacological arguments, is that intestinal noradrenergic innervation is limited to intrinsic neurons. According to this hypothesis, the direct action of norepinephrine on smooth muscle, as demonstrated in rabbit and guinea pig small intestine (118), would be an experimental artifact due to an excess of norepinephrine released by unphysiological activation of sympathetic nerves. It must be stressed, however, that noradrenergic axons are present in the circular muscle coat (108,110,273,303) and, to a lesser extent, in the longitudinal layer (109). These morphological data suggest that the functional importance of the noradrenergic innervation of the smooth muscle is not negligible. Furthermore, in the rabbit duodenum, a weak stimulation of mesenteric nerves inhibits selectively the electrical activity of the circular muscle layer by a noradrenergic mechanism (125). Finally, it must be emphasized that autoreceptors, having a negative feedback function, have been abundantly described in the central and peripheral nervous systems. In the light of such a regulatory mechanism for transmitter release, the functional importance of overflow must be reconsidered.

In conclusion, then, sympathetic inhibition is presumably carried out at both ganglionic and muscular levels, but the relative importance of the two mechanisms has yet to be determined.

Colon

Stimulation and section of parasympathetic nerves. The general scheme of extrinsic nervous control already mentioned for the esophagus, stomach, and small intestine applies also to the colon. As early as the end of the last century, Langley and Anderson (203) showed that stimulation of the distal stump of the divided pelvic nerves elicits a contraction of both colonic muscle layers. These data have been largely confirmed (18,73,115, 120,124,147,185).

The excitatory effect is antagonized by atropine (see 120,124,185). In the presence of atropine, parasympathetic nerve stimulation induces muscle cell hyperpolarization (124,184,185). The parasympathetic inhibitory effect was probably first described by Langley and Anderson (203) who saw that, in some cases, the contraction to pelvic nerve stimulation was preceded by a relaxation. The inhibition is mediated through purinergic nerves and the contraction is the consequence of the postinhibitory rebound excitation. Thus the parasympathetic outflow to the colon contains two kinds of preganglionic axons, one that leads to intramural cholinergic excitatory neurons, and one that connects with

intramural purinergic inhibitory neurons. Both types of preganglionic axons are cholinergic, since they are blocked by hexamethonium (124,184,185).

In contrast to stimulation of the parasympathetic nerves to the small intestine, single shock stimuli evoke muscle responses consisting either of a depolarization (Fig. 20) (an excitatory junction potential, or EJP) (107, 111,120,124,185) or of a hyperpolarization (an inhibitory junction potential, or IJP) (111,124,184,185). These responses have long latencies: from 400 to 600 msec to 1 sec for IJPs. Such a long latency is due in part to intramural transmission mechanisms and in part to the low conduction velocity of the unmyelinated preganglionic axons (72,73). In cat, pelvic efferent axons synapse within extramural ganglia located on the distal colon and rectum serosal surface (73). Synaptic transmission in these ganglia is blocked by TEA and by GABA (73). Parasympathetic outputs from both the right and left pelvic nerves converge on all the intramural excitatory neurons (121).

In humans, it is generally accepted that the ascending and transverse colon are innervated by the vagus, but the actual importance of this innervation is not determined (325). For current laboratory animals, except the rabbit (see 184), the existence of a motor vagal supply to the colon is not well established (18,147). In cat, it is not possible to evoke EJPs on proximal colon by vagal stimulation (124). Pelvic nerves section does not modify greatly colonic motility in acute cats (147), but reflex contractions are markedly decreased (73); this is particularly true for the rectum. In humans, when efferent parasympathetic fibers to the colon are damaged, defecation is impeded (325).

Stimulation and section of sympathetic nerves. Lumbar colonic nerve stimulation inhibits colonic motility in dogs and cats (18,111,113,115,120,121,147,203). In rabbits, the distal part of the colon receives its sympathetic inhibitory innervation from lumbar colonic nerves (185). The proximal colon (the segment presenting haus-

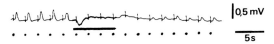

FIG. 20. Effect of lumbar colonic nerve (LCN) stimulation on excitatory junction potentials (EJPs) evoked on rabbit distal colon in response to pelvic nerve stimulation. Electrical recording obtained from *in vitro* experiments using extracellular pressure electrodes. Under the electrical tracing, *dots* indicate pelvic nerve stimulation (single shocks, 1 msec); they correspond with the brief, small-sized stimulation artifacts which can be seen on the recording itself. The *black bar* indicates LCN stimulation (trains of pulses 20 Hz, 1 msec). Pelvic nerve stimulation evokes EJPs. The stimulation of LCN produces both a smooth muscle membrane hyperpolarization which is not maintained on this recording due to the small time constant of the amplifier (0.3 sec) and a disappearance of EJPs. They reappear a few seconds after the end of LCN stimulation. EJP disappearance is due to the interruption of synaptic transmission, on the nerve pathway from extrinsic parasympathetic nerve fibers to smooth muscle cells, by norepinephrine released in intramural ganglia. From Jule and Gonella (185).

trations) is innervated by splanchnic nerves (184). As in the small intestine, the norepinephrine released by lumbar colonic nerve stimulation blocks synaptic transmission (Fig. 20) in intramural ganglionic synapses, and hyperpolarizes smooth muscle cells (111,185). Similar results can be obtained in rabbit proximal colon by splanchnic nerve stimulation (184). In acute cats, section of lumbar colonic nerves is followed by increased colonic motility lasting several hours (111,113,124,206). This suggests that, before nerve section, the colon received permanent inhibitory inputs from the lumbar colonic nerves. Another consequence of this disinhibition is a facilitation of neural transmission from parasympathetic preganglionic axons to intramural excitatory neurons of smooth muscle.

Origin of the sympathetic inhibitory firing to the colon. There is a good deal of evidence that the spinal cord is the source of tonic neural inhibition of the colon. Patients with lumbar spinal cord lesions have colonic hypermotility (59). In acute cats, lumbar spinal cord section between L-1 and L-3 decreases sympathetic inhibitory tone to the colon (Fig. 21). De Groat and Krier (75) recorded simultaneously, in cats, colonic motility and lumbar colonic nerve activity. After lumbar ventral root section or spinal cord removal, there was a decrease in lumbar colonic nerves' efferent firing and a parallel increase in colonic motility. Their results suggest that the efferent discharge is generated in the lumbar cord between T-13 and L-5. It is not abolished by dorsal root section in the corresponding segment. De Groat and Krier propose that lumbar efferent firing to the colon might be due either to intraspinal autorhythmic neurons [preganglionic neurons (see 218) or interneurons] or to a reflex arc whose afferent limb would pass (together with the efferent limb) in the lumbar ventral roots (see 54). The spinal cord is probably not the only source for efferent traffic in the lumbar colonic nerves; indeed, colonic motility is enhanced after lumbar colonic nerve section, even in animals with the thoracolumbar cord previously removed (75). This result suggests that prevertebral ganglia can also be a source of inhibitory inputs to the colon, at least in the cat. This idea is supported by the recent findings of Jule and Szurszewski

who demonstrate the existence of tonically discharging neurons in the cat inferior mesenteric ganglion (186). Differences between species exist, since no spontaneous discharge has been found in the guinea pig prevertebral ganglionic neurons (329).

The existence of any supraspinal control on lumbar inhibitory outflow to the colon has yet to be shown. Clinical observations of Connell et al. (59) indicate that patients with a high cord transsection and an intact cord below the lesion have reduced colonic motility when compared to normal subjects. This would suggest the existence of a supraspinal center having a facilitatory influence on the spinal inhibitory center. The observations of De Groat and Krier on anesthetized cats indicate that the supraspinal influences are weak if not nonexistent. Caution is certainly needed when comparing clinical observation with experimental results on anesthetized animals, but the existence of supraspinal influences cannot be ruled out.

Extrinsic Reflexes

Intestino-Intestinal, Intestino-Colic, and Colocolic Reflexes

The first report of these reflexes is the observation of Bayliss and Starling (17) that handling of an intestinal loop reflexively inhibits the whole intestine. This inhibitory reflex is abolished by extrinsic nerve section. In 1934 Hermann and Morin (140) observed, in chloralosed dogs, that distension of the small intestine with an intraluminal balloon inhibits contractions and decreases tone of other intestinal segments. They called this the intestino-intestinal inhibitory reflex. One year later, Morin (244) reported that inhibition induced by small intestinal distension affects also the large intestine (intestino-colic inhibitory reflex) and the stomach. He showed that bilateral vagotomy does not suppress this reflex and that bilateral splanchnicotomy abolishes it (245). These results were confirmed in dogs with Thiry fistulas (337). The existence of an intestino-colic inhibitory reflex (Fig. 22) has been demonstrated in cats (111,

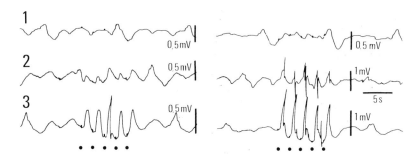

FIG. 21. Facilitation of EJPs evoked by stimulation of the second sacral ventral root (VS-2) after spinal cord section in L2. Cat previously spinalized in C-1–C-2. In left and right panels, 1, 2, and 3 represent stimultaneous recordings of colon EMG performed on proximal colon (1) and distal colon (2 and 3) with extracellular suction electrodes. Left panel, before the section; right panel, after transsection of the lumbar cord in L-2. Before cord section VS-2 stimulation (*dots*) evokes EJPs of small amplitude, whereas after cord section EJP amplitude increases, each EJP giving rise to a spike potential (notice the change in EMG amplification after the section). The facilitation of parasympathetic response after cord section is due to the suppression of efferent inhibitory sympathetic discharge, which has a depressor effect on transmission in the parasympathetic pathway at the intramural ganglionic level. From Gardette and Gonella (111).

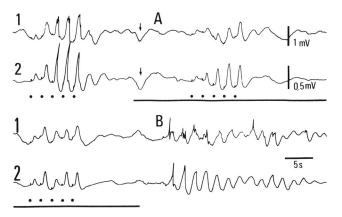

FIG. 22. Inhibitory intestino-colic reflex on spinal cat transsected in C-1–C-2. Recordings B follow recordings A without interruption. 1 and 2 represent the EMG of the distal colon recorded at 10 and 8 cm from the rectum, respectively. Ileal distension (7 ml air) is indicated by the bar under EMG. Stimulation of the second ventral sacral root (*dots*) evokes EJPs, the amplitude of which is decreased during ileal distension. Notice, at the onset of distension, hyperpolarization (*arrows*) on both traces due to the release of norepinephrine in muscle layers. This inhibitory enterocolic reflex disappeared either after lumbar colonic nerve section or in the presence of guanethidine. From Gardette and Gonella (111).

147). A colocolonic reflex (Fig. 23) has been described in guinea pigs (197).

Much literature has been devoted to these reflexes, especially to the intestino-intestinal reflex, and to their nervous pathways (see 108,337). This last matter generated a long controversy as to whether the reflex is exclusively spinal or if it can still occur after prevertebral ganglia decentralization.

Recent findings (64,197,198,313,315), by providing a better understanding of prevertebral ganglia, have greatly clarified the extramural reflexes engaged in the regulation of gut motility. It has been demonstrated (197) that colocolonic inhibitory reflexes can be elicited, *in vitro,* from a proximal to a distal segment (or the reverse) in the guinea pig colon with the attached prevertebral ganglia (celiac, superior and inferior mesenteric) and their

connecting nerves (Fig. 23). Electrophysiological studies of prevertebral ganglionic neurons with intracellular microelectrodes show that prevertebral ganglia with their various neural connections possess a nervous circuitry that is able to mediate extramural reflexes. These data confirm earlier results of Kuntz and Saccomano (202) showing that intestino-intestinal inhibitory reflex can be obtained through decentralized extramural ganglia, and that this reflex is abolished by painting the solar plexus with nicotine (see 337).

In the guinea pig, most of the neurons located in the inferior mesenteric ganglion receive synaptic inputs from both peripheral and central origins (Fig. 24), from mechanoreceptors situated in the colon by axons running in the colonic nerves, and from preganglionic sympathetic neurons located in the spinal cord, by axons running in the splanchnic nerves (313,315). The summation of subthreshold excitatory postsynaptic potentials (EPSPs) produced by peripheral and central nerve pathway activation initiates a spike potential in the postganglionic neuron. That is, postganglionic sympathetic neurons located in prevertebral ganglia are the sympathetic final common pathway integrating information coming from the periphery and the central nervous system. It must be emphasized that "spinal and peripheral reflex pathways do not exist as separate neural circuits, but must be considered to be functionally integrated" (315).

The functioning of the prevertebral ganglia is perhaps still more complicated than it appears now. Immunocytochemical data (*see* 145) indicate the presence in prevertebral ganglia of guinea pig, rat, and cat of nerve cells or nerve processes containing vasoactive intestinal polypeptide, enkephalins, substance P, and somatostatin. Figure 25 summarizes the possible connections of the inferior mesenteric ganglion with the spinal cord and the intestinal wall by peptide-containing neurons. The functional significance of these peptides is unknown. It is highly probable that they play an important

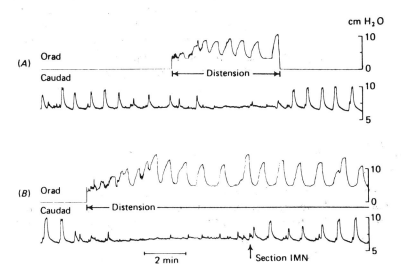

FIG. 23. Effect of distension of orad segment of guinea pig colon on contractions in caudad segment. The intraluminal pressure in the orad segment was zero before and after distension. In **A** and **B**, distension of the orad segment inhibits contractions in the caudad segment. After intermesenteric nerve (IMN) section, caudad segment is no longer inhibited. From Kreulen and Szurszewski (197).

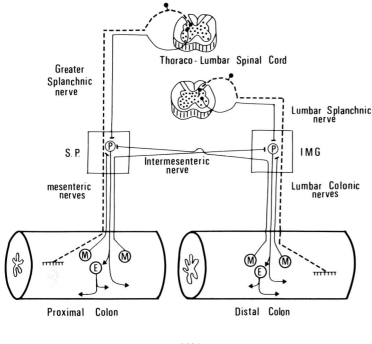

FIG. 24. Schematic representation of possible neural connections of proximal and distal segments of guinea pig colon with prevertebral ganglia and spinal cord. SP, solar plexus; IMG, inferior mesenteric ganglion; P, postganglionic sympathetic neurons; E, cholinergic excitatory intramural neurons; M, mecanoreceptors. The interrupted lines represent the direct afferent connections from gut wall to the spinal cord. Drawn after Szurszewski (313).

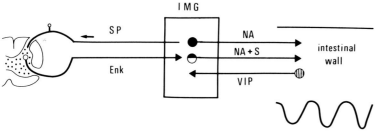

FIG. 25. Diagram illustrating the possible peptidergic and noradrenergic connections between spinal cord, inferior mesenteric ganglion (IMG), and intestinal wall, respectively. E, enkephalin; SP, substance P; VIP, vasoactive intestinal polypeptide; NA, noradrenaline; NA + S, postganglionic neuron containing noradrenaline plus somatostatin. Drawn from Hökfelt (145).

role in prevertebral ganglia synaptic transmission. Preliminary results of Krier (quoted after Szurszewski, 314) show that substance P at very low concentrations (10^{-8} M) increases the excitability of guinea pig prevertebral ganglionic neurons in such a way that subthreshold EPSPs generate spike potentials, or, in the absence of excitatory inputs, postganglionic neurons give rise to a tonic discharge of spike potentials. The prevertebral ganglia can no longer be regarded as simple synaptic relay stations on the pathways of nerve impulses from the spinal cord to the effector.

Extrinsic Parasympathetic Reflexes of the Colon

Mechanical stimulation of the colon or of the rectum elicits a coordinated reflex contraction of the rectum that may be followed by defecation (114,147,295). Section or lesions of the parasympathetic outflow to the colon or of the sacral cord impede defecation (78,325). Little is known about the nature of the pelvic efferent outflow to the colon during reflex evoked contractions. De Groat and Krier (74) recorded simultaneously colon contractions and nerve discharge in small nerve bundles running along the serosal surface of the cat colon. They recorded an efferent firing in parasympathetic axons

even which can be greatly increased by very weak colonic distension (Fig. 26A). This nervous discharge which even can be greatly increased by very weak colsacral dorsal roots (Fig. 26B). These data indicate that the parasympathetic afferent discharge is responsible for the reflex-elicited colonic contractions. This result is in agreement with unpublished observations of Gonella and Jule, who recorded the electrical activity of parasympathetic preganglionic neurons in the spinal cord with extracellular microelectrodes (Fig. 26C). The spontaneous and relatively phasic colonic contractions are elicited by short phasic bursts of the preganglionic neurons. The parasympathetic colocolonic reflex persists after transsection of the spinal cord in T-10 to T-12. It is mediated by afferent and efferent unmyelinated fibers (74).

Gastroileal Reflex, Gastrocolic Reflex

A so-called gastroileal reflex consisting of an enhancement of distal ileal motility in response to feeding has been described (90). There is, however, virtually no evidence that this reflex is mediated by extrinsic nerves (see 194).

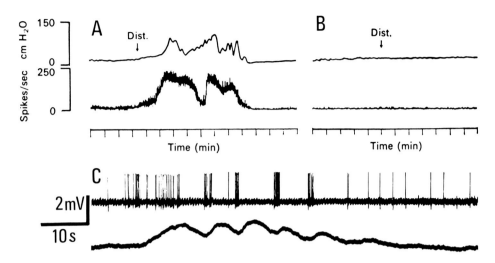

FIG. 26. **A** and **B**: Correlation between colonic motility and firing in parasympathetic efferent nerves to the colon, following distension of the distal colon on chloralosed cat. *Upper traces* represent intraluminal pressure, *lower traces* integration of the neural discharge obtained with a rate-meter (time constant: 1 sec). In record **A**, distension of the distal colon by injection of 2 ml fluid into the recording balloon induced proximal colon contractions and an increase in the neural discharge. Record **B** represents the response to distension in the same experiment after bilateral section of the sacral dorsal and ventral roots. From De Groat and Krier (74). **C**: Correlation between the pelvic preganglionic neuron discharge and the colon contractions in a cat spinalized in C-1–C-2. *Upper trace* represents the neuron discharge recorded with an extracellular microelectrode. The neuron was localized in the intermedio-lateral part of the spinal cord gray matter, between the emergence of S-2 and S-3 spinal roots. *Lower trace* represents the intraluminal pressure recorded with a balloon throughout the length of the colon and filled with 10 ml air. Colonic contractions are preceded by bursts of the preganglionic parasympathetic neuron. From J. Gonella and Y. Jule (*unpublished*).

As to the gastrocolic reflex, published reports indicate that this reflex, characterized by an increase in distal colon motility after feeding, may be partly mediated through extrinsic nerves (194). The investigations performed in order to show the nerve pathways involved in colonic activation, using mainly nerve section, are not conclusive since not only motility but probably also nerve-mediated gut hormone secretion are affected. The fact that the gastrocolic reflex is present in patients with a thoracolumbar spinal cord transsection suggests that an eventual extrinsic neural component of this reflex would be discrete (see 194).

Reflexes of Somatic and Visceral Origin

This section deals with reflexes elicited by noxious stimuli that affect not only the gut but also visceral effectors such as the heart and urinary bladder (290,337). These reflexes are generally produced by somatic or visceral stimuli. Somato-digestive reflexes consist of an inhibition of gastric and intestinal motility in response to skin pinching in various regions of the body (291). Inhibition persists after bilateral vagotomy and is abolished by splanchnic nerve section. Inhibition of motility depends on stimulus localization: Abdominal skin stimulation affects the duodenum whereas that of the skin of the chest or neck does not (291). This reflex seems to have a segmental organization and an important propriospinal component, but a supraspinal component is not excluded. The existence of somato-gastric reflexes has also been reported (189). In vagotomized animals,

pinching of the hind paw inhibits gastric motility, whereas the same stimulus on animals after splanchnicotomy increases gastric motility (189). The efferent limb of the gastric facilitatory reflex is the vagus nerve, whereas the afferent one is spinal in nature, since cervical cord transsection abolishes the reflex (189). The finality of such somato-visceral reflexes has yet to be determined, but they indicate clearly that somatic afferent pathways are connected with vegetative central neurons involved in the control of gut motility.

Noxious stimulation of various organs such as the genitourinary tract, kidney, and gallbladder inhibits gut motility (337). All these reflexes are mediated through sympathetic nerves. However, as was pointed out by Furness and Costa (108), for a great number of experiments the release of epinephrine by the adrenal medulla has not been taken into account. In these conditions, the contribution of the sympathetic innervation remains ill-defined.

EXTRINSIC CONTROL OF ILEOCECAL AND ANAL SPHINCTERS

Ileocecal Sphincter

The ileocecal sphincter is thought to control transit from the small to the large intestine. This sphincter has a sympathetic and a parasympathetic innervation. The parasympathetic preganglionic axons run in the vagus. The sympathetic innervation is mediated by splanchnic and lumbar colonic nerves. Pahlin and Kewenter (257,

258), using chloralosed cats with ligated adrenal arteries and vein to exclude any effect due to variation in levels of circulating catecholamines, demonstrated that sphincteric smooth muscle has a sympathetic and a parasympathetic innervation distinct from that of adjacent ileal and colonic muscle. Thus sphincter contractions can occur independently from those of the ileum and colon.

Stimulation of the distal stump of the divided splanchnic nerve elicits sphincter contraction (258,306, 307). A similar excitatory effect is observed upon stimulation of the distal cut end either of nerve strands running along the superior mesenteric artery or of lumbar colonic nerves. This excitatory effect, blocked by phenoxybenzamine, is mediated through alpha-adrenergic receptors. The sympathetic innervation seems to have also an inhibitory beta effect on ileocecal sphincter motility (258).

Sympathetic motor action on the ileocecal sphincter is markedly reduced by atropine (258), as is that of the lower esophageal sphincter. However, the mechanism of this antagonistic effect of atropine has not been investigated in the ileocecal sphincter.

Stimulation of the distal cut end of the vagus elicits sphincter contraction through a cholinergic mechanism antagonized by atropine. The response to vagal stimulation is impaired by guanethidine (257). However, since it has not been investigated whether or not other sympatholytic drugs, such as alpha or beta blockers, antagonize vagal excitatory effects, the parasympatholytic effect of guanethidine remains unclear.

Internal Anal Sphincter

Extrinsic Nerve Supply

The internal anal sphincter represents the thickened terminal part of the circular smooth muscle coat of the rectum. Its proximal part is continuous with rectal circular muscle, whereas its distal part is attached to the perianal skin. The internal anal sphincter contributes mainly to the pressure recorded inside the anal canal (22,295). It receives a sympathetic innervation issuing from the lumbar spinal cord through the lumbar splanchnic nerves and from the inferior mesenteric ganglion through the hypogastric nerves (146). The parasympathetic supply comes from the sacral spinal cord through the pelvic nerves. Preganglionic parasympathetic axons have synaptic relays within intramural ganglia. In contrast to other segments of the gut, the intramural ganglionic cell bodies are not located in the sphincteric area, but presumably in the distal rectum (109; J. Gonella and M. Bouvier, *unpublished*). Sympathetic motor effect on the internal anal sphincter has been known since the pioneer work of Langley and Anderson (203), and has been confirmed more recently

(112). The sympathetic excitatory effect is noradrenergic in origin. It is antagonized by alpha antagonists (112). A sympathetic beta-inhibitory effect has also been described in the presence of alpha blockers (112). The clearest effect observed by stimulating parasympathetic nerves is relaxation of the sphincter (112,294, 295), presumably due to activation of preganglionic axons synapsing with the intramural purinergic neurons (112, 295).

Reflex and Central Control of the Internal Anal Sphincter

Rectoanal inhibitory reflex. Transient rectal wall distension induces a short-duration relaxation of the internal anal sphincter, as illustrated in Fig. 27 (77,294). In fact, distension induces, in some cases, a contraction in the region of the distending balloon. It is then questionable whether sphincter relaxation is due to an extrinsic reflex or solely to an intrinsic reflex. Strong arguments in favor of the latter hypothesis do exist (77, 105,232,294), so that it is obvious that intrinsic neural circuits are sufficient to initiate sphincter relaxation by rectal distension. However, Meunier and Mollard (232), using weak rectal distension in normal human subjects, obtained sphincter relaxation without rectal contraction. This result demonstrates that the sphincter relaxation reflex has a lower threshold than the rectal contraction reflex. It has yet to be demonstrated whether the low-threshold reflex-induced relaxation is extrinsic

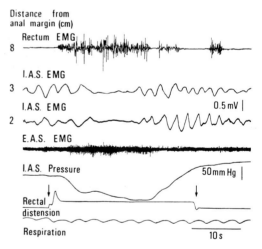

FIG. 27. Responses of internal and external anal sphincters to a rectal distension in man. A transient rectal distension (between arrows), obtained by inflating a balloon with 40 ml air, induces a contraction of the rectum corresponding to the discharge of spike potentials on rectum EMG. At the same time, internal anal sphincter (IAS) EMG, whose electrical response activity consists of slow time course variations of smooth muscle cell membrane potential, is inhibited. A fall in pressure in the anal canal (IAS pressure) corresponds to the inhibition of sphincteric electrical activity. During internal anal sphincter relaxation, the external anal sphincter contracts. This contraction corresponds to the discharge of spike potentials appearing on external sphincter (EAS) EMG. From Monges et al. (242).

in nature or not. However, the participation of an extrinsic parasympathetic pathway in the internal anal sphincter relaxation cannot be completely excluded, since pelvic nerve stimulation induces sphincter relaxation (105,112). Whether the reflex is purely intrinsic or has an extrinsic component, the sphincter relaxation is presumably due to the activation of intramural purinergic neurons (112,243).

Vesicoanal reflex. Garrett et al. (112) described, in anesthetized cats, strong internal anal sphincter contractions during both urinary bladder compression and spontaneous micturition. Although the authors do not give any information about nerve pathways involved in this reflex, it is highly probable that it depends on extrinsic nerve pathways.

Central control. Section of the hypogastric or pelvic nerves in anesthetized cats decreases intraluminal anal pressure (112). The interpretation of these results is that, at rest, both types of nerves convey tonic excitatory influences to the internal anal sphincter (112), but we lack information concerning the nature of their efferent firing and functional role.

Experimental and clinical data indicate that impairment of the hypogastric nerves (112) or anesthesia of the spinal cord between T-6 and T-12 (105) decreases sphincteric tone substantially, but in animals the recovery of tone begins about 30 min after nerve section. The latter result would indicate that the extrinsic nerve control is not essential for the maintenance of sphincter tone. The most puzzling result is the fall in tone observed in cats after pelvic nerve section, especially because these nerves seem mainly to inhibit the sphincter. More accurate experiments are needed to clarify the actions of the central nervous system on the internal anal sphincter.

On the basis of clinical observations, it was concluded that supraspinal centers do not influence sphincteric tone, since intraluminal pressure, in patients with high cord section, does not differ significantly from that in normal human subjects. Another and probably more plausible explanation would be that, after spinal cord section, the remaining nervous structures could adapt to the new situation to maintain a virtually normal sphincteric tone.

External Anal Sphincter

The external anal sphincter, a striated muscle, receives its innervation from the sacral cord via the pudendal nerves (*see* 25,214,294). Its contraction depends exclusively on efferent firing of its motoneurons. The external anal sphincter is paralyzed by the pudendal nerve section. This sphincter is in a state of tonic activity that is subjected to important fluctuations; like skeletal striated muscle, it is under voluntary control (103). The external anal sphincter motoneurons are located in the lateral part of the ventral horn, in the same area as those motoneurons innervating the external urethral sphincter (214,336). The efferent axons as well as afferent pathways are contained mainly in the second sacral roots. Mackel (214) has shown that only about half of sphincter motoneurons can be activated monosynaptically by anal sphincter motor nerve stimulation. Monosynaptic afferent axons, originating probably from the sphincteric muscle spindles, have a high conduction velocity. In contrast with hind limb motoneurons, anal sphincter motoneurons have no recurrent inhibition. A similar observation has been made in external urethral sphincter motoneurons.

Some of the external anal sphincter motoneurons can be reflexly activated by stimulation of afferent axons running in pudendal nerve branches that innervate the external urethral sphincter. This type of connection is generally polysynaptic and excitatory, but inhibitory responses have also been observed (214). These nervous cross-connections between external anal sphincter and urinary tract may explain the relationships between micturition and defecation (see 294).

CENTRAL NERVOUS STRUCTURES INVOLVED IN THE REGULATION OF INTESTINAL MOTILITY

There is relatively limited information about the supraspinal control of gut motility. It is based on experiments that used stimulation or, to a lesser extent, lesions of central nervous structures. A general feature of the effects of stimulation of central nervous structures is their nonspecificity: stimulation of central nervous system areas modifying intestinal motility also generally causes motility changes of the stomach, urinary bladder, and uterus and causes variations in blood pressure (281, 282,318). For example, orbital and anterior cingulate gyrus stimulation induces a decrease in stomach, colon, urinary bladder, and uterus motility, and a fall in arterial pressure (282). Even when pure gut motility effects are provoked by central stimulation, ambiguity still persists as to the nature of the effect observed. For example, anterior sigmoid gyrus stimulation inhibits gastric motility (92) and increases the small intestine movements (282), but it is not clear if intestine activation is due to a primary intestinal excitation or to the inhibition of gastric motility which would, in turn, release intestinal motility (see 65,234). It must also be pointed out that activation of afferences from the gastrointestinal tract can modify the activity of the brain (200,206).

Effects of Bulbar and Mesencephalic Stimulation

In chloralosed dogs, stimulation of the dorsal vagal nucleus or of the nucleus ambiguus induce contractions of the small intestine (1). This excitation is presumably vagal in nature since the vagal efferent neurons are localized in these structures. From the functional standpoint, one of the most accurate studies concerning the effects of central control of intestinal motility is that of Johansson et al. (182,183). They showed, in anesthetized and vagotomized cats, that stimulation of the posterior part of the floor of the fourth ventricle suppresses the intestino-intestinal inhibitory reflex. This effect is presumably due to activation of a descending nerve pathway exerting a depressor effect on synaptic transmission in propriospinal circuits mediating the intestino-intestinal inhibitory reflex (182). The same authors showed that after intercollicular brainstem transsection the threshold of the intestino-intestinal inhibitory reflex is enhanced (183). This means that the section has interrupted descending facilitatory influences. If the spinal cord is then transsected at the cervical level, there is a fall in intestinal tone that can be restored by anesthesia of the spinal cord or of the mesenteric nerves (183). The former result indicates that spinal section has released spinal intestino-inhibitory centers from tonic bulbar inhibitory influences. The latter result shows that the decrease in intestinal tone after cervical transsection is due to an active efferent nervous inhibitory firing. These data confirm the existence of a bulbar inhibitory center for spinal inhibitory center (182) whose existence was postulated by Kewenter (192).

Effects of Diencephalic and Telencephalic Stimulation

Rostad (281) has described excitatory effects of hypothalamic stimulation. These effects are blocked by atropine. They are attributed to the activation of parasympathetic mechanisms mediated via pelvic nerves since they persist after section of the vagus. The same author has also described, on stimulation of various hypothalamic areas, a colonic excitation that disappears after lumbar colonic nerve section and is abolished in the presence of guanethidine (281). The explanation proposed by Rostad (281) of a noradrenergic excitatory effect is not convincing. In the light of the results of Johansson et al. (182), one should attribute the sympathetically mediated excitatory effect of Rostad's result to a withdrawal of inhibition: a depressor effect of hypothalamic structures on the spinal sympathetic inhibitory center, rather than to a primary sympathetic excitatory effect (181,182).

Inhibition of colonic motility by stimulation of various hypothalamic areas (ventromedial nucleus, medial forebrain bundle) has also been described. This inhibition is abolished by guanethidine or by splanchnic and lumbar colonic nerve section (281).

Excitatory responses, parasympathetic in nature, have been obtained in cat colon by stimulation of various cortical areas, the parietal cortex, the anterior part of the ectosylvian gyrus, and the anterior part of the lateral sulcus (282). These responses seem to be mediated through the vagus. Colonic contractions have also been obtained in response to stimulation of the olfactory bulb and olfactory tract; these are abolished by vagus and pelvic nerve section (282). Inhibitory responses mainly mediated via lumbar colonic nerves have been obtained by stimulation of anterior sigmoid, orbital, and anterior cingulate gyri (282). A general feature of this catalog of effects lies in the fact that responses are often neither clear-cut nor reliable; for this reason it is difficult to form any idea of their real functional significance.

Another structure whose stimulation gives colonic contraction is the amygdaloid complex nuclei (188,282). Defecations have been obtained in acute animals by stimulation of the amygdala (188). However, the most significant result from the functional standpoint is that obtained by Gastaut et al. (116) in conscious cats with chronically implanted stimulating electrodes in the amygdaloid complex. These authors sometimes observed uncontrolled defecations, but in most cases defecation occurred during a pattern of motor behavior that led to the characteristic posture of the animal during defecation. These data suggest that amygdala is really engaged in specific control of gut motility at least for its distal part.

Effects of Cerebellar Stimulation

An increase in stomach, small intestine, and colon motility has been obtained by Lisander and Martner (211) in response to stimulation of the fastigial nucleus. This excitation is presumably due to a disinhibition by a depressor effect on the spinal sympathetic inhibitory center of the gut.

REFERENCES

1. Abbadessa, S., Catier, J., and Corriol, J. (1967): Structures bulbaires et motricité duodénojejunale. *Arch. Int. Physiol. Biochem.*, 75:707–722.
2. Abe, S. (1959): On the histology and the innervation of the esophagus and the first forestomach of the goat. *Arch. Histol. Jpn.*, 16:109–129.
3. Abrahamsson, J. (1973): Studies on the inhibitory nervous control of gastric motility. *Acta Physiol. Scand. [Suppl. 390]*, 88:1–38.
4. Aeberhard, P., and Bedi, B. S. (1977): Effects of proximal gastric vagotomy (PGV) followed by total vagotomy (TV) on post prandial and fasting myoelectrical activity of the canine stomach and duodenum. *Gut*, 18:515–523.
5. Allen, G. L., Poole, E. W., and Code, C. F. (1964): Relationship between electrical activities of antrum and duodenum. *Am. J. Physiol.*, 207:906–910.
6. Alvarez, W. C. (1948): *An Introduction to Gastroenterology*, Ed4. Paul B. Hoeber, New York.
7. Andrew, B. L. (1956): The nervous control of cervical oesophagus of the rat. *J. Physiol. (Lond.)*, 134:729–740.
8. Andrews, C. J. H., and Andrews, W. H. H. (1971): Receptors activated by acid in the duodenal wall of rabbits. *Q. J. Exp. Physiol.*, 56:221–230.

9. Arimori, M., Code, C. F., Schlegel, J. F., and Sturm, R. E. (1970): Electrical activity of the canine esophagus and gastro-esophageal sphincter: Its relation to intraluminal pressure and movement of material. *Am. J. Dig. Dis.*, 15:191–208.

10. Armitage, A. K., and Dean, A. C. B. (1966): The effects of pressure and pharmocologically active substances on gastric peristalsis in a transmurally stimulated rat stomach-duodenum preparation. *J. Physiol. (Lond.,)*, 182:42–56.

11. Atanassova, E. (1970): On the mechanism of correlation between the spike activities of the stomach and duodenum. *Bull. Inst. Physiol. Acad. Sci. Bulg.*, 13:229–242.

12. Babkin, B. P., and Kite, W. C., Jr. (1950): Central and reflex regulation of motility of pyloric antrum. *J. Neurophysiol.*, 13:321–334.

13. Babkin, B. P., and Speakman, T. J. (1940): Cortical inhibition of gastric motility. *J. Neurophysiol.*, 13:55–63.

14. Bailey, P., and Sweet, W. H. (1940): Effects on respiration, blood pressure and gastric motility of stimulation of orbital surface of frontal lobe. *J. Neurophysiol.*, 3:276–281.

15. Bartlet, A. L. (1968): The effect of vagal stimulation and eserine on isolated guinea-pig oesophagus. *Q. J. Exp. Physiol.*, 53:170–174.

16. Baumgarten, H. G., and Lange, W. (1969): Adrenergic innervation of the oesophagus in the cat *(Felis domestica)* and rhesus monkey. *Z. Zellforsch.*, 95:529–545.

17. Bayliss, W. M., and Starling, E. H. (1899): The movements and innervation of the small intestine. *J. Physiol. (Lond.)*, 24:99–143.

18. Bayliss, W. M., and Starling, E. H. (1900): The movements and innervation of the large intestine. *J. Physiol. (Lond.)*, 26:107–118.

19. Bayliss, W. M., and Starling, E. H. (1901): The movements and innervation of the small intestine. *J. Physiol. (Lond.)*, 26:125–138.

20. Beani, L., Bianchi, C., and Crema, A. (1971): Vagal non-adrenergic inhibition of guinea-pig stomach. *J. Physiol. (Lond.)*, 217:259–279.

21. Bedi, B. S., and Code, C. F. (1972): Pathway of coordination of postprandial antral and duodenal action potentials. *Am. J. Physiol.*, 222:1295–1298.

22. Bennett, R. C., and Duthie, H. L. (1964): The functional importance of the internal anal sphincter. *Br. J. Surg.*, 51:355–357.

23. Berger, T., Ceder, L., Hampelt, A., and Meurling, S. (1976): Effect of highly selective vagotomy on gastric emptying. *Scand. J. Gastroenterol.*, 11:829–832.

24. Binder, H. J., Bloom, D. L., Stern, H., Solitaire, G. B., Thayer, W. R., and Spiro, H. M. (1968): The effect of cervical vagectomy on esophageal function in the monkey. *Surgery*, 64:1075–1083.

25. Bishop, B., Garry, R. C., Roberts, T. D. M., and Todd, J. K. (1956): Control of the external sphincter of the anus in the cat. *J. Physiol. (Lond.)*, 134:229–240.

26. Bulbring, E., and Gershon, M. D. (1967): 5-Hydroxytryptamine participation in the vagal inhibitory innervation of the stomach. *J. Physiol. (Lond.)*, 192:823–846.

27. Burgess, J. N., Schlegel, J. F., and Ellis, F. H., Jr. (1972): Effect of denervation on feline esophageal function and morphology. *J. Surg. Res.*, 12:24–33.

28. Burnstock, G. (1972): Purinergic nerves. *Pharmacol. Rev.*, 24:509–581.

29. Burnstock, G. (1975): Purinergic transmission. In: *Handbook of Psychopharmacology, Vol. 5, Synaptic Modulators*, edited by L. L. Iverson, S. D. Iverson, S. H. Snyder, pp. 131–194. Plenum, London.

30. Burnstock, G., and Costa, M. (eds.) (1975): *Adrenergic Neurons. Their Organization, Function and Development in the Peripheral Nervous System.* Chapman Hall, London.

31. Campbell, G. (1966): Nerve mediated excitation of the guinea-pig caecum. *J. Physiol. (Lond.)*, 185:148–159.

32. Campbell, G. (1966): The inhibitory nerve fibres in the vagal supply to the guinea-pig stomach. *J. Physiol. (Lond.)*, 185:600–612.

33. Campbell, G. (1970): Autonomic nervous supply to effector tissues. In: *Smooth Muscle*, edited by E. Bülbring, A. F. Brading, A. W. Jones, and T. Tomita, pp. 451–495. Edward Arnold, London.

34. Campbell, G., and Burnstock, G. (1968): Comparative physiology of gastrointestinal motility. In: *Handbook of Physiology, Section 6: Alimentary canal, Vol. 4*, edited by C. F. Code, pp. 2213–2266. American Physiological Society, Washington, D.C.

35. Cannon, W. B. (1907): Esophageal peristalsis after bilateral vagotomy. *Am. J. Physiol.*, 19:436–444.

36. Cannon, W. B., and Lieb, C. W. (1911): The receptive relaxation of the stomach. *Am. J. Physiol.*, 29:267–273.

37. Car, A. (1970): La commande corticale du centre déglutiteur bulbaire. *J. Physiol. (Paris)*, 62:361–386.

38. Car, A. (1973): La commande corticale de la déglutition. I: Sa voie d'expression. *J. Physiol. (Paris)*, 66:531–551.

39. Car, A., and Roman, C. (1965): Etude des vitesses de conduction des fibres nerveuses motrices de l'oesophage. *C. R. Soc. Biol.*, 159:1767–1770.

40. Car, A., and Roman, C. (1970): Déglutitions et contractions oesophagiennes réflexes produites par la stimulation du bulbe rachidien. *Exp. Brain Res.*, 11:75–92.

41. Car, A., and Roman, C. (1970): L'activité spontanée du sphincter oesophagien supérieur; ses variations au cours de la déglutition et de la rumination. *J. Physiol. (Paris)*, 62:505–511.

42. Carlson, A. J., Boyd, T. E., and Pearcy, J. F. (1922): Studies on the visceral sensory nervous system. XII: The innervation of the cardia and the lower end of the esophagus in mammals. *Am. J. Physiol.*, 61:14–41.

43. Carter, D. C., Whitfield, H. N., and Mac Leod, I. B. (1971): The effect of vagotomy on gastric adaptation. *Gut*, 13:874–879.

44. Carveth, S. W., Schlegel, J. F., Code, C. F., and Ellis, F. H. (1962): Esophageal motility after vagotomy, phrenicotomy, myotomy, and myomectomy in dogs. *Surg. Gynecol. Obstet.*, 114:31–42.

45. Castell, D. O. (1975): The lower esophageal sphincter: Physiologic and clinical aspects. *Ann. Intern. Med.*, 83:390–401.

46. Chauveau, A. (1862): Du nerf pneumogastrique considéré comme agent excitateur et comme agent conducteur des contractions oesophagiennes dans l'acte de la déglutition. *J. Physiol. Homme Anim.*, 5:190–226.

47. Christensen, J. (1970): Pharmacological identification of the lower esophageal sphincter. *J. Clin. Invest.*, 49:681–690.

48. Christensen, J. (1975): Pharmacology of the esophageal motor function. *Annu. Rev. Pharmacol.*, 15:243–258.

49. Christensen, J., and Lund, G. F. (1969): Esophageal responses to distension and electrical stimulation. *J. Clin. Invest.*, 48:408–419.

50. Ciampini, G., and Jean, A. (1980): Rôle des afférences glosso-pharyngiennes et trigéminales dans le déclenchement et le déroulement de la déglutition: I. Afférences glossopharyngiennes. *J. Physiol. (Paris)*, 76:49–60.

51. Ciampini, G., and Jean, A. (1980): Rôle des afférences glosso-pharyngiennes et trigéminales dans le déclenchement et le déroulement de la déglutition: II. Afférences trigéminales. *J. Physiol. (Paris)* 76:61–66.

52. Clark, G. C., and Vane, J. R. (1961): The cardiac sphincter in the cat. *Gut*, 2:252–262.

53. Clarke, G. D., and Davison, J. S. (1978): Mucosal receptors in the gastric antrum and small intestine of the rat with afferent fibres in the cervical vagus. *J. Physiol. (Lond.)*, 284:55–67.

54. Clifton, G. L., Coggeshall, R. E., Vance, W. H., and Willis, W. D. (1976): Receptive field of unmyelinated ventral root afferent fibres in the cat. *J. Physiol. (Lond.)*, 256:573–600.

55. Code, C. F., and Marlett, J. A. (1975): The interdigestive myoelectric complex of the stomach and small bowel of dogs. *J. Physiol. (Lond.)*, 246:289–309.

56. Code, C. F., and Schlegel, J. F. (1968): Motor action of the esophagus and its sphincters. In: *Handbook of Physiology, Section 6, Alimentary Canal, Vol. 4*, edited by C. F. Code, pp. 1821–1839. American Physiological Society, Washington, D. C.

57. Coggeshall, R. E., Coulter, J. D., and Willis, W. D. (1973): Unmyelinated fibres in the human L4 and L5 ventral roots. *Brain Res.*, 57:229–233.

58. Cohen, S., Ryan, J., Matarazzo, S., and Snape, W. J., Jr. (1977): Nervous control of esophageal motor activity. In: *Nerves and the Gut.* edited by F. P. Brooks and P. W. Evers, pp. 207–222. C. B. Slack, Inc., Thorofare.

59. Connell, A. M., Frankel, H., and Guttmann, L. (1963): The motility of the pelvic colon following complete lesions of the spinal cord. *Paraplegia,* 1:98–115.

60. Cooke, A. R. (1975): Control of gastric emptying and motility. *Gastroenterology,* 68:804–816.

61. Cooke, A. (1977): Localization of receptors inhibiting gastric emptying in the gut. *Gastroenterology,* 72:875–880.

62. Cooke, A., and Clark, E. (1976): Effect of first part of duodenum on gastric emptying in dogs: Response to acid, fat, glucose and neural blockade. *Gastroenterology,* 70:550–555.

63. Creamer, B., and Schlegel, J. (1957): Motor response of esophagus to distension. *J. Appl. Physiol.,* 10:498–504.

64. Crowcroft, P. J., and Szurszewski, J. H. (1971): A study of the inferior mesenteric and pelvic ganglia of guinea-pigs. *J. Physiol. (Lond.),* 219:421–441.

65. Daniel, E. E. (1977): Nerves and motor activity of the gut. In: *Nerves and the Gut,* edited by F. P. Brooks and P. W. Evers, pp. 154–196. C. B. Slack, Inc., Thorofare.

66. Daniel, E. E., and Irwin, J. (1968): Electrical activity of gastric musculature. In: *Handbook of Physiology, Section 6, Alimentary Canal, Vol. 4,* edited by C. F. Code, pp. 1969–1984. American Physiological Society, Washington, D. C.

67. Daniel, E. E., and Irwin, J. (1971): Electrical activity of the stomach and upper intestine. *Am. J. Dig. Dis.,* 16:602–610.

68. Daniel, E. E., and Sarna, S. K. (1976): Distribution of excitatory vagal fibres in canine gastric wall to control motility. *Gastroenterology,* 71:608–613.

69. Daniel, E. E., and Wiebe, G. E. (1966): Transmission of reflexes arising on both sides of the gastroduodenal junction. *Am. J. Physiol.,* 211:634–642.

70. Davison, J. S. (1972): Response to single vagal afferent fibres to mechanical and chemical stimulation of the gastic and duodenal mucosa in cats. *Q. J. Exp. Physiol.,* 57:405–416.

71. Davison, J. S., and Grundy, D. (1978): Modulation of single vagal efferent fibre discharge by gastrointestinal afferents in the rat. *J. Physiol. (Lond.),* 284:69–82.

72. De Groat, W. C., and Krier, J. (1975): Preganglionic C. fibres: A major component of the sacral autonomic outflow to the colon of the cat. *Pfluegers Arch.,* 359:171–176.

73. De Groat, W. C., and Krier, J. (1976): An electrophysiological study of the sacral parasympathetic pathway to the colon of the cat. *J. Physiol. (Lond.),* 260:425–445.

74. De Groat, W. C., and Krier, J. (1978): The sacral parasympathetic reflex pathway regulating colonic motility and defecation in the cat. *J. Physiol. (Lond.),* 76:481–500.

75. De Groat, W. C., and Krier, J. (1979): The central control of the lumbar sympathetic pathway to the large intestine of the cat. *J. Physiol. (Lond.),* 289:449–468.

76. Delbro, D., and Lisander, B. (1977): The interrelations between hypothalamically induced changes in sympathetic discharge to gastrointestinal and cardiovascular systems. *Acta Physiol. Scand.,* 101:165–175.

77. Denny-Brown, D., and Robertson, G. E. (1935): An investigation of the nervous control of defecation. *Brain,* 58:256–310.

78. Devroede, G., and Lamarche, J. (1974): Functional importance of extrinsic parasympathetic innervation to the distal colon and rectum in man. *Gastroenterology,* 78:208–224.

79. Diamant, N. E. (1974): Electrical activity of the cat smooth muscle esophagus: A study of hyperpolarizing responses. In: *Proceedings of the 4th International Symposium on Gastrointestinal Motility,* edited by E. E. Daniel, pp. 593–605. Mitchell Press, Vancouver.

80. Diamant, N., and Akin, A. (1972): Effect of gastric contractions on lower esophageal sphincter. *Gastroenterology,* 63:38–44.

81. Diamant, N. E., and El Sharkawy, T. Y. (1977): Neural control of esophageal peristalis, a conceptual analysis. *Gastroenterology,* 72:546–556.

82. Diamant, N. E., Hall, K., Mui, H., and El Sharkawy, T. Y. (1980): Vagal control of the feeding motor pattern in the lower esophageal sphincter, stomach, and small intestine of dog. In: *Gastrointestinal Motility,* edited by J. Christensen, pp. 365–370. Raven Press, New York.

83. Di Marino, A. J., and Cohen, S. (1974): The adrenergic control of lower esophageal function. In: *Proceedings of the 4th International Symposium on Gastrointestinal Motility,* edited by E. E. Daniel, pp. 623–630. Mitchell Press, Vancouver.

84. Dodds, W. J., Christensen, J., Dent, J., Wood, J. D., and Arndorfer, R. C. (1978): Esophageal contractions induced by vagal stimulation in the opossum. *Am. J. Physiol.,* 235:E392–E401.

85. Dodds, W. J., Christensen, J., Wood, J. D., and Arndorfer, R. C. (1977): Effect of pharmacologic agents on primary esophageal peristalsis in the opossum. *Gastroenterology,* 72:1050 (abst.).

86. Dodds, W. J., Stef, J. J., Stewart, E. T., Hogan, W. J., Arndorfer, R. C., and Cohen, E. B. (1978): Responses of feline esophagus to cervical vagal stimulation. *Am. J. Physiol.,* 235:E63–E73.

87. Doty, R. W. (1968): Neural organization of deglutition. In: *Handbook of Physiology, Section 6, Alimentary Canal, Vol. 4,* edited by C. F. Code, pp. 1861–1902. American Physiological Society, Washington, D. C.

88. Doty, R. W., Richmond, W. H., and Storey, A. T. (1967): Effect of medullary lesions on coordination of deglutition. *Exp. Neurol.,* 17:91–106.

89. Dougherty, R. W., Habel, R. E., and Bond, H. E. (1958): Esophageal innervation and eructation reflex in sheep. *Am. J. Vet. Res.,* 19:115–128.

90. Douglas, D. M., and Mann, F. C. (1940): The gastro-ileal reflex: further experimental observations. *Am. J. Dig. Dis.,* 7:53–57.

91. Dubner, R., Sessle, B. J., and Storey, A. T. (eds.) (1978): *The Neural Basis of Oral and Facial Function.* Plenum Press, New York.

92. Eliasson, S. (1952): Cerebral influences on gastric motility in the cat. *Acta Physiol. Scand. [Suppl. 95],* 26:1–70.

93. Eliasson, S. (1953): Activation of gastric motility from the brain stem of the cat. *Acta Physiol. Scand.,* 30:199–214.

94. El Ouazzani, T., and Mei, N. (1979): Mise en évidence électrophysiologique des thermorécepteurs vagaux dans la région gastro-intestinale. Leur rôle dans la regulation de la motricité digestive. *Exp. Brain Res.,* 34:419–434.

95. El Sharkawy, T. Y., Morgan, K. G., and Szurszewski, J. H. (1978): Intracellular electrical activity of canine and human gastric smooth muscle. *J. Physiol. (Lond.),* 279:291–307.

96. El Sharkawy, T., and Szurszewksi, J. H. (1978): Modulation of canine antral circular smooth muscle by acetylcholine, noradrenaline and pentagastrin. *J. Physiol. (Lond.),* 279:309–320.

97. Euler, C. Von (1959): Autonomic neuroeffector transmission. In: *Handbook of Physiology, Section 1, Neurophysiology, Vol. 1,* edited by H. W. Magoun, pp. 215–237. American Physiological Society, Washington, D. C.

98. Falempin, M., Mei, N., and Rousseau, J. P. (1978): Vagal mechanoreceptors of the inferior thoracic oesophagus, the lower oesophageal sphincter, and the stomach in sheep. *Pfluegers Arch.,* 373:25–30.

99. Farrell, J. I., and Ivy, A. C. (1926): Studies on the motility of the transplanted gastric pouch. *Am. J. Physiol.,* 76:227–228.

100. Finkleman, B. (1930): On the nature of inhibition in the intestine. *J. Physiol. (Lond.),* 70:145–157.

101. Fleshler, B., Hendrix, I. R., Kramer, P., and Ingelfinger, F. J. (1959): The characteristics and similarity of primary and secondary peristalsis in the esophagus. *J. Clin. Invest.,* 38:110–116.

102. Floyd, K. (1973): Cholinesterase activity in sheep oesophageal muscle. *J. Anat. (Lond.),* 116:357–373.

103. Floyd, W. F., and Walls, E. W. (1953): Electromyography of the sphincter ani externus in man. *J. Physiol. (Lond.),* 122:599–609.

104. Folkow, B., and Rubinstein, E. H. (1965): Behavioural and autonomic patterns evoked by stimulation of the lateral hypothalamic area in the cat. *Acta Physiol. Scand.,* 65:292–299.

105. Frenckner, B., and Ihre, T. (1976): Influence of autonomic nerves on the internal anal sphincter in man. *Gut,* 17:306–312.

106. Fukuda, H. (1968): On the relationship of the inhibitory neurone concerned with the intestinal intrinsic reflexes with vagal inhibition. *J. Physiol. Soc. Jpn.,* 30:702–709.

107. Furness, J. B. (1969): An electrophysiological study of the innervaton of the smooth muscle of the colon. *J. Physiol.,* 205:549–562.

108. Furness, J. B., and Costa, M. (1974): The adrenergic innervation of the gastrointestinal tract. *Ergebn. Physiol. Biol. Chem. Exp. Pharmacol.,* 69:1–51.

109. Gabella, J. (ed.) (1976): *Structure of the Autonomic Nervous System.* Chapman and Hall, London.
110. Gabella, J., and Costa, M. (1969): Adrenergic innervation of the intestinal smooth musculature. *Experientia,* 25:395-396.
111. Gardette, B., and Gonella, J. (1974): Etude electromyographique in vivo de la commande nerveuse orthosympathique du colon chez le chat. *J. Physiol. (Paris),* 68:671-692.
112. Garrett, J. R., Howard, E. R., and Jones, W. (1974): The internal anal sphincter in the cat: A study of nervous mechanisms affecting tone and reflex activity. *J. Physiol. (Lond.),* 243:153-166.
113. Garry, R. C. (1933): The responses to stimulation of the caudal end of the large bowel in the cat. *J. Physiol. (Lond.),* 78:208-244.
114. Garry, R. C. (1933): The nervous control of the caudal region of the large bowel in the cat. *J. Physiol. (Lond.),* 77:422-431.
115. Garry, R. C., and Gillespie, J. S. (1955): The responses of the musculature of the colon of the rabbit to stimulation, in vitro, of the parasympathetic and of the sympathetic outflows. *J. Physiol. (Lond.),* 128:557-576.
116. Gastaut, H., Vigouroux, R., Corriol, J., and Badier, M. (1951): Effet de la stimulation électrique (par électrodes à demeure) du complexe amygdalien chez le chat non narcosé. *J. Physiol. (Paris),* 43:740-746.
117. Gerhardt, D. C., Shuck, T. J., Bordeaux, R. A., and Winship. D. H. (1978): Human upper esophageal sphincter. Response to volume, osmotic, and acid stimuli. *Gastroenterology,* 75:268-274.
118. Gershon, M. D. (1967): Inhibition of gastrointestinal movement by sympathetic nerve stimulation: The site of action. *J. Physiol. (Lond.),* 189:317-327.
119. Getz, B., and Sirnes, T. (1949): The localization within the dorsal motor vagal nucleus. *J. Comp. Neurol.,* 90:95-110.
120. Gillespie, J. S. (1962): The electrical and mechanical responses of intestinal smooth muscle cells to stimulation of their parasympathetic nerves. *J. Physiol. (Lond.),* 162:76-92.
121. Gillespie, J. S. (1968): Electrical activity in the colon. In: *Handbook of Physiology, Section 6, Alimentary Canal, Vol. 4.,* edited by C. F. Code, pp. 2093-2120. American Physiological Society, Washington, D. C.
122. Gillespie, J. S., and Khoyi, M. A. (1977): The site and receptors responsible for the inhibition by sympathetic nerves of intestinal smooth muscle and its parasympathetic motor nerve. *J. Physiol. (Lond.),* 267:767-789.
123. Gonella, J. (1964): Etude de l'activité électrique des fibres musculaires longitudinales du duodenum in vivo. Action de la stimulation des nerfs vagues. *C. R. Soc. Biol.,* 158:2409-2413.
124. Gonella, J., and Gardette, B. (1974): Etude électromyographique in vivo de la commande nerveuse extrinsèque parasympathique du colon. *J. Physiol. (Paris),* 68:395-413.
125. Gonella, J., and Lecchini, S. (1971): Inhibition de l'activité électrique de la couche circulaire du duodenum de lapin in vitro par stimulation des fibres sympathiques per-artérielles du mésentère. *C. R. Acad. Sci. [D] (Paris),* 273:214-217.
126. Gonella, J., Niel, J. P., and Roman, C. (1977): Vagal control of lower oesophageal sphincter motility in the cat. *J. Physiol. (Lond.),* 273:647-664.
127. Gonella, J., Niel, J. P., and Roman, C. (1979): Sympathetic control of lower oesophageal sphincter motility in the cat. *J. Physiol. (Lond.),* 287:177-190.
128. Gonella, J., Niel, J. P., and Roman, C. (1980): Mechanism of the noradrenergic motor control on the lower oesophageal sphincter in the cat. *J. Physiol. (Lond.),* 306:251-260.
129. Goyal, R. K., and Rattan, S. (1975): Nature of the vagal inhibitory innervation to the lower esophageal sphincter. *J. Clin. Invest.,* 55:1119-1126.
130. Goyal, R. K., and Rattan, S. (1978): Neurohumoral, hormonal and drug receptors for the lower esophageal sphincter. *Gastroenterology,* 74:598-619.
131. Greenwood, R. K., Schlegel, J. F., Code, C. F., and Ellis, F. H., Jr. (1962): The effect of sympathectomy, vagotomy and esophageal interruption on the canine gastroesophageal sphincter. *Thorax,* 17:310-319.
132. Gruber, H. (1968): Über Struktur und Innervation der quergestreiften Muskulatur des Oesophagus der Ratte. *Z. Zellforsch.,* 91:236-247.
133. Guimaraes, S. (1969): Alpha excitatory, alpha inhibitory and beta inhibitory adrenergic receptors in the guinea-pig stomach. *Arch. Int. Pharmacodyn. Ther.* 179:188-201.
134. Haffner, J. F. W., and Stadaas, J. (1972): Pressure response to cholinergic and adrenergic agents in the fundus, corpus and antrum of the isolated rabbit stomachs. *Acta Chir. Scand.,* 138:713-719.
135. Harding, R., and Titchen, D. A. (1975): Chemosensitive vagal endings in the oesophagus of the cat. *J. Physiol. (Lond.),* 247:52-53P.
136. Heazell, M. A. (1977): A non-adrenergic inhibitory innervation in the rat stomach. *Arch. Int. Pharmacodyn.,* 226:109-117.
137. Hellemans, J., Janssens, J., Vantrappen, G., Pelemans, W., and Valembois, P. (1974): The role of a bolus in the persistaltic contraction of the esophagus. In: *Proc. 4th International Symposium on Gastrointestinal Motility,* edited by E. E. Daniel, pp. 573-584. Mitchell Press, Vancouver.
138. Hellemans, J., and Vantrappen, G. (1974): Physiology. In: *Diseases of the Esophagus, Handbuch der Inneren Medizine,* edited by H. Schwiegk, pp. 40-102. Springer-Verlag, Berlin.
139. Hellemans, J., Vantrappen, G., and Janssens, J. (1974): Electromyography of the esophagus. In: *Diseases of the Esophagus, Handbuch der Inneren Medizine,* edited by H. Schwiegk, pp. 270-285. Springer-Verlag, Berlin.
140. Hermann, H., and Morin, G. (1934): Mise en evidence d'un réflexe inhibiteur intestino-intestinal. *C. R. Soc. Biol.,* 115:529-531.
141. Hesser, F. H., and Perret, G. E. (1960): Studies on gastric motility in the cat. II. Cerebral and infracerebral influence in control, vagectomy and cervical cord preparations. *Gastroenterology,* 38:231-246.
142. Higgs, B., and Ellis, F. H. (1965): The effect of bilateral supranodosal vagotomy on canine esophageal function. *Surgery,* 58:828-834.
143. Higgs, B., Kerr, F. W. L., and Ellis, F. H. (1965): The experimental production of esophageal achalasia by electrolytic lesions in the medulla. *J. Thorac. Cardiovasc. Surg.,* 50:613-625.
144. Hirst, G. D. S., Holman, M. E., and Mc Kirky, H. C. (1975): Two descending nerve pathways activated by distension of guinea-pig small intestine. *J. Physiol. (Lond.),* 244:113-127.
145. Hokfelt, T. (1979): Polypeptides: localization. *Neurosci. Res. Program. Bull.,* 17:424-443.
146. Howard, E. R., and Garrett, J. R. (1973): The intrinsic innervation of the hind gut and accessory muscles of defecation in the cat. *Z. Zellforsch,* 136:31-44.
147. Hulten, L. (1969): Extrinsic nervous control of colonic motility and blood flow. *Acta Physiol. Scand. [Suppl.],* 335:1-166.
148. Hunt, J. N., and Knox, M. T. (1968): Regulation of gastric emptying. In: *Handbook of Physiology, Section 6, Alimentary Canal, Vol. 4,* edited by C. F. Code, pp. 1917-1935. American Physiological Society, Washington, D. C.
149. Hunt, J. N., and Knox, H. T. (1969): The slowing of gastric emptying by nine acids. *J. Physiol. (Lond.),* 201:161-179.
150. Hunt, J. N., and Knox, H. T. (1972): The slowing of gastric emptying by four strong acids and three weak acids. *J. Physiol. (Lond.),* 222:187-208.
151. Hwang, K. (1954): Mechanism of transportation of the content of the esophagus. *J. Appl. Physiol.,* 6:781-796.
152. Hwang, K., and Grossman, M. I. (1953): A note on the innervation of the cervical portion of the human esophagus. *Gastroenterology,* 25:375-377.
153. Hwang, K., Grossman, M. I., and Ivy, A. C. (1948): Nervous control of cervical esophagus. *Am. J. Physiol.,* 154:343-357.
154. Iggo, A. (1955): Tension receptors in the stomach and urinary bladder. *J. Physiol. (Lond.),* 128:593-607.
155. Iggo, A. (1957): Gastrointestinal tension receptors with unmyelinated afferent fibres in the vagus of the cat. *Q. J. Exp. Physiol.,* 42:130-143.
156. Iggo, A. (1957): Gastric mucosal chemoreceptors with vagal afferent fibres in the cat. *Q. J. Exp. Physiol.,* 42:398-409.
157. Ingelfinger, F. J. (1958): Esophageal motility. *Physiol. Rev.,* 38:533-584.
158. Interone, C. V., Del Finado, J. E., Miller, B., Bombeck, C. T., and Nyhus, L. M. (1971): Parietal cell vagotomy: studies of gastric emptying and observations of protection from histamine induced ulcer. *Arch. Surg.,* 102:43-44.

159. Itoh, Z., Honda, R., Hiwatashi, K., Takeuchi, S., Aizawa, R., Takayanagi, R., and Couch, E. F. (1976): Motilin induced mechanical activity in the canine alimentary tract. *Scand. J. Gastroenterol. [Suppl. 39]*, 11:93–110.

160. Itoh, Z., Takayanagi, R., Takeuchi, S., and Isshiki, S. (1978): Interdigestive motor activity of Heindenhain pouches in relation to main stomach in conscious dog. *Am. J. Physiol.*, 234:E333–E338.

161. Jabonero, V. (1958): Mikroskopische Studien über die Innervation des Verdauungstraktes. Teil 1 (oesophagus). *Acta Neuroveget.*, 17:308–353.

162. Jabonero, V. (1962): Nuevas observaciones sobre la fina inervacion del esofago. *Trab. Inst. Cajal Invest. Biol.*, 54:37–92.

163. Jacobowitz, D. (1965): Histochemical studies of the autonomic innervation of the gut. *J. Pharmacol. Exp. Ther.*, 149:358–364.

164. Jacobowitz, D., and Nemir, P. (1969): The autonomic innervation of the oesophagus of the dog. *J. Thorac. Cardiovasc. Surg.*, 58:678–684.

165. Jahnberg, T. (1977): Gastric adaptative relaxation. Effects of vagal activation and vagotomy. An experimental study in dogs and in man. *Scand. J. Gastroenterol. [Suppl. 46]*, 12:5–32.

166. Janssens, J. (ed.) (1978): *The Peristaltic Mechanism of the Esophagus.* Acco, Lewen.

167. Janssens, J., De Wever, I., Vantrappen, G., and Hellemans, J. (1976): Peristalsis in smooth muscle esophagus after transection and bolus deviation. *Gastroenterolgy,* 71:1004–1009.

168. Janssens, J., Valembois, P., Hellemans, J., Pelemans, W., and Vantrappen, G. (1974): Studies on the necessity of a bolus for the progression of secondary peristalsis in the canine esophagus. *Gastroenterology,* 67:245–251.

169. Janssens, J., Valembois, P., Vantrappen, G., Hellemans, J., and Pelemans, W. (1973): Is the primary peristaltic contraction of the canine esophagus bolus dependent? *Gastroenterology,* 65:750–756.

170. Jansson, G. (1969): Extrinsic nervous control of gastric motility. An experimental study in the cat. *Acta Physiol. Scand. [Suppl.],* 326:5–42.

171. Jansson, G. (1969): Effect of reflexes of somatic afferents on the adrenergic outflow to the stomach in the cat. *Acta Physiol. Scand.,* 77:17–22.

172. Jansson, G., and Lisander, B. (1969): On adrenergic influence on gastric motility in chronically vagotomized cats. *Acta Physiol. Scand.,* 76:463–471.

173. Jansson, G., Lisander, B., and Martinson, J. (1969): Hypothalamic control of adrenergic outflow to the stomach in the cat. *Acta Physiol. Scand.,* 75:176–186.

174. Jansson, G., and Martinson, J. (1966): Studies on the ganglionic site of action of sympathetic outflow to the stomach. *Acta Physiol. Scand.,* 68:184–192.

175. Jean, A. (1972): Localisation et activité des neurones déglutiteurs bulbaires. *J. Physiol. (Paris),* 64:227–268.

176. Jean, A. (1972): Effet de lésions localisées du bulbe rachidien sur le stade oesophagien de la déglutition. *J. Physiol. (Paris),* 64:507–516.

177. Jean, A. (1978): *Contrôle bulbaire de la déglutition et de la motricité oesophagienne.* Thèse de Doctorat ès-Sciences, Faculty of Sciences, Marseille.

178. Jean, A. (1978): Localisation et activité des motoneurones oesophagiens chez le mouton. *J. Physiol. (Paris),* 74:737–742.

179. Jean, A., and Car, A. (1979): Inputs to the swallowing medullary neurons from the peripheral afferent fibers and the swallowing cortical area. *Brain Res.,* 178:567–572.

180. Jefferson, N. C., Kuroyanagi, Y., Arai, T., Geisel, A., and Necheles, H. (1965): Extravagal gastric motor innervation. *Surgery,* 58:420.

181. Jennewein, H. M., Hummelt, H., Meyer, U., Siewert, R., Koch, A., and Waldeck, F. (1976): The effect of vagotomy on the resting pressure and reactivity of the LES in man and dog. In: *Proceedings of the 5th International Symposium on Gastrointestinal Motility,* edited by G. Vantrappen, pp. 186–189. Typoff Press, Herentals.

182. Johansson, B., Jonsson, O., and Ljung, B. (1965): Supraspinal control of the intestino-intestinal inhibitory reflex. *Acta Physiol. Scand.,* 63:442–449.

183. Johansson, B., Jonsson, O., and Ljung, B. (1968): Tonic supraspinal mechanisms influencing the intestino-intestinal inhibitory reflex. *Acta Physiol. Scand.,* 72:200–204.

184. Jule, Y. (1975): Modification de l'activité électrique du colon proximal du lapin in vivo par stimulation des nerfs vagues et splanchniques. *J. Physiol. (Paris),* 70:5–26.

185. Jule, Y., and Gonella, J. (1972): Modifications de l'activité électrique du colon terminal de lapin par stimulation des fibres nerveuses pelviennes et sympathiques. *J. Physiol. (Paris),* 64:599–621.

186. Jule, Y, and Szurszewski, J. H. (1979): Occurrence of spontaneous oscillatory neurons in the cat inferior mesenteric ganglia: relationship to ileus? *Gastroenterology,* 76:1163.

187. Jurica, E. J. (1926): Motility of denervated mammalian esophagus. *Am. J. Physiol.,* 77:371–384.

188. Kaada, B. R. (1951): Somato-motor, autonomic and electrocorticographic responses to electrical stimulation of rhinencephalic and other structures in primates, cat and dog. *Acta Physiol. Scand. [Suppl. 83],* 24:1–285.

189. Kametani, H., Sato, A., Sato, Y., and Simpson, A. (1979): Neural mechanisms of reflex facilitation and inhibition of gastric motility to stimulation of various skin areas in the rat. *J. Physiol. (Lond.),* 294:407–418.

190. Kantrowitz, P. A., Siegel, C. I., and Hendrix, T. R. (1966): Differences in motility of the upper and lower esophagus in man and its alteration by atropine. *Johns Hopkins Med. J.,* 118:476–491.

191. Kelly, K. A., and Code, C. F. (1969): Effect of transthoracic vagotomy on canine gastric electrical activity. *Gastroenterology,* 57:51–58.

192. Kewenter, J. (1965): The vagal control of the duodenal and ileal motility and blood flow. *Acta Physiol. Scand.,* 65 [Suppl.], 251:1–68.

193. Knight, G. C. (1934): Relation of the extrinsic nerves to the functional activity of the esophagus. *Br. J. Surg.,* 22:155–168.

194. Kosterlitz, H. W. (1968): Intrinsic and extrinsic nervous control of motility of the stomach and the intestines. In: *Handbook of Physiology, Section 6, Alimentary Canal, Vol. 4,* edited by C. F. Code, pp. 2147–2171. American Physiological Society, Washington, D. C.

195. Kowalewski, K., and Zajac, S. (1975): Electrical and mechanical activity of the isolated canine stomach perfused with homologous in vitro oxygenated blood. *Pharmacology,* 13:448–457.

196. Kowalewski, K., Zajac, S., and Kolodof, A. (1975): The effect of drugs on the electrical and mechanical activity of the isolated porcine stomach. *Pharmacology,* 13:86–95.

197. Kreulen, D. L., and Szurszewski, J. H. (1979): Reflex pathways in the abdominal prevertebral ganglia: evidence for the colo-colonic inhibitory reflex. *J. Physiol. (Lond.),* 295:21–32.

198. Kreulen, D. L., and Szurszewski, J. H. (1979): Nerve pathways in celiac plexus of the guinea-pig. *Am. J. Physiol.,* 237:E90–E97.

199. Kronecker, H., and Meltzer, S. (1881): On the propagation of inhibitory excitation in the medulla oblongata. *Proc. R. Soc. Lond. [Biol.],* 33:27–29.

200. Kukorelli, T., and Juhasz, G. (1976): Electroencephalic synchronization induced by stimulation of small intestine and splanchnic nerves in cats. *Electroencephalogr. Clin. Neurophysiol.,* 41:491–500.

201. Kuntz, A. (ed.) (1947): *The Autonomic Nervous System.* Lea & Febiger, Philadelphia.

202. Kuntz, A., and Saccomano, J. (1944): Reflex inhibition of intestinal motility mediated through decentralized prevertebral ganglia. *J. Neurophysiol.,* 7:163–170.

203. Langley, J. N., and Anderson, H. K. (1895): The innervation of the pelvic and adjoining viscera. *J. Physiol. (Lond.),* 18:67–105.

204. Langley, J. N., and Anderson, H. K. (1896): The innervation of the pelvic and adjoining viscera. *J. Physiol. (Lond.),* 20:372–406.

205. Lawn, A. M. (1964): The localization, by means of electrical stimulation, of the origin and path in the medulla oblongata of the motor nerve fibres of the rabbit oesophagus. *J. Physiol.,* 174:232–244.

206. Learmonth, J. R., and Markowitz, J. (1930): Studies on the innervation of the large bowel. *Am. J. Physiol.,* 94:501–504.

207. Liedberg, G., Nielsen, K. G., Owman, C. H., and Sjoberg, N. O. (1973): Adrenergic contribution to the abdominal vagus nerves in the cat. *Scand. J. Gastroenterol.*, 8:177-180.

208. Lind, J. F., Crispin, J. S., and Mc Iver, D. K. (1968): The effect of atropine on the gastroesophageal sphincter. *Can. J. Physiol.*, 46:233-238.

209. Lind, J. F., Duthie, H. C., Schlegel, J. F., and Code, C. F. (1961): Motility of gastric fundus. *Am. J. Physiol.*, 201:197-202.

210. Lisander, B. (1975): The hypothalamus and vagally mediated gastric relaxation. *Acta Physiol. Scand.*, 93:1-9.

211. Lisander, B., and Martner, J. (1974): Influences on gastrointestinal and bladder motility by the fastigial nucleus. *Acta Physiol. Scand.*, 90:792-794.

212. Longhi, E. H., and Jordan, P. H., Jr. (1971): Necessity of the bolus for propagation of primary peristalsis in the canine esophagus. *Am. J. Physiol.*, 220:609-612.

213. Lundberg, J., Ahlman, H., Dahlstrom, A., and Kewenter, J. (1976): Catecholamine-containing nerve fibres in the human abdominal vagus. *Gastroenterology*, 70:472-474.

214. Mackel, R. (1979): Segmental and descending control of the external urethral and anal sphincters in the cat. *J. Physiol. (Lond.)*, 294:105-122.

215. McSwiney, B. A. (1931): Innervation of the stomach. *Physiol. Rev.*, 11:478-514.

216. Mann, C. V., Code, C. F., Schlegel, J. F., and Ellis, F. H., Jr. (1968): Intrinsic mechanisms controlling the mammalian gastro-oesophageal sphincter deprived of extrinsic nerve supply. *Thorax*, 23:634-639.

217. Mann, C. V., and Shorter, R. G. (1964): Structure of the canine esophagus and its sphincters. *J. Surg. Res.*, 4:160-164.

218. Mannard, A., and Polosa, C. (1973): Analysis of background firing of single sympathetic preganglionic neurons of cat cervical nerve. *J. Neurophysiol.*, 36:398-408.

219. Marik, F., and Code, C. F. (1975): Control of the interdigestive myoelectrical activity in dogs by the vagus nerves and pentagastrin. *Gastroenterology*, 69:387-395.

220. Marinesco, G., and Parhon, C. (1907): Recherches sur les noyaux d'origine du nerf pneumogastrique et sur les localisations dans les noyaux. *J. Neurol.*, 13:61-77.

221. Martinson, J. (1964): The effect of graded stimulation of efferent vagal nerve fibres on gastric motility. *Acta Physiol. Scand.*, 62:256-262.

222. Martinson, J. (1965): Studies on the efferent vagal control of the stomach. *Acta Physiol. Scand. [Suppl. 255]*, 65:1-23.

223. Martinson, J., and Muren, A. (1963): Excitatory and inhibitory effects of vagus stimulation on gastric motility in the cat. *Acta Physiol. Scand.*, 57:309-316.

224. Meek, W. J., and Herrin, R. C. (1934): The effect of vagotomy on gastric emptying time. *Am. J. Physiol.*, 109:221-231.

225. Meeroff, J. C., Go, V. L. W., and Phillips, S. F. (1975): Control of gastric emptying by osmolality of duodenal contents in man. *Gastroenterology*, 68:1144-1151.

226. Mei, N. (1970): Mécanorecepteurs digestifs chez le chat. *Exp. Brain Res.*, 11:502-514.

227. Mei, N. (1978): Vagal glucoreceptors in the small intestine of the cat. *J. Physiol. (Lond.)*, 282:485-506.

228. Mei, N., Aubert, M., Crousillat, J., and Ranieri, F. (1974): Sensory innervation of the lower oesophagus of the cat. Comparison with the other parts of the digestive system. In: *Proceedings of the 4th International Symposium of Gastrointestinal Motility*, edited by E. E. Daniel, pp. 585-591. Mitchell Press, Vancouver.

229. Meltzer, S. J. (1899): On the causes of the orderly progress of the peristaltic movements in the oesophagus. *Am. J. Physiol.*, 2:266-272.

230. Meltzer, S. J. (1907): secondary peristalsis of the oesophagus. A demonstration on a dog with a permanent fistula. *Proc. Soc. Exp. Biol. Med.*, 4:35-37.

231. Meltzer, S. J., and Auer, J. (1906): Vagus reflexes upon oesophagus and cardia. *Br. Med. J.*, 2:1806-1807.

232. Meunier, P., and Mollard, P. (1977): Control of the internal sphincter (manometric study with human subjects). *Pfluegers Arch.*, 370:233-239.

233. Miller, F. R., and Sherrington, C. S. (1916): Some observations on the buccopharyngeal stage of reflex deglutition in the cat. *Q. J. Exp. Physiol.*, 9:147-186.

234. Miolan, J. P. (1974): *La motricité de l'estomac et du sphincter oesophagien inférieur: Etude electromyographique; rôle de l'innervation extrinsèque*. Theses Doctorat IIIe Cycle, Faculty of Sciences, Marseille.

235. Miolan, J. P., and Roman, C. (1971): Modification de l'électromyogramme gastrique du chien par stimulation des nerfs extrinsèques. *J. Physiol. (Paris)*, 63:561-576.

236. Miolan, J. P., and Roman, C. (1973): Décharge des fibres vagales efférentes destinées au cardia du chien. *J. Physiol. (Paris)*, 66:171-198.

237. Miolan, J. P., and Roman, C. (1974): Décharge unitaire des fibres vagales efférentes lors de la relaxation receptive de l'estomac du chien. *J. Physiol., (Paris)*, 68:693-704.

238. Miolan, J. P., and Roman, C. (1978): Activité des fibres vagales efférentes destinées à la musculature lisse du cardia du chien. *J. Physiol. (Paris)*, 74:709-723.

239. Miolan, J. P., and Roman, C. (1978): Discharge of efferent vagal fibers supplying gastric antrum: indirect study by nerve suture technique. *Am. J. Physiol.*, 235:E366-E373.

240. Mitchell, G. A. G., and Warwick, R. (1955): The dorsal vagal nucleus. *Acta Anat. (Basel)*, 25:371-395.

241. Mohiuddin, A. (1953): Vagal preganglionic fibres to the alimentary canal. *J. Comp. Neurol.*, 99:289-318.

242. Monges, H., Salducci, J., Naudi, B., Ranieri, F., Gonella, J., and Bouvier, M. (1980): Electrical activity of internal anal sphincter. A comparative study in man and cat. In: *Gastrointestinal Motility*, edited by J. Christensen, pp. 495-502. Raven Press, New York.

243. Monges, H., Salducci, J., and Roman, C. (1968): Etude EMG de la contraction oesophagienne chez l'homme normal. *Arc. Fr. Mal. App. Dig.*, 57:545-560.

244. Morin, G. (1935): L'Automatisme intestinal des vértebres et sa régulation. Thèse Doctorat ès-Sciences, Faculty of Sciences, Lyon.

245. Morin, G., and Vial, J. (1934): Sur les voies et les centres du réflexe inhibiteur intestino-intestinal. *C. R. Soc. Biol.*, 116:536-538.

246. Mosso, A. (1876): Ueber die Bewegungen der speiseröhre. *Untersuch. Z. Natur.*, 11:327-349.

247. Mukhopadhyay, A., and Weisbrodt, N. W. (1975): Neural organization of esophageal peristalsis: Role of vagus nerve. *Gastroenterology*, 68:444-447.

248. Muren, A. (1957): Influence of the vagal innervation on gastric motor responses to adrenaline and noradrenaline. *Acta Physiol. Scand.*, 39:195-202.

249. Muryobayashi, T., Mori, J., Fujiwara, M., and Shimamoto, K. (1968): Fluorescence histochemical demonstration of adrenergic nerve fibres in the vagus nerve of cats and dogs. *Jpn. J. Pharmacol.*, 18:285-293.

250. Nakayama, S. (1965): Effects of stimulation of the vagus on the movements of the small intestine. *Jpn. J. Physiol.*, 15:243-252.

251. Nakazato, Y., Saito, K., and Ohga, A. (1970): Gastric motor and inhibitor response to stimulation of the sympathetic nerve in the dog. *Jpn. J. Pharmacol.*, 20:131-141.

252. Neya, T., Watanabe, K., and Yamasoto, T. (1974): Localization of potentials in medullary reticular formation relevant to swallowing. *Rendic. R. Gastroenterol.*, 6:107-110.

253. Niel, J. P., Gonella, J., and Roman, C. (1980): Localisation par la technique de marquage à la péroxydase des corps cellulaires des neurones ortho et parasympathiques innervant le sphincter oesophagien inférieur du chat. *J. Physiol. (Paris)*, 76:591-599.

254. Norberg, K. A. (1964): Adrenergic innervation of the intestinal wall studied by fluorescence microscopy. *Int. J. Neuropharmacol.*, 3:379-382.

255. Ohga, A., Nakazato, Y., and Saito, K. (1970): Considerations of the efferent nervous mechanism of the vago-vagal reflex relaxation of the stomach in the dog. *Jpn. J. Pharmacol.*, 20:116-130.

256. Ohkawa, H. (1976): Evidence for alpha excitatory action of catecholamines on the electrical activity of the guinea-pig stomach. *Jpn. J. Physiol.*, 26:41-52.

257. Pahlin, P., and Kewenter, J. (1976): The vagal control of the ileocecal sphincter in the cat. *Acta Physiol. Scand.*, 96:433-442.

258. Pahlin, P., and Kewenter, J. (1976): Sympathetic control of the cat ileocecal sphincter. *Am. J. Physiol.,* 231:296–305.

259. Paintal, A. S. (1954): A study of gastric stretch receptors, their role in the peripheral mechanism of satiation of hunger and thirst. *J. Physiol. (Lond.),* 126:255–270.

260. Paintal, A. S. (1957): Responses from mucosal mechanoreceptors in the small intestine of the cat. *J. Physiol. (Lond.),* 139:353–368.

261. Paintal, A. S. (1973): Vagal sensory receptors and their reflex effects. *Physiol. Rev.,* 53:159–227.

262. Papazova, M., and Atanassova, E. (1972): Changes in the bioelectric activity of the stomach after bilateral transthoracal vagotomy. *Bull. Inst. Physiol.,* 14:121–133.

263. Paton, W. D. M., and Vane, J. R. (1963): An analysis of the responses of the isolated stomach to electrical stimulation and to drugs. *J. Physiol. (Lond.),* 165:10–46.

264. Pedersen, S. A., Nielsen, P. A., and Sörensen, H. R. (1971): The effect of atropine and hexamethonium in combination on the lower espohageal sphincter. *Scand. J. Gastroenterol. [Suppl.],* 9:43–47.

265. Peeters, T. L., Vantrappen, G., and Janssens, J. (1980): Fluctuations of motilin and gastrin levels in relation to the interdigestive motility complex in man. In: *Gastrointestinal Motility,* edited by J. Christensen, pp. 287–288. Raven Press, New York.

266. Preisich, P., and Adam, G. (1964): La discrimination non consciente des stimuli duodenaux: le test de différenciation d'habituation électroencéphalographique. *Acta Gastroenterol. Belg.,* 27:625–629.

267. Quigley, J. P. (1943): A modern explanation of the gastric emptying mechanism. *Am. J. Dig. Dis.,* 10:418–421.

268. Quigley, J. P., and Louckes, H. S. (1951): The effects of complete vagotomy on the pyloric sphincter and the gastric evacuation mechanism. *Gastroenterology,* 19:533–537.

269. Quigley, J. P., and Louckes, H. S. (1962): Gastric emptying. *Am. J. Dig. Dis.,* 7:672–676.

270. Quigley, J. P. and Meschan, I. (1938): The role of vagus in the regulation of the pyloric sphincter and adjacent portion of the gut with special reference to the process of gastric evacuation. *Am. J. Physiol.,* 123:166.

271. Ranieri, F., Mei, N., and Crousillat, J. (1973): Les afférences splanchinques provenant des mécanorécepteurs gastrointestinaux et péritonéaux. *Exp. Brain Res.,* 16:276–290.

272. Rattan, S., and Goyal, R. K. (1974): Neural control of the lower esophageal sphincter. *J. Clin. Invest.,* 54:899–906.

273. Read, J. B., and Burnstock, J. (1969): Adrenergic innervation of the gut musculature in vertebrates. *Histochemie,* 17:263–272.

274. Roman, C. (1966): Côntrole nerveux du péristaltisme oesophgien. *J. Physiol. (Paris),* 58:79–108.

275. Roman, C. (1967): La commande de la motricité oesophagienne et sa régulation. These Doctorat ès Sciences, Faculty of Sciences, Marseille.

276. Roman, C., and Car, A. (1967): Contractions oesophagiennes produites par la stimulation du vague on du bulbe rachidien. *J. Physiol. (Paris),* 59:377–398.

277. Roman, C., and Car, A. (1970): Déglutitions et contractions oesophagiennes réflexes obtenues par la stimulation des nerfs vague et laryngé supérieur. *Exp. Brain Res.,* 11:48–74.

278. Roman, C., Gonella, J., Niel, J. P., Condamin, M., and Miolan, J. P. (1975): Effets de la stimulation vagale et de l'adrénaline sur la musculeuse liss du bas oesophage du chat. In: *Smooth Muscle Pharmacology and Physiology,* edited by M. Worcel and G. Vassort, pp. 415–422. Coll. INSERM, Paris.

279. Roman, C. and Tieffenbach, L. (1971): Motricité de l'oesophage à musculature lisse après bivagotomie: étude electromyographique (EMG). *J. Physiol. (Paris),* 63:733–762.

280. Roman, C., and Tieffenbach, L. (1972): Enregistrement de l'activité unitaire des fibres motrices vagales destinées à l'oesophage du Babouin. *J. Physiol. (Paris),* 64:479–506.

281. Rostad, H. (1973): Colonic motility in the cat. IV. Peripheral pathways mediating the effect induced by hypothalamic and mesencephalic stimulation. *Acta Physiol. Scand.,* 89:154–168.

282. Rostad, H. (1973): Colonic motility in the cat. V. Influence of telencephalic stimulation and the peripheral pathways mediating the effects. *Acta Physiol. Scand.,* 89:169–181.

283. Roze, C., Couturier, D., Chariot, J., and Debray, C. (1977): Inhibition of gastric electrical and mechanical activity by in-

284. Ruckebusch, Y., and Bueno, L. (1975): Electrical activity of the ovine jejunum and changes due to disturbances. *Am. J. Dig. Dis.,* 20:1027–1035.

285. Ruckebusch, Y., and Bueno, L. (1977): Migrating myoelectric complex of the small intestine. An intrinsic activity mediated by the vagus. *Gastroenterology,* 73:1309–1314.

286. Ryan, J. P., Snape, W. J., and Cohen, S. (1977): Influence of vagal cooling on esophageal function. *Am. J. Physiol.,* 232:E159–E164.

287. Samarasinghe, D. D. (1972): Some observations on the innervation of the striated muscle in the mouse oesphagus. An electron microscope study. *J. Anat. (Lond.),* 112:173–184.

288. Sarna, S. K., and Daniel, E. E. (1975): Vagal control of gastric electrical activity and motility. *Gastroenterology,* 68:301–308.

289. Sato, A., Sato, Y., Shimada, F., and Torigata, J. (1975): Changes in gastric motility produced by nociceptive stimulation of the skin in rats. *Brain Res.,* 87:151–159.

290. Sato, A., and Schmidt, R. F. (1973): Somatosympathetic reflexes: Afferent fibres central pathways discharge characteristics. *Physiol. Rev.,* 53:916–947.

291. Sato, Y., and Terui, N. (1976): Changes in duodenal motility produced by nervous mechanical stimulation of the skin in rat. *Neurosci. Lett.,* 2:189–193.

292. Satomi, H., Yamamoto, T., Ise, H., and Takatama, H. (1978): Origins of parasympathetic preganglionic fibers to the cat intestine as demonstrated by the HRP method. *Brain Res.,* 151:571–578.

293. Schapiro, H., and Woodward, E. R. (1959): Pathway of enterogastric reflex. *Proc. Soc. Exp. Biol. Med.,* 101:407–409.

294. Schuster, M. M. (1968): Motor action of rectum and anal sphincters in continence and defecation. In: *Handbook of Physiology, Section 6, Alimentary Canal, Vol. 4,* edited by C. F. Code, pp. 2121–2146. American Physiological Society, Washington, D. C.

295. Shepherd, J. J., and Wright, P. G. (1968): The response of the internal anal sphincter in man to stimulation of the presacral nerves. *Am. J. Dig. Dis.,* 13:421–427.

296. Selverston, A. I. (1976): Neuronal mechanisms for rhythmic motor pattern generation in a simple system. In: *Neural Control of Locomotion,* edited by R. M. Herman, S. Grillner, P. S. G. Stein, and D. G. Stuart, pp. 377–399. Plenum Press, New York.

297. Semba, T., Fujii, K., and Fujii, Y. (1970): The response of gastric motility and their location by stimulating the thoracic cord of the dog. *Hiroshima J. Med. Sci.,* 19:73–85.

298. Semba, T., and Hiraoka, T. (1957): Motor response of the stomach and small intestine caused by stimulation of the peripheral end of the splanchnic nerve, thoracic sympathetic trunk and spinal roots. *Jpn. J. Physiol.,* 7:64–71.

299. Semba, T., Kimura, N., and Fujii, K. (1969): Bulbar influence on gastric motility. *Jpn. J. Physiol.,* 19:521–533.

300. Semba, T., and Mizonishi, T. (1978): Atropine-resistant excitation of motility of the dog stomach and colon induced by stimulation of the extrinsic nerves and their centers. *Jpn. J. Physiol.,* 28:239–248.

301. Semba, T., Noda, H., and Fujii, K. (1963): On splanchnic motor responses of stomach movements produced by stimulation of the medulla oblongata and spinal cord. *Jpn. J. Physiol.,* 13:466–478.

302. Siegel, C. I., and Hendrix, T. R. (1961): Evidence for the central mediation of secondary peristalsis in the esophagus. *Johns Hopkins Med. J.,* 108:297–307.

303. Silva, D. G., Ross, G., and Osborne, L. W. (1971): Adrenergic innervation of the ileum of the cat. *Am. J. Physiol.,* 220:347–352.

304. Sinclair, W. J. (1971): Role of the pharyngeal plexus in the initiation of swallowing. *Am. J. Physiol.,* 221:1260–1263.

305. Skinner, D. B., and Camp, T. F. (1968): Relation of esophageal reflux to lower esophageal pressures decreased by atropine. *Gastroenterology,* 54:543–551.

306. Smets, W. (1936): L'activité réflexe de la valvule iléo-caecale. *C. R. Soc. Biol. (Paris),* 123:106–107.

307. Smets, W. (1936): La contraction de la valvule iléo-caecale. *C. R. Soc. Biol. (Paris),* 122:739–795.

traduodenal agents in pigs and effects of vagotomy. *Digestion,,* 15:526–539.

308. Spassova, J. (1959): Uber die afferent Innervation an speiseröhre des Menschen. *S. Mier.-Anat. Forsch Dtsch.,* 65:327.

309. Strom, G., and Uvnäs, B. (1950): Motor responses of gastrointestinal tract and bladder to topical stimulation of the frontal lobe, basal ganglia and hypothalamus in the cat. *Acta Physiol. Scand.,* 21:90–104.

310. Sumi, T. (1964): Neuronal mechanisms in swallowing. *Arch. Ges. Physiol.,* 278:467–477.

311. Sumi, T. (1969): Some properties of cortically evoked swallowing and chewing in rabbits. *Brain Res.,* 15:107–120.

312. Szurszewski, J. H. (1969): A migrating electric complex of the canine small intestine. *Am. J. Physiol.,* 217:1757–1763.

313. Szurszewski, J. H. (1977): Toward a new view of prevertebral ganglion. In: *Nerves and Gut,* edited by F. P. Brooks and P. W. Evers, pp. 244–260. C. B. Slack, Inc., Thorofare.

314. Szurszewski, J. H. (1979): Transmission in ganglia. *Neurosci. Res. Program Bull.,* 17:447–449.

315. Szurszewski, J. H., and Weems, W. A. (1976): Control of gastrointestinal motility by prevertebral ganglia. In: *Physiology of Smooth Muscle,* edited by E. Bülbring and M. F. Shuba, pp. 313–319. Raven Press, New York.

316. Takeshima, T. (1971): Functional classification of the vagal afferent discharges in the dog's stomach. *Jpn. J. Smooth Muscle Res.,* 7:19–27.

317. Thomas, J. E. (1957): Mechanics and regulation of gastric emptying. *Physiol. Rev.,* 37:453–474.

318. Thomas, J. E., and Baldwin, M. V. (1968): Pathways and mechanisms of regulation of gastric motility. In: *Handbook of Physiology, Section 6, Alimentary Canal, Vol. 4,* edited by C. F. Code, pp. 1937–1968. American Physiological Society, Washington, D. C.

319. Thomas, J. E., and Crider, J. O. (1935): Rhythmic changes in duodenal motility associated with gastric peristalsis. *Am. J. Physiol.,* 111:124–129.

320. Thomas, J. E., Crider, J. O., and Morgan, C. J. (1934): A study of reflexes involving the pyloric sphincter and antrum and their role in gastric evacuation. *Am. J. Physiol.,* 108:683–700.

321. Thomas, P. A., and Earlam, R. J. (1974): The effect of the gastrointestinal polypeptide hormones on the electrical activity and pressure of the isolated perfused canine gastro-oesophageal sphincter. In: *Proceedings of the 4th International Symposium on Gastrointestinal Motility,* edited by E. E. Daniel, pp. 243–250. Mitchell Press, Vancouver.

322. Thomas, P. A., Kelly, K. A., and Go, V. L. W. (1980): Hormonal regulation of gastrointestinal interdigestive motor cycles. In: *Gastrointestinal Motility,* edited by J. Christensen, pp. 267–268. Raven Press, New York.

323. Tieffenbach, L., and Roman, C. (1972): Role de l'innervation extrinsèque vagale dans la motricité de l'oesphage à musculeuse lisse: étude électromyographique chez le chat et le Babouin. *J. Physiol. (Paris),* 64:193–226.

324. Toyama, T., Yokoyama, I., and Nishi, K. (1975): Effects of hexamethonium and other ganglionic blocking agents on electrical activity of the esophagus induced by vagal stimulation in the dog. *Eur. J. Pharmacol.,* 31:63–71.

325. Truelove, S. C. (1966): Movements of the large intestine. *Physiol. Rev.,* 46:457–512.

326. Ueda, M., Schlegel, J. F., and Code, C. F. (1972): Electric and motor activity of innervated and vagally denervated feline esophagus. *Am. J. Dig. Dis.,* 17:1075–1088.

327. Vizi, E. S. (1976): The role of α-adrenoceptors situated in Auerbach's plexus in the inhibition of gastrointestinal motility. In: *Physiology of Smooth Muscle,* edited by E. Bülbring and M. F. Shuba, pp. 357–367. Raven Press, New York.

328. Waddel, W. R., and Wang, C. C. (1953): Effect of vagotomy on gastric evacuation of high fat meals. *J. Appl. Physiol.,* 5:705–711.

329. Weems, W. A., and Szurszewski, J. H. (1977): Modulation of colonic motility by peripheral neural imputs to neurons of the inferior mesenteric ganglion. *Gastroenterology,* 39:417–448.

330. Weisbrodt, N. W., and Christensen, J. (1972): Gradients of contractions in the opossum esophagus. *Gastroenterology,* 62:1159–1166.

331. Weisbrodt, N. W., Copeland, E. M., Moore, E. P., Kearly, R. W., and Johnson, L. R. (1975): Effect of vagotomy on electrical activity of the small intestine of the dog. *Am. J. Physiol.,* 228:650–654.

332. Wilbur, B. G., and Kelly, K. A. (1973): Effects of proximal gastric, complete gastric and truncal vagotomy on canine gastric electric activity, motility and emptying. *Ann. Surg.,* 178:295–303.

333. Wingate, D. L., Ruppin, H., Green, W. E. R., Thompson, H. H., Domschke, W., Wunsch, E., Demling, L., and Ritchie, M. D. (1976): Motilin-induced electrical activity in the canine gastrointestinal tract. *Scand. J. Gastroenterol. [Suppl. 39],* 11:111–118.

334. Yamamoto, T. (1960): Histological studies on the innervation of the esophagus in formosan Macaque. *Arch. Histol. Jpn.,* 18:545–564.

335. Yamamoto, T., Satomi, H., Hiromi, I., and Takahashi, K. (1977): Evidence of the dual innervation of the cat stomach by the vagal dorsal motor and medial solitary nuclei as demonstrated by the horseradish peroxidase method. *Brain Res.,* 122:125–131.

336. Yamamoto, T., Satomi, H., Ise, H., Takatama, H., and Takahasi, K. (1978): Sacral spinal innervations of the rectal and vesical smooth muscle and the sphincteric striated muscles as demonstrated by the horseradish peroxidase method. *Neurosci. Lett.,* 7:41–47.

337. Youmans, W. B. (1968): Innervation of the gastrointestinal tract. In: *Handbook of Physiology, Section 6, Alimentary Canal, Vol. 4,* edited by C. F. Code, pp. 1655–1663. American Physiological Society, Washington, D. C.

338. Zeller, W., and Burget, G. E. (1937): A study of the cardia. *Am. J. Dig. Dis.,* 4:113–120.

339. Zfass, A. M., Prince, M., Allen, F. N., and Farrar, J. T. (1970): Inhibitory beta adrenergic receptors in the human distal esophagus. *Am. J. Dig. Dis.,* 15:303–310.

Physiology of the Gastrointestinal Tract, edited by
Leonard R. Johnson. Raven Press, New York © 1981.

Chapter 10

Fluid Mechanics of Gastrointestinal Flow

*Enzo O. Macagno and **James Christensen

Fluid flow in the cardiovascular system is a well-studied process; fluid flow in the gut has been neglected. The system involved in cardiovascular flow resembles familiar physical arrangements of pumps and conduits; that of the gut has no everyday analogue.

Flow in the gut seems to be complex. Components of retrograde flow are contained within a net antegrade flow. In the intestine there is the requirement for both a complete internal circulation of the luminal contents and a mucosal access to all parts of the fluid. These flows arise from wall motions, and they are modified by resistances both at the mucosal surface and within the fluid itself. An analysis of gastrointestinal flow thus requires a detailed description of both the wall movements and the character of the fluid. Even a superficial look indicates that both the wall and the rheology of the fluid differ greatly from one region of the gut to another.

This chapter constitutes a review of the analysis that has been made of the fluid mechanics of flow in the gut. This has been done mainly for the small intestine. Since some of the basic principles of fluid mechanics may be unfamiliar to those who are trained mainly in physiology, a nontechnical exposition of some fundamentals of fluid flow is first presented.

KINEMATICS OF FLUIDS

Geometry is usually considered to be a part of mathematics because of the high degree of abstraction attained in geometry since Euclid. But geometry is also the first chapter of physics, and kinematics is really the second chapter. Kinematics is geometry with the added variable of time. Kinematics, the science of motion, is also the science of flow, since any system in which particles are moving through space with some freedom is showing some state of flow, or flux. The study of fluid kinematics without regard to the driving and retarding forces might appear to be a wholly academic undertaking. A glance through the many publications on flow visualization, however, will show that this is actually a practical activity. This section uses a nonmathematical approach to fluid kinematics, retaining mathematical expressions and methods mainly when they are needed to describe accurately the properties and features of fluid flow, or when the topic requires illustration by calculation.

METHODS FOR THE DESCRIPTION OF FLOW

There are different ways to describe fluid flow; they emerged as the science of fluid mechanics became a modern discipline. Hints of such methods are found in the writings of Leonardo da Vinci, but their precise formulation and mathematical application came almost three centuries later when Euler and Lagrange made their fundamental contributions to fluid mechanics (6). Custom has honored these two men by giving their names to the two basic methods used to describe fluid flow. The Lagrangian point of view is that in which the individual fluid particles (large groups of molecules in fact, rather than individual molecules) are followed and their whereabouts established. A common Lagrangian technique to analyze fluid flow is to use direct flow visualization, obtained by marking fluid particles that are photographed to discover their paths through space. The Eulerian point of view is that in which one describes flows as velocity vector fields. A common Eulerian technique is to observe velocity in gases with anemometers or in bodies of water with current meters.

Meteorologists use both methods in daily weather reports. Figures 1A and 1B contrast the Lagrangian and the Eulerian views. Figure 1A shows air pathlines over the North American continent, while Fig. 1B summarizes the velocity field of the wind over the same area. Similar simplified mappings of flows can be made for the stomach (Figs. 1C and 1D). There are obvious differences in the fluid and flow properties between the atmosphere and the stomach, but both systems are so large as compared to molecules and molecular displacements that the fluid kinematics can be similarly described. Kinematics, like geometry, has almost no scale restrictions in its applicability. So long as the fluid can be described as a geometric continuum (like the lines,

surfaces, and volumes of geometry) that can be deformed in time, the methods of kinematics remain universal. Dynamic effects may force a more restricted view so that scaling becomes less simple, but the concepts of kinematics of continua span almost all scales in the universe.

Figure 1 illustrates another important feature common to both geophysical and biological phenomena: a strong dependence on time. The difference between the continent and the stomach in the spatial scales is large; the difference in the temporal scales is small; frequent temporal changes in flow occur in both cases. Flows that change with time are much more difficult to study than those that do not. Figure 1 does not reflect variability with time; it assumes the extremely rare instance of a steady flow condition. But, of course, Pacific air does not necessarily go straight to the Atlantic, nor does food entering the stomach proceed directly to the pylorus (Fig. 1D). The actual pathlines can be very complicated. The flow field (which is Eulerian) is usually a much simpler representation than a display of pathlines (which is Lagrangian). In these statements, there is a condensed expression of the difference in difficulty of application that is intrinsic in the two methods. In the fluid mechanics of the alimentary canal both Eulerian and Lagrangian methods are needed. In most sections of the conduit, complex and unsteady flows related to mixing and absorption occur so that the Lagrangian method is the more informative.

LAGRANGIAN DESCRIPTION OF FLOWS

Single-Particle Motion

With the Lagrangian method, one observes what happens to individual particles. The theory of motion of a single particle can be extended to the motion of a system of particles, if one takes particle interaction into account. What we call a particle is a theoretical unit, a relatively small portion of fluid rather than a single molecule. Fluid mechanics is only rarely based on the kinetic theory of gases or liquids; it is instead based on observed statistical behavior of these so-called fluid particles. In common flow visualizations, used in connection with the Lagrangian point of view, the portion of fluid that is marked to be photographed is often a sphere of about 1 mm in diameter. Where special techniques are used such as the laser type of visualization, the particles observed can be made smaller, but they are still very large compared with molecular size. To describe the motion of such particles, one specifies the coordinates of its cetroid as functions of time. Figure 2 shows a portion of a line described by a particle that moved from an initial point at coordinates x_o, y_o, z_o. Such a line is called the path of the particle, the particle pathline.

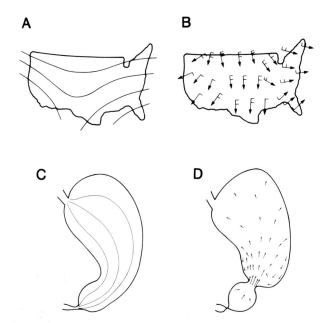

FIG. 1. Diagrams to contrast Lagrangian and Eulerian points of view. The diagrams in **A** and **B** compare these views with respect to air flow. In **C** and **D**, analogous diagrams refer to fluid flow in the stomach.

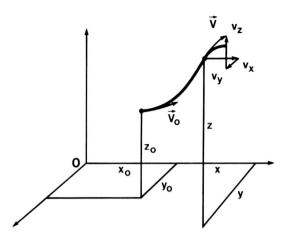

FIG. 2. Motion of a particle in space. The initial position (x_0, y_0, z_0) is shown as well as a generic position (x, y, z). The line described by the particle is the pathline. The velocity vector, $\vec{V}$, is shown with its three components (v_x, v_y, v_z).

As a very simple example of pathline, we can consider the case in which the coordinates x, y, z are linear functions of time:

$$x = x_0 + V_1t$$
$$y = y_0 + V_2t \qquad [1]$$
$$z = z_0 + V_3t$$

Herein, V_1, V_2, V_3 are constant values and define a vector $\vec{V}_0$, such that

$$\vec{r} = \vec{r}_0 + \vec{V}_0t \qquad [2]$$

where $\vec{r}$ is the position vector of the particle, and $\vec{r}_0$ is the value of $\vec{r}$ at time t = 0. If one introduces the definition of velocity as the time rate of change of the position vector:

$$\vec{V} = \frac{d\vec{r}}{dt} \qquad [3]$$

then the vector of components V_1, V_2, V_3 represents the velocity in the motion given by Eqs. 1 or 2. Also the

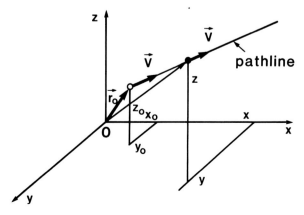

FIG. 3. Motion of a particle in space. The pathline is shown for a particle when the position vector varies linearly, $\vec{r} = \vec{r}_0 + \vec{V}t$.

vector $\vec{r} - \vec{r}_0$ represents the displacement of the particle and it is parallel to $\vec{V}_0$; this means that the particle decribes a straight line through the point of coordinates x_0, y_0, z_0, which is parallel to the vector $\vec{V}_0$ (Fig. 3).

If one expands Eq. 3 into its Cartesian components, one gets

$$v_x = \frac{dx}{dt}, \ v_y = \frac{dy}{dt}, \ v_z = \frac{dz}{dt} \qquad [4]$$

The magnitude of the velocity can be obtained by application of the Pythagoras theorem:

$$V = (v_x^2 + v_y^2 + v_z^2)^{1/2}$$

The time rate of change of the velocity is called the acceleration:

$$\vec{A} = \frac{d\vec{V}}{dt} = \frac{d^2\vec{r}}{dt^2} \qquad [5]$$

Application of the same definition to Eq. 4 gives the expressions for the Cartesian components of the acceleration. A fundamental result of vector calculus shows that the acceleration vector has, in general, two components: one is parallel to the velocity (corresponding to the change in magnitude of the vector $\vec{V}$), and the other is normal to the velocity and contained in the osculating plane of the pathline (corresponding to the change in direction of the vector $\vec{V}$).

Circular Pathlines

Equation 2 represents an open pathline; in many cases, closed pathlines are found. Among closed pathlines, the circular ones are the simplest. The motion on such an orbit may be accomplished with either variable or uniform speed. (Note the tacitly introduced difference between velocity and speed). Circular orbits appear in vortices with either straight or circular axes. They may also be components of other motions, as in the case of helical pathlines. For a circular orbit in the x-y plane the equations may be

$$x = r_0\cos\omega t$$
$$Y = r_0\sin\omega t \qquad [6a]$$

or

$$r = r_0$$
$$\theta = \omega t \qquad [6b]$$

where Eqs. 6a give the path in Cartesian coordinates, and Eqs. 6b give it in plane polar coordinates. To get only the shape of the pathline, eliminate the time parameter in Eqs. 6a; to get $x^2 + y^2 = r_0^2$, the equation of a circle of radius r_0. Note that Eqs. 6a, which are the parametric equations of the circle, contain more information than the preceding Cartesian equation of the circle $(x^2 + y^2 = r_0^2)$. With Eqs. 6a one can represent

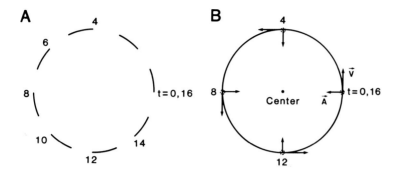

FIG. 4. Circular pathlines. **A:** Diagram shows the time-labeled pathline for a circular motion with uniform speed. **B:** Diagram shows a circular orbit with a velocity vector $\vec{V}$ (that varies with time) and an acceleration vector, $\vec{A}$ (that also varies with time). At each of the 4 points on the circular orbit, the pairs of vectors are different because they have a different direction.

both the circle and the particle in its successive positions in terms of a series of values of the time t (Fig. 4). The use of time-labeled lines gives much more information about the flow. It is convenient to show the displacements of the particle over equal time intervals, as in Fig. 4A. One can then immediately recognize a circular orbit traversed at uniform speed.

While the Cartesian equations (Eqs. 6a) emphasize the periodic nature of the circular uniform motion, the **polar equations (Eqs. 6b)** show immediately that the orbit is circular with the angular coordinate increasing steadily with time. The time rate of change of the angular coordinate is $d\theta/dt = \omega$, the angular speed. To obtain the linear speed, one must form the differential quotient $(rd\theta)/dt = \omega r$. The period can be obtained from that of the trigonometric functions in Eqs. 6b or from the function $\theta = \omega t$ when experiencing an increase of 2π. Hence the period is $T = 2\pi/\omega$. From Eqs. 6a, the components of the velocity and the acceleration vectors can be obtained. Thus one can verify that the magnitude of the velocity is ψr. And one can also find that the two vectors are themselves periodic, rotating full circle with period T. In addition, one can see that the acceleration is a vector with is purely centripetal and has a magnitude, $\psi^2 r_o = v^2/r_o$ (Fig. 4B). In dynamics, the acceleration is important to know. If one knows the acceleration and the mass of a fluid particle, one can determine the force acting on it. Knowledge of the forces acting on the fluid particles allows one to determine the pressure and stress fields acting on the fluid.

Parabolic Pathlines

Parabolic pathlines are very common. Particles moving in the field of the earth's gravity tend to describe second-degree parabolas if the resistance due to the surrounding field is small. The denser the particle, the more likely it is to give a parabolic pathline. It is common knowledge that the acceleration of gravity is nearly constant over a small region of space; this leads to a simple differential equation for the z-coordinate of the particle:

$$\frac{d^2 z}{dt^2} = g \qquad [7]$$

Here the z-axis is assumed to be directed vertically downward. When a motion is given by a differential equation, one must determine it by using the initial and/or the boundary conditions. In this case, if the particle is at the origin of coordinates and is let fall without initial velocity, two successive integrations of Eq. 7 lead to

$$v_z = gt; \quad z = 1/2gt^2 \qquad [8]$$

The time-labeled pathline, a straight line, is shown in Fig. 5 along the z-axis. If the particle is given an initial velocity U in the horizontal direction (x-axis), the coordinates of the particles will be

$$\begin{aligned} x &= Ut \\ z &= 1/2gt^2 \end{aligned} \qquad [9]$$

Elimination of the time t between the two Eqs. 9 leads to $z = gx^2/2U^2$, the equation of a second-degree para-

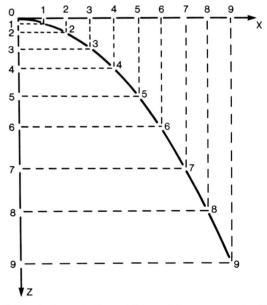

FIG. 5. Typical parabolic pathline and its components. The Z-axis shows the time-labeled pathline in the case when gravity influences the particles in the absence of an initial velocity given to the particle. The X-axis shows the time-labeled pathline when there is no effect of gravity but only an initial velocity. The combined action of the initial velocity and a gravity yields a parabolic pathline.

bola with the vertex at the origin of coordinates. One such parabola, drawn using Eqs. 9, is shown in Fig. 5. That figure also shows the x-component of the motion. Since g is constant, one can easily obtain pathlines for different values of U by changing the length of the segments along the x-axis.

Groups of Particles

The study of simple particulate systems is a useful introduction to fluid flow. Fluids are usually considered as continuum systems, not as discrete systems, in analyses of flow. But in flow visualization one looks, in reality, at a small number of particles. The relationship between systems of particles and continua is illustrated by a look at jet-like motions of groups of particles. Thus, if identical solid particles are ejected from a given point with identical velocities (Fig. 6), they will describe identical parabolas. A similar simultaneous motion of many particles can be described as a jet; sand used in sandblasting is a jet, as is the stream of sugar particles coming from a sugar dispenser.

Of course, there are differences between jets of solid particles and those of fluids, but there are virtues in the analogies. When the ejection of particles is modeled from several points rather than one point, the particulate analog can be made to generate a variety of "flows". One needs only to vary the initial-velocity distribution. Figure 7 shows a relatively wide jet in which the particles have been given different initial velocities (increasing from 1 to 5). Besides simulating a wide jet, this figure shows kinematic features of fluid flow that are difficult to see without a view of what the individual particles do. There are lines of particles that remain straight and parallel to themselves in this flow. The fluid analogs of these lines are fluid lines. There are horizontal lines in Fig. 7 that become longer as the flow pro-

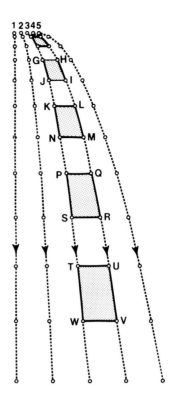

FIG. 7. Jet analog demonstrating linear and angular deformations and volume changes in fluid flow.

ceeds; the separation between lines of particles becomes progressively larger. Also, the distances between particles aligned along the parabolas increase. The material lines dilate in two directions, so that there is an increase in the volume represented by any group of particles. The particles are shown at positions corresponding to a uniform time sequence, so that after any basic time interval, new particles again occupy the same positions occupied by previous particles. For example, in Fig. 7, note the increase in the volume KLMN which, after two time intervals, becomes PQRS. This model using particulate streams seems more like an expanding gas than a liquid in which there is conservation of volume. In a liquid, the distance between particles may vary widely, but if we consider those particles which form a certain volume at any instant, a constraint must be put on such a group of particles: they must continue to embrace the same volume as they move through space. The liquid may undergo great deformations but no volume dilation or compression, since these are observable only when the liquid undergoes very great changes in pressure, a circumstance not found in liquids in biosystems.

This analog is useful to represent flows that vary with time, including the case in which the change is due to the reversal of a sequence of causes. By ejecting particles at a point with variable initial velocity, one can generate the analog of a jet of variable shape with time. Figure 8 shows a group of 10 particles ejected with increasing initial horizontal velocity. Each particle describes a parabola, but the material line formed by the

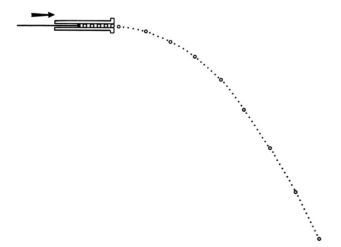

FIG. 6. Jet analog ejecting particles at a constant initial speed. Since initial speed and gravity are both constants, all particles follow the same pathline.

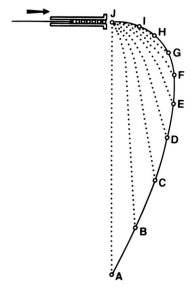

FIG. 8. Jet analog ejecting particles at increasing speed. This is an instantaneous view at the instant when the 10th particle in the series, particle J, initiates its parabolic path. *Dotted lines* are all parabolas.

particles is not a parabola, and has a shape which varies with time. But, if one then begins ejecting particles at constant speed, the upper part of the jet will become stationary and will take the shape of a parabola. Figure 9 illustrates such a case. There was initially a vertical jet that is not indicated. The velocity of the particles was changed instantaneously in steps, thus producing a series of variations in the shape of the jet. If this causal process is reversed, by reducing initial velocity in instantaneous steps through a reversed sequence of the same values, the original verticle jet (due to initial velocity zero) will ultimately be recovered, but the shapes of the jet do not go through the same intermediate phases.

This is shown in Fig. 10. This demonstration brings up the matter of reversibility and irreversibility in flows, an important matter in biological flow processes. It is necessary to find out when reversal of a sequence of causes will generate an exact reverse of the sequence of effects, and when it will generate a different sequence.

EULERIAN DESCRIPTION OF FLOWS

Steady Flows

The Lagrangian method is very direct and intuitive; it will therefore be used first to describe some flows which can then be considered from the Eulerian point of view.

Flows which do not vary with time are called steady flows. The simplest flows of this kind are those in which all particles describe parallel straight lines (Fig. 11A). Time-labeled pathlines can be used to depict steady flows with parallel pathlines. Figure 11B shows a flow in which the velocity is uniform both along the pathlines and across the flow; this would be the flow in a free liquid jet with no resistance on its lateral surface. Figure 11C shows a flow with a velocity that is uniform along each pathline, but that varies across the flow. This flow is found in conduits and channels with fixed walls, where the velocity is maximum at the centerline and zero at the walls. In Figs. 11B and 11C, the flow has been illustrated by examining a number of particles initially located across a given cross section. Another way to show the flow is to mark particles or emit tracers at a given cross section at uniform intervals of time. This method generates strings of particles which make the flow visible by means of material lines, called streaklines (Fig. 12). The flow represented in Figs. 11C and 12 is the same. Figures 11C and 12 appear to be almost

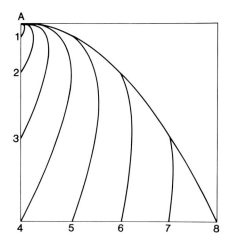

FIG. 9. A jet of fluid that was initially vertical, directed downward along the y-axis, is given progressively greater velocity in the direction of the x-axis. This gradual modification produced by increasing the horizontal component of liquid velocity leaving the nozzle at A gives a series of different lines that culminates in a parabolic line, A-8, when the horizontal component has become maximal.

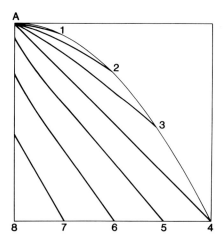

FIG. 10. The reverse sequence to that shown in Fig. 9. Here, a parabolic jet is converted to a vertical jet by a gradual reduction in the initial horizontal velocity component of the liquid. The shapes of the jet in the direct sequence do not go through the same intermediate forms as they do in the reverse.

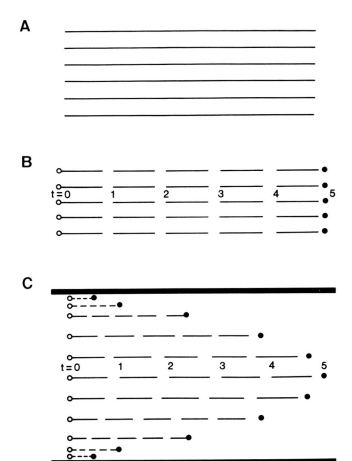

FIG. 11. Two ways to diagram flows with parallel pathlines. **A**: One cannot tell if the flow is steady or unsteady. Time-labeled pathlines are needed for a precise depiction. **B**: Time-labeled pathlines depict paralled steady flow with uniform displacements (and hence velocity) along the pathlines and across the flow. These pathlines could be those of a free liquid jet. **C**: Time-labeled pathlines appear for conduit flow. Displacements and velocities are not uniform across the flow, being reduced to zero at the boundaries of the conduit.

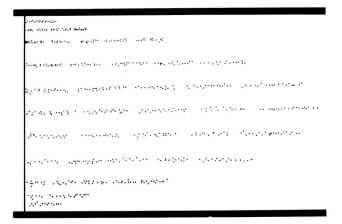

FIG. 12. Streaklines. Conduit flow is represented here by means of lines of fine tracers released at several points across the flow. If emission of tracers is interrupted for a short time every unit of time, a depiction similar to that of time-labeled pathlines results. These are streaklines. The walls of the conduit are drawn as thick lines: flow is from left to right.

identical but they really show quite different events. Figure 11C could result from illumination of the particles with regular interruptions (assuming a unit time interval, illumination would occur during 0.8 of the time). A photograph taken with the shutter open during five such time intervals would produce Fig. 11C. To obtain Fig. 12, one would release particles over a line crossing the flow during part of five time intervals and then take a snapshot.

A variation of the streak technique is to introduce a strip of tracer across the flow and then to see how the strip is changed by the flow. This is illustrated for serveral elementary flows in Fig. 13. In all these flows, the volume of the fluid portion that was originally marked does not change during the flow. Direct observation of the whereabouts of such marked fluid portions is useful in many ways. One that has already been suggested is in the determination of conservation (or variation) of volume. Keeping track of certain fluid volumes is also useful to see the variations in the lines and surfaces separating different regions of the fluid that may have different properties. A change in the length of the line or in the area of the interface between two different fluids may greatly affect the diffusional processes between the fluids. In the analysis of mixing in fluids, therefore, this method is very useful.

Lagrangian observations depend much on flow visualizations, which are cumbersome at best, and almost impossible when there is turbulence. The Eulerian point of view consists in measuring velocities at fixed stations, a technique applicable to turbulent flow. In a study of traffic flow this would be like measuring the speed of passing cars at a number of stations, rather than determining what each car does. From Eulerian observations one can get the corresponding Lagrangian data, and the reverse is also true. This is easy in simple cases. Thus Fig. 14A shows the Eulerian version of Fig. 11B, and Fig. 14B shows that of Fig. 11C. In more complex

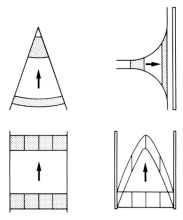

FIG. 13. Examples of the streak technique to demonstrate flow in 4 elementary flows. In each case, one volume of fluid is labeled at one instant and the shape of the volume is shown at a later instant.

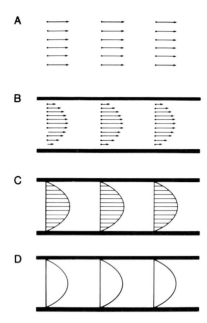

FIG. 14. Eulerian representations of various flows. **A**: Flow is described by its velocity field. This is the Eulerian version of parallel steady flow with uniform displacements along the pathlines and across the flow. **B**: A Eulerian representation, by means of a vector field, of conduit flow. **C**: Another way of representing conduit flow. **D**: Velocity profiles, a convention in which the assumption is implicit that the segments shown in **C** are "seen" by the viewer.

flows, passage from Lagrangian to Eulerian views and vice versa can be extremely difficult.

The Eulerian representations in Figs. 14A and 14B show the velocity vectors to emphasize that they describe a view in which a vector field gives the flow. But other more simplified (or more abstract) forms can be used instead. One may show only the velocity profiles in either of the forms depicted in Figs. 14C and 14D; no vectors are shown, but one could easily draw them. The difference between Fig. 14B and Figs. 14C and 14D may seem trivial, but it is not when more complex flows (two-dimensional or three-dimensional) are represented with velocity profiles for one component rather than with the velocity vector field directly. This point is illustrated by the flow from a reservoir, or from a large tube to a tube of small diameter. At some distance before the inlet to the small tube, the flow tends to be like that converging toward a sink that is far from any solid boundary: it is a flow with uniform velocity over spherical surfaces with their centers at the sink. This spherical uniformity of the flow will be assumed to be valid up to the entrance section of the tube. From there on, the fluid particles near the channel walls are retarded, while those near the centerline have their velocities increased. To make the study of this flow simpler, it can be assumed that the conduit is two-dimensional, i.e., in a plane, rather than in a cylindrical tube. Plane and axisymmetric flows are very similar: since the former are easier to study than the latter, they are commonly used to obtain a qualitative idea of the latter.

The flow at the entrance of a two-dimensional conduit is shown in three Eulerian descriptions. The information is the same in these descriptions if one knows how to relate Figs. 15A, 15B, and 15C. Figure 15A shows the vector field; the magnitude and direction of the velocity are given at each point. Figure 15B shows only the x-component of the velocity; one can determine the other component through volume flux calculations. Figure 15C shows only the velocity profile, with the understanding that it is for the x-component; if needed, the segments shown in Fig. 15B can be drawn easily on Fig. 15C. But other much more meaningful lines can be drawn if one holds the information given in figures such as Fig. 15C. By subdividing the area (or the volume, in three-dimensional flows) under the velocity profile, one can define the streamlines of the flow. The most obvious one is the centerline in Fig. 16 which can be drawn simply on the basis of symmetric partition of the flow. The velocity vector is tangent to the line (i.e., without a component normal to the line). Therefore, the streamlines of a vector field which does not vary with time are also the pathlines, and also the streaklines in such a flow. But the three types of lines, although identical in shape in such a flow, are conceptually different. For

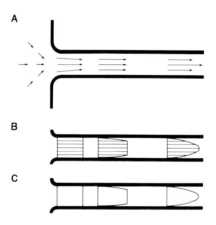

FIG. 15. Flow at the entrance to a two-dimensional conduit, as represented by Eulerian descriptions. **A**: Vector field is shown in flow from a reservoir into a channel. **B**: Velocity profiles in the entrance region of the channel, showing the component in the direction of the channel. **C**: Same velocity profiles as those in **B**. It is always understood that they represent the longitudinal component of the velocity.

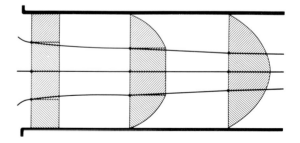

FIG. 16. Subdivision of the area under a velocity profile to determine the streamtubes that carry equal volume fluxes.

instance, the streamlines cannot be sectionalized by time-labeling as the pathlines can be (Fig. 17); also, if one tries to obtain streamlines, streaklines, and pathlines through experimental techniques, the techniques are different, although they are always coincidental lines in steady flows. A flow in which turbulence is absent is called laminar; this type of flow is what is illustrated by the flow visualization in Fig. 17.

Unsteady Flows

The difference between Lagrangian and Eulerian views of flows is striking when the flow configuration is time dependent. Before we consider a truly variable flow, the intermediate case of unsteady flow in which the streamlines remain invariant should be briefly discussed. A simple instance of such a flow is the oscillation of the fluid column in a U-tube manometer (Fig. 18); streamlines, pathlines, and streaklines are still coincident in such a flow. Note that the streamlines extend

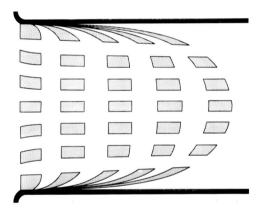

FIG. 17. A Lagrangian depiction of flow at the entrance to a two-dimensional conduit. The visualization of flow is based on a technique in which certain portions of the fluid are marked alternately in space and time so that the history of certain volumes of the fluid can be seen. Such a technique demonstrates several properties of the flow. This is a laminar flow, from left to right.

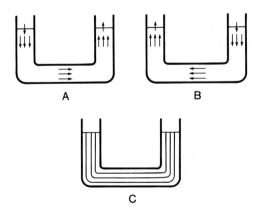

FIG. 18. An oscillatory flow in a U-tube as shown by means of the flow field and by means of streamlines. **A** and **B** show velocity vectors which change with the oscillation; the streamlines, shown in **C**, do not show the oscillation: that is, they are invariant.

from one end of the fluid column to the other, whereas pathlines and streaklines are only segments of the streamlines. An interesting question about such back-and-forth fluid motions is whether or not they proceed along the same lines when flow direction is reversed. In respiration, for example, the external flow is along much different lines during expiration and inspiration (Fig. 19). Note that the natural way to illustrate this point is Eulerian rather than Lagrangian. One would use a Lagrangian description to emphasize that the air entering in each cycle is different from that being expelled. Irreversibility ensures the supply of fresh air in each inspiration.

For a simple case of generally unsteady flow, assume that the wind over a given region changes in direction while having a common direction at each instant of time. Suppose that the wind comes from the west for 1 hr starting at 8 a.m., for instance, then successively from the north, east, and south for periods of 1 hr each, thus making a full circle in 4 hr. A balloon suspended in the air without motion across the wind would return to the starting point after describing a square. But the map of the wind would show four successive pictures in which the flow appears to be uniform with straight streamlines. If the wind were to change with a constant rate of rotation of its direction, then the instantaneous flow pattern (Eulerian) would continue to show parallel flow with straight parallel streamlines (Fig. 20). The pathlines in this case of constant rate of rotation would be circles of equal radius as drawn for the balloon in Fig. 20; these circles would intersect each other and give a confusing—although true—description (Lagrangian) of what happens to fluid particles. To complete the picture of this time dependent flow, the streaklines should be considered. To perceive them more easily, we must assume that there is little diffusion (either molecular or turbulent) and that an idealistic laminar wind exists during the 4 hr. To visualize the streaklines one may suppose that smoke started to be emitted from a smokestack precisely at the moment the rotation of the wind began. Then the smoke trace would appear as an arc of a circumference which rotates with the wind. After 1 hr, we will see a quarter of a circumference. The length of the arc increases with time, as the entire streak rotates

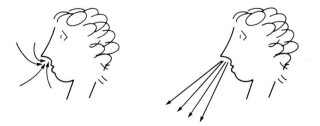

FIG. 19. Flow patterns of external air in inspiration and expiration. Inspiratory flow is like flow toward a sink; expiratory flow is a jet. This illustrates the possibility of different patterns in a case of oscillatory flow with relatively high inertial forces.

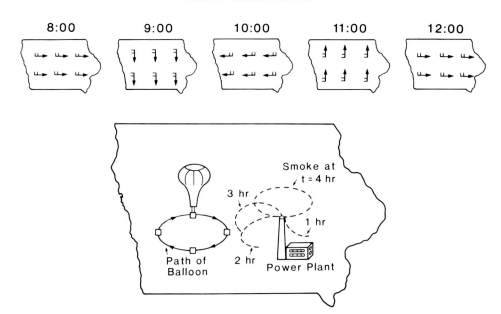

FIG. 20. A simple case of generally unsteady flow illustrating the differences between streamlines, pathlines, and streaklines. At the top is a hypothetical set of weather maps showing hourly shifts in wind direction (in which velocity is constant). Below is shown the effect of the change in wind direction on the distribution of smoke that began to emerge from the smokestack at 8:00. Also, there is shown the effect of the change in wind direction on the path of a balloon. The arrows on the weather maps suggest streamlines, straight parallel lines. The path of the balloon is a pathline. The changing trail of the smoke represents, at each instant, a streakline.

in space. After 4 hr a full circle will be completed. At the smokestack, the streakline is tangent to the velocity vector; i.e., has the instantaneous direction of the wind.

The three types of lines introduced in the example of the regularly turning wind are encountered in all flows which are truly variable with time; i.e., truly unsteady (1,2,5). Use of pathlines, streaklines, and streamlines is dictated in each specific flow phenomenon under analysis by the need to emphasize certain aspects rather than others. Thus, in the example, pathlines are essential to balloonists, whole streamlines may interest airplane pilots. Streaklines are of interest to the environmental engineer or the concerned ecologist. In biofluid mechanics, the specific question may again determine which lines are most useful.

One must be cautious in drawing conclusions about any flow that is unsteady if only Eulerian views of the flow have been examined. Transport properties, mixing features, and circulation patterns are difficult to predict with a view of the streamline alone, and pressure fields and stress fields are difficult to visualize. The transfer from the Eulerian description to the Lagrangian when the flow is generally unsteady (with streamlines different from one time to another) is a painstaking process that is rarely performed and for which techniques are poorly developed. Computerization may soon simplify this conversion.

KINEMATICS OF WALLS

When fluids flow past rigid bodies or inside rigid conduits, the kinematics of the interface between the solid and the fluid is simple, even when the boundary moves. But when that interface is deformable, either passively or actively, one must examine its kinematics carefully. Both the stomach and the intestine are tubes with movable boundaries. The cross-sectional shape and dimensions of the tube can exhibit both long-term and short-term variations. Only the latter will be considered here since they produce most of the flow patterns of concern.

The wall movements can be described by a simple model in which it is assumed that the tube possesses a rest position, and that each particle at the wall moves over a closed orbit through the duration of a given local movement. A wall will be considered that is assumed to be a segment of a circular cylinder. To represent a temporary constriction of the segment, suppose that the wall particles move over elliptical orbits. This allows enough parameters to change so that a number of movements that are acutally observed can be modeled. The first wall movement to be illustrated is one in which the ellipses can be made to degenerate into segments of straight lines, making one of the principal axes of the ellipse of zero dimension (Fig. 21A). Points on the wall are assumed to execute harmonic motions from the rest position toward the axis of the cylinder and back to the rest position. This represents a symmetric transverse contraction of the tube. The contractions represented in Figs. 21A and 21B are occlusive since the central orbit has a large diameter equal to the radius of the tube. These contractions model the classic idea of segmenting contractions in the intestine. But studies show (7) that contractions follow a pattern which is propagative rather than stationary as in Fig. 21C.

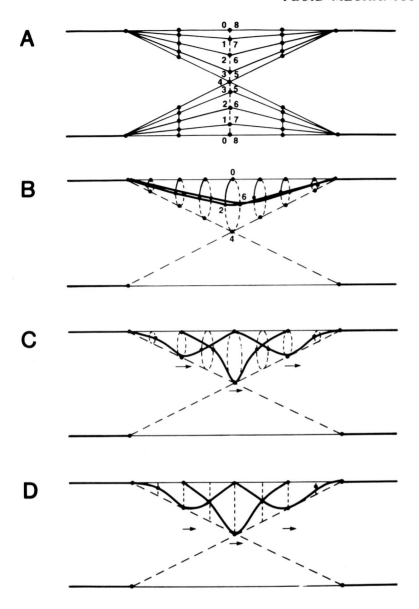

FIG. 21. Various models of a temporary constriction of a conduit segment. **A**: Simultaneous orbits of particles along the walls are represented as straight segments. **B**: Simultaneous orbits are elongated ellipses. **C**: The same elliptical orbits are depicted with a phase lag from left to right. **D**: Flattened elliptical orbits are drawn to depict a propagative transverse contraction produced by the phase lag in orbital motion.

In Fig. 21C the orbits are elliptical with the smaller diameter in the direction of the tube axis. One of the characteristics of this model is a phase lag along the direction of the conduit axis. In Fig. 21B no phase lag has been introduced, but the sense of motion along each orbit introduces a small propagative effect. The contraction phase is not exactly mirrored by the relaxation phase: there is a difference between the shape of the wall halfway toward the axis and the shape of the wall halfway toward the rest position.

In Fig. 21C a phase lag has been introduced along the wall. Each particle accomplishes a cycle and then stops. One can see a wave propagating from left to right. Of course, this could be done also with the degenerated ellipses like those in Fig. 21A to produce a purely transverse contraction that is propagative (see Fig. 21D).

Figures 22A and 22B represent contractions in which there is a predominance of the orbital displacement in the axial or longitudinal direction. Figure 22B shows purely longitudinal movement. In this case, the different configurations have been displayed separately (for three different times), for it would be impossible otherwise to visualize this type of contraction.

These illustrations of the varieties of kinematic models of wall movements have made use of the simplest geometric figures and kinematic functions. As knowledge about muscle movements improves, more realistic orbits and functions could be used. Figure 22C illustrates the law adopted for the orbital motion over the different types of ellipses used in the previous figures. This is based on uniform motion on a circular orbit, as shown. The detail shown on the lower halves of the orbits has been suppressed in the upper halves.

FLOW INDUCED BY DEFORMABLE WALLS

Kinematics alone will not yield answers to all questions about fluid flow; more powerful methodology is

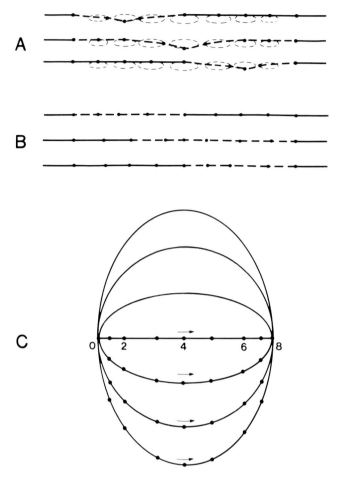

FIG. 22. Contractions of the wall of a segment of a tubular conduit in which there is a predominance of the orbital displacements of wall particles in either the longitudinal or axial direction. **A**: Elliptical orbits have been elongated in the longitudinal direction. **B**: Transverse axis of each ellipse has been reduced to zero to depict a propagative longitudinal contraction. **C**: Uniform motion on the circular orbit is projected on elliptical orbits to illustrate the law adopted in modeling.

needed in which the forces acting on the fluid particles are considered. Some of the general properties of the flow induced by moving boundaries are purely kinematical, however, and these should be examined before the methods of dynamics of fluids are used.

There are two basic types of boundary movements: transverse and longitudinal. Longitudinal motions of the boundary do not produce a change in volume, and without consideration of shear stresses in the fluid, it is impossible to discuss the kinematics of the induced flow in such a case. Purely transverse boundary movements produce volume displacements that can be determined if the law of motion of the boundary is known; by assuming that the fluid is incompressible, one can determine flow rates at other places in the fluid. To illustrate this point, two cases of moving walls will be considered that are simple enough to allow reasonably good conjectures about the flow induced by the moving boundaries.

Consider first a spherical reservoir which contracts radially in a simple manner, following a sine-square law, for instance, so that the velocity is zero at the beginning and at the end of the contraction. If the flow is slow, it can be assumed to be laminar, and then its streamlines can be conjectured without gross errors. Figure 23A is a definition sketch of a contracting spherical reservoir connected to a rigid tube that is open at the other end. If v_w is the velocity of the reservoir wall at any instant of time, the volume flux produced (the rate of change of the reservoir volume displaced) will be approximately $Q = (4\pi R^2 - \pi r^2)V_w$, if R and r are, respectively, the radii of the sphere and of the tube. Five cross sections are shown in Fig. 23A; the volume flux Q through each of them must be constant, hence $Q_1 = Q_2 = Q_3 = Q_4 = Q_5$ applies. Otherwise, somewhere along the flow the specific volume of the fluid would be varying through either compression of dilation. The flow field velocities along the boundaries are known and can be estimated along the centerline. Along the centerline, symmetry assures a knowledge of the direction of the flow field, at least. An assumption of maximum simplicity of the lines can also be made, but this assumption is less reliable than that of symmetry. But if the flow is very slow, simplicity may be confirmed by experiments or calculations. The velocities that are known are shown in Fig. 23B; the conjectural flow pattern is shown in Fig. 23C. What is shown is really a view of the expected streamlines.

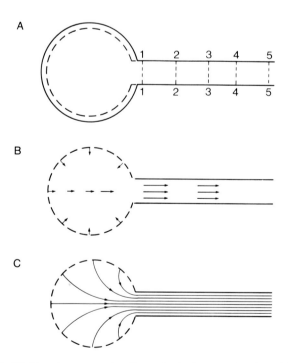

FIG. 23. Flow from a contracting spherical reservoir into a rigid tube that is open at the other end. **A**: Definition sketch showing the contracting spherical surface and control sections. **B**: Parts of the velocity field that are known. **C**: Conjecture about the flow due to the contracting spherical reservoir.

As a second case, consider the same system of reservoir and attached tube, but with a reservoir which is contracting and a tube which is dilating, both radially (Fig. 24A). Again, one can specify the velocities at the boundaries, and assume symmetric flow in a symmetric conduit that is undergoing symmetric displacements. In contrast to the first case, assume one more condition, that the end of the tube is closed. Conservation of volume requires now that $(4\pi R^2 - \pi r^2)v_w - \pi r^2 L V_w$, where L is the length of the tube and V_w its wall velocity. Neglecting longitudinal deformation of the tube, one will find that the volume flux through control sections 1 through 5 is given, respectively, by Q, (3/4)Q, (1/2)Q, (1/4)Q, O. Figure 24B shows what is known of the flow field (with estimates of the magnitude of the velocity along the centerline within the reservoir), and Fig. 24C shows the conjectural streamlines of this flow. In this

figure and in Fig. 23C the velocity of the fluid has been assumed to be coincident with that of the wall particle in contact with the fluid particle at the wall; this is the so-called no-slip condition. This condition is generally applicable in real fluid flow.

Flows with Internal Jets

So far, only very slow flows with boundary geometries that do not favor flow separation from the walls and formation of jets have been considered (except for the example illustrated in Fig. 19). The geometry of the biological conduit may cause fluid particles to separate from the boundary at some point because the forces acting on such particles may not give enough change in momentum to force the particle to make a very sharp turn. This is the case in Fig. 19, where the air coming from the nostrils continues in a jet away from the nose. Jets may be either turbulent or nonturbulent (i.e., laminar). A jet remains laminar if the relationship between jet diameter D, jet velocity V, and the kinematic viscosity of the fluid v (v being dynamic viscosity/mass density), in the form of VD/v, constitutes the criterion to establish laminar or turbulent jets. If this number, the Reynolds number, remains below a value of about 200, steady jets are laminar. When the Reynolds number is larger, steady jets are turbulent. The Reynolds number is usually not the sole determinant of laminar flow. Geometry and time dependency of the flow are also important.

Examples of flow with a submerged jet appear in Figs. 25 and 26. In Fig. 25 a constriction has been introduced at the point of connection of the tube to the spherical contractile reservoir. The sharp orifice ensures the formation of a jet. A well-rounded constriction would tend to give a fluctuating jet, whereas a refined steamlining of the expansion could prevent the formation of the jet and the surrounding vortex (4). This vortex between the jet and the wall is a captive vortex and it could increase mixing of the flowing fluid. In Fig. 26, there appears a depiction of a traveling constriction. This could also produce a jet as indicated by the streamlines.

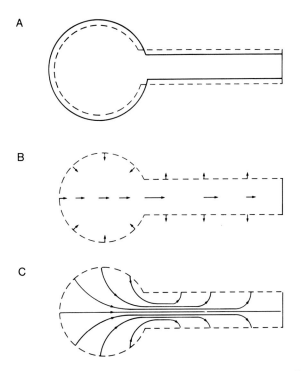

FIG. 24. Kinematics of a flow induced by radial contraction of a reservoir with dilatation of a connected tube.

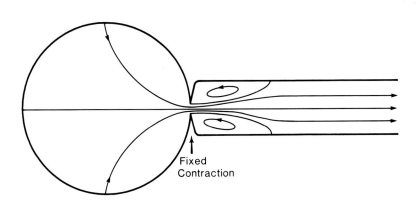

FIG. 25. A contractile spherical reservoir discharges into a conduit through a constriction. Streamlines are shown to depict the consequent jet and captive vortex in this two-dimensional representation.

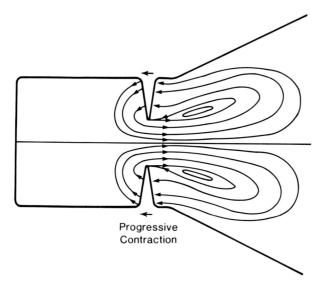

FIG. 26. Traveling constriction moving toward a closed end. For appropriate Reynolds numbers, this flow may generate a transient jet and a captive eddy.

DYNAMICS OF FLUIDS

Forces in Viscous Fluids

The kinematics of fluids is concerned only with the description of flow, not with its accurate prediction. Prediction is possible only through application of the fundamental law of mechanics, the so-called Newton's second law. This law states that the time rate of change of the momentum of any material mass is equal to the sum of the forces acting on it. In the case of a fluid, the calculation of the momentum may require integration over the volume occupied by the fluid mass under analysis, but this is a standard procedure, even if the flow is given in an Eulerian manner. The time rate of change of momentum in Lagrangian form is related to the Eulerian by the Reynolds theorem. It is sometimes a crucial operation to determine the expressions for the forces acting on the fluid, and to evaluate their relative importance. All fluids are subject to gravity, a force identified long ago, and there is no problem in taking it into account. A similar situation exists for the internal pressure of the fluid, which is also easily accounted for. The main difficulty which still exists is the formulation of the internal viscous stresses, or internal friction. Rheology is a discipline that evolved to consider this problem for fluids that show complex behavior. Little is known about the rheology of the contents of the alimentary canal, so the simple linear relationship established by Newton to represent the behavior of common fluids will be used here as a first approximation.

Newton's law for viscous stresses can be formulated as a relationship valid for a simple viscometer, and then extended to more complex flow patterns. Reference will be made to the viscometer that consists of coaxial cyl-

inders (Fig. 27). Assume that the gap between the two cylinders is very small. The outer cylinder rotates with speed U at its inner surface and the inner cylinder remains at rest. After a steady flow pattern has been achieved, the velocity profile can be represented approximately by a linear function $u = (U/a)y$, where a is the gap, and y is the radial local coordinate. Newton postulated a linear relationship between the shear stress τ in the fluid and the quantity U/a, the rate of deformation of the fluid. Thus

$$\tau = \mu(U/a) \qquad [8]$$

The coefficient μ, a property of the fluid in question, is called dynamic viscosity, or simply, viscosity. Once it was noted that $U/a = du/dy$, a generalization was soon introduced to represent viscous shear stresses when the velocity profile is not linear. Thus the present form of Newton's law is

$$\tau = \mu \frac{du}{dy} \qquad [9]$$

Much more general formulations of viscous stresses were introduced by Navier, Saint-Venant, and Stokes (6), but Newton's formula (see Eq. 9) provides a good basis for elementary discussions.

Viscous Flow in a Tube

To illustrate the methods of dynamics, consider the flow in a horizontal circular conduit of a fluid of vis-

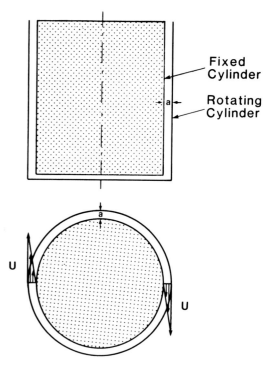

FIG. 27. Definition sketch for fluid subject to shear. The gap (a) is assumed to be small, so that the velocity profile can be approximated by a linear distribution of the velocity.

cosity μ that has reached a steady flow condition with streamlines parallel to the axis of the conduit, and with the same velocity profile section after section. Thus the flow away from an entrance region is considered (Fig. 28). In this case, one should realize that each fluid particle performs rectilinear uniform motion; therefore, there is no change in momentum for each particle, and this is true for the entire fluid cylinder between any two control cross sections. Such a fluid cylinder as the one depicted in Fig. 29 is therefore subject to a system of forces which must have a sum equal to zero; i.e., the system for forces is in equilibrium. The forces acting on the cylinder of radius r (Fig. 29) consist of pressure forces at the ends 1 and 2, and a shear force acting over the lateral surface of cylinder:

$$\pi r^2 p_1 - \pi r^2 p_2 - (2\pi r dx)\,\tau = 0 \qquad [10]$$

In the above equation, we can replace τ by $\mu dr/dr$, assuming that Newton's law can be extended to this case, and du/dy can be replaced by du/dr. This substitution leads to a differential equation for u as a function of r:

$$\left(-\frac{dp}{dx}\right) = \frac{2\mu}{r}\frac{du}{dr} \qquad [11]$$

Integration of this equation, assuming symmetry and the no-slip condition at the wall ($u = 0$ at $r - R$), leads to

$$U = U_m\left(1 - \frac{r^2}{R^2}\right) \qquad [12]$$

as the velocity distribution. This is the velocity distribution for laminar flow of Newtonian fluids in circular tubes in terms of the maximum velocity U_m and the radius r. One can see that a different relationship for the

shear stress, as a function of rates of deformation in the fluid, must lead to other laws for the velocity variation across the tube. In fluids in which the stresses depend on the history of deformations, the solution would be time dependent even if all other conditions were held steady; i.e., even if a constant pressure gradient dp/dx were applied.

Flows Induced by Longitudinally Moving Walls

The viscous fluid flow just considered results from a pressure gradient as the driving force; the viscous shear stress gave rise to a resistive force that was exactly in balance with the driving force. There are cases, however, in which the driving force may be purely a viscous stress, transmitted through the fluid, that in turn may or may not originate a pressure gradient. This will be illustrated by considering two flows due to rigid moving walls. This may seem only remotely related to the study of the flow induced by deformable boundaries, but an understanding of the effects of rigid moving walls is helpful in grasping the possible effects of deformable walls.

Flow Due to a Single Moving Wall

Figure 30 shows two parallel plates with a viscous liquid in the space between them. The upper plate is assumed to start moving at a certain moment with velocity U that is maintained for an indefinite time. Through viscous stresses, i.e., viscous transfer of momentum, layer after layer of the fluid is set into motion. If the lower plate is maintained at rest, the fluid layer in contact with that plate will also remain at rest. The equation governing this flow, which is unsteady (i.e., time dependent), can be established by considering a fluid volume of dimensions dx, dy, dz to which shear stresses τ and $\tau = \partial \tau / \partial x\, dx$ are applied, giving a difference that tends to increase the momentum of the fluid. This leads to the momentum equation

$$\frac{\partial(\varrho u dx dy dz)}{\partial t} + \left(\frac{\partial \tau}{\partial y}dy\right)dx dz \qquad [13]$$

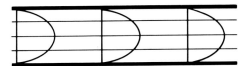

FIG. 28. Eulerian depiction, by the use of velocity diagrams, of uniform flow of a viscous fluid in a conduit.

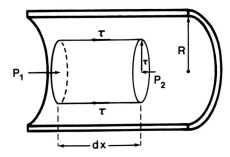

FIG. 29. Diagram of the forces acting on a cylindrical volume of fluid flowing through a tube.

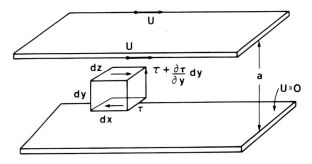

FIG. 30. Flow induced in a viscous fluid by movement of one wall of a two-dimensional channel. Shear forces acting on the fluid element dxdydz are shown.

that in turn yields the following differential equation

$$\varrho \frac{\partial \mu}{\partial t} = \mu \frac{\partial^2 \mu}{\partial y^2}$$ [14]

This is a classic differential equation for diffusional processes, and its integral in a variety of cases is well known.

The results shown in Fig. 31 for the flow induced by a moving plate (8) can be used to estimate the time it takes for the moving wall to produce a certain amount of flow in the fluid which it is entraining. The diagram shows an infinite time for the establishment of the steady flow, but if one considers times needed to attain a fraction of the final flow, the results give finite times which are small as compared to the time scale of this phenomenon. The time scale can be defined as that time which makes the variable t dimensionless in the equation governing this flow (a standard procedure). Such a scale is a^2/v. Using the graph in Fig. 31, one can determine that half the final volume flux is attained in a time given by $0.3a^2/v$. In a liquid of viscosity $v = 0.1$ cm²/s between two plates at a distance $a = 1$ cm, the time is 3 sec.

Walls moving longitudinally can cause circulation of fluid in different ways. One is that in which the fluid is prevented from flowing unidirectionally. Thus, if the fluid is confined between walls arranged to form a box, and one or two walls move, circulation will result, because near the moving wall a current is formed and then flow must extend somehow to the rest of the fluid to satisfy the conservation of volume. This is the case illustrated in the model shown in Fig. 32 in which two parallel walls can move while the other two remain fixed. The most plausible pattern of flow is suggested by the arrows, assuming that the flow will be symmetric. The ratio of length to width is given an intermediate value so that the fluid flow will not break into cells (as it could for ratios which are either too small or too large). The flow in the central portion (away from the fixed walls) can then be modeled as a purely parallel flow. The flow near the corners is curvilinear and much more difficult to determine. The analysis of the assumed uniform flow in the central portion of the model shown in Fig. 33A is instructive because it gives an idea about how fluid mechanics operates. At the wall, there is a specified velocity U (Fig. 33A) and a shear stress τ of unknown magnitude, but which determines a shearing action of the fluid. Through Newton's law, we can establish that (du/dy) wall = τ/μ. This du/dy must adjust itself to produce a velocity profile that results in a certain central volume flux that is equal and opposite to that directly generated by the plates. One can conjecture an approximate velocity profile as shown in Fig. 33B. From the momentum equation one can determine this profile exactly. Assuming uniform flow, there is a zero net momentum flux, and the sum of forces on an element of dimensions dx, 2y must be zero, i.e.:

$$(p_1 - p_2)(2y) - \tau(2dx) - 0$$ [15]

If we assume that $\tau = \mu du/dy$, the preceding equation leads to a differential equation for u:

$$\frac{du}{dy} = \left(-\frac{dp}{dx}\right)\frac{y}{\mu}$$ [16]

Integration, taking into account the boundary conditions, gives

$$u = U\left(1 - \frac{3}{2}\frac{y^2}{a^2}\right)$$ [17]

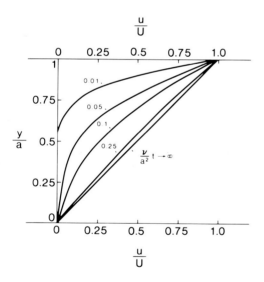

$$\frac{u}{U}$$

FIG. 31. Velocity profiles as a function of time for the flow induced in a viscous fluid by a moving wall. The flow is assumed to be laminar. The diagram, by virtue of being dimensionless, is of universal application.

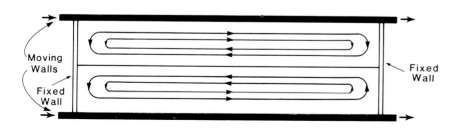

FIG. 32. Approximate flow pattern produced by slowly moving walls. The flow arises from shear stresses exerted by the walls moving at a constant velocity. A pressure gradient is also generated in this flow.

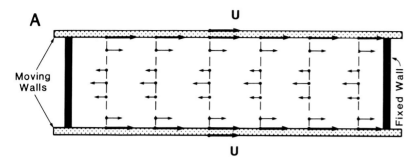

A

B

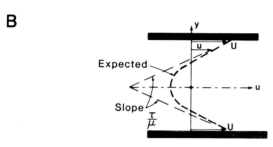

FIG. 33. Two-dimensional flow caused by moving walls. **A**: A box is formed with two fixed walls and two moving walls. Velocity, U, is prescribed for the walls. The fluid velocity vectors (*arrows*) are conjectural, but they could be determined by integration of the equations of conservation of volume and momentum. **B**: Sketch of the expected fluid velocity profile on the basis of the known wall velocity, U, and of Newton's law for shear stresses.

The pressure gradient can be determined from the condition of conservation of volume

$$\int_{-a}^{a} u\,dy = 0 \qquad [18]$$

One obtains

$$\frac{dp}{dx} = \frac{6\mu U}{a^2} = \frac{6\varrho\nu U}{a^2}$$

Therefore, the longitudinal wall motion can generate not only circulation of the fluid but also pressure variation. It is interesting to estimate the order of magnitude of the pressure that may be generated in this manner. Thus, if $a = 1$ cm, $U = 1$ cm/s, $\nu = 1$ cm²/s, the drop in pressure per centimeter is only 0.006 cm of water column! This raises the question of what is important in analyzing the flow. Pressure differences and shear stresses may be almost insignificant; what is most important is the flow that is generated and the consequences of such flow in terms of functions such as transport or mixing.

FLOW INDUCED BY DEFORMABLE WALLS: APPLICATIONS TO THE INTESTINAL FLOW

Duodenal Flow

There are few studies of flow induced by the deformable walls of the alimentary canal (3). The duodenum has been studied in recent years, mainly by the use of simple models, and some insight has been gained about the flow patterns it should ideally generate. The duodenum is a tubular organ with muscular walls that contains a liquid of complex and varied properties, the chyme. The flow of chyme is determined by the movements of muscle layers which perform complicated contractions. The ideal approach to the prediction of duodenal flow—or any other flow in the alimentary canal—should be formulation of the equations that govern muscle movement and chyme rheology. The wall movements should vary with the nature of the chyme. We are, however, far from understanding the correlations between muscle movements and properties of the chyme. The student of fluid mechanics of the intestine must begin with simplified simulations of the wall geometry and kinematics using simple functions that represent the essential features. He must avoid complexities that are still either ill-defined or unknown. One of the essential features that is well established for the intestine in an animal that has been fed is that the intestinal wall, when observed over short enough segments of the tube, shows organized movements, contractions that occur at intervals of small multiples of the period of the electrical slow wave. Seldom does a regular train of contractions sweep more than a few centimeters along the intestine; usually little correlation of contractions along the intestine can be detected during the fed state. The movements of the duodenum are complex, and it appears that an eclectic interpretation (9) that postulates different modes of behavior and combines them statistically may be valid for that organ. Until the wall movements are more clearly established, one must use a model of wall kinematics flexible enough to represent either stationary or propagative contractions. Both simplified stationary and propagative contractions are represented in Fig. 34. Figure 34A can be interpreted as representing both annular and longitudinal contractions. For the representation of longitudinal contractions, one must consider the ordinates in Fig. 34B as a diagram for longitudinal rather than radial displacements. Of course, this

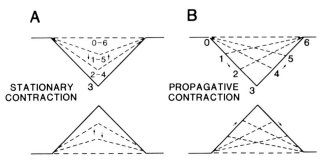

FIG. 34. Two ways to idealize ring contractions of a tubular organ such as the duodenum. Numbers refer to 7 successive stages in the development and recession of the contraction. **A**: Stationary contraction. **B**: Propagative contraction. The ordinates indicate displacements; these can be interpreted as either transverse or longitudinal (relative to the axes of the cylindrical organ).

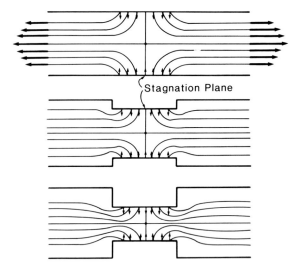

FIG. 35. Eulerian description of flow due to cylindrical contraction in a tube. Streamlines are shown at different times. During relaxation, the same streamlines are obtained. The flow is fully reversible; that is, all fluid particles return to their initial positions.

requires a specification of the scale for the displacements, which should not exceed the possible change in length compatible with the reasonable range of the change in length of the muscle. Another important feature of duodenal contractions is that, although they must be described statistically, each individual contraction is a highly organized event that tends to occur with a high degree of isolation and with a relatively slow motion. All this is important because it offers a good basis for a deterministic treatment of the flow induced by each contraction. The assumption of creeping flow appears to be acceptable as a first approximation. This assumption will be used here to discuss flow in the duodenum. The hypothesis of creeping flow makes an elementary discussion of intestinal flow relatively easy, especially if the fluid is assumed to be Newtonian (i.e., having a linear relationship between shear stresses and rates of deformation). Accurate theoretical solutions are, however, difficult, so the exact flow patterns may still be quite different from those obtained by simplified analyses. This appears to be particularly the case for flows induced by deformable walls. The results of simplified analyses are only a means to gain a basic understanding of the flow mechanisms in the intestine, not a means to predict flow patterns in detail.

Flow Induced by Annular Contractions

A single annular or ring contraction of stationary type produces a flow during the first phase (0 to 3 in Fig. 34A) that is exactly reversed during the second phase (3 to 6 in Fig. 34A). For a segment of tube with a cylindrical contraction occurring in the middle and with no pressure differential between the ends, it is easy to visualize the flow configuration at three different times (Fig. 35). Because of symmetry, a stagnation plane can be drawn centrally, where the axial velocity will be zero during the entire cycle. The boundary velocity is assumed to be known at any instant. Over any cross section we know then the volume flux, and if we

assume a plausible velocity profile for the axial velocity, the velocity field is known in detail; the streamlines can then be drawn. In Fig. 34 we show the flow field at different times; no attempt has been made to attain high accuracy, since this is only a descriptive depiction. During decontraction, the flow just considered reverses exactly so that the fluid returns to its initial configuration. This flow, to some extent, favors contact with walls and to some degree increases diffusion in the fluid: this can be seen from an examination of the interaction between convective and diffusional processes through the equations for mass transfer in fluids. But more effective flow patterns are actually produced by other types of contractions. For instance, two stationary symmetric contractions that are adjacent and occur with a phase lag can produce more effective results, and also accomplish a definite transport of fluid in a certain direction. This can be demonstrated using elementary considerations.

Two stationary symmetric contractions, occurring with a lag in phase, produce flow in a certain direction. This can be shown by considering in a simplified manner the flow in a short conduit connecting two reservoirs with the same liquid level (Fig. 36). Each contraction is assumed to be cylindrical with a length equal to half the length of the connecting tube. The contractions are slow enough that inertial effects and resistive effects in the liquid can be disregarded. Then the flow can be discussed on purely kinematical grounds, including conservation of volume since the flow involves a liquid. The different phases are shown in the figure along with the volumetric displacements. If V represents the volume displaced by a single complete contraction and symmetry relative to a stagnation plane exists because of negligible inertia and resistance, the first phase introduces a volume $V/2$ in each reservoir; the second phase intro-

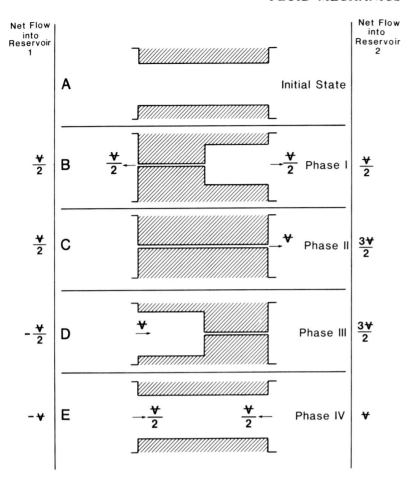

Net Flow into Reservoir 1

Net Flow into Reservoir 2

A — Initial State

$\frac{\Psi}{2}$ — B — $\frac{\Psi}{2} \leftarrow$ $\rightarrow \frac{\Psi}{2}$ Phase I — $\frac{\Psi}{2}$

$\frac{\Psi}{2}$ — C — $\rightarrow \Psi$ Phase II — $\frac{3\Psi}{2}$

$-\frac{\Psi}{2}$ — D — $\Psi \rightarrow$ Phase III — $\frac{3\Psi}{2}$

$-\Psi$ — E — $\rightarrow \frac{\Psi}{2}$ $\frac{\Psi}{2} \leftarrow$ Phase IV — Ψ

FIG. 36. Two cylindrical contractions having a phase lag in a tube that connects two reservoirs. **A** and **E** show the resting positions with both contraction units in the rest stage. **B, C,** and **D** show, respectively, the three steps of the cycle, first with only the left-hand unit occluded, then with both units occluded, and finally with only the right-hand unit occluded. The columns at the left and right indicate the fraction of the volume of the tube (Ψ) that has been displaced both to the left and to the right. The full cycle displaces one volume to the right.

duces an additional Ψ into the right-hand reservoir. At the end of the third phase, $\Psi/2$ has been taken from the left-hand reservoir and introduced into the tube. At the end of the fourth phase, an additional $\Psi/2$ enters the tube from the left-hand reservoir, and a $\Psi/2$ enters from the right-hand reservoir. Therefore a volume Ψ has left the left-hand reservoir and a volume Ψ has entered the right-hand reservoir. No wall particle has been displaced except radially; however, something has "moved" in the direction that the net volume flux occurred. Something at the wall has in fact propagated much in the way a wave propagates, or a change in shape propagates.

The preceding simplified analysis has been confirmed by much more exact calculations and by experiments, and it is basically correct (9). The preceding analysis can be extended to a case of contractions in which the same net flow is produced but in which the frequency of contractions is different in the two contracting parts of the tube. Assume now that the operation described in Fig. 35 is performed with a time period of 10 sec, the actual duration of the movements taking only 5 sec; during the remaining 5 sec one of the halves of the tube undergoes an additional contraction. This additional contraction produces no additional net flow. Therefore, there is twice the frequency of contractions in one of the segments as in the other, but the net volume flux is the

same. This should dispel the misconception that the direction of flow in the intestine is due only to differences in the frequency of contractions. It is asserted that in the presence of a gradient of contraction frequency along the intestine, the flow is directly related to such a gradient: "flow would happen from a region of high frequency towards one of low frequency." This misconception is similar to another often expressed about pressure gradients: "a fluid flows always from regions of high pressure to regions of low pressure." If this were true, water in a tank could not be at rest because the pressure is higher at the bottom than at the surface!

To illustrate the interaction between the flow induced by contractions and that driven by a pressure differential in a horizontal tube, a contraction will be assumed to occur in the middle of a tube connecting two reservoirs. The pressure difference between the ends of the tube will supposedly be due to different liquid levels in the reservoirs. The contractile segment will occupy the middle tier of the tube (Fig. 37); the other two tiers will be assumed to be rigid. The contraction is assumed to be cylindrical, to make the calculations and drawings simpler. During a period of time T, the contraction is supposed to follow some simple law like $r = R\sin 2\pi t/T$ for the variable radius r of the contractile segment. In Fig. 36, the wall is supposed to be moving inward

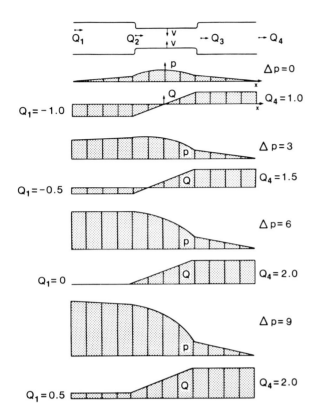

FIG. 37. Pressure diagrams and flux diagrams in a tube with a central segment that is undergoing contraction. Pressure (p) and volume (Q) have been made dimensionless. Δp is the difference in pressure imposed by the difference in fluid elevation in the two reservoirs that are connected by the tube.

and forcing fluid out to the adjacent tube segments. The use of an elementary model for the flow with parabolic velocity distribution, and the assumption that Newton's law for stresses is applicable, allow the determination of pressure variation along the tube. The volume flux is governed by conservation of volume and is easy to determine for the different cross sections. These elementary calculations have provided the results necessary to obtain the flow and pressure diagrams shown in Fig. 37. When the pressure differential is zero, the flow is symmetric as shown in Fig. 35. The pressure line, partly parabolic and partly linear, is also symmetric. One should note in this case that the volume flux varies from zero at the stagnation plane to a maximum at the ends of the contractile segment. The variation is linear, and so also must be both the shear stress at the wall and the pressure gradient. But if dp/dx is linear, a simple integration will show that the pressure p must vary as the axial distance x to the second power. In the rigid portions of the tube, the flux is constant and so is the pressure gradient; therefore the pressure varies linearly in those segments. When there is a difference in pressure between the two ends of the tube, the calculations are rather more complicated, since one must determine the position of the stagnation plane. It is found that the stagnation plane moves toward one of the ends as Δp increases. The limiting position is attained when the

flow in one of the segments is arrested. This occurs for a dimensionless Δp which is equal to 6 in the present case. For higher values of Δp, the flow is unidirectional; the pressure difference, Δp, then becomes the predominant driving force, as opposed to the pressure generated by the contraction.

It should be realized that the diagrams in Fig. 37 are valid only at a given instant of time; as the wall continues to move, they change. Similar calculations are possible for any number of contractions along a tube. In fact, by decomposing other shapes of contractions in short cylindrical components, one can extend the method to almost any shape of contraction. Computer programs can be used in such cases to investigate the flow. This methodology was used by Singerman (9) to study intestinal flow. But Singerman first tested the simplified theory in a physical model in which contractions could be produced under computer control. Figure 38 shows the results of his measurements and calculations for the physical model with two contractile segments working in a form similar to that depicted in Fig. 36.

When this model was applied to contractions which, like those of the duodenum, could be described only by using a stochastic scheme, the result was quite encouraging, since a flow of the order of those observed in the human duodenum was obtained through calculation. Much more work is still needed, but there is now some basic understanding of average flow of fluid in the intestine which can be derived from a rather simple model. More detailed information can be obtained only through much more advanced models.

Flow Induced by Longitudinal Contractions

It is difficult to illustrate in any elementary manner the flows induced by longitudinal contractions, as compared to those due to ring contractions. The wall motion is such that no volume is displaced by it; there is no positive, piston-like motion in the case of purely longitudinal contractions. The wall generates flow only

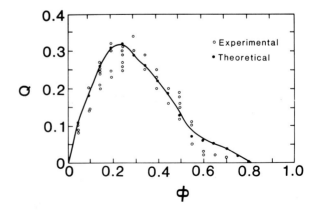

FIG. 38. Theoretical and experimental data for a set of two contractions with a phase lag, φ. The graph shows next flux, Q, as a function of the phase lag between the two contractions, φ.

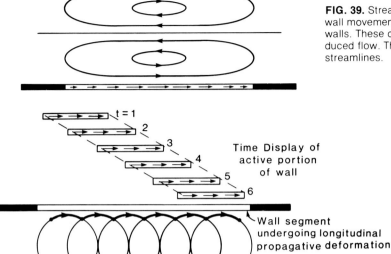

FIG. 39. Streamlines that would be generated by longitudinal axial wall movements. Displacements are indicated by the arrows in the walls. These displacements change with time, as does also the induced flow. The particle pathlines will be very different from these streamlines.

Time Display of active portion of wall

FIG. 40. Sketch of a series of hypothetical circular streamlines that could give a particular fluid particle a purely forward pathline. Actual calculations, of course, give much more complicated results, but they support this purely kinematical model.

Wall segment undergoing longitudinal propagative deformation

Centerline

through tangential diffusion of momentum, and the idea that this can cause a flow with closed streamlines is not easy to prove, but it may be supported by a heuristic argument based on a physical analysis of the flow. A case was considered before in which circulational streamlines were introduced as the only way of making the flow possible (see Fig. 33). In that example, only a minimal pressure gradient was generated. It appears quite possible, then, that local movements of the wall that are purely longitudinal may easily produce a circulatory flow pattern, the flow field tending to close on itself rather than tending to go to infinity. Of course, closed streamlines do not mean closed pathlines in temporary flows. Thus, even if one is ready to accept that longitudinal contractions may easily generate streamlines like those depicted in Fig. 39, one must still show that a transport may result if the contraction is propagative.

In Fig. 40, a propagative contraction is shown for which it is relatively easy to visualize how a particle may be transported over a certain distance, and not return to its initial position. The segment that is contracted is represented in a time display. The rest of the tube, at the left-hand side, is assumed to expand so that the wall particles may return to their initial positions. We assume that under the contractile segment, the flow can be represented by a circular streamline which is valid for a short interval of time during which the particle shown advances over a small arc. For one particle, at least, successive steps in the direction of propagation will be accomplished. Once the contraction has completed its cycle, the particle will be in a position different from the initial one. This is enough to show that the flow is irreversible, no matter how little is known about the other particles. Irreversibility is very important in connection with transport and mixing.

RESEARCH RESULTS

Flow Patterns

The formulation of the partial differential equations of fluid flow and their solution by analytical or computational methods allow reliable predictions of laminar flow. This has been done recently for two-dimensional channels in which a finite part of the wall accomplished finite amplitude displacements that simulated intestinal stationary and propagative contractions. For instance, the streamlines induced by a stationary longitudinal contraction were determined analytically and are shown in Fig. 41. This result supports the hypothesis that local wall motion may result in local fluid motion that does not extend far from the moving segment of the walls.

Streamlines due to a propagative transverse wall motion like the one depicted in Fig. 34B, as determined by computer integrative methods, are shown in Fig. 42 (10). Note that the streamlines change all the time in this

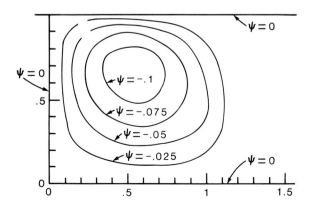

FIG. 41. Calculated streamlines produced by a stationary longitudinal contraction. Only half the flow field needs to be shown because of symmetry.

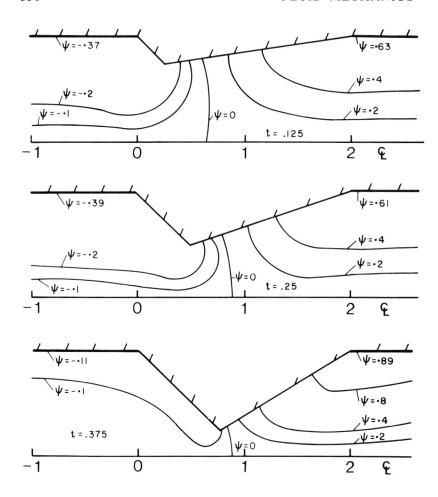

FIG. 42. Calculated streamlines for a transverse propagative contraction. Because of the way the wall moves, the near side of the shape is a part of the boundary streamline.

case. This should be expected since a changing shape propagates along the channel walls. In Fig. 40 the flow pattern is invariant; hence, as the wall returns to the initial configuration, the fluid particles must return to their initial positions, tracing backward the same pathline which they followed during the forward phase of the movement.

In Fig. 42, there is a propagative wall movement; and although the wall particles all return to their initial positions, the fluid particles are transported. They do not execute simple motions and there is usually a forward component and a backward component; but these two components differ from one another, and there is usu-

ally a net transport of particles for each complete contractile cycle. This effect is shown in Fig. 43 for a centerline particle. Since such a particle remains on the centerline, it is somewhat difficult to visualize its back-and-forth movements unless each movement is represented on a different level. One must imagine, in looking at Fig. 42, that the several movements are executed all on a single line.

TRANSPORT AND MIXING

In a flowing liquid, the rates of transfer processes and reactions are affected by the flow properties. A flow

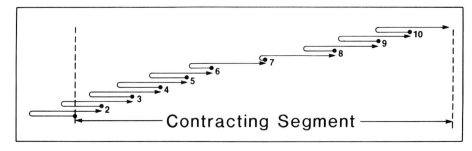

FIG. 43. Sketch showing the stepwise displacements of a fluid particle along the centerline of a tubular conduit that are caused by propagative transverse contraction. The data arise from a computational model.

that is purely uniform, amounting to a simple translation of the fluid, is not different from a fluid at rest in this respect; but a flow in which the fluid is sheared so that patterns of circulatory flow are established may greatly accelerate transfer processes and reactions. This is reflected in the convective and diffusive terms as well as in the source-sink terms in the governing equations, all terms that can increase their contributions if the flow has favorable velocity distributions. Convective mixing of chyme has been recognized as one of the functions accomplished by intestinal motility. It is therefore important to understand how mixing and transport processes can be initiated and accelerated by favorable flow patterns induced by moving walls. This is best done in an elementary manner by making some reference to analogies outside the field of fluid mechanics. The basic motion to be developed is that of mixing through orderly motions.

MIXING THROUGH ORDERLY MOTIONS

It is usually thought that without chaotic motion, or turbulence, it is difficult to accomplish substantial mixing, perhaps because it is believed that thorough mixing is a chaotic arrangement which requires a chaotic motion to be achieved. However, in a perfect mix of two substances that were initially perfectly separated, the final state is fully as orderly as the initial one. There is, therefore, nothing to prevent the achievement of perfect mixing by orderly motions if such motions are possible. Card players, when dividing the deck of cards into two equal groups and shuffling them in such a way that each card from one group slides between two from the other group, accomplish an efficient mixing in an orderly manner (Fig. 44). There is no chaotic motion involved. In a simple case like two batches of cards, one yellow and the other blue, for instance, one can easily verify that in the first such shuffling operation the mixing is already the maximum possible. In fact, if the shuffling is repeated systematically (dividing always the given set into two equal groups and shuffling in the same order), one will proceed to "demix" completely the mixed deck. These results, involving the consequence of such operations with a small number of cards, are illustrated in Fig. 44.

These examples of mixing of cards may be taken as a typical case of mixing in a one-dimensional space. One can similarly consider mixing of two-dimensional and three-dimensional objects, such as squares and cubes. The mixing of fluids requires, of course, a different kinematics than that which may be appropriate for discrete objects of fixed shape and dimensions. The kitchen may provide better inspiration than the living room for modeling the mixing of fluids. Many of the flows in culinary operations are, in fact, laminar.

Laminar Mixing

A mixing of two fluids that is accomplished without turbulence is called laminar mixing. Laminar mixing is a case of mixing through orderly motions. That laminar mixing can be accomplished effectively and by rather simple procedures can be illustrated by considering an idealized mixer not too different from some kitchenware, or from a classic viscometer. In Fig. 45 two coaxial cylinders are represented, of which the external one can be rotated. Between the two cylinders there is a viscous fluid which has been marked half dark and half light. The motion induced in the fluid by rotating one cylinder can easily be predicted; the figure shows the result after one turn, and again after two turns. It can be seen that after one turn there are already three layers, and after two turns, five layers have resulted. The law is simple: if n is the number of turns, the number of layers will be $2n + 1$. Of course, the wall motion in this example is very different from that of the intestinal wall. Moreover, if one turns back the cylinder to restore

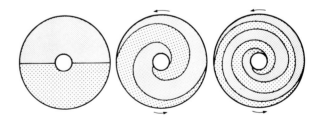

FIG. 45. Laminar mixing caused by tangential wall motion. The degree of mixing depends on the distribution of fluids at the outset: no mixing would result if the two fluid volumes were initially placed concentrically.

FIG. 44. Card shuffling as an example of orderly mixing. Two decks of 6 cards are shuffled by alternation (**B**), and the process is repeated by dividing the stack of 12 and alternating the cards again. Perfect mixing is achieved only after the first shuffle (**B**). Further shuffling causes lesser degrees of mixing as shown after the second (**C**), fourth (**D**), and fifth (**E**) shuffles. In this example, the two decks are perfectly separated after the 10th shuffle.

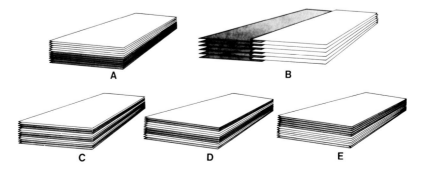

initial positions of wall particles, there is perfect reversibility in the fluid; the mixing is undone, or demixing occurs. But, as discussed above, the flow induced by propagative wall movements of a tube induces irreversible displacements in the fluid inside the tube. Laminar mixing of the type illustrated in Fig. 45 may be accomplished in the intestine, and may last long enough to accelerate transport processes and reactions. This possibility of acceleration is due to the addition of convective mixing, on which molecular diffusion is also superimposed.

The laminar mixing induced by longitudinal contractions of a propagative type is illustrated in Fig. 46 (10). The fluid is marked with variable shading to try to represent a variation in concentration of a substance in the

fluid. The Lagrangian description is presented, which was obtained from Eulerian calculation through a process of numerical integration. The actual workings of the duodenum, for which these calculations were assumed to be valid, may be much more complicated, but the fact remains that, in principle, longitudinal wall movements are able to induce laminar mixing in the fluid inside a tube; it remains to investigate the details of such processes in the intestine.

ACKNOWLEDGMENTS

This work was supported in part by Research Grant AM 08901 from the National Institutes of Health.

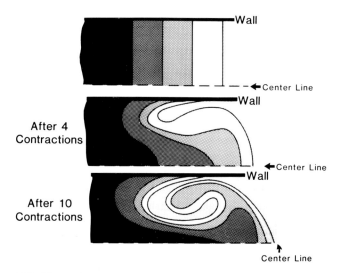

FIG. 46. Laminar mixing caused by longitudinal propagative contractions in a tubular conduit with open ends. In this computational model, the contraction is propagative from left to right. The spread of initially thick layers into thin convoluted layers elongates interfaces between fluid volumes so that diffusional mixing would be accelerated, while also directly producing convective mixing.

REFERENCES

1. Kline, S. J. (1972): Pathlines, streaklines, streamlines and timelines in steady flows. FM 47. National Committee for Fluid Mechanics Films.
2. Kline, S. J. (1972): Pathlines, streaklines and streamlines in unsteady flow. FM 48. National Committee for Fluid Mechanics Films.
3. Macagno, E. O., and Christensen, J. (1980): Fluid mechanics of the duodenum. *Annu. Rev. Fluid Mech.*, 12:139-158.
4. Macagno, E. O., and Hung, T. K. (1967): Computational and experimental study of a captive annular eddy. *J. Fluid Mech.*, 28(Part 1):43-64.
5. National Committee for Fluid Mechanics Films (1972): *Illustrated Experiments in Fluid Mechanics.* MIT Press, Cambridge, MA.
6. Rouse, H., and Ince, S. (1957): *History of Hydraulics.* Iowa Institute of Hydraulic Research, Iowa City, IA.
7. Sancholuz, A. G. (1974): A statistical study of the spike bursts on the slow wave in the duodenum. M.S. thesis, University of Iowa, Iowa City, IA.
8. Schlichting, H. (1979): *Boundary-Layer Theory, Ed. 7.* McGraw-Hill, New York.
9. Singerman, R. B. (1974): Fluid mechanics of the duodenum. Ph.D. thesis, University of Iowa, Iowa City, IA.
10. Stavitsky, D. (1979): Flow and mixing in a contracting channel with applications to the human intestine. Ph.D. thesis, University of Iowa, Iowa City, IA.

Physiology of the Gastrointestinal Tract, edited by
Leonard R. Johnson. Raven Press, New York © 1981.

Chapter 11

Motility of the Pharynx, Esophagus, and Esophageal Sphincters

Raj K. Goyal and Blaine W. Cobb

There are several excellent reviews that deal with physiology and regulation of motor activity in the pharynx and the esophagus (10,40,47,48,49,60,61,62,65,74,92, 109,124,125,146,158,181,187,255,256,339). Many of these reviews provide an in-depth analysis of certain aspects of pharyngoesophageal physiology. The purpose of this chapter is to provide an overview of current concepts regarding the physiology of the pharynx and esophagus as it relates to digestive functions. This review does not provide an unbiased cataloging of all the available data. Rather, we have attempted to synthesize the available data in a critical way. Our own conclusions are stated.

The actual quantitative data pertain primarily to humans. Quantitative animal data is included whenever appropriate. Minor species differences have been ignored; however, when major differences exist, they are pointed out. The review is organized in three segments: a) neuromuscular anatomy, b) motor activity, and c) control of motor activity.

NEUROMUSCULAR ANATOMY

Musculature

Pharynx

The pharynx is 12 to 14 cm in length, extending from the base of the skull to the lower border of the cricoid cartilage (285,343). It is predominantly a muscular structure, although the epiglottic, arytenoid, cuneiform, corniculate, and cricoid cartilages are present in the anterior wall of the hypopharynx. In addition, the thyroid and cricoid cartilages supply solid support for the anterior attachment of muscles. There are four openings that are in communication with the pharynx and are involved in deglutition: the velopharyngeal canal (62), which lies between the posterior aspect of the soft palate and the posterior pharyngeal wall, the oral cavity, the laryngeal inlet, and the opening into the esophagus. Traditionally, the pharynx has been divided into three components (255,285,343).

a. The nasopharynx, extending for approximately 3 cm between the basilar portion of the occipital bone and the soft palate.

b. The oropharynx, measuring approximately 5 cm from soft palate to the upper border of the epiglottis. Some investigators (255) consider the base of the valleculae to represent the lower border of the oropharynx; this definition is actually preferable, in the sense that with swallowing the epiglottis becomes horizontal, resulting in a different longitudinal dimension for the oropharynx and hypopharynx.

c. The laryngeal pharynx (hypopharynx), extending for 5 to 6 cm, from the base of the valleculae to the lower border of the cricoid cartilage.

The musculature of the pharynx is all striated and can be divided into intrinsic and extrinsic components for descriptive purposes.

Extrinsic muscle contributions to the functional pharyngeal anatomy include (343): (a) levator veli palatini, tensor veli palatini, and palatopharyngeus, which act in concert to raise and tense the soft palate and uvula; (b) geniohyoid, mylohyoid, digastric, stylohyoid, stylopharyngeus, salpingopharyngeus, and thyrohyoid, which cause elevation and forward displacement of the larynx and pharynx; and (c) thyroarytenoid, aryepiglottic, and oblique arytenoid muscles, which close the larynx.

Intrinsic musculature of the pharynx is represented by the superior, middle, and inferior pharyngeal constrictors. The superior pharyngeal constrictor (SPC) originates anteriorly from the pterygoid hamulus, pterygomandibular raphe, mandible, and tongue. From their origin, the fibers course posteriorly and medially, their insertion being in the median raphe. The middle pharyngeal constrictor (MPC) originates from the hyoid bone and the lower part of the stylohyoid ligament; its fibers fan out posteriorly and insert in the median raphe. It overlaps fibers from the SPC on the posterior aspect. The inferior pharyngeal constrictor (IPC) has two anatomic components, the thyropharyngeus and the cricopharyngeus. The thyropharyngeus arises from the thyroid cartilages laterally and extends posteriorly, medially, and slightly superiorly, and joins the median raphe. These fibers overlap the posterior surface of the middle constrictor. The cricopharyngeus muscle has oblique and horizontal components (255,256,343). The oblique cranial component courses posteriorly, medially, and superiorly, with its insertion in the median raphe. The horizontal component has no median raphe (255,343), and fibers arise from one side of the lower third of the cricoid cartilage, inserting on the other side, thus creating a horizontal loop of muscle. A triangular area of scanty muscle fibers is formed between the oblique and horizontal components. This area, called Killian's triangle, is the site of Zenker's diverticulum (333). For

pathophysiological purposes, only the horizontal component of the cricopharyngeus is called the cricopharyngeus (CP) muscle, whereas its oblique component along with the thyropharyngeus is considered the inferior pharyngeal constrictor; this nomenclature will be followed in our review.

When calcified, the laryngeal cartilages may be visible on plain-film radiographs. A lateral radiograph shows an air column in the nasopharynx, oropharynx, and upper part of the laryngopharynx (62). The bottom of the air column corresponds to the lower border of the laryngeal opening. The hypopharynx below it is devoid of air. A small amount of air may be seen in the esophagus. When the pharyngeal walls are coated with barium or other radiopaque material, the posterior pharyngeal wall is smooth. The anterior wall is irregular in outline, owing to the posterior nasal apertures, soft palate, oral cavity, tongue, valleculae, epiglottis, laryngeal vestibula, and the posterior surface of the cricoid cartilage (14).

Upper Esophageal Sphincter

The term upper esophageal sphincter (UES) is an operational definition given to an intraluminal zone of high pressure that exists between the pharynx and the esophageal body. Anatomically, the pharynx is continuous with the esophagus and there is no well-defined UES. The UES may include muscles of the pharynx, the esophagus, or both (8,117,256,310,339,359). The length of the upper high-pressure zone (UHPZ) is 2–4 cm (11,61, 117,136,162,256,310,339). Although all investigators seem to agree upon the cricopharyngeus (anatomical horizontal component of cricopharyngeus) as a part of the HPZ, this muscle is only approximately 1 cm in width (18,27,61,117) and, therefore, cannot of itself account for the entire HPZ. Four explanations for the discrepancy have been advanced: (a) Levitt et al. (221) consider the HPZ to be artifactually wider than the CP, because of catheter motion. (b) Other investigators (117,359) are of the opinion that a zone of circular esophageal fibers below the CP comprises the remainder of the HPZ. (c) Yet others (8) have suggested that the inferior pharyngeal constrictor, along with the CP, is responsible for the HPZ. (d) Both CP and upper fibers of the esophagus may contribute to UHPZ (61,187).

It appears that one good way to resolve the issue is simultaneously to record pressure and identify the actual anatomic structures that cause the elevated pressure. Electromyography of pharyngeal and esophageal muscle in opossums has been performed in an attempt to resolve this issue (7). A tonically contracted striated sphincter muscle should be associated with continuous electrical spike potentials, which the cricopharyngeus does show at rest (2,8,38,170,221,302). In addition, the inferior pharyngeal constrictor muscle also demonstrated continuous spike activity at rest (8). Esophageal fibers just distal to the cricopharyngeus were quiet at rest. Moreover, the manometric HPZ extended from the lower level of the cricoid cartilage to the lower border of the laryngeal opening. The muscles involved are the cricopharyngeus and IPC. These studies suggest that the UHPZ, at least in the opossum, may be anatomically a pharyngeal structure. In man, careful manometric studies have shown that the wider manometric HPZ cannot be explained by the respiratory axial movement of the narrower cricopharyngeus muscle (62). Moreover, cricopharyngeal myotomy in humans reduces but does not abolish the high pressure (180,182). Indirect evidence suggests that cricopharyngeus and inferior pharyngeal constrictor muscles may constitute the UES in man as well.

The area that extends from the laryngeal opening (bottom of the air column on a lateral X-ray of pharynx) to the lower border of cricoid cartilage is approximately 3.2 cm. The arytenoid and interarytenoid muscles extend vertically down 0.75 cm from the laryngeal opening (255). The cricoid lamina spans 2.5 cm in vertical extent below that (285), and the cricopharyngeus muscle (horizontal component) spans is present in the lower one third of the cartilage. If the UHPZ extends for ~3 cm below the air column (62), it would appear that the hypopharynx can fully account for the upper HPZ without incriminating part of the cervical esophagus. Mucosal squeeze alone may explain the small elevation of pressure extending further into the esophagus.

At rest, the anterior and posterior walls of the lower hypopharynx are closely opposed, so that plain films cannot delineate the lumen of the UES (339). With contrast material, such as barium, certain anatomic features occurring during the swallowing phase may be seen. Along the anterior wall, the uppermost portion of the cricoid cartilage (lamina) may produce an anterior indentation commencing at the C5 to C6 vertebral level. There may be an impression at the lower border of the cricoid cartilage caused by the postcricoid venous plexus (258). The posterior wall of the pharynx is smooth in the upper part. In the lower part, the cricopharyngeus muscle may sometimes form a posterior indentation termed "hypo-pharyngeal bar" at the level of C6 to C7 (33,299, 304,322). Frequently the CP is obliquely oriented and appears below the level of the lower border of the cricoid cartilage (207). This appearance is produced by upward displacement of the cricoid associated with swallowing.

Esophageal Body

Anatomically, the body of the esophagus is 20 to 22 cm long (61,220,339) and begins at the inferior border of the cricopharyngeus, extending caudally to an unclear end point, the cardiac orifice. From a functional standpoint the esophageal body extends from the lower border of the UES to the upper border of the lower esophageal sphincter (LES). In adults the upper level of the esophageal body is approximately 18 cm from the incisors; the lower level is at 40 cm (range 36–50) in males and at 37 cm (range 22–41) in females (220).

In its proximal extent, the human esophagus is composed of striated muscle in both inner circular and outer longitudinal layers. The longitudinal fibers arise from the superior aspect of the median ridge on the dorsal surface of the cricoid cartilage and are joined by muscle bundles from the cricopharyngeus and posterolateral cricoid cartilage on each lateral aspect. Fibers course dorsally and caudally to join approximately 3 cm below the cricoid cartilage posteriorly. A triangular shaped area devoid of longitudinal muscle is thus formed; this region is called Laimer's triangle (215). Laterally, the longitudinal muscle is somewhat thicker than it is on the anterior and posterior aspects (339); this discrepancy becomes less apparent as the muscle proceeds caudally. Striated muscle is replaced by smooth muscle beginning ~4 cm (range 2-6 cm) from the proximal end of the esophageal body (4,327,339). At 4 to 8 cm from the upper end, smooth and striated muscles are present in equal amounts. This mixed striated and smooth muscle extends to a point 10 to 13 cm from the lower border of the cricopharyngeus such that the distal one-half to one-third of the esophagus is entirely smooth muscle in both inner circular and outer longitudinal coats (61,220,296). Very rarely, striated muscle may extend the length of the entire esophagus (4,187). In addition, a poorly developed oblique layer (bracket fibers of Laimer) may be present internal to the inner circular muscle layer in the distal esophagus (220,360).

It has been suggested that both striated and smooth muscle have an orientation like an apolar screw system (138), but factual data are lacking. Lerche (220) describes an orientation of circular fibers which varies at different levels of the esophagus. The fibers are mostly elliptical in the upper two-thirds of the esophageal body and are arranged in spirals in the terminal part.

Although the muscle distribution in the esophageal body is similar among primates, cats, and opossum, significant differences are present when other species are examined. In the dog, rabbit, sheep, cow, guinea pig, rat, horse, and giraffe, the esophageal body is entirely striated muscle, whereas in amphibians, birds, and reptiles, it is exclusively smooth muscle (187). Such differences in anatomical composition are important in interpreting physiological data, and make inter-species extrapolation hazardous. However, histologically comparable muscle behaves with remarkable similarity in different species.

Lower Esophageal Sphincter

Like the UES, the LES is a functional structure found at the gastroesophageal junction, and can be readily identified by manometric studies as a zone of high pressure at rest. However, the anatomic structures that constitute the sphincter are not known with certainty. The junction of esophagus and stomach is called the cardiac orifice, but its anatomic landmarks are uncertain (134).

A confusing verbiage describing LES landmarks and subdivisions has been generated by anatomists, radiologists, and physiologists (134,220,225,356,360). A single scheme for correlating anatomic, radiographic, and manometric nomenclatures is shown in Fig. 1. For years, anatomists have sought an area of thickened circular muscle containing some kind of dilator fibers in the lower esophagus that could be considered the anatomic lower esophageal sphincter, but such an anatomic lower sphincter does not exist (220). Thickened muscle seen in the LES at autopsy is related to contraction; the muscle thickening disappears if the sphincter segment is distended to a size comparable to the esophageal body. After distension, a 2- to 3-mm annular band of muscle can be identified in some specimens (150,153,220). This band of circular muscle has been called the inferior esophageal sphincter (220). The inferior esophageal sphincter is covered by squamous epithelium and is located 2 to 3 cm proximal to the sling fibers which are present in the esophagogastric angle on the left side of the stomach (150). Although direct evidence is lacking, indirect studies support the view that the inferior esophageal sphincter forms the uppermost part of the LES, and its distal extent may be marked by the upper portion of the sling fibers. Radiographically, the inferior esophageal sphincter may correspond to a muscular ring (150, 153), and the squamocolumnar junction may be identified in association with a mucosal ring. The location of squamocolumnar junction and mucosal ring in relation to lower esophageal sphincter has been a topic of considerable controversy (58,147,150,211,255). Liebermann-Meffert et al. (222) found an area of muscle thickening (which they termed the gastroesophageal ring—GER)

approximately 3 cm wide on the greater curvature and 2.3 cm wide along the lesser curve. Asymmetry in thickness and width was noted. This "ring" is similar to the "collar of Helvetius" described by earlier investigators (255). That region is covered by columnar mucosa, the squamocolumnar junction being located 2.5 cm proximally. Studies using simultaneous manometric and potential difference recordings or mucosal biopsies (to identify the squamocolumnar junction) do not lend support to the view that the squamocolumnar junction is located 2.5 cm proximal to the LES (115,345).

Electron microscopic studies of the sphincter muscle show that the muscle fibers have irregular surfaces and evaginations, which are not seen in the circular muscle of the esophageal body. The surface evaginations may be related to the tonically contracted state of the sphincter muscle (300).

The longitudinal muscle in the lower esophagus shows no distinctive features. Laterally, the fibers follow the greater curvature on the left and lesser curvature on the right. Anteriorly and posteriorly, however, the muscle bundles turn upward, in the direction of the fundus, and interlace with fibers of the inner circular layer (222,255). Obliquely oriented "bracket fibers" similar to those seen in the terminal esophageal body can be found inside the circular muscle layer; such fibers do not extend into the stomach (150,220).

Innervation

Efferent Innervation

Pharynx and upper esophageal sphincter.

Motor neurons supplying the pharynx are located in five major groups (343,346): the trigeminal motor nu-

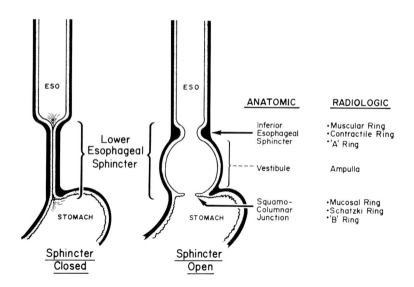

FIG. 1. Suggested scheme for anatomic and radiologic landmarks of the lower esophageal sphincter. From Goyal, ref. 146.

cleus; the facial nucleus; the nucleus ambiguous of the vagus; the hypoglossal nucleus; and spinal cord segments C1 to C3. Cranial nerves are involved in delivery of motor fibers peripherally. The trigeminal nerve innervates the mylohyoid, tensor veli palatini, and digastricus muscles; the facial nerve supplies the stylohyoid and the posterior belly of the digastricus; the glossopharyngeal nerve innervates the stylopharyngeus; the vagus supplies the levator veli palatini, IPC, MPC, SPC, palatopharyngeus, salpingopharyngeus, thyroarytenoid, and arytenoid muscles; and the hypoglossal nerve innervates the thyrohyoid and geniohyoid muscles. (Innervation of the CP is discussed separately.) The accessory nerve actually contains the roots of motor fibers destined for the palatine musculature, but these fibers join the vagus a short distance past their emerging from the medulla with the accessory nerve and, hence, have been grouped with the vagus (343).

Pharyngeal muscles are very richly innervated. The nerve-muscle fiber innervation ratio for pharyngeal muscles has been determined in rabbits (113) and is in the range of 1:4 to 1:6 for the IPC and 1:2 to 1:4 for SPC and MPC. These figures contrast with a ratio of 1:2000 for human gastrocnemius (122). The nerve-muscle fiber ratio for pharyngeal muscles is higher than the ratio (1:9) for extraocular eye muscles (122). This is appropriate for the very "fine" control achieved in pharyngeal muscle response.

Because of the special sphincteral function assigned to the CP, its innervation has aroused special interest. The CP is innervated by vagal fibers. In the dog and the cat, a separate branch of the vagus, the pharyngoesophageal nerve, supplies motor innervation to the CP (186, 208,233,249), but similar fibers have not been identified in humans (234,235). In the past, some observers claimed that CP was innervated by autonomic nerves (208). Parasympathetic fibers were thought to arise from cell bodies in the dorsal motor nucleus of the vagus and reach the CP via the recurrent laryngeal nerves. Sympathetic nerves were also thought to innervate CP and to cause tonic contraction. These suggestions have not been supported. It is likely that the cell bodies of the motor fibers to CP are located in the nucleus ambiguus and the motor fibers are carried in the vagus nerves.

Esophageal body.

Striated muscle. The striated muscle part of the esophagus, like other skeletal muscles, is innervated by somatic motor fibers (109,138,346). These nerve fibers make direct contact with individual muscle fibers at motor end plates. No synapse or second-order neuron is involved in the pathway. Cell bodies of somatic efferents that innervate the skeletal muscle of the proximal esophagus, like those for the pharynx, are located in the nucleus ambiguus (109,217,218). Efferent fibers are car-

ried in the vagus nerves, and these fibers are myelinated. Acetylcholine is the neurotransmitter involved at the neuromuscular junction, and its effects are mediated by nicotinic receptors. Curare and succinyl choline block the neuromuscular transmitter (48,183).

Smooth muscle. The smooth muscle part of the esophagus is supplied by autonomic nerves. The autonomic path consists of efferent axons that reach the esophageal wall and make contacts with cell bodies present in the wall of the esophagus. It is therefore convenient to describe this autonomic pathway in terms of extrinsic and intrinsic nerves.

Extrinsic innervation. Vagal and sympathetic fibers comprise the extrinsic nervous system of the esophagus. Preganglionic parasympathetic fibers destined for the esophageal body take their origin in cell bodies located in the dorsal motor nucleus, located in the floor of the fourth ventricle of the medulla oblongata (3). As the vagi course through the thorax, branches leave to innervate the lung and heart; vagal fibers also distribute themselves over the esophageal body in a plexiform arrangement. Fibers regroup 1 to 4 cm above the diaphragm, forming the anterior and posterior gastric nerves (257). Branches from the esophageal plexus innervate the esophagus. The sympathetic nerve supply to the esophageal body arises from cell bodies in the intermediolateral cell columns of spinal segments T5 and T6 (346). Preganglionic fibers enter the cervical ganglia and ganglia in the thoracic sympathetic chain. Postganglionic branches accompany blood vessels; a few fibers join the vagus and reach the esophagus. Most of the axons terminate in the myenteric plexus (19,190), but a supply to the submucosal plexus has also been demonstrated (138). Very few of these branches are distributed directly to the muscle layers.

Intrinsic innervation. Intramural neurons and their extensions make up the intrinsic innervation of the esophagus. Nerves are arranged in layers, of which the myenteric plexus (Auerbach's) and submucosal plexus (Meissner's) are the major networks. Auerbach's plexus has been found as high as 1 cm from the cricopharyngeus in the esophageal body of humans (296). The function of intramural ganglia located in the striated muscle segment is not known. They are sparse in that location and may supply innervation to esophageal glands, or they may be involved in sensory function. The intramural ganglia are similar in arrangement throughout the gut, but in the esophagus intramural neurons are fewer in number and more haphazard in arrangement than elsewhere in the gut (137,308).

Intramural neurons have been classified on the basis of morphologic, histochemical, functional, and electrical differences (149). Their affinity for silver stains divides these neurons into two types. Five to twenty percent of all enteric neurons are argyrophilic as they stain well with silver stains; argyrophobes, which do not stain well with silver, comprise 80-95% (308). Axons from the intramural nerves extend to smooth muscle cells and other effector cells. Multiple branches take off en route to the effector cells, where synaptic contact is signaled by the appearance of varicosities in the fibers. The varicosities are filled with neurotransmitter granules. Based upon their size and other morphological characteristics, the vesicles have been classified into small agranular, small granular, and large opaque vesicles. Small agranular, small granular, and large opaque vesicles are believed to contain acetylcholine, norepinephrine, and noncholinergic, nonadrenergic neurotransmitter respectively. The noncholinergic, nonadrenergic neurotransmitter may be ATP or a related purine (purinergic) or a neuropeptide (peptidergic). Small granular and large opaque vesicles are frequently present in different proportions in the same varicosity (300).

Lower esophageal sphincter.

The extrinsic nerves to the LES have parasympathetic and sympathetic representation. Parasympathetic fibers originate in the dorsal motor nucleus of the vagus and reach the LES through the vagus to synapse with intramural neurons. Sympathetic nerves influencing the LES have cell bodies in intermedio-lateral cell columns T6 to T10. Their preganglionic axons course in the greater splanchnic nerves, synapsing with postganglionic nerves in the celiac ganglia (19,131). These fibers reach the LES with blood vessels destined for this region, and most of them are connected to intramural ganglia; a few fibers may supply direct innervation to the sphincter muscle. It is not known if the distribution of intrinsic neural elements in the LES is similar to that in the esophageal body. It is also not known whether the neurons in the LES are morphologically or chemically different from those in the esophageal body.

Afferent Innervation

Sensory receptors in the pharynx have not been well characterized; however, a gamma-efferent system is not present, except perhaps in the tensor veli palatini (109). Afferent fibers project to the spinal tract of the trigeminal nerve and to the fasciculus and nucleus solitarius. Trigeminal fibers descend to enter the solitary nucleus in monkey, cat, and rat (325). Vagal and glossopharyngeal nerves carry afferent fibers directly to the nucleus solitarius (260); some may cross and enter the contralateral nucleus solitarius and some enter the commissural nucleus of Cajal (31,206,325). Projections beyond these locations are obscure; presumably, relays to the so-called deglutition center culminate in input to the motor nuclei and reflex action.

Sensation from the upper esophagus is carried by parasympathetic fibers. Sympathetic fibers accompany afferent nerves from the lower esophagus (346). Most fibers are myelinated; their mode of transmission and distribution is, however, largely unknown. Mechanoreceptors have been demonstrated in the wall of the cat esophagus (240), and indirect evidence suggests that other sensory receptors, such as osmoreceptors and free nerve endings may be present in the UES, LES, and esophageal body of humans (75,135,139,179,193,194, 200,230,342). However, the precise nature of the receptors and their extrinsic connections is not known.

MOTOR ACTIVITY

Methods of Study

Pharyngoesophageal activities have been studied in several ways. First, intraluminal pressure can be monitored by use of water-filled catheters, catheter-tip miniature transducers, or small balloons. Because of technical problems, balloons are no longer used (103,279,301). In the past, the catheters employed were unperfused or had poor compliance. Such systems were particularly unsuitable for recording high-frequency events in the pharynx, and led to underestimation of the amplitude of pressure transients (98,103,279). Low-compliance, perfused catheter systems (6,157,353) or catheter-tip transducers are currently the most frequently used recording methods. A sleeve catheter for long-term recording (88) and other catheter modifications (340) for recording sphincter pressure have been described.

The intraluminal pressures obtained in a hollow tube like the esophagus, which is potentially open at either end, have a significance different from that of pressures measured in closed fluid-filled cavities, such as cardiac chambers or blood vessels. The intraluminal pressures in the esophagus are due to direct squeeze by the esophageal muscle on the pressure-sensitive catheter tip, whereas in the heart, for instance, pressure is transmitted to the catheter via the relatively incompressible fluid component (blood). Therefore, intraluminal pressure reflects the squeeze due to tension that is developed in the circular muscle.

In most circumstances, the pressures reflect isometric changes in muscle tone. The magnitude of isometric tone in the circular muscle is related to its length. The mechanical properties (151) and length-tension relationships have been explored for esophageal body and lower esophageal sphincter (25,26) and will be described later in this chapter.

Second, passage of a bolus of swallowed barium can be followed on pictures made in rapid succession by cineradiography (11,55,62,287); thus, the time sequence of events can be determined. Simultaneous manometric and pressure studies show that peristaltic contractile activity follows the tail of the barium bolus (62). Movement through the sphincters occurs while they are relaxed. Therefore, at the time of recorded manometric contraction, the bolus of barium has already passed the segment of the gullet under study. After a barium swallow, radiographic activity may persist for ~10 sec but manometric activity lasts up to ~20 sec. Recently, a scintigraphic technique for quantitating esophageal transit has been described (204,324).

Third, myoelectrical activity can be recorded using bipolar or monopolar electrodes (5,44,168,169,170,221, 281,283). In experimental animals, electrodes are sewn to the outside of the esophagus after dissection (59,140). Electrical activity can also be recorded intraluminally by means of bipolar electrodes; however, the recordings with such a system are not very satisfactory. In any case, electrical recordings generally provide a more precise measure of onset of muscle activity than the peristaltic pressure wave itself, because other pressure changes such as those transmitted by a bolus or arising in extrinsic structures may precede the actual peristaltic wave. In the striated muscle, electrical activity and mechanical activity are practically coincident. Electrical activity in these muscles is present throughout the period of contraction and the intensity of spike activity is related to the strength of the contraction. In the smooth muscle, also, electrical and mechanical contractions are generally coupled. However, electromechanical dissociation may sometimes occur (140).

Electrical activity in the smooth muscle segment leads the mechanical activity by a small latency interval (140). Moreover, spike activity ceases at or near the peak of muscle contraction (339); the descending phase of the peristaltic contraction is not associated with spike activity (140).

Fourth, peristaltic propulsive force (i.e., the force with which a solid bolus in the esophagus is moved along the longitudinal axis during peristalsis) has been studied by using an intraluminal, fixed balloon attached to a device that measures pull (184,295,355). The peristaltic propulsive force may be related to an aborally directed force on the stationary distending object in the esophagus. This force appears soon after distension of a fixed balloon in the esophagus and has also been called the esophageal propulsive force. It is converted into a propagated propulsive wave which propels the distending balloon when the latter is allowed to dislodge.

Resting Phase

At rest, the pharynx functions as a conduit for the passage of air into and out of the tracheobronchial tree. The upper esophageal sphincter remains closed and prevents entrance of inspired air into the esophagus (162).

The esophageal body remains quiescent and may contain small amounts of air and secretions. The LES also remains closed and guards against reflux of gastric contents into the esophagus (127).

Pharynx

The resting pressure in the upper pharynx is near atmospheric. Slight changes in pharyngeal pressure, from +1.4 mm Hg with expiration to -0.2 mm Hg with inspiration, reflect pressure variations during inflow of atmospheric air into the lungs during inspiration and outflow of expired gas during expiration (162,339).

Several pharyngeal muscles are active in breathing. This activity is best demonstrated with electromyography. The stylopharyngeus, cricothyroid, and sternothyroid muscles "fire" during inspiration (2). Asphyxia results in recruitment of the palatopharyngeus, geniohyoid, and MPC to the inspiratory effort (110).

Upper Esophageal Sphincter

The UES is closed at rest. The closure pressure varies somewhat with the experimental circumstances in which measurements are made. The high pressure zone (HPZ) begins immediately below the hypopharyngeal air column and extends caudally for 2 to 4 cm (11,61,117,136, 162,207,256,310,346). The pressure profile along the HPZ shows a sharp ascent in the upper part and a more gradual decline in its lower portions (162,310).

The pressure profile of the UES shows marked radial and axial asymmetry (8,349,352). The peak pressures are much higher when the catheter tip faces either the anterior or posterior walls than when the tip is oriented laterally. Welch and colleagues (349) constructed a three-dimensional pressure profile during suspended breathing, using a manometric catheter with multiple radially arranged holes at the same level withdrawn at a fixed speed across the upper HPZ. This three dimensional profile of the human UES depicts the radial and axial asymmetries very clearly (Fig. 2). Peak pressure occurs below the beginning of the HPZ 1 cm anteriorly and 2 cm posteriorly. Radial and axial asymmetry was not observed after laryngectomy, suggesting that the relatively rigid cartilages of the larynx forming the anterior wall of the UES were responsible for the asymmetric pressures (349).

When a manometric catheter is positioned at various levels in the UES and the patient is breathing quietly, baseline pressure fluctuations are observed. Near the peak in the HPZ the pressure increases with inspiration, whereas on either side of the peak, the pressure falls with inspiration (162). The average increase in peak pressure with inspiration in an unoriented catheter system is approximately 6.5 mm Hg (162). Axial movement

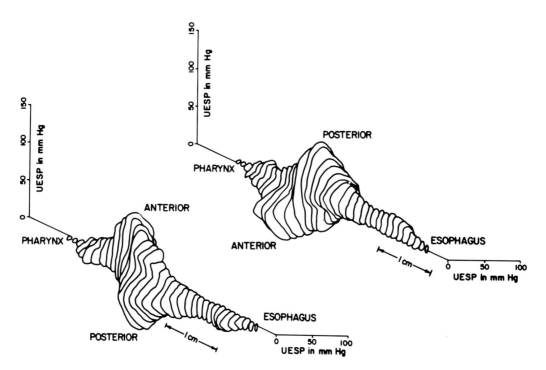

FIG. 2. Three-dimensional pressure profiles of the upper esophageal sphincter pressure. Note that pressures are higher in arterio-posterior orientation than on the sides. From Welch, ref. 349.

of the larynx during respiration does not appear to cause major modifications of UES pressure.

It is difficult to provide a single value for resting UES pressure because the recorded value may vary with: the location of the catheter tip within the UES with regard to its radial orientation and axial location; respiratory phase; diameter of catheter assembly, size of the pressure sensing hole, and to some extent, the fidelity of the recording system; spontaneous and reflex alterations in UES tone; and characteristics of the "normal" subjects used for studies.

In healthy normal medical personnel, anterior and posterior pressures during suspended respiration were approximately 100 mm Hg in one study (352) and 130 mm Hg in another study (349). Laterally, the pressures were one-third as much.

Using a non-oriented intraluminal strain gauge system or high fidelity perfused recording systems, UES pressures have been reported as being approximately 35 mm Hg (98). Older, hospitalized patients admitted for "other than esophageal disease" are likely to have much lower pressures.

Electromyographic studies show continuous spike activity in the cricopharyngeus (2, 8, 38, 221, 302, 339) and the inferior pharyngeal constrictor (8). A brief increase in spike activity lasting ~0.2 sec and corresponding to the brief inspiratory effort associated with swallowing may be observed (38, 339). The intensity of spike activity is directly proportional to the intraluminal pressure.

Esophageal Body

The pressure in the esophageal body varies with respiration. These pressures vary from -5 to -15 mm Hg with inspiration to -2 to $+5$ mm Hg with expiration (61,181). The intraesophageal pressures closely reflect intrapleural pressures, and pulmonary physiologists have long made estimates of intrapleural pressure from measurements of intraesophageal pressures. In general, however, intraesophageal pressures are slightly higher than intrapleural pressures at the same site.

Manometric recordings from the esophagus may also demonstrate extrinsic pressures caused by the aorta and heart (328). Aortic pulsations observed in the middle and lower third of the esophagus, including LES, are caused by the aortic arch and descending aorta respectively. Left atrial and ventricular pulsation may also be transmitted. These extraesophageal events are best seen in balloon recordings. Cardiovascular pressure events affecting the esophageal pressure measurement can be easily recognized by the frequency of pressure elevations. Electromyographically, the esophageal body is quiescent at rest. Sometimes rhythmic activity with each inspiration may be observed.

Lower Esophageal Sphincter

The lower esophageal sphincter (LES) is kept closed at rest and creates a zone of high pressure. A profile of LES pressure, including its length and peak amplitude, can be made conveniently during suspended breathing by withdrawing the manometric catheter with a motorized system at a fixed speed across the LES. The high pressure zone due to LES pressure distribution has a bell-shaped configuration. The total length of the HPZ varies from 2 to 4 cm.

If multiple catheters with openings oriented in different directions are used, it is found that the LES pressure is also asymmetrical but the asymmetry is not as marked as in the UES. The sphincter is fairly symmetrical in its upper half but in the lower half shows higher pressures on the left side (350,351).

The cause of the radial pressure asymmetry in the LES is not fully understood. Part of this asymmetry is clearly related to mechanical factors. For example, the terminal esophagus is not aligned with the axis of the rest of the esophagus but is angled like a hockey stick as it joins the stomach. Moreover, the diaphragm makes an impression on the terminal esophagus which is directed downward and to the right. These factors may be responsible for the higher pressure recorded on the left side of the LES.

Some asymmetry exists even after the influence of the diaphragm is excluded, as in patients with hiatal hernia or animals with an entirely intraabdominal LES. The cause of this residual asymmetry is not fully explained but may be related to the spiral nature of the circular fibers in the LES. The other possibility is that the gastric sling fibers may pull on the left side of the LES, which may explain the higher pressures recorded there. Such an arrangement may be analogous to that of a torus with one wall under tension.

If a catheter tip is positioned at a single site in the LES and recordings are made for a period of time, it becomes clear that LES pressure is not a steady line. The recorded pressures show rhythmic variations. The most prominent pressure fluctuations are those related to the respiratory cycle. In humans, the pressures in the upper and lower halves of the LES are affected by respiration in opposite ways. In the lower part, inspiration causes an increase in pressure, whereas in the upper part, a fall in pressure with inspiration is observed. The point at which this respiratory pressure transition occurs is called the point of respiratory reversal (PRR) or the pressure inversion point (PIP). Frequently, respiratory reversal occurs over a wider region which shows biphasic pressure changes with respiration. This zone is ~0.5 cm wide and usually is located in the middle of the HPZ, but its precise location is variable (167).

The terminal esophagus moves up and down with respiration, moving down with inspiration and up with expiration (29, 105). Because of the bell-shaped profile of the LES high pressure zone the measured pressure changes as a result of movement of different LES sites in relation to the catheter hole. This phenomenon may explain in part inspiratory increase in pressure in the lower part, and an inspiratory reduction in pressure in the upper part of the sphincter.

The PRR may be related to: a) the diaphragm, which separates thoracic from abdominal cavities that provide opposing pressure environments during respiration, b) axial movement of LES, c) the LES, as it separates intraesophageal from intragastric pressure, or d) some combination of the above factors.

In addition to the axial movement, a normally intrahiatally placed LES may be influenced by the contraction of the diaphragmatic sling. Transient peaks or contractions with inspiration are frequently observed in relation to the esophageal hiatus. The pressure inversion point, usually present in the region of the HPZ, is also related to the esophageal hiatus. The lower esophageal sphincter pressure (LESP) is influenced by the environmental pressure within which it resides. In patients with hiatus hernia, double respiratory reversal may be observed. It seems that the esophageal hiatus can produce a respiratory reversal in absence, destruction, or displacement of the LES but the LES itself may also be associated with a respiratory reversal (167). Under normal circumstances, both the axial movement of the LES and the esophageal hiatus may contribute to the point of respiratory reversal.

In experimental animals, respiration-related increases in LESP may occur that are related neither to axial movement nor to extrinsic pressure changes (9).

In addition to respiration-related pressure changes, the LES also shows rhythmic pressure changes that occur at a slow rate of 3 to 4 per min. These pressure changes are clearly observed during long term recordings in animals (159) and they also occur in humans (Goyal, *unpublished observations*). These pressure changes can sometimes be confused with swallow related LES relaxation. This error can be easily avoided by keeping the phenomenon in mind. In addition to these variations, phasic elevations in pressure related to the migrating myoelectrical complex have also been described (189).

Because of pressure fluctuations related to respiration and other variables, it is hard to validate a single value for LESP. Moreover, there are variations due to recording methods, diameter of the recording catheter, fidelity of the recording system, and difficulty in ensuring complete elimination of axial motion artifact caused by movement of the LES in relation to the recording tip. Furthermore, characteristics of the "normal" controls may vary in different studies.

Several different scoring methods have been proposed to obtain a "single" reliable value for sphincter pressure. Some observers suggest using rapid pull through (RPT) in which the manometric catheter is rapidly pulled across the LES during suspended respiration. The major problem with this technique is that it records the LESP only at a single point in time. It would not record any changes in pressure due to variations in the intrinsic tone of the LES muscle. Furthermore, the phase and depth of the respiratory cycle at which RPT is performed cannot be precisely controlled. Also, the technique fails to record LES relaxations. In addition, if the patient happens to swallow or have a secondary peristalsis at the time of the pull through, the contraction in the esophageal body may spuriously be taken as the high pressure. Recent studies have shown that this technique produces great variability in LESP value when repeated measurements are made in the same subject. It is not surprising that the results obtained with this technique correlate poorly with other scoring methods for LESP (350).

The standard station pull through (SPT) technique, in which pressures are measured at each 0.5 cm station by pulling the catheter out 0.5 cm at a time, or the slow, motorized, continuous pull through method show sphincter pressure profiles with respiration related fluctuations in pressure. In such a tracing measurement can be made at the point of respiratory reversal, at the highest peak pressure or the highest mean pressure. In general, the results obtained by these methods correlate reasonably well with each other and have coefficients of variation superior to those obtained with rapid pull through (350). Scoring of peak pressures is convenient, and it has a low interobserver variability as compared to the determination of pressures at respiratory reversal (350).

From a practical standpoint, the axial movement of the HPZ in relation to recording device will allow scanning of the high pressure peak as it moves across the pressure sensitive tip. This peak would be scanned by the sensor as long as the sensor is within .5 to 1 cm above or below the peak (105,351).

It is generally not possible to identify the LES radiographically even with the use of radioopaque material. This is because swallow of radioopaque material or esophageal placement of radioopaque material causes relaxation and opening of the LES. The LES may, however, be located on radiographs in patients with achalasia and in other patients with transient abnormalities in relaxation.

Electromyographic studies have shown that the opossum LES has continuous spike activity which is inhibited during LES relaxation (9). The role of spike activity in the genesis of LES pressure is described later.

Active Phase

Deglutition Reflex: Primary Peristalsis

The action of swallowing is preceded by the delivery of an appropriate size and amount of food from the oral cavity after mastication and mixing with saliva. The bolus of food is positioned on the middle of the dorsum of the tongue. The swallowing process is then ready to start. This process can be divided into voluntary and involuntary components. The voluntary component or oral phase consists of transport of the bolus to the oropharynx. This is achieved by a wave-like contraction that starts from the anterior part of the tongue and moves backward, squeezing the bolus against the hard palate and propelling it toward the oropharynx. The posterior part of the tongue is depressed to form a grooved chute. As the bolus moves backwards, sensory receptors are activated which initiate the involuntary phase of the deglutition reflex.

Deglutition is a reflex which, once initiated, is completed involuntarily. The motor expression of the deglutitive reflex is called primary peristalsis and begins with the onset of mylohoid activity. Deglutitive activity in different pharyngoesophageal segments is described below.

Pharynx.

The nasopharynx shows no intraluminal pressure change with deglutition. However, apposition of soft palate and posterior pharyngeal wall causes a single contractile wave with a peak of ~160 mm Hg. This contraction in the velopharyngeal tunnel lasts over .9 sec (98). This contraction is the beginning of the peristaltic wave. The contraction of the posterior pharyngeal wall is called the Passavant's ridge. The peristaltic wave travels down the oropharynx and hypopharynx at an approximate speed of 15 cm/sec to reach the UES in approximately 0.67 sec (98).

In the oropharynx, the peristaltic wave is immediately preceded by a pressure transient called t-wave which is due to propulsion of the bolus by the tongue into the oropharynx (62,339). The magnitude of this wave depends upon the volume of the bolus and may not be seen with a "dry" swallow. This wave is seen approximately 0.3 sec after onset of a swallow and appears as a small peak on the ascending limb of peristaltic contraction. The peristaltic wave itself has a peak amplitude of 110 ± 60 mm Hg and lasts 0.9 sec in the oropharynx.

The hypopharyngeal area may show two distinct pressure events during swallowing apart from the main peristaltic wave (62,339). Presence of these waves may also be dependent on the size and type of bolus. First, a pressure wave of small magnitude (~10 mm Hg) and duration (0.2 sec) occurs concomitantly with elevation of the larynx; it has therefore been called an e-wave. However, this is also the period during which brief inspiratory effort accompanying the onset of swallowing takes place. The e-wave, therefore, may be related to inspiratory contraction of hypopharyngeal muscles. Next, a second wave of pressure increase is seen. This wave corresponds to movement of the bolus into the pharynx due to the action of the tongue and it occurs approximately .3 sec after onset of the swallow, nearly simultaneous with the t-wave in the oropharynx.

The hypopharyngeal peristaltic wave has a peak amplitude of around 200 ± 150 mm Hg with a mean duration of 0.3 to 0.5 sec (98). Note that these durations of contractions are shorter than those observed in the upper part of the pharynx. In the upper part of the pharynx, the longer duration is probably due to the fusion of the t-wave with the peristaltic wave.

Radiographic phenomena in the pharynx have been documented carefully (62). The radiographically-derived time sequences correlate closely with those observed with manometric and electromyographic studies (Table 1). The bolus usually reaches the cricopharyngeus around 0.3 sec (0.13 to 0.63 sec) after the onset of swallowing and is usually cleared by 0.5 to 1 sec. The velocity of the bolus ejected from the pharynx is dependent upon the volume that is swallowed (123) and gravity (188).

As far as electrical activity is concerned, the first detectable action in swallowing is believed to be activity in the mylohyoid muscle. The onset of activity in mylohyoid precedes that in other muscles by 30 to 40 milliseconds (110). Sometimes other muscles of deglutition that are innervated by the trigeminal nerve start simultaneously with the mylohyoid activity (109). Subsequently, there is activity in other suprahyoid muscles (geniohyoid palatopharyngeus, palatoglossus, superior constrictor, and posterior tongue) (110,202). These muscles constitute the "leading complex" of the motor component of deglutition (28). The total duration of activity in the muscles of the leading complex varies with an average of 0.5 sec. The pharyngeal constrictors fire in overlapping sequence. The action in the middle con-

strictor starts 0.2 sec and in the inferior constrictor it starts 0.5 sec after the onset of deglutition. The duration of activity in pharyngeal constrictors is around .5 sec (17). The total duration of pharyngeal activity is around one second. The electrical events are somewhat faster than manometric and radiographic events. This may be related to differences in experimental conditions.

Upper esophageal sphincter.

The upper sphincter opens with each swallow to allow passage of the bolus into the esophagus. Pressure recordings demonstrate a fall in UES pressure soon after the onset of swallowing (136). Pressure may reach subatmospheric levels (11,136,310) but does not reach intraesophageal levels. Occasionally a short period (0.2s) of slight increase in UES tone may precede the deglutitive relaxation (38,136). The significance of this is unclear, but such a pattern may commonly be recorded in laryngectomized humans (302). This may be related to inspiratory contraction of the cricopharyngeus. The nadir in UES pressure may be interrupted by a brief increase in pressure which corresponds to the backward movement of the tongue (t-wave). The manometrically recorded relaxation lasts 0.5 to 1.0 sec (187) and afterward is followed by a contraction which produces an elevation in pressure approximately two times the resting levels which persists for another one second (61). Resting UES pressure then resumes.

Electromyographically, inhibition in CP activity starts 0 to 0.2 sec after deglutition and persists for 0.5 (0.2-0.8) sec. This is followed by a spike burst that lasts for 1 sec. (338,339). Tonic UES firing returns to resting levels after this burst (Fig. 3).

Esophageal body.

The initial pressure change that accompanies a swallow is a negative deflection beginning around 0.2 sec after onset of swallowing and lasting for 0.3 to 0.5 sec (337,338). This wave is 5 to 10 mm Hg in amplitude. It occurs simultaneously with a drop in pleural pressure and is best recorded in the proximal esophageal body. It is not seen with all swallows and is more frequently recorded in elderly individuals than in younger subjects. Because of the concomitant decrease in intrathoracic pressure, it is felt that a short inspiration immediately preceding swallowing, called "schluckatmung," accounts for this initial negative wave.

After this initial negative deflection a positive pressure change is seen in 87% of the swallows (35). This small positive wave is recorded best in the proximal esophagus and is attributed to transmission of pharyngeal pressures through the swallowed bolus and may be more prominent with liquid swallows. It occurs 0.5 to 1 sec after the onset of swallowing. This wave may occur as a discrete peak or may plateau into a second positive

TABLE 1. *Timing of movement of deglutition as observed cinefluorographically in man*

Movement	Sec Range	(Mean)
First contact of bolus with posterior pharynx	.03–.10	(.05)
Maximal elevation of larynx	.07–.57	(.20)
Start of pharyngeal contraction wave	0.7–.53	(.20)
First contact of tongue with posterior pharynx	.10–.50	(.23)
Bolus reaches cricopharyngeus	.13–.63	(.30)
Start of descent of larynx	.27–1.00	(.54)
Bolus fully past cricopharyngeus	.33–1.00	(.67)
Disappearance of pharyngeal contraction	.36–1.03	(.67)
Larynx in position of rest	.40–1.07	(.74)

Based on data of Christrup (55) as cited by Doty (109).
Appearance of bolus below mandible taken as time zero.
Calculated from frames at 30 per sec.

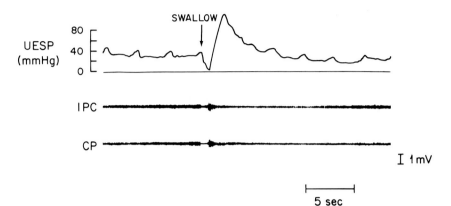

FIG. 3. Simultaneous manometric and electromyographic recordings from opossum upper esophageal sphincter. Note that swallowing is associated with fall in UES pressure and inhibition of ongoing spike activity in the cricopharyngeus (CP) and inferior pharyngeal constrictor (IPC) muscles. Also note increased activity following inhibition as the corresponding increase in pressure. From Asoh and Goyal (*unpublished*).

wave. The second positive pressure component is best demonstrated in the distal esophageal body and is rarely, if ever, recorded in the proximal third. Approximately 33% of the swallows may reveal this waveform. Its incidence can be increased by obstructing the gastroesophageal opening with a tube before swallowing (337). This wave begins 1 to 2 sec after the onset of swallowing. This observation, along with its site of occurrence, is felt to be evidence that the wave is produced by compression of the lower esophageal segment between the advancing bolus and LES. This point needs further investigation.

The third or terminal esophageal pressure wave accompanying deglutition is a larger positive signal which represents the main peristaltic wave. This deflection corresponds to esophageal contraction and as such is the single constant pressure correlate of esophageal deglutitive activity. The amplitude, velocity, and duration of this wave varies with the esophageal segment from which the recording is obtained. The average speed of peristalsis is ~4 cm/sec, but it varies in different esophageal segments. Peristaltic speed is approximately 3 cm/sec in the upper esophagus, accelerates to 5 cm/sec and then slows again to 2.5 cm/sec just above the LES (178). The peristaltic wave reaches the LES in 5 to 6 sec after swallowing (178). The duration of the pressure wave is 2–4 sec and it increases down the esophagus. Peristaltic pressure wave amplitude has been assigned a wide range of values by various investigators due in part to differing recording methods. Using an intraesophageal transducer system, lower esophageal pressure peaks of 69.5 ± 12.1 (SE) mm Hg, mid-esophageal values of 35.0 ± 6.4 mm Hg, and upper esophageal values of 53.4 ± 9.0 mm Hg were found (178). The peristaltic pressure trough was in the region corresponding to the junction of striated and smooth muscle.

The amplitude and propagation of the peristaltic wave may be influenced by several factors. Within the same individual, peristaltic amplitude remains reasonably constant when examined serially (251). In elderly patients, however, amplitude may be diminished (177).

Bolus volume (101,176) and temperature (86,354), intraabdominal pressure (102), recording fidelity (103), and site all significantly influence recorded pressure amplitude and speed of propagation. Electromyographic recordings show that electrical spikes correlate well with esophageal contractions with some variations between smooth and striated muscle (169,339).

Lower esophageal sphincter.

Deglutition causes relaxation of the lower esophageal sphincter. The relaxation may start with the onset of deglutition so that both upper and lower sphincters relax almost simultaneously. Sometimes, relaxation may be preceded by a brief increase in pressure in the area below the respiratory reversal and a brief fall in pressure above the point of respiratory reversal. This phenomenon corresponds with the phenomenon of schluckatmung described earlier. Usually, however, LES relaxation is delayed for 2 to 3 sec after the initiation of swallowing. At this time, the swallowed bolus is usually in the esophagus and the peristaltic contraction following the bolus is in the cervical esophagus. In the upright position, a swallowed bolus may reach the LES very fast due to the action of gravity. When this happens, there may be a transient delay at the LES before passage into the stomach. The LES relaxation may last 5 to 10 sec; subsequently, the upper part of the sphincter shows an after-contraction which is in peristaltic continuity with the peristalsis in the esophageal body. The after-contraction lasts 7 to 10 sec. The lower part of the LES does not show after contractions and the sphincter pressure simply returns to the resting level. Electromyographic studies show LES relaxation is associated with cessation of continuous spike activity (9).

Swallow-Related and Other Pharyngoesophageal Activities

The pharynx participates in a variety of activities. Some of these are swallowing, breathing and speaking. The pharynx is also involved in various activities such as gagging and gargling. The pharynx and esophagus also participate in a variety of swallow related events involved in aboral food transport such as drinking, beer guzzling and secondary peristalsis. In addition, these organs may be involved in retrograde transport of gastric or esophageal contents, as occurs in vomiting, retching, eructation, and esophageal speech.

Drinking

Drinking is merely repetitive swallowing in rapid succession. Each swallow during drinking has a full oropharyngeal component. In humans, swallows may occur from 1 every 3 sec, up to 1 per sec while drinking (109). Because of deglutitive inhibition, the striated as well as smooth muscle segment of the esophagus remains quiescent and the LES remains relaxed. The last of the swallows, however, is associated with a peristaltic wave in the esophagus and upper LES; pressure in the lower LES then returns to its resting level (7,214,291). The process of drinking demonstrates dissociation of pharyngeal and esophageal activities.

Beer Guzzling

A characteristic and highly integrated sequence of pharyngeal, UES and esophageal action has been noted in beer guzzlers (262). These individuals have developed a mechanism of fluid ingestion whereby large volumes can pass through the upper gullet in a fraction of the time required by normal subjects to drink the same amount. The head and neck are extended to take advantage of gravity; the rate of pouring is adjusted to maintain a fluid level flush with the lower lip. The larynx, pharynx and hyoid descend approximately 1 vertebral body in extent much as occurs in yawning. The tongue and soft palate move forward and backward in alternate fashion at a rate of 1/sec, propelling fluid aborally through the pharynx. The UES opens and stays so until the last liquid has passed. Esophageal peristalsis is likewise delayed until the last fluid has entered the upper esophagus; a typical stripping wave then occurs. In contrast to drinking, beer guzzling has no pharyngeal phase of swallowing.

Secondary Peristalsis

Food left behind in the esophagus after primary peristalsis is cleared by secondary peristalsis. Similarly, when reflux of gastric contents occurs in the esophagus it is cleared by secondary peristalsis.

The term secondary peristalsis has been used to describe different things and hence has led to some confusion. Some investigators call secondary peristalsis the deglutition reflex initiated by esophageal distension.

With this definition there is no difference between primary and secondary peristalsis except for its mode of initiation. In this general sense, the response may be observed in the striated muscle esophagus of the cat or dog. In these species, this type of secondary peristalsis is a centrally mediated reflex as it is abolished by vagotomy. More commonly, however, secondary peristalsis is defined as the esophageal response without the oropharyngeal component which is seen with esophageal stimulation. Secondary peristalsis observed in the smooth muscle part of the esophagus is mainly a local reflex and may not require central mediation. Sometimes a central reflex involving the vagus may also participate in the secondary peristaltic response in the smooth muscle part of the esophagus. In this instance, a contraction in the striated muscle also occurs. Such central participation is by no means essential for a response to occur in the smooth muscle portion. Secondary peristalsis is similar to the primary peristaltic response in amplitude and velocity (129,305).

Tertiary contraction is a term used by clinicians to denote a variety of phenomena. This terminology is sometimes applied to simultaneous contractions in the esophageal body. These may occur in response to swallowing or esophageal distension. Frequently the onset of contractions is not exactly simultaneous but there is a very high speed of propagation. It may simply be a variant of primary and secondary peristalsis. Others use this term to describe spontaneous contractions occurring simultaneously at different levels without swallowing or esophageal distension. These spontaneous contractions are usually of small amplitude. In barium studies, they appear as small, nonlumen occluding, ripple-like contractions in the esophageal wall and are localized to the smooth muscle part of the esophagus. Some observers use the term aperistalsis to describe nonperistaltic (nonpropagated) contractions. Unfortunately, aperistalsis is also used to describe absence of contraction. Absence of contraction may be very different from nonperistaltic contractions in terms of pathophysiological significance. The term aperistalsis should not be used without proper qualification, if it must be used at all. Spontaneous contractions may be evoked by acoustical stimuli (312). They also occur in patients with diffuse esophageal spasm (65,187).

Rumination

Rumination is a reflex process by which certain animals such as cows transport previously swallowed food from stomach back to the mouth, where the food is chewed again and swallowed once more. This reflex event begins with contraction of stomach and forceful inspiration against a closed nasopharynx (315,316). This causes a drop in esophageal and increase in intragastric pressure. The LES relaxes and the gastroesophageal gradient causes flow of gastric contents into the esophagus. An antiperistaltic wave moving in retrograde fashion starts. The UES is opened and the material is transported to the mouth. Manometric studies show two distinct pressure peaks: a) associated with reflux of food into the stomach; and b) a reverse peristaltic wave. In the cow, the speed of antegrade peristalsis is 42 cm/sec and that of retrograde peristalsis is twice as fast—a remarkable 80 cm/sec (315)!

Vomiting and Retching

Vomiting is a reflex process by which gastric contents are forcefully expelled through the mouth (231,309). The process can be divided into four phases. Initially, the thoracic cage contracts while the diaphragm descends and the glottis remains closed. The result is negative intrathoracic and intraesophageal pressure. After 0.07 to 0.53 sec (339), the abdominal wall forcefully contracts and gastric contents are propelled through the LES. The LES is lifted up into the thoracic cavity by longitudinal esophageal contraction as it opens. During this period the thoracic cage expands, causing further reduction in intrathoracic pressure and producing a greater gastroesophageal gradient. During the period of abdominal contraction, the gastric antrum also contracts; this helps to deliver gastric contents to the gastric fundus. The esophageal body functions as a passive tube in the orad propulsion of gastric contents (231,309). Afterward, material remaining in the esophagus may be cleared by primary or secondary peristalsis.

The contractile activity of the UES functionally distinguishes retching from vomiting. The UES remains closed in retching so that the regurgitated material does not enter the pharynx. In retching, the LES relaxes and gastric contractions arising in the antrum force stomach contents into the esophageal body. In vomiting the UES is opened and gastric material is propelled orally. As yet it has not been determined whether UES opening is accompanied by termination of spike activity in the UES musculature or whether the high gastric pressures generated simply overcome continued tonic UES contractile activity.

Belching and Esophageal Eructation

Expulsion of gas from the stomach (belching or eructation) involves opening of the LES, relaxation of the UES, and contraction of somatic abdominal musculature to create the necessary pressure differential for gas flow in an oral direction (61,239). The esophageal body musculature acts as a passive conduit in the process. In the absence of UES opening, distension of the esopha-

gus by gas initiates a secondary peristaltic contraction wave which returns the gas to the stomach (239). Certain individuals can eructate at will by swallowing air, straining slightly to increase intraabdominal pressure and thereby retaining gas in the esophagus, and finally opening the UES while continuing to strain, forcing the air out (61). This has been termed esophageal eructation to distinguish it from belching, which implies exit of gas from the stomach as opposed to the esophagus.

Esophageal Speech

Laryngectomized patients may learn to speak by utilizing the phenomenon of esophageal speech. In this process patients swallow air that is accumulated in the esophagus (290). The LES remains closed. Esophageal air is then expelled out against the cricopharyngeus or the cricopharyngeal mucosal fold, which produces speech.

Glossopharyngeal Breathing

In patients afflicted with poliomyelitis complicated by ventilatory failure, a learned breathing technique in which pharyngeal contraction forces air through the glottis may significantly increase their ventilatory function (78). Vital capacities of ~40% of normal may be realized. Initially, the mouth is opened, filling the oropharyngeal cavity with air. Next, the mouth closes and the soft palate rises. The floor of the oral cavity, jaw and larynx then elevate, opening the glottis, and air is forced into the lung by pharyngeal contraction. The UES stays closed throughout the procedure in contrast to the opening seen in deglutition.

CONTROL OF MOTOR ACTIVITY

Initiation of Swallowing Reflex

Sensitive areas that will initiate the deglutitive reflex are present on the base of the tongue, tonsils, anterior and posterior pillars of the fauces, soft palate, uvula, and posterior pharyngeal wall (61,259). The relative sensitivity of these areas in initiating the deglutition reflex varies in different species. In man the anterior and posterior tonsillar pillars and posterior wall of the pharynx are optimal sites for initiation of the reflex (259). Afferents for the deglutitive reflex are carried in the maxillary branch of the trigeminal nerve, glossopharyngeal nerve and the superior laryngeal branch of the vagus nerve (29,260,325).

Swallowing can be initiated voluntarily from the cerebral cortex (37) but it is difficult if the pharynx is anesthetized or if there is no bolus. Esophageal distension may also cause swallowing. In sheep and other animals with only skeletal muscle in the esophageal wall, the peristaltic wave seen with balloon distension of the esophagus is due to activation of the deglutition reflex (61,184,281). In experimental animals, electrical stimulation of the superior laryngeal nerve is a popular method of inducing swallowing. However, stimulation of superior laryngeal nerve (SLN) causes gagging as well as swallowing (108). In the opossum, stimulation of SLN causes reflex contraction of CP which is reminiscent of the gagging reflex (8). However, with continued stimulation CP inhibition associated with swallowing is also induced (8).

Central Organization of Swallowing Reflex

"Swallowing center" is a descriptive concept that includes a well organized central nervous mechanism that executes the deglutition reflex. It exists as two half-centers, one lying on each side 1.5 mm from the midline in the reticular substance at a level 1 to 3 mm dorsal to the superior pole of the inferior olive in the medulla oblongata (111). Connection between the two half-centers is extensive, so that unilateral afferent stimulation can activate both half-centers (195). Each center activates ipsilateral deglutitive muscles except for the middle and inferior pharyngeal constrictors which are stimulated contralaterally. With longitudinal splits in the midline that sever connection between two halves of the center, "unilateral swallowing" may be produced with SLN stimulation (105). Although electrical stimulation of certain cortical and subcortical areas can instigate deglutition (37,320,321), the muscle firing sequence and completion of the swallowing act proceeds independent of cortical influence. In the human, swallowing occurs in the 12-week-old fetus. Near birth, the fetus swallows approximately 500 ml amniotic fluid per day. Normal adults swallow approximately 600 times daily, 350 times during waking activity, 50 times during night sleep, and 200 times while eating (219). Increases in heart rate, inhibition of penile erection, and abolition of hiccoughs have also been found in association with deglutition (242).

Sucking, breathing, and swallowing in infants are coupled in a relatively fixed 1:1:1 relationship (109). In cats, licking and swallowing show a similar linkage. The relationship of swallowing and respiration is of great significance. In humans, approximately 88% of solid swallows and 71% of liquid swallows occur during expiration (109). A respiratory pause averaging 2.5 sec follows each swallow (57). Electromyographic recordings in cats demonstrate inhibition of firing in phrenic motoneurons with SLN stimulation at any phase of the respiratory cycle (98). Furthermore, the SLN threshold for respiratory inhibition is lower than for swallowing (110,216). In contrast to this inhibitory respiratory cor-

relate of swallowing, a brief burst of spikes in diaphragm and intercostal muscles may be recorded 0.2 to 0.3 sec after onset of mylohyoid activity in deglutition (109,319). This marks the brief inspiratory movement which may accompany swallowing. Phrenic nerve section or destruction of the respiratory center abolishes this activity (109). These observations suggest a complex interplay between various medullary "centers" and the swallowing center. The deglutition center modulates the activities of other centers so that they do not interfere with each other. All seem capable of directing pharyngeal contractile activity with their own pattern of activation simultaneous with an inhibition of other centers. The pharynx thus is a tool responding in command to a fixed pattern of output from whichever medullary center is active at a particular point in time.

The efferent link of the deglutition reflex is very stable and exhibits a stereotypic, fixed sequence of contractile events upon stimulation irrespective of the manner or the type of afferent activation. The precise mechanism and the sequences of inhibition and excitation in the swallowing center are not known. The complex command of the swallowing center is executed via the activation of motor nuclei of cranial nerves that innervate muscles of deglutition.

Control of Pharyngeal Phase

The pharyngeal component of swallowing is a complicated process due to the number of muscles involved and the millisecond precision required for normal function.

The pharyngeal component of swallowing fulfills three objectives pertinent to normal deglutitive function (287): a) elevation and forward displacement of laryngeal structures, thereby opening the UES: b) closure of nasal, laryngeal and oral apertures to channel the bolus in the proper direction; and c) active propulsion of material from oral cavity to esophagus.

All these objectives are performed in concert. Moreover, any deviations from this integrated activity lead to major problems such as nasal regurgitation of food, laryngeal aspiration, or dysphagia. These objectives are achieved by integration of swallowing with other activities such as respiration and speaking.

In lesions of the twelfth cranial nerve, the tongue may be paralyzed. Patients so afflicted may learn to push the bolus of food with their finger toward the oropharynx. The bolus then initiates the swallowing reflex and the bolus is normally propelled to the stomach.

Usually, oral and pharyngeal phases are integrated on a one-to-one basis. Beer guzzling may have an oral phase of activity but the pharynx remains inhibited. In the phenomenon of glossopharyngeal breathing, swallow-like activity of the pharynx is utilized for breathing.

Control of Upper Esophageal Sphincter

Genesis of UES pressure, its relaxation (opening), and reflex modulation of pressure have been controversial for a long time. It is generally assumed that basal LES pressure must be due to continuous tonic activity of the cricopharyngeus and other muscles that are responsible for the UES. Indeed, several studies have shown that the cricopharyngeus muscle shows continuous electrical spike activity (2,8,170,221,249,302). In an extensive review of the literature, Doty (109) concluded that UES closure may be entirely due to passive forces caused by elasticity in the wall with measured intraluminal pressures due to stretching of these structures. He argued that such an activity was an artifact caused by reflex stimulation. It is also possible that both active muscle contraction and passive forces contributed to the resting LESP. In order to resolve these issues, simultaneous manometry of the UES and electromyography has been performed in the opossum (8). These studies revealed that a major component of the UES pressure was due to active muscle contraction, as resting tone was inhibited when muscle activity ceased (Fig. 3). The continuous spike activity was shown not to be an artifact caused by reflex stimulation of the recording device as the continuous spike activity was also observed with chronically implanted electrodes without any manometric device (8). However, a small amount of pressure (~10 mm Hg) was measured even when all muscle activity had ceased. This amount of UES pressure could be due to passive forces exerted on the UES wall (see Fig. 4). Thus, both active and passive factors may contribute to resting UESP, in contrast to the LESP, which has no passive component at rest.

Some early studies (208,249) had suggested that tonic contraction of cricopharyngeus is due to tonic sympathetic nerve activity and that the vagus carries inhibitory fibers to the cricopharyngeus muscle. This does not appear to be the case, however. In the opossum, vagal stimulation causes contraction of UES muscles and vagal section abolishes their activity (8). The activity is also abolished by curare-like drugs (8). These studies show that tonic lower motor neuron activity is responsible for tonic CP activity.

UES pressure may be dependent upon the diameter of the recording device and the intensity of activity in the sphincter muscles. The activity is depressed during deep sleep and during deep anesthesia (8,221,302). Sometimes the activity increases during inspiration (2,38, 202,221).

Reflex increases in UESP occur with esophageal distension (76,120,163) and with esophageal acid infusion (139) and gastroesophageal reflux (314). Reflux increases in UES pressure occur during gagging and upon stimulation of SLN (108). The Valsalva maneuver performed against closed mouth and nose (as opposed to glottis) is associated with a reflex contraction of the CP. Increased UESP has been reported in patients with globus sensation (344).

Relaxation and opening of the UES occur during deglutition, rumination, vomiting and several other activities. During swallow-induced relaxation of UES, continuous spike activity of cricopharyngeal (CP) and inferior pharyngeal constrictor (IPC) ceases (2,8,38, 302). The cessation is due to central inhibition rather than to the activity of peripheral inhibitory nerves, in contrast to the LES. In fact, no striated muscles are known that have inhibitory fibers. The inhibition of muscle activity is, however, not sufficient to open the UES, and slight (~10 mm Hg) pressure persists even after cessation of all CP activity. The opening of the UES with abolition of residual pressure is brought about by the anterior displacement of the larynx by suprahyoid muscles (Fig. 4).

The larynx, including the cricoid cartilage, is pulled forward and upward during deglutition. This is brought about by the activation of mylohyoid, geniohyoid, stylohyoid, thyrohyoid and stylo- and salpingopharyngeus muscles. The laryngeal movement is an early event in swallowing. In fact, mylohyoid activity is the first activity to appear in response to swallowing (110). The suprahyoid muscles can be considered as dilator fibers of the UES. Their role is further emphasized by the fact that geniohyoid contraction may open the UES and re-

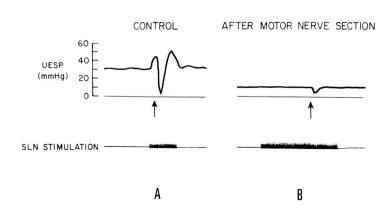

FIG. 4. Effect of motor nerve section on UESP and the influence of SLN stimulation on UESP before and after section of motor nerve to UES muscles. SLN stimulation activated deglutition reflex as marked by *arrows*. Note that during the control period, the resting UESP is approximately 30 mm Hg, and increases transiently during SLN stimulation. When deglutition reflex is activated, the UES relaxes. Also note that after motor nerve section, a residual pressure of ~10 mm Hg remains in the UES. However, activation of deglutition reflex by SLN causes drop in this residual pressure. This drop is due to opening of the UES by the suprahyoid muscles. From Asoh and Goyal, ref. 9.

duce UESP to nearly zero even when the cricopharyngeus continues to fire (8). Under normal circumstances, however, cessation of activity in the CP and contraction of the suprahyoid muscle coordinate to ensure efficient opening of the UES. Paralysis of suprahyoid muscles may impair UES opening even when the cricopharyngeus functions normally (8,15,182,207). This abnormality can be recognized by impaired laryngeal movement during swallowing. On the other hand, in the presence of abnormal relaxation of the cricopharyngeus, contraction of suprahyoid muscles may cause considerable opening of the UES despite continued cricopharyngeal contraction. Because the UES opening is related to two factors it may be useful to distinguish between UES relaxation and UES opening. Inhibition of activity in UES muscle would cause UES relaxation but opening of the UES is due to active contraction of suprahyoid muscles. Such a phenomenon may be responsible for the prominent cricopharyngeal "bar" or so called cricopharyngeal achalasia (33,304,322). Contraction of suprahyoid muscles without CP relaxation may produce such a roentgenographic appearance.

It has been suggested that manometrically observed relaxation may be related to catheter movement during swallowing. However, relaxation of UES with induced swallowing is observed in experimental animals when the manometric catheter assembly is anchored in the UES (8).

Contractile activities of the UES, thus, may display a variety of relationships with pharyngeal and esophageal motor activity. In swallowing, there is a 1:1:1 relationship between pharyngeal, UES, and esophageal contractile patterns. In drinking, the pharyngeal response exceeds that in the UES and esophagus in terms of number of contractions. Furthermore, in glossopharyngeal breathing, there is no motor correlate in the UES or esophagus despite a clear-cut pharyngeal activity. Last, increments in UES activity, such as those produced by esophageal distension or acid infusion, as well as the UES relaxation which occurs in vomiting and belching may be seen without associated pharyngeal or esophageal body activity. These observations reveal the importance of specific control of UES in integrating the various motor events.

Control of Esophageal Body Activity

Striated Muscle Segment

Striated muscle of the esophagus, like any other striated muscle, is dependent entirely on excitatory nerve activity (lower motor neuron). The major control of the skeletal muscle segment resides in the central nervous system. The cell bodies of the lower motor neurons that innervate the skeletal muscle part of the esophagus are located in the dorsal aspect of the rostral part of the nucleus ambiguus (217,218). In the rabbit, stimulation of the rostral part of the nucleus ambiguus causes contraction of the striated esophageal muscle exclusively (217).

The sequential pattern of excitation of motor neurons destined for the various levels of the striated muscle esophagus is responsible for peristalsis in that segment. In his now classical experiments, Roman (281) transplanted vagus into sternomastoid muscle and found that activation of the deglutitive reflex caused sequential contraction of muscle fibers, simulating a peristaltic contraction. In animals with striated muscle predominating in the esophagus, bilateral vagotomy at the cervical level results in abolition of peristalsis (39,173,185, 331,339). It is important to section the vagus high up in the neck to include pharyngoesophageal branches which supply innervation to the most proximal esophageal musculature. Unilateral vagal nerve section has no effect on peristalsis (281).

Peristalsis in the striated muscle segment of the esophagus initiated by esophageal distension has been reported in dogs (184) and sheep (281) but has not been confirmed in humans. This particular reflex is similar to primary peristalsis and should not be confused with secondary peristalsis in the smooth muscle segment due to a local reflex. The skeletal muscle peristaltic response with esophageal distension is abolished by vagotomy (183).

Bolus volume (101,193,194,200,230) and temperature (86,354) may also affect the motor response in striated esophageal musculature. In the baboon, vagal efferent firing is modified in response to afferent input (284). These findings suggest that the peripheral sensory system in the esophagus is capable of influencing the contractile response in a quantitative fashion, whereas the qualitative features of primary peristalsis are unchanged. These modifications require CNS connections for their execution.

Striated muscle esophagus responds on a one-to-one basis, with each pharyngeal phase of swallowing. However, in drinking, esophageal activity is inhibited until the last of the swallows, whereas oropharyngeal activity accompanies each deglutition. The inhibition is centrally mediated. A similar inhibitory effect is exerted during beer guzzling, vomiting, eructation, and esophageal speech.

Reverse peristalsis is observed in ruminants. All ruminants have striated muscle in the esophagus and it appears that only striated muscle is capable of reverse peristalsis (109). Reverse peristalsis is centrally mediated and abolished by vagotomy (112,316). Recently, however, reverse peristalsis has been found to occur in the smooth muscle part of the opossum esophagus in response to certain parameters of stimulation of vagal efferents (59).

Striated muscle of the esophagus also shows reflex

contraction proximal to luminal balloon distension (76,120,184). The degree of contraction is directly related to the volume of distension. A propagated wave during or following balloon deglutition has not been demonstrated in humans. Moreover, this reflex contraction is seen with distension in the more proximal part as compared to the distal part of the esophagus. The pathway for this reflex is not defined. However, it may be important in preventing pharyngeal aspiration of material that has refluxed into the esophagus.

Smooth Muscle Segment

Genesis and control of peristalsis in the smooth muscle segment is more complicated than in the striated muscle part and it has received increasing attention in recent years (46,59,64,89,90,92,96,346).

Role of swallowing center.

Activation of the swallowing center clearly activates peristalsis in the smooth muscle portion of the esophagus (192,323). Central control is responsible for the peristaltic sequence involving the muscles of the pharynx and the striated muscle segment of the esophagus. It is not clear whether a similar central sequence of activation occurring in the vagal nucleus is responsible for peristalsis in the smooth muscle part of the esophageal body. Several lines of evidence suggest that organized central sequences are not essential for peristalsis in the smooth muscle segment. For example, electrical stimulation of the distal end of the cervical vagus in a vagotomized animal should instantaneously activate vagal efferents to all levels of the esophagus, but a peristaltic sequence nevertheless occurs in the smooth muscle part of the esophagus (104,247). In contrast, the skeletal muscle part shows contractile activity which is simultaneous and continuous throughout the period of electrical stimulation.

The swallowing center can, however, modify the ongoing activity in the smooth muscle segment of the esophagus. Closely induced successive swallows inhibit or forestall anticipated esophageal contraction due to a previous swallow (103). That is what happens during drinking. The esophageal body remains quiescent during repeated swallows and only the final swallow is associated with peristaltic sequence in the esophageal body. If esophageal obstruction exists and esophageal propulsive force is being exerted on the obstructing balloon, swallowing causes inhibition of this activity (355). Similarly, ongoing tertiary contractions are also inhibited with swallowing.

Secondary peristalsis produced by balloon distension in the smooth muscle segment is not affected by bilateral vagotomy (212,281) or vagal cooling (289). This finding provides evidence for peripheral control of the esophageal smooth muscle.

Peripheral regulation.

Peripheral control of the smooth muscle segment of the esophagus is related to the phenomenon of temporal dissociation of stimulus and circular muscle response. In the smooth muscle, the response to a stimulus occurs after a latency (43,50,91,104,119,347). It is the gradient of the latency of response that is the determinant of peristalsis. This relationship holds with vagal (50,59,104, 282), intramural (54,59) or circular smooth muscle strip (43,46,52,119,347) preparation. In contrast, the responses in the skeletal muscle coincide in onset and duration with the period of motor nerve stimulus.

Types of responses. Several terms have been used to describe the responses of the esophageal smooth muscle to stimulation. Some of these terms are "off," "rebound," "duration," "on," "intrastimulus," or "poststimulus" responses. Confusion regarding these terms arises because they are used to describe different types of responses (electrical or mechanical responses), and responses elicited with different methods of stimulation (extrinsic nerve stimulation, intramural nerve stimulation, or direct muscle stimulation).

Mechanical contraction in the circular esophageal muscle is usually associated with electrical spike burst. However, dissociation between the electromechanical activities can occur. Lower frequencies of stimulation may be associated with electrical spike burst without mechanical contraction, whereas higher frequency of vagal stimulation may cause mechanical contraction without associated spike burst (140).

Off or poststimulus response is so called because it occurs after the termination of stimulation (46,50,54, 104,232,347). This is seen with vagal stimulation (59, 104), *in situ* local intramural stimulation (54), balloon distension (54), and transmural stimulation of circular muscle strips (46,92,119,232,347). This response is neurogenic as it is antagonized by tetrodotoxin (46,232). The electrical off response is depolarization and this is usually associated with a burst of spike activity.

The poststimulus response is explained on the basis of a single or a two transmitter hypothesis. According to the single neurotransmitter hypothesis, the transmitter (which is neither cholinergic nor adrenergic) causes initial hyperpolarization which is then followed by a rebound depolarization with associated spikes causing contraction. According to the two-neurotransmitter hypothesis (92), an inhibitory and an excitatory transmitter are released simultaneously or sequentially by one or more neurons (92). The inhibitory effect predominates during stimulation; upon termination of the stimulus, the inhibitory transmitter effect is terminated and the excitatory neurotransmitter then exerts its action.

There are several intrastimulus responses that can be observed. Duration response is so called because it coincides with the duration of stimulation (54). This response begins at the onset of stimulation, continues through its duration, and terminates with the stimulus. Esophageal longitudinal muscle shows a mechanical duration response. The mechanical duration response is, of course, most characteristic of striated esophageal muscle. The duration response occurs with excitatory motor nerve stimulation or direct muscle stimulation. The electrical duration response in the circular esophageal muscle is a hyperpolarization which may be associated with inhibition of mechanical activity, as in the LES.

The on response is so called because it is seen at or close to the onset of stimulation but does not persist the duration of stimulation (46,96,104,232). The on response as described in circular muscle strips *in vitro* appears with no latency between it and the stimulus. This response seems to be due to direct activation of circular muscle as it is not antagonized by tetrodotoxin (232).

The contraction does not last the duration of stimulation, presumably because of simultaneous neural release of neurotransmitter causing hyperpolarization of smooth muscle membrane.

Sometimes the term, "on response" is also applied to a contraction that occurs during the early period of stimulation. However, this response does not occur precisely at the onset of stimulation and there is a latency between the onset of stimulation and the onset of the response. This "early" response can be seen with vagal efferent stimulation, or local stimulation. Vagal stimulation of over 6 seconds is generally required to show both the "early" and "off" responses (96,104). With shorter duration of vagal stimulation, the distinction between the early and the off responses of mechanical type may not be possible. The "early" response is neurogenic as it is antagonized by tetrodotoxin (TTX). This response may be selectively elicited by vagal stimulation with certain stimulus parameters (96,104) and selectively antagonized by certain modifications (atropine and hexamethonium may antagonize the response) (95,96,104). Sometimes, multiple responses may be observed during a period of prolonged vagal stimulation. The "early" response may be mediated by cholinergic excitatory pathway, whereas the "off" response may be mediated by the inhibitory nerve activation (92,96,119). Further studies are needed to resolve these issues.

Mechanism of peristalsis.

There has been considerable discussion regarding the response involved in peristalsis. Christensen (49,54) suggested it was the off or poststimulus response that was related to peristalsis seen with swallowing. Dodds et al. (96) suggested that an intrastimulus early response rather than off response was involved in peristalsis.

However, the support for such a hypothesis was not convincing (96).

Latency gradient. Weisbrodt and Christensen (347) showed that circular muscle in different levels of the esophagus possesses a characteristic regional latency of response. In general, there is an aboral gradient of latency (Fig. 5). This latency gradient determines the speed of peristalsis in the circular smooth muscle. Using supramaximal stimulus parameters, the calculated speed of peristalsis from these circular muscle strips *in vitro* was 7.7 cm/sec which is much greater than the speed of peristalsis observed *in vivo* upon swallowing.

Determinants of latency gradient. It has been shown (50) that the duration of electrical stimulation may determine the latency gradient in the circular muscle strips *in vitro*. The latency gradient is inversely proportional to the duration of stimulation of circular smooth muscle strips.

Dodds et al. (96) showed that with 8 sec of stimulation of the cervical vagus, the latency gradient with early responses gave a peristaltic speed of 2.66 cm/sec, and the off response gave a much greater speed of peristalsis

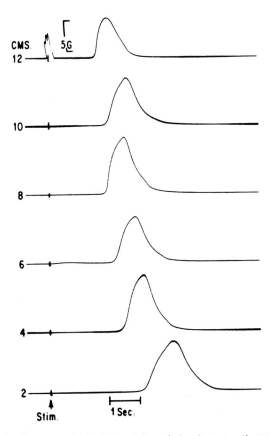

FIG. 5. Response to isolated strips of circular smooth muscle from different levels of opossum esophagus. *Arrow* indicates time of electrical stimulation. Distance is in centimeters from gastroesophageal junction. The delay between the end of the transmural stimulation and the contraction (off-response) of the circular muscle strip gradually increases along the esophagus. From Weisbrodt and Christensen, ref. 347.

at approximately 10 cm/sec. They suggested that the intrastimulus (early) mechanical response to vagal stimulation may be related to peristalsis during swallowing.

Recent studies have shown that parameters of vagal stimulation exert a major influence on latency gradients of off responses. Stimulus parameters may not only determine the speed of peristalsis but certain stimulus parameters may also cause reverse peristalsis, while others may produce esophageal responses resembling those occurring with swallowing (59,140).

The speed of peristalsis as measured by mechanical responses is also different from that measured by electrical response. In general, the mechanical response occurs with a certain delay after the electrical response. Moreover, there is an aborally increasing gradient of electromechanical delay. The speed of peristalsis calculated from mechanical responses is faster than that calculated from electrical responses (140).

Polarity of propagation. When a certain area of the smooth muscle segment is electrically stimulated intramurally, action potentials may be propagated in the aboral direction. However, they do not usually conduct orally (54,59). Thus, it appears that there is a preferred polarity of conduction. This response is neurogenic and tetrodotoxin sensitive. It suggests that the intramural neural circuitry is responsible for this polarity. This neurogenic response is different from the tetrodotoxin resistant myogenic contraction that is observed with high intensity stimulation and is propagated in both oral and aboral directions (292).

Genesis of latency and its gradient. The latency of response may be explained by a one- or two-transmitter hypothesis. The possible causes of latency based on these presumptions could be as follows:

a) A single neurotransmitter initially causes inhibition and cell membrane hyperpolarization which is followed by depolarization and contraction. The latency gradient could be related to regional differences in neurotransmitter release, metabolism, or binding. Another possibility is that, progressively greater amounts of inhibitory neurotransmitter are available in the distal parts of the esophagus. This would cause a progressively greater degree of hyperpolarization and subsequent depolarization would require more time, producing a gradient of latency.

b) Another possibility is that the amount of available neurotransmitter may be the same at each level and the latency gradient may be related to regional properties of the esophageal smooth muscle (298). Thus, the progressively more distal muscle may respond by generating progressively longer lasting hyperpolarization to the same amount of neurotransmitter.

c) In accordance with the two-transmitter model (92), latency is due to either sequential release of inhibitory followed by excitatory neurotransmitter or simultaneous release of the two transmitters with the action of the excitatory transmitter lasting beyond that of the inhibitory.

The gradient of latency thus could be related to a temporal gradient of inhibition relative to excitation. Alternatively, it could be due to a gradient of availability and effectiveness of inhibitory and excitatory neurotransmitters dependent in turn on amounts released, metabolism or transmitter binding.

The effect of various drugs on the motility of esophageal smooth muscle has been reviewed by Christensen (48,52). As yet the identity of the neurotransmitter(s) involved in the poststimulus off response is unknown. Although TTX blocks this response, atropine, hexamethonium, methysergide, propranolol, phenoxybenzamine, tolazoline, nicotine, curare, and succinylcholine are without effect, implying that a noncholinergic, nonadrenergic, postganglionic transmitter is involved. Ganglionic blocking drugs may antagonize vagal stimulated esophageal responses (326). The early response as described by Dodds et al. (95,96) appears to be atropine and hexamethonium sensitive. Other drugs and hormones have been described as decreasing (atropine, isoproterenol) or increasing (gastrin, acetylcholine) contraction amplitude and force velocity relationships in the esophageal smooth muscle *in vitro* (68,69).

Junctional Zone

There are fundamental differences in the mechanisms of latency gradients in the striated and smooth muscle segment, yet *in vivo* there is a smooth transition; the peristaltic wave sweeps over the junctional area without any indication that different mechanisms are involved. For this to occur, the latency gradient in the central nervous system must be precisely matched with the peripheral latency gradient in the smooth muscle.

At 2 to 6 cm below the UES, spikes of the striated muscle type occur with a latency gradient and duration that coincide with the spikes of the smooth muscle type which also appear with a similar latency. The latency gradients of striated muscle and smooth muscle spikes match so that there is no discontinuity. Spikes are recorded from the longitudinal striated muscle first and then from the deeper circular smooth muscle layer (169, 283). The spike characteristics obtained from skeletal muscle are different from those obtained from smooth muscle (5,168,331). The coupling of striated and smooth muscle activation in the transitional segment is not fully understood. Vagotomy results in loss of orderly spike activity in the longitudinal (striated) layer (283) (denervation potentials) while the inner circular muscle (smooth) response is unaltered (283).

Anticholinergic agents (atropine) may disrupt the normal sequence. Atropine delays the appearance of smooth muscle spikes and manometrically a transient delay in peristalsis may be observed in the junctional segment (201).

In monkeys, bolus distension in the transitional zone is followed by spike potentials only in smooth muscle and the striated muscle remains electrically silent (192). There is, therefore, no evidence that a striated muscle contribution exists in the secondary peristaltic response of the junctional esophagus.

Unfortunately, very little is known about the relationship of contractile events between striated and smooth muscle in this region of the esophagus. This smooth orchestration in the transitional zone is certainly a phenomenon worthy of careful scrutiny.

Control of Lower Esophageal Sphincter

Genesis of Basal Sphincter Pressure

In vivo sphincter pressure is dependent upon the mechanical factors and the basal tone in the muscle.

Mechanical factors.

When a manometric device is inserted within the lumen of the sphincter to measure sphincter pressure, the true resting state is modified, as the sphincter is then stretched. At present, there are no reliable methods for measuring sphincter pressure without violating the lumen. The manometrically-derived LESP seems to provide a physiologically useful measurement, however. It correlates well with the force required to pull a Teflon ball across the sphincter (70). LES pressures have been measured with different probe diameters to obtain pressure diameter curves (25,26) which are then utilized to obtain tension-diameter (25) and force of closure-diameter (26) relationships in the LES. These studies reveal that: a) the diameter at which active tension is developed in the LES is smaller than that in the esophageal body; b) tension-diameter curves of LES are steeper than in the esophageal body, and c) the diameter at which maximal tension is developed occurs at a large diameter and not at the diameter of sphincter closure. These biomechanical characteristics may explain the ability of the LES to keep closed at rest with a small tension requirement and to be able to generate fairly stable pressures over a wide range of luminal diameters (25).

At zero diameter and hence zero length, no muscle can generate active tension. Normally, however, the circular muscle of the sphincter is stretched by folds of mucosa with submucosa and muscularis mucosa. These folds (mucosal plug) may play an important role in the basal LESP *in vivo*.

In vitro studies also demonstrate that length tension curves of circular muscle from the LES are steeper than those from the esophageal body (51,53,227). The sphinc-

ter muscle is also more sensitive than the esophageal body in its response to excitatory agents such as gastrin and bethanechol (45,227,293).

The above mentioned characteristics of the sphincter muscle are important but they cannot by themselves generate sphincter pressure at rest as this requires the existence of resting tone in the muscle.

Basal sphincter tone.

Smooth muscles may have tone related to active contraction or, perhaps, to passive tone (286). Passive tone may be due to plastic or viscoelastic properties or to so-called catch phenomena. Manometric studies which show that LES pressure may be abolished with nerve stimulation or with certain relaxant drugs provide evidence against plastic or viscoelastic tone and support the presence of active tone. Passive tone, however, may be revealed at large diameters which cause marked stretching of the LES. The continuous resting tone in the LES may be related to catch phenomena. This phenomenon occurs in certain "catch" muscles and does not require expenditure of energy (286). Studies on LES, however, show that it is an energy requiring active process and that it can be actively relaxed (348).

The genesis of active tone in the LES may be an electrogenic or a nonelectrogenic phenomenon (286). Recent studies show that opossum LES shows continuous spike activity at rest (9). These spikes occur at a rate of 20 to 50 per min. LES relaxation is associated with disappearance of spike activity (Fig. 6). However, a considerable part of basal LES persists in the absence of any spike activity. The spike-related LESP, thus, may represent tetanic contraction associated with repetitive spike activity. Other investigators have not been able to identify continuous spike activity in the LES of cat or dog. It is not clear if these differences are related to technical factors or species differences.

The genesis of the major component of LESP that is spike independent is not clear. This may represent muscle contractions due to slow depolarizations in the transmembrane potential. One unpublished study reported that the resting transmembrane potential difference may be lower in the circular muscle of the LES than in the esophageal body (82). Further studies are needed to explore this possibility. Tone could also be due to nonelectrogenic pharmacomechanical coupling (311). No information on this point is available at the present time.

Active tone in the LES may be due to continuous stimulation of the muscle by a) a tonic excitatory nerve activity, b) a circulating hormone, c) a local hormone or autocoid, d) inherent self-stimulating properties of the smooth muscle cell, or e) a combination of several of these factors.

Tonic excitatory nerve activity.

Tonic vagal or parasympathetic nerves are generally

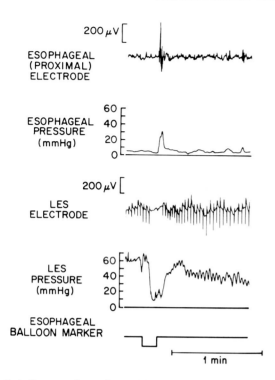

FIG. 6. Influence of esophageal balloon inflation on the electrical activity and pressures in the esophageal body and LES. Balloon distension caused cessation of spike activity and fall in LES pressure. Balloon deflation caused spike activity which preceded the peristaltic contraction in the esophageal body. As the LES pressure returned toward the baseline, spike activity reappeared in the LES. From Asoh and Goyal, ref. 9.

believed to exert an excitatory effect on smooth muscle by the postganglionic cholinergic neurons. Some observers accept the view that vagus nerves may exert a tonic excitatory influence on the sphincter muscle and provide a basal tone, which maintains sphincter closure at rest. According to this concept LES relaxation could be due to cessation of the tonic excitatory activity. Recent studies have shown, however, that in all the species examined the vagus carries inhibitory fibers to the LES (56,104,143,212,236, 264). Ironically, the extent of cholinergic excitatory influences carried in the vagus to the LES has been found to be variable in different species examined. In the opossum, bilateral cervical vagotomy causes either no changes in resting sphincter pressure or a transient increase in LESP. Moreover, electrical stimulation of vagal efferents cause LES relaxation at all stimulation parameters. If excitatory fibers to the LES are carried in the vagus, these fibers are not demonstrable (264).

In the cat, the vagus may carry both excitatory and inhibitory fibers to the LES (56,143). Data of Gonella et al. (143) show that considerable sphincter pressure was observed even after bilateral vagotomy and atropine administration. They did not quantitate numerical change in LESP with vagotomy. Other investigators have found that bilateral cervical vagotomy does not

modify basal LESP (22,130,131). Moreover, vagal stimulation causes frequency dependent relaxation of LES. None of the frequencies of stimulation show contraction (131). In spite of the conclusions by Gonella, there is no clear evidence that tonic vagal excitatory influence is the major determinant of basal closure of LES.

In the dog, cervical vagotomy is thought to abolish basal LESP acutely, but it tends to recover over a period of days and weeks (196). Sympathovagal cooling caused a drop in 2 of 3 animals (261). High abdominal vagotomy does not modify LESP in dogs (223). Stimulation of vagal efferents at certain frequencies causes contraction of LES in the dog. Vagal efferent stimulation in the neck also causes relaxation of LES after thoracic vagotomy, suggesting an intramural path taken by inhibitory fibers (196).

In humans, the influence of cervical or high thoracic vagotomy is not known. However, high abdominal truncal vagotomy causes no influence on basal LESP.

The resting sphincter tone may be due to tonic sympathetic activity. Studies with direct manipulation of sympathetic nerves show that stimulation of sphincteric efferents causes contraction of LES that is atropine sensitive (131). Other observers report that LES contraction caused by sympathetic nerve stimulation is blocked by phentolamine (22). In any event, sympathetic nerve section does not modify the resting LESP (130,131). These studies do not demonstrate a role for tonic splanchnic nerve activity in the genesis of basal LESP.

It is possible that certain excitatory intramural neurons may be active at rest and cause continuous release of neurotransmitters which cause tonic LES contraction. This tonic intramural neuron activity could occur, at least in theory, without the activity of extrinsic nerves. Intramural nerves are difficult to destroy mechanically. However, their activity can be abolished by a puffer fish poison called tetrodotoxin. Tetrodotoxin blocks sodium-dependent conducted action potentials in nerves but does not affect smooth muscle activity. Antagonism of all neural activity in the LES with tetrodotoxin does not modify resting LESP in the opossum (157). These studies are consistent with the view that tonic neural activity is not responsible for tonic LES closure. In one unpublished study, tetrodotoxin has been shown to cause a 25% reduction in LESP in the cat (22). Effects of tetrodotoxin on LESP in other species have not been examined.

Slow spontaneous neurotransmitter release may not be antagonized by tetrodotoxin. To reveal the role of specific excitatory neurotransmitters, the influence of selective antagonists on LESP needs to be examined. Cholinergic neurons are one type of excitatory neurons that may be present in LES. It has been suggested that circulating gastrin provides tonic stimulation to the cholinergic excitatory neurons in the LES (67,229). Ironically, the studies that suggested that gastrin acted by stimulating intramural cholinergic neurons also showed that tonic cholinergic neuron activity could not be responsible for resting LESP (145). Subsequent studies show that gastrin may act directly on the sphincter muscle rather than indirectly by stimulating cholinergic neurons (199,263,288).

The view of tonic excitatory cholinergic influence on the LES is supported by the observation that muscarinic agents cause contraction of LES in animals and in man (280), and LES has muscarinic cholinergic receptors demonstrated by binding studies (278). Atropine, however, does not antagonize resting LESP in opossums (97,263) and monkeys, but it lowers it in dogs (361). Interestingly, in dogs cholinergic blockade with cholinesterase inhibitors produces a picture of achalasia (166). The pressure lowering effect of atropine and anticholinergic agents on the LES is controversial in cat and man (23,97,205,224). In no animal species examined does atropine completely abolish basal LESP. A recent study that took into account radial asymmetry of the LES pressure found that atropine caused a drop in LESP in leftward orientation but not in other orientations (277). The effect of atropine on the left side may be related to the influence of atropine on the sling fibers. Gastric sling fibers appear to have prominent cholinergic innervation. The role of tonic cholinergic nerve activity in the genesis of resting LES tone remains unclear.

Pharmacologic studies have shown alpha adrenergic receptor stimulation causes LES contraction. Adrenergic neuron destruction with 6-hydroxydopamine has been shown to cause reduction in LESP (94), but others have found that catecholamine depletion with reserpine does not substantially modify the basal LESP in the opossum. Similarly, alpha adrenergic antagonism causes a fall in LESP by 25% in opossum and cat. Frequently, however, these antagonist effects are transient and the LESP soon returns to normal levels even when antagonism of adrenergic stimulatory drugs can be demonstrated. These observations do not support the view of tonic alpha-adrenergic activity as a cause of basal LES tone.

Local hormones or autocoid activity.

Tonic LES tone may be due to the activity of some autocoid or local hormones. The autocoid may be an endogenous amine (5-hydroxytryptamine, histamine, and dopamine), a polypeptide (substance P, enkephalin, bombesin, kinin), or a lipid (prostaglandin).

Pharmacologic studies show that dopamine causes a fall in LESP (83,248,266), whereas histamine (16,84, 152,213,269) and 5-HT (16,267), have complex effects on LESP. However, selective antagonists of their effects on the sphincter muscle do not abolish basal LESP. Prostaglandins have attracted special attention as deter-

minants of the basal LESP (148). Daniel et al. suggested that endogenous prostaglandins may be responsible for LES tone *in vitro* (79,80). *In vivo,* however, exogenous prostaglandins E_1, E_2, or arachidonic acid administered intraarterially cause inhibition of LES (81,93,155,160, 246). $PGF_{2\alpha}$ causes contraction of LES (93,274). However, indomethacin which is a potent inhibitor of prostaglandin synthatase, either does not modify basal LESP (272) or causes a small increase in sphincter pressure (93). These observations do not support the view of an important role for endogenous prostaglandins in the genesis of LESP. The role of neuropeptides or kinins in the genesis of basal LESP is not known at the present time. It should be noted, however, that substance P (244), metenkephalin (273), and bombesin (245) cause contraction of LES.

Excitatory circulating hormone activity.

Some years ago, great excitement was generated over the proposal that basal LESP was due to circulating hormone gastrin (42,63,72,171,227,228). Other hormones such as secretin (21), cholecystokinin (126), and glucagon were thought to exert their effects on the sphincter by interacting with gastrin receptors (72,126, 191). Modification in LESP with feeding and antacids was thought to be mediated by changes in circulating gastrin. Moreover, various disorders of LES function were explained on the basis of changes in levels and sensitivity of gastrin (73,121).

Evidence for the physiological role of gastrin in LESP was as follows: Initially, administration of exogenous pentagastrin or gastrin was shown to cause contraction of LES (141). Subsequently, it was reported that instillation of acid in the stomach lowered the LESP and gastric alkalinization increased the LESP. These alterations in LESP were thought to be due to changes in gastrin levels (41). Gastric acidification was believed to lower the LESP by lowering the circulating gastrin and gastric alkalinization was thought to increase the LESP by increasing the circulating gastrin. Such studies in humans or other animals appeared to provide a convincing role for gastrin in the genesis of basal LESP. Further evidence supporting this hypothesis was provided by studies in the opossum. It was reported that the administration of gastrin antiserum selectively bound the circulating gastrin and caused an 80% fall in the basal LESP (228). Moreover, the antiserum was reported to block the rise in LESP following gastric deacidification presumably by binding all the gastrin released (228). However, there are several problems with this hypothesis (317): a) the effect of exogenous administration of gastrin was very short lived, compared with its effect on acid secretion; b) Grossman (164) calculated that the dose of gastrin required to produce LES contraction gave much higher gastrin levels than those found in the physiological state; c) continuous infusion of pentagastrin or gastrin, which gave a half-maximal stimulation of acid secretion, produced only a small increase in the LESP in humans (133,341); d) the bulk of gastrin circulating in the basal state is big gastrin which appears to have little biological activity; e) there is no correlation between basal gastrin levels and LES pressures (77,99,237,238, 358); f) endogenously released gastrin may not be associated with increase in LESP (209,210); and g) finally, a double-blind controlled study failed to show a decrease in basal LESP after neutralization of opossum circulating gastrin with high-titer antiserum (154). In summary, at present, it appears unlikely that gastrin is a major determinant of basal LESP in animals or man.

There are other circulating hormones and other endogenous polypeptides, such as bovine pancreatic polypeptide (270), motilin (114,165,189,197,241), and bombesin (245) that may contract LES. None of the known hormones are currently thought to exert a tonic influence on LES to keep it contracted (114,245,270). Considerable tone in sphincter strips exists even *in vitro* (53), thus it is unlikely that circulating hormones would be the basis of LES tone. The circulating hormones may, however, exert a modulating role on the LESP.

Self-stimulated circular muscle activity.

It is possible that the LES muscle remains tonically contracted because of its own unique property. The sphincter muscles may be self-stimulated rather than by some outside influence. Definitive studies to establish the existence of self-stimulated circular muscle activity of the LES are not available at present. Indirect studies, however, point to this possibility by exclusions.

Ca^{2+} ions are known to play an important role in contractions of all muscles including smooth muscles. On the basis of the selectivity of the actions of calcium antagonists, sodium nitroprusside and verapamil, existence of tonic and phasic calcium activation systems was suggested by Golenhofen (142). These two systems were believed to be in parallel rather than in series. The LES tone is very sensitive to antagonism by sodium nitroprusside *in vitro* as well as *in vivo* (85,132,159). Nitroprusside and verapamil, however, antagonize both tonic and phasic activities of the sphincter in the opossum *in vivo* (159). Preliminary studies of calcium distribution do not show any major difference in the LES and esophageal body circular muscle (294; Rattan, Weiss, and Goyal, unpublished observations).

Modulation of Resting LESP

Reduction in LES tone may occur as a sustained phenomenon or as a transient phenomenon in response to reflex activation of inhibitory neurons, e.g., the LES response to swallowing or esophageal distension. For physiological purposes, it may be convenient to relegate the term LES relaxation to the reflex described above. A sustained reduction in LESP is a part of modulation of LESP and it may or may not involve the inhibitory reflex. This distinction between transient and sustained inhibition of the sphincter tone, however, must be considered arbitrary. The increases in LESP may also be transient or sustained.

Sustained Pressure Modulations

Studies have shown that extrinsic nerves, intrinsic nerves, neuropeptides, autocoids and circulating hormones can modify basal LESP. Some of the agents that did not quite measure up as the determinant of the resting LESP may provide modulatory roles in regulating the resting LESP. Thus, nerves, hormones and other endogenous bioactive agents may exert tonic modulatory influences, some of which may be excitatory and others inhibitory. In such a system of excitatory and inhibitory influences it is not appropriate to assign a certain proportion of the basal LESP to a given excitatory mechanism. For example, atropine may cause 30% reduction in LESP, but this may not mean that 30% of LESP at rest is due to a cholinergic mechanism. This is due to the fact that in the absence of tonic cholinergic influences, the counterbalancing inhibitory influence may cause unopposed reduction in LESP.

Circulating hormones may also modulate basal LESP. Excitatory hormones are gastrin, motilin, and bovine pancreatic polypeptide. These agents do not appear to be major modulators of basal LESP (114,209,237,270). Inhibitory agents are secretin (21), cholecystokinin (20, 276,318), VIP (106,275), glucagon (175,191,198) and gastric inhibitory peptide (307). Similarly excitatory and inhibitory autocoids may also act to modulate basal LESP. Somatostatin may antagonize LESP modulation by hormones by inhibiting their release (36).

Protein meal (252), intraduodenal peptone (210), and gastric pH (174,203) have been reported to cause contraction of LES. In addition, acid in the esophagus and ingestion of a fatty meal (252,254) have been shown to cause a reduction of LESP.

Pregnancy (225,250,334) and menstrual cycle-associated (336) lower esophageal sphincter hypotension is thought to be mediated by the action of female sex hormones (128,297,335). LES hypotension associated with experimental esophagitis in cats is thought to be mediated by endogenous prostaglandins (32,148,172).

LES pressure is reported to be modified by the type of food. Protein meals (12,252) increase while fatty meals reduce LESP (253,254). Body protein may also modify LESP (13), but hiatus hernia does not influence LESP (71,223). Smoking lowers the sphincter pressure (87, 313) and this may be related to the effect of nicotine

(265). Chocolate may lower LESP (357) related to xanthine (155). Coffee and caffein may also modify LESP (66). Many neurohumoral agents cause modifications in LES tone. The final effect of these agents is often a sum total of opposing component effects on the LES tone (158).

Transient Reflex Contractions or Relaxations

The basal tone in the LES, unlike the UES, is not dependent upon tonic neural activity; the inhibition of LES tone is an active inhibitory phenomenon (157,264). As the active tension is abolished, the walls of the LES may still stay in apposition. The actual sphincter dilation or opening occurs largely by the ingested bolus as it appears in the LES lumen.

Reflex contraction of LES may occur with abdominal compression or in association with contractions in the stomach (100,226,332). The reflex contractions may be mediated by cholinergic excitatory nerves (224).

Reflex relaxation of the LES occurs in association with swallowing or esophageal distension. It is generally agreed that such a relaxation is a neurally mediated reflex. LES relaxation is very sensitive and may occur in the absence of peristaltic activity in the esophagus. The inhibition of LES activity, however, is not due to central inhibition of ongoing activity in the CNS as in the UES. This inhibition is an active process brought about by the release of inhibitory neurotransmitter at the neuromuscular site, through activation of inhibitory neurons. This is also true in human sphincter strips (116,243). Indirect evidence suggests that LES relaxation may be mediated by cyclic AMP (155).

The nature of the neurotransmitter released by the inhibitory neurons is not known. However, it is neither a cholinergic nor an adrenergic substance. Hence, this neurotransmitter is dubbed noncholinergic nonadrenergic neurotransmitter (156,329). There is evidence against this neurotransmitter being histamine (269), 5-hydroxytryptamine (267,268), dopamine (266), or prostaglandin (81,272). Prostaglandins, however, may mediate tetrodotoxin-resistant relaxation in LES strips caused by transmural stimulation (79). The possibility that these neurons may be purinergic has been examined (34,64,271). Consistent with this view, relaxation of sphincter muscle strips was shown to be augmented by dipyridamole which acts to antagonize uptake of adenosine by smooth muscle (64). More detailed *in vivo* studies do not support the view of the purinergic nature of the inhibitory neuron (271). These nerves may be peptidergic (330). VIP has been suggested as a possible neurotransmitter (1,275,306). Further evidence for VIP as a possible inhibitory neurotransmitter is provided by a recent study showing that a high titre VIP antiserum causes antagonism of vagal stimulated LES relaxation (161).

The postganglionic inhibitory neurons possess receptors for a variety of endogenous bioactive substances and drugs such as acetylcholine, norepinephrine, histamine, and 5-hydroxytryptamine (158). However, vagal stimulated synaptic neurotransmission appears to involve only the nicotinic and the muscarinic receptors (156) and possibly the serotonergic receptors (268). The neurotransmitter released by the preganglionic fibers in the vagus appears to be largely acetylcholine (156) (Fig. 7).

The postganglionic inhibitory neurons also receive input from afferents in the esophageal body. This pathway is responsible for LES relaxation with esophageal distension in the presence of bilateral vagotomy in animal species with smooth muscle in the lower esophagus. In the dog, bilateral vagal cooling abolished balloon induced relaxation of LES (261). The neurotransmitter involved in this synaptic transmission is not known. A combination of hexamethonium and atropine does not fully antagonize LES relaxation in response to balloon distension in the esophageal body. This suggests that non-cholinergic transmission may be involved. The vagal inhibitory activity is antagonized by splanchnic nerve stimulation and by cholinergic (130,131,144) and dopamine receptor stimulation (107).

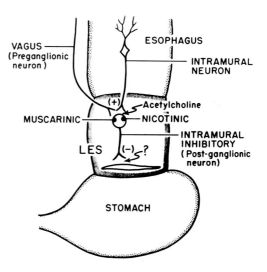

FIG. 7. Schematic representation of the major vagal inhibitory pathway to the LES. The vagi carry preganglionic neurons which synapse with postganglionic inhibitory neurons. The synaptic transmission involves both nicotinic and muscarinic transmission. Both of these pathways of synaptic transmission are substantial, and only when both are blocked does antagonism of synaptic transmission become obvious, particularly at the higher frequencies of stimulation. The nicotinic and muscarinic receptors may be present on different or same postganglionic neurons but, as shown in this model, we consider the latter possibility more likely. The postganglionic inhibitory neurons are neither adrenergic nor cholinergic; their neurotransmitter is not known at present. From Goyal and Rattan, ref. 156.

REFERENCES

1. Alumets, J., Fahrenkrug, J., Hakanson, R., Schaffalitzky, De Muckadell, Sundler, F., Uddman, R. (1979): A rich VIP nerve supply characteristic of sphincters. *Nature*, 280:155–156.

2. Andrew, B. L. (1955): The respiratory displacement of the larynx: a study of the innervation of accessory respiratory muscles. *J. Physiol. (Lond.)*, 130:474–487.

3. Andrew, B. L. (1956): The nervous control of the cervical oesophagus of the rat during swallowing. *J. Physiol. (Lond.)*, 134:729–740.

4. Arey, L. B., and Tremaine, M. J. (1933): The muscle content of the lower oesophagus of man. *Anat. Rec.*, 56:315–320.

5. Arimori, M., Code, C. F., Schlegel, J. F., Sturm, R. E. (1970): Electrical activity of the canine esophagus and gastroesophageal sphincter. *Am. J. Dig. Dis.*, 15:191–208.

6. Arndorfer, R. C., Stef, J. J., Dodds, W. J., Linehon, J. H., Hogan, W. J. (1977): Improved infusion system for intraluminal esophageal manometry. *Gastroenterology*, 73:23–27.

7. Ask, P., Tibbling, L. (1980): Effect of time interval between swallows on esophageal peristalsis. *Am. J. Physiol.*, 1: G485–G490.

8. Asoh, R., Goyal, R. K. (1978): Manometry and electromyography of the upper esophageal sphincter in the opossum. *Gastroenterology*, 74:514–520.

9. Asoh, R., and Goyal, R. K. (1978): Electrical activity of the opossum lower esophageal sphincter *in vivo*. *Gastroenterology*, 74:835–840.

10. Atanassova, E., and Papasova, M. (1977): Gastrointestinal motility. In: *International Review of Physiology, Gastrointestinal Physiology*, Vol. 12, edited by R. K. Crane, pp. 35–69. University Park Press, Baltimore, Maryland.

11. Atkinson, M., Kramer, P., Wyman, S. M., Ingelfinger, A. J. (1957): The dynamics of swallowing. I. Normal pharyngeal mechanisms. *J. Clin. Invest.*, 36:581–588.

12. Babka, J. C., and Castell, D. O. (1973): On the genesis of heartburn—the effect of specific foods on the lower esophageal sphincter. *Am. J. Dig. Dis.*, 18:391–397.

13. Babka, J. C., Hager, G. W., Castell, D. O. (1973): The effect of body position on lower esophageal sphincter pressure. *Am. J. Dig. Dis.*, 18:441–442.

14. Bachman, A. L. (1959): The radiologic study of some normal and abnormal swallowing mechanisms: aspiration pneumonia and cricopharyngeus spasm. *Laryngoscope*, 69:947–967.

15. Baker, A. B., Mutzke, H. A., Brown, J. R. (1950): Poliomyelitis. III. Bulbar poliomyelitis; a study of medullary function. *Arch. Neurol. Psychiat.*, 63:257–281.

16. Bartlet, A. L. (1968): Action of 5-HT and histamine on the neural structures and muscularis mucosae of the guinea pig oesophagus. *Br. J. Pharmacol. Chemother.*, 33:184–192

17. Basmajian, J. V., and Dutta, C. R. (1961): Electromyography of the pharyngeal constrictors and levator palati in man. *Anat. Rec.*, 139:561–563.

18. Batson, O. V. (1955): The cricopharyngeus muscle. *Ann. Otol. Rhinol. Laryngol.*, 64:47–54.

19. Baumgarten, M. G., and Lange, W. (1969): Adrenergic innervation of the oesophagus in the cat (Felis domestica) and rhesus monkey (Macacus rhesus). *Z. Zellforsch.*, 95:529–545.

20. Behar, J., and Biancani, P. (1977): Effect of cholecystokinin-octapeptide on lower esophageal sphincter. *Gastroenterology*, 73:57–61.

21. Behar, J., Field, S., Marin, C. (1979): Effect of glucagon, secretin and vasoactive intestinal polypeptide on the feline lower esophageal sphincter: mechanisms of action. *Gastroenterology*, 77:1001–1007.

22. Behar, J., Kerstein, M., Biancani, P. (1977): Neural control of lower esophageal sphincter (LES) closure. *Gastroenterology*. (*abstr.*) 72:1029.

23. Behar, J., and Kastendieck, J. (1974): Studies on sphincter incompetence. *Gastroenterology*, (*abstr.*) 66:834.

24. Benjamin, S. B., Gerhardt, D. C., Castell, D. O. (1979): High amplitude peristaltic esophageal contractions associated with chest pain and/or dysphagia. *Gastroenterology*, 77:478–483.

25. Biancani, P., Goyal, R. K., Phillips, A., Spiro, H. M. (1973): Mechanics of sphincter action. Studies on the lower esophageal sphincter. *J. Clin. Invest.*, 52:2973–2978.

26. Biancani, P., Zabinski, M. P., Behar, J. (1975): Pressure, tension, and force of closure of the human lower esophageal shincter and esophagus. *J. Clin. Invest.*, 56:476–483.

27. Bosma, J. F. (1953): A correlated study of the anatomy and motor activity of the upper pharynx by cadaver dissection and by cinematic study of patients after maxillofacial surgery. *Ann. Otol. Rhinol. Laryngol.*, 62:51–72.

28. Bosma, J. F. (1957): Deglutition: pharyngeal stage. *Physiol. Rev.*, 37:275–300.

29. Botha, G. S. M. (1962): *The gastro-oesophageal junction: clinical application to oesophageal and gastric surgery.* Little, Brown, Boston.

30. Brand, D. L., Martin, D., Pope, C. E. (1977): Esophageal manometry in patients with angina-like chest pain. *Am. J. Dig. Dis.*, 22:300–304.

31. Brodal, A. (1947): Central course of afferent fibers for pain in facial, glossopharyngeal and vagus nerves. *Arch. Neurol. Psychiat.*, 57:292–306.

32. Brown, F., Beck, B., Fletcher, J., Castell, D., Eastwood, G. (1977): Evidence suggesting prostaglandins mediate lower esophageal sphincter (LES) incompetence associated with inflammation. *Gastroenterology*, (*abstr.*) 72:1033.

33. Brunner, H. (1952): Cricopharyngeal muscle under normal and pathological conditions. *Arch. Otolaryngol*, 56:616–634.

34. Burnstock, G. (1979): Past and current evidence for the purinergic nerve hypothesis. In: *Physiological and Regulatory Function of Adenosine and Adenine Nucleotides*, edited by H. P. Baer and G. I. Drummond. Raven Press, New York.

35. Butin, J. W., Olsen, A. M., Moersh, H. J., Code, C. F. (1953): A study of esophageal pressures in normal persons and patients with cardiospasm. *Gastroenterology*, 23:278–293.

36. Bybee, D. E., Brown, F. C., Georges, L. P., Castell, D. O., McGuigan, J. E. (1979): Somatostatin effects on lower esophageal sphincter function. *Am. J. Physiol.*, 237:E77–E81.

37. Car, A. (1970): La commande corticale du centre deglutition bulbaire. *J. Physiol. (Paris)*, 62:361–386.

38. Car, A., and Roman, C. (1970): L' activite spontanee du sphincter oesophagier chez le mouton. Ses variations au cours de la deglutition et de la rumination. *J. Physiol. (Paris)*, 62:505–511.

39. Carveth, S. W., Schlegel, J. F., Code, C. F. (1962): Esophageal motility after vagotomy, phrenicotomy, myotomy, and myomectomy in dogs. *Surg. Gynecol. Obstet.*, 114:31–42.

40. Castell, D. O. (1975): The lower esophageal sphincter: physiologic and clinical aspects. *Ann. Intern. Med.*, 83:390–401.

41. Castell, D. O., and Levine, S. M. (1971): A new mechanism for treatment of heartburn with antacids: lower esophageal sphincter response to gastric alkalinization. *Ann. Intern. Med.*, 74:223–227.

42. Castell, D. O., and Harris, L. D. (1970): Hormonal control of gastroesophageal sphincter strength *N. Engl. J. Med.*, 282:886–889.

43. Chan, W. W., and Diamant, N. E. (1966): Electrical off response of cat esophageal smooth muscle: an analog simulation. *Am. J. Physiol.*, 230:233–238.

44. Christensen, J. (1967): Electrical activity of the esophagus. *Gastroenterology*, 52:903–904.

45. Christensen, J. (1970): Pharmacologic identification of the lower esophageal sphincter. *J. Clin. Invest.*, 49:681–691.

46. Christensen, J. (1970): Patterns and origin of some esophageal responses to stretch and electrical stimulation. *Gastroenterology*, 59:909–916.

47. Christensen, J. (1975): Pharmacology of esophageal motor function. *Annu. Rev. Pharmacol.*, 15:243–258.

48. Christensen, J. (1976): Effects of drugs on esophageal motility. *Arch. Intern. Med.*, 136:532–537.

49. Christensen, J. (1978): The innervation and motility of the esophagus. *Front. Gastrointest. Res.*, 3:18–32.

50. Christensen, J., Arthur, C., Conklin, J. L. (1979): Some determinants of latency of off-response to electrical field stimulation in circular layer of smooth muscle of opossum esophagus. *Gastroenterology*, 77:677–681.

51. Christensen, J., Conklin, J. L., Freeman, B. W. (1973): Physiologic specialization at the esophagogastric junction in three species. *Am. J. Physiol.*, 225:1265–1270.

52. Christensen, J., and Daniel, E. E. (1968): Effects of some

autonomic drugs on circular esophageal smooth muscle. *J. Pharmacol. Exp. Ther.*, 159:243–249.

53. Christensen, J., Freeman, B. W., Miller, J. K. (1973): Some physiological characteristics of the esophagogastric junction in the opossum. *Gastroenterology*, 64:1119–1125.

54. Christensen, J., and Lund, G. F. (1969): Esophageal responses to distention and electrical stimulation. *J. Clin. Invest.*, 48:408–419.

55. Christrup, J. (1964): Normal swallowing foodstuffs of pasty consistence. A cinefluorographic investigation of a normal material. *Dan. Med. Bull.*, 11:79–91.

56. Clark, C. G., and Vane, J. R. (1961): The cardiac sphincter in the cat. *Gut*, 2:252–262.

57. Clark, G. (1920): Deglutition apnea. *J. Physiol. (Lond.)*, 54:59.

58. Clark, M. D., Rinaldo, J. A., Eyler, W. R. (1970): Correlation of manometric and radiologic data from the esophagogastric area. *Radiology*, 94:261–270.

59. Cobb, B. W., Gidda, J. S., Goyal, R. K. (1980): Mechanism of esophageal peristalsis: Latency gradients and slow electrical response due to vagal and intramural stimulation. *Gastroenterology*, (abstr.) 78:1150.

60. Code, C. F., Creamer, B., Schlegel, J. F., Olsen, A. M., Donoghue, F. E., Andersen, H. A. (1958): *An atlas of esophageal motility in health and disease.* Charles C Thomas, Springfield, Illinois.

61. Code, C. F., and Schlegel, J. F. (1968): Motor action of the esophagus and its sphincters. In: *Handbook of Physiology. Section 6. Alimentary Canal. Vol. IV. Motility*, pp. 1821–1839. American Physiological Society, Washington, D. C.

62. Cohen, B. R., Wolf, B. S. (1968): Cineradiographic and intraluminal correlations in the pharynx and esophagus. In: *Handbook of Physiology. Section 6. Alimentary Canal. Volume IV. Motility*, pp. 1841–1860. American Physiological Society, Washington, D.C.

63. Cohen, S. (1973): Hypogastrinemia and sphincter incompetence. *New Engl. J. Med.*, 289:215–217.

64. Cohen, S. (1974): Augmentation of the neural inhibitory response of the lower esophageal sphincter. *Proc. Soc. Exp. Biol. Med.*, 145:1004–1007.

65. Cohen, S. (1979): Motor disorders of the esophagus. *N. Engl. J. Med.*, 301:184–192.

66. Cohen, S., and Booth, G.H. (1975): Gastric acid secretion and lower esophageal sphincter pressure in response to coffee and caffeine. *New Eng. J. Med.*, 293:897–899.

67. Cohen, S., Fisher, R., Lipshutz, W. (1972): The pathogenesis of esophageal dysfunction in scleroderma and Raynaud's disease. *J. Clin. Invest.*, 51:2663–2668.

68. Cohen, S., and Green, F. (1973): The mechanics of esophageal muscle contraction evidence of an inotropic effect of gastrin. *J. Clin. Invest.*, 52:2029–2040.

69. Cohen, S., and Green, F. (1974): Force velocity characteristics of esophageal muscle: effect of acetylcholine and norepinephrine. *Am. J. Physiol.*, 226:1250–1256.

70. Cohen, S., and Harris, L. D. (1970): Lower esophageal sphincter pressure in an index of lower esophageal sphincter strength. *Gastroenterology*, 58:157–162.

71. Cohen, S., Harris, L. D. (1971): Does hiatus hernia affect competence of the lower esophageal sphincter? *N. Engl. J. Med.*, 284:1053–1056.

72. Cohen, S., and Lipshutz, W. (1971): Hormonal regulation of human esophageal sphincter competence: Interaction of gastrin and secretin. *J. Clin. Invest.*, 50:449–454.

73. Cohen, S., Lipshutz, W., Hughes, W. (1971): Role of gastrin supersensitivity in the pathogenesis of lower esophageal sphincter hypertension in achalasia. *J. Clin. Invest.*, 50:1241–1247.

74. Cohen, S., Long, W. B., Snape, W. J., Jr. (1979): Gastrointestinal motility. In: *International Review of Physiology, Volume 19. Gastrointestinal Physiology III.* Edited by Robert K. Crane., pp. 107–149. University Park Press, Baltimore, Maryland.

75. Corazziari, E., Pozzessere, C., Dani, S., Anzini, F., Torsoli, A. (1978): Intraluminal pH and esophageal motility. *Gastroenterology* 75:275–277.

76. Creamer, B., Schlegel, J. (1957): Motor responses of the esophagus to distention. *J. Appl. Physiol.*, 10:498–504.

77. Csendes, A., Oster, M., Brandsborg, O., Moller, J., Bransborg, M., Amdrup, E. (1978): Gastroesophageal sphincter pressure and serum gastrin: Reaction to food stimulation in normal subjects and in patients with gastric or duodenal ulcer. *Scand. J. Gastroenterol.*, 13:363–368.

78. Dail, C. W., Affeldt, J. E., Collier, C. K. (1955): Clinical aspects of glossopharyngeal breathing-report of use by one-hundred post poliomyelitis patients. *J. Am. Med. Assoc.*, 158:445–449.

79. Daniel, E. E., Crankshaw, J., Sarna, S. (1979): Prostaglandins and tetrodotoxin-insensitive relaxation of opossum lower esophageal sphincter. *Am. J. Physiol.*, 235:E153–E172.

80. Daniel, E. E., Crankshaw, J., Sarna, S. (1979): Prostaglandins and myogenic control of tension in lower esophageal sphincter *in vitro. Prostaglandins*, 17:629–639.

81. Daniel, E. E., Sarna, S., Waterfall, W., Crankshaw, J. (1979): Role of endogenous prostaglandins in regulating the tone of opossum lower esophageal sphincter *in vivo. Prostaglandins*, 17:641–647.

82. Daniel, E. E., Taylor, G. S., Holman, M. E. (1976): The myogenic basis of active tension in the lower esophageal sphincter. *Gastroenterology*, (*Abstr.*) 70:874.

83. De Carle, D. J., and Christensen, J. (1976): A dopamine receptor in esophageal smooth muscle of the opossum. *Gastroenterology*, 70:216–219.

84. De Carle, D. J., and Christensen, J. (1976): Histamine receptors in esophageal smooth muscle of the opossum. *Gastroenterology*, 70:1071–1075.

85. De Carle, D. J., Christensen, J., Szabo, A. C., Templeman, D. C., McKinley, D. R. (1977): Calcium dependence of neuromuscular events in esophageal smooth muscle of the opossum. *Am. J. Physiol.*, 232:E547–E552.

86. De Carle, D. J., Szabo, A. C., Christensen, J. (1977): Temperature dependence of responses of esophageal smooth muscle to electrical field stimulation. *Am. J. Physiol.*, 1(4):E432–E436.

87. Dennish, G., Castell, D. O. (1971): Effect of smoking on lower esophageal sphincter pressure. *N. Engl. J. Med.*, 284:1136–1137.

88. Dent, J. (1976): A new technique for continuous sphincter pressure measurement. *Gastroenterology*, 71:263–267.

89. Diamant, N. E. (1974): Electrical activity of the cat smooth muscle esophagus: a study of hyperpolarizing responses. In: *Proceedings of the Fourth International Symposium on Gastrointestinal Motility,* edited by E. E. Daniel. Mitchell Press Ltd., Vancouver.

90. Diamant, N. E. (1977): How now esophageal peristalsis? *Gastroenterology*, 73:1453–1454.

91. Diamant, N. E., and Chan, W. W. L. (1975): The electrical off response of cat circular esophageal smooth muscle: the effect of stimulus frequency on its timing. In: *Proceedings of the Fifth International Symposium on Gastrointestinal Motility.* Typoff Press, Herentals, Belgium.

92. Diamant, N. E., and El-Sharkawy, T. Y. (1977): Neural control of esophageal peristalsis. *Gastroenterology*, 72:546–556.

93. Dilawari, J. B., Newman, A., Poleo, J., Misiewicz, J. S. (1975): Response of the human cardiac sphincter to circulating prostaglandins $F_{2\alpha}$ and E_2 and to antiinflammatory drugs. *Gut*, 16:137–143.

94. Dimarino, A. J., Cohen, S. (1973): The adrenergic control of lower esophageal sphincter function: an experimental model of denervation supersensitivity. *J. Clin. Invest.*, 52:2264–2271.

95. Dodds, W. J., Christensen, J., Dent, J., Arndorfer, R. C., Wood, J. D. (1979): Pharmacologic investigation of primary peristalsis in smooth muscle portion of opossum esophagus. *Am. J. Physiol.*, 237:E561–E566.

96. Dodds, W. J., Christensen, J., Dent, J., Wood, J. D., Arndorfer, R. C. (1978): Esophageal contractions induced by vagal stimulation in the opossum. *Am. J. Physiol.*, 235:E392–E401.

97. Dodds, W. J., Dent, J., Hogan, W. J., Arndorfer, R. C. (1978): The effect of atropine on esophageal motor function in man. *Gastroenterology*, (abstr.) 74:1028.

98. Dodds, W. J., Hogan, W. J., Lyden, S. B., Stewart, E. T., Stef, J. J., Arndorfer, R. C. (1975): Quantitation of pharyngeal motor function in normal human subjects. *J. Appl. Physiol.*, 39:692–696.

99. Dodds, W. J., Hogan, W. J., Miller, W. N., Barreras, R. F., Arndorfer. R. C.. Stef. J. J. (1975): Relationship between serum gastrin concentration and lower esophageal sphincter pressure. *Am. J. Dig. Dis.*, 20:201-207.

100. Dodds, W. J., Hogan, W. J., Miller, W. N., Stef, J. J., Arndorfer, R. C., Lyden, S. B. (1975): Effect of increased intra-abdominal pressure on lower esophageal sphincter pressure. *Am. J. Dig. Dis.*, 20:298-308.

101. Dodds, W. J., Hogan, W. J., Reid, D. P., Stewart, E. T., Arndorfer, R. C. (1973): A comparison between primary esophageal peristalsis following wet and dry swallows. *J. Appl. Physiol.*, 35:851-857.

102. Dodds, W. J., Hogan, W. J., Stewart, E. T., Stef, J. J., Arndorfer, R. C. (1974): Effects of increased intra-abdominal pressure on esophageal peristalsis. *J. Appl. Physiol.*, 37:378-383.

103. Dodds, W. J., Stef, J. J., Hogan, W. J. (1976): Factors determining pressure measurement accuracy by intraluminal esophageal manometry. *Gastroenterology*, 70:117-123.

104. Dodds, W. J., Stef, J. J., Stewart, E. T., Hogan, W. J., Arndorfer, R. C., Cohen, E. B. (1978): Responses of feline esophagus to cervical vagal stimulation. *Am. J. Physiol.*, 235: E63-73.

105. Dodds, W. J., Stewart, E. T., Hodges, D., Zboralske, F. F. (1973): Movement of the feline esophagus associated with respiration and peristalsis. *J. Clin. Invest.*, 52:1-13.

106. Domschke, W., Lux, G., Domschke, S., Strunz, U., Bloom, S. R., Wunsch, E. (1978): Effects of vasoactive intestinal peptide on resting and pentagastrin stimulated lower esophageal sphincter pressure. *Gastroenterology*, 75:9-12.

107. Doody, P. T. (1976): Adrenergic modulation of vagal inhibitory action: evidence for dopamine receptors. *Gastroenterology,* (abstr.) 70:997.

108. Doty. R. W. (1951): Influence of stimulus pattern on reflex deglutition. *Am. J. Physiol.*, 166:142-158.

109. Doty, R. W. (1968): Neural organization of deglutition. In: *Handbook of Physiology. Section 6. Alimentary Canal. Volume IV. Motility*, pp. 1861-1902. American Physiological Society, Washington, D.C.

110. Doty, R. W., and Bosma, J. F. (1956): An electromyographic analysis of reflex deglutition. *J. Neurophysiol.*, 19:44-60.

111. Doty, R. W., Richmond, W. H., Storey, A. T. (1967): Effect of medullary lesions on coordination of deglutition. *Exp. Neurol.*, 17:91-106.

112. Duncan, D. L. (1953): The effects of vagotomy and splanchnotomy on gastric motility in the sheep. *J. Physiol. (Lond.)*, 119:156-169.

113. Dutta, C. K., and Basmajion, J. V. (1960): Gross and histological structure of the pharyngeal constrictors in the rabbit. *Anat. Rec.*, 137:127-134.

114. Eckhardt, V., and Grace, N. D. (1967): Lower esophageal sphincter pressure and serum motilin levels. *Am. J. Dig. Dis.*, 21:1008-1011.

115. Eckhardt, V. F., Adami, B., Hucker, H., Leeder, H. (1980): The esophagogastric junction in patients with lower esophageal mucosal rings. *Gastroenterology*, 79:426-430.

116. Ellis, F. G., Kauntze, R., Trounce, J. R. (1960): The innervation of the cardia and lower oesophagus in man. *Br. J. Surg.*, 47:466-472.

117. Ellis, F. H. (1971): Upper esophageal sphincter in health and disease. *Surg. Clin. North. Am.*, 51:553-565.

118. Ellis, F. H., Jr., Schlegel, J. F., Lynch, V. P., Payne, W. S. (1969): Cricopharyngeal myotomy for pharyngoesophageal diverticulum. *Ann. Surg.*, 170:340-349.

119. El-Sharkawy, T. Y., and Diamant, N. E. (1976): Contraction patterns of esophageal circular smooth muscle induced by cholinergic excitation. *Gastroenterology*, (Abstr.) 70:969.

120. Enzmann, E. R., Harell, G. S., Zboralske, F. F. (1977): Upper esophageal responses to intraluminal distention in man. *Gastroenterology*, 72:1292-1298.

121. Farrell, R. L.. Castell, D. O.. McGuigan, J. E. (1974): Measurements and comparisons of lower esophageal sphincter pressures and serum gastrin levels in patients with gastroesophageal reflux. *Gastroenterology*, 67:415-422.

122. Feinstein, B. B., Lindegard, B., Nyman, E., Wohlfart, G.

123. Fisher, M. A., Hendrix, T. R., Hunt, J. N., Murrills, A. J. (1978): Relation between volume swallowed and velocity of the bolus ejected from the pharynx into the esophagus. *Gastroenterology*, 74:1238-1240.

124. Fisher, R. S., and Cohen, S. (1975): Disorders of the lower esophageal sphincter. *Annu. Rev. Med.*, 26:373-390.

125. Fisher, R., Cohen, S. (1976): The influence of gastrointestinal hormones and prostaglandins on the lower esophageal sphincter. *Clin. Gastroenterol.*, 5:29.

126. Fisher, R. S., Dimarino, A. J., Cohen, S. (1975): Mechanism of cholecystokinin inhibition of lower esophageal sphincter pressure. *Am. J. Physiol.*, 228:1469-1473.

127. Fisher, R. S., Malmud, L. S., Roberts, G. S., Lobis, I. F. (1976): The lower esophageal sphincter as a barrier to gastroesophageal reflux. *Gastroenterology*, 72:19-22.

128. Fisher, R. S., Roberts, G. S., Grabowski, C. J., Cohen, S. (1978): Inhibition of lower esophageal sphincter circular muscle by female sex hormones. *Am. J. Physiol.*, 234:E243-E247.

129. Fleshler, B., Hendrix, T. R., Kramer, P., Ingelfinger, F. J. (1959): The characteristics and similarity of 1° and 2° peristalsis in the esophagus. *J. Clin. Invest.*, 38:110-116.

130. Fournet, J., Snape, W. J., Cohen, S. (1979): Modulation of lower esophageal sphincter relaxation in the opossum. *Am. J. Physiol.*, 237:E481-E485.

131. Fournet, J., Snape, W. J., Cohen, S. (1979): Sympathetic control of lower esophageal sphincter function in the cat. Action of direct cervical and splanchnic nerve stimulation. *J. Clin. Invest.*, 63:562-570.

132. Fox, J. E. T., and Daniel, E. E. (1979): Role of calcium in genesis of lower esophageal sphincter tone and other active contractions. *Am. J. Physiol.*, 237:E163-E171.

133. Freeland, G. R., Higgs, R. H., Castell, D. O., McGuigan, J. E. (1976): Lower esophageal sphincter (LES) and gastric acid (GA) responses to intravenous infusion of synthetic human gastrin heptadecapeptide I (HGH). *Gastroenterology*, 71:570-574.

134. Friedland, G. W., Melcher, D. H., Berridge, F. R., Gresham, G. A. (1966): Debatable points in the anatomy of the lower oesophagus. *Thorax*, 21:487-498.

135. Freiman, J. M., and Diamant, N. E. (1976): Upper esophageal sphincter (UES) response to esophageal distention and acid, and its alteration with nerve blockade. *Gastroenterology*, 70:970 (Abstract).

136. Fyke, F. E., and Code, C. F. (1955): Resting and deglutition pressures in the pharyngoesophageal region. *Gastroenterology*, 29:24-34.

137. Gabella, G. (1976): *Structure of the Autonomic Nervous System*. Chapman and Hall, London.

138. Geboes, K., Desmet, V. (1978): Histology of the esophagus. In: *Front. Gastro. Intest. Res. Vol. 3*, pp. 1-17. Karger, Basel.

139. Gerhardt, D. C., Shuck, T. J., Bardeaux, R. H., Winship, D. H. (1978): Human upper esophageal sphincter. Responses to volume, osmotic and acid stimuli. *Gastroenterology*, 75: 268-274.

140. Goyal, R. K.. and Gidda, J. S. (1981): Relationship between electrical and mechanical activity in the opossum esophagus. *Am. J. Physiol. (in press)*.

141. Giles, G. R., Mason, M. C., Humphries, C., Clark C. G. (1969): Action of gastrin on the lower oesophageal sphincter in man. *Gut*, 10:730-734.

142. Golenhofen, K. (1976): Theory of P and T systems for calcium activation in smooth muscle. In: *Physiology of Smooth Muscle*, edited by E. Bulbring and M. F. Shuba, pp. 197-202. Raven Press, New York.

143. Gonella, J., Niel, J. P., Roman, C. (1977): Vagal control of lower esophageal sphincter motility in the cat. *J. Physiol. (Lond.)*, 273:647-664.

144. Gonella, J., Niel, J. P., Roman, C. (1979): Sympathetic control of lower esophageal sphincter motility in the cat. *J. Physiol., (Lond.)*, 287:177-190.

145. Goyal, R. K. (1974): Does gastrin act via cholinergic neurons to maintain basal lower esophageal sphincter pressure? *N. Eng. J. Med.*, 291:849-850.

(1955): Morphological studies of motor units in normal human muscles. *Acta. Anat.*, 23:127-142.

146. Goyal, R. K. (1976): The lower esophageal sphincter. *Viewpoints Dig. Dis.*, Vol. 8.

147. Goyal, R. K. (1977): Location of the squamocolumnar junction. *Gastroenterology*, (letter) 73:194-195.

148. Goyal, R. K. (1980): Deleterious effects of prostaglandins on esophageal mucosa. *Gastroenterology*, 78:1085-1086.

149. Goyal, R. K. (1978): Neurology of the Gut. In: *Gastrointestinal Disease, 2nd edition*, edited by Sleisenger and Fordtran, pp. 150-178. W. B. Saunders Co., Philadelphia.

150. Goyal, R. K., Bauer, J. L., Spiro, H. M. (1971): The nature and location of the lower esophageal ring. *N. Engl. J. Med.*, 284: 1175-1180.

151. Goyal, R. K., Biancani, P., Phillips, A., Spiro, H. M. (1971): Mechanical properties of the esophageal wall. *J. Clin. Invest.*, 50:1456-1465.

152. Goyal, R. K., Castell, D. O., Christensen, J., Cohen, S., Pope, C. E. II (1978): Round table discussion on gastroesophageal reflux disease. *Gastroenterology*, 74:449-452.

153. Goyal, R. K., Glancy, J. J., Spiro, H. M. (1970): Lower esophageal ring. *N. Engl. J. Med.*, 282:1298-1305.

154. Goyal, R. K., and McGuigan, J. E. (1976): Is gastrin a major determinant of basal lower esophageal sphincter pressure. A double-blind controlled study using high titer gastrin antiserum. *J. Clin. Invest.*, 57:291-300.

155. Goyal, R. K., and Rattan, S. (1973): Mechanism of the lower esophageal sphincter relaxation. Action of prostaglandin E_1 and theophylline. *J. Clin. Invest.*, 52:337-341.

156. Goyal, R. K., and Rattan, S. (1975): Nature of vagal inhibitory innervation to the lower esophageal sphincter. *J. Clin. Invest.*, 55:1119-1126.

157. Goyal, R. K., and Rattan, S. (1976): Genesis of basal sphincter pressure: effect of tetrodotoxin on lower esophageal sphincter pressure in opossum *in vivo*. *Gastroenterology*, 71:62-67.

158. Goyal, R. K., and Rattan, S. (1978): Neurohumoral, hormonal, and drug receptors for the lower esophageal sphincter. *Gastroenterology*, 74:598-619.

159. Goyal, R. K., and Rattan, S. (1980): Effects of sodium nitroprusside and verapamil on lower esophageal sphincter. *Am. J. Physiol.*, 1(1):G40-G44.

160. Goyal, R. K., Rattan, S., Hersh, T. (1973): Comparison of the effects of prostanglandins E_1, E_2 and A_1, and of hypovolemic hypotension on the lower esophageal sphincter. *Gastroenterology*, 65: 608-612.

161. Goyal, R. K., Said, S., Rattan, S. (1979): Influence of VIP antiserum on lower esophageal sphincter relaxation: possible evidence for VIP as the inhibitory neurotransmitter. *Gastroenterology*, 76:1142.

162. Goyal, R. K., Sangree, M. H., Hersh, T. (1970): Pressure inversion point at the upper high pressure zone and its genesis. *Gastroenterology*, 59:754-759.

163. Gray, J. E., Lockard, O., Shuck, T. J., Winship, D. H. (1979): Response of the upper esophageal sphincter and upper esophagus to intraluminal esophageal balloon distention. *Gastroenterology*, 76:1143 (abstract).

164. Grossman, M. I. (1973): What is physiological? *Gastroenterology*, 65:994.

165. Gutierrez, J. G., Thanik, K. D., Chey, W. Y., Yajima, H. (1977): The effect of motilin on the lower esophageal sphincter of the opossum. *Am. J. Dig. Dis.*, 22:402-405.

166. Harris, L. D., Ashworth, W. D., Ingelfinger, F. J. (1960): Esophageal aperistalsis and achalasia produced in dogs by prolonged cholinesterase inhibition. *J. Clin. Invest.*, 39:1744-1751.

167. Harris, L. D., and Pope, C. E. II (1966): The pressure inversion point: its genesis and reliability. *Gastroenterology*, 51:641-648.

168. Hellemans, J., Vantrappen, G. (1967): Electromyographic studies of canine esophageal motility. *Am. J. Dig. Dis.*, 12: 1240-1255.

169. Hellemans, J., Vantrappen, G., Valembois, P., Janssens, J., Vandenbrouche, J. (1968): Electrical activity of striated and smooth muscle of the esophagus. *Am. J. Dig. Dis.*, 13:320-339.

170. Hellemans, J., Vantrappen, G., Vandenbrouche, J. (1970): The electrical activity of human esophagus. *Gastroenterology*, 58:959.

171. Henderson, J. M., Lidgard, G., Osborne, D. H., Carter, D. C.,

Heading, R. C. (1978): Lower oesophageal sphincter response to gastrin—pharmacological or physiological? *Gut*, 19:99-102.

172. Higgs, R. H., Castell, D. O., Eastwood, G. L. (1976): Studies on the mechanism of esophagitis-induced lower esophageal sphincter hypotension in cats. *Gastroenterology*, 71:51-57.

173. Higgs, B., Ellis, F. H., Jr. (1965): The effect of bilateral supranodosal vagotomy on canine esophageal function. *Surgery*, 58:828-834.

174. Higgs, B., Smyth, R. D., Castell, D. O. (1974): Gastric alkalinization. Effect on lower esophageal sphincter pressure and serum gastrin. *N. Engl. J. Med.*, 291:486-490.

175. Hogan, W. J., Dodds, W. J., Hoke, S. E., Reid, D. P., Kalkhoff, R. K., Arndorfer, R. C. (1975): Effect of glucagon on esophageal motor function. *Gastroenterology*, 69:160-165.

176. Hollis, J. B., and Castell, D. O. (1975): Effect of dry and wet swallows of different volumes on esophageal peristalsis. *J. Appl. Physiol.*, 38:1161-1164.

177. Hollis, J. B., and Castell, D. O. (1974): Esophageal function in elderly men. *Ann. Intern. Med.*, 80:371-374.

178. Humphries, T. J., and Castell, D. O. (1977): Pressure profile of esophageal peristalsis in normal humans as measured by direct intraesophageal transducers. *Am. J. Dig. Dis.*, 22:641-645.

179. Hunt, P. S., Connell, A. M., Smiley, T. B. (1970): The cricopharyngeal sphincter in gastric reflux. *Gut*, 11:303-306.

180. Hurwitz, A. L., and Duranceau, A. (1978): Upper esophageal sphincter dysfunction. Pathogenesis and treatment. *Am. J. Dig. Dis.*, 23:275-281.

181. Hurwitz, A. L., Duranceau, A., Haddad, J. K. (1979): *Disorders of Esophageal Motility*. W. B. Saunders Co., Philadelphia.

182. Hurwitz, A. L., Nelson, J. A., Haddad, J. K. (1975): Oropharyngeal dysphagia: Manometric and cineesophagographic findings. *Am. J. Dig. Dis.*, 20:313-324.

183. Hwang, K. (1953): Nervous control of the esophagus and cardia with observations on experimental cardiospasm. *Ph.D. Thesis.* University of Illinois, Chicago.

184. Hwang, K. (1954): Mechanism of transportation of the content of the esophagus. *J. Appl. Physiol.*, 6:781-796.

185. Hwang, K., Essex, H. E., Mann, F. C. (1947): A study of certain problems resulting from vagotomy in dogs with special emphasis to emesis. *Am. J. Physiol.*, 149:429-448.

186. Hwang, K., Grossman, M. I., Ivy, A. C. (1948): Nervous control of the cervical portion of the esophagus. *Am. J. Physiol.*, 154:343-357.

187. Ingelfinger, F. J. (1958): Esophageal motility. *Physiol. Rev.*, 38: 533-584.

188. Ingervall, B., and Lantz, B. (1973): Significance of gravity on the passage of bolus through the human pharynx. *Arch. Oral Biol.*, 18:351-356.

189. Itoh, I., Aizawa, I, Honda, R, Hivatashi, H., Couch, E. F. (1978): Control of lower esophageal sphincter contractile activity by motilin in conscious dogs. *Am. J. Dig. Dis.*, 23:341-345.

190. Jacobowitz, D., and Nemir, P. (1969): The autonomic innervation of the esophagus of the dog. *J. Thorac. Cardiovasc. Surg.*, 58:678-684.

191. Jaffer, S. S., Makhlouf, G. M., Schorr, B. A., Zfass, A. M. (1974): Nature and kinetics of inhibition of lower esophageal sphincter by glucagon. *Gastroenterology*, 67:42-46.

192. Janssens, J., De Never, I., Vantrappen, G., Hellemans, J. (1976): Peristalsis in smooth muscle esophagus after transection and bolus deviation. *Gastroenterology*, 71:1004-1009.

193. Janssens, J., Valembois, P., Hellemans, J., Vantrappen, G., Pelemans, W. (1974): Studies on the necessity of a bolus for the progression of secondary peristalsis in the canine esophagus. *Gastroenterology*, 67:245-251.

194. Janssens, J., Valembois, P., Vantrappen, G., Hellemans, J., Pelemans, W. (1973): Is the primary peristaltic contraction of the canine esophagus bolus-dependent? *Gastroenterology*, 65: 750-756.

195. Jean, A. (1972): Localisation et activité des neurones déglutiteurs bulbaires. *J. Physiol.*, 64:227-268.

196. Jennewein, H. M., Hummelt, H., Meyer, U., Siewert, R., Koch, A., Waldeck, F. (1975): The effect of vagotomy on the resting pressure and reactivity of the lower esophageal sphincter (LES)

in man and dog. G. Vantrappen, (editor) Proc. of the Fifth International Symposium on Gastrointestinal Motility. Leuven, Belgium, September.

197. Jennewein, H. M., Hummelt, H., Siewert, R., Wuldeck F. (1975): The motor-stimulating effect of natural motilin on the lower esophageal sphincter, fundus, antrum, and duodenum in dogs. *Digestion*, 13:246-250.

198. Jennewein, H. M., Waldeck, F., Siewert, R., Weiser, F., Thimm, R. (1973): The interaction of glucagon and pentagastrin on the lower esophageal sphincter in man and dogs. *Gut*, 14:861-864.

199. Jensen, D. M., McCallum, R., Walsh, J. H. (1978): Failure of atropine to inhibit gastrin-17 stimulation of the lower esophageal sphincter in man. *Gastroenterology*, 75:825-827.

200. Jordon, P. H., and Longhi, E. H. (1971): Relationship between size of bolus and the act of swallowing on esophageal peristalsis in dogs. *Proc. Soc. Exp. Biol. Med.*, 137:868-871.

201. Kantrowitz, P. A., Siegel, C. I., Hendrix, T. R. (1966): Differences in motility of the upper and lower esophagus in man and its alteration by atropine. *Bull. Johns Hopkins Hosp.*, 118:476-491.

202. Kawasaki, M., Ogura, J. H., Takenouchi, S. (1964): Neurophysiologic observations of normal glutition. I. Its relationship to the respiratory cycle. II. Its relationship to allied phenomena. *Laryngoscope*, 74:1747-1780.

203. Kaye, M. D. (1979): On the relationship between gastric pH and pressure in the normal human lower esophageal sphincter. *Gut*, 20:59-63.

204. Kazem, I. (1972): A new scintigraphic technique for the study of the esophagus. *Am. J. Roentgenol. Radium. Ther. Med.*, 115:681-688.

205. Kelly, M. L., and Friedland, H. L. (1967): Gastroesophageal sphincteric pressure before and after oral anticholingeric drug and placebo administration. *Am. J. Dig. Dis.*, 12:823-833.

206. Kerr, F. W. L. (1962): Facial, vagal and glossopharyngeal nerves in the cat. *Arch. Neurol.*, 6:264-281.

207. Kilman, W. J., and Goyal, R. K. (1976): Disorders of pharyngeal and upper esophageal sphincter motor function. *Arch. Intern. Med.*, 136:592-601.

208. Kirchner, J. A. (1958): The motor activity of the cricopharyngeus muscle. *Laryngoscope*, 68:1119-1159.

209. Koelz, H. R., Hollinger, A. P., Sauberli, H., Largiarder, F., Siewert, R., Blum, A. L. (1978): Effect of gastric antrum on regulation of lower esophageal sphincter pressure in dog. *Am. J. Physiol.*, 234:E157-E161.

210. Koelz, H. R., Lepsien, G., Hollinger, A. P., Sauberli, H., Largiarder, F., Arnold, R., Blum, A. L., Siewert, R. (1978): Effect of intraduodenal peptone on the lower esophageal sphincter pressure in the dog. *Gastroenterology*, 75:283-285.

211. Kramer, P. (1977): Location of the squamocolumnar junction. *Gastroenterology*, 73:194 (letter).

212. Kravitz, J. J., Snape, W. J., Cohen, S. (1966): Effect of thoracic vagotomy and vagal stimulation on esophageal function. *Am. J. Physiol.*, 238:233-238.

213. Kravitz, J. J., Snape, W. J., Jr., Cohen, S. (1978): Effect of histamine and histamine antagonists on human lower esophageal sphincter function. *Gastroenterology*, 74:435-440.

214. Kronecker, H., and Metzer, S. J. (1883): Der schluckmechanism seine erregung und seine hemmung. *Arch. Physiol. (Suppl.)*, 7:328-332.

215. Laimer E. (1883): Beitrag zur anatomic des oesophagus. *Med. Jobrbucher. Jahrg.*, pp. 333-338, Wien.

216. Larrabee, M. G., Hodes, R. (1948): Cyclic changes in the respiratory center revealed by the effects of afferent impulses. *Am. J. Physiol.*, 155:147-164.

217. Lawn, A. M. (1964): The localization, by means of electrical stimulation of the origin and path in the medulla oblongata of the motor nerve fibers of the rabbit esophagus. *J. Physiol. (Lond.)*, 174:232-244.

218. Lawn, A. M. (1966): The localization, in the nucleus ambiguous of the rabbit of the cells of origin of motor nerve fibers in the glossopharyngeal nerve and various branches of the vagus nerve by means of retrograde degeneration. *J. Comp. Neurol.*, 127:293-306.

219. Lear, C. S., Flanagan, J. B., Moorrees, C. F. (1965): The frequency of deglutition in man. *Arch. Oral Biol.*, 10:83-99.

220. Lerche W. (1950): *The Esophagus and Pharynx in Action.* Charles C Thomas, Springfield, Illinois.

221. Levitt, M. N., Dedo, H. H., Ogura, J. H. (1965): The cricopharyngeus muscle, an electromyographic study in the dog. *Laryngoscope*, 75:122-136.

222. Liebermann-Meffert, D., Allgower, M., Schmid, P., Blum, A. L. (1979): Muscular equivalent of the lower esophageal sphincter. *Gastroenterology*, 76:31-38.

223. Lind, J. F., Cotton, D. J., Blanchard, R., Crispin, J. J., Dimopolos, G. E. (1969): Effect of thoracic displacement and vagotomy on the canine gastroesophageal junctional zone. *Gastroenterology*, 56:1078-1085.

224. Lind, J. F., Crispin, J. S., McIver, D. K. (1968): The effect of atropine on the gastroesophageal sphincter. *Can. J. Physiol. Pharmacol.*, 46:233-238.

225. Lind, J. F., Smith, A. M., McIver, D. K., Coopland, A. T., Crispin, J. J. (1968): Heartburn in pregnancy—a manometric study. *Can. Med. Assoc. J.* 98:571-574.

226. Lind, J. F., Warrian, W. G., Wankling, W. J. (1966): Responses of the gastroesophageal junction zone to increases in abdominal pressure. *Can. J. Surg.* 9:32-38.

227. Lipshutz, W. H., Cohen, S. (1971): Physiological determinants of lower esophageal sphincter function. *Gastroenterology*, 61:16-24.

228. Lipshutz, W. H., Huges, W., Cohen, S. (1972): The genesis of lower esophageal sphincter pressure: its identification through the use of gastric antiserum. *J. Clin. Invest.*, 51:522-529.

229. Lipshutz, W., Tuch, A. F., Cohen, S. (1971): A comparison of the site of action of gastrin I on lower esophageal sphincter and antral circular smooth muscle. *Gastroenterology*, 61:454-460.

230. Longhi, E. H., Jordon, P. H. Jr., (1971): Necessity of a bolus for propagation of primary peristalsis in the canine esophagus. *Am. J. Physiol.*, 220:609-612.

231. Lumsden, K., and Holden, W. S. (1969): The act of vomiting in man. *Gut*, 10:173-179.

232. Lund, C. F., Christensen, J. (1969): Electrical stimulation of esophageal smooth muscle and effects of antagonists. *Am. J. Physiol.*, 217:1369-1374.

233. Lund, W. S. (1965): The function of the cricopharyngeal sphincter during swallowing. *Acta Otolaryngol.*, 59:497-510.

234. Lund, W. S. (1965): A study of the cricopharyngeal sphincter in man and in the dog. *Ann. R. Coll. Surg. Engl.*, 37:225-246.

235. Lund, W. S., and Ardran, G. M. (1964): The motor nerve supply of the cricopharyngeal sphincter. *Ann. Otol. Rhinol. Laryngol.*, 73:599-617.

236. Matarazzos, S., Snape, W., Jr., Ryan, J., Cohen, S. (1976): The relationship of cervical and abdominal vagal activity in lower esophageal sphincter function. *Gastroenterology*, 71:999-1003.

237. McCall, I. W., Harvey, R. F., Owens, C. J., Clendinnen, B. C. (1975): Relationship between changes in plasma gastrin and lower esophageal sphincter pressure after meals. *Br. J. Surg.*, 62:15-18.

238. McCallum, R. W., and Walsh, J. H. (1979): Relationship between lower esophageal sphincter pressure and serum gastrin concentration in Zollinger-Ellison syndrome and other clinical settings. *Gastroenterology*, 76:76-81.

239. McNally, E. F., Kelly, J. E., Ingelfinger, F. J. (1964): Mechanism of belching effects of gastric distention with air. *Gastroenterology*, 46:254-259.

240. Mei, N., Aubert, M., Crousillat, J., Ranieri, F. (1974): Sensory innervation of the lower esophagus of the cat. Comparison with the other parts of the digestive system. In: *Proceedings of the Fourth International Symposium on Gastrointestinal Motility*, edited by E. E. Daniel, pp. 585-591. Mitchell Press Ltd., Vancouver.

241. Meissner, A. J., Bowes, K. L., Zwick, R., Daniel, E. E., (1976): Effect of motilin on the lower esophageal sphincter. *Gut*, 17:925-932.

242. Meltzer, S (1883): Die Irradiationen des Schluckcentrum und ihre allgemeine Bedeutung. *Arch. Physiol.*, 7:209-238.

243. Misiewicz, J. J., Waller, S. L., Anthoney, P. P., Gummer, J. W. P. (1969): Achalasia of the cardia: pharmacology and histo-

pathology of isolated cardiac sphincter muscle from patients with and without achalasia. *Q. J. Med.*, 38:17-30.

244. Mukhopadhyay, A. K. (1978): Effect of substance P on the lower esophageal sphincter of the opossum. *Gastroenterology*, 75:278-282.

245. Mukhopadhyay, A. K., and Kunnemann, M. (1979): Mechanism of lower esophageal sphincter stimulation by Bombesin in the opossum. *Gastroenterology*, 76:1409-1414.

246. Mukhopadhyay, A., Rattan, S., Goyal, R. K. (1975): Effect of prostaglandin E$_2$ on esophageal motility in man. *J. Appl. Physiol.*, 39:479-481.

247. Mukhopadhyay, A. K., and Weisbrodt, N. W. (1975): Neural organization of esophageal peristalsis: role of the vagus nerve. *Gastroenterology*, 58:444-447.

248. Mukhopadhyay, A. K., and Weisbrodt, N. W. (1977): Effect of dopamine on esophageal motor function. *Am. J. Physiol.*, 232: E19-E24.

249. Murakami, Y., Fukuda, H., Kirchner, J. A. (1972): The cricopharyngeus muscle, an electrophysiological and neuropharmacological study. *Acta Otolaryngol. (Suppl.) (Stockh.)*, 311: 1-19.

250. Nagler, R., and Spiro, H. M. (1961): Heartburn in late pregnancy. Manometric studies of esophageal motor function. *J. Clin. Invest.*, 40:954-970.

251. Nagler, R., and Spiro, H. M. (1961): Serial esophageal motility studies in asymptomatic young subjects. *Gastroenterology*, 41: 371-380.

252. Nebel, O. T., and Castell, D. O. (1972): Lower esophageal sphincter pressure changes after food ingestion. *Gastroenterology*, 63:778-783.

253. Nebel, O. T., and Castell, D. O. (1973): Inhibition of the lower esophageal sphincter by fat—a mechanism for fatty food intolerance. *Gut*, 14:270-274.

254. Nebel, O. T., and Castell, D. O. (1973): Kinetics of fat inhibition of the lower esophageal sphincter. *J. Appl. Physiol.*, 35:6-8.

255. Netter, F. H. (1971): Digestive disease tract. In: *The Ciba Collection of Medical Illustrations*. Vol. 3, Part I, Section II, Plate 5. E. Oppenheimer, editor. Ciba Pharmaceutical Company, New York.

256. Palmer, E. D. (1976): Disorders of the cricopharyngeus muscle: a review. *Gastroenterology*, 71:510-519.

257. Peden, J. K., Schneider, M. D., Bickel, R. D. (1950): Anatomic relations of the vagus nerves to the esophagus. *Am. J. Surg.*, 80: 32-34.

258. Pitman, R. G., and Fraser, G. M. (1965): The post-cricoid impression on the esophagus. *Clin. Radiol.*, 16:34-39.

259. Pommerenke, W. T. (1928): A study of the sensory areas eliciting the swallowing reflex. *Am. J. Physiol.*, 84:36-41.

260. Porter, R. (1963): Unit responses evoked in the medulla oblongata by vagus nerve stimulation. *J. Physiol. (Lond.)*, 168: 717-735.

261. Price, L. M., El-Sharkawy, T. Y., Mui, H. Y., Diamant, N. E. (1979): Effect of bilateral cervical vagotomy on balloon-induced lower esophageal sphincter relaxation in the dog. *Gastroenterology*, 77:324-329.

262. Ramsey, G. H., Watson, J. S., Gramiak, R., Weinberg, S. A. (1955): Cinefluorographic analysis of the mechanism of swallowing. *Radiology*, 64:498-518.

263. Rattan, S., Coln, D., Goyal, R. K. (1976): The mechanism of action of gastrin on the lower esophageal sphincter. *Gastroenterology*, 70:828-835.

264. Rattan, S., and Goyal, R. K. (1974): Neural control of the lower esophageal sphincter influence of the vagus nerves. *J. Clin. Invest.*, 54:899-906.

265. Rattan, S., and Goyal, R. K. (1975): Effect of nicotine on LES—studies on the mechanisms of action. *Gastroenterology*, 69:154-159.

266. Rattan, S., and Goyal R. K. (1976): Effect of dopamine on the esophageal smooth muscle *in vivo*. *Gastronenterology*, 70: 377-381.

267. Rattan, S., and Goyal, R. K. (1977): Effects of 5-hydroxytryptamine on the lower esophageal sphincter *in vivo*. *J. Clin. Invest.*, 59:125-133.

268. Rattan, S., and Goyal, R. K. (1978): Evidence for possible

5-hydroxytrptamine (5-HT) participation of the vagal inhibitory pathway to the lower esophageal sphincter. *Am. J. Physiol.*, 234:E273-E276.

269. Rattan, S., and Goyal, R. K. (1978): Effect of histamine on the lower esophageal sphincter *in vivo*: evidence for action at three different sites. *J. Pharmacol. Exp. Ther.*, 204:334-342.

270. Rattan, S., and Goyal, R. K. (1979): Effect of bovine pancreatic polypeptide on the opossum lower esophageal sphincter. *Gastroenterology*, 77:672-676.

271. Rattan, S., and Goyal, R. K. (1980): Evidence against purinergic inhibitory nerves in the vagal pathway to the opossum lower esophageal sphincter. *Gastroenterology*, 78:898-904.

272. Rattan, S., and Goyal, R. K. (1980): Role of prostaglandins in the regulation of lower esophageal sphincter. In: *Gastrointestinal Motility*, edited by J. Christensen. Raven Press, New York.

273. Rattan, S., and Goyal, R. K. (1980): Effect of morphine and endogenous opiates on the opossum lower esophageal sphincter. *Gastroenterology, (abstr.)* 78:1241.

274. Rattan, S., Hersh, T., Goyal, R. K. (1972): Effect of prostaglandin F$_{2\alpha}$ and gastrin pentapeptide on the lower esophageal sphincter. *Proc. Soc. Exp. Biol. Med.*, 141:573-575.

275. Rattan, S., Said, S. I., Goyal, R. K. (1977): Effect of vasoactive intestinal polypeptide (VIP) on lower esophageal sphincter pressure (LESP). *Proc. Soc. Exp. Biol. Med.*, 155:40-43.

276. Resin, H., and Stern, D. H., Sturdevant, R. A. L., Isenberg, J. I. (1973): Effect of the C-terminal octapeptide of cholecystokinin on lower esophageal sphincter pressure in man. *Gastroenterology*, 64:946-949.

277. Richardson, B. J., and Welch, R. W. (1980): Regional differences in the effect of atropine on lower esophageal sphincter pressure (LESP). *Gastroenterology*, (abstr.) 78:1243.

278. Rimele, T. J., Rogers, W. A., Gaginella, T. S. (1979): Characterization of muscarinic cholinergic receptors in the lower esophageal sphincter of the cat: binding of [^{3}H] quinuclidinyl benzilate. *Gastroenterology*, 77:1225-1234.

279. Rinaldo, J. A., and Levey, J. F. (1968): Correlation of several methods for recording esophageal sphincter pressures. *Am. J. Dig. Dis.*, 13:882-890.

280. Roling, G. T., Farrell, R. L., Castell, D. O. (1972): Cholinergic response of the lower esophageal sphincter. *Am. J. Physiol.*, 222:967-972.

281. Roman, C. (1966): Nervous control of peristalsis in the esophagus. *J. Physiol. (Paris)*, 58:79-108.

282. Roman, C., and Car, A. (1967): Esophageal contractions produced by stimulation of the vagus or medulla oblongata. *J. Physiol. (Paris)*, 59:377-397.

283. Roman, C., and Tieffenbach, L. (1971): Motricite de l'oesophage musculeuse lissé après bivagotomie: Etude electromyographique. *J. Physiol. (Paris)*, 63:733-761.

284. Roman, C., and Tieffenbach, L. (1972): Enregistrement de l'activite unitaire des fibres motrices vagales destine a l'oesophagus du baboun. *J. Physiol. (Paris)*, 64:479-506.

285. Romanes, G. J., editor (1972): *Cunningham's Textbook of Anatomy*. Oxford University Press, London.

286. Ruegg, J. C. (1971): Smooth muscle tone. *Physiol. Rev.*, 51:201-248.

287. Rushner, R. F., and Hendron, J. A. (1951): The act of deglutition: A cinefluorographic study. *J. Appl. Physiol.*, 3:622-630.

288. Ryan, J. P., and Duffy, K. R. (1978): LES pressure response to pentagastrin: effect of cholinergic augmentation and inhibition. *Am. J. Physiol.* 243:E301-E305.

289. Ryan, J. P., and Snape, W. J., Cohen, S. (1977): Influence of vagal cooling on esophageal function. *Am. J. Physiol.* 232(2): 159-164.

290. Samuel, P., and Adams, F. G. (1976): The role of oesophageal and diaphragmatic movements in alaryngeal speech. *J. Laryngol. Otol.*, 90:1105-1111.

291. Sanchez, G. C., Kramer, P., Ingelfinger, F. J. (1953): Motor mechanisms of the esophagus, particularly of its distal portion. *Gastroenterology*, 25:321-332.

292. Sarna, S. K., Daniel, E. E., Waterfall, W. E. (1977): Myogenic and neural control systems for esophageal motility. *Gastroenterology*, 73:1345-1352.

293. Schenck, E. A., and Frederickson, E. L. (1961): Pharmacologic

evidence for a cardiac sphincter mechanism in the cat. *Gastroenterology*, 40:75–80.

294. Schlipert, W., Schulze, K., Forker, E. L. (1979): Calcium in smooth muscle from the opossum esophagus. *Proc. Soc. Exp. Biol. Med.*, 162:354–358.

295. Schoen, H. J., Morris, D. W., Cohen, S. (1977): Esophageal peristaltic force in man: response to mechanical and pharmacological alterations. *Am. J. Dig. Dis.*, 22:589–597.

296. Schofield, G. C. (1968): Anatomy of muscular and neural tissues in the alimentary canal. In: *Handbook of Physiology. Sect. 6: Alimentary Canal. Vol. IV.* pp. 1579–1627. American Physiological Society, Washington, D.C.

297. Schulze, K., Christensen, J. (1977): Lower sphincter of the opossum esophagus in pseudopregnancy. *Gastroenterology*, 73:1082–1085.

298. Schulze, K., Conklin, J. L., Christensen, J. (1977): A potassium gradient in smooth muscle segment of the opossum esophagus. *Am. J. Physiol.*, 232(3):E270–E273.

299. Seaman, W. B. (1966): Cineroentgenographic observations of the cricopharyngeus. *Am. J. Roentgenol.*, 96:922–931.

300. Seelig, L. L., Jr., Goyal, R. K. (1978): Morphological evaluation of opossum lower esophageal sphincter. *Gastroenterology,* 75:51–58.

301. Sheperd, J. K., Diamant, N. E. (1972): Mecholyl test: comparison of balloon kymography and intraluminal pressure measurement. *Gastroenterology*, 63:557–563.

302. Shipp, T., Deatsch, W. W., Roberston, K. (1970): Pharyngoesophageal muscle activity during swallowing in man. *Laryngoscope*, 80:1–16.

303. Sicular, A., Cohen, B., Zimmerman, A., Kark, A. E. (1967): The significance of an intra-abdominal segment of canine esophagus as a competent anti-reflux mechanism. *Surgery*, 61:784–790.

304. Siebert, T. L., Stein, J., Poppel, M. H. (1959): Variations in the roentgen appearance of the "esophageal lip" *Am. J. Roentgenol. Radium. Ther. Nucl. Med.*, 81:570–575.

305. Siegel, C. I., Hendrix, T. R. (1961): Evidence for the central mediation of secondary peristalsis in the esophagus. *Bull. Johns Hopkins Hosp.*, 108:297–307.

306. Siegel, S. R., Brown, F. C., Castell, D. O., Johnson, L. R., Said, S. I. (1979): Effects of vasoactive intestinal polypeptide (VIP) on the lower esophageal sphincter in awake baboons: comparison with glucagon and secretin. *Dig. Dis. and Sci.*, 24:345–349.

307. Sinar, D. R., O'Dorisio, T. M., Mazzaferri, E. L., Mekhjian, H. S., Caldwell, J. H., Thomas, F. B. (1978): Effect of gastric inhibitory polypeptide on lower esophageal sphincter pressure in cats. *Gastroenterology*, 75:263–267.

308. Smith, B. (1976): The autonomic innervation of the oesophagus. In: *Clinics in Gastroenterology*, 5:1–13.

309. Smith, C. C., and Brizzee, K. R. (1960): Cineradiographic analysis of vomiting in the cat. *Gastroenterology*, 40:654–664.

310. Sokol, E. M., Heitmann, P., Wolf, B. S., Cohen, B. R. (1966): Simultaneous cineradiographics and manometric study of the pharynx, hypopharynx and cervical esophagus. *Gastroenterology*, 51:960–974.

311. Somylyo, A. V., and Somylyo, A. P. (1968): Electrochemical and pharmacomechanical coupling in vascular smooth muscle. *J. Pharmacol. Exp. Ther.*, 159:129–145.

312. Stacher, G., Schmierer, G., Landgraf, M. (1979): Tertiary esophageal contractions evoked by acoustical stimuli. *Gastroenterology*, 77:49–54.

313. Stanciu, C., and Bennett, J. R. (1972): Smoking and gastro-oesophageal reflux. *Br. Med. J.*, 3:793–795.

314. Stanciu, C., and Bennett, J. R. (1974): Upper esophageal sphincter yield pressure in normal subjects and in patients with esophageal reflux. *Thorax*, 29:459–462.

315. Stevens, C. E., and Sellers, A. F. (1960): Pressure events to bovine esophagus and reticularumen associated with eructation, deglutition, and regurgitation. *Am. J. Physiol.*, 199:598–602.

316. Stevens, C. E., and Sellers, A. F. (1968): Rumination. In: *Handbook of Physiology. Section 6. Alimentary Canal. Volume V*, American Physiological Society, pp. 2699–2704. Washington, D.C.

317. Sturdevant, R. A. L. (1974): Is gastrin the major regulator of lower esophageal sphincter pressure? *Gastroenterology*, 67:551–553.

318. Sturdevant, R. A. L., and Kun, T. (1974): Interaction of pentagastrin and the octapeptide of cholecystokinin on the human lower esophageal sphincter. *Gut*, 15:700–702.

319. Sumi, T. (1963): The activity of brain-stem respiratory neurons and spinal respiratory motoneuron during swallowing. *J. Neurophysiol.*, 26:466–477.

320. Sumi, T. (1969): Some properties of cortically evoked swallowing and chewing in rabbits. *Brain Res.*, 15:107–120.

321. Sumi, T. (1972): Role of pontine reticular formation in the neural organization of deglutition. *Jap. J. Physiol.*, 22:295–314.

322. Templeton, F. E., and Kredel, R. H. (1943): The cricopharyngeal sphincter: a roentgenologic study. *Laryngoscope*, 53:1–12.

323. Tieffenbach, L., and Roman, C. (1972): The role of extrinsic vagal innervation in the motility of the smooth muscled portion of the esophagus: electromyographic study in the cat and baboon. *J. Physiol. (Paris)*, 64:193–226.

324. Tolin, R. D., Malmud, L. S., Reilley, J., Fisher, R. S. (1979): Esophageal scintigraphy to quantitate esophageal transit (quantitation of esophageal transit). *Gastroenterology*, 76:1402–1408.

325. Torvik, A. (1956): Afferent connections to the sensory trigeminal nuclei, the nucleus of the solitary tract and adjacent structures—an experimental study in the rat. *J. Comp. Neurol.*, 106:51–141.

326. Toyama, T., Yokoyama, I., Nishi, K. (1975): Effect of hexamethonium and other ganglionic blocking agents on electrical activity of the esophagus induced by vagal stimulation in the dog. *Eur. J. Pharmacol.*, 31:63–71.

327. Treacy, W. L., Baggenstoss, H. H., Slocumb, C. H., Code, C. F. (1963): Scleroderma of the esophagus. A correlation of histologic and physiologic findings. *Ann. Intern. Med.*, 59:351–356.

328. Trop, D., Peeters, R., Woestijne, K. P. (1970): Localization of recording site in the esophagus by means of cardiac artifacts. *J. Appl. Physiol.*, 29:283–287.

329. Tuch, A., Cohen, S. (1973): Neurogenic basis of lower esophageal sphincter relaxation. *J. Clin. Invest.*, 52:14–20.

330. Uddman, R., Alumets, J., Edvinsson, L., Hakanson, R., Sundler, F. (1978): Peptidergic (VIP) innervation of the esophagus. *Gastroenterology*, 75:5–8.

331. Ueda, M., Schlegel, J. F., Code, C. F. (1972): Electric and motor activity of innervated and vagally denervated feline esophagus. *Am. J. Dig. Dis.*, 17:1075–1088.

332. Vanderstappen, G., Texter, E. C., Jr. (1964): Response of the physiologic gastroesophageal sphincter to increased intra-abdominal pressure. *J. Clin. Invest.*, 43:1856–1868.

333. Van Overbeck, J. J. M. (1977): The Hypopharyngeal Diverticulum. Endoscopic treatment and manometry. *Van Corcum Assen.,* Amsterdam.

334. Van Thiel, D. H., Gavaler, J. S., Joshi, S. N., Sara, R. K., Stremple, J. (1977): Heartburn of pregnancy. *Gastroenterology*, 72:666–668.

335. Van Thiel, D. H., Gavaler, J. S., Stremple, J. (1976): Lower esophageal sphincter pressure in women using sequential oral contraceptives. *Gastroenterology*, 71:232–235.

336. Van Thiel, D. H., Gavaler, J. S., Stremple, J. F. (1979): Lower esophageal sphincter pressure during the normal menstrual cycle. *Am. J. Obstet. Gynecol.*, 134:64–67.

337. Vantrappen, G., Hellemans, J. (1967): Studies on the normal deglutition complex. *Am. J. Dig. Dis.*, 12:255–266.

338. Vantrappen, G., Hellemans, J. (1970): Esophageal motility. *Rendic. R. Gastroenterology*, 2:7–19.

339. Vantrappen, G., Hellemans, J. (1974): *Diseases of the Esophagus*. Springer Verlag, New York.

340. Waldeck, F. (1972): A new procedure for functional analysis of the lower esophageal sphincter (LES). *Pflugers Arch.*, 335:74–84.

341. Walker, C. O., Frank, S. A., Manton, J., Fordtran, J. S. (1975): Effect of continuous infusion of pentagastrin on lower esophageal sphincter pressure and gastric acid secretion in normal subjects. *J. Clin. Invest.*, 56:218–225,

342. Wallin, L., Boesby, S., Madsen, T. (1978): The effect of HCl infusion in the lower part of the esophagus on the pharyngo-oe-

sophageal sphincter pressure in normal subjects. *Scand. J. Gastroenterology*, 13:821-826.

343. Warwick, R., Williams P. L., editors (1973): *Gray's Anatomy*. W. B. Saunders Co., Philadelphia.

344. Watson, W. C., Sullivan, S. N. (1974): Hypertonicity of cricopharyngeal sphincter: Cause of globus sensation. *Lancet*, 2: 1417-1418.

345. Weinstein, W. M., Bogoch, E. R., Bowes, K. L. (1975): The normal human esophageal mucosa: a histologic reappraisal. *Gastroenterology*, 68:40-44.

346. Weisbrodt, N. W. (1976): Neuromuscular organization of esophageal and pharyngeal motility. *Arch. Intern. Med.*, 136: 524-531.

347. Weisbrodt, N. W., Christensen, J. (1972): Gradient of contractions in the opossum esophagus. *Gastroenterology*, 62: 1159-1166.

348. Weisbrodt, N. W., Lee, S. J. (1977): Metabolic factors which influence esophageal smooth muscle. *Gastroenterology (abst.)*. 72:A-125.

349. Welch, R. W., Luckmann, K., Ricks, P. M., Drake. S. T., Gates, G. A. (1979): Manometry of the normal esophageal sphincter and its alteration in laryngectomy. *J. Clin. Invest.*, 63: 1036-1041.

350. Welch, R. W., Drake, S. T. (1980): Normal lower esophageal sphincter pressure: a comparison of rapid vs. slow pull through techniques. *Gastroenterology*, 78:1446-1451.

351. Welch, R. W. (1980): The influence of breathing on human lower esophageal sphincter pressure (LESP). *Gastroenterology*, (abstr.) 78:1289.

352. Winans, C. S. (1972): The pharyngoesophageal closure mechanism: a manometric study. *Gastroenterology*, 63:768-777.

353. Winans, C. S., and Harris, L. D. (1967): Quantitation of lower esophageal sphincter competence. *Gastroenterology*, 52: 773-778.

354. Winship, D. H., DeAndrade, S. R., Zboralske, F. F. (1970): Influence of bolus temperature on human esophageal motor function. *J. Clin. Invest.*, 49:243-250.

355. Winship, D. H., and Zboralske, F. F. (1967): The esophageal propulsive force: esophageal response to acute obstruction. *J. Clin. Invest.*, 46:1391-1401.

356. Wolf, B. S. (1970): The inferior esophageal sphincter. Anatomic, roentgenologic and manometric correlation, contradiction and terminology. *Am. J. Roentgenol.*, 110:260-277.

357. Wright, L. E., and Castell, D. O. (1975): The adverse effect of chocolate on lower esophageal sphincter pressure. *Am. J. Dig. Dis.*, 20:703-707.

358. Wright, L. E., Slaughter, R. L., Gibson, R. G., Hirschowitz, B. I. (1975): Correlation of lower esophageal sphincter pressure and serum gastrin level in man. *Am. J. Dig. Dis.*, 20:603-606.

359. Zaino, C., Jacobson, H. G., Lepow, H., Ozturk, C. H. (1970): *The Pharyngeal Sphincter*. Charles C Thomas, Springfield, Illinois.

360. Zaino, C., Poppel, M. H., Jacobson, H. G., Lepow, H. (1963): *Lower Esophageal Vestibular Complex*. Charles C Thomas, Springfield, Illinois.

361. Zwick, R., Bowes, K. L., Daniel, E. E., Sarna, S. K. (1976): Mechanism of action of pentagastrin on the lower esophageal sphincter. *J. Clin. Invest.*, 57:1644-1651.

Physiology of the Gastrointestinal Tract, edited by
Leonard R. Johnson. Raven Press, New York © 1981.

Chapter 12

Motility of the Stomach and Gastroduodenal Junction

Keith A. Kelly

The objectives of this chapter are to describe the motility of the stomach and gastroduodenal junction and to show how these motor events determine the orderly pattern of gastric emptying of chyme. The chapter should be read in conjunction with the work of Cannon (16) and the reviews by Thomas (101), Hunt and Knox (50), and Code (22).

OVERVIEW

Motor events in the stomach have a key role in upper gastrointestinal physiology. The proximal stomach receives and stores boluses of food from the esophagus. Its slow, sustained contractions gradually press the ingested content toward the distal stomach and duodenum. The peristaltic waves of the distal stomach aid in the aboral propulsion of the content and mix it with gastric juice. The liquids in chyme are permitted to pass readily into the duodenum, but the solids are retained by the terminal antrum and gastroduodenal junction. Powerful terminal antral contractions grind the solids into particles about 0.1 mm in size, which are then emptied from the stomach with the liquids. Once gastric content has been emptied into the duodenum, the gastroduodenal junction prevents its reflux back into the

stomach. The rate of gastric emptying is carefully controlled by feedback from small intestinal receptors, so that the rate is commensurate with digestion and absorption in the small intestine. In contrast to the liquids and digestible solids in chyme, indigestible solids larger than about 1 mm are held in the stomach throughout the postprandial period, after which they are emptied by cyclically recurring bursts of interdigestive gastric contractions.

GASTRIC MOTOR REGIONS

The stomach accomplishes its motor tasks by the interaction of two distinct motor regions, a proximal region and a distal region. The line of division between the two regions does not correspond to the usual anatomic division of the stomach into fundus, corpus, antrum, and pylorus. The proximal motor region includes all of the gastric fundus and about the oral one-third of the gastric corpus, whereas the distal motor region includes the remaining aboral two-thirds of the gastric corpus, the antrum, and the gastroduodenal junction (Fig. 1). The dividing line between the two regions begins at a point on the greater curve of the stomach approximately one-third the distance between the esophagogastric junc-

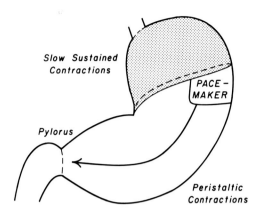

FIG. 1. Proximal (*shaded area*) and distal gastric motor regions (63).

tion and the gastroduodenal junction and then follows an oblique course around both anterior and posterior gastric walls to a point on the lesser curve approximately one-half the distance between the esophagogastric junction and the gastroduodenal junction.

The dividing line between the two gastric regions has been established by myoelectric and motor criteria. Aborally propagated, cyclical changes in potential which phase the onset of peristaltic waves are present in the distal stomach, whereas the proximal stomach has no such changes in potential and no peristaltic waves (66, 91). The characteristic myoelectrical activity of the proximal stomach is a slow depolarization of membrane potential of small amplitude, which triggers a sustained or "tonal" contraction (79,83).

The proximal stomach and the distal stomach have unique motor roles. The proximal stomach is primarily concerned with the receipt and storage of food and the transfer of liquified gastric chyme from the stomach to the duodenum, whereas the distal stomach is primarily concerned with retention and trituration of solids, and the prevention of duodenal-gastric reflux.

Proximal Stomach

The proximal stomach receives and stores ingested boluses of food from the esophagus. Its slow, sustained, tonal contractions exert a steady pressure on the proximal gastric content, gradually pressing it toward the distal stomach and duodenum. By regulating intragastric pressure and, hence, the gradient in pressure between the stomach and the duodenum, the tonal contractions of the proximal stomach have a major role in controlling gastric emptying of liquids.

Anatomy

The smooth muscle of the proximal part of the stomach is not as clearly separated into three distinct muscular layers as is the smooth muscle of the distal stomach. The smooth muscle in the fundus and orad corpus interlaces and cannot be easily separated into an outer

longitudinal layer, a median circular layer, and an inner oblique layer, except near the cardia. However, the muscle is innervated by both parasympathetic neurons via the vagi and sympathetic neurons via the splanchnic nerves and celiac plexus, as is true for the distal stomach.

Electrical Activity

Intracellular recordings. Intracellular recordings from the smooth muscle cells of the proximal stomach show that the cells have a steady, nonfluctuating transmembrane potential when at rest (79,83). The spontaneous cyclical changes in potential characteristic of the cells of the distal stomach are not found. Contractions in the proximal stomach result from small, slow depolarizations of the membrane without spikes. Repolarization occurs as the muscle relaxes. A complete description of the transmembrane electrical events of these smooth muscle cells is found in Chapter 7.

Extracellular recordings. *In vivo* recordings of the tunica muscularis of the proximal stomach made through the use of extracellular techniques have also shown a steady resting potential with no spontaneous fluctuations, at least in dog and man (43,66). When phasic contractions are present, however, some workers have recorded bursts of spiking changes in potential (85). The bursts occur just preceding and during the contractions. Other workers have not been able to distinguish clearly such changes in potential from background noise, and no one has recorded extracellularly the electrical events that precede proximal gastric tonal contractions.

Contractions

The contractions of the proximal stomach are of two types: slow, sustained contractions and more rapid, phasic contractions (Fig. 2). The slow, sustained contractions result in changes in intragastric pressure with durations of 1 to 3 min and amplitudes of 10 to 50 cm H_2O. In contrast, the rapid, phasic contractions cause changes in intragastric pressure with amplitudes of 5 to 15 cm H_2O and durations of about 10 to 15 sec. An

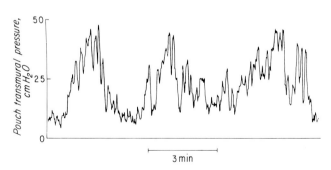

FIG. 2. Contractions of a vagally innervated proximal gastric pouch (62).

additional phasic contraction, termed the fundal wave, also sometimes occurs in the proximal stomach (69). It results in a change in intragastric pressure with an amplitude greater than 50 cm H_2O and a duration of about 1 min. The phasic contractions are usually superimposed upon the sustained contractions, but either type of contraction can occur in the absence of the other.

The entire tunica muscularis of the proximal stomach acts as an encompassing muscular net that alternatively compresses the content of the proximal stomach and relaxes its compression. The contractions are stationary and do not migrate from one section of the proximal stomach to another.

Regulation of Contractions

The lack of spontaneous depolarization of the proximal gastric smooth muscle means that the activation of contractions of the muscle is dependent on external controls. The controls appear to influence most areas of the proximal stomach simultaneously, facilitating the action of the entire proximal stomach as a single contractile unit. The controls are neural, hormonal, and possibly paracrine in nature.

Neural. The vagal nerves have neurons that carry both excitatory and inhibitory messages to the proximal stomach (1). The excitatory vagal neurons release acetylcholine from their postganglionic nerve terminals, which in turn stimulates the smooth muscle cells of the proximal stomach to contract. The inhibitory vagal neurons release a transmitter from their postganglionic nerve terminals, which inhibits the contractions of the proximal gastric smooth muscle cells. The chemical nature of this transmitter is unknown, but it is noncholinergic and nonadrenergic. The sympathetic nerves also release a transmitter from their neurons which inhibits proximal gastric contractions; viz., norepinephrine.

Recent evidence indicates that other transmitters or modulators of gastric contractions may be released by vagal or other neurons in the proximal gastric wall, viz., dopamine (106) and enkephalin (70). Dopamine may have an inhibitory role and enkephalin a stimulatory one, but the physiologic significance of these substances is unknown.

Both excitatory and inhibitory responses are activated by extrinsic or intrinsic reflex activity. For example, inhibitory reflexes are brought into play by deglutition or by distention of the stomach or small intestine. Such reflexes inhibit contractions of the proximal stomach and enhance gastric accommodation. Once the stomach is distended, the inhibitory influences decline, and proximal gastric contractions appear that promote distal propulsion of chyme.

Hormonal. A number of hormones also influence contractions in the proximal stomach. Motilin stimulates proximal gastric contractions, and gastrin, chole-

cystokinin, secretin, gatric inhibitory polypeptide, glucagon, vasoactive intestinal peptide, and somatostatin inhibit proximal gastric contractions (79,83,105,107, 112,115). Motilin probably exerts its action in part by enhancing release of acetylcholine from the cholinergic neurons of the proximal stomach (79), whereas gastrin probably acts by augmenting release of the vagal inhibitory transmitter (83). The sensitivity of the proximal stomach to both motilin and gastrin is decreased by vagotomy (32,85). Of all these hormones, the only one that has been shown to influence proximal gastric motility, when given in physiological doses, is cholecystokinin (31).

Paracrine. Substances may be released locally that act locally to influence proximal gastric contractions. For example, histamine and serotonin, both of which are found in the wall of the proximal stomach, enhance contractions of smooth muscle, and they may do so in the proximal stomach. However, there is little evidence to date to document this.

Consequences of Contractions

The contractions of the proximal stomach have a major role in regulating its motor functions.

Receipt of food. The proximal stomach has an important property, called receptive relaxation, which enables it to receive readily boluses of food from the esophagus. With the onset of deglutition and before the arrival of the bolus from the esophagus, the pressure within the lumen of the proximal stomach decreases (Fig. 3). The proximal stomach relaxes to receive the entering bolus; hence, the term *receptive relaxation.* This property allows the stomach to fill without large increases in intragastric pressure occurring with each swallowed bolus. Receptive relaxation is a reflex mediated by inhibitory neurons in the vagal nerves, for when the vagal nerves to the stomach are divided, receptive relaxation is abolished (1,18).

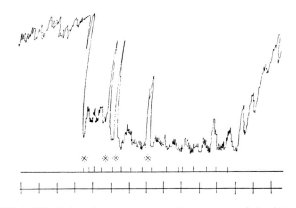

FIG. 3. Effect of swallowing on intragastric pressure. Animal movements (*asterisks*), swallowing (*middle line*), and time in half-minutes (*bottom line*) are shown. (From Cannon and Lieb, ref. 18, with permission.)

Storage. The proximal stomach stores the boluses of ingested food. The solid portions of the food form a mass in the proximal stomach. Successive boluses add to the external diameter of the mass, which gradually enlarges as more and more solid food is taken. Swallowed liquids, however, flow readily around the outside of the mass, and pass into the distal stomach and duodenum. Gastric juice, secreted in response to the meal, also flows around the outside of the mass and into the distal corpus and antrum. The pH in the center of the mass remains near neutrality. As a consequence, the continued enzymatic breakdown of starches in the center of the mass by salivary amylase continues even though the food is in the stomach (10,16).

The storage of food in the proximal stomach is facilitated by another property of the proximal stomach, accommodation. Accommodation is that property of the proximal stomach that allows it to be distended to a large size with little change in intragastric pressure. For example, as the proximal stomach of a dog is gradually distended from 0 ml to 300 ml with an intragastric balloon, the pressure within the gastric lumen increases from 0 cm H_2O to about 10 cm H_2O (Fig. 4). However, with continuing distention from 300 ml to 700 ml, little further increase in intragastric pressure occurs. The stomach adapts or accommodates to the increasing distention without increasing intragastric pressure. Accommodation and receptive relaxation are largely properties of the proximal stomach. They are found to a lesser extent in the distal corpus and occur little if at all in the antrum.

Regulation of intragastric pressure. The slow sustained contractions of the proximal stomach have a major role in regulating intragastric pressure. The phasic contractions of the proximal stomach result in local disturbances of the chyme in the gastric lumen at the site of the contractions, but they do not alter greatly intragastric pressure. However, the sustained pressure of the tonal proximal gastric stomach contractions maintains a steady, continuing compression of the gastric content. Thus, increases or decreases in intragastric pressure are mainly brought about by increases or de-

creases in the strength of tonal proximal gastric contractions.

Propulsion. The slow, sustained contractions of the proximal stomach gradually press proximal gastric content toward the distal stomach and duodenum. Proximal gastric contractions do not churn the content or mix it with gastric juice; rather, they exert a steady pressure on it. In carnivores, the behavior of the proximal stomach has been likened to that of a hopper, delivering its content steadily to more distal sites (16).

Emptying of liquids. The steady pressure exerted on the gastric content by the sustained contractions of the proximal stomach has a major role in controlling gastric emptying of liquids. Increases in the strength of the contractions increase intragastric pressure and speed gastric emptying of liquids. Decreases in the strength of the contractions decrease intragastric pressure and slow gastric emptying of liquids. To illustrate, resections and/or vagotomy of the proximal stomach impair its ability to accommodate to distention (Fig. 5). Intragastric pressure increases greatly with gastric distention after these operations, and gastric emptying of liquids is rapid (11,111,113). In contrast, gastrin and cholecystokinin inhibit proximal gastric contractions, decrease intragastric pressure, and slow gastric emptying of liquids (21,31,35,54,112). Also, when intragastric pressure is set arbitrarily at various levels using a gastric barostat while intraduodenal pressure and resistance to flow across the pylorus are not altered, the rate of gastric emptying increases linearly as intragastric pressure increases, at least when large volumes are present in the stomach (99).

In contrast to its major role in regulating gastric emptying of liquids, the proximal stomach has a minor role in gastric emptying of solids. The latter function is reg-

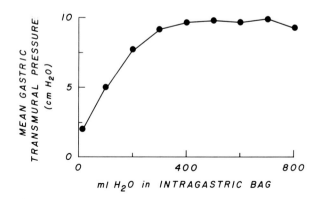

FIG. 4. Accommodation of canine stomach to distension (63).

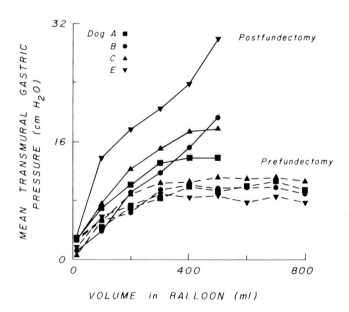

FIG. 5. Effect of gastric fundectomy on accommodation of canine stomach to distension (113).

ulated primarily by the distal stomach and gastroduodenal junction.

Distal Stomach

The peristaltic waves of the distal stomach aid propulsion of gastric content toward the pylorus. Liquids pass readily through the distal stomach and pylorus into the duodenum, but solids are retained in the distal stomach, where they are mixed with gastric juice and triturated into particles about 0.1 mm in size.

Anatomy

The distal stomach includes the distal two-thirds of the gastric corpus as well as the entire gastric antrum. Its tunica muscularis consists of three distinct layers: an outer longitudinal layer, an inner circular layer, and an innermost oblique layer (104). The longitudinal layer is most prominent over the lesser and greater curvatures of the distal stomach and thins out in the mid portions of the anterior and posterior gastric walls. The circular layer gradually thickens as the gastroduodenal junction is approached. Moreover, near the junction it is gathered into two bands or slings that intermingle over a distance of about 1.5 cm on the lesser curvature and that fan out over a distance of 2 to 5 cm on the greater curvature. The oblique layer is best seen along the lesser curvature in the proximal portion of the distal stomach. In the distal portion, the oblique fibers assume a more transverse direction and are not easily differentiated from the underlying circular muscular fibers. The tunica muscularis of the distal stomach, like that of the proximal stomach, receives vagal excitatory and vagal inhibitory fibers as well as sympathetic inhibitory fibers.

Electrical Activity

Much more is known about the electrical activity of the distal stomach than of the proximal stomach. Intracellular recordings from distal gastric smooth muscle cells reveal well-defined, slow, cyclic changes in potential that consist of an upstroke potential and a plateau potential, with or without spikes (see Chapter 7). Extracellular recordings detect these changes in potential as pacesetter potentials (slow waves, electrical control activity, basic electrical rhythm) and action potentials (spike potentials, burst potentials, or electrical response activity). A major effect of these electrical phenomena is to coordinate the activities of the millions of distal gastric smooth muscle cells, so that a regular series of peristaltic waves sweeps aborally through the distal stomach.

Pacesetter potentials. The cycles of the pacesetter potentials are found throughout the distal stomach, but they are not detected in the proximal stomach (3,66). In fact, their presence establishes the physiological motor division between the two gastric regions. Each cycle consists of an initial triphasic complex and a second isopotential segment (Fig. 6). The initial positive deflection of the triphasic complex gives way to a larger negative deflection, which then returns to the base line, usually with a slight overshoot. The amplitude of the negative deflection is smallest in the orad corpus (0.1–0.5 mV) and gradually increases as the gastroduodenal junction is approached, so that the amplitude in the terminal antrum is 2 to 4 mV. The duration of the triphasic complex in humans is 2 to 4 sec; the duration of the second component of the cycles, the isopotential segment, is about 14 to 16 sec. The end of one cycle occurs with the onset of the triphasic complex of the next cycle. The cycles have a regular rhythm and a frequency of about 3/min in humans and 4 to 5/min in dogs.

The pacesetter potentials originate in an area of tunica muscularis along the greater curve of the stomach near the junction of the orad and middle thirds of the gastric corpus (65,92,108). The cycles are then propagated from their site of origin circumferentially and distally to the pylorus, moving as a ring down the gastric wall. The velocity of propagation is slow in the corpus (0.5 cm/sec), but the cycles accelerate as they move distally, reaching speeds of up to 4 cm/sec in the terminal antrum. The velocity is slightly faster along the greater curve of the stomach than along the lesser curve, so that each cycle arrives at the pylorus simultaneously. The cycles are generated and propagated by the longitudinal smooth muscle of the tunica muscularis, but their amplitude is reinforced and increased by the circular muscle. Neural transmitters and hormones may modify, but are not essential to, the generation and propagation of the cycles.

The longitudinal smooth muscle cells in the tunica

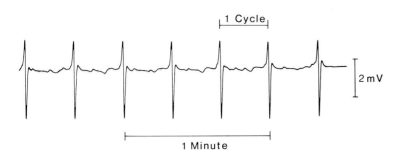

FIG. 6. Human gastric pacesetter potential (43).

muscularis of all parts of the distal stomach have the intrinsic ability to generate pacesetter potentials. However, the frequency with which they can do so progressively declines from the orad corpus to the gastroduodenal junction, as well as from the greater to the lesser curve (92). For example, the intrinsic frequency of the cells in the canine orad corpus is about 5 cycles/min along the greater curve and about 4.5 cycles/min along the lesser curve, whereas those cells near the gastroduodenal junction oscillate at a frequency of only about 1 cycle/min. The fastest beating area, the area in the orad corpus along the greater curve, acts as the pacemaker, and drives or entrains the more distal areas to its own frequency. Entrainment of the distal areas by the pacemaker is facilitated by the greater excitability of the distal areas. The antrum reaches threshold with stimuli of smaller strength and duration than the corpus and has a shorter refractory period than the corpus. These properties allow the antrum to be more readily driven (61,90).

Because the pacemaker entrains the entire distal stomach, the frequency of the pacesetter potentials in any part of the distal stomach is identical. However, if portions of the distal stomach are separated from the pacemaking area, as, for example, by transverse transection, the frequency of the separated cells decreases to the slower intrinsic frequency of that area. A new group of smooth muscle cells within the separated region then assumes the pacemaking role, generating pacesetter potentials which are also propagated distally, but the frequency of the new pacemaker is slower than that of the orad corporeal pacemaker (108).

The tunica muscularis of the distal stomach is a functional syncytium allowing pacesetter potentials to spread in all directions from a site of generation. For example, the pacesetter potentials in all parts of the distal stomach can be driven to more rapid frequencies by electrical stimuli given at a single site (Fig. 7). The maximum driven frequency is about 30 to 50% faster than the intrinsic frequency and is slower in the corpus than in the

antrum (67,89). These pacesetter potentials generated by the stimuli spread in aborad, circumferential, and orad directions from the site of stimulation to other parts of the distal stomach. The spontaneous cycles of the unstimulated stomach, however, usually spread in a caudad direction from the orad corporeal pacemaker, because the pacemaker generates the cycles at the fastest frequency. Neither spontaneous cycles nor cycles generated by electrical stimuli spread into the proximal stomach.

Thus, the distal stomach behaves like a series of bidirectionally coupled relaxation oscillators and has been so modeled using computer simulation (91–93). The intrinsic frequency of individual oscillators declines from the orad corpus to the gastroduodenal junction as well as from the greater to the lesser curve, with the oscillator of dominant frequency being in the area of the pacemaker. The fastest oscillator entrains the next adjacent oscillator, which in turn entrains the next, and so on from the orad corpus to the pylorus. The coupling factors facilitating entrainment are greater for the greater curve than for the lesser curve.

Current evidence indicates that the cycles of the pacesetter potential are omnipresent in the distal stomach regardless of the presence or absence of contractions (24). As they sweep distally through the gastric wall, the cycles bring the distal gastric smooth muscle cells closer to the threshold for the generation of action potentials, but they usually do not bring the cells to the threshold. In contrast, recent experiments in which highly sensitive recording apparatus was used suggest that the pacesetter potentials do bring the gastric smooth muscle cells to the threshold for generation of contractions each time they sweep through the distal gastric wall. The threshold is exceeded briefly (1 sec or less) at the peak of the initial depolarization of the pacesetter potential (82). The resulting contractions are of correspondingly short duration and small amplitude. However, both recent and past experiments support the view that excitatory stimuli, such as neural transmitters or hormones,

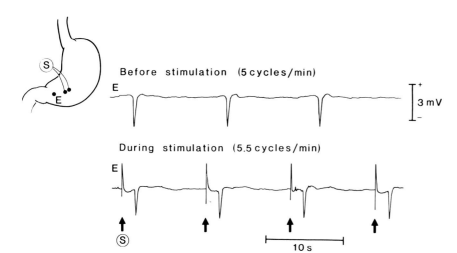

FIG. 7. Electric pacing of canine gastric pacesetter potential. Bipolar stimulating electrode(S); recording electrodes(E); stimulus artifact (*arrows*).

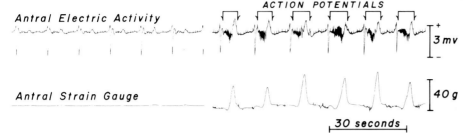

FIG. 8. Relationship between antral action potentials and antral contractions (64).

are also needed before threshold is reached for longer periods, action potentials (spike potentials) are generated, and more prolonged, stronger contractions occur. Moreover, the frequency, direction of propagation, and velocity of propagation of all the resulting contractions are set by the pacesetter potentials; hence their name (66,68).

Action potentials. Action potentials are electrical phenomena associated with distal gastric contractions. They are superimposed on the cycles of the pacesetter potential and always appear just after the triphasic complex (Fig. 8). They usually consist of rapid, spiking changes in potential with amplitudes of 0.1 to 1 mV and durations of 5 to 50 msec. They may occur singly or as a train of spikes. However, action potentials may also consist of slow, negative depolarizations of 0.5 to 2 mV that slowly return to the base line, usually with an overshoot. The spiking type of action potentials are often more clearly found in the antrum than in the corpus.

The time of onset of the action potentials is phased by the pacesetter potentials, and the action potentials in turn result in contractions (Fig. 8). The greater the amplitude and duration of the burst of action potentials, the greater the strength and duration of the resulting contractions (66).

Contractions

The characteristic contraction of the distal stomach is the peristaltic wave. Peristaltic waves are circular rings of contraction that sweep distally through the distal gastric wall. They bring about changes in intraluminal pressure that range in amplitude from a few centimeters of water to over 100 centimeters of water and in duration from 1 to 4 sec. They usually occur at a frequency of about 3/min in humans and about 5/min in the dog. Their amplitude and velocity of propagation increase as they approach the antrum, but their frequency does not (Fig. 9).

Pacesetter potentials phase the onset of action potentials, which in turn bring about the peristaltic waves. However, not every pacesetter potential initiates action potentials; and if one does so, it may not do so throughout the entire sweep of the distal stomach. Therefore peristaltic waves may begin in the pacemaking area and sweep all the way to the gastroduodenal junction. In other instances, however, the waves may not reach the gastroduodenal junction or may begin at a more distal site. The site at which peristaltic waves begin depends on the "tone" of the distal gastric wall and on the magnitude of the intragastric pressure (17). The greater the intragastric pressure, the more distal the site at which the waves begin. Local factors, such as the degree of stretch of the gastric tunica muscularis, the release of neurotransmitters, and the presence of hormones or paracrine substances, determine whether or not a contraction will appear at a given site as the pacesetter potential sweeps by.

Peristaltic waves move through the corpus and antrum at a frequency and a velocity set by the pacesetter potentials. As the peristaltic waves sweep distally, their

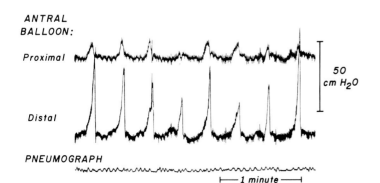

FIG. 9. Human antral contractions during fasting (63).

velocity of propagation increases, so that in the distal antrum the entire gastric wall appears to contract simultaneously. This distal antral systole has been called the terminal antral contraction (19). The lumen of the stomach is smallest at the gastroduodenal junction, so that, with the onset of the terminal antral contraction, the pylorus closes prior to the obliteration of the lumen in the more proximal terminal antrum.

Postprandial gastric peristaltic waves usually do not occlude the gastric lumen. They propel chyme near the gastric wall toward the pylorus but allow content more centrally located in the gastric lumen to pass backwards through their central orifice toward the more proximal stomach (16). However, peristaltic waves occurring during fasting at times occlude the gastric lumen entirely. When this occurs, all of the gastric content distal to such waves is swept through the pylorus into the duodenum (94).

Regulation of Contractions

Neural. Afferent nerves responsive to stretch as well as to mechanical and pH perturbations are present in the wall of the distal stomach. Nerve impulses from these afferent nerves activate efferent neurons, which, in turn, augment or inhibit contractions of the distal stomach. For example, vagal efferent fibers of the cholinergic variety enhance contractions of the distal stomach, whereas other vagal efferent neurons and the sympathetic fibers inhibit these contractions.

Hormonal. Several hormones can alter contractions in the distal stomach. Gastrin has two major effects. It increases the frequency of oscillation of the gastric pacemaker by about 20%; i.e., by about 1 cycle/min. In addition, gastrin stimulates the appearance of action potentials and medium amplitude contractions with every cycle of the pacesetter potential (60,80). Cholecystokinin has an action similar to gastrin (81). Motilin also stimulates distal gastric contractions (79). In contrast, secretin, glucagon, gastric inhibitory polypeptide, vasoactive intestinal peptide, and somatostatin have an inhibitory effect (13,82,97). Of these hormonal actions, only those of gastrin have been shown to occur when physiologic doses of the hormone are given (80,98).

Paracrine. Histamine, serotonin, and substance P also enhance contractions in the distal stomach, but their importance as physiologic regulators is unclear.

Consequences of Contractions

Trituration. The main effects of the peristaltic contractions are to mix gastric chyme with gastric juice and to triturate gastric solids. Gastric chyme is propelled by the peristaltic waves from the corpus through the an-

trum toward the pylorus. Liquids in chyme are allowed to pass through the gastroduodenal junction into the duodenum, but the solids are retained. With the onset of the terminal antral contraction, the pylorus closes, trapping the remaining liquids and the solids in the terminal antrum. Antral systole then forcefully compresses the antral content, grinding the solids together. Unable to pass forward, the antral content is retropelled in a retrograde fashion from the terminal antrum back into the corpus. The sequence of propulsion, squeezing, and retropulsion occurs over and over in the distal stomach thoroughly mixing the gastric content with gastric juice and triturating the solids into smaller pieces. (Fig. 10).

Emptying of solids. Once the solids have been broken into particles about 0.1 mm in size, they become suspended in the liquid phase of gastric chyme and are then allowed to pass with the liquids through the gastroduodenal junction into the duodenum (76).

The operation, distal antrectomy and gastroduodenostomy, illustrates the importance of the antrum in retention, mixing and grinding, and gastric emptying of solids (36). In this experimental preparation, only the distal portion of the antrum and the pylorus are excised. The operation abolishes retention of solids, destroys antral trituration, and results in premature and rapid gastric emptying of solids of large size (Fig. 11).

Emptying of liquids. In contrast to its major role in gastric emptying of solids, the antrum has a less essential role in the propulsion of liquids. Although distal gastric peristaltic waves most likely aid propulsion of liquid from the stomach into the duodenum, liquids empty promptly from the canine stomach regardless of the presence or absence of such contractions (95). In humans, few or no changes in intraluminal pressure are found in the distal stomach during gastric emptying of liquids (88). The human distal gastric lumen remains open to allow ready egress of the liquids. Such contractions as do occur probably serve more of a mixing than a propelling function and perhaps even retard the

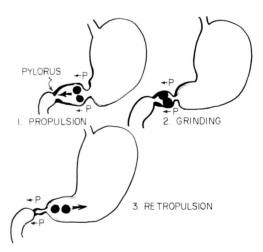

FIG. 10. Consequences of antral peristalsis (P).

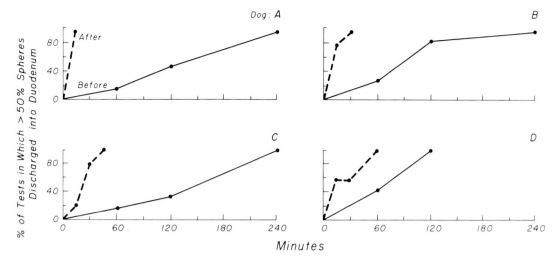

FIG. 11. Effect of distal antrectomy on gastric emptying of solid spheres (63).

emptying of liquids. Cholecystokinin and gastrin, which enhance distal gastric contractions, actually slow gastric emptying of liquids (32,54). Resections or extrinsic denervations of the distal stomach, which abolish or markedly decrease the strength of distal gastric contractions, have little effect on the rate of gastric emptying of liquids (36,84). Even propping open the lumen of the distal antrum and pylorus with a noncompressible cylinder does not alter the rate of liquid emptying (30).

Gastroduodenal Junction

The gastroduodenal junction, or pylorus, relaxes to allow liquids to empty and contracts to provide continence for gastric solids and to prevent reflux of duodenal content back into the stomach. The gastroduodenal junction acts as an integral part of the terminal antrum

and probably is not a distinct autonomous sphincter, such as the gastroesophageal or internal anal sphincter.

Anatomy

The tunica muscularis at the gastroduodenal junction shows a marked thickening of the circular layer which narrows the lumen of the stomach just at the junction with the duodenum (Fig. 12). About one-fourth of the longitudinal muscle fibers of the distal part of the stomach pass across the gastroduodenal junction into the duodenum, whereas about three-fourths of the longitudinal muscle turn luminalward into the circular muscle at the gastroduodenal junction to separate the circular muscle by a series of septa. The circular muscle projects as a distinct bulge into the lumen at the gastroduodenal junction, and the bulge, together with the

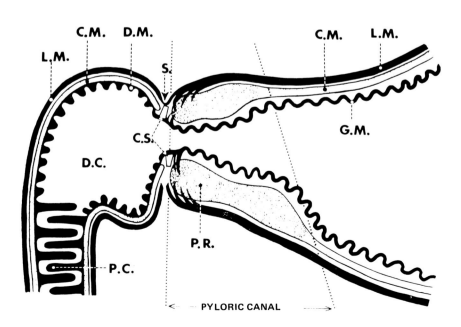

FIG. 12. Diagram of gastroduodenal junction in the human being. C.M., circular muscle; C.S., connective tissue septum; D.C., duodenal cap; D.M., duodenal mucosa; G.M., gastric mucosa; L.M., longitudinal muscle; P.C., plicae circulares; P.R., pyloric ring or sphincter. (From Edwards, and Rowlands, ref. 37, with permisssion.)

overlying mucosa, protrudes slightly into the duodenum like a circular lip (22,37). A connective tissue septum separates the gastric circular muscle from the duodenal circular muscle at the pylorus. Some have descirbed this septum as an electric insulator (8). The gastroduodenal junction receives both vagal excitatory and inhibitory fibers as well as sympathetic inhibitory fibers.

Electrical Activity

The electrical activity of the gastroduodenal junction is similar to that of the more proximal antrum. Pacesetter potentials occur at a frequency of 3/min in humans and 5/min in dogs. The pacesetter potentials phase the onset of action potentials which in turn result in contractions. The pylorus contracts in sequence with the terminal antral contraction.

Contractions

There is little evidence that a sphincter is present at the gastroduodenal junction. Most investigators have not found a zone of increased pressure at the pylorus when pressure-sensitive devices are pulled through the resting pylorus from the duodenum into the stomach (4, 6,37,59), although some groups have (12,41). The increase in pressure recorded by the latter groups was small, however, and may have resulted from drawing a recording device of relatively large diameter through an area of the gastrointestinal tract where the lumen is small and the tract curves. Thus, the bulk of evidence shows that the lumen of the gastroduodenal junction remains open and patent when the stomach is at rest. In doing so, the pylorus of the resting stomach does not provide a barrier to the flow of liquid content from the stomach into the duodenum, or vice versa.

The phylorus does close, however, when contractions appear in the distal stomach. As the peristaltic waves sweep down the corpus and through the antrum to end in the terminal antral contraction, the pylorus closes in sequence with the contraction, after which it relaxes (19). Thus, the pylorus is ordinarily closed only during the brief period when the peristaltic wave arrives at the pylorus. The opening of the pylorus may be aided by the contraction to those longitudinal muscle fibers which dip down into the circular muscle at the pylorus. When these longitudinal muscle fibers contract, they likely pull the pylorus open (C. F. Code, 1968, *personal communication*).

Regulation of Contractions

Neural.

Vagal excitatory and vagal inhibitory fibers augment and inhibit contractions of the pylorus respectively (5, 78). In addition, the sympathetic fibers also inhibit contractions of the gastroduodenal junction. The inhibitory fibers may be dominant, for, when the nerves of the pyloric region are stimulated electrically, the predominant effect is inhibition.

Hormonal.

Cholecystokinin and secretin enhance the contractions of the gastroduodenal junction (42). In contrast, gastrin does not alter the contractions, although it does block the response to cholecystokinin and secretin (42). Whether these actions are physiological is unknown. At any rate, the action of individual hormones on pyloric motility is strikingly different from their action on distal gastric motility, which, in turn, differs from their action on proximal gastric motility (Table 1).

Paracrine.

Little is known regarding the function of paracrine substances in the regulation of pyloric contractions.

Consequences of Contractions

Continence for solids.

The small diameter of the gastric lumen at the gastroduodenal junction provides continence of gastric solids. As solids are swept into the distal stomach by the peristaltic wave, the gastroduodenal junction contracts, closes, and prevents their entrance into the duodenum. The ability of the gastroduodenal junction to perform

TABLE 1. *Effect of hormones on gastric motility*

| Hormone | Proximal stomach | | Distal stomach | | Pylorus |
	Action potentials	Contractions[a]	Action potentials	Contractions[a]	Contractions
Gastrin	−	−	+	+	0
Cholecystokinin	nt	−	+	+	+
Motilin	+	+	+	+	nt
Secretin	nt	−	−	−	+
Glucagon	nt	−	−	−	nt

(−) Inhibits; (+) stimulates; (0) no effect; (nt) not tested.
[a] Gastric inhibitory polypeptide, vasoactive inhibitory peptide, and somatostatin also inhibit.

this function is quite remarkable in that over 90% of the particles passing through the gastroduodenal junction are less than 0.25 mm in size (76). Almost no particles larger than 2 mm are allowed to leave the stomach.

Prevention of reflux. The gastroduodenal junction also remains closed while contractions are occurring in the proximal duodenum. The consequence of the closure is that duodenal content does not usually re-enter the stomach when the proximal duodenum contracts. The content must move distally toward the jejunum.

The closure of the pylorus just after chyme enters the duodenum from the stomach is brought about in part by the hydrogen ions in the chyme. The hydrogen ions trigger receptors in the duodenum which in turn probably activate both neural and hormonal pathways that enhance pyloric closure (12). The closure occurs so quickly that neural pathways likely have the more important role.

GASTRIC EMPTYING

Physics of Emptying

Determinants of Emptying. The rate of gastric emptying of chyme (dv/dt) is a function of the difference in pressure between the stomach (P_S) and the duodenum (P_D), as well as of the resistance to flow across the gastroduodenal junction (R_P):

$$dv/dt = (P_S - P_D)/R_P$$

The stomach does not drain by gravity but empties only when there is a sufficient difference in pressure between the gastric and duodenal lumens to overcome the resistance to flow at the pylorus and drive content from the stomach into the duodenum.

The implications of this relationship are that the rate of gastric emptying of liquids is primarily dependent on the gradient in pressure between the stomach and the duodenum, because the resistance to the flow of liquids across the gastroduodenal junction is small. Moreover, the magnitude of the gradient varies directly with the intragastric pressure. Because proximal gastric contractions are the major regulator on intragastric pressure, they are a major regulator of gastric emptying of liquids. The duodenal contractions are another major regulator by virtue of their effect on intraduodenal pressure and the gastroduodenal pressure gradient.

In contrast, the rate of gastric emptying of solids, because of their large size, is largely determined by the resistance to their flow across the pylorus. Even though big gradients in pressure might exist between the stomach and the duodenum, the resistance at the gastroduodenal junction to the flow of solids is so large that the movement of solids from the stomach to the duodenum does not occur. Solids are retained in the stomach. Because antral and pyloric contractions determine the magnitude of the resistance at the gastroduodenal junction, they have a major role in regulating gastric emptying of solids.

Gastroduodenal motor coordination. During gastric emptying, a sequence of contractile events occurs in the stomach, gastroduodenal junction, and proximal duodenum which facilitates emptying (19,110). As content is propelled into the distal stomach, the antrum, pylorus, and proximal duodenum relax and allow the liquids in the content to pass readily into the duodenum. The terminal antrum then contracts, further aiding propulsion of the liquids. With the development of the terminal antral contraction, the pylorus closes, and emptying from the stomach ceases. After the pylorus is closed, the proximal duodenum contracts, moving the content just emptied from the stomach into the distal duodenum and jejunum. The antrum, pylorus, and proximal duodenum then relax, and the sequence begins again.

This coordination of contractions at the gastroduodenal junction is fundamental to the process of gastric emptying. For example, if duodenal contractions were occurring during gastric emptying, gastic emptying would be impeded. Moreover, if duodenal contractions were occurring when the pylorus was open, gastroduodenal reflux would result, and the distal movement of content from the proximal duodenum to the distal duodenum would be impaired.

The electrical basis for gastroduodenal motor coordination has, in part, been defined. The coordination is not due to a triggering of duodenal pacesetter potentials by gastric pacesetter potentials. No temporal relationship exists between the pacesetter potentials of the antrum and those of the duodenum. However, postprandial duodenal action potentials and contractions are temporally related to the antral pacesetter potentials (2). Duodenal action potentials appear with the first or second duodenal pacesetter potential that follows an antral pacesetter potential. The pathway that provides the coordination between the duodenal action potentials and the antral pacesetter potentials travels through the wall of the bowel at the gastroduodenal junction, for when the wall is completely divided by transverse transection, the coordination is lost (9). A neural mechanism is probably involved.

Postprandial Patterns

The stomach has the remarkable ability to selectively empty different constituents of a meal at different rates even though these constituents are ingested simultaneously (Fig. 13). Liquids are rapidly emptied, digestible solids are emptied more slowly, and indigestible solids are nearly completely retained throughout the postprandial period.

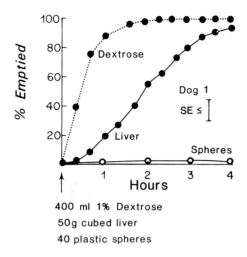

FIG. 13. Patterns of canine gastric emptying of a liquid, a digestible solid, and an indigestible solid after their concurrent ingestion (44).

Liquids.

The rate of gastric emptying of simple crystalline solutions is rapid. For example, the time required for one-half of a 500ml load of isotonic saline solution to empty (T½) is about 12 min in humans (47) and about 20 min in the dog (36). The pattern of emptying of a simple solution like 3.5% sucrose with pectin or 154 mм NaCl is such that the square root of the volume of instillate remaining in the stomach declines linearly with time (Fig. 14) (45). However, the pattern varies depending on the effect of the solution on the small intestinal braking mechanisms. For example, the volume of hyperosmolar, calorically dense solution, such as an instillate of homogenized liver and 10% dextrose, declines nearly linearly with time (44).

Digestible solids.

Digestible solids empty more slowly than liquids. The T½ for emptying of 50 g of solid food is in the range of

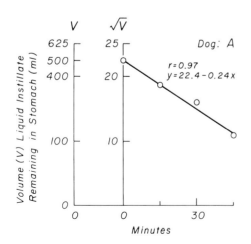

FIG. 14. Pattern of canine gastric emptying of 500 ml, 154 mM NaC1 solution (63).

2 hr. The amount of digestible solids emptied decreases linearly with time (44,71,72).

Indigestible solids.

In contrast to both liquids and digestible solids, large indigestible solids are not emptied from the stomach during the postprandial period. For example, solid spheres with a diameter of 7 mm remain within the canine gastric lumen, whereas liquids and digestible solids are emptied (Fig. 13).

Modifying Factors

Gravity. In the intact stomach, gravity ordinarily has a small influence on the rate of gastric emptying of either liquids or solids. Liquids that do not activate duodenal braking mechanisms are emptied faster when human subjects lie on the right side as opposed to when they are sitting or lying on their left side, but the rate of emptying of liquids that activate the braking mechanisms is not much influenced by gravity (15,52). In contrast, in the vagotomized stomach, the rate of gastric emptying of liquids is much faster in the upright position than in the supine position (74), presumably because the vagotomy has disrupted the pathway whereby the duodenal braking mechanisms slow the emptying.

Temperature. The temperature of the gastric content is important in its rate of emptying. The rate of emptying of solutions that are colder or warmer than body temperature is slower than that of fluids at body temperature.

Volume. The rate of gastric emptying of liquid is faster when larger volumes are ingested. The greater the volume of liquid in the stomach, the more rapid its rate of emptying in terms of milliliters emptied per minute (55). In contrast, the rate of gastric emptying of digestible solids does not vary greatly with the volume ingested. The emptying of solids follows a linear pattern.

Composition of Chyme.

Type of foodstuff. Carbohydrates generally empty faster than proteins, which in turn empty faster than fats (16). However, when the kilocalories per gram of each foodstuff are considered, isocaloric amounts of fat, protein, and carbohydrate empty at similar rates (56). Simple sugars, such as glucose, empty at the same rate as most amino acids, providing that the osmolarities of the two solutions containing each of the materials are identical. An exception is the amino acid tryptophan which empties at a slower rate than would be predicted from the osmolarity (96).

Acidity. Gastric contents at pH 7.0 empty more rapidly than those that are more acidic. In fact, the greater the concentration of acid in gastric chyme the slower the chyme empties (50,51). The effectiveness of an acid in slowing gastric emptying decreases as the square root of its molecular weight increases.

Osmolarity. As the osmolarity of a solution increases, the rate of its emptying decreases, with but few exceptions. The exceptions are solutions of sodium salts with impermanent anions, urea, and glycerol. Isomolar solutions of these substances empty more rapidly than those that are hyposmolar or hyperosmolar (47,48,53). However, the retardation in the rate of gastric emptying when these substances are given as hyposmolar solutions is small.

Viscosity. The viscosity of gastric chyme has little influence on its rate of emptying. Viscous solutions tend to empty at the same rate as those that are less viscous (46).

Energy density. When meals of different energy density are ingested, the rate of gastric emptying of each is such that the number of calories delivered to the duodenum tends to be constant over time (20). However, when foods of great energy density are eaten, more calories are delivered per unit time than when foods of moderate energy density are ingested (56).

Small Intestinal Regulation

The rate of gastric emptying is controlled by receptors present in the small intestine. The receptors sense the nature of the just-emptied gastric chyme and activate mechanisms which in turn slow or speed gastric emptying appropriately (26,50).

Specificity of Receptors.

The receptors are sensitive to the titratable acidity of the chyme, to its osmolarity, and to its content of fatty acids and tryptophan.

Acidic receptors. Acidic solutions empty more slowly from the stomach than neutral solutions because of the presence of small intestinal receptors sensitive to the acids (51). The receptors detect the acids and activate mechanisms which in turn slow gastric emptying. The strength of acids in slowing gastric emptying decreases as their molecular weight increases, but the strength is independent of the fat solubility of the acid and its pK value, if the pK value is below pH 5.0. The receptor for acids appears to act as a titration apparatus to pH 6.5.

Osmo-receptors. Receptors sensitive to the osmolarity of the just-emptied gastric chyme also influence gastric emptying (50). The osmo-receptors are postulated to act in response to a change in their volume brought about by the osmotically active particles. In general, the more hyperosmolar the solution, the slower the emptying, but isosmolar solutions of NaCl empty at the fastest rate. A model has been constructed to explain these findings (50). The model postulates that when chyme is hyperosmolar, the osmo-receptors shrink in size and thereby activate mechanisms designed to slow gastric emptying. In contrast, when chyme is hyposmolar, the receptor increases in size, leading to a speeding of gastric emptying. Certain solutes, such as NaCl, might be actively transported inside the receptor, thus allowing the receptor to increase to a size even larger than that resulting from pure water. This could explain why isosmolar NaCl solutions empty more rapidly than pure water.

Fatty acid receptors. Small intestinal receptors sensitive to fatty acids, as well as to mono- and diglycerides, are also present (50). Unsaturated fats slow emptying more than saturated fats. The chain length of the fatty acids is important in determining the degree of gastric slowing that results from the activation of the fatty acids receptors (Fig. 15). The greatest slowing is brought about by fatty acids with chain lengths of 14 carbon atoms. Less slowing is brought about by fatty acids with a chain length of 16 to 18 carbon atoms, whereas little to no slowing is brought about by fatty acids with a chain length of 2 to 10 carbon atoms. Fats empty more slowly than the aqueous component of a meal when both are ingested simultaneously (28). However, if the fatty component and the aqueous component are homogenized prior to ingestion, both empty at the same rate, a rate slower than that of the aqueous component alone (29).

Tryptophan receptors. Receptors sensitive to L-tryptophan are able to detect physiologic concentrations of this amino acid in chyme and activate an inhibitory feedback mechanism that slows gastric emptying (96). L-tryptophan is the only amino acid known to date that has such a specific effect. Other amino acids slow gastric emptying only in pharmacologic quantities, an effect exerted via the osmo-receptors (96) or via the acidic receptors (40).

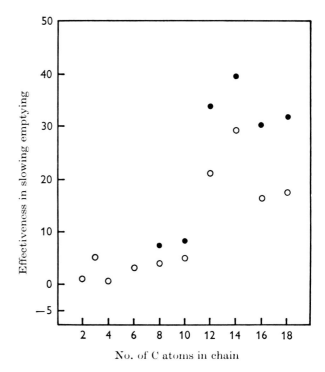

FIG. 15. Effect of chain length on the ability of fatty acids to slow gastric emptying. (From Hunt and Knox, ref. 49, with permission.)

Site of Receptors.

Osmo-receptors are located in the duodenum of humans and in the jejunum of dogs (27,75). Solutions containing osmotically active particles delivered directly into the human duodenum or the canine jejunum slow gastric emptying in a fashion similar to that which occurs when the solutions are taken first into the stomach. Receptors sensitive to acid and tryptophan are also present in the duodenum and jejunum of the dog, with those acidic receptors in the proximal duodenum having an especially powerful effect (25). In contrast, fatty acid receptors have not been identified in the canine duodenum but are present in the canine jejunum.

The receptors for osmotically active particles are positioned in the small intestine deep to the "brush border." The site is thought to be deep to the brush border because when isocaloric solutions of starch and glucose are given, they empty from the stomach at nearly the same rate. The osmolarity of the starch solution in the stomach is less than that of the glucose solution. However, when the starch enters the small intestine, it is cleaved into its component monosaccharides by the brush border enzymes. The resulting monosaccharides then pass deep to the brush border enzymes and exert an osmotic effect on the receptors similar to that of the glucose (50). Some have postulated that the receptors may be located in the lateral intercellular spaces around the enterocytes (7). Proteins are also emptied at a rate consistent with the products of hydrolysis of the proteins stimulating osmo-receptors in the duodenum (14).

Feedback Pathways.

The receptors relay their messages back to the stomach by feedback pathways, the exact natures of which are unknown. However, it seems likely that they are both neural and hormonal. The braking effect caused by the fatty acid receptors occurs with such rapidity that it is unlikely to be entirely a hormonal mechanism (50). On the other hand, meals containing fats and hydrogen ions release cholecystokinin and secretin, respectively, substances which could result in a slowing of gastric emptying by virtue of their ability to inhibit proximal gastric contractions. Fats do inhibit contractions of autotransplanted gastric pouches, so that hormones must be involved (39). Tryptophan also likely acts in part by a hormonal mechanism, since it is a potent releaser of cholecystokinin (31). Tryptophan may also release other inhibitory hormones or excite an inhibitory neural reflex.

Interdigestive Patterns

Myoelectric cycles. During fasting the stomach is ordinarily empty, aside from swallowed saliva, a small basal secretion of mucus, and cellular debris that collects in the gastric lumen. In addition, there may be particles of indigestible solid content left over from the previous meal. A special mechanism exists to empty this fasting content, called the interdigestive myoelectric complex (23).

The interdigestive myoelectric complex has four phases (23). During phase 1 which lasts 45 to 60 min, few or no action potentials or contractions occur in the gastric wall (Fig. 16). Phase 2 has intermittent action potentials and contractions and lasts about 30 to 45 min. The incidence of action potentials and contractions gradually increases during phase 2, culminating in the onset of phase 3. During phase 3, intense bursts of action potentials occur with each pacesetter potential, and these action potentials result in powerful distal gastric peristaltic contractions. Strong proximal gastric tonal contractions occur as well (102). This phase lasts 5 to 15 minutes. Phase 4 follows and is a 5-min transition phase between the intense activity of phase 3 and the quiescence of phase 1, the onset of the next cycle. The period of one entire cycle is about 2 hr.

Each phase of the cycle migrates distally from the stomach to the duodenum and thence down the small intestine to the colon. The migration takes about 2 hr, so that, for example, when one phase 3 is arriving at the colon, another is beginning in the stomach.

Fasting

Phase 1   duration 45-60 min.

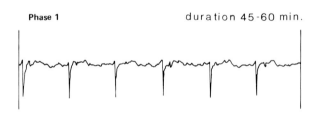

Phase 2   duration 30-45 min.

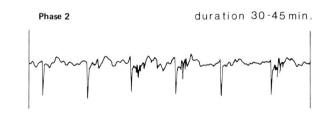

Phase 3   (activity front)   duration 5-15 min.

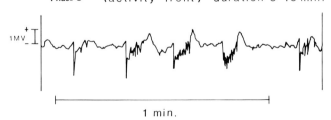

⊢————————————————————⊣
1 min.

FIG. 16. Phases of canine gastric interdigestive myoelectric activity (84).

Function of the cycles. The powerful contractions that occur in the stomach during phase 2 and phase 3 of the interdigestive myoelectric complex have a role in emptying the stomach of its fasting content and indigestible debris (84,94). The emptying begins during phase 2 and is completed by phase 3. The interdigestive contractions that occur during these periods occlude or nearly occlude the gastric lumen as they sweep the fasting content toward the pylorus. The pylorus does not close with the approach of the interdigestive waves, as it does when digestive waves approach, but remains open. Thus, both liquid and solid gastric content are propelled past the pylorus and into the duodenum (Fig. 17). The ability of phase 3 to completely empty the stomach of its residue is so striking that phase 3 has been called the "interdigestive housekeeper" of the gastrointestinal tract (100).

Regulation of the cycles. The initiation of the interdigestive cycles appears to be controlled by a "clock mechanism," which some have postulated may be located in the central nervous system (114). The "clock" must initiate the cycles, at least in part, by releasing a hormonal messenger. The cycles appear at regular intervals in an autotransplanted pouch of proximal stomach, the extrinsic neural connections of which have been entirely divided (Fig. 18) (102). Motilin may be the hormone released by the clock. The concentration of motilin in the plasma varies cyclically during fasting, reaching peaks at about 2-hr intervals (57). The peaks coincide with the onset of phase 3 in the stomach. Exogenous infusions of motilin increase the frequency of the fasting gastric cycles (58).

In contrast, migration of the cycles from the proximal stomach to the distal stomach and thence to the small intestine is not regulated solely by hormones and requires intact extrinsic and intrinsic innervation (84,109). Vagal neurons fire with increasing frequency as the sequence of gastric interdigestive phases progresses from phase 1 to phase 3 (77). Pharmacologic blockade with hexamethonium, atropine, or guanethidine disrupts the regular appearance of the fasting cycles in the stomach (86). Acute cooling of the cervical vagi or complete extrinsic denervation of the distal stomach abolishes the appearance of the interdigestive cycles in the distal stomach and results in gastric retention of indigestible solid materials (34,84). Division of the intrinsic plexi of the bowel, as in the construction of a Thiry-Vella loop, disturbs the rhythmicity of the cycles in the isolated segment even though the extrinsic nerves are intact (87).

Abolition of the fasting cycles occurs promptly with feeding (Fig. 18). Both nerves and hormones have a role in the abolition. After truncal vagotomy the transition from a fasting to a fed pattern occurs more slowly (73). Cooling the vagi in the neck results in a premature reconversion from a fed to a fasted pattern (33). Gastrin inhibits gastric interdigestive cycles and induces in their

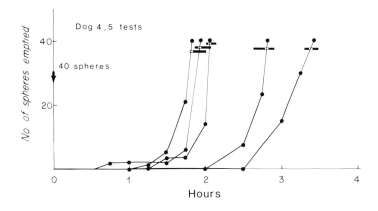

FIG. 17. Pattern of canine gastric emptying of plastic spheres (diameter, 7 mm) during fasting. Occurrence of phase 3 of the gastric interdigestive myoelectric complex (*horizontal bars*) is indicated (84).

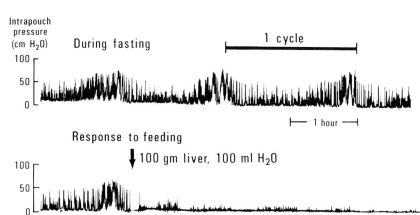

FIG. 18. (*Top*) Cyclical variations of intrapouch pressure in an autotransplanted canine proximal gastric pouch during fasting. (*Bottom*) Abolition of cycles after feeding (102).

place a steady series of medium-amplitude peristaltic contractions in the distal stomach (60,103). It is likely that other hormones besides gastrin also have a role in inhibiting the interdigestive cycles (38).

ACKNOWLEDGEMENT

Helpful critique from J. N. Hunt is gratefully acknowledged. This work was supported in part by U. S. Public Health Service N. I. H. grant AM 18278.

REFERENCES

1. Abrahamson, H. (1973): Studies on the inhibitory nervous control of gastric motility. *Acta Physiol. Scand. (Suppl.),* 390:1–38.
2. Allen, G. L., Poole, E. W., and Code, C. F. (1964): Relationships between electrical activities of antrum and duodenum. *Am. J. Physiol.,* 207:906–910.
3. Alvarez, W. C., and Mahoney, L. J. (1922): Action currents in stomach and intestine. *Am. J. Physiol.,* 58:476–493.
4. Andersson, S., and Grossman, M. I. (1965): Profile of pH, pressure and potential difference at gastroduodenal junction in man. *Gastroenterology,* 49:364–371.
5. Anuras, S., Cooke, A. R., and Christensen, J. (1973): An inhibitory innervation of the gastroduodenal junction. *J. Clin. Invest.,* 54:529–535.
6. Atkinson, M., Edwards, D. A. W., Honour, A. J., and Rowlands, E. N. (1957): Comparison of cardiac and pyloric sphincters. *Lancet,* 2:918–922.
7. Barker, G. R., Cochrane, A. McL., Corbett, G. A., Dufton, J. F., Hunt, J. N., and Kemp Roberts, S. (1978): Glucose, glycine, and diglycine in test meals as stimuli to a duodenal osmoreceptor slowing gastric emptying. *J. Physiol. (Lond.),* 283:341–346.
8. Bass, P., Code, C. F., and Lambert, E. H. (1961): Electric activity of gastroduodenal junction. *Am. J. Physiol.,* 201:587–592.
9. Bedi, B. S., and Code, C. F. (1972): Pathway of coordination of postprandial, antral, and duodenal action potentials. *Am. J. Physiol.,* 222:1295–1298.
10. Beazell, J. L. (1941): A reexamination of the role of the stomach in the digestion of carbohydrate and protein. *Am. J. Physiol.,* 132:42–50.
11. Brandsborg, O., Brandsborg, M., Løvgreen, N. A., Mikkelsen, K., Moller, B., Rokkjaer, M., and Amdrup, E. (1977): Influence of parietal cell vagotomy and selective gastric vagotomy on gastric emptying rate and serum gastrin concentration. *Gastroenterology,* 72:212–214.
12. Brink, B. M., Schlegel, J. F., and Code, C. F. (1965): The pressure profile of the gastroduodenal junctional zone in dogs. *Gut,* 6:163–171.
13. Brown, J. C., Dryburgh, J. R., Moccia, P., and Pederson, R. A. (1975): The current status of G.I.P. In: *Gastrointestinal Hormones,* edited by J. C. Thompson, pp. 537–547. University of Texas Press, Austin.
14. Burn-Murdock, R. A., Fisher, M. A., and Hunt, J. N. (1978): The slowing of gastric emptying by proteins in test meals. *J. Physiol. (Lond.),* 274:477–485.
15. Burn-Murdock, R., Fisher, M. A., and Hunt, J. N. (1980): Does lying on the right side increase the rate of gastric emptying? *J. Physiol. (Lond.),* 302:395–398.
16. Cannon, W. B. (1911): *The Mechanical Factors of Digestion.* Edward Arnold and Co., London.
17. Cannon, W. B. (1911): The nature of gastric peristalsis. *Am. J. Physiol.,* 29:250–266.
18. Cannon, W. B., and Lieb, C. M. (1911): The receptive relaxation of the stomach. *Am. J. Physiol.,* 29:270–273.
19. Carlson, H. C., Code, C. F., and Nelson, R. A. (1966): Motor action of the canine gastroduodenal junction: a cineradiographic, pressure, and electric study. *Am. J. Dig. Dis.,* 11:155–172.
20. Chaddock, T. E., Carlson, G. M., Hamilton, C. L. (1974): Gastric emptying of a nutritionally balanced liquid diet in the rhesus monkey. In: *Proceedings of the Fourth International Symposium on Gastrointestinal Motility,* edited by E. E. Daniel, pp. 515–522. Mitchell Press, Vancouver.
21. Chey, W. Y., Hitanant, S., Hendricks, J., and Lorber, S. H. (1970): Effect of secretin and cholecystokinin on gastric emptying and gastric secretion in man. *Gastroenterology,* 58:820–827.
22. Code, C. F. (1970): The mystique of the gastroduodenal junction. *Rendic. R. Gastroenterol.,* 2:20–37.
23. Code, C. F., and Marlett, J. A. (1975): The interdigestive myoelectric complex of the stomach and small bowel of dogs. *J. Physiol. (Lond.),* 246:289–309.
24. Code, C. F., Szurszewski, J. H., Kelly, K. A., and Smith, I. B. (1968): A concept of control of gastrointestinal motility. In: *Handbook of Physiology, Section 6, Volume 5: Alimentary Canal,* edited by C. F. Code and W. Heidel, pp. 2881–2896. American Physiological Society, Washington, D.C.
25. Cooke, A. R. (1974): Duodenal acidification: role of first part of duodenum in gastric emptying and secretion in dogs. *Gastroenterology,* 67:85–92.
26. Cooke, A. R. (1975): Control of gastric emptying and motility. *Gastroenterology,* 68:804–816.
27. Cooke, A. R. (1977): Localization of receptors inhibiting gastric emptying in the gut. *Gastroenterology,* 72:875–880.
28. Cortot, A., Phillips, S. F., and Malagelada, J. R. (1978): Gastric emptying of lipids after mixed meals in man. *Gastroenterology,* 74:1021.
29. Cortot, A., Phillips, S. F., and Malagelada, J. R. (1979): Gastric emptying of lipids after ingestion of a homogenized meal. *Gastroenterology,* 76:939–944.
30. Crider, J. O., and Thomas, J. E. (1937): A study of gastric emptying with the pylorus open. *Am. J. Dig. Dis.,* 4:295–300.
31. Debas, H. T., Farooq, O., and Grossman, M. I. (1975): Inhibition of gastric emptying is a physiological action of cholecystokinin. *Gastroenterology,* 68:1211–1217.
32. Debas, H. T., Yamagishi, T., and Dryburgh, J. R. (1977): Motilin enhances gastric emptying of liquids in dogs. *Gastroenterology,* 73:777–780.
33. Diamant, N. E., Hall, K., Mui, H., and El-Sharkawy, T. Y. (1980): Vagal control of the feeding motor patterns in the lower esophageal sphincter, stomach, and upper small intestine of the dog. *Gastrointestinal Motility,* edited by J. Christensen, pp. 365–370. Raven Press, New York.
34. Diamant, N. E., Mui, H., El-Sharkawy, T. Y., and Hall, K. (1979): The vagus controls the lower esophageal sphincter and gastric components of the migrating motor complex in the dog. *Gastroenterology,* 76:1122.
35. Dozois, R. R., and Kelly, K. A. (1971): Effect of a gastrin pentapeptide on canine gastric emptying of liquids. *Am. J. Physiol.,* 221:113–117.
36. Dozois, R. R., Kelly, K. A., and Code, C. F. (1971): Effect of distal antrectomy on gastric emptying of liquids and solids. *Gastroenterology,* 61:675–681.
37. Edwards, D. A. W., and Rowlands, E. N. (1968): Physiology of the gastroduodenal junction. In: *Handbook of Physiology, Section 6, Volume 4: Alimentary Canal,* edited by C. F. Code and W. Heidel, pp. 1985–2000. American Physiological Society, Washington, D.C.
38. Eeckhout, C., DeWeuer, I., Peters, T., Hellemans, J., and Vantrappen, A. (1978): Role of gastrin and insulin in postprandial disruption of migrating complex in dogs. *Am. J. Physiol.,* 4:E666–E669.
39. Farrel, J. I., and Ivy, A. C. (1926): Studies on the motility of transplanted gastric pouch. *Am. J. Physiol.,* 76:227–228.
40. Fisher, M., and Hunt, J. N. (1977): Effects of hydrochlorides of amino acids in test meals on gastric emptying. *Digestion,* 16:18–22.
41. Fisher, R. S., and Cohen, S. (1973): Physiological characteristics of the human pyloric sphincter. *Gastroenterology,* 64:67–75.

42. Fisher, R. S., Lipshutz, W., and Cohen, S. (1973): The hormonal regulation of pyloric sphincter function. *J. Clin. Invest.,* 52:1289–1296.

43. Hinder, R. A., and Kelly, K. A. (1977): Human gastric pacesetter potential. Site of origin, spread, and response to gastric transection and proximal gastric vagotomy. *Am. J. Surg.,* 133:29–33.

44. Hinder, R. A., and Kelly, K. A. (1977): Canine gastric emptying of solids and liquids. *Am. J. Physiol.,* 233:E335–E340.

45. Hopkins, A. (1966): The pattern of gastric emptying: a new view of old results. *J. Physiol. (Lond.),* 182:144–149.

46. Hunt, J. N. (1954): Viscosity of a test meal, its influence on gastric emptying and secretion. *Lancet,* 1:17–18.

47. Hunt, J. N. (1956): Some properties of an alimentary osmoreceptor mechanism. *J. Physiol. (Lond.),* 132:267–288.

48. Hunt, J. N. (1963): The duodenal regulation of gastric emptying. *Gastroenterology,* 45:149–156.

49. Hunt, J. N., and Knox, M. T. (1968): A relation between the chain length of fatty acids and the slowing of gastric emptying. *J. Physiol. (Lond.),* 194:327–336.

50. Hunt, J. N., and Knox, M. T. (1968): Regulation of gastric emptying. In: *Handbook of Physiology, Section 6, Volume 4: Alimentary Canal,* edited by C. F. Code and W. Heidel, Chapt. 94. American Physiological Society, Washington, D.C.

51. Hunt, J. N., and Knox, M. T. (1972): The slowing of gastric emptying by four strong acids and three weak acids. *J. Physiol. (Lond.),* 222:187–208.

52. Hunt, J. N., Knox, M. T., and Oginski, A. (1965): The effect of gravity on gastric emptying of various meals. *J. Physiol. (Lond.),* 178:92–97.

53. Hunt, J. N., and Pathak, J. D. (1960): The osmotic effects of some simple molecules and ions on gastric emptying. *J. Physiol. (Lond.),* 154:254–269.

54. Hunt, J. N., and Ramsbottom, N. (1967): Effect of gastrin II on gastric emptying and secretion during a test meal. *Br. Med. J.,* 4:386–387.

55. Hunt, J. N., and Spurrell, W. R. (1951): The pattern of emptying of the human stomach. *J. Physiol. (Lond.),* 113:157–168.

56. Hunt, J. N., and Stubbs, D. F. (1975): The volume and energy content of meals as determinants of gastric emptying. *J. Physiol. (Lond.),* 215:209–225.

57. Itoh, Z., Takeuchi, S., Aizawa, I., Mori, K., Taminato, T., Seino, Y., Imura, H., and Yanaihara, N. (1978): Changes in plasma motilin concentrations and gastrointestinal contractile activity in conscious dogs. *Am. J. Dig. Dis.,* 23:929–935.

58. Itoh, Z., Takeuchi, S., Aizawa, I., and Takayanagi, R. (1977): Effect of synthetic motilin on gastric motor activity in conscious dogs. *Am. J. Dig. Dis.,* 22:813–819.

59. Kaye, M. D., Mehta, S. J., and Showalter, J. P. (1976): Manometric studies of the human pylorus. *Gastroenterology,* 70:477–480.

60. Kelly, K. A. (1970): Effect of gastrin on gastric myo-electric activity. *Am. J. Dig. Dis.,* 15:399–405.

61. Kelly, K. A. (1974): Differential responses of the canine gastric corpus and antrum to electric stimulation. *Am. J. Physiol.,* 226:230–234.

62. Kelly, K. A. (1974): Canine gastric motility and emptying: electric, neural, and hormonal controls. In: *Proceedings of the Fourth International Symposium on Gastrointestinal Motility,* edited by E. E. Daniel, pp. 463–470. Mitchell Press, Vancouver.

63. Kelly, K. A. (1974): Gastric motility after gastric operations. *Surg. Annu.,* 6:103–123.

64. Kelly, K. A. (1976): Gastric motility in health and after gastric surgery. *Viewpoints on Dig. Dis.,* 8:1–4.

65. Kelly, K. A., and Code, C. F. (1971): Canine gastric pacemaker. *Am. J. Physiol.,* 220:112–118.

66. Kelly, K. A., Code, C. F., and Elveback, L. R. (1969): Patterns of canine gastric electrical activity. *Am. J. Physiol.,* 217:461–470.

67. Kelly, K. A., and La Force, R. C. (1972): Pacing the canine stomach with electric stimulation. *Am. J. Physiol.,* 222:588–594.

68. Kelly, K. A., and La Force, R. C. (1972): Role of the gastric pacesetter potential defined by electrical pacing. *Can. J. Physiol. Phamacol.,* 50:1017–1019.

69. Lind, J. F., Duthie, H. L., Schlegel, J. F., and Code, C. F. (1961): Motility of the gastric fundus. *Am. J. Physiol.,* 201:197–202.

70. Lundberg, J. M., Hökfelt, T., Kewenter, J., Pettersson, G., Ahlman, H., Edin, R., Dahlström, A., Nilsson, G., Terenius, L., Uvnäs-Wallensten, K., and Said, S. (1979): Substance P-, VIP- and enkephalin-like immunoreactivity in the human vagus nerve. *Gastroenterology,* 77:468–471.

71. Macgregor, I. L., Martin, P., and Meyer, J. H. (1977): Gastric emptying of solid food in normal man and after subtotal gastrectomy and truncal vagotomy with pyloroplasty. *Gastroenterology,* 72:206–211.

72. Malagelada, J. -R. (1977): Quantification of gastric solid-liquid discrimination during digestion of ordinary meals. *Gastroenterology,* 72:1264–1267.

73. Marik, F., and Code, C. F. (1975): Control of the interdigestive myoelectric activity in dogs by the vagus nerves and pentagastrin. *Gastroenterology,* 69:387–395.

74. McKelvey, S. T. D. (1970): Gastric incontinence and post-vagotomy diarrhea. *Br. J. Surg.,* 57:741–747.

75. Meeroff, J. C., Go, V. L. W., and Phillips, S. F. (1975): Control of gastric emptying by osmolality of duodenal contents. *Gastroenterology,* 68:1144–1151.

76. Meyer, J. H., Thomson, J. B., Cohen, M. B., Shadchehr, A., and Mandiola, S. A. (1979): Sieving of solid food by the canine stomach and sieving after gastric surgery. *Gastroenterology,* 76:804–813.

77. Miolan, J. -P., and Roman, C. (1978): Discharge of efferent vagal fibers supplying gastric antrum: indirect study by nerve suture technique. *Am. J. Physiol.,* 235:E366–E373.

78. Mir, S. S., Telford, G. L., Mason, G. R., and Ormsbee, H. S. III (1979): Noncholinergic nonadrenergic inhibitory innervation of the canine pylorus. *Gastroenterology,* 76:1443–1448.

79. Morgan, K. G., Go, V. L. W., and Szurszewski, J. H. (1980): Motilin increases the influence of excitatory myenteric plexus neurons on gastric smooth muscle *in vitro.* In: *Gastrointestinal Motility,* edited by J. Christensen, pp. 365–370. Raven Press, New York.

80. Morgan, K. G., Schmalz, P. F., Go, V. L. W., and Szurszewski, J. H. (1978): Effects of pentagastrin, G_{17}, and G_{34} on the electrical and mechanical activities of canine antral smooth muscle. *Gastroenterology,* 75:405–412.

81. Morgan, K. G., Schmalz, P. F., Go, V. L. W., and Szurszewski, J. H. (1978): Electrical and mechanical effects of molecular variants of CCK on antral smooth muscle. *Am. J. Physiol.,* 235:E324–E329.

82. Morgan, K. G., Schmalz, P. F., and Szurszewski, J. H. (1978): The inhibitory effects of vasoactive intestinal polypeptide on the mechanical and electrical activity of canine antral smooth muscle. *J. Physiol. (Lond.),* 282:437–450.

83. Morgan, K. G., Schmalz, P. F., and Szurszewski, J. H. (1979): Action of pentagastrin on nonadrenergic inhibitory intramural nerves of the canine orad stomach. *Gastroenterology,* 76:1206.

84. Mroz, C. T., and Kelly, K. A. (1977): The role of the extrinsic antral nerves in the regulation of gastric emptying. *Surgery,* 145:369–377.

85. Okike, N., and Kelly, K. A. (1977): Vagotomy impairs pentagastrin-induced relaxation of the canine gastric fundus. *Am. J. Physiol.,* 232:E504–E509.

86. Ormsbee, H. S. III, Telford, G. L., and Mason, G. R. (1979): Required neural involvement in control of canine migrating motor complex. *Am. J. Physiol.,* 237:E451–E456.

87. Ormsbee, H. S. III, Telford, G. L., and Mason, G. R. (1979): Mechanism of propagation of canine migrating motor complex—a reappraisal. *Gastroenterology,* 76:1212.

88. Rees, W. D. W., Go, V. L. W., and Malagelada, J. -R. (1979): Antroduodenal motor response to solid-liquid and homogenized meal. *Gastroenterology,* 76:1438–1442.

89. Sarna, S. K., and Daniel, E. E. (1973): Electrical stimulation of gastric electrical control activity. *Am. J. Physiol.,* 225:125–131.

90. Sarna, S. K., and Daniel, E. E. (1974): Threshold curves and refractoriness properties of gastric relaxation oscillators. *Am. J. Physiol.,* 226:749–755.

91. Sarna, S. K., Daniel, E. E., and Kingma, Y. J. (1972): Simulation of the electric-control activity of the stomach by an array of relaxation oscillators. *Am. J. Dig. Dis.,* 17:299–310.

92. Sarna, S. K., Daniel, E. E., and Kingma, Y. J. (1972): Effects of partial cuts on gastric electrical control activity and its computer model. *Am. J. Physiol.,* 223:332–340.

93. Sarna, S. K., Daniel, E. E., and Kingma, Y. J. (1972): Premature control potentials in the dog stomach and in the gastric computer model. *Am. J. Physiol.,* 222:1518–1523.

94. Schlegel, J. F., and Code, C. F. (1975): The gastric peristalsis of the interdigestive housekeeper. In: *Proceedings of the Fifth International Symposium on Gastrointestinal Motility,* edited by G. Vantrappen, p. 321. Typoff Press, Herentals.

95. Stemper, T. J., and Cooke, A. R. (1975): Gastric emptying and its relationship to antral contractile activity. *Gastroenterology,* 69:649–653.

96. Stephens, J. R., Woolson, R. F., and Cooke, A. R. (1975): Effects of essential and nonessential amino acids on gastric emptying in the dog. *Gastroenterology,* 69:920–927.

97. Stoddard, C. J., and Duthie, H. L. (1976): Effect of vagotomy on the response of gastric myoelectrical activity to glucagon and food. *Scand. J. Gastroenterol. (Suppl. 42),* 11:77–83.

98. Strunz, U. T., Code, C. F., and Grossman, M. I. (1979): Effect of gastrin on electrical activity of antrum and duodenum of dogs. *Proc. Soc. Exp. Biol. Med.,* 161:25–27.

99. Strunz, U. T., and Grossman, M. I. (1978): Effect of intragastric pressure on gastric emptying and secretion. *Am. J. Physiol.,* 235:E552–E555.

100. Szurszewski, J. H. (1969): A migrating electric complex of the canine small intestine. *Am. J. Physiol.,* 217:1757–1763.

101. Thomas, J. E. (1957): Mechanics and regulation of gastric emptying. *Physiol. Rev.* 37:453–474.

102. Thomas, P. A., and Kelly, K. A. (1979): Hormonal control of interdigestive motor cycles of canine proximal stomach. *Am. J. Physiol.,* 237:E192–E197.

103. Thomas, P. A., Schang, J. C., Kelly, K. A., and Go, V. L. W. (1980): Can endogenous gastrin inhibit canine interdigestive gastric motility? *Gastroenterology,* 78:716–721.

104. Torgersen, J. (1942): The muscular build and movements of the stomach and duodenal bulb. *Acta Radiol. (Suppl.) (Stockh),* 45:1–191.

105. Valenzuela, J. E. (1976): Effect of intestinal hormones and peptides on intragastric pressure in dogs. *Gastroenterology,* 71:766–769.

106. Valenzuela, J. E. (1976): Dopamine as a possible nerve transmitter in gastric relaxation. *Gastroenterology,* 71:1019–1022.

107. Valenzuela, J. E., and Grossman, M. I. (1975): Effect of pentagastrin and caerulein on intragastric pressure in the dog. *Gastroenterology,* 69:1383–1384.

108. Weber, J., Jr., and Kohatsu, S. (1970): Pacemaker localization and electrical conduction patterns in the canine stomach. *Gastroenterology,* 59:717–726.

109. Weisbrodt, N. W., Copeland, E. M., Thor, P. J., Mukhopadhyay, A. K., and Johnson, L. R. (1975): Nervous and humoral factors which influence the fasted and fed patterns of intestinal myoelectrical activity. In: *The Proceedings of the Fifth International Symposium on Gastrointestinal Motility,* edited by G. Vantrappen, pp. 82–87. Typoff Press, Herentals.

110. Weisbrodt, N. W., Wiley, J. N., Overholt, B. F., and Bass, P. (1969): A relation between gastroduodenal muscle contractions and gastric emptying. *Gut,* 10:543–548.

111. Wilbur, B. G., and Kelly, K. A. (1973): Effect of proximal gastric, complete gastric, and truncal vagotomy on canine gastric electric activity, motility and emptying. *Ann. Surg.,* 178:295–303.

112. Wilbur, B. G., and Kelly, K. A. (1974): Gastrin pentapeptide decreases canine gastric transmural pressure. *Gastroenterology,* 67:1139–1142.

113. Wilbur, B. G., Kelly, K. A., and Code, C. F. (1974): Effect of gastric fundectomy on canine gastric electrical and motor activity. *Am. J. Physiol.,* 226:1445–1449.

114. Wingate, D. (1976): The eupeptide system: a general theory of gastrointestinal hormones. *Lancet,* 1:529–532.

115. Yamagishi, T., and Debas, H. T. (1978): Cholecystokinin inhibits gastric emptying by acting on both proximal stomach and pylorus. *Am. J. Physiol.,* 234:E375–E378.

Physiology of the Gastrointestinal Tract, edited by
Leonard R. Johnson. Raven Press, New York © 1981.

Chapter 13

Motility of the Small Intestine

Norman W. Weisbrodt

SMALL INTESTINE

Approximately 6 to 12 liters of partially digested foodstuffs, water, and secretions are delivered to the small intestine each day. Of this amount, only about 1500 ml are passed on to the colon. Thus, most nutrients, electrolytes, and water are absorbed as they are transported through the small bowel. Absorption and transit are brought about by activities of the absorptive cells of the mucosa and by coordinated contractions of the smooth muscle cells of the muscularis externa. Contractions of these muscle layers bring about (a) mixing of the foodstuffs with digestive enzymes, (b) circulation of the contents so that they come into contact with the absorptive cells of the mucosa, and (c) net aboral movement of the contents (chyme). The smooth muscle cells of the muscularis mucosae may play a role in one or more of these functions; this possibility, however, will not be discussed in this chapter.

History and Methods

It is difficult to determine when the first studies of intestinal motility were conducted. According to previous reviews (2,3,20,46,61,66,78,96,199,200), detailed investigations began about the middle of the last century. Many of these early studies dealt with direct observation of the bowel through abdominal hernias and fistulas, or in anesthetized animals whose abdomens were opened. These techniques allowed for long-term observations and for descriptions of various types of contractions; they suffered, however, from the fact that quantification was difficult and that no permanent records could be made.

Radiographic techniques were introduced by Cannon (38) around the turn of the century. By mixing subnitrate of bismuth with canned salmon and feeding it to cats, he was able to describe the patterns of movement of the bismuth within the intestine of conscious animals. Many of the terms and descriptions from his classic paper still are in use today. Radiography has the advantages that movement of material within the gut lumen can be followed and that experiments can be performed in conscious, minimally restrained animals. It suffers from the fact that contractions of the musculature cannot be viewed directly and cannot be quantified. Also, overlying loops of small bowel make it difficult to study all areas of the intestine. Initially, permanent records could not be obtained and there were dangers of overexposure to radiation. However, these problems have been overcome with the advent of cineradiography with video taping and image intensifiers.

Graphic methods for measuring contractions of the intestines in anesthetized animals were also introduced in the late nineteenth century. The technique of introducing a balloon into the intestinal lumen in order to record contractions of the circular muscle layer was popularized by the classic work of Bayliss and Starling (14). This technique has the advantages that contractions can be quantified and a permanent record obtained. Also, various modifications of the technique allowed for measurements at more than one site and from unanesthetized animals, including humans. The major disadvantages of balloon recording are that the sensors must be placed within the lumen where they may elicit abnormal patterns of motility, and that little can be learned about the effects of the contractions on intestinal contents.

During the last 20 years, much interest has centered on methods of monitoring contractions of the musculature by placing sensors on the serosal surface. Both myoelectrical and mechanical activities have been recorded. Alvarez and Mahoney (4) recorded electrical activity from the musculature of the gut around 1920. However, it wasn't until the introduction of improved electronic recorders that interest in this method blossomed (9). Electromyography has the advantages that sensors can be placed on the serosa, thus avoiding stimulation of mucosal receptors; the electrodes are inexpensive and small so they can be implanted easily in most species; many electrodes can be implanted at one time so that multiple areas of the gut can be monitored simultaneously; recordings can be made from chronic as well as acute preparations; and electrical recordings yield information about the noncontracting as well as the contracting muscle. A particular disadvantage of electrical recordings is that the relationship, or lack thereof, between electrical recordings and contractions must be either assumed or determined separately. Two basic types of sensors for recording mechanical activity have been developed; one measures the force of contraction and the other the displacement of the muscle walls (78,129). Strain-gage transducers are used widely to record the force of contraction. These units are sewn to the organ in question and can be oriented to record contractions mainly of one or the other of the two muscle layers. These units have many of the advantages of electrodes except that they are more expensive. They have the additional advantage that they record contractions directly. Displacement transducers have not been used extensively. These units monitor distances between two sensors and thus should prove particularly useful in studying various sphincters. However, problems with exact placement of the sensors and with calibration make their use difficult.

Propulsive activities of the intestine can be studied by placing a tracer substance in the lumen and then following its progress. Various experimental preparations and markers have been used. At one extreme, humans have swallowed mixtures which contain charcoal or another marker and appearance in the stool of the substance noted (55,92,117,140). At he other extreme, radioactive isotopes have been placed in the small intestine of animals, the animals sacrificed at certain times later, and the distribution of isotope within the bowel determined (191). There are many advantages and disadvantages to each technique. Advantages of the first are simplicity and safety for the subject. However, the technique is not precise. Only total transit, not that of each organ, is measured. Also, the results are difficult to quantify. Advantages of the second are that transit through only one organ can be determined and the results can be quantified. The disadvantages are that devices to deliver the marker into the bowel must be implanted beforehand, and that the animals must usually be sacrificed to complete the experiments. All techniques that monitor only propulsion suffer from the fact that little to nothing is learned about the types and patterns of contractions that bring about the propulsion. Also, only the movements of the marker can be followed. Movements of foodstuffs have to be inferred. Thus, when intestinal transit after ingestion of various foods is being studied, what actually is being determined is the effect of these foods on the movement of the marker and not the transit of the foods themselves.

From the discussion above, it is obvious that many techniques can be used to study small intestinal motility *in vivo*. Each one has its own distinct advantages and disadvantages, and each is chosen or not depending on the question to be answered and on the animal preparation to be used. If possible, more than one method can be used simultaneously to yield more information. For example, measurements of intraluminal pressures have been combined with radiography to provide information about the propulsive functions of various types and patterns of contractions (83). Obviously, other combinations could and should be used.

Often, the question being asked cannot be answered by using whole animal preparations. In those instances, segments of intestine have been removed from the appropriate animal and placed in a physiological salt solution. Such *"in vitro"* preparations of intestine appear to have been first used by Magnus nearly a century ago (2). Propulsion, contractions of the musculature, and electrical activity of the muscle and nerves can be measured in such preparations (159). *In vitro* techniques have the advantage that the tissue is readily accessible; the influence of extrinsic nerves, chemical transmitters, and other organs or part of the same organ are eliminated; and it is easier to manipulate the environment of the tissue. The major disadvantage of *in vitro* techniques is that it is difficult to relate what is seen *in vitro* to what occurs in the intact animal.

Anatomical Considerations

The small intestine is a long tubular structure that extends from the stomach to the cecum (181). Its absolute length varies from species to species, but it generally makes up 80% to 90% of the entire gut length. In humans, lengths of 18 to 24 feet have been reported. This length is accommodated in the abdominal cavity, since most of the intestine is loosely suspended by the mesentery so it is looped upon itself. Its diameter varies from species to species and is less than that of the large intestine, hence the adjective small. The diameter is not constant; there is a gradual decrease from proximal to distal. Although the small intestine is a continuous structure, it often is regarded as being composed of three parts—the duodenum, jejunum, and ileum. The duodenum constitutes the first 10 to 12 inches and the jejunum and ileum make up the next two-fifths and three-fifths of bowel length, respectively.

The intestine at every level is composed of four layers—mucosa, submucosa, muscularis externa, and serosa. The mucosa is the innermost layer and comes into contact with the ingested materials. It is concerned primarily with the processes of digestion and absorption. The mucosa does contain organized smooth muscle cells, the muscularis mucosae, but the function and control of this muscle is not clear. The submucosa, as its name indicates, lies just under the mucosa and is composed mainly of connective, lymphatic, and vascular tissue. The muscularis externa is composed of two muscle layers, a thicker inner layer in which the long axis of the cells is oriented in the circular direction and an outer thinner layer in which the long axis of the cells is oriented in the longitudinal direction. Both are composed of smooth muscle cells and both extend throughout the entire length of the bowel. Each smooth muscle cell is spindle shaped, being about 20 to 40μm in length and 2 to 8μm in diameter. The cells are rather tightly packed, with little connective tissue being present in either layer. Many cells within a given layer make various types of contacts to allow for electrical coupling among the cells (64,65,93). Although the two layers are separated by the myenteric plexus (see below), they are linked to each other by connective tissue bridges (197). These bridges have been implicated as the means of communication between the two layers. The outermost layer, the serosa, is composed of a thin sheet of epithelial cells and connective tissue.

Neural tissue and cells that contain various hormones, paracrines, and autocoids also are present in the bowel. Nerve cell bodies and fibers are found in various plexuses (84,181). From the standpoint of contractions, the two most important plexuses are the myenteric (Auerbach's) and submucosal (Meisner's). The myenteric plexus is found between the two muscle layers of the muscularis externa. This plexus has nodes of neurons which are connected to one another by nerve fibers. The entire structure resembles anatomically an intrinsic nerve net. These intrinsic nerves communicate with structures outside the myenteric plexus. Additionally, fibers run between the myenteric plexus and the other plexus as well as the mucosa and muscularis externae. Extrinsic nerves not only impinge upon the myenteric plexus, there are some which appear to extend directly to the other layers of the intestine (227). The relationship between the cells that contain various biologically active chemicals and the other structures of the gut are less clear. However, various peptides, esters, and amines have been found in the nerve plexuses and mucosa (217). Surprisingly few potential chemical mediators have been found in the muscularis externa.

Movements of Intraluminal Contents

The actual movement of material within the lumen of the intestine is complex, and it has received rather little study. As stated above, material must be mixed, circulated locally, and transported in a net aboral direction. All of these functions must be performed in a system in which the conduit and the pump are the same. Thus, contractions of the musculature all along the bowel provide the forces for propulsion. This is in contrast to the cardiovascular system, in which the force for propulsion of blood through the conduits (the arteries) is supplied by a separate pump (the heart). Propulsion in the intestine is further complicated by the fact that secretion of material into and absorption of material from the intestine is taking place along its entire length. Also, the composition of what is being propelled is a complex mixture of water and lipid-soluble and -insoluble components.

Since the manner in which material is moved may depend upon its volume and composition, knowledge of these characteristics is needed. Unfortunately, little is known about the volume and composition of the chyme at various levels of the intestine. What is known is that contents are more voluminous and less viscous in the duodenum than in the ileum. In human beings, approximately 6 to 10 liters/day of material is presented to the duodenum, whereas the ileum passes only 1 to 2 liters/day on to the colon. The details of what happens in between are virtually unknown. What is known is that contractile activity is altered whenever volume within a given area of intestine is increased above normal.

From the time of Cannon's original observation (38), studies have shown that intestinal contents move in both oral and aboral directions from moment to moment. However, net movement of intestinal contents is in an aboral direction. The velocity of this net aboral movement varies among species and from one area of the bowel to another in the same species. For example, a nonabsorbable isotope or dye placed in the upper small intestine of a nonfasted conscious rat is propelled rapidly through the duodenum and jejunum (160,191) (Fig. 1). Around 20 min is all that is required for 50% of the small bowel to be transversed (a velocity of approximately 2.5 cm/min). Transit through the remaining half of the bowel is much slower. More than 1 hr is required for movement from 50% to 80% of bowel length (a velocity of approximately 0.5 cm/min). In dogs and sheep that have been recently fed, velocities of transit in the upper small bowel are around 10 to 25 cm/min and 5 to 18 cm/min, respectively (26). Some estimates have been made in humans, but these are difficult to interpret, since the marker often was ingested, so that the variable of gastric emptying influenced the results (92,117,140) Also, it often was difficult to determine just where the marker was in the bowel at any given time. Nevertheless, all such studies show gradients in velocity down the bowel (55).

In certain species the velocity of transit depends on the feeding state of the animal. In fasted rats and dogs, the velocity is highly variable (167,182,190). For example, in dogs velocity in the upper intestine can vary from 0.2 to 16 cm/min. When viewed radiographically, a bolus of material may either sit undisturbed for many minutes, or it may move back and forth, or it may be propelled rapidly in an aboral direction. The reason for this variability in velocity is now clear; it is related to a changed pattern of contractions that exists in the fasted animal, a pattern that will be described later in this chapter.

Transit through the small bowel also is influenced by a variety of neurohumoral and pharmacological agents. Although a number of studies on the effects of drugs on transit have been performed, many of them are difficult to interpret, since the marker was placed in the stomach rather than in the small bowel. Thus, it often is not clear whether or not the agent was influencing intestinal transit by altering gastric emptying. Also, in many studies the small bowel was being perfused with fluid, a procedure which in itself could alter contractions. Nevertheless, in those studies in which the variable of gastric emptying was avoided, it appears that agents which interfere with cholinergic nerve activity decrease velocity of transit (60,178,191). One notable exception is that atropine has little effect on intestinal transit in the rat (173). Other important agents that inhibit transit include adrenergic amines, morphine, and certain gastrointestinal hormones (157,188,191). Few agents have been found to accelerate transit (191,203). In human beings, motilin and cholecystokinin (CCK) appear to do so (16,156,172). Transit has been noted to be increased in certain pathological states (e.g., after

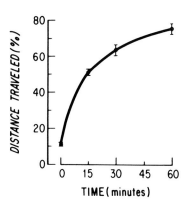

FIG. 1. Percentage of small intestine traversed by the front of a bolus of ^{51}Cr at various times after injection of the isotope into the lumen of the upper duodenum. (From Summers et al. ref. 191, with permission.)

irradiation of the bowel), in certain diseased states (191), and during the acute stages of infection with the parasite *Trichinella spiralis* (43).

Mixing and local circulation of intestinal contents has received less study than has transit. Hard data are lacking, but it has been inferred that localized contractions do cause localized flow of intestinal contents. Although there is mixing of contents at a given level of bowel, there does not appear to be appreciable exchange of material among various levels of bowel. In one study, two different markers were alternatively infused into the duodenum of conscious rats (91). The marker being infused was alternated at varying intervals from 2 hr to 20 min. After infusion, each animal was sacrificed and the distribution of markers determined. As long as the time between changing markers was greater than 20 min, there was little mixing of the markers at any one locus of the bowel.

The pattern of transit through the bowel is complex. As first described by Cannon (38), material may lie motionless in the bowel for some time. Then it is segmented into small pieces that are pushed to and fro over short distances; they are combined with other pieces, only to be divided again. Finally, some pieces may be gathered together and whisked either rapidly or slowly for some distance down the bowel. Then, the process may start over again. Thus, the net aboral progression of chyme is not a smooth, uniform process. The reasons for this complex movement of chyme will become clearer after consideration of the contractile activity of the intestinal musculature.

Contractions and Patterns of Contractions

Although the neuromuscular composition of the bowel appears to be similar along its entire length, there is no fundamental reason to assume that motility will be qualitatively and quantitatively identical at all areas.

Indeed, since the fluid loads presented to the intestine differ along its length, and since different digestive and absorptive processes are occurring at different areas along its length, there may be reasons to expect differences in motility. In spite of this, many studies fail to mention what area of the intestine is being studied; many investigators tend to extrapolate results from one area of the bowel to explain events that are occurring in another area. Many studies, especially in humans, involve recording only from the upper intestine (which can be approached by way of the stomach) or from the lower intestine (which can be reached through an ileostomy).

Contractions of Circular Versus Longitudinal Muscle

Contractions of either or both layers of the intestinal musculature could conceivably cause movement of the intestinal contents. Thus, information should be sought about both layers. Unfortunately, rather little is known about the *in vivo* contractile activity of the longitudinal muscle layer. In fact, what few studies there are of the contractions of this layer, especially in relation to contractions of the circular layer, have often yielded conflicting data. It appears that both layers are capable of independent contractile activity. In anesthetized animals and certain preparations *in vitro,* prominent contractions of the longitudinal layer can be recorded. These may occur either independently or along with contractions of the circular muscle layer (21,41,87,138,139, 159). Such results have been obtained by using such diverse techniques as the enterograph, strain gage transducers, subserosal markers, and measurements of forces of unidirectional contractions of isolated segments of gut. On the other hand, similar techniques have been used to show that contractions of the longitudinal layer are minimal and if they do occur are 180° out of phase with contractions of the circular layer (13,196,225). Some results have even been interpreted as showing that the longitudinal muscle is passively elongated by forceful contractions of the circular layer (225). Many of these data have been obtained from studies on unanesthetized animals. It seems likely that the results obtained have been influenced by the methods used and by the preparation studied. Contractions of longitudinal muscle that occur alone or simultaneously with contractions of the circular muscle will be recorded whenever forceful contractions of the circular layer are absent. Such is the case in anesthetized animals and in most preparations *in vitro*. In those preparations in which forceful contractions of the circular muscle occur, however, as in unanesthetized dogs, contractions of the longitudinal muscle are masked and may even be obscured to the point where the muscle appears to be relaxing. This cannot be the entire explanation, since results from some studies (with the same preparation)

show at times simultaneous contractions of circular and longitudinal muscles, and at other times, contractions of the circular muscle with relaxation of the longitudinal muscle (159).

Since there is confusion as to the relative activities of the two muscle layers and the timing of their contractions, it is not surprising that the relative contributions of the two layers to movement of chyme also is not clear. Contractions of either layer could cause mixing and local circulation. Eccentric and concentric contractions of circular muscle can move material to and fro and thus cause mixing (83). Contractions of longitudinal muscle theoretically can create patterns in which contents flow between the core and the periphery of the intestine, especially if the chyme is viscous (138). Although the picture for mixing and local circulation is very unclear, there is general agreement that contractions of the circular muscle layer are of utmost importance for net aboral propulsion. Combined radiographic and intraluminal pressure recordings indicate that most movements of chyme take place during contractions which increase intraluminal pressure around the sensor (83). Other studies have shown that increases in intraluminal pressure occur when there is contraction of the circular muscle (11,12). Results from experiments *in vitro* also point to a major role for the circular muscle and a minor one for the longitudinal muscle. Segments of bowel can be held at constant length so that the longitudinal muscle cannot shorten. Even under these conditions, contraction of the circular muscle results in propulsion of intraluminal contents (120). Since circular muscle contractions have been studied much more thoroughly, and since they appear to be the more important, the rest of this chapter will deal with contractions of that layer. This is not to say that contractions of the longitudinal layer are unimportant for transit. Indeed, by contracting and thus changing the length of the bowel, the longitudinal muscle could greatly influence propulsion as well as mixing and local circulation of chyme.

Contractions at One Locus

Contractions of the circular muscle at any one locus can be complex (15,50,67,81,82,115). First, contractions may be concentric and occlude the bowel lumen or they may be eccentric and shallow. Second, the length of intestine involved in a local contraction may vary from less than 1 cm to more than 4 cm. Third, the amplitude or force of contraction may vary from barely perceptible to several hundred mm Hg. Fourth, the duration of the contraction may vary from several seconds to several minutes, and at times more than one type of contraction may be present.

Eccentric contractions have been visualized in radiographic studies in humans (83) and have been recorded myoelectrically from the isolated duodenum of the cat (175). In the duodenum of the cat, 75% of the contractions at a given planar section of bowel exhibited some degree of eccentricity. Concentric contractions also have been visualized radiographically and have been recorded myoelectrically from conscious dogs (10). During periods of moderate to intense contractile activity, the majority of contractions in conscious animals appear to be concentric. This is so because, in the conscious dog, there is an excellent relationship between myoelectric events that indicate contraction at a given locus and intraluminal pressure at that locus (12). If the contractions were not concentric, there would probably be little to no increase in intraluminal pressure.

It is difficult to determine the length of a contracting segment. The small bowel can be viewed as an infinite number of overlapping contractile units. Thus, the length of a contracting segment will depend on how many of these overlapping units are active simultaneously. As explained below, smooth muscle cells of the intestine exhibit potential changes across their membranes which act to control muscle excitability. These changes in potential are synchronous over varying numbers of cells so that a relatively long segment of intestine may be capable of being excited simultaneously. The length of that segment may depend upon several variables, including the species and the region of intestine studied. Thus, it should be possible to predict the length of a contracting segment. However, the fact that a region of muscle is capable of being excited to contract does not necessarily mean that it will contract. Therefore, it is possible to predict only the maximum length that could be contracting simultaneously, not the length actually involved. Attempts have been made to measure actual lengths of contraction. Electrodes placed less than 1 cm apart on the jejunum of conscious cats have recorded independent contractions (211). These revealed that the line between a contracting and noncontracting segment can be very sharp. Likewise, both cineradiographic and intraluminal pressure studies have recorded contractions involving less than 2 cm of bowel length (48,83). On the other hand, simultaneous contractions involving lengths of greater than 2 cm also have been seen (83).

The absolute force of circular muscle contraction and the amplitudes of intraluminal pressure developed by the contraction likewise are hard to determine. The values obtained depend both on the technique of recording that is used and on the species and conditions of experiments used. For example, it has been shown clearly that the absolute pressure obtained from the lumen of the contracting esophagus depends on the size and the compliance of the recording device (71). Since various investigators use different methods, absolute values are hard to compare; however, relative values can be assessed. Not all contractions of the bowel are equal in

force. In conscious dogs, contractions of duodenal circular muscle as measured by strain gages vary from 5 g force or less to 80 g force or more (13,40,164). Likewise, in humans, intraluminal pressures recorded from the upper small bowel vary from just detectable (less than 5 mm Hg) to over 50 mm Hg (81,115).

Contractions and intraluminal pressure changes are of two basic types, phasic and tonic. Phasic contractions are usually defined as having definite beginnings and endings, smooth contours, and durations of only a few seconds. Tonic contractions, on the other hand, usually consist of elevations in base-line force or pressure, the beginnings and endings of which are hard to determine and which last from several seconds to several minutes. In conscious dogs and in humans, the majority of contractions are phasic. Each contraction in the dog duodenum lasts about 3 sec (105,164), whereas those in the human duodenum last about 5 sec (81). An infrequently occurring phasic wave which lasts for up to 2 min has been recorded from the distal small intestine of both the dog (164) and the human (50). Tonic contractions may last from as little as 10 sec to as long as 8 min (50,81). These waves seldom occur alone; most often they are accompanied by superimposed phasic contractions. Tonic contractions have not received much attention lately. This may be due to difficulties in recording and in assigning a function to them. Tonic contractions are seen most often in recordings of intraluminal pressure. They seldom are seen in recordings made with strain gages and are not recognized in myoelectric recordings. Tonic contractions once were thought to be necessary for propulsion of intraluminal contents. Now, however, it is recognized that properly timed and oriented phasic contractions are all that are needed for propulsion (46,83). Tonic contractions may reflect long lasting changes in the diameter of the intestinal lumen, which may in turn affect mixing and propulsion. However, this possibility has not been examined.

Because various amplitudes and durations of contractions can be recorded from the small bowel, some investigators have attempted to classify these waves. One popular classification system is a modification of that developed by Templeton and Lawson (198) for description of contractions recorded from the large bowel. Basically, the short-lasting phasic contractions are designated type 1 contractions. The tonic contractions with superimposed phasic contractions are called type 3. Type 2 contractions are anything between types 1 and 3. Type 4 is assigned to the large, long-lasting phasic contractions seen primarily in the lower small bowel. Not only were waves classified as such, but also functions were assigned to each type. Types 1 and 2 were thought to be concerned with mixing, whereas types 3 and 4 were assigned propulsive functions. Such classifications and assignment of function have fallen out of use. Some investigators find it impossible to make clear-cut distinctions among the recorded contractions. Also, the assignment of such precise functions to the different waves has not been supported (55,199). It now appears that the temporal and spatial relationships of the waves are more important for mixing and propulsion than are the amplitudes and durations of each wave. Although there appears to be a current loss of interest in the types of contractions and more interest in the patterns of contractions, one should not forget that the intestine is capable of various forms of contractions. These various forms may play important roles in normal movement of chyme as well as in abnormal movement seen in certain pathological states.

Contractions at Adjacent Loci

Contractions of the small intestine do not occur at only a single locus. As mentioned above, the bowel can be viewed as an infinite number of overlapping contractile units. Thus, contractions occur at multiple sites along the bowel. The effects of these contractions on intestinal contents depend on the spatial and temporal distributions of contractions at adjacent loci.

If a 1- to 4-cm segment of bowel contracts and relaxes during a time when there is inactivity in the segments oral and aboral to that segment, chyme will be displaced in both directions. If localized areas of contractions with intervening noncontracting areas occur over a long segment of bowel, the chyme will be divided into segments with little net propulsion. Then if the contracted areas relax and the relaxed areas contract, new segments of chyme will be formed from the existing ones. This type of activity was the most common one which Cannon (38) observed in conscious fed cats. He called it rhythmic segmentation. Studies that combined cineradiography with measurements of either intraluminal pressure or myoelectric activity have confirmed that indeed such short-lasting phasic contractions do occur and do cause such segmenting movements of contents (51,83).

If contractions occur at adjacent loci but in an oral to aboral sequence, propulsion of chyme will occur. This is the second major type of contraction seen in the small intestine. Both Bayliss and Starling (14) and Cannon (38) observed such contractions and assigned the name *peristalsis*. Bayliss and Starling felt that such propulsion was due to a reflex. When a distending bolus was placed in the bowel, it elicited contraction above the bolus and relaxation below; the peristaltic reflex. Whether or not peristalsis involves such descending inhibition is still debated. It is clear, however, that sequential contractions at adjacent loci do occur. The exact type of contraction associated with peristalsis is not known. Combined studies of propulsion and contractile or myoelectric activity indicate that the same short-lasting phasic waves seen during segmentation also can

cause peristalsis (26,190). However, in other studies, propulsion is seen to be accompanied by tonal (type 3) waves (83) as well as by long-lasting phasic (type 4) waves (50). The significance of propulsion being caused by several types of waves is not known.

Some confusion exists over the terms *peristalsis, peristaltic contractions,* and *peristaltic reflex. Peristalsis* sometimes is used to describe the overall contractile activity of the gut. On historical grounds, this probably is not correct. *Peristaltic contractions* is used to describe events that lead to propulsion of chyme. This is peristalsis as described by Cannon (38). The term *peristaltic reflex* is used to decribe the contraction that is elicited by stimulation of the bowel. In view of this confusion, it is best to describe what is meant rather than to fall back on one of these terms. Other types of contractions also have been described but not so definitively as rhythmic segmentation and peristalsis. One notable example is pendular movement. Confusion about pendular movements probably result from the fact that different accounts have been used to describe them and the contractile events associated with such movements have not been identified (46).

Patterns of Contractions

Migrating motility complex.

Early investigators were concerned mainly with the shape and propulsive effects of individual contractions and with the number of contractions that occurred over short periods of time. Seldom were recordings or observations made over periods of hours in order to observe long cycles of activity. However, even in these early experiments, many investigators noted that activities of the bowel were not uniform over time (18,42,89, 162). For example, Douglas and Mann (72) reported in 1939 that "the bowel of the fasting animal (dog), on the contrary, showed long periods of quiescence alternating with periods of activity. It was at the end of one of these periods of activity in the fasting animal that rhythmic contractions were most commonly observed." Although such cyclical activity was noted, only a few investigators before the 1960s made attempts fully to describe and quantify the patterns. Perhaps the best and most quantitative early description of cyclic activity was provided by Boldyreff (18) in 1911. The illustration on page 186 of his article (18) shows periods of gastric contractions occurring every 80 min. Although not documented with a figure, he stated that similar periodic activity also occurred in the intestine of the fasted dog.

Renewed interest in such cyclical activity began around 20 years ago. In 1963, Jacoby et al. (105) used strain gage transducers to record contractions of the duodenum of conscious dogs. They noted that the patterns of contractions differed between fasted and fed dogs and that the pattern seen in fasted animals was cyclical in nature. Reinke et al. (164) and Carlson et al. (40) further refined the method used by Jacoby et al. and described more fully the patterns that were seen. Basically, four types of contractile activity could be recorded (Fig. 2). One type, intermediate, was seen in the recently fed animal. It consisted of seemingly randomly occurring contractions of varying amplitude. The three other types—basal, preburst, and burst—were seen in dogs that had been fasted for 12 hr or more. These types occurred in a cyclical manner. Basal activity was characterized by complete lack of contractions for approximately 54 min. This was followed by preburst activity characterized by contractions which increased in number and amplitude over a period of approximately 11 min. A period of burst activity then was seen. Bursts consisted of large amplitude contractions which occurred at the maximum frequency seen in the duodenum. These contractions lasted for approximately 14 min then ceased abruptly, to be followed by another period of basal activity.

In 1969, Szurszewski (193) verified these observations in his studies on myoelectric activity recorded from numerous sites on the small intestine of the conscious, fasted dog. As in the mechanical studies cited above, he found cyclical activity at each site on the intestine. There were periods of time (approximately 60 min) when no myoelectrical evidence of contraction (action or spike potentials) was recorded. This was followed by a period of 15 to 40 min when random spike potentials were present. Then a period of 4 to 8 min occurred during which there was myoelectrical evidence of intense activity. This intense activity (which he called an electric complex) appeared to begin in the duodenum and upper jejunum and to migrate down the bowel. The migration was such that as one complex reached the terminal ileum another one had begun on the upper bowel. Thus, the interval between complexes at any one site and the time for migration from upper to lower small bowel was sim-

ilar, being 115 to 183 min depending on the dog studied. Not all complexes migrated over the entire bowel. Of 37 complexes observed to begin in the upper small bowel, 30 reached the terminal ileum. The velocity of migration along the bowel was not constant. In the orad 10% of bowel, velocity ranged from 6.1 to 3.5 cm/min; in the caudad 10%, velocity ranged from 1.9 to 1.2 cm/min.

The description of these cyclical events was refined by Carlson et al. (39) and by Code and Marlett (49). They called the entire cycle of activity seen in the fasted dog the interdigestive myoelectric complex and divided each complex into four phases. Phase 1 was the period in which no spike potentials (hence contractions, see below) were seen. Phase 2 was the period when seemingly random spike potential activity was seen. Phase 3 was characterized by the occurrence of myoelectric activity characteristic of maximum contractile activity. It was the most notable phase and the easiest to identify and corresponds to the electric complex described by Szurszewski. Phase 3 was followed by phase 4, a short period during which the activity returned to that seen during phase 1 (Fig. 3). Code and Marlett observed that all phases of the complex migrated down the bowel and that they involved the stomach as well as the small bowel.

Since several hours of recordings must be obtained in order to characterize adequately the cyclical patterns, data reduction and presentation are important considerations. One of the more popular ways of handling the data is to divide a recording into short intervals of time (e.g., 2 min). Then the number of contractions, or myoelectric events that indicate contractions, are counted during each interval. These data can then be used to construct histograms. Figure 4 illustrates data obtained from a dog before and after feeding. The ordinate shows the percentage of slow waves that were accompanied by spike potentials during each 2-min interval. The abscissa shows the time of recording in 2-min in-

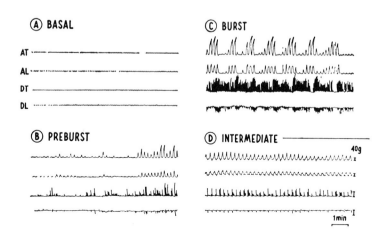

FIG. 2. Gastric antral and duodenal contractile activity during fasting (**A, B,** and **C**) and after feeding (**D**). Recordings were made with strain-gage transducers. AT, antrum transverse (circular); AL, antrum longitudinal; DT, duodenum tranverse (circular); DL, duodenum longitudinal. (From Carlson et al., ref. 40, with permission.)

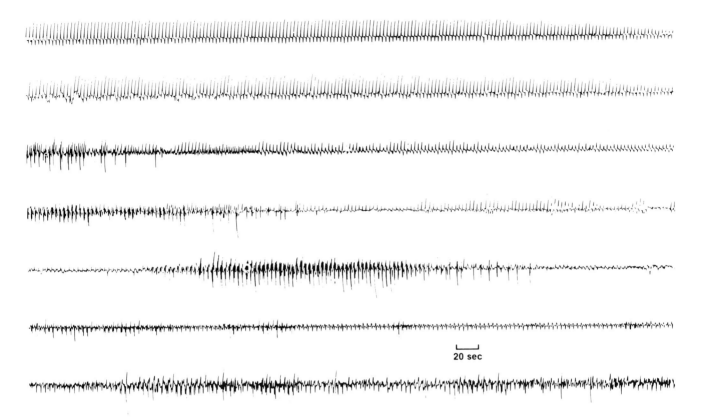

FIG. 3. Electrical activity of small intestine of the conscious dog. Traces show electromyograms from seven electrodes placed equidistant along the intestine. Dog had been fasted for 18 hr. The top two traces show slow waves only (phase 1 activity). Traces 3 and 4 show phase 3, 4, and 1 activity. Phases 2, 3, and 4 are seen on trace 5. The bottom two traces show phase 2 activity.

20 sec

tervals. Recordings from three electrodes, one on the proximal, one on the mid, and one on the distal small bowel were analyzed. During fasting, the cycle of activity described above is evident. Feeding disrupts this pattern (see below). Some investigators have automated the processs so that the number of spike potentials per unit time are summed electrically and histograms are printed by computer (125,218). This reduces the error and subjectivity of manual interpretations and allows for closer inspection of the data.

The measurements of the velocity of migration made by Carlson et al. and by Code and Marlett differed somewhat from those obtained by Szurszewski. They did, however, observe a similar gradient in the velocity of migration. Differences in measured velocities from one study to another should not be totally unexpected. Velocity measurements depend on knowledge of the distance between two points on the small intestine. This knowledge is difficult to obtain, since there is no definite "resting length" of the bowel. Thus, one can measure the distance between the sensors when they are sewn to the gut wall; however, there is no guarantee that that distance will remain the same once the animal has recovered from anesthesia and surgery. Likewise, a tube placed in the lumen of the gut has a definite distance between any two openings in the tube. However, the

length of bowel spanned by the openings does not remain constant. Telescoping of the bowel over an intraluminal probe has been observed (98).

Shortly after the description by Szurszewski of the events that take place in the dog intestine, Grivel and Ruckebusch (90) reported that similar cycles of contractile activity occurred in rabbits and sheep. In both of these species, complexes occurred at intervals of approximately 90 min, the same interval that they observed in dogs. Although complex frequency was the same in all three species, there were some major difference in the events recorded. The velocity of migration was around 10 times faster in the sheep. Hence, even though the small bowel of the sheep is very long, the time taken for the complex to traverse the bowel was similar in dogs, rabbits, and sheep. A second major difference was that the complex occurred in the dog only in the fasted state, whereas complexes occurred in sheep and rabbits that were feeding *ad lib*. Thus, the term *fasted pattern* is not universal but applies only to certain species.

Over the past 6 years, similar cyclical activity has been recorded from a number of other animals including rats, guinea pigs, pigs, cattle, and horses (167,168,170). In some of these species, the ruminents and the pigs, complexes are seen in both fasted animals and those

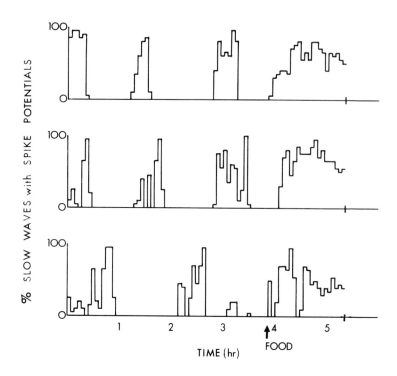

FIG. 4. Temporal distribution of spike potentials at three sites in a fasted dog (*top,* duodenum; *middle,* jejunum; *bottom,* ileum). The percentage of slow waves that were accompanied by spike potentials is on the ordinate; time in 2-min intervals is on the abscissa. Periods of no spike potentials correspond to phase 1 and periods of 100% activity correspond to phase 3 of the MMC. Note how the complexes recurred at each site and how each phase of each complex appeared to migrate aborally. Also note that the pattern changed when the dog was fed.

feeding *ad lib.* In the rat, complexes are seen only during the fasted state. They occur more frequently than in the dog, every 15 to 30 min and are not so regular. The complexes do migrate down the bowel; however, about one-third do not traverse its entire length. One species that may not show this migrating type of cyclical activity is the cat. Periodic activity does occur in the cat but it is of a different type (see below).

Recordings of both mechanical and electrical activities have shown that migrating complexes do indeed occur in the small intestine of the human being (Fig. 5).

Vantrappen et al. (205) placed perfused catheters in the upper small bowel of normal subjects and recorded all phases of the complex. Complexes occurred every 84 to 112 min and migrated along the upper bowel at a velocity of around 6 to 8 cm/min. Not all complexes began at the uppermost recording site. Thus, in humans in contrast to dogs, the site of initiation of the complex may not be constant. Fleckenstein (79) placed an assembly of 11 pairs of electrodes into the lumen of the small intestine of five healthy subjects in such a way that myoelectric activity of the entire small bowel could be

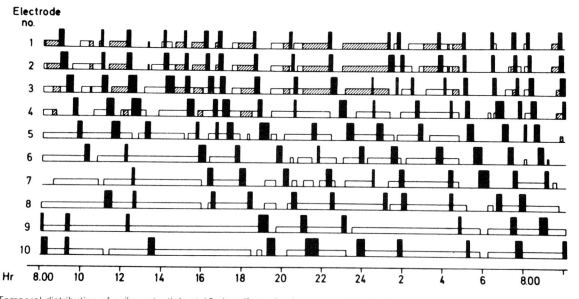

FIG. 5. Temporal distribution of spike potentials at 10 sites (from duodenum to ileum) in a fasted human. The various phases of the MMC that occurred at each site over a 24-hr period are shown: (*solid line*) phase 1; (*open bar*) phase 2; (*closed bar*) phase 3; (*hatched bar*) minute-rhythm. Note how the complexes recurred at each site and how many of the complexes appeared to migrate aborally. (From Fleckenstein and Oigaard, ref. 80, with permission.)

recorded. He found that migrating complexes occurred with an average period of 144 min. In a companion paper, Fleckenstein and Oigaard (80) reported that most of the complexes migrated along the entire small bowel.

Practically all the studies on cyclical contractile activity of the small bowel have been performed on adult animals. However, Bueno and Ruckebusch (32) recently reported on the perinatal development of motility in dogs and sheep. Electrodes were implanted on the bowel of fetuses *in utero* as well as in newborn animals. The recordings they obtained after the animals had recovered from surgery were of one of three patterns (Fig. 6). Before 0.8 of term in sheep and up to 5 days before term in dogs, an unorganized pattern of spike potentials was seen. Between 0.8 and the last 10 days of term in sheep and between 5 to 15 days in the neonatal dog, cyclical periods of 3 to 4 min of intense spike activity occurred every 10 to 20 min. From 10 days prior to birth in sheep and from 15 days after birth in dogs, the normal adult pattern of migrating motor complexes was seen. Thus, complexes develop quite early in life and there are differences in development among species. What is responsible for development of the complexes is unknown.

As with other activities recorded from the small intestine, different investigators have used different terms to describe the patterns of motility characterized by cyclical periods of inactivity and activity. This can create confusion, since several names are being applied to the same event and since the same name is being used to describe different events. Since any attempts to standardize the nomenclature would be futile, it must suffice to list the terminologies used and to try to clarify some points of confusion.

The first clearly described cyclical activities were recorded from fasted dogs. Thus, the term interdigestive myoelectric (or motor) complex (or pattern) was applied. However, recordings from other species have shown that similar cyclical activities can be recorded from some species that are feeding *ad lib*. Thus the general term interdigestive cannot be used. Also, the complexes can be recorded mechanically as well as myoelectrically. Thus the general term myoelectric is not always appropriate. A better general term is migrating motility complex (MMC). Migrating is appropriate, since no matter how recordings are made, the complexes do appear to migrate down the intestine. Motility is appropriate, since it is a general term to describe contractile activity of the gut no matter how it is recorded. Complex is appropriate, since the event is composed of many elements. The term migrating motility complex should be applied to the entire cycle of events, not to just one phase of the cycle. Also, if periods of inactivity do not alternate with periods of intense activity and if the periods do not appear to migrate, then the term migrating motility complex should not be used.

The MMC is composed of definitely three and perhaps four distinct phases. Each phase has been recognized by numerous investigators, but not every investigator has used the same term to describe each phase. Table 1 lists some of the more popular synonyms for each of the phases.

Fed Pattern. In several species, MMCs are seen only in the fasted state. Feeding is followed by interruption of the complex and by the appearance of a different pattern. Although early observations (42,72,89,136,162) indicated that small bowel motility in dogs and humans differed in the fasted and fed states, only after adequate characterization of the MMC could precise comparisons be made. Jacoby et al. (105), Reinke et al. (164), and Carlson et al. (40) recorded what they called an intermediate pattern of contractions from the recently fed dog. The activity consisted of "varying-amplitude, ungrouped contractions, often superimposed on low-amplitude tone changes." Myoelectrically, the fed pattern consists of seemingly random bursts of spike potentials. Similar changes in patterns after eating a normal meal have been recorded in the rat (167) and in the human (205).

The fed pattern is not so easy to identify as the MMC. There are no distinct phases and it is impossible to predict the sequence of contractions at any one locus or between any two adjacent loci. Some attempts have been made to describe the fed pattern. In humans fed 16 oz of skimmed milk, contractions at any one site of the duodenum occurred at multiple intervals of 5 sec (48). The predominant activity consisted of groups of 1 to 3 sequential contractions separated by periods of 5 to 40 sec. Similar analyses have not been made in the dog, but when contractile activity is analyzed in 2-min periods, a fairly uniform distribution of contractions over time is evident (Fig. 4).

In the dog, the number of contractions per unit time seen during the fed pattern depends on the physical and chemical composition of the food ingested. McCoy and Baker (136) observed an increase in spike potential activity with feeding of either canned dog food or milk. However, activity remained higher over the next 4 hr after canned dog food than after milk. Moore et al. (142) fed dogs equicaloric meals of canned dog food and an elemental diet and recorded small bowel myoelectrical activity. They recorded about one-half the number of bursts of spike potentials with the elemental diet as with the canned food. The effects of specific food components were studied by Schang et al. (180). Saline had little effect on the number or pattern of spike potentials when infused into the duodenum at a rate of 0.7 ml/kg-min. Glucose, casein hydrolysate, and medium chain triglycerides infused singly all disrupted the MMC. Of the three, glucose caused the largest number of bursts of spike potentials. The peptides were next, with lipids actually causing a decrease below that seen during fasting.

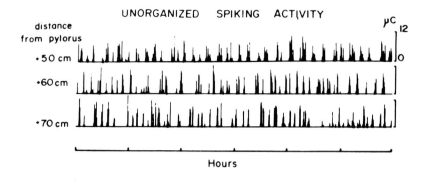

UNORGANIZED SPIKING ACTIVITY

Hours

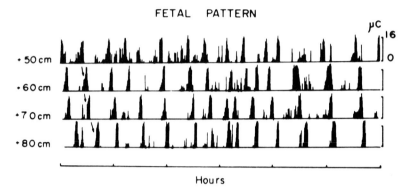

FETAL PATTERN

Hours

FIG. 6. Temporal distribution of spike potentials at three sites on the jejunum in fetal lamb at 0.7 (unorganized) and 0.9 (fetal pattern) of term, and at 2 days before birth (MMC pattern). The intensity of spike activity is indicated on the ordinate, time in 20-sec intervals is on the abscissa. Level of spike activity increased progressively and aboral migration of some phases was evident at 0.9 of term. Near term, all phases were present, thus resembling the MMCs seen in the adult. (From Bueno and Ruckebusch, ref. 32, with permission.)

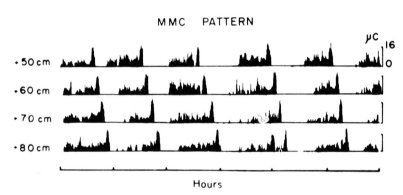

MMC PATTERN

Hours

TABLE 1. *Nomenclature of the components that constitute the MMC*

Author	Period of no or minimal activity	Period of seemingly random activity	Period of intense activity	Period of declining activity
Jacoby et al. (105)	Basal	Intermediate	Burst	
Reinke et al. (164)	Basal	Intermediate	Burst	
Carlson et al. (40)	Basal	Preburst	Burst	
Code and Marlett (49)	Phase 1	Phase 2	Phase 3 or activity front	Phase 4
Bueno et al. (26)	Inactivity	Irregular spike activity	Regular spike activity	
Vantrappen et al. (205)	Phase 1	Phase 2	Phase 3 or activity front	
Fleckenstein (79)	Phase 1	Phase 2	Phase 3 or active phase	

There was little difference in the level of activity caused by 7.5 and 15 kcal/kg of any one substance. The ingestion of any two of the substances mixed together caused an increase in activity above that seen with fasting, and the increase was similar regardless of which two substances were given.

The duration of the fed state depends on the species studied, and on the amount of food ingested as well as on the physical and chemical composition of that food. In dogs with pancreatic fistulas, small amounts of canned dog food did not disrupt the MMC (214). More than 12 g/kg had to be given before a clear-cut change occurred. Code and Marlett (49) reported that oral administration of 400 ml of saline to the dog resulted in disruption of the MMC for only one cycle; 400 ml of milk, on the other hand, induced a fed pattern for 2.5 to 4 hr. DeWever et al. (68) found that in any one dog, there was a linear relationship between the quantity of food ingested orally and the duration of disruption of the MMC. A similar relationship between the amount of food and the duration of disruption of the MMC was observed by Schang et al. (180) for nutrients infused into the duodenum. Thus, gastric emptying does not account for the relationship. Both Schang et al. and DeWever et al. also found that equicaloric amounts of carbohydrate, protein, and lipids induced fed patterns of unequal length. For example, intraduodenal instillation of 15 kcal/kg of peptides, glucose, and medium chain triglycerides caused fed patterns of 165, 285 and 450 min., respectively. Mixing the nutrients together yielded some interesting results. When DeWever et al. administered 30 kcal/kg of protein and 30 kcal/kg of lipid, the duration of the fed pattern was reduced to almost half that seen with 30 kcal/kg of lipid alone. Thus, the effects of a mixed meal do not represent a simple summation of the effects of its individual components. These results could yield much information on the factors that control the fed pattern of motility if more were known about the location and time of intestinal digestion and absorption of the foodstuffs when given alone or in combination, the hormonal response to these foodstuffs, and the reflexes excited by the various foodstuffs. Although studied in much less detail, the period of disruption in humans appears to be much shorter. Vantrappen et al. (205) found that a mixed meal of 450 kcal resulted in a disruption of only 3.5 hr.

Although several species do not exhibit a "fed" pattern when feeding normally, such a pattern can be induced by forcing a change in the animals' dietary habits. When pigs were fed their daily ration in one meal per day, MMCs were disrupted for about 6 hr (170). The disruption lasted 2 to 3 hr after each meal when the animals were fed twice a day. Similar results were found in sheep that were allowed to overeat (169). Flow rates of intestinal contents were measured simultaneously with motility in several of these experiments. The results indicate a direct correlation between flow rates and disruption of the MMC. It is difficult to determine if the patterns of motility induced by altering diets are identical to the fed patterns seen in dogs, humans, and rats, since precise descriptions of the fed pattern are not available.

Other Patterns. Most of the recent studies have emphasized the MMC and the fed pattern. Other patterns, however, have been noticed. In the fasted cat, a species that does not appear to exhibit MMCs, 4- to 16-sec prolonged bursts of spike potentials are seen (209,211). These bursts appear to migrate down the bowel; neither their timing nor their sites of initiation and termination, however, are constant. Although seen during phase 2 of the MMC in the human being, Fleckenstein and Oigaard (80) have described a pattern which they call the "minute rhythm." This pattern consists of a few bursts of spike potentials which appear in the upper jejunum and migrate for varying distances. They occur at intervals of around 1 min and migrate rapidly (2 cm/sec). Such a pattern has been recorded from healthy dogs and sheep (90); however, not all who have recorded from healthy animals have reported such activity. Thus, it is not certain whether the method of recording (via an intraluminal catheter) used by Fleckenstein and Oigaard may have induced the rhythm or whether others have missed seeing or reporting the pattern.

In addition to the patterns seen in normal healthy animals, certain other patterns have been described in animals in various pathological states. Ruckebusch and Bueno (30,169) fed sheep a diet of excess grain until the sheep developed diarrhea. The MMC was disrupted in these animals and a pattern of irregular activity appeared. Atchison et al. (8) administered castor oil, or ricinoleic acid, to fasted dogs in doses that induced catharsis. Changes in intestinal motility were seen within 40 to 60 min of drug administration. The MMC pattern was disrupted and recurrent groups of 3 to 15 spike potential bursts occurred at each site. These groups of spike bursts migrated aborally along the jejunum at an apparent velocity of 0.7 cm/sec. Oleic acid, or triolein, caused disruption of MMCs but did not induce the pattern seen during diarrhea. Administration of the parasite *T. spiralis* to dogs caused diarrhea during the intestinal phase of the infection (179). During this phase, bursts of spike potentials occurred in a pattern similar to that described by Atchison et al. (8) (Fig. 7). In anesthetized rabbits, Mathias et al. (134) found that cultures of *Vibrio cholerae* and cholera enterotoxin induced a series of organized migrating action potential complexes (MAPCs) in a loop of ileum (Fig. 8). These complexes resulted in movement of fluid. Studies on other organisms indicate that other bacteria and/or their toxins as well as ricinoleic acid can induce similar abnormal patterns of motility (110,208). Recently, Burns et al. (35) identified another pattern, which was induced by an in-

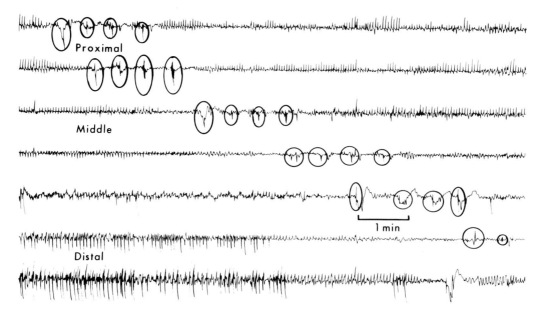

FIG. 7. Myoelectric activity recorded from a fasted dog 3 days after infection with *T. spiralis* larvae. Traces are from seven areas of the bowel. Note alterations in shape of slow waves (compare to Fig. 3). Also note relatively rapid movement of bursts of spike potentials down the bowel. These bursts (circled for easier identification) were never seen before infection. (From Schanbacher et al., ref. 179, with permission.)

vasive strain of *Escherichia coli* (IEC). Ileal loops infected with IEC demonstrated repetitive bursts of action potentials at each location. Such bursts were not seen in loops infected with noninvasive bacteria.

Another specific pattern of motility has been seen in cats, dogs, and perhaps humans shortly before emesis (1,101,141,185,211). This pattern consists of one or more contractions, which begin in the middle or distal small bowel and migrate orally (Fig. 9). Stewart et al. (186) recorded from conscious cats and found that an intense burst of spike potentials lasting 4 to 5 sec occurred at most of the electrode sites. This burst first

appeared at the more distal electrode some 20 to 60 sec before emesis and spread orally at a velocity of 2 to 3 cm/sec. The burst reached the upper duodenum just seconds before the animal began to retch and vomit.

Correlations Between Patterns of Contractions and Movements of Intraluminal Contents

The relationship between individual contractions and the flow of intraluminal fluid has been studied over the past 80 years or so. More recently, studies have concentrated on the patterns of contractions and flow.

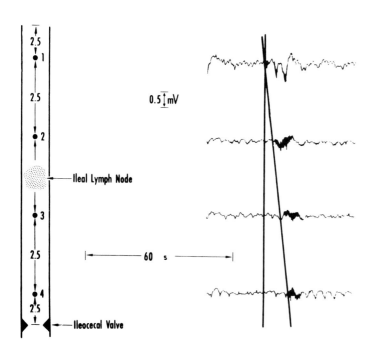

FIG. 8. MAPC recorded from a loop of ileum in an anesthetized rabbit. *Left:* Electrode placement illustrated schematically. Note the prolonged burst of action potentials which appears to migrate aborally. (From Mathias et al., ref. 134, with permission.)

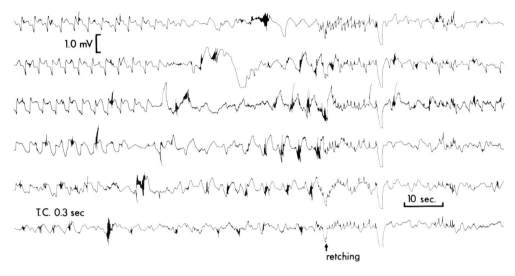

FIG. 9. Spike potential activity induced by the subcutaneous injection of morphine. The six tracings show myoelectrical activity from sites. 10, 20, 35, 50, 65, and 80 cm from gastroduodenal junction. Note that the spike burst appears first at the most distal electrode and spreads orally.

Reinke et al. (164) reported that burst activity (phase 3) in the fasted dog was correlated with the expulsion of mucus from a cannula that was placed in the small bowel. Szurszewski and Code (193) interpreted their data about the migrating complex in light of Reinke et al.'s observation as indicating that the MMC may serve as an "intestinal housekeeper" that rapidly moves interdigestive contents down the small intestine into the colon. Shortly after this interpretation, Code and Schlegel (51) combined cineradiography with recording of myoelectric activity to show that indeed intestinal contents were propelled ahead of the advancing front of the phase 3 activity. Also, any material injected into the lumen of a loop of bowel that was in phase 3 was immediately propelled distally at high velocity. If material was injected during phase 1, however, no movement was detected. Thus, they felt that phase 3 was the housekeeper. Bueno et al. (26) followed the movement of a nonabsorbable marker through the intestine of dogs and sheep while recording myoelectric activity from the same animals. They obtained essentially the same results as Code and Schlegel did in the fasting dog and in sheep fed *ad lib;* that is, the time it took for a bolus to traverse a segment of the intestine depended on the phase of the MMC during which it was placed in the bowel lumen. It took four times as long when the marker was injected during phase 1 as when it was injected during phase 2. Thus, they felt that the main period of propulsive activity was phase 2 (irregular activity). In the fed dog, propulsive activity was similar to that seen during phase 2 of the MMC in fasted dogs. Summers et al. (190) followed the appearance and disappearance of a bolus of a radioactive isotope in dogs that were prepared with Biebl loops. Additionally, myoelectric activity was recorded both from above the loop and on the loop itself. In fasted dogs, there was marked variability in the time

of appearance of the isotope in the loop (Fig. 10). This time was shown to be correlated with the phase of the MMC in which the isotope was administered. Appearance was quick when injected during phase 2 or 3 and slow when injected during phase 1. In fed animals, appearance was quick and there was little variability. Sim-

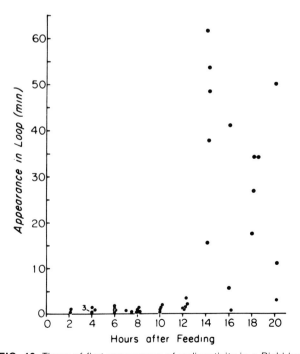

FIG. 10. Times of first appearance of radioactivity in a Biebl loop after injection of an isotope into the lumen of the small bowel at a site orad to the loop. Each point represents one experiment. When tested from 2–12 hr after feeding, transit was rapid and uniform. Transit was variable, however, when tested from 14–20 hr after feeding. Variability in transit was shown to be due to the variable nature of the MMC. (From Summers et al., ref. 190, with permission.)

ilar results have been obtained in rats (167). The velocity of transit was greater when a bolus was administered before phase 3 of an MMC than after. Also, velocity was rapid and uniform in recently fed rats. Pharmacological agents also have been used to alter motility patterns and transit. The injection of low doses of glucagon and cerulein changed the MMC pattern of anesthetized rats to one similar to the fed pattern (182). This resulted in a more rapid transit of intestinal contents. Higher doses of the agents caused an overall reduction in contractions and a decrease in transit. Similar decreases in contraction and transit have been reported after administration of morphine sulphate (192).

Thus, the pattern of contractions has a marked influence on intestinal transit and presumably on such other functions as digestion and absorption. Another interesting proposal is that the propulsive phases of the MMC are necessary to prevent bacterial overgrowth of the small intestine during fasting. In support of this proposal, Vantrappen et al. (205) found that of 12 patients possibly having bacterial overgrowth of the small intestine, 5 had gross disorders of the MMC patterns. Presumably, other diseases associated with abnormalities of intestinal transit [e.g., intestinal pseudo-obstruction (123) and diarrhea] will be characterized by abnormalities in one or more of these motility patterns.

Regulation of Intestinal Contractions

The contractions of the wall of the small intestine are a consequence of changes in length of the smooth muscle cells that make up the tunica muscularis. Thus, the temporal and spatial patterns of intestinal contractions depend on factors that influence these smooth muscle cells. These factors include the intrinsic properties of the smooth muscle cells themselves, the activities of nerves that constitute the intrinsic nerve plexuses such as the myenteric plexus, the influence of the extrinsic sympathetic and parasympathetic nerves that are distributed to the muscle and intrinsic nerves, and the influences of the various chemicals (hormones, autocoids, and paracrines) that reach the nerves and muscles of the gut.

Intrinsic Muscular Control

Contractions of smooth muscle of mammalian small intestine, like contractions of most other muscle, are preceded by changes in electrical potential of the muscle cells (20,56,66,161,204). In 1922, Alvarez and Mahoney (4) reported that slow potential changes could be recorded from the surface of the small intestine. These action currents, as they called them, occurred at a constant frequency at any one site and were present even if the bowel was not contracting. Additionally, they found that the frequency was not the same at all sites,

but that it decreased from the duodenum to the ileum. In 1932, Peustow (162), studying loops of dog intestine *in vivo,* recorded two types of electrical potentials. Potential changes such as those seen by Alvarez and Mahoney were recorded when the bowel was not contracting. When the bowel was contracting, these slow potential changes were accompanied by superimposed rapid oscillations in electrical potential. Thus, the presence of the two main types of electrical activity of the bowel was established. Since 1932, many investigators have added to our knowledge regarding the myoelectric activity of the bowel.

The two types of electrical activity go by many different names. The slower, omnipresent signal has been called slow wave, basic electric rhythm (BER), pacesetter potential, and electrical control potential. The more rapid potential change which is associated with contractions has been called the action potential, spike potential, burst potential, spike burst, and electrical response activity. In this chapter the terms *slow wave* and *spike potential* will be used.

Slow waves are generated by the smooth muscle cells themselves. In mammals, they are virtually unaltered in the presence of nerve blocking agents or in the presence of antagonists of the various known and postulated neurohumoral transmitters (66,161). One possible exception is in the guinea pig intestine, where atropine has been reported to abolish them (161). Slow waves appear to be generated by smooth muscle cells of the longitudinal muscle layer. Microelectrode recordings from sheets of isolated longitudinal muscle show periodic depolarizations of around 13 mV at a frequency that is characteristic of the intact bowel. Sheets of the isolated circular muscle layer show no such regular potential changes. However, in intact muscularis externa containing both muscle layers, slow waves with amplitudes of around 27 mV can be recorded from either layer (56, 57,118). Thus, there is an electrical coupling between the two muscle layers in the intact bowel. The basis of the coupling is not clear; interstitial cells and fibroblasts, however, may be responsible (197).

The mechanism for generation of slow waves is not agreed upon. Two proposals have received the most recent attention. One idea is that there is an electrogenic sodium pump that is turned on and off periodically (59). The other is that there are periodic changes in conductance to various ions, primarily sodium and chloride (77). Also, the role of the circular muscle layer is not clear. One view is that slow waves are generated in the longitudinal layers and then spread electrotonically into the circular muscle (19). Another view is that slow waves, once generated in the longitudinal layer, are amplified within the circular layer so that the final form of the waves is influenced by both layers (57,118).

Whatever the mechanism of production of the slow waves, they are recorded from all areas of the small intestine. Thus, it may be that every individual longitudinal smooth muscle cell is capable of generating slow waves. Although slow waves can be recorded from all areas, neither the frequency nor the timing of the wave is the same at all areas of the intact bowel. As pointed out by Alvarez and Mahoney (4), there is a gradient in slow-wave frequency, decreasing from duodenum to ileum. Later studies have shown that the gradient is not a simple one. For example, the slow-wave frequency is the same in dogs, around 18 cpm, over the orad 30% to 50% of the intestine. Hence, there is a frequency plateau over the proximal bowel. Beyond the plateau, frequency falls. This fall has been reported to be both a linear decrease (177) and a series of short frequency plateaus (33,69,194). Whatever the pattern of decrease, the frequency in the ileum is only about 60% to 70% of that in the duodenum.

Although the slow-wave frequency is the same all along the frequency plateau, slow waves do not occur simultaneously at all loci. There is a phase lag such that the waves appear to be propagated distally from a point near the pylorus (10,69,94,137). Thus, the occurrence of slow waves at one locus of the bowel appears to influence their occurrence at other loci. Further support for this influence comes from studies in which the bowel has been transected (33,69,94,177). Cutting the bowel in the region of the frequency plateau causes a fall in frequency below the cut. Slow waves do not disappear below the cut; rather, they no longer appear to be linked to those above the cut. If enough cuts are made, slow-wave frequency will appear to decrease in a more or less linear fashion from the proximal duodenum to the distal ileum. Thus, even though all areas of the small bowel can generate slow waves, in the intact bowel the slow waves at any one locus influence the slow waves at other loci. Obviously some form of coupling must exist and there must be some mechanism for this coupling. The pattern of coupling can be modeled by a series of relaxation oscillators (33,145,177). Relaxation oscillators with small differences in intrinsic frequencies will oscillate at the same frequency when capacitatively coupled. Although frequency will be the same, there will be a phase lag with the oscillator with the highest frequency in the lead. This mimics the frequency plateau. Oscillators whose frequencies are not close to that of the lead oscillator will not be able to follow. Even though their activity will be influenced by those in the plateau, their frequency will be less. Thus, these oscillators mimic the gradient that is seen beyond the frequency plateau. The exact nature of the coupling of smooth muscle cells that allows for the frequency plateau and gradient and for the spread of slow waves along the plateau are not clear. It is generally agreed that some form of contacts must exist among the smooth muscle cells to allow for the spread of influence. However, the exact types of contacts are not clear. Some reports in-

dicate that true fusions of cell membranes (nexuses) can be found in both muscle layers (197). Others, however, indicate that true nexuses exist only in circular muscle and that other types of close contacts occur in longitudinal muscle (64,65,93). Also, the role of the circular muscle in the spread of slow waves is not clear. Some studies indicate that slow waves are generated and propagated solely within the longitudinal layer (20). Other studies indicate that the potential change must spread from the longitudinal layer into the circular layer and back into the longitudinal layer before its influence can be propagated distally (57,58).

Spike potentials, like slow waves, also are generated by the smooth muscle cells themselves (20,66,161,204). Unlike slow waves, however, spike potentials occur in isolated sheets of both muscle layers, are not present at all times, and do lead to contractions of the muscle (12, 56,118,161). Spike potentials are rapid depolarizations and repolarizations of the smooth muscle cell membrane. Their durations vary from preparation to preparation but are of the order of tens of milliseconds. Their amplitudes vary, with most reports giving values of around 30 mV. Microelectrode recordings indicate that during spikes, transmembrane potentials seldom reach or surpass 0 mV. Studies of the ionic requirements for these signals indicate that the current required for the depolarization phase of the potential is carried in large part by calcium. This differs from the action potential seen in most nerves and striated muscle but is similar to what has been reported in other mammalian smooth muscles. Spike potentials are not always present and their occurrence depends upon neurohumoral influences (12,66,67). For example, cholinergic agents enhance spike potential activity, whereas adrenergic amines inhibit it. Also, spike potentials do not appear to be propagated for any distance (10,174,175). When spike potentials do occur, they lead to contractions of the activated muscle. Thus, they are very similar to the action potentials seen in striated muscle. The link between the spike potential and activation of the contractile proteins, as in the other muscles, appears to involve calcium ions. The mechanism of calcium activation of the proteins in smooth muscle, however, may differ from that described in striated muscle (see Chapter 7).

Although slow waves do not in themselves directly induce contractions, their presence greatly influences the pattern of contractions. Puestow (162) found that oscillations (spike potentials) only occurred during the positively altered phase of the slow wave. Later studies with both extracellular and intracellular electrodes clearly demonstrated that spike potentials only occur near the peak of depolarization of the slow wave (9,20,54). It is as if the slow wave had to bring the membrane potential near a threshold in order that spikes could be generated. Since spike potentials (and hence contractions) can develop only during a short phase of the slow-wave cycle, slow waves control the timing of contractions at any one locus (9, 174). Thus, it was not surprising to find that contractions of the human duodenum occurred at multiple intervals of 5 sec, since the slow-wave frequency at this locus is 12 cpm (45,48).

This relationship of spike potentials to slow waves also dictates that those contractions associated with spike potentials will be phasic and not tonic. Tonic contractions must be due to either a breakdown in this relationship between slow waves and spike potentials or else to mechanisms set into motion by events other than spike potentials.

Slow waves not only control the pattern of contractions at any one locus, they also influence the patterns at adjacent loci. As mentioned above, spike potentials are not propagated very far. They only occur at a given locus if neurohumoral conditions are conducive, and then only during a specific phase of the slow-wave cycle. If, however, neurohumoral conditions are optimal for spike potentials to occur over a long length of bowel, then a seemingly propagated contraction along the frequency plateau will occur as the depolarization phase of the slow wave occurs at each locus. Thus, this contraction will appear to be propagated at the same velocity as the slow wave (49,90,166,193). Such a condition is seen during phase 3 of the MMC. In the dog, the length of bowel simultaneously exhibiting phase 3 activity varies from 5 to 62 cm (49). During this time sequential contractions are taking place that are propulsive in nature. The timing and velocity of propulsion of these contractions and the length of bowel involved are set by the slow wave.

Thus, the temporal and spatial relationships of contractions, when contractions occur, are largely determined by the pattern of slow wave activity. However, whether or not contractions will occur depends on other factors. The MMC and fed patterns appear to be due to neural and humoral factors that work through the normal relationships of slow waves and spike potentials. Other patterns, such as those seen in certain disease states, may involve not only neural and humoral influences but also abnormalities in the relationship of slow waves to spike potentials.

Intrinsic Neural Control

As discussed above, many nerve cell bodies, nerve trunks, and nerve endings are present in the wall of the small intestine. Although their presence was noted and their function surmised many years ago, their study has proven difficult. For the purposes of this chapter, it is necessary to touch lightly on the functions of these nerves.

The organization of neurons of the myenteric plexus into nodes that are interconnected and innervated by extrinsic nerves gives rise to the possibility that the myenteric plexus represents the postganglionic component of the parasympathetic nervous system, a kind of substation. However, anatomical, physiological, and pharmacological evidence indicates that the plexus is much more complex (223,224). It is clear that several different types of cells exist. These cell types differ in appearance, in spontaneous electrical activity, and in their response to electrical and chemical stimulation. Also, it is evident that there is polarity in the input and output of the neurons. All these factors point to the fact that the neurons of the myenteric plexus may have an important effect in regulating the contractions of the small bowel.

Some of the most convincing arguments for an influence of these nerves comes from studies in which they have been inhibited or activated. A segment of the small intestine of the cat placed in an organ bath contracts irregularly. When tetrodotoxin, an agent that blocks action potentials in nerves but not in smooth muscle, is added, the preparation contracts vigorously at the frequency of the slow wave (17,22,222). Recordings from neurons within the myenteric plexus showed that many of them were active during those periods when the bowel was not contracting and that tetrodotoxin blocked activity of these neurons (146,147). Thus, it appears that there are tonic inhibitory nerves in the plexus that actively suppress contractions of the circular muscle. Further evidence for this possibility comes from studies on aganglionic segments of bowel. These segments lack a normal myenteric plexus and are tonically contracted (222). Electrical or chemical stimulation of the nerves within the myenteric plexus also affects contractions of the muscle (95,223,224). Transmural electrical stimulation of guinea pig ileum activates cholinergic nerves to release acetylcholine and so to cause contraction of the longitudinal muscle. Other preparations can be stimulated such that inhibitory nerves are activated to suppress contractions of the circular muscle.

Polarity within the small intestine was demonstrated over 80 years ago. Perhaps the most widely quoted description of this polarity was provided by Bayliss and Starling (14). Their "law of the intestine" states that stimulation at a locus of small bowel induces contraction above and relaxation below the point of stimulation. Whether this polarity is due to the muscle, to the intrinsic nerves, or to both is not clear. As pointed out above, there is a polarity in the muscle in that slow waves are propagated distally. However, slow-wave propagation cannot explain everything (e.g., descending inhibition of activity). Polarity within the myenteric plexus has been demonstrated only recently (99,100, 226). Stimulation of a node of the myenteric plexus has been shown to produce hyperpolarization of the smooth muscle aboral to the node and depolarization oral to the node. Thus, the peristaltic reflex probably is mediated primarily by way of the myenteric neurons.

Activity of the intrinsic nerves could control many of the patterns of motility seen in the small intestine (124, 223,224). Tonic inhibitory output could prevent spike potentials, and hence contractions, from occurring. Momentary lifting of this inhibition could allow each slow wave at a particular locus to lead to generation of spikes and contraction of the muscle of that locus. If lifting of inhibition was local, a segmenting contraction would occur. If lifting was sequential, at adjacent sites, a peristaltic contraction could result. Whether or not inhibition is lifted and whether or not the lifting will be local or sequential depends on sensory information received by the plexal neurons and on the integrative capacities of the neurons. That such integrative capacities within the intrinsic nerves are possible is discussed in Chapter 1. Recent studies of isolated segments of bowel and of extrinsically denervated loops of bowel *in vivo* have demonstrated cyclical activity recurring at intervals of several minutes (28,207). Thus, activity of the intrinsic nerves could control some of the cyclical recurring patterns seen in fasted and fed animals.

Extrinsic Neural Control

As mentioned above, the small intestine receives an extrinsic innervation from both divisions of the autonomic nervous system, parasympathetic and sympathetic. Although early studies demonstrated clearly that nervous pathways between the central nervous system and the intestine exist, the extent and organization of these pathways are far from being understood.

Early studies on the effects of nerve stimulation and transection on intestinal contractions demonstrated, in general, that activation of the parasympathetic nerves increased contractions and activation of the sympathetic nerves decreased contractions (114,116,119). Also, these studies demonstrated that certain reflexes depended on integrity of extrinsic innervation (86,88,107,108,122, 163). The primary reflex studied was the intestinal inhibitory reflex which is characterized by inhibition of intestinal contractions at all adjacent loci during marked distension of an area of bowel. This reflex appeared to depend on integrity of the sympathetic nerves. Some studies implicated participation of the brain and spinal cord, since sectioning of the splanchnic nerves abolished the reflex. Other studies, however, suggested that the reflex involved only the prevertebral ganglia, since the reflex persisted after splanchnic section but not after ganglionectomy.

Recently, several studies have been designed to determine the neural pathways between the intestine and the prevertebral ganglia (121,122,195). Both afferent and efferent fibers have been demonstrated electrophysiologically. Also, an intestino-intestinal reflex has been observed in a preparation *in vitro* that contained only the colon, the prevertebral ganglia, and interconnecting nerves (122). Thus, reflex arcs contained solely within the intrinsic and prevertebral ganglia do exist and they are functional. These studies were performed on preparations of colon. Ideally, similar studies should be performed using the small intestine.

The spinal and supraspinal influences on the intestine are well documented (119). Those studies that indicate that certain reflexes and patterns of motility can be expressed in preparations devoid of central nervous connections should not be interpreted as showing that central nervous connections are not needed or do not influence these patterns of motility. There are areas within the brain that when stimulated cause either an increase or a decrease in intestinal contractions (see Chapter 10). Thus, higher centers can alter activity of other neural and muscular tissue. Also, pharmacological agents injected into the cerebral ventricles alter contractions and intestinal propulsion (31,186–188). Such activation of structures within the brain is thought to elicit a response by way of the autonomic nervous system. However, there are data to indicate that in some instances a humoral substance may be involved.

The site of action of the extrinsic nerves could be either on the smooth muscle cells themselves or on the nerves of the myenteric plexus (84,227). Structural and physiological studies indicate that extrinsic nerves end at the level of the myenteric plexus. This is true for both sympathetic as well as parasympathetic nerves. A few adrenergic nerve terminals can be found within the muscle layers themselves, but their function is not clear. Therefore, extrinsic nerves probably function to regulate and modulate activity of the intrinsic nerves, which in turn affect the intrinsic activity of the intestinal smooth muscle.

Chemical Control

The nerves and smooth muscle of the intestine are responsive and sensitive to a wide variety of chemicals (7,60,74,176). Among these chemicals are the neurotransmitters acetylcholine and norepinephrine; many suspected neurotransmitters such as ATP, serotonin, and various peptides; many hormones and paracrines such as gastrin, CCK, and the enkephalins; and many pharmacological agents. The effects of many of these agents are discussed above and in other chapters of this volume.

Since acetylcholine and norepinephrine are believed to be important neurotransmitters, many studies have concentrated on the effects of these agents on various intestinal preparations. Responses to cholinergic agents are complex and depend on the particular chemical and intestinal preparation being used (60). In general, those analogs of acetylcholine which act predominantly on muscarinic receptors on smooth muscle cells cause a stimulation of contractions of any intestinal preparation. Responses to cholinergic agents that act on nicotinic receptors can cause either stimulation or inhibition. For example, in intact unanesthetized dogs, intravenous injections of nicotine cause inhibition of contractions because of activation of the sympathetic nervous system (40). However, if nicotine is injected intraarterially into either *in situ* or isolated loops of intestine, stimulation of contractions is seen (41,60). Supposedly this stimulation is due to the actions of the drug on intrinsic stimulatory nerves. The response to catecholamines, characterized by norepinephrine, is generally one of inhibition of contraction (60,119). The site of action could be at one or more of several sites. Intestinal smooth muscle cells appear to possess adrenergic receptors of both the alpha and the beta type. Activation of either receptor type leads to inhibition of contractions. In addition to the receptors on muscle, the intrinsic nerves appear to have adrenergic receptors as well. In certain preparations, norepinephrine appears to inhibit contractions by decreasing the release of acetylcholine from these intrinsic nerves. Thus, the physiological site of norepinephrine action may be on these intrinsic nerves. This view is even more plausible in light of the fact that most postganglionic sympathetic nerves end on the myenteric plexus and not on the smooth muscle cells themselves.

Other postulated neurotransmitters receiving attention recently are serotonin and the "nonadrenergic inhibitory" transmitter. Responses to serotonin are complex, but in most preparations stimulation of contractions is observed (60). Serotonin acts on nerve cells and/or smooth muscle cells to induce contractions. Recent interest in serotonin has been stimulated by the observation that there may be serotonergic nerves in the myenteric plexus and that there are intrinsic nerves that respond to both exogenously administered and endogenously released serotonin (224). For years, physiological evidence has existed for the presence of an inhibitory transmitter that is not an adrenergic amine. Excitation of intrinsic nerves in many preparations leads to an inhibition of contractions, inhibition that is not antagonized by any of the conventional blockers of known receptors. Since the inhibition is blocked by local anesthetics and tetrodotoxin, it is thought to be due to liberation of a neurotransmitter. However, the identity of the neurotransmitter has remained elusive. A body of evidence has been advanced that suggests the transmitter may be a purine metabolite such as ATP (37). Many of the inhibitory responses can be mimicked by the application of ATP and ATP is released upon nerve stimulation. However, not all the data fit the idea of

purines being the inhibitory transmitter. Many tissues require large amounts of ATP to induce relaxation, much more than could be released endogenously (62). More importantly, some tissues respond to purines with contractions rather than relaxation (34). Thus, the presence and role of "purinergic nerves" is far from clear. Nonetheless, there are more data on purinergic nerves than for the other postulated inhibitory substances. Most recently, the possibility has been raised that the inhibitory substance may be a peptide (63). Support for this idea comes from studies that have identified many peptides in the myenteric plexus and from studies that demonstrate that some peptides, such as vasoactive intestinal polypeptide, inhibit contractions of gastrointestinal smooth muscle.

Many hormones and candidate hormones affect contractions of the small intestine (56,109,143). Generally, the ones most often studied are the ones that are found in the gastrointestinal tract. All of these appear to exert an effect when injected or infused intravenously in intact unanesthetized animals. Although they have an effect, it is not clear if any of the effects are physiological or how the hormones are acting to produce the effects. Early studies with these compounds usually employed bolus injections and examination of the immediate effects. These studies showed, in general, that gastrin, motilin, and CCK would stimulate contractions. Secretin, glucagon, vasoactive intestinal polypeptide (VIP), and gastric inhibitory polypeptide (GIP), on the other hand, inhibited contractions. Postulated mechanisms of action range from a direct effect on the smooth muscle cells to an action on intrinsic nerves to release acetylcholine. More recently, the effects of these hormones on patterns of contraction have been determined during intravenous infusion or during endogenous release. These studies are discussed below.

Integration of Controlling Influences

As described above, there are many potential mechanisms for control of intestinal motility. In all likelihood, all the mechanisms are operating simultaneously to produce the various patterns of contractions seen in intact animals. Not only are they operating simultaneously, but probably their operations are integrated with one another. A simple scheme for these actions and interactions is presented in Fig. 11. The primary unit of contractile activity is the smooth muscle cell. This unit can contract on its own, and, because of the intrinsic behavior of its membrane, its contractions can be quite regular. However, contractions of the smooth muscle cells are modulated by at least two other factors; circulating and locally released chemicals, and neurotransmitters released by intrinsic (and perhaps extrinsic) nerves. But reciprocal effects occur as well. Receptors within the intestine can be activated by contractions of

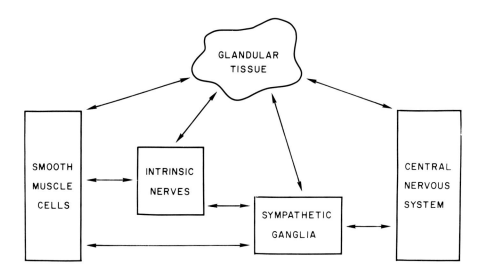

FIG. 11. Schematic of those factors that control intestinal motility. See text for explanation.

the smooth muscle cells and by the presence of intraluminal contents. These receptors can have a direct influence on the intrinsic (and perhaps extrinsic) nerves. Both excitatory and inhibitory influences have been described. It also is becoming clear that neuronal circuits between the intrinsic nerves and muscle layer and within the intrinsic nerves themselves have the capacity to integrate and produce various patterns of contractions.

Intrinsic nerves and muscle are in turn influenced by extrinsic nerves (autonomic ganglia and the central nervous system) and circulating and locally released chemicals. This influence at times is stimulatory and at times inhibitory; and as with the intrinsic nerves, the influence is bi-directional. Stimulation of receptors within the intestine affects activities of the extrinsic nerves. Of course, the integrative capacity of the extrinsic nerves is enormous, since they also receive neural and chemical input from all other areas of the body and the environment.

The concept of several discrete units whose activities are integrated to produce patterns of intestinal contraction may seem simple. However, the operation of each of these units, isolated or integrated with the other units, is very complex. So long as these units are described as "black boxes," illustrations such as Fig. 11 point out only the potential complexities of the system and our ignorance of them. It is only by studying the behavior of these units, both isolated and in the presence of other units, that we can ever gain an understanding of what controls intestinal motility.

Regulation of Patterns of Contraction

Migrating Motility Complex

For purposes of this discussion, there are three basic characteristics of MMCs that must be regulated by one or more factors: (a) MMCs recur in the stomach and

upper small bowel at fairly regular intervals, (b) each MMC is composed of definitely three, and perhaps four, distinct phases, and (c) each phase of each MMC appears to migrate aborally along the bowel.

Factors possibly controlling cycle length have been studied primarily in dogs and humans. Since phase 3 (the period of regular activity) is the most distinct, most investigators used the time between successive phase 3s as an indicator of cycle length. It did not matter if the other phases were altered as long as recognizable phase 3s were present. Under these criteria, a role for the humoral control of MMC initiation has been postulated.

About a decade ago, Brown et al. (23) isolated the putative hormone motilin and found that it would stimulate contractions of the stomach. They postulated a role for this substance in the control of motility. Some years later Itoh et al. (102,104) reported that motilin would initiate premature MMCs in fasted dogs. Intravenous infusion of 0.1 to 2.7 $\mu g/(kg\ hr)$ begun just after the appearance of phase 3 activity in the stomach and upper small intestine induced a second period of phase 3 activity within 20 min. The pattern of response to motilin was independent of dose; however, the larger the dose the sooner the initiation of the second complex. The premature complexes were similar to the naturally occurring ones in both appearance and migration. Also, if initiation of the infusion was delayed, less motilin had to be infused to initiate a complex. Thus, it appeared that a relative refractory period existed. Motilin had no effect on the patterns that were induced by either feeding or the infusion of pentagastrin. Similar results in the dog were obtained by Wingate et al. (221). Ormsbee and Mir (149) found that a bolus injection of motilin also induced a premature phase 3 when injected 30 min after a naturally occurring phase 3 had passed the duodenum. Additionally, they found that the next naturally occurring complex was delayed so that a compensatory pause appeared likely. Vantrappen et al. (206) found that in humans motilin, 0.4 to 6.4 pmoles/(kg min), infused for

30 min, starting 1 to 2 min after a period of phase 3 activity in the upper intestine, induced a complex within 46 min. This was well before the next naturally occurring complex was due. Thus, motilin is also effective in humans. In agreement with the results found in the dog, the premature complex in the human being seemed normal in appearance and in migration, and there was no dose-response relationship; however, in disagreement with the results found in the dog, the time of appearance of the premature complex was not dependent on dose. The reasons for this difference are not clear.

The physiological significance of motilin has been tested by observing the effect of endogenously released motilin and by correlating endogenous plasma levels of motilin to the various phases of the MMC. Brown et al. (24) found that infusion of alkali into the duodenum of the dog would stimulate contractions of a gastric pouch. This same treatment also would release motilin (73). Lee et al. (126,127) reported that intraduodenal infusion of Tris buffer increased plasma motilin levels and induced phase-3-like activity in the duodenum. Thus it appears that endogenously released motilin is effective in stimulating contractions. The ability of motilin released endogenously to initiate specifically an MMC needs further study. Lewis et al. (128) found that in humans acid can induce an MMC on the small bowel; however, the premature MMC differed from a normal one in that phase 3 activity was not seen in the stomach. Motilin is released by acidification of the duodenum, but the amount of acid used did not appear to cause a consistent release of motilin (53). Thus, in humans acid may induce an MMC-like pattern that is not mediated by motilin. Alternatively, acid may act on other neural and humoral mechanisms to modify and cloud the effect of motilin. At any rate, the results with endogenously released motilin are far from being clear or complete. The more convincing evidence for a role of motilin comes from studies in which plasma levels of motilin have been monitored along with contractile activity. Lee et al. (127), Itoh et al. (103), and Thomas et al. (201) have drawn blood from dogs during various phases of the MMC. All three studies have shown cyclical changes in plasma levels of motilin. Highest concentrations were found just before or during phase 3 activity of the stomach or upper duodenum. Lower concentrations were found during phase 1 activity at the same loci. Vantrappen et al. (206) report similar data for humans. Phase 3 activity in the upper small bowel was preceded by peak plasma levels of motilin that were 25 pmoles/liter higher than the lowest level which occurred during phase 1 activity. Thus, these authors proposed the possibility that the increased levels of motilin could be initiating the MMCs. However, as they point out, the correlation of events does not necessarily mean cause and effect. Also, recent data of Collins et al. (53) suggest that under certain conditions there may not be cycles of

motilin levels correlated with motility. Even if initiation of MMCs is convincingly shown to be due to cyclical fluctuations in plasma motilin levels, the question of what controls cyclical release of motilin will still remain.

How motilin induces MMCs has received some study. Strunz et al. (189) and Wingate et al. (221) found that isolated muscle segments from the upper gastrointestinal tract are much more sensitive to the effects of motilin than is the rest of the bowel. Thus, this differential sensitivity may explain how motilin can induce a complex in the upper bowel without affecting the lower bowel. The fact that exogenously administered motilin is effective only after a "refractory period" could be due to periodic increases and decreases in sensitivity of the upper gut to motilin. This changing sensitivity could be the result of excitatory and inhibitory nervous input. For example, inhibitory input initiated by phase 3 activity present in the small bowel could prevent very premature complexes from propagating. This would be in keeping with the observation by Itoh et al. (102) that a premature complex would die out if a previous period of phase 3 activity were present in the upper 70% of small bowel (an observation I have also made). Whether the actions of motilin are exerted directly on the muscle or upon extrinsic and/or intrinsic nerves is not clear. Strunz et al. (189) thought that the effects of the substance on isolated intestinal segments were due to direct effects on the muscle, since they were not altered by various antagonists. In vivo, however, motilin's effects are antagonized by hexamethonium and atropine (149). Thus, preganglionic and postganglionic cholinergic neurons may be involved. If nerves are involved, connections with the central nervous system do not appear to be vital. In a recent experiment, Thomas et al. (201) found that motilin could initiate phase 3 activity in autotransplanted gastric pouches. These pouches contain intrinsic nerves but are totally devoid of extrinsic innervation. It is not known if the effects of motilin on the small intestine are similarly independent; however, it is known that the actions of motilin on the small bowel are seen in dogs that have undergone bilateral thoracic vagotomy (149).

Initiation of MMCs also is affected by other hormones. Somatostatin has been reported to both increase and decrease their formation. Thor et al. (202) infused fasted dogs with 0.6 μg/kg-hr and found that the interval between MMCs was reduced by about one-half. On the other hand, Ormsbee et al. (148) found that 5 μg/kg-hr would inhibit spontaneously occurring MMCs as well as those induced by infusion of motilin. The reasons for these differences could lie in the dosages or preparations of somatostatin used. Whether somatostatin was acting by altering the release of motilin or not was not clear. However, the fact that the actions of exogenously administered motilin were blocked indicates an action other than on motilin release. Other hormones, such as secretin, insulin, CCK, and gastrin, also disrupt MMCs (29,130,143,144,213). Whether or not any of these actions are physiologically important and whether or not their actions have anything to do with motilin is not known.

Inititation of MMCs does not appear to depend critically on intact extrinsic innervation. Complexes still occurred in humans, dogs, and sheep after bilateral truncal vagotomy (29,44,130,171,212). Although MMCs still occur, there is minor disagreement on whether or not timing of the complexes is altered. In humans and sheep there appeared to be no change. In dogs, two reports indicated no change, the others indicated either a decrease in cycle length from 89 to 71 min or an increase in cycle length variability. Interruption of the sympathetic nerves also does not abolish initiation of MMCs (131). However, both splanchnicotomy and celiac combined with superior mesenteric ganglionectomy altered their timing. Splanchnic nerve section increased the interval from 77 to 108 min. Ganglionectomy made the interval variable. Administration of guanethidine disrupted the pattern such that it was difficult to determine if MMCs were present. Probably the best evidence that extrinsic nerves are not required for MMC initiation comes from Thomas et al. (201). They found that an autotransplanted gastric pouch developed MMCs which were in phase with those on the rest of the stomach and upper small bowel.

The fact that the extrinsic nerves do not seem to be required for normal initiation of MMCs does not mean that these nerves cannot affect their formation. Bueno et al. (25,27) performed various operative procedures on rats, dogs, and sheep. In many cases they found that MMC initiation was inhibited but that the inhibition could be prevented by sectioning the splanchnic nerves. Thus adrenergic nerves were involved in suppressing MMC initiation. Less direct evidence for involvement of extrinsic factors is provided by drugs that supposedly act primarily within the central nervous system. The general anesthetic, ether, depressed MMCs in the rat (25). On the other hand, morphine appeared to enhance initiation of MMCs (44).

In summary, initiation of MMCs appears to be primarily under humoral control. The substance involved has not been elucidated fully; however, there is a strong case for a controlling effect of motilin. The role of extrinsic and intrinsic nerves is not clear. Extrinsic nerves are not vital, yet extrinsic reflexes can alter MMC initiation. The role of intrinsic nerves has received little study.

As mentioned earlier, each cycle of a MMC is made up of several phases. Thus, it is possible for two cycles to have the same duration but yet be composed of phases of different lengths. Recently investigators have noted this and have designed experiments to determine influences on the individual phases (29,49,130,151,168,

170,171). In general, these studies demonstrated that phase 3 activity was fairly constant and was altered only by those manipulations that completely abolished MMCs. The other phases, however, vary, with durations of phases 1 and 2 being related inversely on one another. Phase 2 activity seems to be influenced by nerve activity and by intraluminal contents. After vagotomy in both dogs and sheep, the mean duration of phase 2 (irregular activity) decreased by about 30% (171). After splanchnicotomy and celiac and superior mesenteric ganglionectomy, phase 2 activity increased in duration (131). Furthermore, atropine decreased and guanethidine enhanced this same activity. These data suggest that cholinergic nerves enhance and adrenergic nerves suppress phase 2 activity. In sheep, an animal that normally exhibits MMCs all the time, phase 2 activity was shown to be proportional to flow of contents through the bowel (30). The more intraluminal contents, the longer the duration of phase 2. Such a relationship also may be true in the dog. By closely following phase durations in subsequent cycles during fasting, Ruckebusch and Bueno (171) found that the duration of phase 2 decreased with time. They also found that total parenteral nutrition was accompanied by a decrease in duration of phase 2 activity.

Each phase of the MMC occurs in sequence such that complexes appear to be initiated in the stomach and upper small bowel and then migrate aborally. Such an occurence could come about in a number of ways: (a) there could be a controller (analogous to the swallowing center for the pharynx and esophagus) that sends out sequential impulses to progressively more distal areas of the intestine; (b) there could be a series of signals that originate in the stomach and small bowel and then spread down the bowel via the intrinsic and/or extrinsic nerves, (c) each area of the small bowel could generate all phases of the MMC on its own, and activity in each area could be coordinated by having differential latencies of response to a humoral substance such as motilin; (d) each area could possess autonomy but yet be influenced by reflexes in either the intrinsic or the extrinsic nerves; or (e) there could be any combination of the above possibilities.

The first experiments to specifically test any of these possibilities were carried out by Carlson et al. (39) and by Grivel and Ruckebusch (90). Carlson et al. provided dogs with Thiry-Vella loops and found that the majority of the complexes migrated down the bowel to the point of anastomosis, jumped over onto the loop, migrated along the loop, then jumped back onto the bowel below the anastomosis, and finally migrated along the rest of the bowel. Grivel and Ruckebusch prepared loops in sheep and obtained similar results, except that only 30% of the complexes behaved in this manner. Additionally, they prepared dogs with reversed segments of bowel and found that about 30% to 40% of the complexes passed along the reversed segments as if they were in normal orientation. These experiments demonstrated that neither continuity of the bowel wall (intrinsic nerves and muscle) nor propulsion of intraluminal contents were needed for coordinated migration of the MMC. Furthermore, they suggested that coordinated migration was brought about by way of the extrinsic nerves. Although these experiments emphasized the importance of extrinsic factors, they did not rule out a role for intrinsic factors, since many complexes would either die out or else pass over anastomotic sites without passing over the loop. Further evidence for a role of extrinsic nerves was obtained with the demonstration that extrinsic denervation of a Thiry-Vella loop abolished MMCs in the loop but not in the rest of the bowel (214). However, these data were complicated by the fact that the loops became very active after denervation, so that it was difficult to tell if MMCs were present.

More recently, experimental results have indicated an important need for continuity of the bowel in order for normal migration to occur. Bueno et al. (28) found that after transection and reanastomosis of the small bowel in dogs, 38% of the MMCs failed to cross the anastomosis. Those that did appear to cross did so only after a delay and only after skipping over the area immediate to the anastomosis. It appeared as though the complex died out and then a new one re-formed below. Double transection caused an even greater decrease in the number of MMCs that migrated. The authors also found that Thiry-Vella loops often behaved like those described above; however, phase 3 activity often would pass from above to below without passing over the loop. Also, many complexes appeared to begin on the loop and then to pass over the distal bowel. This resulted in there being more MMCs distal to the anastomosis than above. These data as well as those of others indicate that activity in Thiry-Vella loops is not always coordinated with that on the rest of the bowel (150,158). Thus extrinsic connections are often not enough. An important role for intrinsic connections also was indicated by the fact that extrinsic denervation of an *in situ* segment of bowel did not totally disrupt migration of MMCs over the segment. Many passed with only a slight delay.

The above data indicate that migration can occur (although not always normally) with only intrinsic or extrinsic connections. However, one or the other must be required, since activity of an extrinsically denervated loop of bowel (either placed under the skin or fashioned into a Thiry-Vella loop) exhibited activity which was not coordinated with the rest of the bowel at any time (Fig. 12). MMC-like activity was recorded from loops placed under the skin, but the cycle lengths were very short and variable. Of the five possibilities listed at the beginning of this section, the scheme that may best explain the data is that intrinsic factors at each level of the bowel

can independently initiate activity that resembles MMCs. However, reflexes within the intrinsic and/or extrinsic nerves are necessary to coordinate activity at adjacent and distant sites.

Fed Pattern

In dogs, rats, and humans there is a change in intestinal motility brought about by eating. This change has not received a great deal of study partly because it does not occur in all species and partly because the "fed" pattern is not discrete and is harder to describe. Thus, some investigators refer to it as the period of disruption of MMCs caused by foods. However, there is a change; therefore, eating must somehow influence motility.

Ingestion of food causes an increase in intraluminal contents and an increase in circulating products of digestion. Either one or both of these factors could be responsible for disruption of MMCs; most data, however, indicate that neither is involved. Early experiments on loops of bowel placed under the skin indicated that contractions of the loops were altered when the dog ate (42,72,89,162). These results have been confirmed and extended recently. When dogs with Thiry-Vella loops were fed, MMCs on the loops as well as the incontinent bowel were disrupted (158,214). Thus, intraluminal contents are not required. However, intraluminal contents do influence motility (see below), so that the final pattern seen after eating probably is a result of intraluminal and extraluminal factors (76). The influence of circulating products of digestion was examined by maintaining animals on total parenteral nutrition (171, 210,213). Dogs maintained for up to 12 weeks with nothing but water by mouth still demonstrated MMCs. No signs of a fed pattern were evident. However, not all products of digestion have been tested. Most formulas for total parenteral nutrition contain only glucose and amino acids. Effects of other nutrients, such as lipids, need to be determined.

Ingestion of food also alters the release of various hormones; thus, hormones have been implicated in the changes in motility. A case for hormonal control was posed when Marik and Code (130) and Weisbrodt et al. (215) infused pentagastrin 2–6 μg/kg-hr into dogs and found disruption of MMCs. In both instances, the primary effect was a change in pattern rather than an increase in overall activity. This effect of pentagastrin was not due to acid secretion, since acid was drained from the stomach. The pattern induced by pentagastrin somewhat resembled that seen after feeding; thus, the suggestion was made that gastrin may be one of the factors involved in conversion of the pattern caused by feeding. This idea was attractive because eating is known to cause gastrin release. Bueno and Ruckebusch (29) injected insulin, 1 U/kg, into dogs and obtained 4-

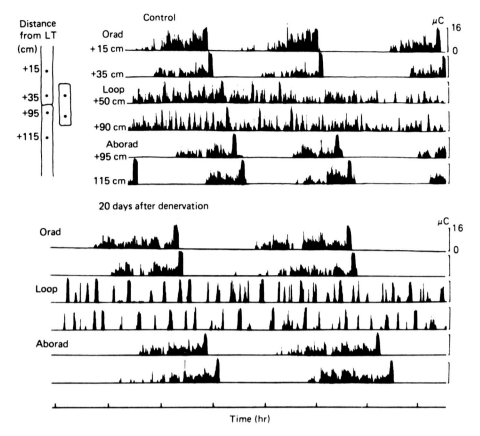

FIG. 12. Temporal distribution of spike potentials from the intact jejunum and a loop of bowel in an unanesthetized dog. Spike activity was integrated at 20-sec intervals. Positions of the electrodes are shown (*top left*). Before denervation, MMCs propagated through the loop as if it were in place. After denervation, activity occurred on the loop, but it was out of phase with that on the rest of the bowel. (From Bueno et al., ref. 28, with permission.)

to 5-hr disruption of MMCs. In these experiments also, the pattern was changed to one resembling the fed pattern; thus, a role for insulin was postulated. This postulate was strengthened by the findings that feeding released insulin and that there was a good correlation between the disruption of MMCs and the serum levels of insulin. In dogs rendered diabetic, both insulin levels and the duration of disruption of MMCs with feeding were reduced. Other gastrointestinal hormones have been shown to have similar effects. The octapeptide of CCK and glucagon produced changes in patterns when infused intravenously into dogs (144,220). The octapeptide in addition to inducing a change in pattern also caused a dose-dependent increase in spike potential activity.

Although a role for these hormones is possible, recent experiments have cast doubt on the importance of some of them. Wingate et al. (219,220) examined closely the patterns of slow waves and spike potentials on the duodenum, jejunum, and distal ileum of dogs during infusion of various hormones and after feeding. They found that even though CCK and pentagastrin did inhibit MMCs, the hormones did not induce patterns that closely mimicked those found after feeding. This was

especially true on the distal ileum, which seemed to be resistant to the hormones but not to feeding. Eeckhout et al. (75) fed various test meals to dogs and monitored motility and serum levels of insulin and gastrin. Test meals of sucrose, 30 kcal/kg, and milk protein, 30 kcal/kg, disrupted MMCs for a short period and increased serum levels of gastrin and insulin. Thus, hormones and motility appeared to be related. However, MMCs returned before serum levels of gastrin and insulin returned to normal. More important, test meals of arachis (peanut) oil, 30 kcal/kg, and medium chain triglycerides, 10 kcal/kg, produced disruption of MMCs for long periods of time, but neither caused any increases in insulin or gastrin. Although these results indicate that insulin and gastrin cannot be responsible for all cases of disruption of MMCs, they do not rule out a role for other hormones. It may be that different nutrients cause disruption by different means. Lipids may act through the liberation of CCK or some other hormone.

Ingestion of food also alters neural activity, thus the conversion of patterns of motility could be under neural control. What few studies have been performed indicate that both extrinsic and intrinsic nerves play minor to major roles. Sham feeding as well as gastric distension had only a slight effect on MMCs (49,171). What effect there was occurred immediately and was altered slightly after vagotomy. Vagotomy also had a slight effect on the response to feeding. MMCs still were disrupted; more food was required, however, and the period of disruption was shorter (29,130,171,212). These experiments are hard to evaluate, since vagotomy is known to alter gastric emptying, which in turn could alter small bowel motility. Most of these results indicate that external connections by way of the vagus play only a minor role. Unfortunately, the role of the sympathetic nerves in response to feeding has not been tested. Testing may prove difficult, as interruption of sympathetic nerves to the intestine will in itself disrupt MMC activity (see above).

Stimulation of intrinsic nerves disrupts MMCs. Eeckhout et al. (76) perfused Thiry-Vella loops in dogs with glucose solutions of various concentrations. They found that solutions of greater than 10% glucose would prevent MMCs from occurring on the loop. Importantly, however, MMCs still appeared on the rest of the bowel. Thus, the disruption was due to local factors and did not include systemic influences such as hormones and/or extrinsic nerves.

The results discussed above indicate that the change in pattern induced by feeding is brought about by several interacting factors. Hormones and/or extrinsic nerves may mediate the change at distant loci of the bowel. This response, however, then may be modified by intraluminal contents, which act via intrinsic nerves and locally released chemicals.

Other Patterns

The other patterns of contractions seen in healthy animals have received little attention. Hence, factors that control the prolonged burst of spike potentials seen in cats and the "minute rhythm" seen by some in humans, dogs, and sheep are unknown.

Some studies have been performed on the mechanisms responsible for the motility patterns seen in certain diarrheal states and/or infections. Results of most of these experiments point to a local mechanism which implicates fluid accummulation and/or mucosal damage. Many of the agents that cause diarrhea do so by increasing fluid secretion by the intestinal epithelia (36, 132,134,135). Thus, any motility change could be secondary to increased fluid. However, Mathias et al. (135) have injected saline into loops of bowel in quantities in excess of that secreted under the influence of castor oil and were unable to elicit MAPCs. More recently, Sinar and Burns (183) injected choleragenoid into loops of rabbit bowel and obtained a change in pattern (characterized by many MAPCs) but no increase in secretion, suggesting that motility changes and fluid secretion may be separable. The second possibility, mucosal damage,

may be responsible for the repetitive bursts of action potentials (RBAPs) seen during certain infections. Burns et al. (35) found that an invasive strain of E. coli but not a toxogenic strain, caused RBAPs in loops of rabbit bowel. These RBAPs were very similar to the potentials recorded from unanesthetized dogs during the intestinal phase of infection with T. spiralis, an organism that causes mucosal inflammation (179). However, results of a study by Weisberg et al. (208) do not fit this scheme. They infected loops of rabbit bowel with various strains of Salmonella typhimurium and found a change in motility only with those strains that caused increased secretion. A strain that caused extensive mucosal damage but yet no secretion did not induce any MAPCs or RBAPs. The differences here are not apparent but may be the result of using different bacteria. Regardless of whether or not the change in motility is due to increased fluid, mucosal damage, or other factors, the change seems to be local. In a preparation with two loops of bowel, MAPCs were observed only in the loops that were treated with cholera toxin (133). This local effect may involve a prostaglandin, since indomethacin, an inhibitor of prostaglandin synthesis, abolished MAPCs that were initiated by cholera (132). On the basis of this observation as well as on the ability of tetrodotoxin, scopolamine, and trimethaphan to block MAPCs, Mathias et al. (133) postulated that a local neural reflex which includes prostaglandin is involved. This interesting proposal deserves further study.

The pattern of contractions that precedes emesis appears to be controlled at least in part by extrinsic nerves. Gregory (88) recorded secretory and motor activity from Thiry and Thiry-Vella loops of intestine in unanesthetized dogs. Subcutaneous injections of apomorphine caused an increase in secretion and motility from these loops before and during emesis. Denervation of the vascular pedicle supplying the loop prevented this increase in secretion and motility. Similar abolition of the response to apomorphine was seen after bilateral thoracic vagotomy but not after section of the splanchnic nerves. Thus, the intestinal motor phase of the emetic response appears to have part of its pathway in the vagus nerve. Stewart et al. (186) recorded intestinal myoelectric activity before and after the injection of emetic drugs into the lateral cerebral ventricle of unanesthetized cats. Epinephrine, apomorphine, and morphine all caused an orally migrating burst of spike potentials on the small intestine, which preceded emesis. Equal doses given peripherally caused no effects. Thus, the drugs acted on structures within the central nervous system. The myoelectric response, but not emesis, was prevented by the subcutaneous injection of atropine. Thus, the intestinal component of the emetic response includes a muscarinic cholinergic receptor. Although nerve sections were not evaluated, results of this study are in keeping with the observations made by Gregory that a vagal pathway may be involved.

ILEOCECAL JUNCTION

Anatomical Considerations

The ileocecal junction is a specialized area which forms the boundary between the small and large intestines (70,152). This boundary is anatomically distinct, although there are variations in structure from species to species. In most animals there is a thickening of the musculature of the last few centimeters of ileum. In several, e.g., human and cat, a portion of the terminal ileum protrudes into the colon and is surrounded by colonic musculature. This feature makes some of the data on this area hard to interpret, since junctional activity can be influenced markedly by colonic activity. Although hard data are meager, it is thought that the myenteric plexus extends into the junction and that extrinsic innervation is supplied by the vagus and by fibers from the superior and inferior mesenteric ganglia.

The function and relative importance of this area are not settled. Alvarez (2) maintained that it served two purposes: to prevent reflux of colonic contents into the small intestine and to prevent rapid passage of contents through the ileum. Rather large pressures have to be exerted in order to get large quantities of material to reflux from the colon into the ileum (165). This indicates that the junction may serve as a barrier. On the other hand, reflux generally is not a problem when the junctional area is removed (184). Thus, normal propulsive activity of the small and large intestines may be all that is necessary to prevent reflux. Also, even in the presence of a normal junction some reflux still occurs. As far as regulation of transit is concerned, removal of the junction has little effect on small intestinal transit in normal animals. In animals with partial bowel resection, however, transit is markedly affected if the junction is removed (184). Hence, in otherwise normal animals, the ileocecal junction appears to be of minor importance. Caution should be exerted in this interpretation, however, until the role of this area on such subtle things as bile salt absorption and localization of microbes is determined.

Movements of Contents and Contractile Activity

Most material has been absorbed by the time the chyme reaches the ileocecal junction; however, a substantial amount still passes on to the colon. In humans, this may be from 1 to 2 liters daily. The pattern of movement has not been studied in detail. Thus, we do not know if contents are moved gradually and uniformly over long periods of time or whether movement occurs in spurts. Also, we do not know if there are any differences in the way material is transported during the fasted as compared to the fed states. This is probably so, since this area is difficult to study in normal, conscious animals and since most studies were performed before recognition of the different patterns of small intestinal motility.

Most studies indicate that the ileocecal junction maintains closure between the small and large intestine (52, 97,102,112). For some time it was debated whether or not this was due to structural or functional properties of the area. Because the small bowel protrudes into the colonic wall, the area has the appearance of a valve. Thus, structure seemed important. This argument was enhanced by studies showing that there is resistance to reflux in animals shortly after death (165). Although structure is important, there also is a case for functional specialization. A zone of high pressure has been detected in this area in several species (52,106,112). This zone has been shown to have the ability to relax under certain circumstances and to contract under others. In unanesthetized dogs with ileal and colonic fistulae, Kelley et al. (113) used balloon manometry to record a mean resting pressure of 66 ± 2.2 cm H_2O. Intermittent distension of the ileum induced junctional relaxation during about 80% of the trials. Relaxation as measured with this technique was not complete, possibly owing to the relatively large size of the balloon. Colonic distension, on the other hand, induced junctional contractions during about 60% of the trials. Responses were not consistent, however; often no response to distension was seen. In humans, Cohen et al. (52) used perfused catheters and recorded mean resting pressures of 20.3 mm Hg. They obtained an average 70% reduction in pressure during ileal distension in about 90% of the trials. Colonic distension induced an increase in pressure in 80% of the trials. Thus, this area exhibits many of the characteristics of a sphincter. Not all investigators have obtained such results. Pahlin and Kewenter (153) monitored flow through the ileocecal junction in anesthesized cats and found that it took rather high pressures to force fluid from the ileum to the colon, suggesting a sphincter or valve. In their study, however, no relaxations could be uncovered. Ileal distension caused an increase in sphincter tone (manifested by a decrease in flow through the junction). Some major differences between this study and those mentioned above are that (a) a different species was used, (b) the state of anesthesia was not the same, and (c) the continuity of the distended intestinal segment was interrupted. Therefore, the results are hard to compare.

More direct evidence for a difference in function of the ileocecal junction comes from studies on muscle strips taken from this area. Studies by Gazet and Jarrett (85) and by Conklin and Christensen (54) showed that strips of circular muscle from this area behave differently than do strips of colonic or ileal muscle. Strips taken from an ileocecal region of cat and oppossum maintained a resting tone and demonstrated steeper length-tension slopes than did strips taken from the colon or more proximal ileum. Likewise, strips of ileal and junctional muscle relaxed during transmural electrical stimulation. Thus, these strips behaved similarly to one taken from the lower esophageal sphincter (47).

All studies cited above used short periods of recording and/or surgically altered intestine. On the other hand, Wienbeck and Janssen (216) recorded for long periods of time from intact unanesthetized cats. They implanted electrodes along the serosal surface of the ileocolonic junction and recorded after the animals had recovered. Organized groups of spike potential activity passed from the ileum over onto the colon. Thus, the ileocecal junction does not serve as a barrier to the passage of certain patterns of motility. Interesting as these observations are, they are hard to interpret without further studies. It is not clear if any of the electrodes were truly on the sphincteric muscle. Also, it would be interesting to know what is happening to the flow of contents and to intestinal pressures between and during these spike potential bursts.

Control of Contractile Activity

As in the rest of the intestine, contractile activity of the ileocecal junction or sphincter is regulated at several levels. Since strips isolated from this area maintain a resting tension, local factors must be at least partially responsible for maintenance of closure of this area *in vivo*. These local factors appear to involve activity of the smooth muscle cells themselves, since resting tension of sphincter strips is not abolished by tetrodotoxin. In fact, Conklin and Christensen (54) found tension to increase in the presence of tetrodotoxin.

Tension produced by the sphincter muscle cells is modulated by intrinsic neural activity. Strips stimulated electrically respond by relaxing, a response blocked by tetrodotoxin (54). Thus, intrinsic inhibitory nerves are present. Whether or not there are reflex arcs within the intrinsic nerves has not been studied directly. However, the relaxation in response to ileal distension may be mediated by such an arc as relaxation was seen in those preparations with intact intestines (52,111,113) and not in those with transected intestines (153).

Results from studies on the influence of extrinsic nerves on the sphincter are not consistent. Extrinsic nerves do not appear to be mandatory for maintenance of closure, since cutting them does not abolish resting tone. Stimulating these nerves, however, can alter sphincteric activity. Most studies agree that stimulation of the sympathetic nerves induces contraction of the sphincter. Hinrichsen and Ivy (97) found that stimulation of the splanchnic nerves and nerve fibers from the superior and inferior mesenteric ganglia caused contractions of the sphincter in anesthetized dogs. Similar results in the cat have been reported by Jarrett and Gazet (106) and by Pahlin and Kewenter (154). Contraction in response to sympathetic stimulation appears to be mediated by catecholamines which act on alpha

adrenergic receptors located on the muscle cells, since it was blocked by guanethidine, an agent which interferes with activity of adrenergic nerves, and by phenoxybenzamine, an alpha adrenergic receptor blocking agent. The muscle cells of the sphincter appear to possess beta adrenergic receptors which when activated (e.g., by isoproterenol) lead to relaxation. These receptors, however, are not activated when the adrenergic nerves are stimulated. Results of vagal nerve stimulation differ from study to study. Hinrichsen and Ivy (97) found variable responses. Stimulation (parameters not given) caused a short relaxation followed by contraction in about 50% of the trials. Jarrett and Gazet (106) obtained similar results, although their data hinted that lower frequencies of stimulation (1 and 5 Hz) favored relaxation. Pahlen and Kewenter (155), on the other hand, obtained only contractions upon vagal stimulation in anesthetized cats. They attempted to bring out a relaxation by stimulating the vagus after tone of the sphincter had been increased, but they were unsuccessful. Contraction in response to vagal stimulation was prevented by atropine; however, in the presence of this drug, no relaxation was seen. Thus, there do not appear to be any nonadrenergic inhibitory fibers to this area.

References

1. Alvarez, W. C. (1925): Reverse peristalsis in the bowel, a precursor of vomiting. *J. A. M. A.*, 85:1051–1054.
2. Alvarez, W. C. (1928): *The Mechanics of the Digestive Tract.* Hoeber, New York.
3. Alvarez, W. C. (1968): Early studies of the movements of the stomach and bowel. In: *Handbook of Physiology, Section 6, Volume 4: Motility,* edited by C. F. Code, pp. 1573–1578. Williams and Wilkins, Baltimore.
4. Alvarez, W. C., and Mahoney, L. J. (1922): Action currents in stomach and intestine. *Am. J. Physiol.*, 58:476–493
5. Anderson, S., Rosell, S., Hjelmquist, U., Chang, D., and Folkers, K. (1977): Inhibition of gastric and intestinal motor activity in dogs by (Gln^4) neurotensin. *Acta Physiol. Scand.*, 100:231–235.
6. Anuras, S., and Cooke, A. (1978): Effects of some gastrointestinal hormones on two muscle layers of duodenum. *Am. J. Physiol.*, 234:E60–E63.
7. Anuras, S., Faulk, D. L., Christensen, J. (1979): Effects of some autonomic drugs on duodenal smooth muscle. *Am. J. Physiol.*, 236:E33–E38.
8. Atchison, W. D., Stewart, J. J., and Bass, P. (1978): A unique distribution of laxative-induced spike potentials from the small intestine of the dog. *Am. J. Dig. Dis.*, 23:513–520.
9. Bass, P. (1968): In vivo electrical activity of the small bowel. In: *Handbook of Physiology, Section 6, Volume 4: Motility,* edited by C. F. Code, pp. 2051–2074. Williams and Wilkins, Baltimore.
10. Bass, P., Code, C. F., and Lambert, E. H. (1961): Electric activity of gastroduodenal junction. *Am. J. Physiol.*, 201:587–592.
11. Bass, P., Code, C. F., and Lambert, E. H. (1961): Motor and electric activity of the duodenum. *Am. J. Physiol.*, 201:287–291.
12. Bass, P., and Wiley, J. N. (1965): Effects of ligation and morphine on electric and motor activity of dog duodenum. *Am. J. Physiol.*, 208:908–913.
13. Bass, P., and Wiley, J. N. (1965): Electrical and extraluminal contractile-force activity of the duodenum of the dog. *Am. J. Dig. Dis.*, 10:183–200.
14. Bayliss, W. M., and Starling, E. H. (1899): The movements and

innervation of the small intestine. *J. Physiol. (Lond.),* 24:99–143.

15. Beck, I. T., McKenna, R. D., Peterfy, G., Sidorov, J., and Strawczynski, H. (1965): Pressure studies in the normal human jejunum. *Am. J. Dig. Dis.,* 10:436–448.
16. Bertaccini, G., and Agosti, A. (1971): Action of caerulein on intestinal motility in man. *Gastroenterology,* 60:55–63.
17. Biber, B., and Fara, J. (1973): Intestinal motility increased by tetrodotoxin, lidocaine and procaine. *Experientia,* 29:551–f552.
18. Boldyreff, W. (1911): Einige heue seiten der tatigkeit des pandreas. *Ergeb. der Physiol.,* 11:121–217.
19. Bortoff, A. (1965): Electrical transmission of slow waves from longitudinal to circular intestinal muscle. *Am. J. Physiol.,* 209:1254–1260.
20. Bortoff, A. (1972): Digestion: Motility. *Annu. Rev. Physiol.,* 34:261–290.
21. Bortoff, A., and Chalib, E. (1972): Temporal relationship between electrical and mechanical activity of longitudinal and circular muscle during intestinal peristalsis. *Am. J. Dig. Dis.,* 17:317–325.
22. Bortoff, A., and Muller, R. (1975): Stimulation of intestinal smooth muscle by atropine, procaine, and tetrodotoxin. *Am. J. Physiol.,* 229:1609–1613.
23. Brown, J. C., Cook, M. A., and Dryburgh, J. R. (1972): Motilin, a gastric motor activity-stimulating polypeptide: final purification, amino-acid composition and C-terminal residues. *Gastroenterology,* 62:401–404.
24. Brown, J. C., Johnson, L. P., and Magee, D. F. (1966): Effect of duodenal alkalinization on gastric motility. *Gastroenterology,* 50:333–339.
25. Bueno, L., Ferra, I-P., and Ruckebusch, Y. (1978): Effects of anesthesia and surgical procedures on intestinal myoelectric activity in rats. *Am. J. Dig. Dis.,* 23:690–695.
26. Bueno, L., Firoamonti, J., and Ruckebusch, Y. (1975): Rate of flow of digesta and electrical activity of the small intestine in dogs and sheep. *J. Physiol. (Lond.),* 249:69–85.
27. Bueno, L., Firoamonti, J. and Ruckebusch, Y. (1978): Postoperative intestinal motility in dogs and sheep. *Am. J. Dig. Dis.* 23:682–689.
28. Bueno, L., Prudbande, F., and Ruckebusch, Y. (1979): Propagation of electrical spiking activity along the small intestine: intrinsic versus extrinsic neural influences. *J. Physiol. (Lond.),* 292:16–26.
29. Bueno, L., and Ruckebusch, M. (1976): Insulin and jejunal electrical activity in dogs and sheep. *Am. J. Physiol.,* 230:1538–1544.
30. Bueno, L., and Ruckebusch, Y. (1977): Migrating myoelectric complexes: disruption, enhancement and disorganization. In: *Gastrointestinal Motility in Health and Disease,* edited by H. L. Duthie, pp. 83–91. MTP Press Ltd., Lancaster.
31. Bueno, L., and Ruckebusch, Y. (1978): Origine centrale de l'action excitomotrice de l'intestin par la morphine. *Comptes rendus Biologie,* 172:972–977.
32. Bueno, L., and Ruckebusch, Y. (1979): Perinatal development of intestinal myoelectric activity in dogs and sheep. *Am. J. Physiol.,* 237:E61–E67.
33. Bunker, C. E., Johnson, L. P., and Nelson, T. S. (1967): Chronic in situ studies of the electrical activity of the small intestine. *Arch. Surg.,* 95:259–268.
34. Burks, T. F., and Grubb, M. N. (1978): Stimulatory actions of adenosine triphosphate in dog intestine. In: *Gastrointestinal Motility in Health and Disease,* edited by H. L. Duthie, pp. 151–159. MTP Press, Ltd., Lancaster.
35. Burns, T. W., Mathias, J. R., Carlson, G. M., and Martin, J. L. (1978): Comparative effects of toxigenic and invasive Escherichia coli on small intestinal motility. *Clin. Res.,* 26:17A.
36. Burns, T. W., Mathias, J. R., Carlson, G. M., Martin, J. L., and Shields, R. P. (1978): Effect of toxigenic Escherichia coli on myoelectric activity of small intestine. *Am. J. Physiol.,* 235:E311–E315.
37. Burnstock, G. (1972): Purinergic nerves. *Parmacol. Rev.,* 54:418–440.
38. Cannon, W. B. (1902): The movements of the intestines studied by means of the roentgen rays. *Am. J. Physiol.,* 6:251–277.
39. Carlson, G. M., Bedi, B. S., and Code, C. F. (1972): Mecha-

nism of propagation of intestinal interdigestive myoelectric complex. *Am. J. Physiol.,* 222:1027–1030.
40. Carlson, G. M., Rudden, R. W., Hug, C. C., and Bass, P. (1970): Effects of nicotine on gastric antral and duodenal contractile activity in the dog. *J. Pharmacol. Exp. Ther.,* 172:367–376.
41. Carlson, G. M., Rudden, R. W., Hug, C. C., Schmiego, S. K., and Bass, P. (1970): Analysis of the site of nicotine action on gastric antral and duodenal contractile activity. *J. Pharmacol. Exp. Ther.,* 172:377–383.
42. Castleton, K. B. (1934): An experimental study of the movements of the small intestine. *Am. J. Physiol.,* 107:641–646.
43. Castro, G. A., Badial-Aceves, F., Smith, J. W., Dudrick, S. J., and Weisbrodt, N. W. (1976): Altered small bowel propulsion associated with parasitism. *Gastroenterology,* 71:620–625.
44. Catchpole, B. N., and Duthie, H. L. (1978): Postoperative gastrointestinal complexes. In: *Gastrointestinal Motility in Health and Disease,* edited by H. L. Duthie, pp. 33–41. MTP Press, Ltd., Lancaster.
45. Christensen, J., Schedl, H. P., and Clifton, J. A. (1964): The basic electrical rhythm of the duodenum in normal human subjects and in patients with thyroid disease. *J. Clin. Invest.,* 43:1659–1667.
46. Christensen, J. (1971): The controls of gastrointestinal movements: some old and new views. *N. Engl. J. Med.,* 285:85–98.
47. Christensen, J., Conklin, J. L., and Freeman, B. W. (1973): Physiologic specialization at esophagogastric junction in three species. *Am. J. Physiol.,* 225:1265–1270.
48. Christensen, J., Glover, J. R., Macagno, E. D., Singerman, R. B. and Weisbrodt, N. W. (1971): Statistics of contractions at a point in the human duodenum. *Am. J. Physiol.,* 221:1818–1823.
49. Code, C. F., and Marlett, J. A. (1975): The interdigestive myoelectric complex of the stomach and small bowel of dogs. *J. Physiol. (Lond.),* 246:289–309.
50. Code, C. F., Rogers, A. G., Schlegel, J., Hightower, N. C., and Bargen, J. A. (1957): Motility patterns in the terminal ileum: studies on two patients with ulcerative colitis and ileac stomas. *Gastroenterology,* 32:651–665.
51. Code, C. F., and Schlegel, J. F. (1974): The gastrointestinal housekeeper. In: *Gastrointestinal Motility,* edited by E. E. Daniel, pp. 631–633. Mitchell Press, Vancouver.
52. Cohen, S., Harris, L. D., and Levitan, R. (1968): Manometric characteristics of the human ileocecal junctional zone. *Gastroenterology,* 54:72–75.
53. Collins, S. M., Lewis, T. D., Track, N., Fox, J., and Daniel, E. E. (1978): Release of motilin. *Gastroenterology,* 74:1020.
54. Conklin, J. L., and Christensen, J. (1975): Local specialization at ileocecal junction of the cat and opossum. *Am. J. Physiol.,* 228:1075–1081
55. Connell, A. M. (1970): Propulsion in the small intestine. *Rendic. R. Gastroenterol.,* 2:38–46.
56. Connor, J. A. (1979): On exploring the basis for slow potential oscillations in the mammalian stomach and intestine. *J. Exp. Biol.,* 81:153–173.
57. Connor, J. A., Kreulin, D., Prosser, C. L., and Weigel, R. (1977): Interaction between longitudinal and circular muscle in intestine of cat. *J. Physiol. (Lond.),* 273:665–689.
58. Connor, J. A., Mangol, A. W., and Nelson, B. (1979): Propagation and entrainment of slow waves in cat small intestine. *Am. J. Physiol.,* 237:C237–C246.
59. Connor, J. A., Prosser, C. L., and Weems, W. A. (1974): A study of pacemaker activity in intestinal smooth muscle. *J. Physiol.,* 240:671–701.
60. Daniel, E. E. (1968): Pharmacology of the gastrointestinal tract. In: *Handbook of Physiology, Section 6, Volume 4: Motility,* edited by C. F. Code, pp. 2267–2324. Williams and Wilkins, Baltimore.
61. Daniel, E. E. (1969): Digestion: motor function. *Annu. Rev. Physiol.,* 31:203–226.
62. Daniel, E. E. (1972): A conceptual analysis of the pharmacology of gastrointestinal motility. In: *International Encyclopedia of Pharmacology and Therapeutics,* edited by G. Peters, pp. 94–187, Section 39a. Pergamon Press, Oxford.

63. Daniel, E. E. (1978): Peptidergic nerves in the gut. *Gastroenterology,* 75:142–145.
64. Daniel, E. E., Daniel, V. P., Duchon, G., Garfield, R. E., Nichols, M., Malhotra, S. K., and Oki, M. (1978): Is the nexus necessary for cell-to-cell coupling of smooth muscle? *J. Membr. Biol.,* 28:207–239.
65. Daniel, E. E., Duchon, G., and Henderson, R. M. (1972): The ultrastructural basis for coordination of intestinal motility. *Am. J. Dig. Dis.,* 17:289–298.
66. Daniel, E. E., and Sarna, S. (1978): The generation and conduction of activity in smooth muscle. *Annu. Rev. Pharmacol. Toxicol.,* 18:145–166.
67. Daniel, E. E., Wachter, B. T., Honour, A. J., and Bogoch, A. (1960): The relationship between electrical and mechanical activity of the small intestine of dog and man. *Can. J. Biochem. Physiol.,* 38:777–801.
68. DeWever, I., Eeckhout, C., Vantrappen, G., and Hellemans, J. (1978): Disruptive effect of test meals on interdigestive motor complex in dogs. *Am. J. Physiol.,* 235:E661–E665.
69. Diamant, N. E., and Bortoff, A. (1969): Nature of the intestinal slow-wave frequency gradient. *Am. J. Physiol.,* 216:301–307.
70. Didio, L. T. A., and Anderson, M. C. (1968): *The "sphincters" of the Digestive System.* Williams and Wilkins, Baltimore.
71. Dodds, W. J., Stef, J. J., and Hogan, W. J. (1976): Factors determining pressure measurement accuracy by intraluminal esophageal manometry. *Gastroenterology,* 70:117–123.
72. Douglas, D. M., and Mann, F. C. (1939): An experimental study of the rhythmic contractions in the small intestine of the dog. *Am. J. Dig. Dis.,* 6:318–322.
73. Dryburgh, J. R., and Brown, J. C. (1975): Radioimmunoassay for motilin. *Gastroenterology,* 68:1169–1176.
74. Dubois, A., and Bremer, A. (1972): Jejunal propulsive motility of the dog. Influence of neostigmine and dihydroergotamine. *Arch. Int. Pharmacodyn. Ther.,* 198:162–172.
75. Eeckhout, C., DeWever, I., Peeters, T., Hellemans, J., and Vantrappen, G. (1978): Role of gastrin and insulin in postprandial disruption of migrating complex in dogs. *Am. J. Physiol.,* 235:E666–E669.
76. Eeckhout, C., DeWever, I., Vantrappen, G., and Hellemans, J. (1979): Local disorganization of the interdigestive migrating motor complex (MMC) by perfusion of a Thiry-Vella loop. *Gastroenterology,* 76:1127.
77. El-Sharkawy, T. Y., and Daniel, E. E. (1975): Ionic mechanisms of intestinal electrical control activity. *Am. J. Physiol.,* 229:1287–1298.
78. Farrar, J. T. (1963): Gastrointestinal smooth muscle function. *Am. J. Dig. Dis.,* 8:103–110.
79. Fleckenstein, P. (1978): Migrating electrical spike activity in the fasting human small intestine. *Am. J. Dig. Dis.,* 23:769–775.
80. Fleckenstein, P., and Oigaard, A. (1978): Electrical spike activity in the human small intestine. *Am. J. Dig. Dis.,* 23:776–780.
81. Foulk, W. T., Code, C. F., Morlock, C. G., and Barzon, J. A. (1954): A study of the motility patterns and the basic rhythm in the duodenum and upper part of the jejunum of human beings. *Gastroenterology,* 26:601–611.
82. Friedman, G., Waye, J. D., Weingarten, L., and Janowitz, H. D. (1964): The patterns of simultaneous intraluminal pressure changes in the human proximal small intestine. *Gastroenterology,* 47:258–268.
83. Friedman, G., Wolf, B. S., Waye, J. D., and Janowitz, H. D. (1965): Correlation of cineradiographic and intraluminal pressure changes in the human duodenum: an analysis of the functional significance of monophasic waves. *Gastroenterology,* 49:37–49.
84. Gabella, G. (1972): Innervation of the intestinal muscular coat. *J. Neurocytol.,* 1:341–362.
85. Gazet, J. C., and Jarrett, R. J. (1964): The ileocolic sphincter. Studies in vitro in man, monkey, cat, and dog. *Br. J. Surg.,* 51:368–370.
86. Gernandt, B., and Zotterman, Y. (1946): Intestinal pain: an electrophysiological investigation on mesenteric nerves. *Acta Physiol. Scand.,* 12:56–72.
87. Gonella, J. (1971): Etude electromyographique des contractions segmentaires et peristaltiques du duodenum de lapin. *Pflugers Arch.,* 322:217–234.

88. Gregory, R. A. (1947): The nervous pathways of intestinal reflexes associated with nausea and vomitting. *J. Physiol. (Lond.),* 106:95–103.
89. Grindlay, J. H., and Mann, F. C. (1941): Effect of liquid and solid meals on intestinal activity. *Am. J. Dig. Dis.,* 8:324–327.
90. Grivel, M-L., and Ruckebusch, Y. (1972): The propagation of segmental contractions along the small intestine. *J. Physiol.,* 227:611–625.
91. Gustavsson, S. (1978): Studies on the transport of small bowel contents. *Ups. J. Med. Sci.,* 83:167–173.
92. Hansky, J., and Connell, A. M. (1962): Measurement of gastrointestinal transit using radioactive chromium. *Gut,* 3:187–188.
93. Henderson, R. M., Duchon, G., and Daniel, E. E. (1971): Cell contacts in duodenal smooth muscle layers. *Am. J. Physiol.,* 221:564–574.
94. Hermon-Taylor, J., and Code, C. F. (1971): Localization of the duodenal pacemaker and its role in the organization of duodenal myoelectric activity. *Gut,* 12:40–47.
95. Hidaka, T., and Kuriyama, H. (1969): Response of the smooth muscle membrane of guinea-pig jejunum elicited by field stimulation. *J. Gen. Physiol.,* 53:471–486.
96. Hightower, N. C. (1968): Motor action of the small bowel. In: *Handbook of Physiology, Section 6, Volume 4: Motility,* edited by C. F. Code, pp. 2001–2024. Williams and Wilkins, Baltimore.
97. Hinrichsen, J., and Ivy, A. C. (1931): Studies on the ileo-cecal sphincter of the dog. *Am. J. Physiol.,* 96:494–507.
98. Hirsch, J., Ahrens, E. H., and Blankendorn, D. H. (1956): Measurement of the human intestinal length in vivo and some causes of variation. *Gastroenterology,* 31:274–284.
99. Hirst, G. D. S., Holman, M. E., and McKirdy, H. C. (1975): Two descending nerve pathways activated by distension of guinea pig small intestine. *J. Physiol. (Lond.),* 244:113–127.
100. Hirst, G. D. S., and McKirdy, H. C. (1974): A nervous mechanism for descending inhibition in guinea-pig small intestine. *J. Physiol. (Lond.),* 238:129–143.
101. Ingelfinger, F. J., and Moss, R. F. (1942): The activity of the descending duodenum during nausea. *Am. J. Physiol.,* 136:561–566.
102. Itoh, Z., Honda, R., Hiwatashi, K., Takeuchi, S., Aizawa, I., Takayanagi, R., and Couch, E. F. (1976): Motilin-induced mechanical activity in the canine alimentary tract. *Scand. J. Gastroenterol. (Suppl. 39),* 11:93–110.
103. Itoh, Z., Takeuchi, S., Aizawi, I., Mori, K., Taminato, T., Seino, Y., Imura, H., and Yanashara, N. (1978): Changes in plasma motilin concentration and gastrointestinal contractile activity in conscious dogs. *Dig. Dis. Sci.,* 23:929–935.
104. Itoh, Z., Takeuchi, S., Aizawa, I., and Takayanagi, R. (1977): Effect of synthetic motilin on gastric motor activity in conscious dogs. *Am. J. Dig. Dis.,* 22:813–819.
105. Jacoby, H. I., Bass, P., and Bennett, D. R. (1963): In vivo extraluminal contractile force transducer for gastrointestinal muscle. *J. Appl. Physiol.,* 18:658–665.
106. Jarrett, R. J., and Gazet, J. C. (1966): Studies in vivo of the ileocaeco-colic sphincter in the cat and dog. *Gut,* 7:271–275.
107. Johansson, B., Jonsson, D., and Ljung, B. (1967): Tonic supraspinal mechanisms influencing the intestino-intestinal inhibitory reflex. *Acta Physiol. Scand.,* 72:200–204.
108. Johansson, B., and Langston, J. B. (1963): Reflex influence of mesenteric afferents on renal, intestinal and muscle blood flow and on intestinal motility. *Acta Physiol. Scand.,* 61:400–412.
109. Johnson, L. R. (1977): Gastrointestinal hormones and their functions. *Annu. Rev. Physiol.,* 39:135–158.
110. Justus, P. G., Mathias, J. R., Carlson, G. M., Martin, J. L., and Formal, S. (1979): The myoelectric activity of the small intestine in response to *Clostridiam difficile* culture filtrates. *Gastroenterology,* 76:1163.
111. Kelley, M. L., and DeWeese, J. A. (1969): Effects of eating and intraluminal filling on ileocolonic junctional zone pressures. *Am. J. Physiol.,* 216:1491–1495.
112. Kelley, M. L., Gordon, E. A., and DeWeese, J. A. (1965): Pressure studies of the ileocolonic junctional zone of dogs. *Am. J. Physiol.,* 209:333–339.
113. Kelley, M. L., Gordon, E. A., and DeWeese, J. A. (1966): Pres-

sure responses of canine ileocolonic junctional zone to intestinal distention. *Am. J. Physiol.,* 211:614-618.

114. Kewenter, J. (1965): The vagal control of the jejunal and ileal motility and blood flow. *Acta Physiol. Scand. (Suppl.),* 251:3-68.

115. Kewenter, J., and Kock, N. G. (1960): Motility of the human small intestine. *Acta Chir. Scand.,* 119:430-438.

116. Kewenter, J., Pahlin, P-E., and Strom, B. (1970): The effects of periarterial nerve stimulation on the jejunal and ileal motility in cat. *Acta Physiol. Scand.,* 80:353-359.

117. Kim, S. K. (1968): Small intestinal transit time in the normal small bowel study. *Radiology,* 104:522-524.

118. Kobayashi, M., Nagai, T., and Prosser, C. L. (1966): Electrical interaction between muscle layers of cat intestine. *Am. J. Physiol.,* 211:1281-1291.

119. Kosterlitz, H. W. (1968): Intrinsic and extrinsic nervous control of motility of the stomach and the intestine. In: *Handbook of Physiology, Section 6, Volume 4: Motility,* edited by C. F. Code, pp. 2147-2171. Williams and Wilkins, Baltimore.

120. Kosterlitz, H. W., Pirie, V. W., and Robinson, J. A. (1956): The mechanism of the peristaltic reflex in the isolated guinea-pig ileum. *J. Physiol. (Lond.),* 133:681-694.

121. Kreulen, D. L. and Szurszewski, J. H. (1979): Nerve pathways in celiac plexus of the guinea pig. *Am. J. Physiol.,* 237:E90-E97.

122. Kreulen, D. L., and Szurszewski, J. H. (1979): Reflex pathways in the abdominal prevertebral ganglia: evidence for a colo-colonic inhibitory reflex. *J. Physiol. (Lond.),* 295:21-32.

123. Kumpuris, D. D., Brannan, P. G., and Goyal, R. K. (1979): Characterization of motor activity in the jejunum of normal subjects and two patients with idiopathic intestinal pseudo-obstruction syndrome (IIPS). *Gastroenterology,* 76:1177.

124. Kuntz, A. (1922): On the occurrence of reflex arcs in the myenteric and submucous plexuses. *Anat. Rec.,* 24:193-210.

125. Latour, A. (1977): Quantitative analysis and measurement of myoelectrical spike activity at the gastroduodenal junction. *Ann. Biol. Anim. Biochem. Biophys.,* 18:1-6.

126. Lee, K. Y., Chey, W. Y., Tay, H. H., Wagner, D., and Yajima, H. (1977): Cyclic changes in plasma motilin levels and interdigestive myoelectric activity of canine antrum and duodenum. *Gastroenterology,* 72:1162.

127. Lee, K. Y., Chey, W. Y., and Yajima, H. (1978): Radioimmunoassay of motilin: validation of studies on the relationship between plasma motilin and interdigestive myoelectric activity of the duodenum of dog. *Am. J. Dig. Dis.,* 23:789-795.

128. Lewis, T. D., Collins, S. M., Fox, J-A. E., and Daniel, E. E. (1979): Initiation of duodenal acid-induced motor complexes. *Gastroenterology,* 77:1217-1224.

129. Louckes, H. S., Quigley, J. P., and Kersay, J. (1960): Inductograph method of recording muscle activity especially pyloric sphincter physiology. *Am. J. Physiol.,* 199:301-310.

130. Marik, F., and Code, C. F. (1975): Control of the interdigestive myoelectric activity in dogs by the vagus nerves and pentagastrin. *Gastroenterology,* 69:387-395.

131. Marlett, J. A., and Code, C. F. (1979): Effects of celiac and superior mesenteric ganglionectomy on interdigestive myoelectric complex in dogs. *Am. J. Physiol.,* 237:E432-E436.

132. Mathias, J. R., Carlson, G. M., Bertiger, G., Martin, J. L., and Cohen, S. (1977): Migrating action potential complex of cholera: a possible prostaglandin-induced response. *Am. J. Physiol.,* 232:E529-E534.

133. Mathias, J. R., Carlson, G. M., DiMarino, A. J., Bartiger, G., and Cohen, S. (1975): The effect of cholera toxin on ileal myoelectric activity: a neural-hormonal mechanism. In: *Proceedings of the 5th International Symposium on Gastrointestinal Motility,* edited by G. Vantrappen, pp. 219-226. Typoff-Press, Herentals, Belgium.

134. Mathias, J. R., Carlson, G. M., DiMarino, A. J., Bertiger, G., Morton, H. E., and Cohen, S. (1976): Intestinal myoelectric activity in response to live Vibrio cholerae and cholera enterotoxin. *J. Clin. Invest.,* 58:91-96.

135. Mathias, J. R., Martin, J. L., Burns, T. W., Carlson, G. M., and Shields, R. P. (1978): Ricinoleic acid effect on the electrical activity of the small intestine in rabbits. *J. Clin. Invest.,* 61:640-644.

136. McCoy, E. J., and Baker, R. D. (1968): Effect of feeding on electrical activity of dog's small intestine. *Am. J. Physiol.,* 214:1291-1295.

137. McCoy, E. J., and Baker, R. D. (1969): Intestinal slow waves: decrease in propagation velocity along upper small intestine. *Am. J. Dig. Dis.,* 14:9-13.

138. Melville, J., Macagno, E., and Christensen, J. (1975): Longitudinal contractions in the duodenum: their fluid-mechanical function. *Am. J. Physiol.,* 228:1887-1892.

139. Mendel, C., Pousse, A., Schang, J. C., Dauchel, J., and Grenier, J. F. (1978): Longitudinal contractions in the jejunum of fasting dogs. In: *Gastrointestinal Motility in Health and Disease,* edited by H. C. Duthie, pp. 61-71. MTP Press Ltd., Lancaster.

140. Menville, L. J., and Ane, J. N. (1932): X-ray study of passage of different food stuffs through small intestine of man. *Radiology,* 18:783-786.

141. Monges, H., Salducci, J., and Naudy, B. (1974): Electrical activity of the gastrointestinal tract in dog during vomiting. In: *Gastrointestinal Motility,* edited by E. E. Daniel, pp. 479-488. Mitchell Press, Vancouver.

142. Moore, E. P., Copeland, E. M., Dudrick, S. J., and Weisbrodt, N. W. (1976): Effect of an elemental diet on the electrical activity of the small intestine in dogs. *J. Surg. Res.,* 20:533-537.

143. Mukhopadhyay, A. K., Johnson, L. R., Copeland, E. M., and Weisbrodt, N. W. (1975): Effect of secretin on electrical activity of small intestine. *Am. J. Physiol.,* 229:484-488.

144. Mukhopadhyay, A. K., Thor, P. J., Copeland, E. M., Johnson, L. R., and Weisbrodt, N. W. (1977): Effect of cholecystokinin on myoelectric activity of small bowel of the dog. *Am. J. Physiol.,* 232:E44-E47.

145. Nelsen, T. S., and Becker, J. C. (1968): Stimulation of the electrical and mechanical gradient of the small intestine. *Am. J. Physiol.,* 214:749-757.

146. Ohkawa, H., and Prosser, C. L. (1972): Electrical activity in myenteric and submucous plexuses of cat intestine. *Am. J. Physiol.,* 222:1412-1419.

147. Ohkawa, H., and Prosser, C. L. (1972): Functions of neurons in enteric plexuses of cat intestine. *Am. J. Physiol.,* 222:1420-1426.

148. Ormsbee, H. S., Koehler, S. L., and Telford, G. L. (1978): Somatostatin inhibits motilin-induced interdigestive contractile activity in the dog. *Am. J. Dig. Dis.,* 23:781-788.

149. Ormsbee, H. S., and Mir, S. S. (1978): The role of the cholinergic nervous system in the gastrointestinal response to motilin in vivo. In: *Gastrointestinal Motility in Health and Disease,* edited by H. L. Duthie, pp. 113-124. MTP Press, Ltd., Lancaster.

150. Ormsbee, H. S., Telford, G. L., and Mason, G. R. (1979): Mechanism of propagation of canine migrating motor complex—a reappraisal. *Gastroenterology,* 76:1212.

151. Ormsbee, H. S., Telford, G. I., and Mason, G. R. (1979): Required neural involvement in control of canine migrating motor complex. *Am. J. Physiol.,* 237:E451-E456.

152. Pahlin, P. E. (1975): Extrinsic nervous control of the ileo-cecal sphincter in the cat. *Acta Physiol. Scand. (Suppl.),* 426:1-32.

153. Pahlin, P.-E., and Kewenter, J. (1975): Reflexogenic contraction of the ileocecal sphincter in the cat following small or large intestinal distension. *Acta Physiol. Scand.,* 95:126-132.

154. Pahlin, P.-E., and Kewenter, J. (1976): Sympathetic nervous control of cat ileocecal sphincter. *Am. J. Physiol.,* 231:296-305.

155. Pahlin, P-E., and Kewenter, J. (1976): The vagal control of the ileo-cecal sphincter in the cat. *Acta Physiol. Scand.,* 96:433-442.

156. Parker, J. G., and Beneventano, T. C. (1970): Acceleration of small bowel contrast study by cholecystokinin. *Gastroenterology,* 58:679-684.

157. Patel, G. K., Whalen, G. E., Soergel, K. H., Wu, W. C., and Meade, R. C. (1979): Glucagon effect on the human small intestine. *Dig. Dis. Sci.,* 24:501-508.

158. Pearce, E. A., and Wingate, D. C. (1979): The role of the myenteric plexuses. *Gastroenterology,* 76:1215.

159. Perkins, W. E. (1971): Method for studying electrical and mechanical activity of isolated intestine. *J. Appl. Physiol.,* 30:768-771.

160. Poulakos, L., and Kent, T. H. (1973): Gastric emptying and

small intestinal propulsion in fed and fasted rats. *Gastroenterology,* 64:962-967.

161. Prosser, C. L. (1974): Smooth muscle. *Annu. Rev. Physiol.,* 36:503-535.

162. Puestow, C. B. (1932): The activity of isolated intestinal segments. *Arch. Surg.,* 24:565-573.

163. Ranieri, F., Mei, N., and Cousillat, J. (1973): Les afferences splanchniques provenant des mechanoreceptours gastrointestinaux et peritoneaux. *Exp. Brain Res.,* 16:276-290.

164. Reinke, D. A., Rosenbaum, A. H., and Bennett, D. R. (1967): Patterns of dog gastrointestinal contractile activity monitored in vivo with extraluminal force transducers. *Am. J. Dig. Dis.,* 12:113-141.

165. Rendleman, D. F., Anthony, Z. E., Davis, C., Buenger, R. E., Brooks, A. J., and Beattie, E. J. (1958): Reflux pressure studies on the ileocecal valve of dogs and humans. *Surgery,* 44:640-643.

166. Rinecker, H., Chaussy, C., and Brendel, W. (1969): The propagation of contractile waves from duodenum to jejunum. *Pflugers Arch.,* 305:210-218.

167. Ruckebusch, M., and Fioramonti, J. (1975): Electrical spiking activity and propulsion in small intestine in fed and fasted rats. *Gastroenterology,* 68:1500-1508.

168. Ruckebusch, Y., and Bueno, L. (1973): The effect of weaning on the motility of the small intestine in the calf. *Br. J. Nutr.,* 30:491-499.

169. Ruckebusch, Y., and Bueno, L. (1975): Electrical activity of the ovine jejunum and changes due to disturbances. *Am. J. Dig. Dis.,* 20:1027-1034.

170. Ruckebusch, Y., and Bueno, L. (1976): The effect of feeding on the motility of the stomach and small intestine in the pig. *Br. J. Nutr.,* 35:397-405.

171. Ruckebusch, Y., and Bueno, L. (1977): Migrating myoelectrical complex of the small intestine. *Gastroenterology,* 73:1309-1314.

172. Ruppin, H., Sturm, G., Westhoff, D., Domschke, S., Domschke, W., Wunsch, E., and Demling, L. (1976): Effect of 13-mle-motilin on small intestinal transit time in healthy subjects. *Scand. J. Gastroenterol. (Suppl. 39),* 11:85-88.

173. Ruwart, M. J., Klepper, M. S., and Rush, B. D. (1979): Evidence of noncholinergic mediation of small intestinal transit in the rat. *J. Pharmacol. Exp. Ther.,* 209:462-465.

174. Sancholuz, A. O., Croley, T. E., Christensen, J., Macagno, E. O., and Glover, J. R. (1975): Phase lock of electrical slow waves and spike bursts in cat duodenum. *Am. J. Physiol.,* 229:608-612.

175. Sancholuz, A. G., Croley, T. E., Glover, J. R., Macagno, E. O., and Christensen, J. (1975): Distribution of spike bursts in cat duodenum. *Am. J. Physiol.,* 229:925-929.

176. Sandors, K., and Ross, G. (1978): Effects of endogenous prostaglandin E on intestinal motility. *Am. J. Physiol.,* 234:E204-E208.

177. Sarna, S. K., Daniel, E. E., and Kingma, Y. J. (1971): Simulation of slow-wave electrical activity of small intestine. *Am. J. Physiol.,* 221:166-173.

178. Scarpollo, J. H., Greaves, M., and Sladen, G. E. (1976): Small intestinal transit in diabetes. *Br. Med. J.,* 2:1225-1226.

179. Schanbacher, L. M., Nations, J. K., Weisbrodt, N. W., and Castro, G. A. (1978): Intestinal myoelectric activity in parasitized dogs. *Am. J. Physiol.,* 234:R188-R195.

180. Schang, J. C., Danchel, J., Sara, P., Angel, F., Bouchet, P., Lambert, A., and Grenier, J. F. (1978): Specific effects of different food components on intestinal motility. *Eur. Surg. Res.,* 10:425-432.

181. Schofield, G. C. (1968): Anatomy of muscular and neural tissues in the alimentary canal. In: *Handbook of Physiology, Section 6, Volume 4: Motility,* edited by C. F. Code, pp. 1579-1627. Williams and Wilkins, Baltimore.

182. Scott, L. D., and Summers, R. W. (1976): Correlation of contractions and transit in rat small intestine. *Am. J. Physiol.,* 230:132-137.

183. Sinar, D. R., and Burns, T. W. (1979): Migrating action potential complexes occur independent of fluid secretion from cholera toxin. *Gastroenterology,* 76:1249.

184. Singleton, A. O., Redmond, D. C., and McMurray, J. E. (1964): Ileocecal resection and small bowel transit and absorption. *Ann. Surg.,* 159:690-694.

185. Smith, C. C., and Brizzee, K. R. (1961): Cineradiographic analysis of vomiting in the cat. *Gastroenterology,* 40:654-664.

186. Stewart, J. J., Burks, T. F., and Weisbrodt, N. W. (1977): Intestinal myoelectric activity after activation of central emetic mechanism. *Am. J. Physiol.,* 233:E131-E137.

187. Stewart, J. J., Weisbrodt, N. W., and Burks, T. F. (1977): Centrally mediated intestinal stimulation by morphine. *J. Pharmacol. Exp. Ther.,* 202:174-181.

188. Stewart, J. J., Weisbrodt, N. W., and Burks, T. F. (1978): Central and peripheral actions of morphine on intestinal transit. *J. Pharmacol. Exp. Ther.,* 205:547-555.

189. Strunz, U., Domschke, W., Mitznegg, P., Domschke, S., Schubert, E., Wunsch, E., Jaeger, E., and Demling, L. (1975): Analysis of the motor effects of 13-norleucine motilin on the rabbit, guinea pig, rat, and human alimentary tract in vitro. *Gastroenterology,* 68:1485-1491.

190. Summers, R. W., Helm, J., and Christensen, J. (1976): Intestinal propulsion in the dog. *Gastroenterology,* 70:753-758.

191. Summers, R. W., Kent, T. H., and Osborne, J. W. (1970): Effects of drugs, ileal obstruction, and irradiation on rat gastrointestinal propulsion. *Gastroenterology,* 59:731-739.

192. Sussman, S. E., Stewart, J. J., Burks, T. F., and Weisbrodt, N. W. (1978): Effects of morphine sulfate on motility of the small intestine. *Fed. Proc.,* 37:640.

193. Szurszewski, J. H. (1969): A migrating electrical complex of the canine small intestine. *Am. J. Physiol.,* 217:1757-1763.

194. Szurszewski, J. H., Elvaback, L. R., and Code, C. F. (1970): Configuration and frequency gradient of electric slow wave over canine small bowel. *Am. J. Physiol.,* 218:1468-1473.

195. Szurszewski, J. H., and Weems, W. W. (1976): Control of gastrointestinal motility by prevertebral ganglia. In: *Physiology of Smooth Muscle,* edited by E. Bulbring and M. F. Shuba, pp. 313-320. Raven Press, New York.

196. Tasaka, K., and Farrar, J. T. (1969): Mechanics of small intestinal muscle function in the dog. *Am. J. Physiol.,* 217:1224-1229.

197. Taylor, A. B., Kreulen, D., and Prosser, C. L. (1977): Electron microscopy of the connective tissues between longitudinal and circular muscle of small intestine of cat. *Am. J. Anat.,* 150:427-442.

198. Templeton, R. D., and Lawson, H. (1931): Studies in the motor activity of the large intestine. *Am. J. Physiol.,* 96:667-676.

199. Texter, E. C. (1963): Motility in the gastrointestinal tract. *JAMA,* 184:640-647.

200. Texter, E. C. (1964): The control of gastrointestinal motor activity. *Am. J. Dig. Dis.,* 9:585-598.

201. Thomas, P. A, Kelly, K. A., and Go, V. L. W. (1979): Does motilin regulate interdigestive gastric motility? *Dig. Dis. Sci.,* 24:577-582.

202. Thor, P., Krol, R., Konturek, S. J., Coy, D. H., and Schally, A. V. (1978): Effect of somatostatin on myoelectric activity of small bowel. *Am. J. Physiol.,* 235:E249-E254.

203. Tinker, J., and Cox, A. G. (1969): Effect of metaclopramide on transport in the small intestine of the dog. *Gut,* 10:986-989.

204. Tomita, T. (1975): Electrophysiology of mammalian smooth muscle. *Prog. Biophys. Mol. Biol.,* 30:185-203.

205. Vantrappen, G., Janssens, J., and Ghoos, Y. (1977): The interdigestive motor complex of normal subjects and patients with bacterial overgrowth of the small intestine. *J. Clin. Invest.,* 59:1158-1166.

206. Vantrappen, G., Janssens, J., Peeters, T. L., Bloom, S. R., Christofides, N. D., and Hellemans, J. (1979): Motility and the interdigestive migrating motor complex in man. *Dig. Dis. Sci.,* 24:497-500.

207. Weems, W. A., and Seygal, G. E. (1978): Intrinsic abilities of the cat intestine to do propulsive work. *Fed. Proc.,* 37:228.

208. Weisberg, P. B., Carlson, G. M., and Cohen, S. (1978): Effect of Salmonella typhimurium on myoelectrical activity in the rabbit ileum. *Gastroenterology,* 74:47-51.

209. Weisbrodt, N. W. (1974): Electrical and contractile activities of the small intestine of the cat. *Am. J. Dig. Dis.,* 19:93-99.

210. Weisbrodt, N. W., Badial-Aceves, F., Copeland, E. M., Dudrick, S. J., and Castro, G. A. (1978): Small-intestinal transit during total parenteral nutrition in the rat. *Am. J. Dig. Dis.,* 23:363-369.

211. Weisbrodt, N. W., and Christensen, J. (1972): Electrical activity of the cat duodenum in fasting and vomiting. *Gastroenterology,* 63:1004–1010.

212. Weisbrodt, N. W., Copeland, E. M., Moore, E. P., Kearley, R. W., and Johnson, L. R. (1965): Effect of vagotomy on electrical activity of the small intestine of the dog. *Am. J. Physiol.,* 228:650–654.

213. Weisbrodt, N. W., Copeland, E. M., Thor, P. J., and Dudrick, S. J. (1976): The myoelectric activity of the small intestine of the dog during total parenteral nutrition. *Proc. Soc. Biol. Med.,* 153:121–124.

214. Weisbrodt, N. W., Copeland, E. M., Thor, P. J., Mukhopadhyay, A. K., and Johnson, L. R. (1976): Nervous and humoral factors which influence the fasted and fed patterns of intestinal myoelectric activity. In: *Proceedings of the 5th International Symposium on Gastrointestinal Motility,* edited by G. Vantrappen, pp. 82–87. Typoff Press, Herentals, Belgium.

215. Weisbrodt, N. W., Moore, E., Kearley, R., Copeland, E. M., and Johnson, L. R. (1974): Effects of pentagastrin on the myoelectric activity of the small intestine. *Am. J. Physiol.,* 227:425–429.

216. Wienbeck, M., and Janssen, H. (1974): Electrical control mechanisms at the ileo-colic junction. In: *Proceedings of the 4th International Symposium on Gastrointestinal Motility,* edited by E. E. Daniel, pp. 97–107. Mitchell Press, Vancouver.

217. Wingate, D. (1976): The eupeptide system: a general theory of gastrointestinal hormones. *Lancet,* 1:529–532.

218. Wingate, D., Barnett, T., Green, R., and Armstrong, J. M. (1977): Automated high speed analysis of gastrointestinal myoelectric activity. *Am. J. Dig. Dis.,* 22:243–251.

219. Wingate, D. L., Pearce, E. A., Hutton, M., Dand, A., Thompson, H. H., and Wunsch, E. (1978): Quantitative comparison of the effects of cholecystokinin, secretin, and pentagastrin on gastrointestinal myoelectric activity in the conscious fasted dog. *Gut,* 19:593–601.

220. Wingate, D. L., Pearce, E., Ling, A., Boucher, B., Thompson, H., and Hutton, M. (1979): Quantitative effect of oral feeding on gastrointestinal myoelectric activity in the conscious dog. *Dig. Dis. Sci.,* 24:417–423.

221. Wingate, D. L., Ruppin, H., Green, W. E. R., Thompson, H. H., Domschke, W., Wunsch, E., Demling, L., and Ritchie, H. D. (1976): Motilin-induced electrical activity in the canine gastrointestinal tract. *Scand. J. Gastroenterol. (Suppl. 39),* 11:111–118.

222. Wood, J. D. (1972): Excitation of intestinal muscle by atropine, tetrodotoxin and Xylocaine. *Am. J. Physiol.,* 222:118–125.

223. Wood, J. D. (1975): Neurophysiology of Auerbach's plexus and control of intestinal motility. *Physiol. Rev.,* 55:307–324.

224. Wood, J. D. (1979): Neurophysiology of the enteric nervous system. In: *Integrative Functions of the Autonomic Nervous System,* edited by C. M. C. Brooks, pp. 177–193. University of Tokyo Press, Tokyo.

225. Wood, J. D., and Perkins, W. E. (1970): Mechanical interaction between longitudinal and circular axes of the small intestine. *Am. J. Physiol.,* 218:762–768.

226. Yokoyama, S., and Ozaki, T. (1978): Polarity of effects of stimulation of Auerbach's plexus on longitudinal muscle. *Am. J. Physiol.,* 235:E345–E353.

227. Youmans, W. B. (1972): Do adrenergic nerves innervate smooth muscle in the intestinal wall? *Gastroenterology,* 62:1278–1279.

ACKNOWLEDGMENTS

During the writing of this chapter I was supported in part by Research Grant AM 19886 and Research Scientist Development Award DA 00022 from the U.S. Public Health Service. I am grateful to Ms. Carla Maywald and Ms. Margaret Freeman for their excellent secretarial support.

Physiology of the Gastrointestinal Tract, edited by
Leonard R. Johnson. Raven Press, New York © 1981.

Chapter 14

Motility of the Colon

James Christensen

The colon has evolved to serve three major functions in mammalian physiology. The extraction of water and electrolytes from the fluid contents of the intestinal lumen, the first function of the colon, was clearly essential for the terrestrial adaptation of animal life and for later adaptation to dry environments. The second function of the mammalian colon is served by the presence of an abundant growth of microorganisms; this flora makes an important contribution to mammalian nutrition in some species, especially in perissodactyls. A third function is related to protection against tracking by scent: the ability of the potential victim of a scent-oriented predator to control the location of his fecal deposition surely has great value for the survival of that species.

The special character of the movements of the colon is responsible for these three special colonic functions. The extraction of water from the fecal mass by the colonic mucosa is slow because it must depend on the diffusion of water, a slow process. Also, the maintenance of a large population of microorganisms in the luminal content of the colon requires that the organ generate flows in the fluid contents to distribute nutrients for those bacteria while not evacuating its contents. The movements of the walls of the colon must be such as to retain the contents, to mix the contents over long periods of time, and to allow their extrusion to be at least partly under voluntary control.

Exactly how colonic contractions are organized to accomplish the normal patterns of flow in the colon is not clear. Our ignorance of colonic motility cannot be attributed to lack of interest, for the colon has not been wholly disregarded by physiologists, physicians, or laymen. Rather, our ignorance in the matter is related to a variety of factors. Among them are the complexity of the subject, the inaccessibility of the colon to study, and the unattractive nature of the organ and its contents. Also, a clear animal model of the human colon is lacking: the obvious and extreme differences among mammals in respect to colonic anatomy imply a degree of variability in physiology, and this makes tenuous the transposition of conclusions derived from the study of one species to another. Finally, it is clear that colonic motions are so slow or recur at such long intervals that they may not be fully appreciated in short-term observations.

This chapter will review the topic of colonic motion, emphasizing evidence that has come forth since the last such reviews (84,171).

ANATOMY

Gross Structure of the Human Colon

The colon, as measured in adult male cadavers, is about 1.5 m long, but it is probably somewhat shorter in life. The colon in man is usually described in terms of eight parts: the appendix, cecum, ascending colon, transverse colon, descending colon, sigmoid colon, rectum, and anal canal. These terms are based upon anatomy, not physiology. The cecum, from which the narrow appendix arises, is that part of the colon that lies upstream from the ileocolic junction. The ascending colon is the segment between the ileocolic junction and the hepatic flexure. The transverse colon extends from the hepatic flexure to the splenic flexure. The descending colon lies between the splenic flexure and the pelvic brim. The sigmoid colon extends from the pelvic brim to the point where the axis of the colon turns at the apex of the rectum. The rectum is the segment from that point to the anal canal, and the anal canal is the last 3 cm or so, ending at the anal verge.

Muscular Walls of the Colon

Throughout most of its length, the human colon is a sacculated organ. Sacculation is achieved in part as a result of specialization of the distribution of the outer (longitudinal) muscle layer. The bundles of this muscle layer are not uniformly distributed around the circumference of the colon as they are in the stomach and small intestine. Instead, the longitudinal layer of muscle is grouped into three thick bands, the three taeniae of the colon. Between the three taeniae, the longitudinal muscle layer is still present, although it is very thin. One of these taeniae is located along the line of the mesenteric insertion. The other two are placed at approximately equal distances from this mesenteric taenia. The saccular appearance of the colon seems also to be a consequence of an elongation of the muscle bundles of the circular muscle coat, so that, in a cross section of the colon, the wall appears to bulge in the three spaces between the three taeniae. These bulges are interrupted at fairly uniform intervals by comparatively tight circular bands, the plicae circulares. These produce the appearance of a chain of pockets, called the haustra. At about the point where the sigmoid colon ends, at the apex of the rectum, the three taeniae broaden and fuse, so that the longitudinal muscle layer is uniformly thick in the circumference of the rectum. At the anal canal, the outer longitudinal muscle layer merges with the external anal sphincter, which is striated muscle, and with the other striated musculature of the pelvic floor. The smooth-muscle internal anal sphincter is a continuation of the inner circular muscle layer of the rectum.

The human colon is suspended from the dorsal body wall by a mesentery, but the breadth of this mesentery varies. The cecum has essentially no mesentery, so that the cecum is quite fixed. The ascending and descending colon have a rather narrow mesentery. The mesentery of the transverse colon and of the sigmoid colon is broad, so that these parts are quite mobile. Throughout the length of the colon there are bundles of smooth muscle within the mesentery, which join the muscular coats of the colon to the dorsal body wall (75). The number and distribution of these bands are highly variable, but they are especially well developed along the cecum.

The colon, like the rest of the gut, contains a layer of mucosal muscle. This consists of an inner circular and an outer longitudinal layer, but the two are tightly fixed together by mixing and intertwining of fiber bundles at the interface of the two layers.

Nerves of the Colon

The laminated nature of the intramural nerve structures of the gut is described elsewhere in this volume. Most of the colon conforms to the rule, having well-developed plexuses at all levels. The appendix and cecum do not, however, for in those regions the ganglion cells are arranged in an apparently irregular pattern within the muscle layers (66). The functional significance of this difference is not known. In the remainder of the colon, the nervous elements constitute the subserous, myenteric, submucous, and mucous plexuses. The neurons of the myenteric plexus seem to be concentrated beneath the taenia and to be relatively sparse between taeniae, where the longitudinal muscle layer is thin. Abundant neurons have been described in the submucous plexus in the colon, particularly in the rectum. These plexuses are connected to the centers of the craniosacral autonomic nerves by way of the vagi in the proximal part of the colon and by way of the pelvic nerves in the distal colon. Sympathetic nerves reach the colon by way of the perivascular plexuses from the superior and inferior mesenteric ganglia.

Comparative Anatomy

Garry (84) was aware of the problem raised by the extreme anatomic variability among mammalian colons and he published a figure to illustrate the variations (Fig. 1). Carnivores, he pointed out, have a colon in which the longitudinal muscle is of uniform thickness all about the circumference, so that the colon has the appearance of the uniform tube. Taeniae and sacculation, a large cecum, and elongation, he believed, were all adaptations of herbivores to their diet. This rule, however, may be something of an oversimplification, for many exceptions occur (100,113,132,155). The colons of the horse and the cow, both herbivores, are quite different from one another. That of the horse is exten-

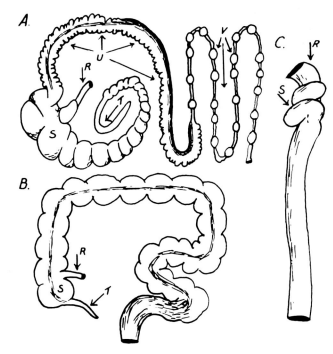

FIG. 1. The morphological variation in the mammalian large bowel. **A:** Rabbit colon. **B:** Human colon. **C:** Dog colon. (**R**) the ileum; (**S**) the cecum; (**T**) the appendix; (**U**) the proximal colon; and (**V**) the distal colon. (From ref. 84, with permission.)

sively taeniated and sacculated, whereas that of the cow is not. The colon of the rat and that of the opossum, both omnivores, resemble very much those of carnivores, whereas the colon of the pig, another omnivore, is elongated, taeniated, sacculated, and equipped with a large cecum.

It seems much more likely that these anatomic variations exist because of variations among species in the place of the colon in the physiological economy. Thus, for example, the fantastic complexity of the colon of horses is probably related to the very important contribution to the nutrition of those animals made by fermentation processes that take place in the cecum. In ruminants, a similar dependence upon intraluminal fermentation as a source of calories evolved, but this fermentation took place in the stomach rather than in the proximal colon, and so it was the stomach that became anatomically complex.

Development of the Colon

There are differences in function of the various parts of the colon, and there may be clues to that in the study of its organogenesis. The proximal part of the colon develops from the midgut and the distal part develops from the hindgut (121). The point at which the two come together is apparently at the point of abutment of the distributions of the superior and inferior mesenteric arteries, usually said to be a point about two-thirds of the way along the transverse colon. The rectum and anal

canal also have an origin distinct from that of the rest of the colon. Those parts develop from a primitive cloaca, being separated from what is to become the urogenital tract by the growth of the urorectal septum across the primitive cloaca. The cecum seems to develop very early in life, being appreciable as a distinct widening in the primitive intestine at least as early as the 7.5-mm embryo (121).

Controversy has existed as to when the haustra and taeniae first appear in the human colon. Various authors report haustra as first appearing as early as the 11th week of fetal life (133) and as late as the 3rd year of life (8), with other reports of intermediate ages. The evidence in favor of the earlier date is compelling, however, for both muscle layers are formed by the middle of the 3rd fetal month and the taeniae can at least be appreciated by the 11th fetal week.

METHODS TO STUDY CONTRACTIONS AND FLOW IN THE COLON

A thorough critique of the methods used to study colonic motility appeared in a previous article (171). This account will briefly survey the methods that have been used. They are many, and all have major shortcomings.

Examination of the colon exposed at operation has the advantage of directness but many disadvantages. First, it can be used in the human colon only rarely. Second, the colon so observed cannot reasonably be considered to be in a normal state, being possibly affected by preoperative fasting, by anesthetic agents and other drugs, by reflexes induced by the opening of the peritoneum, by a subnormal temperature, and by the effects of handling. Third, no permanent record can be obtained, so that conclusions drawn from such methods of observation cannot be made objectively.

Radiographic observations have been used in animals and in humans since the start of the century. They have the advantage that such variables as the actions of drugs, reflexes, and subnormal body temperature are not problems. On the other hand, in radiographic observations one is observing the flow of a luminal content that is chemically very different from normal luminal content, the foreign material is introduced under high pressure, the wall movements themselves are not visualized, and the duration of study is severely limited by considerations of safety in humans. Also, objectivity and quantitation are very hard to achieve.

The recording of intraluminal pressures by balloon kymography is a technique also used for a very long time. Balloons are introduced into the colon, inflated, and connected by a tube to a pressure-sensing device or to a volume recorder so that a contraction of the colon against the balloon is recorded as a rise in pressure or fall in volume within the balloon. Such methods have several disadvantages. First, the balloon, if large enough, evokes a reflex response, so that the bowel cannot be considered to be in its normal state. Second, the balloon may not yield to the contraction in the same way that normal colonic content would. Third, the characteristics of the balloon itself may influence the signals recorded.

Open-ended tubes have been used commonly in the esophagus in recent years and have had some application to the colon as well. They have the advantage that they can be used in animals and in humans with reasonable assurance that the motility of the colon is not being greatly influenced by the method of measurement. They have the major disadvantage that they record pressure in whatever sealed cavity the open end of the tubing happens to lie (Fig. 2). It is difficult if not impossible to know what kinds of wall movement give rise to the pressure changes recorded by open-ended tubes. Also, it is difficult to know precisely where the open end of the tube is along the colon. Considerable shifts in the position of the tube could occur without being appreciated.

Direct recordings of contractions of the colonic wall in experimental animals can be made by the use of chronically implanted strain gauges on the colon wall. Miniature strain gauges have been developed and have been used extensively in the study of contractions of the stomach and small intestine, but the colon has been neglected. Such a method has the advantages of objectivity, ease of quantitation, and, probably, minimal interference with normality of function.

Direct recordings *in vitro* of contractions of colonic muscle taken from experimental animals or from human beings have been made in recent years to a limited extent. The usual methods involve cutting strips of the muscular wall of the colon in either longitudinal or transverse directions, attaching them to a strain gauge and recording their contractions isometrically. Such methods cannot, of course, be used to depict the operation of the whole organ, but the behavior of such strips of muscle can contribute to the perception of how the colon works.

Electromyography, the recording of electrical signals generated by the colonic musculature, has been used in recent years. There have been very few studies made with chronically implanted serosal electrodes *in vivo*, but mucosal electrodes, acutely implanted in the rectal mucosa in humans, have been used to try to record the electromyogram in various diseases. Electromyography of the human colon is in its infancy, but electromyography of the animal colon has done much to provide a picture of colonic motility. Electromyography has advantages, such as ease of application and freedom from observational artifact. Its disadvantage is that the signals recorded are not yet fully interpretable in terms of wall movements and intraluminal flows.

GROSS PATTERNS OF CONTRACTION AND FLOW IN THE COLON

The gross patterns of flow and of contractions in the colon have been appreciated for a long time, for they were clearly set forth in two early papers on the subject.

Cannon (25) in 1902, used the then new methods of radiography to examine colonic motility in the cat. Using bismuth subnitrate as a contrast medium, he observed the movements of the fecal mass over long periods of time. He saw that different patterns of movement could be used to separate the colon into two distinct parts.

"The usual movement of the transverse and ascending colon is antiperistalsis," he observed. By this term, *antiperistalsis,* he meant ring contractions that move cephalad rather than caudad as they do in the small intestine. He saw that there were periods of 2 to 8 min in which cephalad-moving ring contractions would occur at a fundamental frequency of about 5.5 cycles/min. Between these periods, there would be periods of about 10 to 15 min of rest. These periods of retrograde peristalsis would drive the colonic contents into the cecum, but the contents would not pass retrograde through the ileocecal junction. Thus, the colonic content was churned and mixed within a closed compartment constituting the cecum and ascending colon. The entry of a new quantity of intestinal content from the ileum would cause a brief period of strong contractions in the cecum and colon so that some of the content was pushed caudad, but the cephalad-moving ring contractions would soon resume. "Thus, the contents of the colon, instead of being driven immediately toward the rectum by slow peristalsis, as is the general opinion, are first repeatedly pushed toward the cecum by an antiperistaltic action," said Can-

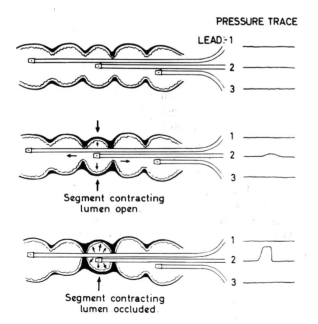

FIG. 2. Diagram showing mechanism of production of localized intracolonic pressure. From: ref. 136a, with permission.

non. He noted that, when they had reached a maximal intensity, these antiperistaltic waves start near the proximal end of the transverse colon and pass without interruption to the end of the cecum.

The other part of the colon that Cannon distinguished constitutes the distal transverse and descending colon. Here, "tonic constrictions appear which separate the contents into a series of globular masses. These rings . . . are in reality moving slowly away from the cecum, pushing the hardening contents before them," said Cannon.

The second of these pioneer papers is that of Elliott and Barclay-Smith (64). These authors studied a variety of animals—cat, rat, guinea pig, rabbit, dog, ferret, and hedgehog. In most cases, the animals were anesthetized, the spinal cord was destroyed, and the abdomen was opened. The colon was left *in situ* but floated in a warm bath of a physiological solution. Colonic movements were excited by putting a ". . . thick yellow gruel—prepared by mixing pea flour with water until the whole was of precisely the same consistency as that of the food in the ileum—through an incision made in the ileum a few centimeters above the ileo-colic sphincter." These authors observed three main types of movement. First, they saw that, in the proximal colon, antiperistalsis was the dominant activity. They described this most clearly in the cat. Here, starting from a point about 7 cm beyond the cecal apex, narrow constrictions slowly traveled toward the cecum at about 1 to 2 mm/sec. These would repel content that had entered the colon from the ileum and would temporarily prevent its caudad movement. These constrictions would follow one another at an interval of about 1 cm at a frequency of 5 to 6 cycles/ min. These waves constituted the main activity of the proximal colon, that is, the cecum and ascending colon. They were seen to be much more prominent in the rabbit (that has a big cecum) than in the dog (that has a small cecum). They were observed to have a pronounced churning or mixing effect on colonic content.

In the middle part of the colon, Elliott and Barclay-Smith noted that the predominant pattern of motion was coordinated peristalsis, tonic contraction rings moving caudad. They observed that this pattern could occur in any part of the colon, but that it was the sole pattern of movement in the middle part of the colon. They saw that these rings would drive the colonic contents toward the anus, and that the contents seemed to stimulate contractions by distention of the colon.

The third region of the colon noted by Elliott and Barclay-Smith was the part corresponding to the sigmoid colon and rectum in the human beings. Here, they observed that the main activity is a strong contraction, a constriction moving slowly caudad that empties the colon. This activity could be excited by stimulation of the pelvic nerves.

Thus, in these early studies, both Cannon and Elliott

and Barclay-Smith observed that greatly different patterns of contraction and flow can be distinguished in the three different parts of the colon. Given the early date and the mutually confirmatory nature of these papers, it is curious that they have not been given more importance in previous reviews of the subject. Furthermore, these observations are quite consistent with other observations made subsequently in humans. For example, simple observation by radiography of the position of fecal shadows in humans suggest that there is a prolonged residence of fecal matter in the right side of the colon. Those who do colonoscopy are well aware of the fact that the right side of the colon seems to retain its content with greater avidity than the left. A systematic study, moreover, has demonstrated that fecal shadows, seen by simple radiographic observation, accumulate in the right side of the abdomen, in the proximal colon, and are displaced from that region by laxatives (45).

Indeed, from studies of transit, the cecum and sigmoid colon can be seen clearly to be major points in delay of mouth-to-anus transit. This transit may require several days (95) and the principal delays occur in the cecum and the sigmoid colon.

During the prolonged residence of intestinal contents in the cecum of the human being, there is an extensive mixing of the contents, just as it was described in animals by Cannon and Elliott and Barclay-Smith. This has been shown clearly by human experiments in which three kinds of radiopaque markers are ingested by subjects at three separate meals, so that marker location can be subsequently monitored. Three different batches of radiopaque disks of three different sizes were ingested at 36, 34, and 12 hr before X-ray examination of the abdomen. Free mixing of the three sizes of disks was observed throughout the colon, with some of the latest ingested lying in advance of some of the earliest ingested (94). This mixing seems to occur mainly in the right colon. Thus, there seems to be general agreement among both laboratory studies in animals and clinical observations in man as to the prolonged residence and mixing of intestinal content in the proximal colon.

The authors of both the early papers suggested that the distal transverse colon and the descending colon tend to exhibit a contraction pattern in which the lumen is divided into fairly uniform segments by contraction rings that tend to move slowly caudad. This pattern, too, is supported by clinical observations in humans. In an early radiographic study, it was noted that such contractions may propel the feces in both directions but over very short distances (12). In another more modern study, Ritchie (144) used time-lapse photography with cineradiography to study movements of segmental contractions in the human colon. He observed that such segmental contractions form, disappear, and re-form with an inconstant relationship to fixed points on the colon wall. These segmental contractions were seen to be quite capable of pushing contents in either antegrade or retrograde directions.

Cannon and Elliott and Barclay-Smith did not mention another pattern of movement, which has, however, subsequently attracted a considerable degree of attention. This has come to be called mass movement. It may even have been described before the time of Hertz (98), but the publication by Holzknecht is often taken as the classic report (105). Holzknecht was a radiologist who in the course of 1,000 radiographic examinations of the colon, observed mass movement only twice. Such a movement was described by Holzknecht as a sudden shift of a column of feces that filled about one-third of the length of the colon to the next empty segment of similar length. This shift was preceded by the disappearance of segmental contractions in the region both in the donating segment and in the receiving segment, but the receiving segment quickly returned to a pattern of segmental contractions after the shift was accomplished. Such a pattern of movement was later reported by others (99). The authors of the latter report saw mass movements rather more frequently than Holzknecht had suggested and believed that such movements tend to be more common during the hours in which meals are taken (99). Modern investigators have likewise seen sudden massive shifts of colonic content. Holdstock et al. (104) used various types of markers, radiopaque shapes, radiotelemeter capsules, capsules containing ^{51}Cr and free ^{51}Cr to observe fecal movement. With all methods they observed that "colonic contents progress distally by a series of infrequent large movements, known as mass movements or mass peristalsis." Ritchie (145) also saw such shifts in a study combining cinefluorography and intraluminal manometry. The colonic contractions that induce these mass movements are very likely the same contractions that Mann and Hardcastle (126) called colonic peristalsis in their manometric study of patients with colostomy. Methods to observe gross movements of the human colon are, of course, much more restrictive than are those that can be used in animals.

Intraluminal Pressure Recording as an Indicator of Rhythmic Contractions

Because of the advantages listed earlier, the recording of intraluminal pressures was used extensively for a time to delineate colonic movements. The work was well reviewed previously (41) and little more has been done since. These manometric methods have made use of a variety of sensing devices—large balloons, small balloons, open-tip perfused catheters, and radiotelemetering capsules. A great deal of the writing on this subject has been devoted to a discussion of the relative merits of these methods and to details of methodology. There has been less concern about interpretation of records.

The interpretation of manometric tracings requires some understanding of the source of the signal and the validity of the method of detecting it. Despite residual uncertainties, however, such tracings have indeed been subjected to interpretation. These interpretations have been of two kinds: interpretations of patterns of contractions and interpretations of quantity (both magnitude and number) of contractions.

Pattern interpretation began with an attempt to classify pressure peaks detected manometrically (169). Manometric tracings were made from the dog colon in vivo using balloons 3 cm in length. Three wave forms were distinguished, called types 1, 2, and 3. The classification has been applied to the human colon (1,38,54, 141,163) and is still alluded to. Yet, others have found this classification of waves inadequate in view of the great irregularity of the patterns seen, both in tracings obtained by large balloons and in those obtained from other sensing devices (29,39,55). The question of the validity of the classification may be considered to be moot, however, for no agreement was ever reached as to what pressure peaks signify beyond the preception that most of them reflect contractions of the muscular walls.

Because of this, more recent students interpret manometric tracings in quantitative terms only, either by counting the number of peaks per time or by some method of integration of amplitude and time. The use of such methods to arrive at an estimate of the "duration of activity" of the colon has yielded a result that might have surprised Holzknecht (105), who thought that the colon was largely motionless except for the rare mass movements he saw. The "duration of activity," that is, the proportion of time during which pressure peaks are being generated by the colon, is quite high. Measurements listed by Connell (41) range from 13% to 59% of time.

Because of its shortcomings, the manometric method alone is unlikely to be useful in completely depicting colonic motility. When combined with cineradiography, however, manometry might be useful in helping to describe colonic movement. A thorough study by these combined techniques was made by Ritchie et al. (146). They examined the sigmoid colon of normal persons using several kinds of pressure-sensing devices, including small balloons and open-tip tubes, while observing movements of the wall of the sigmoid colon by cineradiography. The wall movements that can produce a rise in intraluminal pressure can be exceedingly complex, they found, so that pressure tracings alone cannot be interpreted in terms of either contractions or flow. They found in observations of colonic diameter by cineradiography that great changes could occur with little change in pressure. They proposed a complex classification of colonic contractions. This classification does not, however, appear to have found general use. They observed contractions as being localized or progressive.

The localized ones often recurred quite regularly with a 5-sec period or a 30-sec period. Progressive contractions were also seen, but much less commonly. These traveled from the descending to the sigmoid colon at 2.5 cm/sec in runs of six or more at intervals of 20 sec to 2 min. Other contractions seemed to be provoked by distention of the bowel by contents displaced by upstream contractions. Deller and Wangel (55) also combined intraluminal manometry with cineradiography and reported a considerable discordance. Gross movements of the colonic wall and colonic content could occur, they noted, without recorded pressure changes. Also, they were troubled by a temporal discordance between pressure changes and wall movements. In another recent study combining intraluminal manometry and cineradiography, only two-thirds of pressure waves were associated with some form of movement of the bowel, but when movements were seen, they nearly always produced a pressure peak (92). In light of these papers, it seems doubtful that manometry in the colon can be considered fully reliable either as a major research technique to investigate the physiology of colonic motility or as a diagnostic technique for clinical studies. And, indeed, there are few studies in recent years that make use of manometric methods.

Tonic Contractions

The discussion above has dealt only with periodic or rhythmic contractions. Tone, a contraction maintained at a more-or-less constant level over a long period of time, is a property that has long been attributed to smooth muscle. Attempts have been made to measure tone in the colon *in vivo* by manometric methods. White et al. (178) obtained a plot of pressure against volume during the slow infusion of water to fill the colon. This "colonmetrogram" yielded a plot of values that was different from normal in patients with various neurologic lesions. The limitations of the method are obvious: it is difficult to know how much of the colon is being examined and it is impossible to prevent retrograde flow through the ileocecal junction; even if both these objections did not exist, it would measure that property for all of the colon and one can be reasonably sure that the colon is not a single physiological entity, but probably at least three units. Lipkin et al. (122) overcame these objections by using a latex balloon of such size that, at 400 cm of water pressure, it held 900 ml at the dimensions of 9.7 cm in diameter and 14 cm in length. The collapsed balloon was put into the sigmoid colon and inflated under constant pressure. The elastic distortion of the balloon was minimized and the changes in volume, within the range used in the experiment, reflected mainly the change in volume of the viscus. The method was found to yield reproducible results, and consistent effects of drugs could be recorded. The technique, however, seems not to have found further application.

Such methods seem to measure some property of the bowel wall commonly called tone. This is an ancient and inexact term whose definition has been argued for a long time. Youmans defined tone in terms of the relationship between lumen volume and pressure (185). This seems to be what the aforementioned workers have been examining, but there is no evidence as to what exact property or which element of the colon wall is responsible.

MYOGENIC FACTORS IN COLON CONTRACTIONS

This section will deal with those factors involved in control of contractions of the colon that seem to reside in the smooth muscle itself. Colonic smooth muscle, like other gastrointestinal smooth muscle, generates electrical signals that are related to contractions of the muscle. Thus, the myogenic factors involved in colonic motility include the following: the electrical activities of smooth muscle cells, the communications between cells, the communications between muscle bundles and between muscle layers, the metabolism and transduction of energy in smooth muscle, and the way in which the myoelectrical events are superimposed on the energy metabolism of muscle to produce colonic contractions. Not all of these factors can be discussed for the colon, because of the lack of enough information.

The muscle of the colon, like those of the stomach and small intestine, generates electrical signals that resemble those produced by cardiac muscle. These signals constitute the elements of the electromyogram of the colon. The signals in the colon differ in function in one major respect from those of cardiac muscle. In the heart, the cardiac action potential has two functions, the initiation of contraction in the muscle cells through which it passes, and the integration of contraction, achieved by virtue of the fact that the cardiac action potential appears to spread from one part of the heart to another in a fixed order. In the gastrointestinal viscera in general, these two functions can be assigned to two separate elements of the signal that is recorded on the electromyogram (Fig. 3). Integration of contraction is achieved by a slow electrical transient called the electrical slow wave. Initiation of contraction is accomplished by a burst of much more rapid electrical transients, the spike burst. When records are made from a single point in the gut, the electrical slow waves recur continuously at a constant frequency. The muscle at the electrode site contracts only in relationship to these slow waves, but not to all of them. Contraction only occurs with those slow waves that carry a spike burst. The spike burst always occurs at a fixed position in relation to a slow wave. Thus, the slow wave is a mechanism to re-

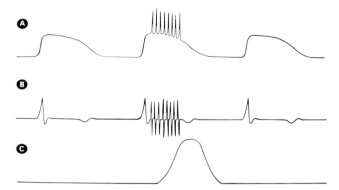

FIG. 3. Diagram of the relationship between electrical slow waves, the spike burst, and contraction. **A:** A sketch of a record of transmembrane potential as recorded in a gastrointestinal smooth muscle cell. **B:** Same signal as it would be recorded by an extracellular electrode. **C:** The tension in the muscle. Three slow-wave cycles are shown. A spike burst and a contraction occur only with the second cycle. From ref. 30a, with permission.

strict a contraction of the muscular wall to a fixed place and time.

When the electromyogram is recorded from several points along the bowel, slow waves can be seen to spread away from a source, as though toward a sink. Since contraction is so closely linked to a slow wave, the pattern of spread of the slow waves determines the pattern of spread of contractions. That is, slow waves coordinate contractions. Thus, they are also called pacesetter potentials, or the electrical control activity.

In the small intestine, the relationship between rhythmic contractions and the electrical slow waves has been recognized for decades. The rhythmicity of contractions in the colon was also recognized long ago. Despite this, the possibility that colonic muscle exhibits electrical slow waves that resemble those of the small intestine and stomach seems not to have been intensely examined until after 1960. Gillespie described electrical potential variations in smooth muscle from the rabbit colon (86, 87). His preparation was a 4-cm length of the terminal colon with the mucosa intact. Records were made by single-cell recording from the outer longitudinal muscle layer. He described three kinds of signals: slow waves, spike bursts grouped on the slow waves, and prepotentials with each spike (86, 87). The spike bursts and contractions were phase-locked to slow waves. The slow waves were of low amplitude and disappeared when the tissue was stretched, and the spiking became continuous.

Recognition of the existence of a system of electrical slow waves in the colon that resemble those of the small intestine has mainly followed a study of 1969 in the cat (33). In this study, strips of the muscularis propria containing both muscle layers were cut from the wall of various parts of the cat colon and arranged for simultaneous recording of contractions by an isometric strain gauge and of the electromyogram by a small surface

electrode. The electromyogram of the inner circular muscle layer was found to generate slow electrical transients very much like those found in recordings from the stomach and small intestine from the longitudinal muscle layer. Similar slow waves had been seen in earlier studies from France (48).

The origin of these slow waves in the inner circular muscle layer was inferred from the fact that they could be better recorded from the circular muscle layer (exposed by removal of the mucosa) than from the serosal surface. Also, they were readily recorded by intracellular recording from the circular muscle layer but not from the outer longitudinal layer of muscle (33). Caprilli and Onori (26) provided even stronger evidence by showing that electrical slow waves were detected in isolated strips of muscle of the circular layer but not from isolated strips of the longitudinal muscle layer. They used a variety of other simple experimental techniques like those that had been used previously in the cat small intestine (117), and the results of these studies all supported the conclusion that the electrical slow waves of the colon are generated in the inner circular muscle layer. These techniques included studies in which, in strips of muscle with both layers attached, the circular layer was removed from half of each strip. Electrodes were then applied to the exposed longitudinal muscle layer at various distances from the cut edge of the circular layer. It was found that slow-wave amplitude declined exponentially with distance from the edge of the circular muscle. Also, strips containing both muscle layers were mounted vertically "on edge," and electrodes were applied at corresponding points on both surfaces—on the serosal surface and on the inner surface of the circular muscle that had been exposed by removal of the mucosa. Electrical slow waves were recorded from both surfaces. The amplitude of the slow waves was much greater in the records from the side of the circular muscle than it was in records from the serosal surface. Also, the slow waves from the circular muscle slightly preceded those in the same cycle recorded from the corresponding point on the longitudinal muscle surface (Fig. 4).

Much effort was devoted to an examination of the patterns of propagation of the slow waves of the cat colon. This was done early because of the evidence from studies of the small intestine that the patterns of spread of slow waves dictate the patterns of spread of contractions. Slow waves were recorded simultaneously from a battery of electrodes spaced at intervals over the inner surface of the circular muscle layer. The use of various configurations of distribution of such extracellular electrodes revealed that slow waves spread in both the x-axis and the y-axis of the plane of the circular muscle layer. This was seen even in the earliest studies that made use of small pieces of the colon wall (33). It was made clearer in subsequent studies that employed large segments, one-third, one-half, or more of the whole co-

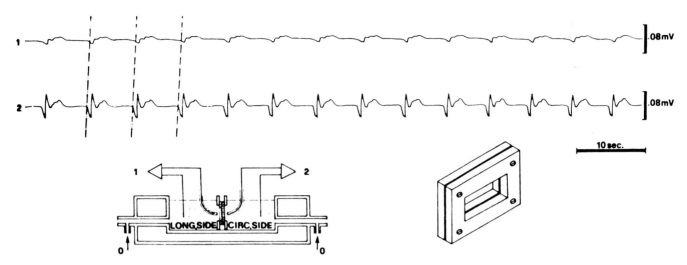

FIG. 4. Electromyogram recorded simultaneously from longitudinal (1) and circular (2) muscle sides of a vertically mounted strip of the muscle wall of the cat colon. **Bottom left:** Diagram of the recording bath. **Bottom right:** Drawing of the clamp in which the segment of the muscular wall is mounted. Slow waves recorded from the circular muscle surface occur earlier and are bigger than those recorded from the longitudinal side. (From ref. 26, with permission.)

lon (35,36). Velocity in the direction of the long axis of the circular muscle cells, along the circumference of the colon, was fast (1.6 cm/sec), whereas velocity across the circular muscle cells, in the long axis of the colon, was slower (1-5 mm/sec). When a 3-cm segment of the colon was studied, the slow waves of that whole segment were seen to be driven from a single pacemaker about two-thirds of the time. The rest of the time, 2, 3, 4, or even more pacemakers could be seen to be operating simultaneously. When only a single pacemaker was operating, it was caudad to the study segment, so that the slow waves tended to be propagated cephalad, toward the cecum. A great deal of subsequent experience suggests that the emergence of multiple pacemakers is a pathological process. Dominance of the proximal colon by a single pacemaker is the normal state. The single pacemaker in the proximal colon is usually situated somewhere near the middle of the length of the colon. The normal pattern is for slow waves to spread from this pacemaker throughout the proximal colon to, but not into, the cecum. The cecum seems not to be invaded by slow waves, at least not in the opossum (9).

The studies discussed above were done only in the ascending colon of the cat. Subsequently, it was seen that electrical slow waves occur throughout the whole of the colon in the cat (180,181). It was concluded that the whole colon should be studied in detail, much as the ascending colon had been, and so a suitable preparation was devised (32). The whole abdominal colon (excluding only the rectum) of the cat was everted over a tube and a strip of the mucosa was removed. Sixteen electrodes were aligned at uniform intervals along the exposed circular muscle and slow waves recorded from each. On the average, slow-wave frequency was found to rise from 4.5 cycles/min in the most proximal 10% of the colon to 6.0 cycles/min in the most distal 10%, with

intermediate values at intermediate points. The colon was then cut between electrodes so that it was divided into rings and the 16 electrodes were reapplied at their former positions. This procedure separated the segments from influences of other parts of the colon, so that the intrinsic frequencies of the electrical slow wave could be determined. The slow-wave frequency of the most proximal 10% of the colon fell with the cutting to 44% of its value in the intact colon *in vitro,* and it declined to 57% and 73% in the next two 10-percentile segments. Frequency was not changed by cutting in the region of the colon that included the fifth to the ninth percentile segments. It rose to 121% of control in the tenth percentile segment (Fig. 5).

Thus, a gradient of intrinsic frequencies for the electrical slow wave was found that is consistent with or accounts for the patterns of spread of slow waves found previously. This gradient is consistent with the distal-to-proximal spread of slow waves in the proximal colon from a pacemaking region in the midcolon. It also shows that in the rest of the colon, slow-wave spread should occur only over very short distances and in either direction. In this study, as in all the others, it was observed that there is considerable lability in the frequency of the electrical slow waves along the colon. This lability of intrinsic frequencies allows slow waves occasionally to pass over rather long distances, for if one pacemaker fires first, it may capture all the others over some distance. It is not known to what extent all these things are true *in vivo.*

In these studies on the electromyogram of the cat colon (33), it was observed that a short burst of rapid electrical transients occurred on some electrical slow waves, and that such a spike burst correlated with a contraction of the circular muscle layer. Thus, it appeared that the slow waves pace contractions in the colon just as they

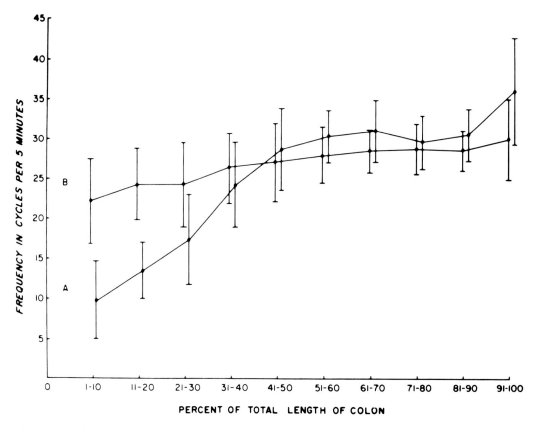

FIG. 5. Average frequencies of electrical slow waves along the colon before (**B**) and after (**A**) division into rings. The ordinate shows frequency in cycles/5 min. The abscissa shows normalized length of the 14 colons, with 0% at the ileocecal junction and 100% at the anal verge. (*Brackets*) 1 SD above and below the mean. (From ref. 32, with permission.)

do in the small intestine. In the study of the whole colon (32), however, another kind of spike burst was seen for the first time. This spike burst was much more prolonged, spanning several slow-wave cycles and seeming to be independent of slow waves (Fig. 6). In the study that made use of 16 electrodes spaced all along the colon, this prolonged spike burst was seen to migrate along the colon, usually migrating caudad but sometimes sweeping cephalad as well. It was periodic, recurring about every 80 sec, and it lasted, at a single point along the colon, about 30 sec, though these values are extremely variable. It migrated at a velocity of about 5 mm/sec. The prolonged spike burst was often weak or absent in the ascending colon, but it was seen to be best developed distal to the hepatic flexure. Within each cycle, each spike in the migrating spike burst seemed to arise from a small sinusoidal signal; at times, only these sinusoidal signals occurred, the superimposed spikes being absent. These migrating spike bursts were found to be associated with powerful and prolonged contractions of the circular muscle layer. It was proposed that the migrating spike burst is the electromyographic appearance of the contraction that accomplishes mass movement, but that idea has not been further investigated.

Some Studies in the Human Colon

The point has been made previously that the profound differences in anatomy of the colon among species warn of differences in function. Virtually all the work referred to on the myogenic factors in colonic motility has been done in the cat, although a few studies have also been reported in other species, the opossum (9), rabbit (111,112), and mouse (183,184).

Many papers have described attempts to record the colonic electromyogram in humans. Most such attempts have been made to record from the most easily reached parts of the bowel—the anal canal, rectum, sigmoid or descending colon. A monopolar electrode technique is often used, but bipolar electrodes have been used as well, the electrodes being suction electrodes or clip electrodes attached to the colonic mucosa. There are problems in these studies that dictate caution in the interpretation of results. First, since no primate colon (including the human colon) has been investigated *in vitro* to the extent that the cat colon has, one does not know exactly what to expect to find in studies *in vivo*. Second, it is assumed that the mucosal electrode is detecting mainly the electrical signals generated by the circular muscle layer, but it is quite possible that these rec-

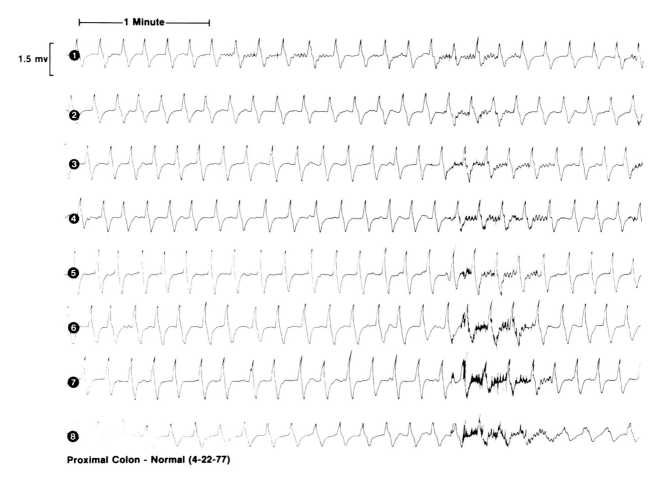

Proximal Colon - Normal (4-22-77)

FIG. 6. Slow waves and one migrating spike burst from cat colon. Numbers at the left indicate electrode position. 1 being at the ileocecal junction and 8 at about the middle of the colon. The regular succession of slow waves is interrupted by a migrating spike burst.

ords also contain signals generated by the mucosal muscle and the longitudinal layer of the muscularis propria; also, there may be contributions from blood flow, movement artifacts, skin potentials, and transmucosal potentials. Third, there is every possibility that the distal colon is different functionally from the more proximal areas and so one cannot blindly project "abnormalities" that are found in the rectum to the whole of the organ; it is quite possible, indeed, that the smooth muscle of the various parts of just the distal colon (the sigmoid colon, rectum, and anal canal) may differ qualitatively from one area to another. Failure to recognize these problems is undoubtedly responsible for much of the disagreement and confusion that still attaches to studies of colonic electromyography in humans.

In many investigations of humans, but not in all, it has been seen that slow-wave activity is not constant, but intermittent. Intermittency is not mentioned in studies of the electromyogram of the anal canal (172,176), but it seems to be much more prominent in recordings from the rectum (48,158). This intermittency of recording of slow waves may be real, but it is equally likely that it is artifactual, arising from an intermittency in electrode contact with the signal source rather than an intermittency in the generation of the signal. In the studies of the anal canal, the electrode is likely to be held very tightly against the sphincter by the action of that sphincter, whereas such close contact is harder to achieve or maintain in the more distensible rectosigmoid or rectum. That would account for the difference in the constancy of the recording of the signals between the rectum and the anal canal. Also, the inconsistency of the reported values for time that slow-wave activity is present supports the idea that its failure to appear on records may be artifactual rather than a failure of generation of slow waves. Thus, Couturier and his colleagues (48) recorded slow waves for only 5% to 20% of the time from the rectosigmoid, and Snape's group (158) reported it to be recorded for 46% of the time from the rectum and 28.5% of the time from the rectosigmoid. Others (168) found slow waves 67% of the time in the lower rectum and 25% of the time in the rectosigmoid. A more recent study (154) lends further support to the idea that inconstancy of detection of slow waves by mucosal electrodes is artifactual. In this study, records were made from human subjects by three methods: from a mucosal suction electrode, from serosal electrodes implanted under the serosal coat of the colon at laparotomy, and from cutaneous electrodes. In the ascending and transverse colon, electrical activity was recorded less than 50% of the time from mucosal electrodes, whereas it was recorded 60% to 85% of the time from the implanted electrodes. This difference would be consistent with the idea that a mucosal electrode loses contact with the signal source more readily than does an implanted electrode. In view of the fact that, in colon muscle *in vitro,* the slow-wave activity is always present both in the cat (9,26,32,33,35,36,180,181) and in the dog (154), and in view of the inconsistencies cited above from studies *in vivo* in man, it seems reasonable to propose that the inconstancy of the slow waves seen in mucosal recordings *in vivo* from man is due to intermittent changes in the electrical contact between the electrode and the slow-wave source, the circular muscle layer. It is possible, also, that the recording of slow waves could be lost temporarily because of asynchrony of slow waves at closely adjacent points.

A much greater variation in slow-wave frequency is noted in colonic slow waves recorded *in situ* in humans than in those recorded *in vitro* in colonic muscle from experimental animals. Normal frequencies in the cat colon *in situ* have been consistently found to lie in the range of 5 to 6 cycles/min (9,26,32,33,35,36,180,181) and the frequency is similar in the muscle of the dog colon *in situ* (154). It has often been noted, in studies *in vitro* in the cat, that the frequency is somewhat labile, but this lability has generally been attributed to tissue damage. Similar transient changes of frequency appear in records from colonic muscle of the dog studied *in vitro.* These frequency changes seen *in vitro* are usually brief and, in the cat at least, they are uncommon. In contrast, the records from the human colon *in situ* seem to display a great variety of frequencies. These records from humans are, without exception, so badly distorted that the visual recognition of the existence of a regular wave form is usually difficult except for short periods. Hence, recent papers attempting frequency analysis have relied on computers to read tape-recorded signals and to analyze the records by such methods as the fast Fourier transform. Wankling et al. (176) reported several frequencies: "ultraslow" waves were found with frequencies of 1 to 2/min; other slow waves had a frequency of 10 to 20/min (average 16.9 ± 0.9) in records from the anal canal by mucosal electrode. Ustach et al. (172) in records from the same region by a similar electrode, found slow waves of 17 cycles/min with a range from about 6 to about 26 cycles/min. They did not see the "ultraslow" waves. In studies from more proximal levels of the colon, similar variations in frequency are reported. Couturier et al. (48) reported frequencies of 8.4 to 10.6 cycles/min in 12 normal subjects in records from the rectosigmoid with mucosal electrodes. Snape et al. (158) reported two frequencies: in records from the rectum, slow waves were detected at 6.5 and 3.4 cycles/min; at the rectosigmoid they were found at 7.3

and 2.9 cycles/min. Taylor et al. (168) also saw two frequencies in the rectum, 3 to 4 cycles/min and 6 to 9 cycles/min. In more recent studies, the presence of two slow-wave frequencies has been repeatedly reaffirmed in reports of records from mucosal electrodes in humans by Snape et al. (159–161), and this idea has been supported by a computer analysis of real-time records (52), though the latter study suggests two very broad ranges of frequencies rather than two discrete frequencies.

The interpretation of such variation in frequency is difficult. Several recent publications suggest that a change in the frequency correlates with the existence of the "functional bowel syndrome" (61,158,160,166). There is agreement that, as compared to records from normal people, records made by a bipolar electrode from the rectosigmoid of patients with this diagnosis show an increase in the fraction of time in which slow waves occur at about 3 cycles/min, as opposed to a frequency about twice as great. Two facts complicate the interpretation of such observations. First, the functional bowel syndrome, or "irritable bowel syndrome," is so poorly defined an entity that patients who carry this diagnosis are very unlikely to constitute a homogeneous group. And second, the limitations of methodology described above make it difficult to know what such changes mean in terms of the basic processes that generate slow waves in the circular muscle layer of the colon. Thus, these correlations remain observations that are uninterpretable both as to their source and to their significance. A recent paper (164) indicates that differences among the computational methods used for data analysis to discover frequency could account for the differing incidences of slow-wave frequencies that are reported in studies of the human colon *in situ.*

Relationship Between Slow Waves, Contractions, and Flows

A part of the problem of interpretation of records of the electromyogram from the colon *in situ* is uncertainty about the degree to which slow waves pace contractions of the circular muscle layer. This uncertainty was emphasized by Daniel (50), who pointed out that the relationships between spikes, slow waves, and contractions in the colon remain to be established as clearly as they have been in the stomach and small intestine. A general correlation between slow waves, spike bursts, and contractions was observed in the earliest report on the study of muscle of the cat colon (33) and the rabbit colon (86,87), and it was suggested then that the relationship is essentially the same as that in the stomach and small bowel. Subsequent studies, including one in the dog (154), have not made use of simultaneous recording of electrical and mechanical activity. In the sole study of humans in which manometry was done at the same time as recording of the myoelectrical activity (161), no attempt was made to establish this point.

Thus, Daniel's statement of 1975 (50) remains true. The need is for simultaneous records from implanted electrodes using strain gauges from the colon in acutely anesthetized and chronically prepared animals. Pending such studies, the degree to which slow waves actually do control contractions in the colon must remain conjectural.

A relationship between slow waves, contractions, and flows is implied in the observations of slow waves made in animals with diarrhea. By chance, colons were prepared for recording of the electromyogram that were taken from animals affected by an epidemic of diarrhea (37). This was presumably of viral etiology, though no cause was sought. It was found that, in such colons, a single pacemaker did not dominate the proximal few centimeters of colon, the normal situation (35,36). Instead, from electrodes spaced only a few millimeters apart, slow waves were detected that were generated essentially independently. This could be looked upon either as the emergence of a great many pacemakers firing independently, or as the uncoupling of the muscle from the single pacemaker that usually dominates it. Healthy animals were then given a laxative, castor oil, in a dose sufficient to induce a diarrheal state, and their colons were removed for recording of the electromyogram of the circular muscle layer in the ascending colon. Other healthy cats were given equal volumes of corn oil. They did not develop diarrhea, but their colons were removed at the same time after treatment as in the cats that had received castor oil. In the cats treated with castor oil, the same anomaly was found, the existence in the muscle of the ascending colon of multiple slow-wave generators operating simultaneously, whereas a single pacemaker tended to dominate the colon in the corn oil-treated animals. In subsequent studies, it was seen that a variety of laxative agents can induce such changes in the colonic electromyogram in vitro. These include sodium ricinoleate, the salt of the laxative principal of castor oil (34), quinine and quinidine (13), and capsaicin (10). The electromyogram in tissues so treated comes to resemble the electrocardiogram in fibrillation. Whether or not the pattern of contraction of the circular muscle is actually altered by such agents remains to be seen.

NEUROGENIC FACTORS IN COLONIC CONTRACTIONS

That motor nerves influence colonic contractions seems to be widely accepted. The nature of the nerves and the way in which they act remain matters of some ignorance and controversy.

Morphologic Studies

Classification of the motor nerves of the colon rests almost entirely upon pharmacological evidence, al-though there have been limited morphological studies in the human and guinea pig. There appear to be four kinds of motor nerves demonstrable in colonic muscle, excitatory nerves that are cholinergic and noncholinergic, and inhibitory nerves that are adrenergic and nonadrenergic (76,78,79).

Adrenergic nerves have been described morphologically in the colon by several investigators (14,18,27, 108). All these studies agree in the conclusion that most of the adrenergic innervation is directed to the ganglion cells rather than to the layers of smooth muscle. The adrenergic nerves, as revealed by catecholamine fluorescence, terminate principally in a synaptic relationship with ganglion cells of the myenteric plexus. Very few fibers seem to enter the muscle layers proper. None of the ganglion cells, at least in most species, exhibit catecholamine fluorescence, but there do appear to be such adrenergic ganglion cells in the distal colon of the guinea pig (78). Thus, important species variations exist. The cholinergic innervation of the colon resides mainly in the ganglion cells of the myenteric plexus (108). Not all these cells exhibit the same degree of activity in the stain for cholinesterase, but the significance of this variability is unknown (82).

The noncholinergic and nonadrenergic nerves in the colon cannot be specifically identified morphologically, and so their existence is inferred from physiological or pharmacological evidence (77).

Peristaltic Reflex in the Colon

The existence of the peristaltic reflex in the colon was claimed by Bayliss and Starling (15) as a result of studies of the colon of the dog. These animals had received castor oil, had received "morphia and A. C. E. mixture," and had the colon separated from the central nervous system either by destruction of the spinal cord below the 10th dorsal vertebra with section of the splanchnic nerves or by extirpation of the inferior mesenteric ganglia with section of the pelvic nerves. In such preparations, a pinch of the colon produced inhibition of the whole colon below the site of the pinch. Contractions above the pinch were difficult to demonstrate. Considerable differences were found in the rabbit, but the authors felt justified in the conclusion that the peristaltic reflex, ascending excitation and descending inhibition in response to a pinch, characterizes the colon in both species. Thirty-four years later, Raiford and Mulinos (142), on the basis of studies of a chronically exteriorized colon in unanesthetized dogs, saw no inhibitory component and restated "the law of the intestine" in the colon to exclude an inhibitory response. They saw only contractions as a consequence of mucosal stroking; contraction of the circular layer occurred above the level of the stimulus and contraction of the longitudinal layer occurred below it. These responses were blocked by application of cocaine to the mucosa.

Twenty-five years later, Hukuhara and Miyaka (109) confirmed the work of Bayliss and Starling in further studies in anesthetized dogs. In addition to this disagreement even as to the description of the reflexes, it is unknown to what degree such reflexes are related to the governance of normal colonic motility. Thus, it is not clear that one can reasonably invoke the reflex in explaining colonic motility.

Tonic Neurogenic Inhibition

The influence of nerves on colonic motility could also be expressed as a tonic effect, a continuously sustained and broadly applied influence as opposed to a localized one brought about only as a reflex response to a stimulus. A high degree of such tonic activity is suggested by experiments in the cat colon in which the colonic muscle is exposed *in vitro* to the neurotoxin, tetrodotoxin, or to a local anesthetic, lidocaine (31). These agents produce excitation of the circular muscle layer; this appears to come about through prolongation of the electromyographic phenomenon called the migrating spike burst. This suggests that there is tonic neurogenic inhibition of the colonic musculature; it also supports the idea that the migrating spike burst is a consequence of periodic removal of this tonic neurogenic inhibition. That is, the migrating spike burst is a consequence of periodic disinhibition. There may be species variation in this matter, however, for tetrodotoxin was not seen to cause excitation of the rabbit colon in a Trendelenburg preparation (125).

Electrical Field Stimulation

Only a few studies have been made of human colonic muscle *in vitro* that shed some light on the nature of the motor nerves to colonic muscle. Crema et al. (49), in electrical field stimulation of both longitudinal and circular strips from human colon, saw that both contractions and relaxations occur. Atropine always converted contractions into relaxations, but it did not affect the relaxations themselves. The stimuli were 1 msec pulses at 1 to 10 Hz. The relaxations were unaffected by adrenergic receptor antagonists and by methysergide, but they were tetrodotoxin-sensitive. The inhibitory response has also been seen in guinea-pig colon where it is not inhibited by reserpine pretreatment, alpha-methyltyrosine, perivascular denervation, or bretylium (21). All the preceding findings indicate that both cholinergic excitatory and nonadrenergic inhibitory nerves are present in both layers of the colon wall.

In human colonic muscle *in vitro*, the release of acetylcholine induced by electrical field stimulation is inhibited by norepinephrine, an observation that is consistent with the view that catecholamines released from adrenergic nerves may act by modulating cholinergic ganglion cell activity. The adrenergic innervation of the colon appears to be mainly inhibitory, for ganglionic stimulants such as nicotine and dimethylphenylpiperazine induce relaxation, an effect that is sensitive both to neurotoxins and to adrenergic antagonists (24,70). The existence of noncholinergic excitatory fibers is suggested by the fact that some contractions induced in human colonic muscle *in vitro* by electrical field stimulation persist in the presence of anticholinergic agents but are tetrodotoxin-sensitive.

The interrelations of these different kinds of motor innervation and their place in the integration of motor activity of the whole colon remains to be worked out. It is noteworthy, also, that very few studies have been done with the technique of electrical field stimulation of colonic muscle; such possible complicating factors as species variation, variability between different parts of the colon, and differences between the two layers of the muscle appear not to have been much explored.

Responses to Autonomic Drugs

The use of agents that act at the selective receptors for autonomic neuroeffectors can, of course, also be helpful in understanding a possible role for nerves in the governing of contractions. In general, cholinergic agents cause colonic muscle to contract *in vitro*, but careful comparisons of sensitivity to such agents from one part of the colon to another have not been made. Norepinephrine, *in vitro*, is inhibitory to colonic muscle through both alpha and beta receptor mechanisms. There is at least one suggestion of an excitatory adrenergic alpha-receptor mechanism (80). Serotonin, or 5-hydroxytryptamine, is usually inhibitory *in vitro* in colonic muscle (20), but excitation may occur as well. Histamine is said also to cause either response (20). In such experiments, excitation refers to the generation of contractions or to an increase in force or frequency of spontaneous contractions, and inhibition means the opposite. It is obvious that autonomic agents could also influence motility through an influence on slow waves, and in this way such agents could affect the duration of contractions, the integration of movements along the colon, or the direction of propagation of contractions. These relatively more subtle actions of the neuroeffectors seem not to have been sought. Also, there is a paucity of data about effects of such naturally occurring neuroeffector substances on colonic motility *in vivo*. An exception is serotonin, concerning which the results of studies *in vivo* generally agree with those *in vitro* (131).

Extrinsic Nervous Control of Colonic Motility

The role of the extrinsic nerves in governing motility seems not to have been very much studied until rather recently. This neglect is probably due to the difficulty in making suitable experimental preparations. The various animal preparations used in the past have been unphysiological, have not lent themselves to studies of long duration, or have used methods to detect contractions that yielded records that are difficult or impossible to interpret in terms of the nature, magnitude, and distribution of wall movements and flows of luminal content. At least some of these methodological problems can be overcome with the use of extraluminal force strain-gauge transducers that are sewn to the serosal surface of the colon. Rostad (147–151) has used such devices on the colon of the cat to examine colonic motility as it is affected by the extrinsic innervation. The devices were always sutured transversely so as to detect mainly circumferential contractions of the colon, with one transducer at the cecum, one in the midcolon, and one on the sigmoid colon. The colon was observed to be seldom quiet except during deep anesthesia. Contractions of two kinds occurred: slow contractions lasting 0.5 to 2.0 min and rhythmic contractions of 4 to 7 cycles/min. Excitatory vagal effects and inhibitory splanchnic effects were shown throughout the colon, although the major effect was in the proximal part. The lumbar sympathetic nerves with both inhibitory and excitatory fibers were found to go to all parts of the colon. Stimulation of the hypothalamus could be either excitatory or inhibitory depending on the part stimulated. In the mesencephalon, also, both excitation of colonic motility (mainly in the proximal colon) and inhibition resulted from stimulation of various regions. Nerve section combined with brain stimulation revealed the peripheral pathways concerned in some of these effects. Excitatory effects of stimulation of the hypothalamic areas pass through both the lumbar sympathetic nerves and the parasympathetic pelvic nerves. Excitation from mesencephalic stimulation is mediated by the lumbar colonic nerves. Guanethidine blocked responses mediated through lumbar nerves, and atropine blocked those of the pelvic nerves. Some of the excitation appears to make use of excitatory alpha-receptors. In the telencephalon, both vagally mediated excitatory responses and inhibition mediated by lumbar nerves was found. These results confirm and extend previous studies on the subject of central control of colonic motility, a literature that is cited by Rostad. It is thus well established that such effects exist. It is not clear, however, that such central control mechanisms are essential in the normal control of colonic motility. It may be that such extrinsic controls are concerned in the integrated colonic activities that are described later in this chapter.

Julé (112) made a study of electromyographic responses of both proximal and distal colon of the rabbit to vagal and splanchnic nerve stimulation. He saw evidence both for parasympathetic nonadrenergic inhibitory nerves and for a sympathetic adrenergic inhibitory innervation in both parts of the colon. Evidence for both kinds of inhibitory nerves has been found in a study of the gerbil colon also (89).

EFFECTS OF DRUGS ON COLONIC CONTRACTIONS

Many drugs are thought to influence colonic motility. For the most part, the effects of these agents, if they have been investigated at all, are difficult to relate directly to colonic motor physiology as a whole.

Anticholinergics. The effect of atropine and similar anticholinergic agents on colonic motility has long been investigated and remains controversial (2,65,115,140). The disagreements might be related to differences in methodology. One must conclude that the inhibitory effect of atropine, if any, is not overwhelming. The effect is variably present and, if present, it is slight and brief, lasting less than 30 min. In view of the variable results reported and the methodological problems concerned with studies *in vivo,* it is difficult to accept that any effect at all exists. *In vitro,* the electromyogram of colonic muscle has been studied as it is affected by atropine (181): the drug has no effect on the electromyogram, including the spike bursts, which are the electromyographic equivalent of contractions. In other unpublished studies of contractions from my laboratory, it has been observed that atropine has no influence on the spontaneous contractions of the circular muscle layer of the cat colon, although the drug depresses contractions of the longitudinal layer.

Polypeptides. Substance P has been reported to cause contractions of the circular muscle layer of the colon (16). Bradykinin inhibits both layers of the colon, but an excitation may be seen at higher concentrations in the longitudinal muscle layer (68). Gastrin heptadecapeptide has little effect on either layer of human colonic muscle *in vitro* (19) or *in vivo* (130). Cholecystokinin is said to stimulate the colon *in vivo* (96). Angiotensin excites contractions in both layers of human colonic muscle (69) *in vitro.*

Prostaglandins. Prostaglandins of the F series (PGFs) contract both layers of the human colon; PGE compounds contract the longitudinal layer but relax the circular layer (17). The physiological significance of these agents and these actions is unknown.

Morphine. In vivo, morphine causes an increase in contractions in the left colon of the human being (135, 136), and this effect may be, in part, cholinergically mediated (51). *In vitro,* in the cat colon, morphine at a concentration of 3μM, had two effects on the electromyogram (181): It increased the intensity of spike activity, suggesting an increase in the force of contractions, and it prolonged slow-wave duration, with no effect on slow-wave frequency.

Laxatives. A wide variety of agents used as laxatives are believed to possess that effect through their ability to affect colonic motility. These are the agents commonly classified as contact or irritant laxatives. With the exception of castor oil (or its active principle, ricinoleic acid), little evidence exists to support the view that these laxatives in fact alter colonic motility. Ricinoleic acid seems to have little effect on the amplitude of contractions of colonic muscle *in vitro*, but it has a pronounced effect on the coupling of the electrical slow waves, as described previously (34,37).

THE ANAL SPHINCTERS

The Internal Anal Sphincter

The internal anal sphincter is a thickening of the circular layer of smooth muscle of the rectum at the level of the dentate line (165,167). The tonic contraction of the internal sphincter is certainly responsible for part of the maintained closure of the anal canal. This conclusion rests on evidence from balloon manometry (101) and on evidence that the division of the internal sphincter with preservation of the external sphincter weakens but does not abolish closure of the anal canal (59,90). The way in which this tone is maintained by this smooth muscle seems not to have been studied. It is sometimes implied that the tone is neurogenic, maintained by an excitatory sympathetic innervation, but there is no evidence for such a view. The internal anal sphincter relaxes in response to rectal distension (56,153). This relaxation is neurogenic, a reflex response that is excited by mechanoreceptors in the rectum that may also be present to some degree in the sigmoid colon (85,153). Exactly how far up the colon these receptors can be found is a question of obvious clinical importance. The pathway of this reflex has been debated. Studies in normal men (85) have suggested that the reflex pathway involves the spinal cord. Garry (83) observed that simple distension of a rectal balloon was ineffective but that rotation or axial movement of a distended balloon in the rectum caused relaxation in the anal canal in either anesthetized, decerebrate, decapitated, or cord-transected cats; the response continued after division of pudendal nerves and after full curarization. The effect was abolished by spinal anesthesia, pelvic nerve section, and mucosal application of cocaine; it was facilitated by division of the lumbar nerves. Garry was cautious in his interpretations but believed that the relaxation of the internal sphincter occurred by way of the spinal cord. A principal cause of uncertainty in these studies arises from the technique of recording from balloons in the anal canal: the ability of this technique to distinguish precisely between the operation of the internal and external sphincters seems at least questionable. Denny-Brown and Robertson (56) studied patients with a variety of neurologic lesions, using balloons both to excite the rectum and to record relaxation of the anal canal. They concluded that the relaxation of the internal sphincter in response to excitation of mechanoreceptors

in the rectum is mediated wholly through the intramural plexuses, as did others (153).

Drugs can be used to answer questions about mechanisms for tonic contraction and relaxation of the internal anal sphincter. Garrett et al. (81) used balloon kymography in the cat treated with succinylcholine to study the effects of drugs and nerves on the internal anal sphincter. The drugs were given intravenously or into a femoral artery. It was observed that the sphincter normally contracts rhythmically 12 to 36 times each minute. Rectal distention caused sphincteric relaxation. Tone was reduced by large doses of pentobarbital. Compression of the urinary bladder and voiding were accompanied by contractions of the sphincter, an effect blocked by dihydroergotamine. Division of the sympathetic hypogastric nerves caused a transient fall in tone, and electrical stimulation of the peripheral stump caused a contraction that was resistant to atropine and hexamethonium. Division of the sacral nerves reduced tone permanently, and electrical stimulation of the distal stump could cause either a contraction or a relaxation; the contractions, when they occurred, were variably affected by atropine; the relaxations were resistant to atropine, hexamethonium, and adrenergic beta-receptor antagonists. Adrenergic alpha-receptor stimulation was excitatory; adrenergic beta-receptor stimulation was inhibitory. Cholinergic agonists were usually excitatory. Sphincteric relaxations with rectal distention was unaffected by dihydroergotamine. Propranolol converted the relaxation to a dihydroergotamine-sensitive contraction; after both propranolol and dihydroegotamine, however, relaxation with rectal distention still persisted. Although this study is impressive, questions are raised by the inconsistency of the results, by the general objections that can be raised to the physiological significance of studies in acutely anesthetized animals, and by the lack of certainty that one can selectively identify the behavior of the internal sphincter by balloon recording from the anal canal.

Many of these objections could be overridden by studies of sphincteric muscle *in vitro*, but this approach seems not to have been fully exploited. Friedman (74) studied human sphincter muscle *in vitro*. They too concluded that adrenergic alpha-receptors are excitatory receptors inhibitory. He noted poor responses to acetylcholine. Responses to nicotine and other ganglionic stimulants were both excitatory and inhibitory; this was interpreted as representing an action on adrenergic nerves to release norepinephrine that would act on either alpha- or beta-receptors. Parks et al. (137) also studied human sphincter muscle *in vitro*. They too concluded that adrenergic alpha-receptors are excitatory and beta-receptors inhibitory in this tissue. They, too, noted the poor responsiveness of the sphincter to the contractile action of acetylcholine, and they observed the catecholamine-mediated actions of nicotine. Another important contribution is that of Costa and Furness (47). They used isolated innervated preparations of the internal sphincter from guinea pigs arranged for selective stimulation of the colonic, pelvic, and pudendal nerves, and for transmural stimulation as well. They identified (a) cholinergic (atropine-sensitive) excitatory nerves from the pelvic plexuses, (b) adrenergic (phentolamine-sensitive) excitatory nerves from the pelvic plexuses and pudendal nerves; and (c) inhibitory nerves (insensitive to antagonists of cholinergic and adrenergic transmission) descending to the sphincter within the gut wall and arising as well from the pelvic plexuses. One might object to the guinea pig as an animal model for all mammals, but very similar observations were made in a study of the internal anal sphincter of the vervet monkey by Rayner (143).

From these studies, it may be concluded that the sphincter has two excitatory innervations, one cholinergic and one adrenergic, and two inhibitory innervations, one adrenergic and the other nonadrenergic. The relative importance of these four kinds of nerves in the operation of the internal sphincter, however, remains to be worked out.

The recent paper of Frenckner and Ihre (73) approached the question of the relative roles of the sympathetic and parasympathetic nerves in determining tone of the internal sphincter. They studied the intact sphincter in patients, using high spinal anesthesia and low spinal anesthesia to block sympathetic and parasympathetic outflows, respectively. They concluded that a tonic excitatory sympathetic discharge to the sphincter exists and accounts for some of the tone, but there is no tonic parasympathetic discharge at all. A second point can be made also from the study of Frenckner and Ihre (73). In their studies, they observed relaxations of the internal anal sphincter in response to rectal distention. These continued both during low spinal anesthesia, the technique used to suppress the parasympathetic supply to the sphincter and during high spinal anesthesia, the technique used to suppress the sympathetic nerve supply. From this, one would conclude that the relaxation is neither sympathetic nor parasympathetic.

The External Anal Sphincter

The external anal sphincter is a striated muscle constituting several muscle bundles that surround the internal sphincter. These several bundles, however, seem to act as a single unit. The external anal sphincter is a voluntary muscle. In manometric studies of the anal canal, it is usually assumed that the external sphincter makes an important contribution to the tonic closure of the canal. It is assumed that this striated muscle maintains a tonic contraction. Evidence for such tone has been obtained by recording the electromyogram from electrodes in the form of disks applied to the skin over

the external sphincter (71). From this study, it was concluded that the external sphincter maintains tone during waking hours, but that tone becomes "minimal" in sleep. The magnitude of tone, indicated by the electromyographic intensity of spike discharges, was seen to rise with any maneuver that raised intra-abdominal pressure, except for straining at defecation, when the tone decreased. Electromyography from needle electrodes in the striated sphincter muscle has confirmed that a continuous discharge of spiking, interpreted as showing tone, is present at rest in this muscle (7,72).

There has been some controversy as to the relative importance of the two sphincters. Gaston (85) said that the internal sphincter ". . . has nothing to do with sphincteric continence." Data from Hill et al. (101) suggests that the internal sphincter contributes most of the pressure recorded on manometry of the anal canal. Frenckner and Euler (72) anesthetized the pudendal nerves during continuous manometry of the anal canal and electromyography of the external sphincter. They concluded that the internal sphincter contributes 85% of anal canal pressure at rest, only 40% after sudden rectal distention and 65% during constant rectal distention. The internal sphincter, they said, is mainly responsible for continence, the external sphincter being important in continence only in the event of sudden substantial rectal distention, a stimulus that makes the internal sphincter relax.

Thus, the evidence supports the idea that the external anal sphincter is most important when it is caused to contract in reflex response to sudden rectal distention (91), a response that, together with the relaxation of the internal sphincter, has been called the inflation reflex (110). In support of that idea, Duthie and Watts (61) found that the striated external sphincter contributes significantly to anal canal pressure only when a body is present in the rectum.

The tone of the external sphincter is a consequence of tonic neural activation. This is evident from the fact that the external sphincter and the puborectalis muscle are innervated only by a somatic innervation from the second, third, and fourth sacral roots, via the pudendal nerves. No autonomic innervation to this striated muscle has been described. Since the only innervation known is an excitatory one, it follows that changes in the level of its contraction, including reflex contractions, must represent changes in the level of continuous activity of these somatic nerves coming from the sacral cord. Thus, reflexes involving the external sphincter must be mediated by extrinsic nerves and centers.

SOME INTEGRATED COLONIC ACTIVITIES

Response of the Colon to Eating

The term, *gastrocolic reflex,* though it has wide usage, is not appropriate to describe this effect for three reasons: the response is not clearly established as neural, the stimulus is not confined to the stomach, and the response is not restricted to the colon. The term should be abandoned.

An effect of eating on motions of the colon is, of course, indirectly evident to laymen, and it was first observed directly decades ago (25,124). Hertz and Newton (99) observed that mass movement tends to occur soon after eating. Although the effect seems to be well-known, it seems not to have been described with any precision, probably because of the deficiencies of the methods to observe colonic motility. The extent and magnitude of the effect are hard to judge. Most studies of the response have made use of the left side of the colon, since that is more accessible to sensing devices used *in vivo*, but a study by the telemetering capsule makes it clear that both proximal and distal colon respond to eating (129). One of the earliest studies described the response as it was seen in the cecum (124). A manometric study in postoperative patients also showed that the whole colon responds to eating, but the response of the sigmoid colon is most marked (118). The magnitude of the effect may be considerable. Measuring magnitudes of responses is difficult, of course, with all methods that use intraluminal sensing devices. The effect, moreover, seems to involve an increase both in the frequency of contractions and in the amplitudes of pressures recorded. Amplitudes of contractions may double (129), but frequency tends to increase less, perhaps only 10% to 25%.

The mechanism of the response has been a matter of conjecture. Macewen (124) thought it was neurally mediated, but more recent investigators have indicated that it may be hormonal. There can be little doubt, though, that some nervous functions are involved, at least in the stimulus. Hertz (99), who seems to have originated the term *gastrocolic reflex,* thought that the chief stimulus was the entry of food into the empty stomach, despite the fact that he reported once seeing a mass movement in a fasted patient who had only just seen the food. Thus, there may be a "cephalic phase" in this effect. Welch and Plaut (177) studied dogs by balloon recording from the colon. They noted no effect if food is introduced into the stomach by fistula. But others (43), as part of a study of movements of the pelvic colon by balloon manometry, deliberately tried to demonstrate the cephalic phase of the colonic effect of eating and failed; they attributed the failure in this one case to the unappetizing nature of the meal offered. Thus, the question of a cephalic phase is not clearly resolved, and convincing evidence for a function of gastric mucosal receptors in initiating the response is lacking. There is one report that a 1,000-calorie meal in humans produced the effect but a 350-calorie meal did not (60). An "intestinal phase" in the response of the colon to eating was postulated by Holdstock and Misiewicz (103), be-

cause they found, in studies of patients, that the response does not require the presence of a stomach, of acid, of antral gastrin, or of an intact vagal innervation.

The pathways involved in transmission of the information from the sensors (wherever they are) to the colon are likewise not clear, apparently because they have not been very thoroughly sought. The effect is said to persist after vagotomy in humans, but the evidence is not cited (41), and it is well known that vagotomy in humans is often far from complete. Furthermore, the effect persists in patients with complete transection of the spinal cord (42). An effect of interruption of the splanchnic innervation in man seems not to have been sought. Studies in experimental animals are scarcely more helpful. Gregory (93), in his study of Thiry-Vella loops of jejunum in conscious dogs, observed that there is an increase in motility in such jejunal loops in association with feeding, that this occurs also in sham-feeding, that it occurs also in response to gastric distention by balloon and to mechanical stimulation of the gastric mucosa, and that vascular denervation of the Thiry-Vella loop abolishes the effect of feeding. But that was in the jejunum. Such thorough animal experiments seem not to have been done to study the effect of eating on the movements of the colon.

Those who propose that the response of the colon to eating is mediated by nerves tend to assume that it represents the activation of the muscle by excitatory cholinergic nerves (162), but the assumption may not be justified. There is better reason to consider the possibility that the response is due to an adrenergic mechanism, as suggested by Gregory's data (93) on the effect of perivascular denervation of the jejunum on the jejunal response to feeding. The mechanism, of course, would be through stimulation of excitatory alpha-receptors. But as good a case can also be made that the response is a disinhibition, a transient suspension of a tonic neurogenic inhibition, and such tonic inhibition has clearly been demonstrated to be present in animals. Also, the ability of even well-established anticholinergic agents to affect colonic motility, as reviewed previously, is certainly not impressive.

The alternative hypothesis is that the mechanism is hormonal. The most obvious first step to challenge this idea, a cross-circulation experiment, either has not been done or has been widely ignored. The absence of such evidence, however, has not prevented speculation. Gastrin, in "physiological" doses, increases colonic motor activity in humans and dogs (46) and increases the spike activity in the human rectum and sigmoid (162), but the timing of the colonic response to eating is apparently not quite right for gastrin to be solely responsible (162). Furthermore, there is evidence to suggest that gastrin itself may excite muscle in part by causing release of acetylcholine from local stores (173), and also atropine can affect the release of gastrin and cholecystokinin

(119,175). Thus, attempts to sort out putative effects of these hormones on colonic contractions from the effects of a cholinergic innervation *in vivo* solely through the use of drugs directed at muscarinic receptors are very likely to be futile.

The response of the colon to eating cannot be fully analyzed until a much more rigorous definition of the whole response is made. Also, it is no longer satisfactory simply to look for an increase or a decrease in activity. Patterns of movements are important. These patterns must be defined and methods developed to allow them to be observed.

Defecation

Our understanding of the complex process of defecation is hampered by the fact that the greater part of the research on the process has been done in humans.

It is clear that the central nervous system is normally involved in the process. This is evident from the fact that such a great variety of actions take place at least briefly in defecation. Some of these, necessary to raise intra-abdominal pressure, are closure of the glottis, descent of the diaphragm, contraction of abdominal wall muscles, and contraction of muscles of the pelvic floor. Others, related to evacuation of the rectum, include relaxation of the sphincters and contraction of the rectal wall. The precise locations of the nervous centers responsible for integration of these movements, which are partly voluntary and partly involuntary, remain unknown.

The process is normally initiated by excitation of mechanoreceptors in the anorectal area. These mechanoreceptors are excited by movements of the rectal mucosa (83) or by rectal distention (153). Their exact location is a matter of debate. Garry thought that they lie on the mucosa, for he observed that the application of cocaine to the rectal mucosa of the cat abolished all responses to balloon movement in the rectum, an experiment that apparently has not been repeated. But other evidence suggests that they are not in the mucosa. Apparently normal defecatory processes return after healing in dogs that have had a rectal reconstruction operation in which there is a total colectomy preserving a rectum in which the seromuscular layers of the rectosigmoid are lined by ileal mucosa (88). Subsequent general clinical experience has confirmed those observations. These receptors, whether in mucosa or muscle, are either more sensitive or more numerous in the distal rectum than more proximally, for progressively smaller degrees of distention are effective as the stimulating balloon is moved caudad along the rectum (153).

The evidence leading to these inconsistent conclusions about the location of the receptors can be reconciled if one proposes that the receptors are mucosal (hence, accessible to cocaine) but not rectal (hence not removed

with the rectal mucosa in the course of ileoanal anastomosis). This would be the case if the receptors are confined to the mucosa in and just above the anal canal. In this situation, they very likely would have been exposed to cocaine in Garry's experiment but might not be fully resected in operations in which the rectal mucosa is stripped. And, in fact, such a distribution is suggested by the results of Goligher's survey (90) of continence after a variety of sphincter-sparing operations of the rectum. He pointed out that an anorectal remnant of at least 6 cm from the anal verge will usually suffice for perfect function. Duthie and Gairns (60) followed up on this observation by applying silver stains to human rectal and anal mucosa to visualize the form and distribution of neural structures in the mucosa. In confirmation and extension of earlier studies cited, they found a profuse innervation, expecially in the region of the anal crypts, and valves with both free intraepithelial nerve endings and organized endings. Only about half of the organized endings are of recognized types, Golgi-Mazzoni, Krause, Meissner, Pacinian, and genital corpuscles. This area extends up to about 1 cm above the anal valves. The perianal skin contains a less dense distribution of nerves with only peritrichial and some free endings, and the rectal mucosa itself is virtually devoid of nerve endings. In human volunteers, the anal canal lining was found to be very sensitive to pain, heat, cold, and light touch. Duthie and Gairns postulated a role for anal canal receptors in continence and defecation. Duthie and Bennett (58) sought to confirm this by plotting the distribution of the sensory area (mapped by plotting the extent of perception of light touch) and the length of the high-pressure area as mapped by pulling a pressure-sensing unit through the sphincter. They found that the sensory zone lies entirely within the high-pressure zone when the rectum is empty; balloon distention of the rectum, however, causes the high-pressure segment to shorten, presumably through relaxation of the internal sphincter, so that the sensory zone now faces the rectal vault. Duthie's hypothesis was further supported by the radiographic studies of Phillips and Edwards (139); they also postulated a flutter-valve mechanism as contributing to the maintenance of closure of the anal canal under conditions of raised intra-abdominal pressure. It seems possible that these anal canal receptors are the only ones involved in the rectoanal reflexes concerned in continence and defecation. Balloon distention of the rectum should secondarily move or displace, to some extent, the mucosa of the anal canal, and that would explain the observation that the sensitivity to rectal distention is more pronounced with more distal placement of the stimulating balloon.

When continence is mentioned it is commonly said that the rectum is empty until the act of defecation is about to occur. This view is not consistent with common clinical experience, for the physician who routinely does digital examination of the anal canal on physical examination usually encounters enough stool at least to check for blood. The conclusion was not confirmed either by a radiographic study directed to the question (94). Besides showing that the rectum is very commonly filled with feces in the absence of the urge to defecate, the study also showed that, in some subjects at least, the whole of the left side of the colon from the splenic flexure downward is emptied in defecation. This indicates that the reflexes involved in defecation must also promote, as a part of the act, a contraction of the muscular wall not only of the rectum itself but also of a part of the descending colon. No one, it appears, has tried to demonstrate or measure these wall movements in more detail, however, so that nothing more can be said of them now.

When continence is discussed, it is usual to speak of sphincteric continence and of rectal continence as two separate functions. Sphincteric continence refers to the actions and properties of the two sphincters and of the anal canal as discussed previously. Rectal continence refers to the capacity of the rectum itself to act as a reservoir. Its ability to do so is related to its ability to allow an increase in volume without a corresponding increase in pressure. One might assume that, like the gastric fundus, the rectum contains a mechanism for receptive relaxation, but this seems, also, not to have been studied. Apparently, there have been no attempts to detail the pressure-volume relationships of the rectum in appropriate animal experiments.

It is a very old observation that defecation, though it may be transiently disturbed, ultimately is reestablished in patients that have had cortical injuries or injuries of the spinal cord above the lumbosacral level (23). From this, it is concluded that the lumbosacral cord alone can sustain the essential reflexes concerned in defecation. Although the conclusion has been amply supported by further observations in such patients, the conclusion seems not to have been pursued with controlled and objective experimentation in animals. Thus, there is insufficient evidence to say exactly what nerves transmit effective inputs to the presumed "defecatory center" of the lumbosacral cord or to identify or characterize the nerves that transmit the outflows from this center.

Effect of Emotions on the Colon

From the studies of Rostad (147–151), it is clear that at least a physiological basis exists for an influence of emotions on the colon. Furthermore, anxiety is assumed widely to affect colonic function. A way to demonstrate such an effect objectively, however, is difficult to find. The experiments that have been done were mainly done in humans in a setting where the stress is produced by conversation. Colonic motility was recorded by ballons while anxiety-producing topics were discussed. The experiments have been largely poorly controlled, and results have been contradictory and unconvincing. The reports of this kind of experiment (3–6,29,33,116) are all more than a decade old, so that this experimental approach has probably been abandoned.

It has been said that sleep depresses colonic motility and this is taken as evidence for an influence of emotions on colonic motility (24). Such a conclusion cannot be considered well founded, for other things may occur in sleep as well. For one thing, most people fast during sleep.

DISORDERED COLONIC MOTILITY

Diverticulosis of the Colon

Diverticulosis of the colon is a clinical entity which, according to much-publicized recent evidence, can now be said with some conviction to be a consequence of disordered motility. The evidence for a disorder of motility can be summarized in the following observations: there is thickening of rings of circular muscle adjacent to the diverticula; this thickening precedes the development of the diverticula; intraluminal pressures in the area of the diverticula are abnormally great when contractions are induced by morphine, by prostigmine, and by eating. All this evidence was generated over a decade ago in a series of studies that have been well reviewed elsewhere (11,134,182). This thickening of the circular muscle is commonly called hypertrophy, despite evidence that the ratio of DNA to nitrogen in the thickened circular muscle next to diverticula is not different from that of normal circular or normal longitudinal muscle. Thus, the thickening represents either hyperplasia of the circular muscle or shortening in the longitudinal axis of the colon (156). There are no ideas as to the direct cause of the thickening, but there may be one small clue in the observation that there is a "plethora of ganglionic tissue" in specimens of the muscular wall that contain diverticula (123). Of course, this plethora may be a result rather than a cause of the thickening. On the basis of epidemiological evidence, the idea has been put forward that diverticulosis is a consequence of prolonged adherence to a low residue diet. The pathophysiology to explain such a causal relationship is obscure, and the few experiments that have been done do not support the idea. Carlson and Hoelzel (28), in life-span studies of rats fed various diets, concluded that colonic diverticula form in aging rats as a consequence of a lack of a suitable kind and volume of roughage in the diet. These diverticula were, however, unlike those of the human disorder in that they were within or close to the cecum. Furthermore, Carlson and Hoelzel did not report muscle thickening, though there is nothing to suggest that they looked for it. Dowling et al. (57) fed rats diets containing large amounts of powdered kaolin; on such a highbulk diet, their animals developed an increase in colon weight due mainly to an increase in the thickness of the muscle coat, a change they attributed to work hypertrophy. Havia and Klossner (97) fed puppies a low-residue diet for 10 months. No diverticula developed. On manometric and fluoroscopic studies, no abnormalities were observed, nor was muscle thickening found.

Aganglionosis of the Colon

Hirschsprung's disease, aganglionosis or congenital megacolon, is a well-established example of a motility disorder of the colon. A neurogenic origin was first proposed in 1946 (62). It may not be, however, a single entity, for a degree of heterogeneity is evident from epidemiological studies (138). There is heterogeneity in the extent of the lesion. In most patients the aganglionic segment goes no further than the rectum and sigmoid colon, but longer segments have been described up to the length of the whole colon. Furthermore, there is variety in the clinical presentation, for some patients may require immediate surgical relief of obstruction in the neonatal period, whereas others with similar lengths of rectum involved present themselves much later in life with only constipation.

Few studies of motility in children with aganglionosis have been reported. The characteristic barium enema X-ray appearance is well known: a narrowed distal segment constituting the rectal or rectosigmoid regions gives way to a dilated proximal colon. Davidson et al. (53) looked for denervation supersensitivity using a triple-lumen nonperfused tube to record intraluminal pressures in response to methacholine from the distal colon of such patients and normal controls. In the normal controls, methacholine relaxed the distal colon in 9 of 20, and it had no effect in the other 11. In the patients with megacolon, the drug relaxed the dilated segment in 4 of 6, had no effect in the other 2, and had no effect in the narrowed segment in any. These workers explained the lack of denervation supersensitivity in the narrow segment on the grounds that the denervation is congenital, not acquired, as it probably is in idiopathic esophageal achalasia. In one of those 6 cases, however, operated on with success because of the clinical diagnosis and the failure of methacholine to make the distal segment relax, the narrowed distal segment was found to contain ganglia. Studies of anal sphincteric responses to balloon distention in 10 children with congenital megacolon (152) revealed that the internal anal sphincter did not relax in response to rectal distention: there was, instead, a contraction. Lawson and Nixon (120), in a more detailed study, used a balloon system to record pressures in the anal canal in 24 normal children and 47 with congenital megacolon. They observed that nor-

mally the internal sphincter is kept closed by rhythmical contractions at 10 to 13/min, relaxing upon a sufficient degree of rectal distention. In Hirschsprung's disease they thought that resting pressures in the intestinal sphincter were somewhat raised with pronounced rhythmic contractions. Rectal distention produced no relaxation and, indeed, in some it tended to raise the base-line pressure and the amplitude of the rhythmic contractions. Similar observations were made by Howard (106). The suggestion that this abnormal response be used as a diagnostic test (120,152) was repeated by Tobon et al. (170).

The neuropathology of the disease, first described by Whitehouse and Kernohan (179), was used to distinguish it from idiopathic megacolon by Bodian et al. (22). They found, in both myenteric and submucosal plexuses, an absence of ganglion cells throughout the narrowed segments and 1 to 5 cm into the dilated segment; the plexuses in the aganglionic segments contained numerous bundles of unusually dense nerve fibrils and interstitial cells. Smith (157) used silver stains in sections cut parallel to the gut wall in 2 adult cases and observed, in the dilated segments above the narrowed zone, a reduced number of ganglion cells, many of them abnormal in appearance, unmyelinated nerve trunks, and a grossly disorganized pattern of nerves. Ehrenpreis et al. (63) applied the catecholamine fluorescence technique to 10 specimens and found that the dilated segment contained normal-appearing basket-like adrenergic networks surrounding ganglion cells; the narrowed segment contained no such synapses. In both segments, a small number of adrenergic terminals was seen in the submucosa, in the circular muscle layer, and at the interface between the circular muscle layer and the taeniae. They concluded that there is adrenergic denervation of the normal segment as well as aganglionosis. Bennett et al. (18) suggested that the numbers of adrenergic nerves in the muscle layers themselves are actually increased. Meier-Ruge (127), using the cholinesterase stain, found an extreme increase in cholinesterase activity in the abnormal dense bundle of nerves in the narrowed segment. He proposed that the sustained contraction represents an increased excitatory cholinergic innervation of the muscle that accompanies the aganglionosis, whereas others have viewed the contraction as a consequence of cholinergic denervation. Garrett et al. (82) used both catecholamine fluorescence and cholinesterase stains. In the circular muscle layer from the aganglionic segment, the number of cholinergic nerves varied; those cases with the most such nerves tended to be those with the most severe clinical presentations; those with the fewest such nerves had the mildest clinical presentation. The number of catecholamine-fluorescent nerves varied widely in the aganglionic segment. In the functional zone between the ganglionic segment and the aganglionic segment there was a deficiency of intramuscular nerves. Garrett et al. concluded that the spasm of the contracted segment represents an unopposed action of cholinergic muscular nerves, that the failure of coordinated contraction and relaxation is due to the aganglionosis, and that deficient muscular nerves in the junctional region lead to deficient propulsive forces at this level. A subsequent electron microscopic study (107,108) supported the previous histochemical studies in indicating a rich supply of intramuscular nerve bundles in the aganglionic segment, without obvious structural abnormality of the constituent axons, and a relative deficiency of these intramuscular nerves at the junction between ganglionic and aganglionic segments.

Thus, there appears to be some degree of heterogeneity in the neuropathology of aganglionosis of the colon. The histology that is reviewed above, taken together with the demonstration that the internal anal sphincter fails to relax and that internal sphincter relaxation in response to rectal distention is nonadrenergic, suggests that at least some of the ganglion cells that are lost are nonadrenergic inhibitory ganglion cells. Wood (183,184) in his study of a strain of mice with an inherited aganglionic megacolon, suggested that the entity is also characterized by an absence of spontaneously active inhibitory neurons from the enteric plexuses. That mouse disease, however, may not be a fully appropriate model of human aganglionosis.

Diarrhea and Constipation

It is commonly held that abnormal colonic motility causes constipation and diarrhea. It is further commonly held that diarrhea is a consequence of a hypermotile state, constipation the consequence of a hypomotile one. Manometric records from the left colon, however, show the opposite to be true: in patients with diarrhea, the number of contractions recorded in the left colon seems to be less than normal, while the opposite is found in patients who are constipated (40,114). Although these studies are now old, they have not been notably extended or elaborated upon. Perhaps the most important subsequent advance in this area has been that diarrhea and constipation have been defined quantitatively (44).

The Irritable Colon Syndrome

The irritable colon syndrome is a very commonly used diagnostic term. Its use suggests that a defined symptom-complex can be blamed on irritability of the colon. That implication is wrong on three counts: the symptom-complex has not been defined, the colon has not been shown to be involved, and irritability has neither been defined nor demonstrated. Nevertheless, many physicians who use the term speak of it as though it applies to a single clinical entity and that it is a psycho-

somatic disorder related to stresses in living and to depression (29,30,102,128,174). Most studies supporting the concept have focused on the attempt to find psychological abnormalities in patients who seem to fit this ill-defined diagnostic category. The observations made seem often uncontrolled or do not seem objective, but these problems are common in attempts to pin down psychological abnormalities. Attempts to demonstrate colonic motor abnormalities in such patients have not always been successful; many of these have been described above in other contexts. A recent attempt (67) to demonstrate abnormalities in urinary epinephrine excretion in such patients showed a higher excretion in patients with the syndrome in which diarrhea was the dominant symptom (as opposed to those in which pain dominated the clinical picture) than did a control population. The diarrhea-predominant patients also showed more evidence for anxiety and neurosis, on objective tests for such character traits, than did the control population. The pain-dominant form of the syndrome did not differ from normal controls in tests for personality dysfunction or in urinary epinephrine excretion. What an increased urinary epinephrine excretion might have to do with colonic motility was not explained.

SUMMARY

Colonic movements are so organized as to produce patterns of flow consistent with three important functions: the conservation of water, the maintenance of an abundant intraluminal bacterial population, and the capacity to control the delivery of feces.

The gross patterns of contraction and flow suggest that the colon constitutes three segments that are functionally distinct. In the proximal part of the colon the major pattern is one in which retrograde annular contractions, constituting rhythmic antiperistalsis, drive the colonic content toward the cecum, where it is retained for long periods. In the middle part of the colon, the major activity constitutes annular contractions that divide the fecal mass and tend to move the feces very slowly toward the rectum. In the most distal segment of the colon the main activity is a strong contraction, oriented to move caudad, that is excited by stimulation of the pelvic nerves.

The patterns of the movements of the colon may be determined by controls of three kinds—myogenic, neurogenic, and hormonal factors. Myogenic factors, properties of the muscle itself, account in part for the contraction patterns of the proximal and middle parts of the colon. In these regions, electrical slow waves (pacesetter potentials or electrical control activity) seem to establish the frequency, velocity, and direction of propagation of rhythmic annular contractions. Neurogenic factors, influences of the autonomic nerves, have a less clearly established place in controlling normal colonic motility in the proximal and middle parts of the colon. There is some evidence to suggest that mass movement is neurogenic and that it may represent disinhibition, transient suppression of tonic neurogenic inhibition. Neurogenic factors are clearly most important in the most distal part of the colon, where the variety of actions that take place in defecation are the consequence of the actions of nerves connected to centers in the central nervous system that are concerned in defecation. The principal excitatory nerves in the colon are cholinergic, and the principal inhibitory ones appear to be nonadrenergic. Adrenergic inhibition is also present and is directed mainly to the cholinergic ganglion cells of the intramural plexuses. An effect of hormones in the normal control of colonic motility remains to be shown.

The enhanced activity of the colonic muscle that results from eating is still of unknown cause. A presumed effect of the emotional state on colonic motor function remains to be shown. Diverticulosis of the colon is clearly a motor disorder, but it is not clear how it comes about. Aganglionosis of the colon is also clearly a motor disorder; in aganglionosis there is a congenital defect in the innervation of the distal colon, a defect that seems to involve cholinergic, adrenergic, and noncholinergic inhibitory nerves. A relationship between abnormal colonic motility and the symptoms of diarrhea and constipation also remain conjectural. A commonly used diagnostic term, the irritable colon syndrome, implies that there is a clinical entity characterized by abnormal colonic contractions, but this idea is not yet supported by convincing evidence.

ACKNOWLEDGMENT

This work was supported in part by Research Grant AM 20448 from the National Institutes of Health.

REFERENCES

1. Adler, H. F., Atkinson, A. J., and Ivy, A. C. (1941): A study of motility of the human colon: an explanation of dysynergia [dyssynergia] of the colon, or of the "unstable colon." *Am. J. Dig. Dis.,* 8:197–202.
2. Adler, H. F., Atkinson, A. J., and Ivy, A. C. (1942): The effect of morphine and Dilaudid on the ileum and of morphine, Dilaudid and atropine on the colon of man. *Arch. Intern. Med.,* 69:974–985.
3. Almy, T. P., Abbot, F. K., and Hinkle, L. E., Jr. (1950): Alterations in colonic function in man under stress. IV. Hypomotility of the sigmoid colon, and its relationship to the mechanism of functional diarrhea. *Gastroenterology,* 15:95–103.
4. Almy, T. P., Hinkle, L. E., Jr., Berle, B. B., and Kern, F., Jr. (1949): Alterations in colonic function in man under stress. III. Experimental production of sigmoid spasm in patients with spastic constipation. *Gastroenterology,* 12:437–449.
5. Almy, T. P., Kern, F., Jr., and Tulin, M. (1949): Alterations in colonic function in man under stress. II. Experimental production of sigmoid spasm in healthy persons. *Gastroenterology,* 12:425–436.
6. Almy, T. P., and Tulin, M. (1947): Alterations in colonic function in man under stress. I. Experimental production of changes simulating the "irritable colon." *Gastroenterology,* 8:616–626.
7. Alva, J., Mendeloff, A. I., and Schuster, M. M. (1967): Reflex and electromyographic abnormalities associated with fecal incontinence. *Gastroenterology,* 53:101–106.
8. Anson, B. J., and Maddock, W. G. (1952): Ileocecal-appendiceal Region. In: *Callander's Surgical Anatomy,* ed. 3, chapt. 15, p. 473. W. B. Saunders, Philadelphia and London.
9. Anuras, S., and Christensen, J. (1975): Electrical slow waves of the colon do not extend into the caecum. *Rendiconti di Gastroenterologia,* 7:56–59.
10. Anuras, S., Christensen, J., and Templeman, D. (1977): Effect of capsaicin on electrical slow waves in the isolated cat colon. *Gut,* 18:666–669.
11. Arfwidsson, S. (1964): Pathogenesis of multiple diverticula of the sigmoid colon in diverticular disease. *Acta Chir. Scand. (Suppl.),* 342:1–68.
12. Barclay, A. E. (1935): Direct x-ray cinematography with a preliminary note on the nature of non-propulsive movements of the large intestine. *Br. J. Radiol.,* 8:652–658.
13. Barker, J. D., and Christensen, J. (1973): Some effects of quinidine and quinine on the electromyogram of the colon. *Gastroenterology,* 65:773–777.
14. Baumgarten, H. G. (1967): Über die verteilung von catecholaminen in darm des menschen. *Z. Zellforsch.,* 83:133–146.
15. Bayliss, W. M., and Starling, E. H. (1900): The movements and the innervation of the large intestine. *J. Physiol. (Lond.),* 26:107–118.
16. Bennett, A. (1975): Symposium on colonic function. Pharmacology of colonic muscle. *Gut,* 16:307–311.
17. Bennett, A., and Fleshler, B. (1970): Prostaglandins and the gastrointestinal tract. *Gastroenterology,* 59:790–800.
18. Bennett, A., Garrett, J. R., and Howard, E. R. (1968): Adrenergic myenteric nerves in Hirschsprung's disease. *Br. Med. J.,* 1:487–489.
19. Bennett, A., Misiewicz, J. J., and Waller, S. L. (1967): Analysis of the motor effects of gastrin and pentagastrin on the human alimentary tract in vitro. *Gut,* 8:470–474.
20. Bennett, A., and Whitney, B. (1966): A pharmacological study of the motility of the human gastrointestinal tract. *Gut,* 7:307–316.
21. Bianchi, C., Beani, L., Frigo, G. M., and Crema, A. (1968): Further evidence for the presence of non-adrenergic inhibitory structures in the guinea-pig colon. *Eur. J. Pharmacol.,* 4:51–61.
22. Bodian, M., Stephens, F. D., and Ward, B. C. H. (1949): Hirschsprung's disease and idiopathic megacolon. *Lancet,* 1:6–11.
23. Boring, E. G. (1915): The sensations of the alimentary canal. *Am. J. Psychol.,* 26:1–57.
24. Bucknell, A., and Whitney, B. (1964): A preliminary investigation of the pharmacology of the human isolated taenia coli preparation. *Br. J. Pharmacol.,* 23:164–175.
25. Cannon, W. B. (1902): The movements of the intestines studied by means of the röntgen rays. *Am. J. Physiol.,* 6:251–277.
26. Caprilli, R., and Onori, L. (1972): Origin, transmission and ionic dependence of colonic electrical slow waves. *Scand. J. Gastroenterol.,* 7:65–74.
27. Capurso, L., Friedmann, C. A., and Parks, A. G. (1968): Adrenergic fibers in the human intestine. *Gut,* 9:678–682.
28. Carlson, A. J., and Hoelzel, F. (1949): Relation of diet to diverticulosis of the colon in rats. *Gastroenterology,* 12:108–115.
29. Chaudhary, N. A., and Truelove, S. C. (1961): Human colonic motility: a comparative study of normal subjects, patients with ulcerative colitis, and patients with the irritable colon syndrome (parts I, II, and III). *Gastroenterology,* 40:1–36.
30. Chaudhary, N. A., and Truelove, S. C. (1962): The irritable colon syndrome: a study of the clinical features, predisposing causes, and prognosis in 130 cases. *Q. J. Med.,* 31:307–322.
30a. Christensen, J. (1971): The controls of gastrointestinal movements; some old and new views. *N. Engl. J. Med.,* 285:85–98.
31. Christensen, J., Anuras, S., and Arthur, C. (1978): Influence of intrinsic nerves on electromyogram of cat colon in vitro. *Am. J. Physiol.,* 234:E641–647.
32. Christensen, J., Anuras, S., and Hauser, R. L. (1974): Migrating spike bursts and electrical slow waves in the cat colon: effect of sectioning. *Gastroenterology,* 66:240–247.

33. Christensen, J., Caprilli, R., and Lund, G. F. (1969): Electric slow waves in circular muscle of cat colon. *Am. J. Physiol.,* 217:771–776.

34. Christensen, J., and Freeman, B. W. (1972): Circular muscle electromyogram in the cat colon: local effect of sodium ricinoleate. *Gastroenterology,* 63:1011–1015.

35. Christensen, J., and Hauser, R. L. (1971): Longitudinal axial coupling of slow waves in proximal cat colon. *Am. J. Physiol.,* 221:246–250.

36. Christensen, J., and Hauser, R. L. (1971): Circumferential coupling of electric slow waves in circular muscle of the cat colon. *Am. J. Physiol.,* 221:1033–1037.

37. Christensen, J., Weisbrodt, N. W., and Hauser, R. L. (1972): Electrical slow waves of the proximal colon of the cat in diarrhea. *Gastroenterology,* 62:1167–1173.

38. Code, C. F., Hightower, N. C., Jr., and Morlock, C. G. (1952): Motility of the alimentary canal in man. Review of recent studies. *Am. J. Med.,* 13:328–351.

39. Connell, A. M. (1961): The motility of the pelvic colon. I. Motility in normals and in patients with asymptomatic duodenal ulcer. *Gut,* 2:175–186.

40. Connell, A. M. (1962): The motility of the pelvic colon. II. Paradoxical motility in diarrhoea and constipation, *Gut,* 3:342–348.

41. Connell, A. M. (1968): Motor action of the large bowel. In: *Handbook of Physiology. A Critical Comprehensive Presentation of Physiological Knowledge and Concepts, Section 6: Alimentary Canal; Volume IV: Motility,* edited by C. F. Code, chapt. 101, pp. 2075–2091. American Physiological Society, Washington, D.C.

42. Connell, A. M., Frankel, H., and Guttmann, L. (1963): The motility of the pelvic colon following complete lesions of the spinal cord. *Paraplegia,* 1:98–115.

43. Connell, A. M., Gaafer, M., Hassanein, M. A., and Khayal, M. A. (1964): Motility of the pelvic colon. III. Motility responses in patients with symptoms following amoebic dysentery. *Gut,* 5:443–447.

44. Connell, A. M., Hilton, C., Irvine, G., Lennard-Jones, J. E., and Misiewicz, J. J. (1965): Variation of bowel habit in two population samples. *Br. Med. J.,* 2:1095–1099.

45. Connell, A. M., Lennard Jones, J. E., and Madanagopalan, N. (1964): The distribution of faecal x-ray shadows in subjects without gastro-intestinal disease. *Proc. R. Soc. Med.,* 57:894–895.

46. Connell, A. M., and Logan, C. J. H. (1967): The role of gastrin in gastroileocolic responses. *Am. J. Dig. Dis.,* 12:277–284.

47. Costa, M., and Furness, J. B. (1974): The innervation of the internal anal sphincter of the guinea-pig. In: *Proceedings of the Fourth International Symposium on Gastrointestinal Motility,* edited by E. E. Daniel, pp. 681–689. Mitchell Press, Vancouver.

48. Couturier, D., Roze, C., Couturier-Turpin, M. H., and Debray, C. (1969): Electromyography of the colon in situ: an experimental study in man and in the rabbit. *Gastroenterology,* 56:317–322.

49. Crema, A., Del Tacca, M., Frigo, G. M., and Lecchini, S. (1968): Presence of a non-adrenergic inhibitory system in the human colon. *Gut,* 9:633–637.

50. Daniel, E. E. (1975): Symposium on colonic function. Electrophysiology of the colon. *Gut,* 16:298–306.

51. Daniel, E. E., Sutherland, W. H., and Bogoch, A. (1959): Effects of morphine and other drugs on motility of the terminal ileum. *Gastroenterology,* 36:510–523.

52. Darby, C. F., Hammond, P., and Taylor, I. (1978): Real time analysis of colonic myoelectrical rhythms in disease. In: *Gastrointestinal Motility in Health and Disease,* edited by H. L. Duthie, pp. 287–294. MTP Press Ltd., Lancaster.

53. Davidson, M., Sleisenger, M. H., Almy, T. P., and Levine, S. Z. (1956): Studies of distal colonic motility in children; nonpropulsive patterns in normal children. *Pediatrics,* 17:807–818.

54. Davidson, M., Sleisenger, M. H., Steinberg, H., and Almy, T. P. (1955): Studies of distal colonic motility in children. III. The pathologic physiology of congenital megacolon—(Hirschsprung's disease). *Gastroenterology,* 29:803–824.

55. Deller, D. J., and Wangel, A. G. (1965): Intestinal motility in man. I. A study combining the use of intraluminal pressure recording and cineradiography. *Gastroenterology,* 48:45–57.

56. Denny-Brown, D., and Robertson, E. G. (1935): An investigation of the nervous control of defaecation. *Brain,* 58:256–310.

57. Dowling, R. H., Riecken, E. O., Laws, J. W., and Booth, C. C. (1967): The intestinal response to high bulk feeding in the rat. *Clin. Sci.,* 32:1–9.

58. Duthie, H. L., and Bennett, R. C. (1963): The relation of sensation in the anal canal to the functional anal sphincter: a possible factor in anal continence. *Gut,* 4:179–182.

59. Duthie, H. L., and Bennett, R. C. (1964): Anal sphincteric pressure in fissure in ano. *Surg. Gynecol. Obstet.,* 119:19–21.

60. Duthie, H. L., and Gairns, F. W. (1960): Sensory nerve-endings and sensation in the anal region of man. *Br. J. Surg.,* 47:585–595.

61. Duthie, H. L., and Watts, J. M. (1965): Contribution of the external anal sphincter to the pressure zone in the anal canal. *Gut,* 6:64–68.

62. Ehrenpreis, T. (1946): Megacolon in the newborn; a clinical and roentgenological study with special regard to the pathogenesis. *Acta Chir. Scand. (Suppl. 112),* 94:1–114.

63. Ehrenpreis, T., Norberg, K.-A., and Wirsén, C. (1968): Sympathetic innervation of the colon in Hirschsprung's disease: a histochemical study. *J. Pediatr. Surg.,* 3:43–49.

64. Elliott, T. R., and Barclay-Smith, E. (1904): Antiperistalsis and other muscular activities of the colon. *J. Physiol. (Lond.),* 31:272–304.

65. Elsom, K. A., and Drossner, J. L. (1939): Intubation studies of the human small intestine. XVII. The effect of atropine and belladonna on the motor activity of the small intestine and colon. *Am. J. Dig. Dis.,* 6:589–593.

66. Emery, J. L., and Underwood, J. (1970): The neurological junction between the appendix and ascending colon. *Gut,* 11:118–120.

67. Esler, M. D., and Goulston, K. J. (1973): Levels of anxiety in colonic disorders. *N. Engl. J. Med.,* 288:16–20.

68. Fishlock, D. J. (1966): Effect of bradykinin on the human isolated small and large intestine. *Nature,* 212:1533–1535.

69. Fishlock, D. J., and Gunn, A. (1970): The action of angiotensin on the human colon in vitro. *Br. J. Pharmacol.,* 39:34–39.

70. Fishlock, D. J., and Parks, A. G. (1963): A study of human colonic muscle in vitro. *Br. Med. J.,* 2:666–667.

71. Floyd, W. F., and Walls, E. W. (1953): Electromyography of the sphincter ani externus in man. *J. Physiol. (Lond.),* 122:599–609.

72. Frenckner, B., and Euler, C. von (1975): Influence of pudendal block on the function of the anal sphincters. *Gut,* 16:482–489.

73. Frenckner, B., and Ihre, T. (1976): Influence of autonomic nerves on the internal anal sphincter in man. *Gut,* 17:306–312.

74. Friedmann, C. A. (1968): The action of nicotine and catecholamines on the human internal anal sphincter. *Am. J. Dig. Dis.,* 13:428–431.

75. Fujita, T. (1952): A fixation muscle system in the human large intestine. *Anat. Rec.,* 114:467–477.

76. Furness, J. B. (1969): The presence of inhibitory nerves in the colon after sympathetic denervation. *Eur. J. Pharmacol.,* 6:349–352.

77. Furness, J. B. (1969): An electrophysiological study of the innervation of the smooth muscle of the colon. *J. Physiol.,* 205:549–562.

78. Furness, J. B. (1970): The origin and distribution of adrenergic nerve fibers in the guinea-pig colon. *Histochemie,* 21:295–306.

79. Furness, J. B. (1970): An examination of nerve-mediated, hyoscine-resistant excitation of the guinea-pig colon. *J. Physiol.,* 207:803–821.

80. Gagnon, D. J., Devroede, G., and Belisle, S. (1972): Excitatory effects of adrenaline upon isolated preparations of human colon. *Gut,* 13:654–657.

81. Garrett, J. R., Howard, E. R., and Jones, W. (1974): The internal anal sphincter in the cat: a study of nervous mechanisms affecting tone and reflex activity., *J. Physiol. (Lond.),* 243:153–166.

82. Garrett, J. R., Howard, E. R., and Nixon, H. H. (1969): Autonomic nerves in rectum and colon in Hirschsprung's disease. A cholinesterase and catecholamine histochemical study. *Arch. Dis. Child.,* 44:406–417.

83. Garry, R. C. (1933): The responses to stimulation of the caudal end of the large bowel in the cat. *J. Physiol. (Lond.)*, 78:208-224.

84. Garry, R. C. (1934): The movements of the large intestine. *Physiol. Res.*, 14:103-132.

85. Gaston, E. A. (1951): Physiological basis for preservation of fecal continence after resection of rectum. *JAMA*, 146:1486-1489.

86. Gillespie, J. S. (1962): Spontaneous mechanical and electrical activity of stretched and unstretched intestinal smooth muscle cells and their response to sympathetic-nerve stimulation. *J. Physiol. (Lond.)*, 162:54-75.

87. Gillespie, J. S. (1962): The electrical and mechanical responses of intestinal smooth muscle to stimulation of their extrinsic parasympathetic nerves. *J. Physiol.*, 162:76-92.

88. Glotzer, D. J., and Sharma, A. N. (1964): Experimental total abdominoperineal colectomy with preservation of the sphincters. *Surg. Gynecol. Obstet.*, 119:338-344.

89. Goldenberg, M. M. (1968): Analysis of the inhibitory innervation of the isolated gerbil colon. *Arch. Int. Pharmacodyn.*, 175:347-364.

90. Goligher, J. C. (1951): The functional results after sphincter-saving resections of the rectum; Hunterian lecture. *Ann. R. Coll. Surg. Engl.*, 8:421-439.

91. Goligher, J. C., and Hughes, E. S. R. (1951): Sensibility of the rectum and colon; its role in the mechanism of anal continence. *Lancet*, 1:543-548.

92. Gramiak, R., Ross, P., and Olmsted, W. W. (1971): Normal motor activity of the human colon: combined radiotelemetric manometry and slow-frame cineroentgenography. *Am. J. Roent. Rad. Ther. Nucl. Med.*, 113:301-309.

93. Gregory, R. A. (1950): Some factors influencing the passage of fluid through intestinal loops in dogs. *J. Physiol.*, 111:119-137.

94. Halls, J. (1965): Bowel content shift during normal defaecation [Summary]. *Proc. Roy. Soc. Med.*, 58:859-860.

95. Hansky, J., and Connell, A. M. (1962): Measurement of gastrointestinal transit using radioactive chromium. *Gut*, 3:187-188.

96. Harvey, R. F., and Read, A. E. (1973): Effect of cholecystokinin on colonic motility and symptoms in patients with the irritable-bowel syndrome. *Lancet*, 1:1-3.

97. Havia, T., and Klossner, J. (1971): The effect of low-residue diet on the canine colonic wall. *Ann. Chir. Gynaecol.*, 60:132-134.

98. Hertz, A. F. (1907): The passage of food along the human alimentary canal. *Guy's Hosp. Rep.*, 61:389-427.

99. Hertz, A. F., and Newton, A. (1913): The normal movements of the colon in man. *J. Physiol. (Lond.)*, 47:57-65.

100. Hill, C. J., Osman, W. G., and Rewell, R. E. (1954): The caecum of monotremes and marsupials. *Trans. Zool. Soc. Lond.*, 28:185-240.

101. Hill, J. R., Kelley, M. L., Schlegel, J. F., and Code, C. F. (1960): Pressure profile of the rectum and anus of healthy persons. *Dis. Colon Rectum*, 3:203-209.

102. Hislop, I. G. (1971): Psychological significance of the irritable colon syndrome. *Gut*, 12:452-457.

103. Holdstock, D. J., and Misiewicz, J. J. (1970): Factors controlling colonic motility: colonic pressures and transit after meals in patients with total gastrectomy, pernicious anaemia or duodenal ulcer. *Gut*, 11:100-110.

104. Holdstock, D. J., Misiewicz, J. J., Smith, T., and Rowlands, E. N. (1970): Propulsion (mass movements) in the human colon and its relationship to meals and somatic activity. *Gut*, 11:91-99.

105. Holzknecht, G. (1909): Die normale Peristaltik des Colon. *Münch. Med. Wochenschr.*, 56:2401-2403.

106. Howard, E. R. (1968): Abnormality of anorectal physiology in Hirschsprung's disease. *Am. J. Dig. Dis.*, 13:432-433.

107. Howard, E. R., and Garrett, J. R. (1970): Electron microscopy of myenteric nerves in Hirschsprung's disease and in normal bowel. *Gut*, 11:1007-1014.

108. Howard, E. R., and Garrett, J. R. (1970): Histochemistry and electron microscopy of rectum and colon in Hirschsprung's disease. *Proc. R. Soc. Med.*, 63:1264-1266.

109. Hukuhara, T., and Miyaka, T. (1959): The intrinsic reflexes in the colon. *Jpn. J. Physiol.*, 9:49-55.

110. Ihre, T. (1974): Studies on anal function in continent and incontinent patients. *Scand. J. Gastroenterol. (Suppl. 25)*, 9:1-64.

111. Julé, Y. (1974): Étude *in vitro* de l'activité electromyographique du côlon proximal et distal du lapin. *J. Physiol. (Paris)*, 88:305-329.

112. Julé, Y. (1975): Modifications de l'activité électrique du côlon proximal de lapin *in vivo*, par stimulation des nerfs vagues et splanchniques. *J. Physiol. (Paris)*, 70:5-26.

113. Kent, G. C. (1965): *Comparative Anatomy of the Vertebrates.* C. V. Mosby Company, St. Louis.

114. Kern, F., Jr., Almy, T. P., Abbot, F. K., and Bogdonoff, M. D. (1951): The motility of the distal colon in non-specific ulcerative colitis. *Gastroenterology*, 19:492-503.

115. Kern, F., Jr., Almy, T. P., and Stolk, N. J. (1951): Effects of certain antispasmodic drugs on the intact human colon with special reference to Banthine (beta-diethylaminoethyl xanthene-9-carboxylate methobromide). *Am. J. Med.*, 11:67-74.

116. Kim, I. C., and Barbero, G. J. (1963): The pattern of rectosigmoid motility in children. *Gastroenterology*, 45:57-66.

117. Kobayashi, M., Nagai, T., and Prosser, C. L. (1966): Electrical interaction between muscle layers of cat intestine. *Am. J. Physiol.*, 211:1281-1291.

118. Kock, N. G., Hultén, L., and Leandoer, L. (1968): A study of the motility in different parts of the human colon. Resting activity, response to feeding and to prostigmine. *Scand. J. Gastroenterol.*, 3:163-169.

119. Konturek, S. J., Tasler, J., and Oblulowicz, W. (1972): Effect of atropine on pancreatic responses to endogenous and exogenous cholecystokinin. *Am. J. Dig. Dis.*, 17:911-917.

120. Lawson, J. O. N., and Nixon, H. H. (1967): Anal canal pressures in the diagnosis of Hirschsprung's disease. *J. Pediatr. Surg.*, 2:544-552.

121. Lewis, F. T. (1912): The development of the large intestine. In: *Manual of Human Embryology, Volume 2*, edited by F. Keibel and F. P. Mall, pp. 393-403. J. B. Lippincott Company, Philadelphia and London.

122. Lipkin, M., Almy, T., and Bell, B. M. (1962): Pressure-volume characteristics of the human colon. *J. Clin. Invest.*, 41:1831-1839.

123. Macbeth, W. A., and Hawthorne, J. H. (1965): Intramural ganglia in diverticular disease of the colon. *J. Clin. Pathol.*, 18:40-42.

124. Macewen, W. (1904): The Huxley lecture on the function of the caecum and appendix. *Lancet*, 2:995-1000.

125. Mackenna, B. R., and McKirdy, H. C. (1972): Peristalsis in the rabbit distal colon. *J. Physiol.*, 220:33-54.

126. Mann, C. V., and Hardcastle, J. D. (1970): Recent studies of colonic and rectal motor action. *Dis. Colon Rectum*, 13:225-230.

127. Meier-Ruge, W. (1968): Das Megacolon: seine Diagnose und Pathophysiologie. *Virchows Arch. (Pathol. Anat.)*, 344:67-85.

128. Mendeloff, A. I., Monk, M., Siegel, C. I., and Lilienfeld, A. (1970): Illness experience and life stresses in patients with irritable colon and with ulcerative colitis. An epidemiologic study of ulcerative colitis and regional enteritis in Baltimore, 1960-1964. *N. Engl. J. Med.*, 282:14-17.

129. Misiewicz, J. J., Connell, A. M., and Pontes, F. A. (1966): Comparison of the effect of meals and prostigmine on the proximal and distal colon in patients with and without diarrhoea. *Gut*, 7:468-473.

130. Misiewicz, J. J., Holdstock, D. J., and Waller, S. L. (1967): Motor responses of the human alimentary tract to near-maximal infusions of pentagastrin. *Gut*, 8:463-469.

131. Misiewicz, J. J., Waller, S. L., and Eisner, M. (1966): Motor responses of human gastrointestinal tract to 5-hydroxytryptamine *in vivo* and *in vitro*. *Gut*, 7:208-216.

132. Nickel, R., Schummer, A., and Sieferle, E. (1973): *The Viscera of Domestic Mammals*, translated and revised by W. O. Sack. Paul Parey, Berlin.

133. Pace, J. L. (1971): The age of appearance of the haustra of the human colon. *J. Anat.*, 109:75-80.

134. Painter, N. S. (1967): Diverticulosis of the colon—fact and speculation. *Am. J. Dig. Dis.*, 12:222-227.

135. Painter, N. S., and Truelove, S. C. (1964): The intraluminal pressure patterns in diverticulosis of the colon (parts I and II). *Gut,* 5:201–213.

136. Painter, N. S., and Truelove, S. C. (1964): The intraluminal pressure patterns in diverticulosis of the colon (parts III and IV). *Gut,* 5:365–373.

136a. Painter, N. S., Truelove, S. C., Ardran, G. M., and Tuckey, M. (1965): Segmentation and the localization of intraluminal pressures in the human colon, with special reference to the pathogenesis of colonic diverticula. *Gastroenterology,* 49:169–177.

137. Parks, A. G., Fishlock, D. J., Cameron, J. D. H., and May, H. (1969): Preliminary investigation of the pharmacology of the human internal anal sphincter. *Gut,* 10:674–677.

138. Passarge, E. (1967): The genetics of Hirschsprung's disease. Evidence for heterogeneous etiology and a study of sixty-three families. *N. Engl. J. Med.,* 276:138–143.

139. Phillips, S. F., and Edwards, D. A. W. (1965): Some aspects of anal continence and defaecation. *Gut,* 6:396–406.

140. Posey, E. L., Jr., Bargen, J. A., Dearing, W. H., and Code, C. F. (1948): The effects of certain so-called antispasmodics on intestinal motility. *Gastroenterology,* 11:344–356.

141. Posey, E. L, Jr., Dearing, W. H., Sauer, W. G., Bargen, J. A., and Code, C. F. (1948): The recording of intestinal motility. *Proc. Staff Mtgs. Mayo Clin.,* 23:297–304.

142. Raiford, T., and Mulinos, M. G. (1934): The myenteric reflex as exhibited by the exteriorized colon of the dog. *Am. J. Physiol.,* 110:129–136.

143. Rayner, V. (1971): Observations on the functional internal anal sphincter of the vervet monkey. *J. Physiol. (Lond.),* 213:27P–28P.

144. Ritchie, J. A. (1971): Movement of segmental constrictions in the human colon. *Gut,* 12:350–355.

145. Ritchie, J. A. (1972): Mass peristalsis in the human colon after contact with oxyphenisatin. *Gut,* 13:211–219.

146. Ritchie, J. A., Ardran, G. M., and Truelove, S. C. (1962): Motor activity of the sigmoid colon of humans. A combined study by intraluminal pressure recording and cineradiography. *Gastroenterology,* 43:642–668.

147. Rostad, H. (1973): Colonic motility in the cat. I. Extraluminal strain gage technique. Influence of anesthesia and temperature. *Acta Physiol. Scand.,* 89:79–90.

148. Rostad, H. (1973): Colonic motility in the cat. II. Extrinsic nervous control. *Acta Physiol. Scand.,* 89:91–103.

149. Rostad, H. (1973): Colonic motility in the cat. III. Influence of hypothalamic and mesencephalic stimulation. *Acta. Physiol. Scand.,* 89:104–115.

150. Rostad, H. (1973): Colonic motility in the cat. IV. Peripheral pathways mediating the effects induced by hypothalamic and mesencephalic stimulation. *Acta. Physiol. Scand.,* 89:154–168.

151. Rostad, H. (1973): Colonic motility in the cat. V. Influence of telencephalic stimulation and the peripheral pathways mediating the effects. *Acta. Physiol. Scand.,* 89:169–181.

152. Schnaufer, L., Talbert, J. L., Haller, J. A., Reid, N. C. R. W., Tobon, F., and Schuster, M. M. (1967): Differential sphincteric studies in the diagnosis of ano-rectal disorders of childhood. *J. Pediatr. Surg.,* 2:538–543.

153. Schuster, M. M., Hendrix, T. R., and Mendeloff, A. I. (1963): The internal anal sphincter response: manometric studies on its normal physiology, neural pathways, and alteration in bowel disorders. *J. Clin. Invest.,* 42:196–207.

154. Shearin, N. L., Bowes, K. L., and Kingma, Y. J. (1978): *In vitro* electrical activity in canine colon. *Gut,* 20:780–786.

155. Sisson, S. (1953): *The Anatomy of the Domestic Animals,* revised by J. D. Grossman, 4th edition, pp. 972. W. B. Saunders Company, Philadelphia.

156. Slack, W. W. (1966): Bowel muscle in diverticular disease. *Gut,* 7:668–670.

157. Smith, B. (1967): Myenteric plexus in Hirschsprung's disease. *Gut,* 8:308–312.

158. Snape, W. J., Jr., Carlson, G. M., and Cohen, S. (1976): Colonic myoelectric activity in the irritable bowel syndrome. *Gastroenterology,* 70:326–330.

159. Snape, W. J., Jr., Carlson, G. M., and Cohen, S. (1977): Human colonic myoelectric activity in response to prostigmine and the gastrointestinal hormones. *Am. J. Dig. Dis.,* 22:881–887.

160. Snape, W. J., Jr., Carlson, G. M., Matarazzo, S. A., and Cohen, S. (1977): Evidence that abnormal myoelectrical activity produces colonic motor dysfunction in the irritable bowel syndrome. *Gastroenterology,* 72:383–387.

161. Snape, W. J., Jr., Matarazzo, S. A., and Cohen, S. (1978): Effect of eating and gastrointestinal hormones on human colonic myoelectrical and motor activity. *Gastroenterology,* 75:373–378.

162. Snape, W. J., Jr., Wright, S. H., Battle, W. M., and Cohen, S. (1979): The gastrocolic response: evidence for a neural mechanism. *Gastroenterology,* 77:1235–1240.

163. Spriggs, E. A., Code, C. F., Bargen, J. A., Curtiss, R. K., and Hightower, N. C., Jr. (1951): Motility of the pelvic colon and rectum of normal persons and patients with ulcerative colitis. *Gastroenterology,* 19:480–491.

164. Stoddard, C. J., Duthie, H. L., Smallwood, R. H., and Linkens, D. A. (1979): Colonic myoelectrical activity in man: comparison of recording techniques and methods of analysis. *Gut,* 20:476–483.

165. Stonesifer, G. L., Jr., Murphy, G. P., and Lombardo, C. R. (1960): The anatomy of the anorectum. *Am. J. Surg.,* 10:666–671.

166. Sullivan, M. A., Cohen, S., and Snape, W. J., Jr. (1978): Colonic myoelectrical activity in irritable-bowel syndrome. Effect of eating and anticholinergics. *N. Engl. J. Med.,* 298:878–883.

167. Swenson, O., and Bill, A. H., Jr. (1948): Resection of the rectum and rectosigmoid with preservation of the sphincter for benign spastic lesions probably megacolon; an experimental study. *Surgery, 24:212–220.*

168. Taylor, I., Smallwood, R., and Duthie, H. L. (1974): Myoelectrical activity in the rectosigmoid in man. In: *Proceedings of the Fourth International Symposium on Gastrointestinal Motility,* edited by E. E. Daniel, pp. 109–119. Mitchell Press, Vancouver.

169. Templeton, R. D., and Lawson, H. (1931): Studies in the motor activity of the large intestine. I. Normal motility in the dog, recorded by the tandem balloon method. *Am. J. Physiol.,* 96:667–676.

170. Tobon, F., Reid, N. C. R. W., Talbert, J. L., and Schuster, M. M. (1968): Nonsurgical test for the diagnosis of Hirschsprung's disease. *N. Engl. J. Med.,* 278:188–194.

171. Truelove, S. C. (1966): Movements of the large intestine. *Physiol. Res.,* 46:457–512.

172. Ustach, T. J., Tobon, F., Hambrecht, T., Bass, D. D., and Schuster, M. M. (1970): Electrophysiological aspects of human sphincter function. *J. Clin. Invest.,* 49:41–48.

173. Vizi, S. E., Bertaccini, G., Impicciatore, M., and Knoll, J. (1973): Evidence that acetylcholine released by gastrin and related polypeptides contributes to their effect on gastrointestinal motility. *Gastroenterology,* 64:268–277.

174. Waller, S. L., and Misiewicz, J. J. (1969): Prognosis in the irritable bowel syndrome: a prospective study. *Lancet,* 2:754–756.

175. Walsh, J. H., Yalow, R. S., and Berson, S. A. (1971): The effect of atropine on plasma gastrin response to feeding. *Gastroenterology,* 60:16–21.

176. Wankling, W. J., Brown, B. H., Collins, C. D., and Duthie, H. L. (1968): Basal electrical activity in the anal canal in man. *Gut,* 457–460.

177. Welch, P. B., and Plaut, O. H. (1926): A graphic study of the muscular activity of the colon, with special reference to its response to feeding. *Am. J. Med. Sci.,* 172:261–268.

178. White, J. C., Verlot, M. G., and Ehrentheil, O. (1940): Neurogenic disturbances of the colon and their investigation by the colon-metrogram; preliminary report. *Ann. Surg.,* 112:1042–1057.

179. Whitehouse, F. R., and Kernohan, J. W. (1948): Myenteric plexus in congenital megacolon; study of 11 cases. *Arch. Intern. Med.,* 82:75–111.

180. Wienbeck, M., and Christensen, J. (1971): Cationic requirements of colon slow waves in the cat. *Am. J. Physiol.,* 220:513–519.

181. Wienbeck, M., and Christensen, J. (1971): Effects of some drugs on electrical activity of the isolated colon of the cat. *Gastroenterology,* 61:470-478.

182. Williams, I. (1968): Diverticular disease of the colon: a 1968 view. *Gut,* 9:498-501.

183. Wood, J. D., (1973): Electrical activity of the intestine of mice with hereditary megacolon and absence of enteric ganglion cells. *Am. J. Dig. Dis.,* 18:477-488.

184. Wood, J. D., (1974): Physiological studies on the large intestine of mice with hereditary megacolon and absence of enteric ganglion cells. In: *Proceedings of the Fourth International Symposium on Gastrointestinal Motility,* edited by E. E. Daniel, pp. 177-194. Mitchell Press, Vancouver.

185. Youmans, W. B. (1949): *Nervous and Neurohumoral Regulation of Intestinal Motility.* Interscience Publishers, Inc., New York.

Physiology of the Gastrointestinal Tract, edited by
Leonard R. Johnson, Raven Press, New York © 1981.

Chapter 15

Motility of the Gallbladder and Biliary Tree

James P. Ryan

The gallbladder performs two distinct but physiologically related functions (14). First, it absorbs most of the water and electrolytes from dilute hepatic bile, thereby producing a smaller volume of viscid, dark bile. Second, during a meal, it contracts and delivers its contents into the small intestine. This chapter will review the factors that regulate the motor activity of the gallbladder and the associated biliary tract.

The physiology of the gallbladder has been studied since the early years of this century. Lin (125) has referred to the first three decades as the golden age of research on the mechanism of bile delivery into the duodenum. Detailed reviews of the studies conducted during this era can be found in the reports of Mann (138) and Ivy (101). Essentially, the early years were characterized by significant advances in technology (14,80,139,143,172,177), experimental design (97,102), and theory (30,101). The advent of biliary tract intubation, manometric recordings systems, and the development of reliable *in vivo* procedures permitted the examination and quantification of parameters that previously evaded critical analysis.

It was during this period also that the concept of the humoral control of gallbladder motility was developed. Studies by numerous investigators demonstrated that the introduction of food (29,156), fat (29,92,155,156,204), egg yolk (92,156), and meat (30) into the duodenum enhanced the evacuation of bile and increased the amplitude of gallbladder contractions. They reported no change in activity, however, when the food products were given intravenously (93,227). Thus, several lines of evidence suggested the existence of a humoral agent, located within the duodenum, whose major function was the initiation of gallbladder motility.

In 1928, Ivy and Oldberg (102) successfully extracted from the upper intestinal mucosa of the hog a substance which, when injected intravenously into dogs, enhanced the evacuation of the gallbladder. They named the substance cholecystokinin (CCK) ("that which excites or moves the gallbladder"). Their cross-circulation experiments, as well as the experiments of Houssay and Rubio (97) with the viviperfused gallbladder, firmly established the hormonal nature of CCK.

In more recent years, the chemical isolation and identification of gastrin (81), secretin (112), and CCK (111,113) has permitted the evaluation of their effect on a number of target organs, including the biliary system. Coupled with improvements in *in vivo* (110,126,127,232) and *in vitro* (5,50,86) experimental design, significant advances have been made in our understanding of the factors that influence the pressures and flows within the biliary tree.

ANATOMY OF THE GALLBLADDER AND BILIARY TRACT

Gallbladder

The biliary tract arises as a series of closed-ended canaliculi formed by the apposition of specialized structures located in the cell membrane of adjacent hepatocytes (67,176). The liver synthesizes and actively secretes bile into the canaliculi, which communicate with numerous interlobular ducts. At the transverse fossa of the liver, the main ducts from the different liver lobes fuse to form the common hepatic duct. The gallbladder is an appendage of the common hepatic duct. After the cystic duct from the gallbladder joins the hepatic duct, the structure is known as the common bile duct (Fig. 1).

The human gallbladder is a pear-shaped sac approximately 7 to 10 cm long and 2 to 3 cm wide, with a storage capacity of 35 to 50 ml (34,211). It is located on the inferior surface of the liver and can be divided into three areas. The fundus is the broad-ended portion, which is palpated when the abdomen is examined. The body comprises the major portion of the gallbladder and terminates at the narrowed S-shaped neck region. Both the neck and the cystic duct are characterized by prominent mucosal foldings, the valves of Heister. Hartmann's pouch, a sacculation at the neck of the gallbladder, is a common site for a gallstone to lodge.

The wall of the gallbladder consists of the following layers: an inner mucous layer characterized by folds with scores of connective tissue analogous to intestinal villi, a lamina propria containing simple tuboaleolvar glands, a layer of irregularly oriented smooth muscle cells, a perimuscular connective tissue layer, and a serous layer that surrounds most of the gallbladder.

The major arterial supply of the gallbladder is by way of the cystic artery. This branch of the hepatic artery is large and demonstrates considerable anatomical variation. The veins of the gallbladder also are variable but tend to drain primarily into the hepatic capillaries. Blood may also drain into the cystic branch of the portal vein. A prominent feature of the gallbladder is its abundance of lymphatic vessels within the lamina propria and the connective tissue layer. The ultimate drainage of these vessels is into the cysterna chyli.

The gallbladder and bile ducts are liberally supplied with branches of the splanchnic sympathetics and the vagus nerve (117). Vagal fibers travel in the hepatic branch of the anterior vagal trunk. Sympathetic fibers come from the celiac plexus. Both afferent and efferent fibers are present. A myenteric plexus occurs in both the submucosa and subserosa layers. Ganglia are small and sparse around the neck of the gallbladder but increase in size and number over the body and fundus. The common duct mucosa contains many single neurons and small ganglia which are closely related to the mucous glands. The density of the plexuses increases in the sphincter of Oddi region.

Choledochoduodenal Junction

The common hepatic duct directs bile from the liver to a point where it joins the cystic duct from the gall-

bladder to form the common bile duct (ductus choledochus) (83). The common bile duct descends behind the first portion of the pancreas. As it passes obliquely through the duodenal wall, it is joined by the main pancreatic duct. The two structures form a common ductal segment and terminate at the ampulla of Vater. Although the name implies an enlargement, such a structure is not common in humans and the termination of the common bile duct and pancreatic duct is more correctly referred to as the papilla of Vater.

The region where the duodenal wall is penetrated by the biliary and pancreatic ducts has been termed the choledochoduodenal junction. For most of their passage through the duodenal wall, the common bile duct, the pancreatic duct, and the papilla are surrounded by a complex arrangement of smooth muscle, the sphincter of Oddi (Fig. 2).

In humans, the sphincter of Oddi can be divided into four sections (26). The first, the sphincter choledochus, is a sheath of circular smooth muscle surrounding the common bile duct from just proximal to its entrance into the duodenal wall (superior sphincter) to its junction with the pancreatic duct (inferior sphincter). The second, the fasiculi longitudinalis, is a grouping of longitudinally arranged muscle that occupies the spaces between the biliary and the pancreatic ducts. The sphincter ampullae, the third segment of the sphincter of Oddi, is a network of muscle fibers encircling the ampulla of Vater and is present in less than 20% of the adult human population. Finally, the sphincter pancreaticus is an arrangement of circular muscle fibers about the pancreatic duct, which may or may not be associated with the sphincter choledochus.

Although it has been almost 100 years since the noted Italian physiologist Rugero Oddi rediscovered Frances Glisson's "locking mechanism" (154), controversy still exists concerning the presence and significance of a truly independent sphincter. Because the muscle fibers encircling the common duct are often interlaced with fibers from the duodenal wall, several investigators have questioned the autonomy of Oddi's sphincter (59,66, 73,74,197). A detailed account of the early arguments and interpretations can be found in the reviews of Mann (138), Ivy (101), and Michels (146).

The majority of opinions support the existence of an anatomically distinct sphincter that is functionally independent of the duodenal musculature (33,83, 89,154,161). The careful anatomical investigations of Boyden and his associates (31–33,66,198) were of paramount importance in confirming the existence of the sphincter of Oddi. Their studies, conducted on several animal species, demonstrated unequivocally that the sphincter of Oddi musculature is anatomically and embryologically distinct from the musculature of the duodenum.

Much of the controversy connected with the sphincter of Oddi can be attributed to the numerous animal

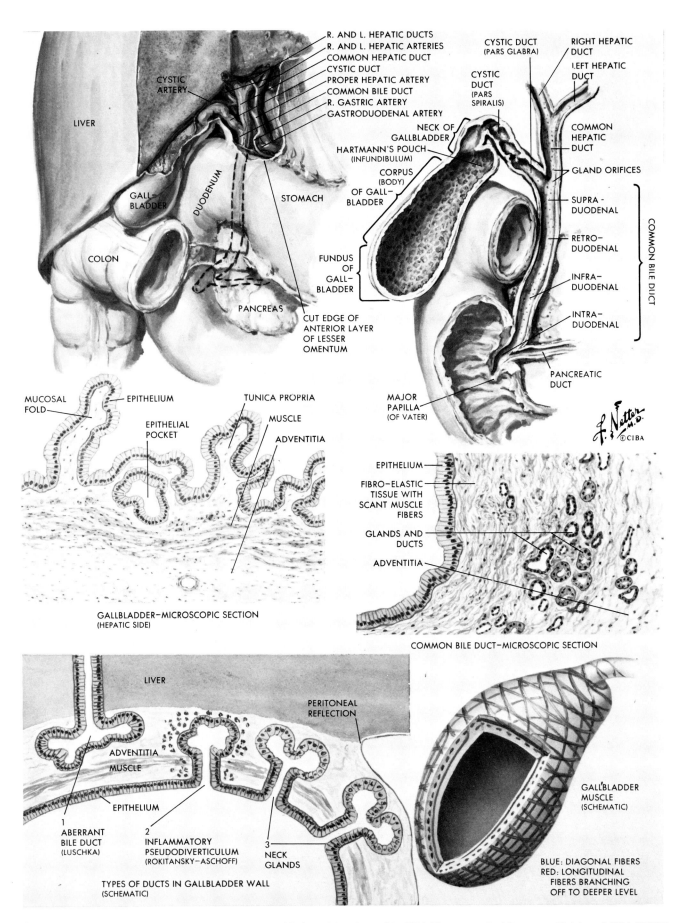

FIG. 1. Gross anatomy of the gallbladder and bile ducts. (© Copyright 1957, 1964 CIBA Pharmaceutical Company, Division of CIBA-GEIGY Corporation. Reproduced with permission, from *The CIBA Collection of Medical Illustrations*, Vol. 3, Part III, by Frank H. Netter. All rights reserved.)

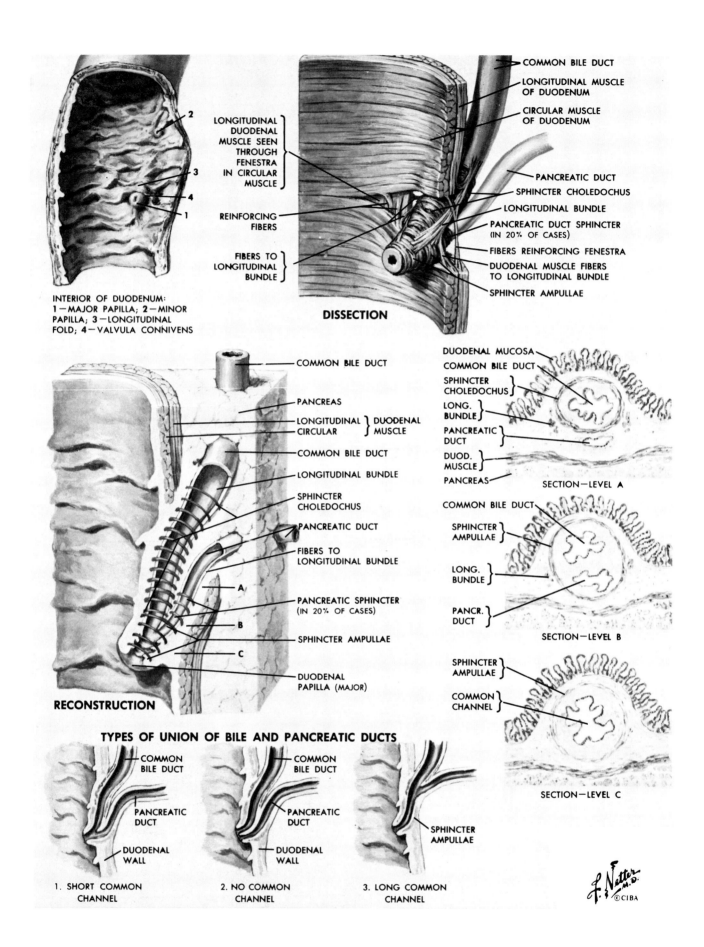

INTERIOR OF DUODENUM:
1—MAJOR PAPILLA; 2—MINOR PAPILLA; 3—LONGITUDINAL FOLD; 4—VALVULA CONNIVENS

LONGITUDINAL DUODENAL MUSCLE SEEN THROUGH FENESTRA IN CIRCULAR MUSCLE

REINFORCING FIBERS

FIBERS TO LONGITUDINAL BUNDLE

COMMON BILE DUCT

LONGITUDINAL MUSCLE OF DUODENUM

CIRCULAR MUSCLE OF DUODENUM

PANCREATIC DUCT

SPHINCTER CHOLEDOCHUS

LONGITUDINAL BUNDLE

PANCREATIC DUCT SPHINCTER (IN 20% OF CASES)

FIBERS REINFORCING FENESTRA

DUODENAL MUSCLE FIBERS TO LONGITUDINAL BUNDLE

SPHINCTER AMPULLAE

DISSECTION

COMMON BILE DUCT

PANCREAS

LONGITUDINAL } DUODENAL
CIRCULAR } MUSCLE

COMMON BILE DUCT

LONGITUDINAL BUNDLE

SPHINCTER CHOLEDOCHUS

PANCREATIC DUCT

FIBERS TO LONGITUDINAL BUNDLE

A

PANCREATIC SPHINCTER (IN 20% OF CASES)

B

SPHINCTER AMPULLAE

C

DUODENAL PAPILLA (MAJOR)

RECONSTRUCTION

DUODENAL MUCOSA
COMMON BILE DUCT
SPHINCTER CHOLEDOCHUS }
LONG. BUNDLE }
PANCREATIC DUCT }
DUOD. MUSCLE }
PANCREAS

SECTION—LEVEL A

COMMON BILE DUCT
SPHINCTER AMPULLAE }
LONG. BUNDLE }
PANCR. DUCT }

SECTION—LEVEL B

SPHINCTER AMPULLAE }
COMMON CHANNEL }

SECTION—LEVEL C

TYPES OF UNION OF BILE AND PANCREATIC DUCTS

COMMON BILE DUCT
PANCREATIC DUCT
DUODENAL WALL

1. SHORT COMMON CHANNEL

COMMON BILE DUCT
PANCREATIC DUCT
DUODENAL WALL

2. NO COMMON CHANNEL

SPHINCTER AMPULLAE

3. LONG COMMON CHANNEL

F. Netter M.D. ©CIBA

FIG. 2. Anatomy of the choledochoduodenal junction. (© Copyright 1957, 1964 CIBA Pharmaceutical Company, Division of CIBA-GEIGY Corporation. Reproduced, with permission, from *The CIBA Collections of Medical Illustrations*, Vol. 3, Part III, by Frank H. Netter. All rights reserved.)

models employed. In a recent review, Delmont (62) has attempted to standardize the vocabulary associated with the various portions of the sphincter. He has suggested that the sphincter of Oddi can be divided into five parts: (a) The sphincter choledochus proprius divides the common bile duct into two portions—an upper, longer, thin-walled, wide-lumened portion and a lower, shorter, thick-walled, narrowed-lumen portion of the common bile duct. It is located proximal to the common bile duct penetration into the duodenal wall and corresponds to Boyden's sphincter choledochus superior (33) and to the notch of Hand (83). (b) The sphincter pancreaticus proprius is analogous to Boyden's (33) musculature of the pancreatic duct. Papamiltiades and Rettori (161) have termed it simply the pancreatic sphincter. (c) The common papillary sphincter refers to the musculature surrounding the termination of the biliary and pancreatic ducts. Boyden (33) has referred to it as the sphincter ampullae or the sphincter papillae. (d) The infundibulum of the common bile duct is the region located between the sphincter choledochus superior above and the common papillary sphincter below. It corresponds to Papamiltiades and Rettori's (161) sphincter choledochus and approximately to Boyden's (33) sphincter choledochus inferius. (e) The pancreatic infundibulum is the structure located between the sphincter pancreaticus and the common papillary sphincter. Regardless of the classification, it is now generally accepted that the motor activity of the sphincter plays a significant role in the delivery of bile into the duodenum.

BILIARY TRACT PRESSURES

The presence of food in the duodenum causes the gallbladder to contract, its internal pressure to rise, and its X-ray shadow to become smaller (134). This forces bile into the common bile duct and, after relaxation of the sphincter of Oddi, bile flows into the duodenum. Although this concept is easily understood, as recently as the 1920s many investigators believed either that all the bile entering the gallbladder was absorbed (214) or that the gallbladder evacuation resulted from respiratory movements and externally applied pressures rather than from contraction of the gallbladder itself (234). The reviews of Ivy (101) and Hallenbeck (82) summarize the extensive data supporting the role of gallbladder contraction and sphincter relaxation in affecting gallbladder emptying.

A knowledge of the factors influencing intrabiliary pressures is important in understanding gallbladder filling and emptying. As in any system that involves the flow of liquid through tubes, biliary pressures depend upon the rate and pressure of bile flow into the system and upon the resistance to flow through the system (12,94).

The maximal secretory pressure of the liver has been determined by numerous investigators for several animal species (90,140,143,202). In general, the pressures vary between 15 and 30 cm bile. Kjellgren (114), using a T tube fitted at one end with a small balloon that could obstruct the bile duct, measured liver secretory pressures in cholecystectomized patients that ranged from 29 to 39 cm bile. The values represent the pressure available to move bile through the biliary system.

Resistance to bile flow through the common bile duct is influenced by several factors, including duct length and diameter. The principal determinant, however, is the contractile state of the sphincter of Oddi (82). Elman and McMaster (68) made the important observation that the resistance of the sphincter of Oddi in the postabsorptive state is greater than that following the ingestion of a meal. In general, under basal conditions, the sphincter of Oddi pressure ranges from 8 to 30 cm water. Bergh (20) reported that the pressure needed to overcome the resistance to flow through the sphincter of Oddi in the human was usually 12 to 15 cm water but ranged from 9 to 23 cm water in different patients.

It is obvious that the pressure in the biliary tract depends on the rate of bile secretion and the resistance to bile flow through the sphincter of Oddi. Potter and Mann (172) were among the first to measure biliary tract pressures in the unanesthetized dog by a method that did not remove the influence of the sphincter of Oddi. They reported a mean common bile duct pressure of 11.7 cm bile, and an average intraluminal gallbladder pressure of 14.1 cm bile. In a more recent study, Gilsdorf (78) monitored the pressure within the gallbladder and common bile duct of the conscious dog during basal conditions and following the ingestion of a meal. Similar to the findings of Potter and Mann (172), there was no significant difference between gallbladder and ductal pressures recorded in the fasted state. Upon feeding, the gallbladder pressure rose 60% and bile flowed freely into the duodenum. Although Gilsdorf (78) did not comment on any change in common bile duct pressure, others have documented that the pressure normally increases above basal levels (21,68,144,147). This increase can be attributed to the enhanced rate of bile flow through the ducts (82,143).

In summary, during the basal (postabsorptive) state the resistance of the sphincter of Oddi is approximately 12 to 15 cm water, and the pressure in the common bile duct is slightly less. The pressure within the common duct exceeds any resistance to flow through the cystic duct, and therefore bile enters the gallbladder. During this period the secretory rate of the liver is minimal, and only occasionally are conditions optimal for the delivery of bile into the duodenum.

With the entrance of chyme into the duodenum, the rate of hepatic bile secretion increases and the gallbladder contracts. Both factors contribute to an increase in common bile duct pressure. At the same time the resistance to bile flow through the sphincter decreases. Each of these events favors the delivery of bile into the duodenum.

GALLBLADDER MOTILITY

Hormonal Control

Cholecystokinin

It was demonstrated very early in this century that the presence of food in the duodenum enhanced gallbladder emptying (101,102,138). In addition, the studies firmly established the humoral nature of the stimulus. Initial attempts by Whitaker (230) and Copher and Illingsworth (46) to identify the humoral agent involved, however, met with little success. In 1928, Ivy and Oldberg (102) extracted from the upper small intestinal mucosa of the hog a substance which, when injected intravenously, caused contraction and evacuation of the gallbladder. Moreover, in a series of carotid-to-carotid cross-circulation experiments, they reported that the introduction of dilute hydrochloric acid into the duodenum of one dog was followed by gallbladder contraction in both animals. Thus, the evidence indicated that a hormone was involved and the authors named the substance cholecystokinin (CCK).

The isolation and purification of CCK was accomplished by Jorpes and Mutt (111–113) in the early 1960s. CCK is a linear polypeptide hormone containing 33 amino acids. It is found in the jejunum, with lesser amounts in the duodenum and ileum (24), and is localized in a specific cell type of the APUD series, the "I" cell (207). Because of the lack of a specific and sensitive radioimmunoassay for CCK, the physiological levels of the hormone have not been determined. CCK is released from the endocrine cells of the small intestine in response to a variety of digestion products, particularly phenylalanine and tryptophan (61), fatty acids (45), and hydrogen ions (142).

During the isolation and purification of CCK, Mutt and Jorpes (149,150) found that the C-terminal octapeptide region of the whole molecule was capable of stimulating the pancreas and the gallbladder. The fragment was later synthesized by Ondetti (157) and subsequently shown to have an even greater contractile effect on the gallbladder than the extracted CCK preparation. Hedner (86), using isolated muscle strips of guinea pig gallbladder, reported that the octapeptide of cholecystokinin (OP-CCK) was about 10 times more active on a weight basis and approximately 3 times more potent on a molar basis than the whole molecule. Rubin and coworkers (178) confirmed Hedner's (86) observation in three animal preparations, the guinea pig gallbladder in vitro and the guinea pig and canine gallbladder in vivo.

The cholecystokinetic activity of CCK and OP-CCK has been established in a number of different species using both in vivo and in vitro preparations. Table 1 lists several of these studies and summarizes the minimal effective dose of hormone needed to elicit contraction of the gallbladder. The wide variation in the reported threshold dose values can be attributed to species differences, the route of hormone administration, the sensitivity of the recording systems, and the purity of the various CCK preparations.

Several investigators have examined the cholecystokinetic activity of CCK in humans (38,136,208,212,223). Although most studies have been performed in vivo, Cameron et al. (38) used an in vitro tissue preparation to demonstrate the dose-related shortening of the gallbladder to varying concentrations of CCK (Fig. 3).

In vivo, several methods for evaluating the gallbladder response to CCK have been designed (40,77,98). The classical and most frequently employed technique in-

TABLE 1. Cholecystokinetic activity of CCK and OP-CCK

Hormone	Species[a]	Threshold dose[b]	Method	Ref.
CCK	Dog	4 ng/(kg·hr)	In vivo	124
CCK	Dog	18 ng/kg	In vivo	225
OP-CCK	Cat	0.25 ng/ml	In vitro	43
CCK	Rabbit	0.006 IDU/ml	In vitro	7
CCK	GP	0.08 ng/ml	In vitro	236
CCK	GP	3 ng/ml	In vitro	178
CCK	GP	300 ng/ml	In vitro	87
OP-CCK	GP	15 ng/ml	In vitro	178
OP-CCK	Opossum	0.05 ng/ml	In vitro	180
OP-CCK	Opossum	0.025 μg/(kg·hr)	In vivo	181
OP-CCK	Human	2.5 ng/kl	In vivo	212
CCK	Human	0.0625 CHR/(kg·min)	In vivo	136
CCK	Human	0.04 IDU/ml	In vitro	38
CCK	Human	0.02 CHR/(kg·min)	In vivo	208

[a]GP, guinea pig.
[b]IDU, Ivy Dog Unit; CHR, Crick-Harper-Raper Unit.

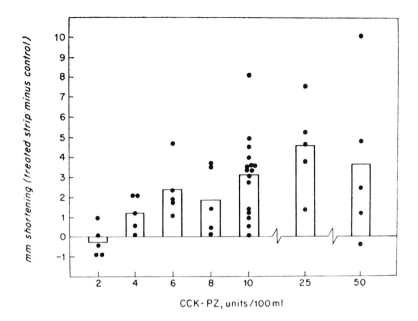

FIG. 3. Dose-response shortening of human gallbladder muscle strips treated for 30 min with different concentrations of cholecystokinin. (From Cameron et al., ref. 38, with permission.)

volves opacification of the gallbladder with an oral cholecystographic agent and the monitoring of the evacuation process with regularly spaced radiographs (31,91,162,203). The volume of the gallbladder is then estimated by planimetric measurement of the radiopaque areas. Edholm (65), using planigraphic measurements of gallbladder length and width, found that there was a prompt and rapid evacuation of the gallbladder in normal fasting human subjects following the injection of 1 Ivy dog unit/kg CCK. On the average, about 38% of the initial volume was emptied within the first 15 min. Sturdevant and his co-workers (212), using 18 healthy male subjects, reported a 44% decrease in gallbladder size following the bolus infusion of 2 ng/kg OP-CCK.

In 1966, Englert and Chiu (69) were the first to monitor gallbladder evacuation by combining a radionuclide that is secreted in bile with continuous external recording by means of a scintillation counter. Using ^{131}I-labeled iopanoic acid, they measured a 32% decrease in the initial gallbladder volume following a bolus injection of CCK. Significantly, the ingestion of a fatty meal or the slow intravenous administration of CCK produced a sustained contraction, which, after about 20 min, resulted in virtually complete gallbladder emptying. Hedner and Lunderquist (87) reported similar findings while examining the effect of bolus and continuous infusions of OP-CCK on gallbladder motility. The incomplete emptying of the gallbladder after a bolus injection of CCK or OP-CCK appears to be related to an excessive contraction of the infundibulum relative to the remainder of the gallbladder (224). The reason for this regional sensitivity is not known.

CCK and OP-CCK act directly on gallbladder smooth muscle. Hedner (86,88) reported that atropine had no effect on the guinea pig gallbladder response to CCK,

either *in vitro* or *in vivo*. Amer and Becvar (5,7), using rabbits, confirmed this finding and extended the observation by demonstrating that CCK-induced gallbladder contractions were unaffected by α- or β-adrenergic blockage. Similarly, the response to CCK is unaltered by depolarizing agents or tetrodotoxin (8,236).

The mechanism through which CCK or OP-CCK excites gallbladder smooth muscle appears to be associated with changes in intracellular cyclic nucleotide concentrations. Amer (5) reported that imidazole, an agent known to alter intracellular cyclic nucleotide levels, acetylcholine, and CCK each contracted isolated muscle strips from the rabbit gallbladder and that the response could be blocked by cAMP and by theophylline and glucagon, known stimulants of cAMP. In a later study, Amer and McKinney (8) found that the excitatory effect of CCK or OP-CCK on rabbit and guinea pig gallbladders was preceded by a significant increase in intracellular phosphodiesterase enzyme activity and a subsequent reduction in cAMP content. Andersson and his associates (10a) also confirmed the relationship between CCK stimulation, intracellular cAMP levels, and phosphodiesterase enzyme activity. They reported a 50% increase in phosphodiesterase activity and a 33% reduction in cAMP content following CCK stimulation. They proposed that the contractile state of the gallbladder depends upon the intracellular levels of cAMP and that CCK-stimulated gallbladder contractions are the direct result of a phosphodiesterase-induced reduction in cAMP content. The authors thought this hypothesis was reasonable, since such a mechanism of action had been described for other hormones (11,166,175).

Not all the data are consistent with the idea that CCK-induced gallbladder contraction results from reductions in intracellular cAMP levels. Amer in a later study (6) failed to measure any significant reduction in gallbladder cAMP content, despite a measurable rise in phosphodiesterase activity. He did report, however, a significant increase in cGMP levels. He interpreted the previously reported reductions in cAMP as unimportant and secondary to cGMP increases. He noted that cGMP had previously been shown to enhance cAMP breakdown in other systems (16,76). In a more recent study, Andersson and his associates (10a) also have reported significant increases in cGMP levels following stimulation with OP-CCK. However, indomethacin, although abolishing the CCK induced rise in cGMP, had no affect on the contractile response. Thus, the exact role of cGMP in CCK-mediated gallbladder contraction remains unsettled.

In summary, CCK-induced gallbladder contractions are unaffected by either cholinergic or α- and β-adrenergic blockade and thus act independently of the autonomic nervous system. On the other hand, the mechanical activity of the gallbladder appears to be associated with alterations in intracellular cyclic nucleotide content. The specific nucleotide involved remains unresolved. The discrepancies in the literature may reflect species differences, insensitive or nonspecific measurement techniques, or might simply reflect the complexity of the CCK–gallbladder interaction.

Gastrin, Caerulein

Structural similarities exist between CCK and the antral hormone, gastrin (63). Each of the peptides share an identical carboxyterminal pentapeptide amide and a tyrosine residue at position 6 (gastrin) or 7 (CCK), counting, unconventionally from the carboxyl terminus. For CCK and OP-CCK, sulfation of the tyrosyl residue is essential for cholecystokinetic activity (157). Rubin et al. (178) noted that the C-terminal tetrapeptide, on both a weight basis and a molar basis, was less potent than CCK and OP-CCK in contracting the guinea pig gallbladder. Similar findings were reported by Vagne and Grossman (225). Ondetti et al. (157) demonstrated that desulfation of the tyrosyl residue or the exchange of the tyrosyl-O-sulfate with aspartic acid at position 6 resulted in a significant decrease in the cholecystokinetic potency of the hormone. On the other hand, gastrin exists in both the unsulfated (gastrin I) and the sulfated form (gastrin II), and both forms are equipotent on most target organs (25).

Because of structural similarities, it should not be surprising that gastrin has been reported to exhibit cholecystokinetic activity (151,173,178,225,236). Vagne and Grossman (225) were the first to demonstrate this activity while examining the potency of several peptides on gallbladder contraction in the unconscious dog. They found that sulfated and unsulfated gastrin were equally effective in contracting the gallbladder. However, on a molar basis, gastrin was only 1/22 as potent as CCK.

This finding was later confirmed by Bertaccini et al. (23) and by Lin and Spray (127). Amer (4) reported that in vitro, gastrin II was 20 to 33 times less potent than CCK in contracting either rabbit or guinea pig gallbladder muscle strips. More recently, Chowdhury and his colleagues (43) demonstrated that gastrin I contracted isolated muscle strips from cat gallbladder. The concentration of gastrin required, however, was 1,000 times greater than the amounts of OP-CCK required to produce an equivalent response. The synthetic analog of gastrin, pentagastrin, also has been shown to have cholecystokinetic activity (151). However, the doses required to elicit a contraction were far in excess of the minimally effective doses of either CCK or OP-CCK. Toouli and Watts (223) reported that gastrin contracted all parts of the canine extrahepatic biliary tract and the common bile duct in man. Their results are difficult to interpret, however, because of the use of impure hormone preparations.

Not all studies confirmed the cholecystokinetic effect of gastrin. Cameron et al. (38) were unable to record any contractions from isolated strips of human gallbladder exposed for 20 min to a bathing solution containing gastrin I. Ryan and Cohen (180,181) were unable to produce gallbladder contraction in the guinea pig, in vitro, or in the opossum, in vivo, while using a broad dose range of gastrin I. It is now commonly believed that the stimulatory effect of gastrin observed in some studes can be attributed to the pharmacological properties rather than to the physiological properties of the hormone (225). The doses required for contraction of the gallbladder far exceed the minimal dose necessary for stimulation of gastric acid secretion. The latter response has been taken as a criterion for evaluating the importance of gastrin on a target organ.

Caerulein, a decapeptide isolated from frog skin, has a carboxyterminal pentapeptide portion identical with that of CCK and gastrin (9). Similar to CCK, it has a sulfated tyrosine residue at position 7. Johnson and Grossman (108) have shown that desulfation of the peptide produced an agonist that was 1/160 as potent as the natural, sulfated peptide in stimulating gallbladder motility. Fara and Erde (72) reported that sulfate caerulein was 75 times more potent than the unsulfated peptide in contracting the guinea pig gallbladder.

Unlike gastrin, caerulein is an extremely potent stimulant of gallbladder motility both in vitro and in vivo (70). Yau et al. (236) reported that, in vitro, caerulein was 2 times as potent as CCK on a molar basis in contracting the guinea pig gallbladder. In vivo, caerulein has been found to be 10 times as active as CCK on a molar basis (23) and 47 times as potent on a weight basis (236). Lin and Spray (127) reported that the intravenous infusion of caerulein at 10 ng/(kg.hr) significantly increased intragallbladder pressure. In the same study, the minimal effective dose of CCK was 40 ng/(kg·hr). Since this peptide is not present in humans, the physiological significance remains obscure. In theory, it may provide a way for future experimentalists and clinicians to stimulate gallbladder motility while avoiding the unwanted side effects that often accompany the administration of large amounts of CCK. The relative cholecystokinetic activity of CCK and structurally related peptides is summarized in Table 2.

Secretin, Vasoactive Intestinal Peptide, Glucagon

Two distinct groups, or families, of gastrointestinal hormones have been identified, the gastrin family and the secretin family. Each group consists of peptides that are both structurally and, in many cases, functionally related (63). Gastrin and CCK comprise the members of the gastrin family. Their effects on gallbladder motility have already been discussed.

Four polypeptides are members of the secretin family: secretin, glucagon, vasoactive intestinal polypeptide (VIP), and gastric inhibitory peptide (GIP). Unlike the gastrin-CCK family, the entire molecule is required for biological activity (63). Secretin, VIP, and glucagon each has been reported to affect gallbladder motility.

The early studies of Boyden (29,30,31), Ivy and Oldberg (102), and others (15,41) established that gallbladder emptying occurred following the instillation of acid into the duodenum. Although it is now known that CCK is released along with secretin in response to a large acid load in the intestine, these investigators felt that secretin played a physiological role in regulating gallbladder motility. The more recent literature, although variable in its findings, does not support this hypothesis.

Stening and Grossman (210), using dogs fitted with chronic gallbladder and gastric fistulas, measured the gallbladder pressure response to exogenously administered and endogenously released secretin. They observed that when secretin was given alone, no change in gallbladder motility could be recorded. They did report, however, that the simultaneous administration of secretin with CCK, or the endogenous release of secretin in association with CCK administration, shifted the CCK dose-response curve to the left. They concluded that endogenously released secretin enhanced the activity of CCK on gallbladder motility. Lin and Spray (127) confirmed that secretin augments the cholecystokinetic action of CCK in conscious dogs and, in addition, found that both natural and synthetic secretin preparations increased intragallbladder pressure. More recently, Vagne and Troitskaja (226) have reported that secretin augments CCK-induced gallbladder contractions in the anesthetized guinea pig. Given alone, however, secretin had no effect on motility. The inability of secretin alone to induce gallbladder contraction *in vivo* also has been reported for the anesthetized cat (105) and opossum (181,182). In the latter studies, secretin had a moderate relaxing effect on basal gallbladder pressures.

Most *in vitro* studies are in agreement with the *in vivo* observations that secretin is ineffective in contracting the gallbladder. Although the initial studies of Toouli and Watts (223) and Cameron et al. (38) suggested a slight cholecystokinetic response to secretin, the authors cautioned against attaching any significance to their findings because of the impure hormone preparations they used. More recent studies, utilizing purer hormone preparations, have failed to measure any contractile response to secretin. Chowdhury et al. (43), however,

TABLE 2. *Relative cholecystokinetic activity of CCK and structurally related peptides*

Hormone	Species[a]	Potency[b]	Method	Ref.
CCK	Dog, GP	1	*In vivo*	225,23
Gastrin I	Dog	1:22	*In vivo*	225,23
Gastrin I	Dog	1:22	*In vivo*	225,23
Pentapeptide	Dog	1:160	*In vivo*	225,23
Pentapeptide	Dog	1:123	*In vivo*	38,124,125
Tetrapeptide	Dog	1:160	*In vivo*	225
Tetrapeptide	Dog	1:132	*In vivo*	124
OP-CCK	Dog	23:1	*In vivo*	178
OP-CCK	GP	128:1	*In vivo*	178
Caerulein	Dog, GP	16:1	*In vitro*	23,225
CCK	GP, rabbit	1	*In vitro*	4,236
Gastrin I	GP	1:630-1,000	*In vitro*	4,23
Gastrin II	GP	1:33	*In vitro*	4
OP-CCK	GP	10:1	*In vitro*	236
Caerulein	GP	2.3:1	*In vitro*	236
Gastrin I	Rabbit	1:420-1,555	*In vitro*	4,23
Gastrin II	Rabbit	1:20	*In vitro*	4

[a]GP, guinea pig.
[b]Relative to CCK.

have also suggested that secretin can potentiate the effect of OP-CCK on gallbladder motor activity.

The physiological significance of secretin-CCK interaction, if any, is not known. The doses of secretin required to demonstrate the augmentation far exceed those required for the stimulation of pancreatic secretion, a known physiological response to secretin. Thus, the effect may be pharmacological. Further studies integrating the plasma levels of secretin and CCK with the contractile state of the gallbladder are needed to confirm this assumption.

VIP, a recently isolated peptide that is chemically related to secretin, exhibits a broad spectrum of biological actions (185–187). One prominent action appears to be a profound inhibition of basal and CCK-stimulated gallbladder motor activity (Fig. 4). Piper et al. (171) were the first to report this inhibition using an isolated superfused guinea pig gallbladder preparation. Later studies on the opossum (184), guinea pig (226), and cat (103,104) in vivo and the guinea pig in vitro (183) confirmed the inhibitory effect of VIP on the gallbladder.

The physiological significance of the inhibitory effect of VIP on resting gallbladder tone must remain speculative until reliable studies can demonstrate the true physiological actions of endogenously released VIP. No release of VIP is seen after a meal and fasting blood levels are extremely low (24). Sundler and his associates (213) recently reported the presence of VIP-containing nerve fibers in the smooth muscle layers of the feline and human gallbladder. This finding is significant, since other authors (35) have postulated that VIP functions as neurotransmitter and since it is known that electrical stimulation of the vagus increases the concentration of VIP in the portal blood (193). It is possible, therefore, that VIP acts locally to modulate the tone of the gallbladder smooth muscle.

Glucagon, another member of the secretin family of hormones, does not exhibit any excitatory or inhibitory effect on the human (38) or guinea pig (225) gallbladder in vitro. In vivo, Lin and Spray (126) reported relaxation of the canine gallbladder following either the subcutaneous or intravenous administration of glucagon. In humans, the size of the gallbladder has been reported to increase significantly following glucagon administration (42). The doses of glucagon required for relaxation of the gallbladder in vivo far exceed those required for glycogenesis. This suggests that a physiological role for glucagon in the regulation of gallbladder motility is unlikely. GIP, the additional member of the secretin family of gut hormones, has not been reported to have any effect on gallbladder motor function.

Hormone Interaction

It is now well appreciated and accepted that the response of a target organ to a particular gut hormone can often times be modified by the presence of additional gut hormones (107). As noted previously, Stening and Grossman (210) reported that both the exogenous administration and the endogenous release of secretin significantly augmented the contractile effect of CCK on the canine gallbladder. Vagne and Troitskaja (226) reported that secretin increased the cholecystokinetic effects of CCK on the gallbladder of the anesthetized guinea pig. Similar findings have also been reported for the feline gallbladder (43).

Not all the studies have confirmed the augmented response to CCK in the presence of secretin. Cameron and his associates (38) were unable to demonstrate any secretin augmentation of CCK in isolated strips of human gallbladder. Similarly, Ryan and Cohen (180–182) have reported that secretin antagonizes the contractile response of the gallbladder to CCK, both in vivo and in vitro. The reasons for the discrepancies in the literature are not readily apparent. The potentiating effect may be due to a pharmacological response of the gallbladder to secretin infusion or to the endogenous release of CCK or some other gut peptide with inherent cholecystokinetic activity.

There is little doubt that VIP relaxes the CCK-stimulated gallbladder both in vivo and in vitro (183,185). Vagne and Troitskaja (226) reported that 1 μg VIP significantly decreased the contractile response of the guinea pig gallbladder to 0.2 units CCK. In a later study, Ryan and Ryave (184) demonstrated that as little as 0.1 μg/ml VIP could significantly reduce the contractile response of the guinea pig gallbladder to 10 ng/ml OP-CCK. In the opossum (183), in vivo, infusion of VIP at 2 μg/(kg·hr) significantly antagonized the gallbladder response to a maximally effective dose of CCK 0.25 μg/(kg·hr). The physiological significance of these observations awaits clarification. The localization

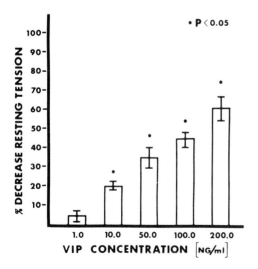

FIG. 4. Effect of VIP on resting tension of isolated gallbladder smooth muscle strips. (From Ryan and Ryave, ref. 184, with permission.)

of a peptide in neurons within the muscular wall of the gallbladder suggests a possible role for the neural modulation of hormonal influences on gallbladder motility.

Both gastrin and CCK have been shown to contract the gallbladder (103,125) and interactions between the two hormones are common (109). However, Ryan and Cohen (180) using isolated strips of guinea pig gallbladder *in vitro* failed to demonstrate any effect of gastrin on CCK-induced contractions. On the other hand, in the opossum *in vivo,* gastrin infusion in dose ranges from 0.125 to 0.50 μg/(kg$\cdot$hr) significantly reduced the expected cholecystokinetic response to 0.25 μg/(kg$\cdot$hr) CCK (181). The degree of inhibition was dose-related. Similarly, Chowdhury et al. (43) reported that the addition of gastrin to an *in vitro* bathing solution containing a maximal dose of OP-CCK decreased the contractile response of the feline gallbladder. The high dose of gastrin used in these studies makes it unlikely that this interaction has any physiological significance.

In summary, a number of gastrointestinal hormones have been shown to have an effect on the contractile state of the gallbladder. In addition, the action of a single hormone can often be altered by the presence of an additional gut peptide. With the exception of CCK, however, the physiological significance of these observations remains speculative. A summary of the different hormone interactions evaluated to date is presented in Table 3.

Neural Control

Parasympathetic Influence

It is well documented that exogenous stimulation of the gallbladder with acetylcholine or other parasympathomimetic drugs increases the tone and motility of the gallbladder (7,88,115,128,180,196,223,234,236). In addition, electrical stimulation of the parasympathetic nerves to the biliary tract increases the pressure within the common bile duct. This pressure rise is due to both an increase in gallbladder motility and an increase in the rate of bile flow (160,221). Despite the obvious effects of acetylcholine and vagal stimulation on biliary pressures, it has been known since the early years of this century that the increased pressures are not associated with any evacuation of the gallbladder (13,101,138). Thus, the physiological significance of the vagal innervation to the gallbladder remains uncertain.

Numerous investigators have reported that total vagotomy produces atony of the gallbladder and bile ducts (27,47,84,95,106,179,231). Johnson and Boyden (106) in 1952 found that complete severence of the vagi in humans resulted in an enlargement of the gallbladder and almost doubled its fasting volume. Rudic and Hutchinson (179) assessed gallbladder function by means of oral cholecystography and intravenous cholangiography and reported that total vagotomy was followed by an almost 100% increase in the fasting volume of the gallbladder. Significantly, anterior selective vagotomy, with preservation of the hepatic branch, had no significant affect on the fasting volume of the gallbladder.

The differences between the effect of total vagotomy and selective vagotomy have been reported by several investigators (3,99,163). Inberg and Vuorio (99) compared the effect of selective vagotomy and total vagotomy on the resting volume of the gallbladder in 68 patients and concluded that dilation of the gallbladder results from sectioning of the anterior hepatic branch of the vagus. Similar studies by Parkin et al. (163) in humans and Amdrup and Griffith (3) in dogs have confirmed the role of the hepatic and celiac vagi in maintaining gallbladder tone.

Not all authors have reported a change in gallbladder tone following complete vagotomy (17,79,116). Glanville and Duthie (79) measured the contractile response of the gallbladder in humans before and after total subdiaphragmatic vagotomy with pyloroplasty. They could demonstrate no change in the mean area of the gall-

TABLE 3. *Effect of gastrointestinal hormones on gallbladder motility in response to CCK*

Hormone pair[a]	Species[b]	Results[c]	Method	Ref.
CCK + secretin	Dog	Enhancement	*In vivo*	210
CCK + secretin	GP	Enhancement	*In vivo*	226
CCK + secretin	Cat	Enhancement	*In vitro*	43
CCK + secretin	Human	No effect	*In vitro*	38
CCK + secretin	GP	Inhibition	*In vitro*	180
CCK + secretin	Opossum	Inhibition	*In vivo*	181
CCK + VIP	GP	Inhibition	*In vivo*	226
CCK + VIP	GP	Inhibition	*In vitro*	184
CCK + VIP	Opossum	Inhibition	*In vivo*	183
CCK + G	GP	No effect	*In vitro*	180
CCK + G	Opossum	Inhibition	*In vivo*	181
CCK + G	Cat	Inhibition	*In vitro*	43

[a]G, gastrin.
[b]GP, guinea pig.
[c]Relative to CCK control response.

bladder when examined within 1 year of the surgical procedure. Similar findings have been reported by Beneventano el al. (17) in acute experiments in dogs. It is now generally agreed that the decreased tone of the gallbladder and the subsequent dilatation that occurs after vagatomy develop slowly but progressively and may not become evident for several months to a year or more. This might explain why some investigators failed to demonstrate any significant change in the resting gallbladder tone (17,79).

The cause of gallbladder dilation following total vagotomy has not been adequately explained but has been linked to an increase in intragallbladder pressure (233). Williams and Huang (233) measured the intraluminal pressure of the gallbladder in 23 dogs both before and following complete truncal vagotomy and noted an almost immediate and significant rise in pressure, which was maintained (Fig. 5). No studies have yet determined the causative factors for the rise in gallbladder pressure. The authors suggested it may be due to alterations in bile flow rate or sphincter of Oddi tone.

Most studies while examining the effect of vagotomy on gallbladder tone also have evaluated the ability of the gallbladder to contract in response to a fatty meal. Although Johnson and Boyden (106) and Rudick and Hutchinson (179) reported a decreased emptying rate following complete vagotomy, most investigators have failed to demonstrate any significant change in evacuation rate. This was true whether or not the authors noted any change in the resting volume of the gallbladder. It appears, therefore, that vagal innervation of the gallbladder is responsible for affecting the tone of the organ, whereas emptying is primarily determined by hormonal (CCK) influences.

Although gallbladder emptying in response to endogenous CCK release appears unaffected by total vagotomy, some investigators have reported a change in sensitivity of the gallbladder to exogenously administered CCK. Tinker and Cox (222) found that a dose of CCK that was uneffective in contracting the gallbladder of humans with intact vagi, produced a 27% reduction in the area of the gallbladder following truncal vagotomy. Isaza and colleagues (100) demonstrated that the intravenous administration of CCK prolonged the duration of gallbladder contractions in dogs subjected to a complete vagotomy. More recently, Malagelada, et al. (135) have shown that the threshold response of the gallbladder to CCK, as measured by bile acid output, was reduced by vagotomy. It should be pointed out that studies on the anesthetized cat (123), dog (2), and rabbit (71) have all failed to demonstrate any enhanced response to CCK following vagotomy. Although the explanation for these different findings is not readily apparent, it might well be related to species differences or to the influence of anesthesia. Table 4 summarizes the effect of complete vagotomy on gallbladder motility.

The increased sensitivity of the gallbladder to CCK after vagotomy has been explained in the context of Cannon's law of denervation supersensitivity (39), in this case to a hormonal stimulus (222). One explanation that has not been considered relates to the recent observation that VIP is found within nerve terminals associated with gallbladder smooth muscle (213) and that the peptide, a potent inhibitor of gallbladder smooth muscle (183,184,186), is released upon extrinsic vagal stimulation (193). Denervation might well be associated with a decreased content or release of VIP. The removal of an inhibitory influence would be expected, therefore, to result in a greater contractile response to a given agonist. This hypothesis must remain speculative until the physiological role of VIP can be determined.

In summary, parasympathetic influences on gallbladder motor activity seem to be of primary importance in maintaining the tone of the gallbladder. Sectioning of the vagal fibers innervating the gallbladder results in a decrease in tone, which is associated with an increase

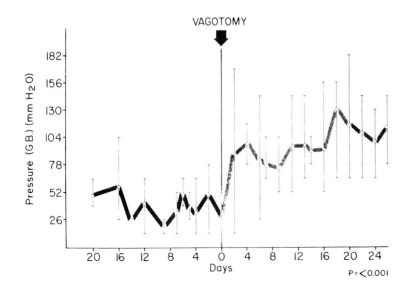

FIG. 5. Effect of vagotomy on the intraluminal pressure of gallbladder in dogs. The difference in pre- and postvagotomy pressures is significant. (From Williams and Huang, ref. 233, with permission.)

TABLE 4. *Effect of total vagotomy on gallbladder tone and motor activity*

Species	Fasting volume	Emptying	Response to CCK	Ref.
Human	Increase	Decrease	—	106
Human	No change	No change	—	79
Human	Increase	No change	—	99
Human	Increase	No change	—	163
Human	Increase	—	—	179
Human	Increase	—	No change	71
Human	—	—	Increase	135
Human	—	—	Increase	222
Dog	Increase	—	—	231
Dog	No change	No change	—	3
Dog	No change	—	No change	100
Dog	Increase	—	No change	2
Cat	Increase	—	Decrease	121
Rabbit	—	—	Decrease	100

in fasting volume. The contractile response induced by the presence of fat in the duodenum, on the other hand, does not seem to be affected by vagotomy.

The augmented response of the gallbladder to exogenous CCK stimulation following vagotomy suggests that neural influences can modify the hormonal input to the gallbladder. Recent observations by Pallin and Skoglund (160), Davison and Fosel (60), and Fosel and Sewing (75) support this idea. These authors demonstrated that subthreshold doses of CCK and gastrin can augment the stimulatory effect of vagal stimulation on gallbladder motility. Thus, the concept that gallbladder emptying results principally from hormonal influences must be tempered with the knowledge that neural influences can modulate the response.

Sympathetic Influence

Although investigations into the role of the sympathetic nervous system in affecting gallbladder motility have produced inconsistent and variable findings, it is now generally accepted that stimulation of the sympathetic nerves or the injection of norepinephrine relaxes the gallbladder (14,48,120,132,137,167,169,230,234). In order for this effect to be obvious, however, the pressure or tension in the gallbladder must be elevated by prior CCK or vagal stimulation (10,160).

Bertaccini et al. (23) were the first to report that norepinephrine relaxed cerulein-stimulated guinea pig gallbladders both *in situ* and *in vitro*. Andersson and colleagues (10) noted relaxation of the OP-CCK stimulated gallbladder following the addition of isoprenaline to the bathing solution. Amer (5), using the rabbit as an animal model, demonstrated a dose-related relaxation of the gallbladder following administration of the β-adrenergic agonist, isoproterenal. The relaxation could be blocked by propanolol. He also noted that the α-adrenergic agonists oxymetazoline and methoxamine contracted the muscle strips and that this effect could be

abolished by phentolamine or phenoxybenzamine. Thus, he provided data that both α- and β-adrenergic receptors existed on the smooth muscle of the gallbladder.

Pallin and Skoglund (159,160), while studying the neurohumoral control of gallbladder emptying in the cat, found that stimulation of the right splanchnic nerves inhibits the contractile effect of CCK. Persson (167,169) confirmed this finding and showed also that norephinephrine produced qualitatively similar results. Using a variety of adrenergic blocking agents, he was able to demonstrate that the gallbladder contains only a small population of excitatory α-receptors and that excitation occurs only when the inhibitory β-receptors have been blocked. Thus, under normal circumstances adrenergic stimulation produces relaxation through activation of numerous β-inhibitory receptors.

The significance of a predominantly adrenergic inhibitory innervation to the gallbladder is not known. Persson (167,169) has suggested it may be important during gallbladder filling. Lechin et al. (120) have recently come to the same conclusion while examining the effects of α-adrenergic blockade on CCK-induced gallbladder emptying in humans. Further studies are needed to determine the validity of this hypothesis.

In summary, smooth muscle of the gallbladder contains both excitatory (α) and inhibitory (β) adrenergic receptors. Under normal circumstances, adrenergic stimulation inhibits gallbladder motility. In order for this effect to be obvious the gallbladder first must be stimulated to contract. The physiological significance of this inhibition remains unanswered.

BILIARY TRACT MOTILITY

Common Bile Duct

The role of the common bile duct in the dynamics of the extrahepatic biliary tract is a point of some controversy. Research has centered on defining whether the common duct serves as a passive conduit or whether it can, by its own intrinsic activity, actively contribute to the propulsion of bile through its lumen.

In several species, including humans, the common bile duct exhibits a well-defined spontaneous rhythmical activity *in vitro* (130,223). In addition, several investigators have reported peristaltic contraction of the common bile duct *in vivo* (37,55,64,141,201,219,229). McDonald (141) in 1941 was one of the first to report that peristalsis could occur in the extraduodenal portion of the duct in humans. Burnett and Shields (37) later confirmed this observation and reported the presence of 3 to 5 waves/min, each with a duration of 1 to 3 sec.

Several investigators have questioned the presence or significance of peristaltic contractions in the common bile duct (56,85,145,153,188,209,228). Myers et al. (145) were unable to demonstrate any inherent contractile activity of the common duct in humans. Similarly, Hauge and Mark (85) could not demonstrate common duct peristalsis in the dog and attributed ductal pressure changes to variations in respiratory pattern and sphincter tone. Daniels et al. (56) came to a similar conclusion while cineflourographically monitoring extrahepatic bile duct motility in dogs and humans. Nebesar et al. (153) proposed that the peristalsis observed by some investigators could be explained in terms of duodenal or sphincter pressure fluctuations being reflected backward into the duct. They reasoned that an increase in the motor activity of either area could expand the elastic fibers of the duct wall. Subsequent to sphincter or duodenal relaxation a diffuse, but passive, recoil of the elastic fibers would occur, which would return the duct to its original size and mimic an active contractile response. Stassa and Graffe (209) came to a similar conclusion after an extensive series of studies on the effect of cholecystectomy, sphincterotomy, and vagotomy on biliary tract motility.

Histological examination of the common bile duct reveals that smooth muscle, where present, is oriented primarily in a longitudinal direction. Thus it seems inappropriate to apply the term *peristalsis* to the bile duct in the same manner that it is used to describe intestinal motility. Tansy et al. (219) have concluded that demonstrable fluctuations in bile duct flow and pressure are a function of alterations in the longitudinal muscle. Ludwick (130) has proposed that the musculature of the bile duct is more involved with maintaining the tone in the wall, rather than propulsion of intraluminal contents. He suggested that the tone was a function of the activity of the intrinsic autonomic nervous system of the biliary tree. Although more studies are needed to prove this hypothesis, it seems reasonable to assume that common duct peristalsis is not a requirement for efficient bile transport.

Sphincter of Oddi

Overview

The efficient delivery of bile into the duodenum requires not only gallbladder contraction but also relaxation of the high pressure zone characteristic of the choledochoduodenal junction, i.e., the sphincter of Oddi. Although there has been controversy concerning the anatomic independence of the sphincter (59,73,74), it is now well established that the intrinsic muscle fibers of the sphincter differ from the musculature of the duodenum both in embryological development and in structure (28,32,33).

In addition to the controversy surrounding the anatomic independence of the sphincter, the functional significance in relation to biliary pressures and flow has also been questioned. A review of the early literature reveals that Burget (36), Elman and McMaster (68), and Potter and Mann (172) considered biliary flow and pressures to be solely dependent on changes in duodenal tone and muscular activity. On the other hand, Lueth (131), Bergh and Lane (22), and Long (129) maintained that the sphincter was functionally independent of the duodenal musculature and was responsible for changes in biliary pressures.

In a more recent study, Smith and his associates (205), while perfusing the common bile duct and simultaneously recording pressures, reported that the predominant factor influencing biliary pressures was choledochal sphincter tone. They did observe, however, that alterations in duodenal activity could also affect biliary pressures. These observations have since been confirmed by Caroli et al. (40), Daniels et al. (55), Nebesar et al. (153), Wyatt, (235), Cushieri et al. (54), and Askin et al. (12).

Perhaps the most significant *in vivo* study demonstrating that choledochoduodenal sphincter activity occurs independent of duodenal motility was performed by Ono and his colleagues (158). They investigated the mechanism of bile flow in humans by simultaneously recording both bile flow and the electromyogram of the sphincter and duodenal muscle. From their observations they concluded (a) cessation of bile flow occurs simultaneously with the initiation of electrical activity in the sphincter muscle, (b) bile flow into the duodenum occurs only in the absence of sphincter electrical activity, and (c) there is no correlation between duodenal electrical activity and the delivery of bile into the duodenum. These findings clearly establish the role of sphincter tone in regulating bile flow into the duodenum. However, as noted by Hallenback (82), it seems reasonable to assume that the activity of the duodenal musculature can modify the rate of bile delivery into the duodenum.

In recent years Tansy, and co-workers (215–218,220) have questioned the anatomic existence of a sphincteric mechanism dependent on muscular influences. Their studies have lead them to conclude that the occlusive nature of the choledochoduodenal junction is due entirely to the physical arrangement of the mucosa at the terminal portion of the common bile duct. Furthermore, they noted that the resistance of the "sphincter" could be altered by duodenal contractions, by the localized intraductal administration of vasoactive agents, as well as by changes in central arterial, central venous, and portal venous blood pressures. On the other hand, they provided evidence that the ductal opening pressures were unaffected by direct neural or hormonal influences. They have concluded that the choledochoduodenal junction possesses the physical and functional properties of a passive, nonlinear, and essentially one-way flutter valve. These findings, although intriguing, are difficult to categorize in light of the vast amounts of data supporting the idea of an anatomically distinct and functionally independent sphincter mechanism at the choledochoduodenal junction.

Several investigators have noted that the sphincter of Oddi exhibits spontaneous and rhythmic opening and closing (3,27,100,106,128,135,190,200,234). Wyatt (235) recorded bile duct pressures just proximal to the sphincter in the dog and observed characteristic pressure tracing, occurring 12 to 14 times/min, that varied very little from animal to animal. In the cat, tension changes in the longitudinally mounted sphincter and cyclic changes in resistance to flow through the sphincter can be recorded (123,164,165,168,170). The spontaneous activity of the sphincter appears to be myogenic in origin, since it was not inhibited by phenoxybenzamine, atropine, hexamethonium, or tetrodotoxin (123,164,165). The functional significance of this spontaneous activity is not known. Watts and Dunphy (229) suggested that the rhythmical activity produces a "milking" effect on bile delivery into the duodenum. Nebesar and colleagues (153) supported this idea and described a 60° to 90° angulation of the sphincter as the contraction proceeded. Persson (166), on the other hand, provides ample evidence that the spontaneous activity has no propulsive function but is associated with alterations in resistance to flow through the sphincter. Most investigators support this latter assumption.

Hormonal Influence

Shortly after the identification of CCK by Ivy and Oldberg (102), Sandblom et al. (189) reported that the hormone decreased the resistance to flow through the sphincteric region at the lower end of the common bile duct. This observation has since been confirmed by numerous investigators (44,125,133,206) in a number of different animal species (Fig. 6).

However, not all investigators have reported a decrease in sphincter tone following CCK administration. Toouli and Watts (223) and Watts and Dunphy (229) proposed that in the dog CCK increases the sphincteric activity, and that this increased activity enhances the flow of bile from the common duct into the duodenum through an increase in the milking function of the sphincter. These findings are not supported by the work of Scott and Secord (199) and Lin and Spray (126). In both cases, the authors recorded a relaxation of the sphincter in response to intravenous CCK administration. Lin and Spray (125), in conscious dogs, found that the minimal dose of CCK required for relaxation of the choledochus was 0.025 U/kg. At this dose, sphincter relaxation occurred without any evidence of gallbladder contraction. They concluded that the data provided evidence that sphincter relaxation is a physiological action of CCK. The findings of Toouli and Watts (223) and Watts and Dunphy (229) are difficult to explain but might well be related to the purity of their hormone preparations or the concentrations of CCK infused. At high dose, the increased motor activity of the duodenum might well have overshadowed the relaxation of the sphincter. In a recent study, Sarles et al. (191) reported that CCK and cerulein both produced a marked rise in sphincteric activity when injected intravenously into the rabbit. No explanations are evident to explain these findings but, as the authors suggest, it may illustrate a species difference in the action of the hormone.

The studies of Persson and Ekman (169,170) have added significantly to our understanding of the effect of CCK on the sphincter of Oddi. Their findings have demonstrated very clearly that in the cat, an animal model similar in anatomy to the human, CCK relaxes the sphincter and that the sphincter muscle can respond independent of the duodenal musculature. When vein grafts were implanted into the duodenal wall in an at-

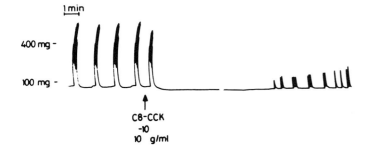

FIG. 6. Relaxing effect of OP-CCK on the isolated sphincter of Oddi. Note also the spontaneous activity of the sphincter. (From Andersson et al., ref. 10b, with permission.)

tempt to measure the intramural pressure within the duodenum, Persson and Ekman (170) found that morphine and noradenaline both contracted the sphincter but relaxed the duodenum. Thus they confirmed the observation of Oddi and others that the sphincter is a functionally distinct entity capable of acting independently of changes in duodenal tone.

The inhibitory effect of CCK on the sphincter, like its excitatory effect on the gallbladder, is a direct action of the hormone on the muscle. Hedner et al. (88) found that in the anesthetized cat the effect of CCK on the sphincter muscle could not be blocked by atropine or by pretreatment with reserpine. Lin and Spray (126) showed that the choledochal action of CCK in the conscious dog was not affected by phenoxybenzamine, propanolol, or atropine at doses that significantly affected gastrin- or histamine-induced gastric acid secretion.

Very little is known concerning the mechanism of action of CCK on the sphincter of Oddi. Andersson et al. (10b) reported that the relaxing effect of OP-CCK on the rabbit sphincter, when fully developed, was associated with a 91% increase in tissue cAMP levels and a 69% increase in phosphodiesterase enzyme activity. They proposed that the elevated levels of cAMP, which occurred despite augmented phosphodiesterase activity, were the result of a simultaneous increase in adenyl cyclase enzyme activity. More studies are needed to confirm this hypothesis.

Other peptides and gastrointestinal hormones also can affect the tone at the choledochus (174). Cerulein has been shown to relax the choledochus in the anesthetized guinea pig (23), the conscious dog (126), and in sheep (19). The low concentrations of the peptide required to demonstrate this effect make it one of the most potent inhibitors of sphincter tone. The mechanisms by which cerulein acts is probably identical to that of CCK. In the conscious dog, neither the cholecystokinetic nor the choledochal-inhibitory effect of the peptide is antagonized by cholenergic, adrenergic, or autonomic ganglia blockade (23,126).

Gastrin, pentagastrin, and the carboxyterminal tetra- and tripeptides of gastrin all have been reported to decrease the resistance of the sphincter of Oddi (124–126). The potency of these substances, however, is considerably less than that of CCK or cerulein. Agosti et al. (1) showed that human gastrin I was only 1/10 to 1/40 as active as CCK in relaxing the sphincter of the anesthetized guinea pig. Evidence that endogenously released gastrin has a physiological role in the regulation of sphincter activity does not exist.

Secretin has been reported to decrease choledochal resistance in the conscious dog (127). The dose range infused was less than that required for the stimulation of bile secretion. As a result, it has been suggested that secretin plays a physiological role in regulating sphincter tone. This view is further supported by the observation that secretin augments CCK's inhibitory effect on the sphincter (127). In addition, the intraduodenal instillation of dilute acid, a known stimulant for secretin release, causes a significant reduction in sphincter resistance (82).

The synergistic effects of secretin and CCK on the choledochus have not been demonstrated *in vitro*. Furthermore, Nebel (152) has shown that in the human being secretin increased intrasphincteric pressure, as assessed by endoscopic cannulation of the ampulla of Vater. Clearly, more studies are needed to determine the existence of possible species differences and to assess the physiological importance of secretin on the choledochus.

In summary, the relaxation of the choledochus following the ingestion of a meal can be attributed to the direct effect of CCK on the sphincter musculature. The physiological importance of secretin (or other as yet unidentified gut peptides) in modifying or augmenting the sphincter's response to CCK remains to be determined. The action of CCK on the sphincter complements the effect on the gallbladder and enhances the delivery of bile into the duodenum.

Neural Influence

Sympathetics. In vitro studies generally support the concept that the sphincter of Oddi contracts in response to adrenergic stimulation. Crema and co-workers (49–53) examined the response of the isolated terminal bile duct to adrenaline and noradrenaline stimulation and reported contraction of both the longitudinal and circular muscle layers, despite relaxation of the adjacent duodenal musculature. They concluded that the sphincter muscle can function independent of duodenal responses and they postulated that the response of the sphincter represented stimulation of α-adrenergic receptors on the muscle. This hypothesis was later tested and confirmed by Persson (164) using three different preparations of isolated sphincter from the cat. In his study, adrenaline and noradrenaline each increased the activity and tonus of the sphincter and decreased duodenal tone. This effect could be blocked by phenoxybenzamine, an α-adrenergic blocking agent. In addition to α-receptors, Persson provided evidence for the presence of β-receptors on the sphincter muscle. Stimulation of this receptor by isoprenaline or terbutaline decreased the spontaneous activity and tonus of the sphincter and diminished the resistance to flow through the sphincter. This response could be demonstrated only by the prior pharmacological blockade of the α-adrenergic receptors.

Unlike the response to adrenergic stimulation *in vitro*, *in vivo* studies have shown both decreases and increases in rate of bile flow through the sphincter. Liedberg and Persson (123) studied the response of the feline sphincter to intravenous administration of adrenaline, nore-adrenaline, isoprenaline, and terbutaline, a specific β-adrenoreceptor agonist. Both adrenaline and noradrenaline increased the resistance to flow through the sphincter and the effect was blocked by α-adrenoreceptor blocking agents. On the other hand, isoprenaline and terbutaline decreased the resistance to flow through the sphincter. This latter response was abolished by propanolol. These results confirmed previous *in vitro* findings that α-adrenoreceptors mediate sphincter contraction and β-adrenoreceptors contribute to relaxation of the muscle.

In a later study, Persson (169) concluded that stimulation of the sympathetic nerves to the sphincter primarily activates α-adrenoreceptors, thereby contracting the muscle. Relaxation of the sphincter was observed only when the α-receptors had been previously blocked with phenoxybenzamine. He proposed that, although both receptor types exist on sphincter smooth muscle, α-adrenoreceptors are the principal receptor mechanism activated following sympathetic nerve stimulation.

In contrast to these findings, Benzi et al. and Crema et al. (18,53) reported that the resistance to flow through the cat sphincter was decreased by nerve stimulation and by noradrenaline. Mori et al. (148) found that in the rabbit, adrenergic stimulation was more often associated with decreases in sphincteric tone. Dardick et al. (57) reported a 32% decrease in sphincter resistance following vagotomy in the dog and contributed the relaxation to the presence of tonically active β-adrenoreceptors. In addition, the intravenous administration of norepinephrine decreased sphincter tone. These findings suggest that β-adrenoreceptor stimulation is the primary response to adrenergic stimulation. The obvious discrepancies in the literature make it impossible to attribute any physiological significance to the sympathetic innervation of the sphincter. This conclusion is supported by the fact that sympathetic blockade has no effect on sphincter dynamics (195).

Parasympathetics. It is well documented that the exogenous administration of parasympathomimetic drugs increases the resistance to bile flow through the sphincter of Oddi. Similarly, several investigators have shown that vagal stimulation is associated with an increase in sphincter tone and a decrease in bile flow through the sphincter (96,192). Sarles et al. (191) reported that, in the rabbit, the reduced bile flow can be associated with an increase in the electromyographic activity of the sphincter.

The effect of vagotomy on sphincter tone is controversial. Stassa and Graffe (209) concluded, on the basis of cineradiographic studies in dogs, that vagotomy has no influence on sphincter dynamics. Liedberg and Halabi (122) also reported that vagotomy had no effect on CCK-induced sphincter relaxation in the cat. In contrast, Schein et al. (194), Beneventano et al. (17), and Dardick and his colleagues (58) found decreases in

sphincter tone following vagotomy. It should be cautioned that these latter studies were acute experiments and that the results might well reflect the transitory atonia that characteristically occurs following vagotomy. In fact, Williams and Huang (233), in a series of chronic experiments with dogs, observed an increase in duct pressure after vagotomy, which they assumed was the result of an increased resistance at the sphincter.

Recently, several studies have defined the neurohistochemical and ultrastructural characteristics of an intrinsic nerve network within the sphincter region of the cat and dog (118,119,215). Extrinsic vagal denervation has been shown to have little or no effect on the integrity of the nerve network. These data, combined with the inconsistent effect of vagotomy, support the idea that the vagus plays no significant role in affecting sphincter tone.

In summary, the smooth muscle of the sphincter of Oddi is responsive to a variety of neural and humoral stimuli. Aside from the physiological importance of CCK in decreasing sphincter tone, however, little quantitative information is available concerning the significance of neural-hormonal and hormone-hormone interactions at the sphincter. In addition, the affect of neural and hormonal influences on the development and maintenance of sphincter tone remains unsettled.

SUMMARY

The movement and direction of bile flow within the biliary tract depends on the regional differences in intraluminal pressures. In the interdigestive period the resistance to bile flow through the sphincter of Oddi exceeds the pressure within the common bile duct and, as a result, bile is diverted into the gallbladder. Because of the large absorptive capacity of the gallbladder, as well as the distensibility of the muscular sac, the intraluminal pressure remains low and only rarely are conditions suitable for the delivery of bile into the duodenum. Despite the numerous studies on the factors affecting gallbladder distensibility and sphincter of Oddi tone, much of the data remain speculative. Although there is little doubt that the vagal input to the gallbladder modifies the distensibility of the organ and that the tone of the sphincter is an intrinsic property of the muscle, the effect of adrenergic and nonadrenergic systems remains unresolved. In addition, the importance of endocrine and paracrine influences is not known.

Following the delivery of chyme into the duodenum, the rate of bile secretion by the liver increases, the gallbladder contracts, and the resistance to bile flow through the sphincter decreases. Each of these changes enhances the delivery of bile into the proximal small intestine. The magnitude of the changes depends on a complex interaction of endocrine, paracrine, and neural influences, very little of which is fully understood.

There is no doubt, however, that the release of CCK from the proximal small intestine is of paramount importance. Numerous studies have already demonstrated that CCK acts directly upon gallbladder and sphincter smooth muscle to enhance gallbladder emptying and sphincter relaxation, respectively. At the present time, the physiological significance of additional neural, neural-hormonal, and hormonal-hormonal interactions remains uncertain. It will be up to future investigators to resolve these questions. The development of reliable immunoscope for CCK and secretin, the identification and quantification of additional gut peptides with cholecystokinetic and choledochal activity, and the design of noninvasive methods for evaluating biliary tract motility should provide valuable information in our quest toward understanding the factors that are of physiological importance in affecting the motility of the gallbladder and biliary tree.

ACKNOWLEDGMENTS

The author would like to thank Mrs. Eleanor Seeds for her editioral and secretarial assistance.

REFERENCES

1. Agosti, A., Mantovani, P., and Mori, L. (1971): Actions of caerulein and related substances on the sphincter of Oddi. *Naunyn-Schmiedlbergs Arch. Pharmacol.,* 208:114–118.
2. Amberg, J. R., Jones, R. S., Moss, A., Gourlay, S., and Goldberg, H. I. (1973): Effect of vagotomy on gallbladder size and contractility in the dog. *Invest. Radiol.,* 8:371–376.
3. Amdrup, B. M., and Griffith, C. A. (1970): The effects of vagotomy upon biliary function in dogs. *J. Surg. Res.,* 10:209–212.
4. Amer, M. S. (1969): Studies with cholecystokinin. II. Cholecystokinetic potency of porcine gastrins I and II and related peptides in three systems. *Endocrinology,* 84:1277–1281.
5. Amer, M. S. (1972): Studies with cholecystokinin in vitro. III. Mechanism of the effect on the isolated rabbit gallbladder strips. *J. Pharmacol. Exp. Ther.,* 183:527–534.
6. Amer, M. S. (1974): Cyclic guanosine 3′, 5′-monophosphate and gallbladder contraction. *Gastroenterology,* 67:333–337.
7. Amer, M. S., and Becvar, W. E. (1969): A sensitive in vitro method for the assay of cholecystokinin. *J. Endocrinol.,* 43:637–642.
8. Amer, M. S., and McKinney, G. R. (1972): Studies with cholecystokinin in vitro. IV. Effect of cholecystokinin and related peptides on phosphodiesterase. *J. Pharmacol. Exp. Ther.,* 183:535–548.
9. Anastasi, A., Erspamer, V., and Endean, R. (1968): Isolation and amino acid sequence of caerulein, the active decapeptide of the skin of *Hyla caerulea. Arch. Biochem. Biophys.,* 125:57–68.
10a. Andersson, K. E., Andersson, R., and Hedner, P. (1972): Cholecystokinetic effect and concentration of cyclic AMP in gallbladder muscle in vitro. *Acta Physiol. Scand.,* 85:511–516.
10b. Andersson, K. E., Andersson, R., Hedner, P., and Pearson, C. G. A. (1972): *Life Sci.,* 11:723–732.
11. Andersson, R., Nilsson, K., Wikberg, J., Johansson, S., Lundholm, E. M., and Lundholm, L. (1975): Gastrointestinal hormones. In: *Advances in Cyclic Nucleotide Research,* edited by G. J. Drummand, P. Greengard, and G. A. Robinson, vol. 5, pp. 491–518. Raven Press, New York.
12. Ashkin, J. R., Lyon, D. T., Shull, S. D., Wagner, C. I., and Soloway, R. D. (1978): Factors affecting delivery of bile into the duodenum in man. *Gastroenterology,* 74:560–565.
13. Bainbridge, F. A., and Dale, H. H. (1906): The contractile mechanism of the gallbladder and its extrinsic nervous control. *J. Physiol.,* 33:138–155.
14. Banfield, W. J. (1975): Physiology of the gallbladder. *Gastroenterology,* 69:770–777.
15. Bassin, A. L., and Whitaker, L. R. (1930): Pharmacodynamic effects upon the gallbladder. *N. Engl. J. Med.,* 202:311–318.
16. Beava, J. A., Hardman, J. G., and Sutherland, E. W. (1971): Stimulation of adenosine 3′,5′-monophosphate hydrolysis by guanosine 3′,5′-monophosphate. *J. Biol. Chem.,* 246:3841–3846.
17. Beneventano, T. C., Rosen, R. G., and Schein, C. J. (1969): The physiological effect of acute vagal section on canine biliary dynamics. *J. Surg. Res.,* 9:331–334.
18. Benzi, G., Berte, F., Crema, A., and Frigo, G. M. (1964): Actions of sympathomimetic drugs on the smooth muscle at the junction of the bile duct and duodenum studied in vitro. *Br. J. Pharmacol.,* 23:101–114.
19. Beretta, C., Calvari, A. R., and Leonardi, L. (1972): Cholecystokinetic action of caerulein in sheep. *Atti Soc. Ital. Sci. Vet.,* 26:230–231.
20. Bergh, G. S. (1942): The sphincter mechanism of common bile duct in human subjects: Its reaction to certain types of stimulation. *Surgery,* 11:299–330.
21. Bergh, G. S. (1942): The effect of food upon the sphincter of Oddi in human subjects. *Am. J. Dig. Dis.,* 9:40–43.
22. Bergh, G. S., and Lane, J. A. (1940): A demonstration of the independent contraction of the sphincter of the common bile duct in human subjects. *Am. J. Physiol.,* 128:690–694.
23. Bertaccini, G., DeCaro, G., Endean, R., Erspamer, V., and Impicciatore, M. (1968): The action of caerulein on the smooth muscle of the gastrointestinal tract and the gallbladder. *Br. J. Pharmacol.,* 34:291–310.
24. Bloom, S. R. (1977): Gastrointestinal Hormones. In: *Gastrointestinal Physiology II,* edited by R. K. Crane, vol. 12, pp. 71–103. University Press, Baltimore.
25. Bloom, S. R., Bryant, M. G., and Cochrane, J. P. S. (1975): Normal distribution and post-prandial release of gut hormones. *Clin. Sci. Mol. Med.,* 49:3P.
26. Bloom, W., and Fawcett, D. W. (1968): The Liver, Bile Ducts, and Gallbladder. In: *A Textbook of Histology,* edited by W. Bloom and D. W. Fawcett, pp. 582–613. W. B. Saunders, Philadelphia.
27. Bouchier, I. A. D. (1970): The vagus, the bile, and gallstones. *Gut,* 11:799–803.
28. Boyden, E. A. (1923): The gallbladder in the cat, its development, its functional periodicity, and its anatomical variation as recorded in twenty-five hundred specimens. *Anat. Rec.,* 24:388–389.
29. Boyden, E. A. (1925): The effect of natural foods on the distension of the gallbladder, with a note on the change in pattern of the mucosa as it passes from distension to collapse. *Anat. Rec.,* 30:333–363.
30. Boyden, E. A. (1926): A study of the human gallbladder in response to the ingestion of food; together with some observation on the mechanism of the expulsion of bile in experimental animals. *Anat. Rec.,* 33:201–255.
31. Boyden, E. A. (1928): Analysis of reaction of human gallbladder to food. *Anat. Rec.,* 40:147–192.
32. Boyden, E. A. (1937): The sphincter of Oddi in man and certain representative mammals. *Surgery,* 1:25–37.
33. Boyden, E. A. (1957): The anatomy of the choledochoduodenal junction in man. *Surg. Gynecol. Obstet.,* 104:641–652.
34. Brooks, F. P. (1976): Anatomy and Physiology of the Gallbladder and Bile Ducts. In: *Gastroenterology,* edited by H. L. Bochus, pp. 611–650. W. B. Saunders, Philadelphia.
35. Bryant, M. G., Polak, J. M., Modlin, I., Bloom, S. R., Albuquerque, R. H., and Pearse, A. G. E. (1976): Possible dual role for vasoactive intestinal peptide as gastrointestinal hormone and neurotransmitter substance. *Lancet,* 1:991–993.
36. Burget, G. E. (1925): The regulation of the flow of bile. *Am. J. Physiol.,* 74:583–589.
37. Burnett, W., and Shields, R. (1958): Movements of common bile duct in man: studies with image intensifier. *Lancet,* 2:387–390.
38. Cameron, A. J., Phillips, S. F., and Summerskill, W. H. (1969): Effect of cholecystokinin, gastrin, secretin, and glucagon on

human gallbladder in vitro. *Proc. Soc. Exp. Biol. Med.,* 131:149–153.

39. Cannon, W. B., and Rosenbleuth, A. (1949): *The Supersensitivity of Denervated Structures.* Macmillan Company, New York.

40. Caroli, J., Porcher, P., Pequignot, G., and Deltare, M. (1960): Contribution of cineradiography to the study of function of the human biliary tract. *Am. J. Dig. Dis.,* 5:677–696.

41. Cheray, M., and Panel, I. (1926): Physiology of the Meltzer-Lyon Test. *Am. J. Med. Sci.,* 172:11–21.

42. Chernish, S. M., Miller, R. E., and Rsoenak, B. D. (1972): Hypotonic duodenography with the use of glucagon. *Gastroenterology,* 63:392–398.

43. Chowdhury, J. R., Berkowitz, J. M., Praissman, M. L., and Fara, J. W. (1975): Interaction between octapeptide-cholecystokinin, gastrin, and secretin on cat gallbladder in vitro. *Am. J. Physiol.,* 229:1311–1315.

44. Cole, W. H. (1978): The Development of cholecystography: The first fifty years. *Am. J. Surg.,* 136:541–560.

45. Cooperman, A. M. (1977): Gastrointestinal hormones and apudomas. *Clev. Clin. Quart.,* 44:83–93.

46. Copher, G. H., and Illingworth, C. F. W. (1928): Mechanism of emptying of the gallbladder and common bile duct. *Surg. Gynecol. Obstet.,* 46:459–463.

47. Cox, H. T., Doherty, J. F., and Kerr, D. F. (1950): Changes in the gallbladder after elective gastric surgery. *Lancet,* 1:764–766.

48. Crandall, L. A., Jr. (1931): Mechanism of the contraction and evacuation of the gallbladder. *Arch. Intern. Med.,* 48:1217–1224.

49. Crema, A., and Benzi, G. (1961): Comportamento in vitro dello sfintere di Oddi di alcuni animali. *Arch. Fisiol.,* 60:374–386.

50. Crema, A., Benzi, G., and Berte, F. (1962): The action of some natural substances on terminal portion of the common bile duct isolate in toto. *Arch. Int. Pharmacodyn. Ther.,* 137:307–317.

51. Crema, A., and Berte, F. (1963): Actions of sympathomimetic drugs on the isolated junction of the bile duct and duodenum. *Br. J. Pharmac. Chemother.,* 20:221–229.

52. Crema, A., Berte, F., Benzi, G., and Frigio, G. M. (1963): Action of sympathomemetic agents on the choledochoduodenal junction "in vitro". *Arch. Int. Pharmacodyn.,* 146:586–595.

53. Crema, A., Berte, F., Benzi, G., and Frigio, G. M. (1964): The response of the sphincterial areas of the extrahepatic biliary tract to stimulation of sympathetic and parasympathetic nerves. *Acta. Physiol. Lat. Am.,* 14:24–32.

54. Cushieri, A., Hughes, J. H., and Cohen, M. (1972): Biliary pressure studies during cholecystectomy. *Brit. J. Surg.,* 59:267–273.

55. Daniels, B. T., McGlone, F. B., Job, H., and Sawyer, R. B. (1961): Changing concepts of common bile duct anatomy and physiology. *JAMA,* 178:394–497.

56. Daniels, B. T., McGlone, F. B., and Shuey, H. E. (1965): Extrahepatic bile duct motility. *Am. J. Gastoenterol.,* 44:198–203.

57. Dardik, H., Schein, C. J., Warren, A., and Gliedman, M. L. (1969): Adrenergic receptors in the canine biliary tract. *Surg. Gynecol. Obstet.,* 128:823–826.

58. Dardik, H., Gliedman, M. L., Christ, R., Koslow, A., and Schein, C. J. (1970): Neuroendocrine influences on the dynamics of the choledochal sphincter. *Surg. Gynecol. Obstet.,* 129:675–678.

59. Dardinski, V. J. (1935): The anatomy of the major duodenal papilla of man, with special reference to its musculature. *J. Anat.,* 69:469–478.

60. Davison, J. S., and Fosel, S. (1975): Interactions between vagus nerve stimulation and pentagastrin or secretin on the guinea pig gallbladder. *Digestion,* 13:251–254.

61. Debas, H. T., and Grossman, M. T. (1973): Pure cholecystokinin: pancreatic protein and bicarbonate response. *Digestion,* 9:469–481.

62. Delmont, J. (1976): An attempt to collate. In: *Third Gastroenterological Symposium,* edited by J. Delmont, pp. 240–255. S. Karger, New York.

63. Dockray, G. J. (1978): Molecular evolution of gut hormones: application of comparative studies on the regulation of digestion. *Gastroenterology,* 72:344–358.

64. DuBois, F. S., and Hunt, E. A. (1932): Peristalsis of the common bile duct in the opossum. *Anat. Rec.,* 53:387–397.

65. Edholm, P. (1960): Gallbladder evacuation in the normal male induced by cholecystokinin. *Acta Radiol.,* 53:257–265.

66. Eickhorn, E. A., Jr., and Boyden, E. A. (1955): The choledochoduodenal junction in the dog: A study of Oddi's sphincter. *Am. J. Anat.,* 97:431–451.

67. Elias, H. (1967): Embryology, Histology, and Anatomy of the Biliary System. In: *The Biliary System,* edited by W. Taylor, pp. 1–13. Blackwell Scientific, Oxford.

68. Elman, R., and McMaster, P. D. (1926): The physiological variation in resistance to bile flow to the intestine. *J. Exptl. Med.,* 44:151–171.

69. Englert, E., Jr., and Chiu, V. S. (1966): Quantitation of human biliary evacuation with a radioisotope technique. *Gastroenterology,* 50:506–508.

70. Erspamer, V., Bertaccini, G., DeCarlo, G., Endean, R., and Impicciatori, M. (1967): Pharmacological actions of caerulein. *Experentia,* 23:702–703.

71. Fagerberg, S., Gravsten, S., Johansson, H., and Krause, U. (1970): Vagotomy and gallbladder function. *Gut,* 11:789–793.

72. Fara, J. W., and Erde, S. M. (1978): Comparison of in vivo and in vitro responses to sulfated and non-sulfated ceruletide. *Eur. J. Pharmacol.,* 47:359–363.

73. Flouget, J., and Coutin, C. (1975): L'anatomie du sphincter d' Oddi. *Acta Endoscop Radiocinemat.,* 5:103–108.

74. Flouget, J., Laurent, J., and Plenat, F. (1976): Is the sphincter of Oddi a reality in man? In: *Proceedings of the Third Gastroenterology Symposium,* edited by J. Delmont, pp. 21–24. S. Karger, New York.

75. Fosel, S., and Sewing, D. F. (1978): Enhancement of electrically stimulated guinea pig gallbladder contraction by subthreshold concentration of gastrointestinal hormones in vitro. *Experentia,* 34:205–206.

76. Franks, D. J., and MacManus, J. P. (1971): Cyclic GMP stimulation and inhibition of cyclic AMP phosphodiesterase from thymic lymphocytes. *Biochem. Biophys. Res. Commun.,* 42:844–849.

77. Gelfand, M. D. (1979): Gallbladder Disease: Diagnostic Guide. *Hospital Medicine,* 15:8–18.

78. Gilsdorf, R. B. (1974): The effect of simulated gallstones on gallbladder pressures and bile flow in response to eating. *Surg. Gynecol. Obstet.,* 138:161–168.

79. Glanville, J. N., and Duthie, H. L. (1964): Contraction of the gallbladder before and after total abdominal vagotomy. *Clin. Radiol.,* 15:350–354.

80. Graham, E. A., and Cole, W. H. (1924): Roentgenologic examination of the gallbladder: preliminary report of new method utilizing intravenous injection of tetrabromophenopthalein. *JAMA,* 82:613–614.

81. Gregory, R. A., and Tracy, H. J. (1964): The constitution and properties of two gastrins extracted from hog antrol mucosa. *Gut,* 5:103–117.

82. Hallenbeck, G. A. (1968): Biliary and pancreatic pressures. In: *The Handbook of Physiology, section 6, The Alimentary Canal, vol. 2, Secretion,* edited by C. F. Code, pp. 1007–1025. American Physiological Society, Washington, D.C.

83. Hand, B. H. (1973): Anatomy and function of the extrahepatic biliary system. In: *Clinics in Gastroenterology,* edited by J. Bouchier, vol. 2, pp. 3–29. W. B. Saunders Co., London.

84. Harkins, H. N., Stavney, L. S., Griffith, C. A., Savage, L. E., Kato, T., and Nyhus, L. M. (1963): Selective gastric vagotomy. *Ann. Surg.,* 158:448–451.

85. Hauge, C. W., and Mark, J. B. (1965): Common bile duct motility and sphincter mechanism. *Ann. Surg.,* 162:1028–1038.

86. Hedner, P. (1970): Effect of the C-terminal octapeptide of cholecystokinin on guinea pig ileum and gallbladder in vitro. *Acta Physiol., Scand.,* 78:232–235.

87. Hedner, R., and Lunderquist, A. (1972): Use of the C-terminal octapeptide of cholecystokinin for gallbladder evacuation in cholecystography. *Am. J. Roentgenol., Rad., Therapy and Nuclear Med.,* 116:320–326.

88. Hedner, R., Persson, H., and Rossman, G. (1967): Effect of cholecystokinin on small intestine. *Acta Physiol. Scand.,* 70:250–254.

89. Hendrickson, W. F. (1898): A study of the musculature of the entire extrahepatic biliary system, including that of the duodenal *portion of the common biliary duct and of the sphincter. Johns Hopkins Hosp. Bull.,* 9:212–232.

90. Herring, R. T., and Simpson, S. (1907): The pressure of bile secretion and the mechanism of bile absorption in obstruction of the bile duct. *Proc. Roy. Soc. Lond. (Biol.),* 79:517–532.

91. Herzog, R. J., and Nelson, J. A. (1976): The role of cholecystokinin in radiographic opacification of the gallbladder. *Invest. Radiol.,* 11:440–447.

92. Higgins, G. M., and Mann, F. C. (1926): Observations on the emptying of the gallbladder. *Am. J. Physiol.,* 78:339–348.

93. Higgins, G. M., and Wilhelmj, C. M. (1929): The effect of intravenous injections of various emulsions of fat on the emptying of the gallbladder. *Am. J. Med. Sci.,* 178:805–813.

94. Hong, S. S., Magee, D. F., and Crewdson, F. (1956): The physiologic regulation of gallbladder evacuation. *Gastroenterology,* 30:625–630.

95. Hopton, D. S. (1973): The influence of the vagus nerves on the biliary system. *Br. J. Surg.,* 60:216–218.

96. Hopton, D., and White, T. T. (1972): Effect of hepatic and celiac vagal stimulation on common bile duct pressure. *Am. J. Dig. Dis.,* 16:1095–1101.

97. Houssay, B. A., and Rubio, H. H. (1932): La function de la vesicula biliar injertada y la hormona duodenocolecistoquintica. *Ren. Soc. Argent. Biol.,* 8:369–378.

98. Howat, H. T. (1965): Tests of Human Gallbladder Function. In: *The Biliary System,* edited by W. Taylor, pp. 249–262. F. A. Davis Co., Phildelphia.

99. Inberg, M., and Vuorio, M. (1969): Human gallbladder function after selective gastric and total abdominal vagotomy. *Acta Chir. Scand.,* 135:625–633.

100. Isaza, J., Jones, D. T., Dragstedt, L. R., and Woodward, E. R. (1971): The effect of vagotomy on motor function of the gallbladder. *Surgery,* 70:616–621.

101. Ivy, A. C. (1934): The physiology of the gallbladder. *Physiol. Rev.,* 14:1–102.

102. Ivy, A. C., and Oldberg, E. (1928): A hormone mechanism for gallbladder contraction and evacuation. *Am. J. Physiol.,* 86:599–613.

103. Jansson, R. (1979): Effects of gastrointestinal hormones on concentrating function and motility in the gallbladder. *Acta. Physiol. Scand. (Suppl.),* 456:1–38.

104. Jansson, R., Steen, G., and Svanvik, J. (1978): Effects of intravenous vasoactive intestinal peptide (VIP) on gallbladder function in the cat. *Gastroenterology,* 75:47–50.

105. Jansson, R., and Svanvik, J. (1977): Effects of intravenous secretin and cholecystokinin net water absorption and motility in the cat. *Gastroenterology,* 72:639–643.

106. Johnson, F. E., and Boyden, E. A. (1952): The effect of double vagotomy on the motor activity of the human gallbladder. *Surgery,* 32:591–601.

107. Johnson, L. R. (1974): Gastrointestinal Hormones. In: *Gastrointestinal Physiology,* edited by E. D. Jacobsen and L. L. Shambour, pp. 1–43. University Park Press, Baltimore.

108. Johnson, L. R., and Grossman, M. I. (1970): Effect of sulfation on the gastrointestinal actions of caerulein. *Gastroenterology,* 58:208–216.

109. Johnson, L. R., and Grossman, M. I. (1970): Analysis of inhibition of acid secretion by cholecystokinin in dogs. *Am. J. Physiol.,* 218:550–554.

110. Jones, D. T., Isaza, J., and Woodward, E. R. (1971): A new method for long-term measurement of gallbladder contraction in the conscious dog. *J. Surg. Res.,* 11:187–190.

111. Jorpes, J. E. (1968): The isolation and chemistry of secretin and cholecystokinin. *Gastroenterology,* 55:157–164.

112. Jorpes, J. E., and Mutt, V. (1961): On the biological activity and amino acid composition of secretin. *Acta Chem. Scand.,* 15:1790–1791.

113. Jorpes, J. E., Mutt, V., and Toczko, K. (1964): Further purification of cholecystokinin and pancreozymin. *Acta Chem. Scand.,* 18:2408–2410.

114. Kjellgren, K. (1960): Persistence of symptoms following biliary surgery. *Ann. Surg.,* 152:1026–1036.

115. Kozoll, D. D., and Necheles, H. (1942): A study of the mechanisms of bile blow. III. Response to pharmacological stimuli. *Surg. Gynecol. Obstet.,* 74:961–967.

116. Kramkoft, J., Balslev, I., Lendahl, F., and Backer, O. G. (1972): Vagotomy and function of the gallbladder. *Scand. J. Gastroenterol.,* 7:109–112.

117. Kune, G. A. (1972): *Current Practice of Biliary Surgery.* Little, Brown & Co., Boston.

118. Kyosola, K. (1974): Cholinesterase histochemistry of the innervation of the smooth muscle sphincters around the terminal intramural part of the ductus choledochus in the cat and the dog. *Acta Physiol. Scand.,* 90:278–280.

119. Kysola, K. (1978): Effect of vagotomy upon the neurohistochemical and ultrastructural integrity of the inbuilt intrinsic nervous apparatus of the choledochoduodenal junction. *Experentia,* 34:82–84.

120. Lechin, F., Van der Dijs, B., Bentolila, A., and Pena, F. (1978): Adrenergic influences on the gallbladder emptying. *Am. J. Gastroenterol.,* 69:662–668.

121. Liedberg, G. (1969): The effect of vagotomy on gallbladder and duodenal pressures during rest and stimulation with cholecystokinin. *Acta Chir. Scand.,* 135:695–700.

122. Liedberg, G., and Halabi, M. (1970): The effect of vagotomy on flow resistance at the choledochoduodenal junction. *Acta Chir. Scand.,* 136:208–212.

123. Liedberg, G., and Persson, C. G. A. (1970): Adrenoreceptors in the cat choledochoduodenal junction studied in situ. *Br. J. Pharmacol.,* 39:619–626.

124. Lin, T. M. (1971): Hepatic, cholecystokinetic and choledochal actions of cholecystokinin, secretin, caerulein and gastrin-like peptides. *Proc. Int. Congr. Physiol. Sci.,* 9:1877.

125. Lin, T. M. (1975): Actions of gastrointestinal hormones and related peptides on the motor function of the biliary tract. *Gastroenterology,* 69:1006–1022.

126. Lin, T. M., and Spray, G. F. (1969): Effect of pentagastrin, cholecystokinin, caerulein and glucagon on the choledochal resistance and bile flow of dogs. *Gastroenterology,* 56:1178.

127. Lin, T. M., and Spray, G. F. (1971): Choledochal, hepatic, and cholecystokinetic action of secretin, potentiation by cholecystokinin. *Gastroenterology,* 60:783.

128. Loddi, L., Pandolfini, A., LeBrun, S. (1951): Ricershe sul meccanismo del diflusso biliare. *Ann. Ital. Chir.,* 28:395–411.

129. Long, H. (1942): Observations on choledochoduodenal mechanics and their bearings on physiology and pathology of biliary tract. *Br. J. Surg.,* 29:422–437.

130. Ludwick, J. R. (1966): Observations on the smooth muscle and contractile activity of the common bile duct. *Ann. Surg.,* 164:1041–1050.

131. Lueth, H. C. (1931): Studies on the flow of bile into the duodenum and the existence of a sphincter of Oddi. *Am. J. Physiol.,* 99:237–252.

132. Mack, A. J., and Todd, J. K. (1968): A study of human gallbladder in vitro. *Gut,* 9:546–549.

133. Magee, D. F. (1946): Some new observations on the pharmacology of the sphincter of Oddi. *Q. J. Pharm.,* 19:38–43.

134. Magee, D. F. (1965): Physiology of Gallbladder Emptying. In: *The Biliary System,* edited by W. Taylor, pp. 233–247. Blackwell Scientific, Philadelphia.

135. Malagelada, J. R., Go, V. L. W., and Summerskill, W. H. J. (1973): Differing sensitivities of gallbladder and pancreas to cholecystokinin-pancreozymin in man. *Gastroenterology,* 64:950–954.

136. Malagelada, J. R., Go., V. L. W., and Summerskill, W. H. J. (1974): Altered pancreatic and biliary function after vagotomy and pyloroplasty. *Gastroenterology,* 66:22–27.

137. Mann, F. C. (1919): A study of the toxicity of the sphincter at the duodenal end of the common bile duct (with special reference to animals without a gallbladder). *J. Lab. Clin. Med.,* 5:107–110.

138. Mann, F. C. (1924): The functions of the gallbladder. *Physiol. Rev.,* 4:251–273.

139. Mann, F. C. (1924): A physiologic consideration of the gallbladder. *JAMA,* 83:829–832.

140. Mann, F. C., and Foster J. P. (1918): The secretory pressure of the liver with special reference to the presence or absence of a gallbladder. *Am. J. Physiol.,* 47:278–282.

141. McDonald, D. (1941): Common bile duct peristalsis; preliminary report. *Surg. Gynecol. Obstet.,* 73:668–673.

142. McGuigan, J. E. (1978): Gastrointestinal hormones. *Annu. Rev. Med.,* 29:307–318.

143. McMaster, P. D., and Elman, R. (1926): On the expulsion of bile by the gallbladder, and a reciprocal relationship with the sphincter activity. *J. Exp. Med.,* 44:173–198.

144. Menguy, R. B., Hallenbeck, G. A., Bollman, J. L., and Grindlay, J. H. (1958): Intraductal pressures and sphincter resistance in canine pancreatic and biliary ducts after various stimuli. *Surg. Gynecol. Obstet.,* 106:306–320.

145. Meyers, R. N., Haupt, G. J., Birkhead, N. C., Deaver, J. M. (1962): Cineflourographic observations of common bile duct physiology. *Ann. Surg.,* 156:442–450.

146. Michels, N. A. (1955): *Blood Supply and Anatomy of the Upper Abdominal Organs.* Lippincott, Philadelphia.

147. Mitchell, W. T., and Stifel, R. E. (1916): The pressure of bile secretions during chronic obstruction of the common bile ducts. *Bull. Johns Hopkins Hosp.,* 27:79–89.

148. Mori, J., Azuma, H., and Fujiwara, M. (1971): Adrenergic innervation and receptors in the sphincter of Oddi. *Eur. J. Pharmacol.,* 14:365–373.

149. Mutt, V., and Jorpes, J. E. (1968): Structure of porcine cholecystokinin pancreozymin. I. Cleavage with thrombin and trypsin. *Eur. J. Biochem.,* 6:156–162.

150. Mutt, V., and Jorpes, J. E. (1968): Chemistry and physiology of cholecystokinin-pancreozymin. *Proc. Int. Union Physiol. Sci.,* 6:193.

151. Nakano, M., McCloy, R. E., Gin, A. C., and Nakano, S. K. (1975): Effect of prostaglandins E_1, E_2, and $F_{2\alpha}$, and pentagastrin on gallbladder pressure in dogs. *Eur. J. Pharmacol.,* 30:107–112.

152. Nebel, O. T. (1975): Effect of enteric hormones on the human sphincter of Oddi. *Gastroenterology,* 68:962.

153. Nebesar, R. A., Pollard, J. J., and Potsaid, M. S. (1966): Cinecholangiography, some physiological observations. *Radiology,* 86:475–479.

154. Oddi, R. (1887): D'une disposition a' sphincter spéciale de l'ouverturé du canal cholidoque. *Arch. Ital. Biol.,* 8:317–322.

155. Oddi, R. (1888): Sulla toniato dello afintere del coledoco. *Arch. Sci. Med.,* 12:333–339.

156. Ohada, S. (1916): On the contractile movement of the gallbladder. *J. Physiol.,* 50:42–46.

157. Ondetti, M. A., Ruben, B., and Engel, I. L. (1970): Cholecystokinin-pancreozymin: recent developments. *Am. J. Dig. Dis.,* 15:149–155.

158. Ono, K. Watanabe, N., Suzuki, K., Tsuchida, H., Sugiyama, Y., and Abo, M. (1968): Bile flow mechanisms in man. *Arch. Surg.,* 96:869–874.

159. Pallin, B., and Skoglund, S. (1961): On the nervous regulation of the biliary system in the cat. *Acta Physiol. Scand.,* 51:187–192.

160. Pallin, B., and Skoglund, S. (1964): Neural and humoral control of the gallbladder emptying mechanism in the cat. *Acta Physiol. Scand.,* 60:358–362.

161. Papamiltiades, M., and Rettori, R. (1957): Architecture musculaire de la junction choledoco-pancreatico-duodenale. *Acta Anat.,* 30:575–600.

162. Park, C. Y., Pae, Y. S., and Hong, S. S. (1970): Radiologic studies on emptying of the human gallbladder. *Ann. Surg.,* 171:294–299.

163. Parkin, G. J. S., Smith, R. B., and Johnston, D. (1973): Gallbladder volume and contractility after truncal, selective and highly selective vagotomy in man. *Ann. Surg.,* 178:581–586.

164. Persson, C. G. A. (1971): Adrenoreceptor functions in the cat choledochoduodenal junction in vitro. *Br. J. Pharmacol.,* 42:447–461.

165. Persson, C. G. A. (1971): Excitatory effect of tetrodoxin on an isolated smooth muscle organ. *J. Pharm. Pharmacol.,* 23:986–987.

166. Persson, C. G. A. (1972): Adrenergic, cholecystokinetic and morphine induced effects on extra-hepatic biliary motility. *Acta Physiol. Scand. (Suppl.),* 383:1–32.

167. Persson, C. G. A. (1972): Adrenoreceptors in the gallbladder. *Acta Pharmacol.,* 31:177–185.

168. Persson, C. G. A. (1972): Resistance to flow through the pancreatic duct by the isolated cat sphincter of Oddi. *Experentia,* 28:276–278.

169. Persson, C. G. A. (1973): Dual effects on the sphincter of Oddi and gallbladder induced by stimulation of the right splanchnic nerve. *Acta Physiol. Scand.,* 87:334–343.

170. Persson, C. G. A., and Ekman, M. (1972): Effect of morphine, cholecystokinin, and sympathamimetics on the sphincter of Oddi and intramural pressure in cat duodenum. *Scand. J. Gastroenterol.,* 7:345–351.

171. Piper, P. J., Said, S. I., and Vane, J. R. (1970): Effects on smooth muscle preparations of unidentified vasoactive peptides from intestine and lung. *Nature,* 225:1144–1146.

172. Potter, J. C., and Mann, F. C. (1926): Pressure changes in the biliary tract. *Am. J. Med. Sci.,* 171:202–217.

173. Praissman, M., Fara, J. W., and Berkowitz, J. N. (1977): Bending characteristics of the C-terminal octapeptide of cholecystokinin and gastrin to cat gallbladder tissue in vitro: comparison with isometric tension development. In: *Hormonal Receptors in Digestive Tract Physiology,* edited by S. Bonfils, P. Fromougeot, and G. Rosselin, pp. 469–462. North Holland, New York.

174. Rey, J. F., and Harvey, R. F. (1977): Hormonal Control of the Sphincter of Oddi. In: *Proceedings of the Third Gastroenterological Symposium,* edited by J. Delmont, pp. 66–71. S. Karger, Basil.

175. Robinson, G. A., Butcher, R. W., and Sutherland, E. W. (1971): *Cyclic AMP.* Academic Press, New York.

176. Rothman, M. N. (1963): Anatomy and Physiology of the Gallbladder and bile ducts. In: *Gastroenterology,* edited by H. L. Bockus, vol. 3, 2nd ed., p. 567. Saunders, Philadelphia.

177. Rous, P., and McMaster, P. D. (1921): The concentrating activity of the gallbladder. *J. Exp. Med.,* 34:47–73.

178. Rubin, B., Engel, S. L., Drungis, A. M., Dzelzkalns, M., Grigas, E. O., Waugh, M. H., and Yiacas, E. (1969): Cholecystokinin-like activities in guinea pigs and in dogs of the C-terminal octapeptide of cholecystokinin. *J. Pharm. Sci.,* 58:955–959.

179. Rudick, J., and Hutchinson, J. S. F. (1965): Evaluation of vagotomy and biliary function by combined oral cholecystography and intravenous cholangiography. *Ann. Surg.,* 162:234–240.

180. Ryan, J., and Cohen, S. (1976): Interaction of gastrin I, secretin, and cholecystokinin on gallbladder smooth muscle. *Am. J. Physiol.,* 230:553–556.

181. Ryan, J., and Cohen, S. (1976): Pressure-volume response to gastrointestinal hormones. *Am. J. Physiol.,* 230:1461–1465.

182. Ryan, J., and Cohen, S. (1976): Interaction of luminal volume and gastrointestinal hormone stimulation on gallbladder motor function. In: *Fifth International Symposium on Gastrointestinal Motility,* edited by G. Vantrappen and H. Agg, pp. 55–63. Tydoff-Press, Belgium.

183. Ryan, J., and Cohen, S. (1977): Effect of vasoactive intestinal peptide on basal and cholecystokinin induced gallbladder pressure. *Gastroenterology,* 73:870–872.

184. Ryan, J., and Ryave, S. (1978): Effect of vasoactive intestinal polypeptide on gallbladder smooth muscle in vitro. *Am. J. Physiol.,* 234:E44–E46.

185. Said, S. I., and Makhlouf, G. M. (1974): Vasoactive intestinal polypeptide. Spectrum of biological actions. In: *Endocrinology of the Gut,* edited by W. Y. Chey and F. P. Brooks, pp. 83–87. C. B. Slack, Inc., New Jersey.

186. Said, S. I., and Mutt, V. (1970): Polypeptide with broad biological activity: isolation from small intestine. *Science,* 169:1217–1218.

187. Said, S. I., and Mutt, V. (1973): Isolation from procine intestinal wall of a vasoactive octacosapeptide related to secretin and glucagon. *Eur. J. Biochem.,* 28:199–204.

188. Salik, J. O., Siegel, C. I., and Mendeloff, A. I. (1973): Biliaryduodenal dynamics in man. *Radiology,* 106:1–11.

189. Sandblom, P., Voegtlen, W. L., and Ivy, I. C. (1935): The effect of CCK on the choledochoduodenal mechanism (sphincter of Oddi). *Am. J. Physiol.,* 93:175–180.

190. Sarles, J. C., Bidant, J. M., Devaux, M. A., Echinard, C., and Castaginini, C. (1976): Actions of cholecystokinin and caerulein on the rabbit sphincter of Oddi. *Digestion,* 14:415–423.

191. Sarles, J. C., Midejean, A., and Devaux, M. A. (1975): Electromyography of the sphincter of Oddi. *Am. J. Gastroenterol.,* 63:221-231.

192. Satler, J. J., Sakikihara, Y., Nussbaum, M., and Tumen, H. J. (1972): The effect of electrical stimulation of the hepatic periarterial nerve on the dynamics of the biliary tract of the dog. *Acta Hepatogastroenterol. (Stuttg.),* 19:234-238.

193. Schaffalitzky, D. M., Fahrenkrug, J., and Holst, J. J. (1977): Release of vasoactive intestinal polypeptide by electrical stimulation of vagal nerves. *Gastroenterology,* 72:373-375.

194. Schein, C. J., Rosen, R. G., Warren, A., and Gliedman, M. L. (1969): A vagal factor in cholecystitis. *Surgery,* 66:345-352.

195. Schein, C. J., Tawil, V. E., Dardick, H., and Beneventano, T. C. (1970): Common duct dynamics in man. The influence of sympathetic block. *Am. J. Surg.,* 119:261-263.

196. Schoetz, D. J., Jr., Birkett, D. H., and Williams, L. F. (1978): Gallbladder motor function in the intact primate: autonomic pharmacology. *J. Surg. Res.,* 24:513-519.

197. Schreiber, H. (1944): Das muskelapparat des duodenalin choledochusendes beim menschen. *Arch. Klin. Chir.,* 206:211-232.

198. Schwegler, R. A., Jr., and Boyden, E. A. (1937): The development of the pars intestinalis of the common bile duct in the human fetus, with special reference to the origin of the ampulla of Vater and the sphincter of Oddi. II. The early development of the muscularis propruis. III. The composition of the muscularis proprius. *Anat. Rec.,* 68:17-41; 193-219.

199. Scott, G. W., and Secord, D. C. (1976): Flow through the sphincter of Oddi. In: *The Sphincter of Oddi,* edited by J. Delmont, pp. 411-419. Karger, Basel.

200. Scott, G. W., Smallwood, R. E., and Rowland, S. (1975): Flow through the bile duct after cholecystectomy. *Surg. Gynecol. Obstet.,* 140:912-918.

201. Sheldamer, J. (1973): Physiology of the bile transport: manometric studies of common bile duct and sphincter of Oddi. *Gastroenterology,* 64:686.

202. Shorter, R. G., Bollman, J. L., and Baggenstoss, H. (1959): Pressures in the common hepatic duct of the rat. *Proc. Soc. Exp. Biol. Med.,* 102:682-686.

203. Siffort, P., and Silva, G. (1949): A simple method for computing the volume of the human gallbladder. *Radiology,* 52:94-102.

204. Silverman, D. N., and Dennis, W. (1928): On relationship of gallbladder emptying to ingested fats. *Radiology,* 11:45-47.

205. Smith, J. L., Walters, R. L., and Beal, J. M. (1952): A study of choledochal sphincter action. *Gastroenterology,* 20:129-137.

206. Snape, W. J. (1948): Studies of the gallbladder in unanesthetized dog before and after vagotomy. *Gastroenterology,* 10:129-133.

207. Solcia, E., Pearse, A. G. E., Grube, O., Kobayashi, S., Bussols, G., Creutzfeldt, W., and Gepta, M. (1973): Revised Weisbaden classification of gut cells. *Rendic. Gastroenterol.,* 5:13-17.

208. Spellman, S. J., Shaffer, E. A., and Rosenthal, L. (1979): Gallbladder emptying in response to cholecystokinin. *Gastroenterology,* 77:115-120.

209. Stassa, G., and Graffe, W. B. (1968): The cineradiographic evaluation of the biliary tract after drug therapy following cholecystectomy, sphincterotomy, and vagotomy. *Radiology,* 91:297-301.

210. Stening, G. F., and Grossman, M. I. (1969): Potentiation of cholecystokinetic action of cholecystokinin by secretin. *Clin. Res.,* 17:528.

211. Sterling, J. A. (1955): *The Biliary Tract.* Wilkins Co., Baltimore.

212. Sturdivant, R. A. L., Stern, D. H., Resin, H., and Isenberg, J. I. (1973): Effect of graded doses of octapeptide of cholecystokinin on gallbladder size in man. *Gastroenterology,* 64:452-456.

213. Sundler, F., Alumets, J., Hakanson, R., Ingemansson, S., Fahrenkrug, J., and Schaffalitzky, O. B. (1977): VIP innervation of the gallbladder. *Gastroenterology,* 72:1375-1377.

214. Sweet, J. E. (1924): The gallbladder: its past, present and future. *Intern. Clin.,* L:187-226.

215. Tansy, M. F., Innes D. L., Martin, J. S., and Kendall (1974): An evaluation of neural influences on the sphincter of Oddi in the dog. *Am. J. Dig. Dis.,* 19:423-437.

216. Tansy, M. F., Innes, D. L., Martin, J. S., and Kendall, F. M. (1974): Vascular influences on the dynamic stability of the choledochoduodenal junction. *Am. J. Dig. Dis.,* 19:1124-1139.

217. Tansy, M. F., Innes, D. L., Martin, J. S., and Kendall, F. M. (1975): Technique for assessment of local effects of substances found in bile upon opening pressure of choledochoduodenal junction. *J. Pharm. Sci.,* 64:1174-1177.

218. Tansy, M. F., Innes, D. L., Martin, J. S., and Kendall, F. M. (1976): A functional description of the canine choledochoduodenal flutter valve. *Am. J. Dig. Dis.,* 21:233-241.

219. Tansy, M. F., Mackowisk, R. C., and Chaffee, R. B. (1971): A vagosympathetic pathway capable of influencing common bile duct motility in the dog. *Surg. Gynecol. Obstet.,* 133:225-236.

220. Tansy, M. F., Salkin, L., Innes, D. L., Martin, J. S., Kendall, F. M., and Litwack, D. (1975): The muscosal lining of the intramural common bile duct as a determinant of ductal opening pressure. *Am. J. Dig. Dis.,* 20:613-625.

221. Tanturi, C. A., and Ivy, A. C. (1938): A study of the effect of vascular changes in the liver and the excitation of its nerve supply on the formation of bile. *Am. J. Physiol.,* 121:61-74.

222. Tinker, J., and Cox, A. G. (1969): Gallbladder function after vagotomy. *Br. J. Surg.,* 56:779-781.

223. Toouli, J., and Watts, J. M. (1971): In vitro motility studies on canine and human extrahepatic biliary tracts. *Aust. NZ J. Surg.,* 40:380-387.

224. Torsoli, A., Ramorino, M. L., Colagrande, C., and Demaio, G. (1961): Experiments with cholecystokinin. *Acta Radiol.,* 55:193-206.

225. Vagne, M., and Grossman, M. I. (1968): Cholecystokinetic potency of gastrointestinal hormones and related peptides. *Am. J. Physiol.,* 215:881-884.

226. Vagne, M., and Troitskaja, V. (1976): Effects of secretin, glucagon, and VIP on gallbladder contraction. *Digestion,* 14:62-67.

227. Voegtlin, W. L., McEwen, E. G., and Ivy, A. C. (1933): On the humoral agents concerned in the causation of gallbladder contraction. *Am. J. Physiol.,* 103:121-130.

228. Wakim, K. G. (1971): Passive role of the bile duct system in the delivery of bile into the intestine. *Surg. Gynecol. Obstet.,* 133:826-828.

229. Watts, J., McK., and Dunphy, J. E. (1966): The role of the common bile duct in biliary dynamics. *Surg. Gynecol. Obstet.,* 122:1207-1218.

230. Whitaker, L. R. (1926): The mechanism of the gallbladder. *Am. J. Physiol.,* 78:411-436.

231. Wilbur, B. G., Gomez, D., and Tompkins, R. K. (1975): Canine gallbladder bile. *Arch. Surg.,* 110:792-796.

232. Williams, R. D., and Huang, T. T. (1969): New technique for experimental repeated long-term measurement of biliary pressure. *Surgery,* 65:454-456.

233. Williams, R. D., and Huang, T. T. (1969): The effect of vagotomy on biliary pressure. *Surgery,* 66:353-356.

234. Winkelstein, A., and Aschner, P. W. (1926): The mechanism of bile flow from the liver into the intestines. *Am. J. Med. Sci.,* 171:104-111.

235. Wyatt, A. P. (1967): The relationship of the sphincter of Oddi to the stomach, duodenum and gallbladder. *J. Physiol.,* 193:225-243.

236. Yau, W. M., Makhlouf, G. M., and Edwards, L. E. (1973): Mode of action of cholecystokinin and related peptides on gallbladder muscle. *Gastroenterology,* 65:451-456.

Physiology of the Gastrointestinal Tract, edited by
Leonard R. Johnson, Raven Press, New York © 1981.

Chapter 16

Actions of Drugs on Gastrointestinal Motility

Thomas F. Burks

The effects of drugs on motility of the digestive organs are studied primarily for two reasons. Drug effects are used as tools to probe physiological systems involved in control of motility. They are also explored within the process of development of new therapeutic agents or they are used to understand actions and side effects of existing agents. Motives for the study of drug effects often affect choice of drugs and design of specific experiments. Unfortunately, drugs are often used as pharmacological tools without adequate appreciation for basic pharmacological principles to be applied. Also, drug studies on gastrointestinal motility as a function of therapeutic development often fail to take into account the physiological relevance of the particular test system chosen. It is the purpose of this chapter to point out some relevant pharmacological principles which should influence experimental design in both types of studies.

Drugs do not create new physiological functions. In terms of gastrointestinal motility, drugs can only modify (increase or decrease) specific physiological influences on smooth muscle cells. Muscle cells of the digestive system receive multipartite control information from neurotransmitters, hormones, autacoids, and other sources. The contractile state of an individual cell at any given time depends on the balance of these influences, that is, on the algebraic sum of stimulatory and inhibitory chemical messages.

Often, the neural influences on a smooth muscle cell are the most important determinants of its excitability. As is illustrated in Fig. 1, the neural influences are themselves subject to considerable modulation and they function against a complex background of other factors

that can alter smooth muscle excitability. Many cells of the gastrointestinal system are primarily under parasympathetic cholinergic control. However, the parasympathetic outflow to smooth muscle cells is subject to a number of modulating influences. These influences can increase or decrease release of neurotransmitter from preganglionic or postganglionic terminals of nerve fibers (presynaptic facilitation or inhibition). Modulatory influences can also be exerted on intramural cholinergic ganglion cells. In most species, the major role

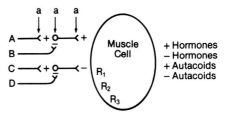

FIG. 1. Schematic representation of chemical influences on a gastrointestinal smooth muscle cell. Neuronal system *A* is characteristic of the conventional excitatory cholinergic innervation; the preganglionic fiber releases an excitatory (+) neurotransmitter to activate ganglia and postganglionic fibers, which release an excitatory transmitter directly onto the smooth muscle cell. Neural, hormonal and autacoid neuroregulatory modulation can be exerted at sites marked *a*. Neuronal system *B* is characteristic of sympathetic innervation and serves mainly to release an inhibitory (−) neurotransmitter at a ganglionic modulatory site. Neuronal system *C* may be characteristic of a nonadrenergic inhibitory innervation, although the presence of a ganglionic synapse is speculative. Neuronal system *D* would be characteristic of a mechanism for producing stimulation by disinhibition (inhibition of an inhibitory system). R_1, R_2, and R_3 represent different neurotransmitter, hormone, and autacoid receptors occurring on the same cell. Individual hormones and autacoids can exert excitatory (+) and inhibitory (−) influences directly on smooth muscle cells.

of the inhibitory sympathetic (adrenergic) innervation is probably to inhibit release of acetylcholine from parasympathetic postganglionic fibers by actions of norepinephrine on cholinergic intramural ganglia. The existence of nonadrenergic, noncholinergic inhibitory neural systems in the gastrointestinal tract has been demonstrated. Although the specific neurotransmitters have not yet been identified, nonadrenergic inhibitory nerves apparently are functionally similar to well-identified neurons in sensitivity to modulating influences.

It is sometimes forgotten that individual muscle cells may contain a variety of receptors that can initiate similar events. For example, an individual smooth muscle cell may contain receptors for acetylcholine, 5-hydroxytryptamine (5-HT), histamine, and substance P, all of which can induce a similar response, usually contraction. Prostaglandins, 5-HT, histamine, and related autacoid substances may be formed locally and exert local hormone effects on smooth muscle cells. The local influences can affect the cell directly or modify neural influences on the cell. Likewise, systemic hormones, including those produced in gastrointestinal tissues, can influence smooth muscle cells directly or can modulate neural influence on individual cells.

Probably all the influences mentioned above are subject to chemical alteration by drugs. Drugs can affect the amount of specific neurotransmitters released, can interact directly with smooth muscle cell neurotransmitter, autocoid, and hormone receptors, and can modify the formation, release, or receptor actions of autacoids and hormones. In view of the potential complexity of these interactions, it is little wonder that we know so little about the mechanisms by which drugs affect gastrointestinal motility!

SPECIAL PHARMACOLOGICAL CONSIDERATIONS

Whether drugs are used as pharmacological tools or as therapeutic agents, a high degree of specificity of action is desirable. *Specificity* implies a restricted effect, usually on a single organ. A highly specific drug would have a single effect on a single organ. For example, a particular specific drug might increase the amplitude of antral contractions without affecting contractions of the intestine or gallbladder and without affecting other organ systems, including bone marrow or brain. Specificity usually requires selectivity of drug action. *Selectivity* implies a single pharmacological action, for example, antagonist actions on a single type of receptor without actions on other types of receptors. Many relatively selective drugs are, in fact, available. Unfortunately, many selective drugs are still not specific. To illustrate, atropine is relatively selective as a muscarinic cholinergic receptor antagonist. Because of the widespread distribution of muscarinic cholinergic receptors and

their physiological importance in regulating function of many organ systems, including the central nervous system, atropine blockade of muscarinic cholinergic receptors is a classic example of nonspecific drug action. Atropine can alter gastrointestinal motility and secretions, pupil size, sweating, contractions of urinary bladder, ganglionic transmission, temperature regulation, thought and behavior, even at dosages that are selective for blockade of muscarinic cholinergic receptors. The problem of specificity is greatly exaggerated for other drugs that are even less selective than atropine. Many drugs can be relatively nonselective in their precise pharmacological actions; these drugs are notoriously nonspecific. Nonspecificity is particularly a problem when drugs are being employed as pharmacological tools. It is especially important to demonstrate in this case the selectivity and specificity of the pharmacological tool under actual experimental conditions.

One method for demonstrating the selectivity and specificity of the drug under investigation is through the use of modalities that will help rule out alternative possibilities. For example, the use of three different control drugs to determine whether intestinal stimulatory effects of morphine could be neurally mediated is illustrated in Fig. 2. In this case, tetrodotoxin was employed as a pharmacological tool to disrupt conduction of neural impulses in isolated intestine (18,60). The rationale for the experiment was that if some portion of the response to morphine is mediated by intramural nerves, tetrodotoxin treatment should reduce responses to morphine. To interpret the results, however, it was necessary to use other control intestinal stimulants. 5-Hydroxytryptamine (5-HT, serotonin), which acts in part by activation of intramural cholinergic nerves and which was proposed to mediate some intestinal actions of morphine, was employed as a control agonist in the absence and presence of tetrodotoxin. Dimethylphenylpiperazinium (DMPP) is a nicotinic cholinergic receptor agonist that produces contractions of intestinal smooth muscle by activation of intramural cholinergic nerves. Bethanechol is a muscarinic cholinergic receptor agonist that acts directly upon intestinal smooth muscle cells to produce contractions. If the concentration of tetrodotoxin employed was adequate to inhibit neural function, it was expected to depress responses to 5-HT and DMPP in a noncompetitive (see below) fashion. If it also depressed responses to bethanechol, however, direct inhibitory effects on smooth muscle cells would be indicated. In fact, tetrodotoxin depressed responses to 5-HT, DMPP, and morphine, without affecting responses to bethanechol. The results indicated that tetrodotoxin was exerting the expected pharmacological actions in this preparation. The specificity of tetrodotoxin action was thus demonstrated in the particular experiment.

For a drug to exert its intended pharmacological ef-

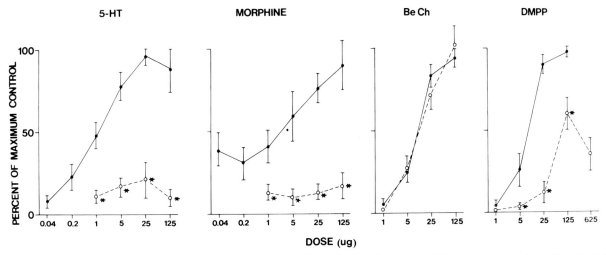

FIG. 2. The use of control agonists to establish specificity of action of tetrodotoxin. Responses of dog vascularly perfused isolated intestine 5-HT, morphine, BeCh, and DMPP were determined in the absence (● — ●) and in the presence (O---O) of 1×10^{-7} g/ml tetrodotoxin. Perfusion with tetrodotoxin inhibited responses to 5-HT, morphine, and DMPP, which have neural stimulatory effects in the intestine, but did not alter responses to BeCh, which acts directly on smooth muscle. (From Burks, ref. 18, with permission.)

fects, it must be present in adequate concentration at its site of action. This simple idea is too often ignored. The concentration of a drug at its site of action depends on the rate and extent of drug delivery to the site and the rate and extent of drug removal mechanisms. In *in vitro* tests, the drug is usually assumed to be present at tissue sites in the same concentration present in the bath fluid after an appropriate period of equilibration. Probably, this dictum is usually true if the drug has an extracellular site of action and if the equilibration period is long enough. If the drug acts intracellularly, the plasma membrane may prevent diffusion of the drug to its intended site of action. Intracellular concentrations in that case may be considerably less than concentration in the bath fluid. If the drug is actively transported into tissue cells, intracellular concentrations may very well exceed the concentration in the bath fluid. Even for drugs with extracellular sites of action, the time required for equilibration between bathing medium and tissue depends on the chemical nature of the drug. Obviously, it is necessary that the drug actually be in solution (not suspended in an insoluble form). Large, polar molecules are not readily soluble in lipid and may require relatively long periods of incubation to reach equilibrium with tissue extracellular spaces.

If the drug is administered *in vivo*, the situation is even more complicated. To avoid the obvious variables of absorption from the digestive system, we will consider only the case of intravenous administration of drug. After intravenous injection, many drugs show biphasic plasma decay curves. The initial, rapid decay (distributive phase) is often associated with redistribution of the drug out of the blood stream into tissues. The second, less rapid phase of the decay curve is known as the postdistributive phase. The slope of the postdistributive phase is largely a measure of drug clear-

ance by metabolism and excretion. As illustrated in Fig. 3, a biological barrier may be interposed between the bloodstream and the phamacological site of action of the drug. Often, the drug does not reach its site of action at the same rate that it peaks in plasma concentration because it is necessary for the drug to diffuse from the blood into its tissue site of action. Presuming that some minimal concentration is necessary for drug effect at its site of action, the critical effective concentration may be achieved only after some finite delay, somewhat exaggerated in Fig. 3 to illustrate the principle. Once equilibrium has been achieved, it generally is cleared from the tissue at the same rate that it is cleared from blood. Experimentalists and clinicians should take into account possible delays in drug distribution to its site of action even after parenteral administration of the drug.

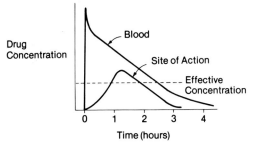

FIG. 3. Drug concentration in blood and at cellular site of action after intravenous administration. Many drugs display a biexponential curve that consists of an initial distributive phase and a later postdistributive phase. The distributive phase represents rapid distribution of drug out of the blood stream into extravascular fluids and tissues. If a biological barrier (e.g., lipid membrane) is interposed between the vascular compartment and the site of drug action, distribution of the drug to its site of pharmacological effect can be delayed (generally less than 1 hr). Because of declining drug concentrations in blood, the presence of a pharmacologically effective concentration of drug at its site of action may be relatively brief.

The relationship between dosage and blood level is illustrated in Fig. 4. With a few exceptions (ethanol, aspirin), most drugs are cleared from the bloodstream by mechanisms that follow first-order kinetics. Thus, the rate of drug clearance is proportional to the plasma concentration of drug. If drug concentration is plotted on a logarithmic scale, the plasma concentration decreases linearly with time. Because of this relationship, the rate of clearance of a drug from the plasma is often expressed in terms of plasma half-life of the drug. Plasma half-life refers to the time required for the plasma concentration of drug to fall to one-half the concentration present at some previous time. The reference time (t_1) can be selected from any linear portion of the plasma decay curve. Plasma half-life will be the time ($t_{1/2}$) required for the plasma level to reach 50% of its value at t_1. It is necessary to keep these relationships in mind because of their impact on duration of drug action. It is incorrect to assume that a drug will exert its particular pharmacological effects when plasma half-life is the sole consideration. As illustrated in Fig. 4, the effective concentration of the drug depends also on the actual dose administered. After a particular dose (curve A) a drug might have a 3-hr effective duration. A smaller dose (curve B) of the same drug with the same plasma half-life may be present in the plasma in an effective concentration for only 1 hr. Experimental protocols which assume that either dosage will be effective for 3 hrs would be acceptable after dosage A but incorrect after dosage B. Thus, both absolute dosage and plasma half-life must be taken into account as determinants of effective duration of drug action.

PHARMACOLOGICAL RECEPTORS

Many drugs that affect gastrointestinal motility do so by interactions with specific pharmacological receptors. Receptors are presumed to be specific sites on macromolecules which offer electrochemical and steric complementarity to drug molecules. In most cases, at least, the natural purpose of receptors is to interact with specific neurotransmitters, autacoids, or hormones. Acti-

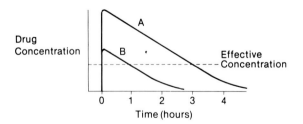

FIG. 4. Concentrations of a drug in blood after intravenous administration of two different dose levels. After injection of dose *A*, blood levels are maintained at effective concentrations for 3 hr. After a smaller dose (*B*), an effective concentration is present for only 1 hr. The slopes of the decay curves are identical (same plasma half-life).

vation of a receptor leads to a specific tissue response; blockade of the receptor does not in itself initiate a response but prevents activation of that specific receptor. The existence of pharmacological receptors was originally deduced from the extreme biological activity of many chemical compounds and by the observation that similar molecules often produce similar effects. The fact that stereoisomers usually differ dramatically in biological activity provides further evidence for the existence of receptors. Finally, the biological effects of competitive antagonists provide compelling evidence for the existence of receptors.

In the simplest terms, a drug molecule interacts with a receptor to produce a biological response. We now know that receptors consist of multiple components. The most proximal component of the receptor system is the recognition or binding site. After a drug molecule binds to the receptor to activate it, a transducing mechanism is necessary to begin the process of biological multiplication. The transducer mechanism may be a simple opening of ion channels or activation of an enzyme system. In some cases the sequence of transducing and multiplication events is fairly well understood. More often, however, little is known about events between receptor binding and biological response. Studies of competition between molecules for binding have provided many new insights into the recognition component of several types of receptors. However, because binding and biological response can rarely be studied in the same experimental preparation, much remains to be learned about the specific events initiated in most cases by receptor activation.

Responses to drugs are nearly always graded or dose-dependent. As binding studies have shown that drug-receptor interactions follow simple mass-action relationships, it can be assumed that the magnitude of the response is directly proportional to the fraction of total receptor sites occupied by the drug molecules. Thus, fractional receptor occupancy is related to magnitude of the response obtained. It follows, then, that treatments that reduce the number of available receptors should somehow interfere with the ability of the drug to induce a response.

A drug that occupies a receptor to bring about a biological response is known as an *agonist*. The biological response may be either an increase or a decrease in organ function. The relative ability of a molecule to bind to a particular receptor is known as *affinity*. The amount of drug required to produce a particular response is known as *potency*. *Efficacy* or *intrinsic activity* is the ability of a drug to produce a maximum biological response. Drugs that can bring about only a partial response, drugs lacking in efficacy or intrinsic activity, are referred to as *partial agonists*. An *antagonist* is a drug that occupies a receptor, but, because it is totally devoid of efficacy or intrinsic activity, cannot initiate a response. An antagonist interferes with ability of agonists to bind with that particular receptor and thus inhibits responses to agonists. Antagonists are generally classified either as *competitive* or *noncompetitive*. As the terms imply, competitive antagonists interact reversibly with the receptor and, following mass-action kinetics, compete with the agonists for occupancy of the receptor binding site. Noncompetitive antagonists interact irreversibly with the binding site or reversibly at another site which prevents expression of the biological response initiated by activation of the receptor.

As dictated by receptor theory, there is a quantitative relationship between receptor activation by agonists and amplitude of the response obtained. This relationship is usually expressed in the form of dose-response curves. It is customary when plotting dose-response curves to express response as the ordinant and dose as the abcissa. Dose is generally expressed on a logarithmic scale and is often called a *log dose-response curve*. Usually, the middle range of the dose-response curve is nearly straight when dose is plotted on a log scale. It is important in studies of dose-response relationships to achieve a maximum response, if possible. In the case of gastrointestinal smooth muscle it is nearly always possible to achieve a maximum response. Dose may be expressed in any convenient units: mg/kg, μg/ml, μM/kg. When comparing potencies of different drugs, it is desirable to express dosage on a molar basis to eliminate the variable of differences in molecular weight.

The use of the log dose-response curve for comparison of different drugs or study of drug interactions is illustrated in Fig. 5. We will first consider that curves A, B, and C in Fig. 5 represent responses to three different drugs. As can be seen, drugs A and C both are capable of producing maximum responses, although different doses are required with each drug to achieve the maximum response. Drug B cannot produce a maximum response. Drug A produces a half-maximal response at a dose of 3 (μg, mg/kg, μM). Drug C requires a dose of over 30 to achieve a half-maximal response.

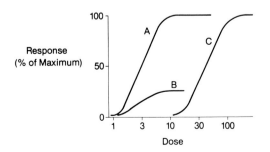

FIG. 5. Hypothetical dose-response curves. Dose is plotted on a log scale, response is plotted as a percentage of the maximum response that can be obtained. Curves may represent responses to three different drugs or responses to the same drug after different treatments (*see text*).

We may conclude that drug A is more potent than drug C in eliciting this particular response. Drug B also requires a dose of 3 to produce its half-maximal response, even though its maximal response is not as great as the maximum responses produced by drugs A and C. The median effective dose (ED_{50}) of drugs A and B are equal and they are of equal potency. Drugs A and C display equal efficacy, which is the ability to elicit a maximum response. Drug B displays less efficacy than either drug A or drug C.

We will assume now that the dose-response curves illustrated in Fig. 5 represent responses to a single agonist under different conditions. First, curve A will represent control responses to an agonist. In this case, curve B would represent responses to agonist A in the presence of a noncompetitive antagonist. Noncompetitive antagonists characteristically reduce the maximum response achieved with the agonist without much change in the ED_{50} dose. Curve C would represent responses to agonist A in the presence of a competitive antagonist. It is a feature of competitive antagonism that the ED_{50} dose of the agonist is increased without significant change in the maximum response achieved. Careful studies of dose-response relationships can thus provide considerable information concerning drug interactions. Note also another feature. If, instead of multiple doses, a single dose of agonist A (100) had been studied under control conditions, after addition of the competitive antagonist, there would be no observable change in response to this supramaximal dose of agonist A, even though the dose-response curve was actually shifted over 10-fold to the right. Obviously, the most sensitive portion of the dose-response curve is the middle range around the ED_{50} dose. It is important in studies of drug interactions to ascertain that submaximal doses are employed.

Finally, we will assume that curve C is the control response to an agonist. In this case, curve A could represent a shift to the left in the dose-response curve induced by a treatment. Curve A, an apparent increase in potency, could be observed as a result of supersensitivity, such as that which occurs after denervation or application of a drug that inhibits inactivation of the agonist (neostigmine and acetylcholine, cocaine and norepinephrine).

Functional inhibition or physiological antagonism can occur with drugs that induce opposite biological responses. For example, simultaneous application to intestinal smooth muscle of acetylcholine, which induces contractions, and epinephrine, which causes relaxation, will result in apparent antagonism between the two agonists, which act on completely different receptors. In this case, dose-response curves constructed for one of the drugs in the absence and presence of the other would give the appearance of noncompetitive antagonism between the two agents.

MECHANISMS OF DRUG ACTION

Ideally, we would like to know the precise molecular mechanism by which any drug produces its biological effect. In the vast majority of cases, the precise mechanisms are not known. Often, in fact, even the site of action may not have been established with precision. It is sometimes tempting to ascribe a site of action anatomically close to the response observed. Because of the ability of neural and hormonal systems to operate across large distances, the site of action of a drug may be quite remote from the response observed. For example, a particular drug may affect intestinal motility *in vivo* mainly by actions in the central nervous system which alter neural outflow to the gastrointestinal smooth muscle. Sometimes drugs may exert similar effects at multiple sites. For example, a particular drug may produce similar motility effects by actions at central sites as well as by means of local effects. Thus, even demonstration of local effects *in vitro* cannot rule out the possibility of other important sites of action in intact animals.

Complex interplay among neural, paracrine, and endocrine systems complicate interpretation of drug actions. For example, inhibition of a particular pattern of contractions by atropine might be attributed to removal of cholinergic influences on the smooth muscle cells responsible for the contractions. In fact, the action of atropine may have been to reduce secretion of a peptide hormone that acted on the smooth muscle to produce the contractions. Similarly, a prostaglandin synthetase inhibitor might be observed to inhibit a particular pattern of contractions. It might be assumed that a prostaglandin was directly responsible for production of the contractions. In fact, the explanation could be considerably more complicated. The prostaglandin might have acted by inhibiting release of neural norepinephrine, which in turn inhibited release of acetylcholine. Prevention of prostaglandin synthesis would remove an inhibitory control on the adrenergic inhibitory neuron, allowing it to cause further inhibition of acetylcholine release. Many drugs can, of course, act directly on smooth muscle cells. To understand the actions of a drug, it is necessary to know its sites of action.

Drugs that act directly upon smooth muscle cells often do so by interactions with specific drug receptors. Activation of the drug receptor initiates a series of intracellular events characterized by production of a second messenger, which activates the intracellular multiplier system. The best known and only well-described second messenger system is that which involves cyclic adenosine monophosphate (cAMP). The importance of a second messenger in pharmacology is that it allows better understanding of the molecular basis of drug action and it provides an additional opportunity to modify cell responses by the use of drugs.

In terms of direct drug effects on smooth muscle cells, the most important effect of the cyclic nucleotide second messenger systems may be their ability to regulate availability of calcium to the contractile elements (17). In general, those chemical agents that stimulate contractions act by raising intracellular levels of calcium, whereas the relaxing agents lower the calcium level by a mechanism which, in some cases, is regulated by cAMP (12).

There is little doubt that the relaxation of gastrointestinal smooth muscle induced by β-adrenergic receptor agonists is associated with an increased intracellular level of cAMP, which stimulates an increase in the calcium binding capacity of the sarcoplasmic reticulum (4,5). The role of cyclic guanosine monophosphate (cGMP) is less clear. cGMP can induce contractions of gastrointestinal smooth muscle, an effect often accompanied by concomitant decreases in cAMP concentration (3,112). However, drugs and neurotransmitters can induce contractions without altering intracellular cGMP levels (142). It is possible that the increases in cGMP concentrations sometimes observed after activation of muscarinic cholinergic receptors results from membrane depolarization and the associated increase in myoplasmic calcium levels (94). The calcium ions may be responsible for stimulation of guanylate cyclase and the resulting increase in cGMP levels. The elevation of cGMP could be a factor of importance for the maintenance of contraction by supporting release of calcium from subcellular pools. There is at present insufficient evidence to state that drugs which induce relaxation of gastrointestinal smooth muscle do so invariably by increasing intracellular concentrations of cAMP. Similarly, there is no compelling evidence that contractions of the smooth muscle are invariably associated with increases in intracellular concentrations of cGMP.

In addition to possible roles under certain circumstances in intestinal smooth muscle, cyclic nucleotides may alter external influences on smooth muscle cells. The probable role of cyclic nucleotides as second messenger mediators of secretory events (80,84) could, through reflex mechanisms activated by luminal distention, alter neural influences on muscle cells. Cyclic nucleotides may function also in neurons to modulate synthesis, storage, and release of neurotransmitter chemicals. β-Adrenergic receptor agonists, for example, may act presynaptically to enhance release of norepinephrine from adrenergic nerve terminals (1,141). This effect may be mediated by cAMP. Many other modulators of neurally mediated norepinephrine release affect cAMP or cGMP levels in nerves. However, there seems to be no completely consistent relationship between the effects of these agents on neural adenylate cyclase or guanylate cyclase and their effects on release of norepinephrine from nerves (156). More convincing evidence is available that cAMP and cGMP serve as essential second messengers in ganglion cells in the genesis of ganglionic synaptic potentials (77,89). Acetylcholine released from preganglionic fibers interacts with ganglion cell nicotinic cholinergic receptors to produce a rapid depolarization of the postsynaptic membrane with subsequent initiation of propagated action potentials. The acetylcholine also acts on ganglion cell muscarinic cholinergic receptors to stimulate increased formation of cGMP, resulting in a late excitatory postsynaptic potential (78). In superior cervical ganglia, the acetylcholine released from the preganglionic fiber also acts on muscarinic cholinergic receptors of dopaminergic interneurons to cause release of dopamine, an adrenergic amine. The dopamine acts on ganglion cell α-adrenergic receptors, causing increased formation of cAMP. The cAMP produces a slow inhibitory postsynaptic potential (74). Thus, ganglionic transmission in the superior cervical ganglion is modulated by a number of cyclic-nucleotide-mediated events that can inhibit or facilitate the transmission process. Similar mechanisms may modulate ganglionic transmission in gastrointestinal tissues. Cyclic nucleotides could be important second messengers, intimately involved in these events.

Many drugs that affect gastrointestinal motility do so by altering the neurotransmission processes that normally regulate cell function. Regardless of the specific type of neuron involved, neurotransmission is a multistep process with many opportunities for drug intervention.

NEUROTRANSMISSION

Nerves communicate with other cells by means of specific chemical neurotransmitter substances. The cells affected by neurally released neurotransmitters may be nerve, gland, or muscle cells. In the periphery, nerve-nerve connections occur primarily in ganglia, including ganglia of the myenteric plexus. Nerve-muscle connections provide the final neural control of muscle function. The neural element that releases the neurotransmitter is commonly called the presynaptic element, the cell on which the neurotransmitter acts is called the postsynaptic element or effector cell. Neurotransmitter chemicals alter function of effector cells, including gastrointestinal smooth muscle cells, by effects on the external surface of the postsynaptic (effector cell) plasma membrane. Whether the neurotransmitter is acetylcholine, norepinephrine, 5-HT, or another substance, the specific processes involved in neurotransmission are remarkably similar. The major steps in the sequence, illustrated in Fig. 6, are neurotransmitter synthesis, storage, release, interaction with postsynaptic receptors, and termination of neurotransmitter action. Each step is subject to modification by drugs.

Neurotransmitter compounds may be synthesized in nerve cell bodies or in nerve axon terminals. Appropri-

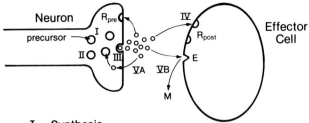

I. Synthesis
II. Storage
III. Release
IV. Interaction with postsynaptic receptors
V. Termination of action
   A. Reuptake
   B. Enzymatic

FIG. 6. Summary of events involved in neurotransmission between a neuron and an effector cell such as a gastrointestinal smooth muscle cell. Neurotransmitter is synthesized (*I*) and stored (*II*) in vesicles in the neuron. In response to invasion of a nerve action potential, neurotransmitter vesicles fuse with the neuronal membrane and their content of transmitter is released (*III*) into the synaptic cleft. Neurotransmitter molecules diffuse across the synaptic space and interact (*IV*) with receptors (R_{post}) on the postsynaptic (effector cell) membrane to initiate a biological response. The neurotransmitter also interacts with presynaptic neural receptors (R_{pre}) to modify secretion of neurotransmitter. Actions of the neurotransmitter are terminated by reuptake (*A*) into the neuron or by enzymatic (*E*) degradation (*B*) into an inactive metabolite (*M*).

ate precursor chemicals are taken up into the nerve for synthesis of the neurotransmitter and the reactions are catalyzed by the appropriate enzymes. Once synthesis has occurred, the neurotransmitter is stored in high concentration in a form that protects it from enzymatic degradation and is held in readiness for release. Storage occurs in membrane-limited vesicles, which usually are concentrated in specific regions of the nerve terminal. At the nerve terminal, arrival of a nerve action potential allows influx of calcium and other ions which promote fusion of vesicle membranes with neuronal membranes. Vesicular contents, including neurotransmitter, are released into the synaptic cleft by exocytosis. The neurotransmitter molecules diffuse across the synaptic space and interact with specific neurotransmitter receptors on the postsynaptic (effector cell) membrane. Activation of the effector cell receptors by binding of the neurotransmitter with receptor recognition sites initiates the intracellular multiplier events which result in the biological response. Interaction of neurotransmitter molecules with receptors is a readily reversible process which follows the law of mass action. Actions of neurotransmitters in the synaptic space are terminated by several different processes which result in removal of the transmitter molecules. For acetylcholine, the major terminating event is hydrolysis into acetate and choline by acetylcholinesterase. The actions of norepinephrine in most tissues are terminated primarily by active reuptake into the presynaptic neural element. The monoamine neurotransmitters, norepinephrine, dopamine, and 5-HT, are also substrates for monoamine oxidase

(MAO), located primarily in mitochondria. MAO catalyzes oxidative deamination to form an aldehyde, which is oxidized by aldehyde dehydrogenase to the corresponding carboxylic acid. Both the aldehyde intermediate and the acid metabolites are physiologically inactive. Many effector cells also contain the enzyme catechol-*O*-methyltransferase (COMT), which inactivates norepinephrine and other catechols by methylation of a ring hydroxyl function. In most tissues, including gastrointestinal tissue, enzymatic degradation by MAO and COMT are relatively unimportant, and norepinephrine actions are terminated mainly by uptake into the presynaptic neuron.

The neurotransmission process can be modulated physiologically in several ways. The most common and important way is by adjustment of the amount of neurotransmitter released in response to volleys of nerve discharge. After release into the synaptic space, neurotransmitter molecules may interact with presynaptic receptors as well as with postsynaptic receptors. After its release, norepinephrine can interact with presynaptic α-adrenergic receptors which inhibit further release of norepinephrine. As calcium influx is required for exocytotic release of norepinephrine, it is thought that activation of presynaptic α-receptors inhibits norepinephrine release through inhibition of calcium influx. Presynaptic inhibition of neurotransmitter release is of considerable physiological importance because drugs, such as phentolamine, that block presynaptic α-adrenergic receptors promote excessive release of norepinephrine in response to nerve stimulation. In the gastrointestinal tract, inhibition of norepinephrine release may also represent an important presynaptic modulating action of prostaglandins. Prostaglandins appear to act on specific neuronal prostaglandin receptors to cause inhibition of norepinephrine release, possibly by increasing intraneuronal levels of cAMP, which facilitates sequestering of the calcium ions required for release of the transmitter (67). Although of great potential importance as mechanisms of drug action, the physiological roles of other types of presynaptic modulating influences have not been well established.

Drugs can act in several different ways to alter the processes responsible for neurotransmission. Theoretically, at least, drugs can enhance neurotransmission by the following mechanisms: increasing neurotransmitter synthesis, increasing neurotransmitter release, mimicking receptor actions of neurotransmitter, or decreasing efficacy of mechanisms responsible for termination of neurotransmitter actions. Conversely, drugs can inhibit neurotransmission processes by interference with synthesis of neurotransmitter, decreasing storage of neurotransmitter, inhibiting release of neurotransmitter, promoting formation of false transmitter molecules, or inhibiting interaction of the neurotransmitter with postsynaptic receptors. Specific drugs that produce effects at these various sites are presented below in the context of each neurotransmitter system.

CHOLINERGIC STIMULANTS AND INHIBITORS

The pharmacologic strategy to be employed in studies of cholinergic neurotransmission depends on the aim of the experiment and the degree of precision required. If the aim of the experiment is to determine whether a particular substance causes intestinal contractions through actions on muscarinic cholinergic receptors, demonstration of antagonism by atropine may be sufficient. However, because atropine may exert nonspecific effects (see below), ample control experiments to demonstrate specificity of atropine action are required for greater precision. Also, use of atropine cannot rule out the possibility of drug actions other than direct agonist effects on muscarinic cholinergic receptors. For example, the test drug may act on neural elements to promote release of acetylcholine, yet the contractions would be blocked at the muscarinic receptors by atropine. In this case, neural effects could be tested by the use of tetrodotoxin, by depletion of neural acetylcholine content, or by potentiation of the response by use of an acetylcholinesterase inhibitor. Obviously, use of atropine alone provides relatively little information. Some prototype drugs that affect cholinergic function are listed in Table 1.

Synthesis of acetylcholine in intestine can be increased by treatment with its metabolic precursor, cho-

TABLE 1. *Drug effects on cholinergic neurotransmission*

Process	Drug	Effect
Acetylcholine synthesis	Choline	Increase
	Hemicholinium	Inhibit
Acetylcholine release	Botulinum toxin	Inhibit
Acetylcholine hydrolysis	Neostigmine	Inhibit
Actions on cholinergic receptors		
Nicotinic	DMPP	Agonist
	Hexamethonium	Antagonist
Muscarinic	Bethanechol	Agonist
	Atropine	Antagonist

line (66,107). Choline alone generally has only minimal effects on gastrointestinal motility. A more effective method for manipulation of acetylcholine synthesis is by use of hemicholinium. Hemicholinium competes with choline for its neural transport mechanism, which results in inadequate intraneuronal supplies of choline to the acetylcholine synthetic machinery (13). In the absence of ongoing cholinergic neurotransmission, hemicholinium will exert no effect on gastrointestinal preparations because intraneuronal stores of acetylcholine are maintained intact under static conditions. Hemicholinium effects can be observed only after continuous cholinergic neural activity, often driven by electrical stimulation. Continuous stimulation leads to exhaustion of neural acetylcholine stores and failure of cholinergic transmission. Two maneuvers are necessary to demonstrate specificity of hemicholinium actions. Direct-acting agonists, such as methacholine or bethanechol, can be applied to determine smooth muscle viability after hemicholinium treatment. This can be coupled with use of a ganglionic stimulant, such as DMPP, which should show greatly diminished activity after neural acetylcholine is depleted. Finally, at the termination of the experiment, the tissue can be exposed to choline, which, by competing with hemicholinium for neural transport mechanisms, can enter the nerve and allow repletion of acetylcholine stores and reestablishment of cholinergic transmission and responses to DMPP.

Neural release of acetylcholine can be inhibited by application of botulinum toxin, causing blockade of cholinergic transmission (75). However, botulinum toxin is difficult to prepare and is extremely hazardous, therefore its use is not recommended.

The transmitter actions of acetylcholine ordinarily are terminated rapidly by the action of acetylcholinesterase. Inhibitors of acetylcholinesterase delay hydrolysis of acetylcholine and increase its concentration in the receptor region. Actions of acetylcholinesterase inhibitors can be of benefit in demonstrating cholinergic links in drug action. With *in vivo* experiments, neostigmine is a popular acetylcholinesterase inhibitor. It is a quaternary amine and does not penetrate effectively into the brain, thus limiting its effects to peripheral sites of action. With *in vitro* preparations, neostigmine may be delayed in penetrating to sites of action because of its highly polar chemical nature. *In vitro*, physostigmine, also known as eserine, which is more lipid-soluble, can be quite useful. As acetylcholinesterase is the enzyme responsible for terminating acetylcholine actions at sites of synaptic transmission, plasma or nonspecific cholinesterases are usually of little consequence to acetylcholine neurotransmission. However, in intact preparations where plasma cholinesterases in circulating blood could affect exogenously administered acetylcholine, drugs that inhibit both plasma cholinesterases as well as acetylcholinesterase can sometimes be of value. The organophosphate cholinesterase inhibitors are effective against both plasma cholinesterases and acetylcholinesterase. The best characterized of the organophosphate cholinesterase inhibitors is diisopropylfluorophosphate (DFP). Because of the hazardous nature of this drug, its use should be strictly limited to those experimental situations where it is essential. If hydrolysis of acetylcholine presents an experimental difficulty, the problem can be solved easily by use of a stable choline ester, such as carbachol.

In laboratory and clinical experiments, receptor agonists and antagonists provide degrees of specificity and selectivity that cannot be achieved through the use of more generalized modalities, such as inhibition of acetylcholinesterase. Gastrointestinal smooth muscle cholinergic receptors are almost exclusively of the muscarinic type. Neural receptors for acetylcholine are generally nicotinic cholinergic receptors, although muscarinic cholinergic receptors may also occur in neural elements. At autonomic ganglia, possibly including to some degree the intramural cholinergic ganglia, muscarinic cholinergic receptors may facilitate ganglionic transmission initiated by the nicotinic cholinergic receptor agonist actions of acetylcholine (78). Muscarinic cholinergic receptors located on nerve terminals may serve to inhibit release of acetylcholine, possibly functioning in a negative feedback mechanism that regulates transmitter release (79). Intestinal cholinergic neurons also contain adrenergic receptors that inhibit release of acetylcholine (45,103) and serve as a major modulatory site of adrenergic influences (9).

Nicotine is the classic nicotinic cholinergic receptor agonist. However, nicotine may exert nonspecific effects in gastrointestinal tissues, including persistent depolarization of neuronal membranes. DMPP is generally regarded as a more selective nicotinic cholinergic receptor agonist. In excessive dosages, DMPP, like nicotine, can also induce persistent depolarization of neural membranes. Tetramethylammonium has sometimes been used as a ganglionic stimulant. Although it can activate nicotinic cholinergic receptors, use of tetramethylammonium should be avoided, as it can also act upon muscarinic cholinergic receptors. Hexamethonium (C_6) is a competitive antagonist at nicotinic cholinergic receptors. In some cases, C_6 will not establish good blockade in isolated tissues in the absence of ongoing cholinergic transmission. In those instances, tetraethylammonium, a depolarizing-type nicotinic cholinergic receptor antagonist, may be employed beneficially. In addition to effects on nicotinic cholinergic receptors, tetraethylammonium also can block potassium conductance. Other nicotinic cholinergic receptor competitive antagonists, such as *d*-tubocurarine, pentolinium, and chlorisondamine, have been employed successfully with gastrointestinal tissues.

When precise specificity of receptor actions is required, receptor specific agents should be employed. Acetylcholine and carbachol act on both nicotinic and muscarinic cholinergic receptors. For this reason, use of these agents *in vivo* is generally undesirable. However, *in vitro*, they often appear to act primarily on muscarinic cholinergic receptors. In any event, the prudent investigator will conduct appropriate control experiments to determine the receptor specificity of the drugs employed. Pilocarpine, generally classified as a muscarinic cholinergic receptor agonist, can sometimes act on nicotinic cholinergic receptors and even adrenergic receptors.

Bethanechol and methacholine are relatively selective muscarinic cholinergic receptor agonists. Bethanechol may have slightly greater selectivity for smooth muscle muscarinic cholinergic receptors and is almost completely resistent to hydrolysis by acetylcholinesterase. Bethanechol, therefore, is often the preferred muscar-

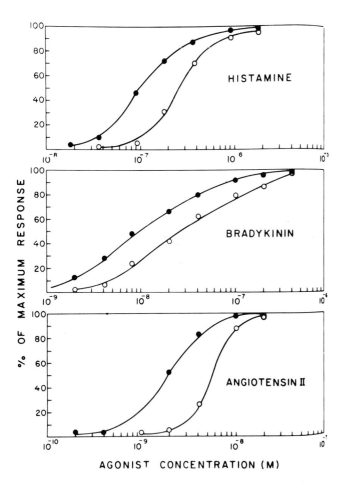

FIG. 7. Probably nonspecific effects of high concentrations of atropine on responses of guinea pig ileum to histamine, bradykinin, and angiotensin. The concentration of atropine (3×10^{-6} M) was sufficient to produce a 4300-fold shift to the right of dose-response curves for acetylcholine and 2–5-fold shifts to the right for the substances illustrated here. (From Paiva et al., ref. 101, with permission.)

inic cholinergic receptor agonist. Atropine is the classic muscarinic cholinergic receptor antagonist. In low concentrations, it is a drug of considerable specificity. To achieve the desired level of antagonism *in vitro*, however, atropine is generally employed in relatively high concentrations which can be much less specific. In the usual *in vitro* concentrations required to produce 95% antagonism of cholinergic transmission, atropine can cause nonspecific inhibition (Fig. 7). The possible nonspecificity of atropine at higher concentrations should caution against over-reliance on this drug to demonstrate cholinergic components in drug action. Atropine and similar agents can be tremendously valuable pharmacological tools, but their utility is enhanced when other parallel experiments are conducted to verify specificity of action. Other muscarinic cholinergic receptor antagonists presumably suffer to varying extents the same flaws. However, some investigators prefer scopolamine (hyoscine) or a quaternary ammonium derivative, such as methylatropine or propantheline. The quaternary ammonium compounds, however, may exhibit modest nicotinic cholinergic receptor antagonism in addition to their effects on muscarinic cholinergic receptors.

ADRENERGIC STIMULANTS AND INHIBITORS

Owing possibly to the previous lack of adequately specific drugs, the actions of adrenergic stimulants and inhibitors have not been adequately explored in terms of gastrointestinal motility. With the development of new, specific drugs and the continuing availability of reliable old drugs, improved definition of adrenergic actions on gastrointestinal motility should now be possible.

The postganglionic sympathetic nerves that innervate much of the gastrointestinal tract probably serve primarily to regulate activity in cholinergic nerves (9,73,133). Most of the adrenergic fibers in the intestine appear to terminate in the region of intramural ganglia or on blood vessels. A few adrenergic fibers penetrate to smooth muscle layers. Whether or not they receive significant adrenergic innervation, gastrointestinal smooth muscle cells have adrenergic receptors and smooth muscle function can be modified by adrenergic and antiadrenergic agents. Prototype drugs that affect adrenergic neurotransmission are listed in Table 2.

In some tissues, synthesis of norepinephrine can be enhanced by exogenously applied dihydroxyphenylalanine (DOPA), its metabolic precursor. As the rate-limiting step in the synthesis of norepinephrine is activity of tyrosine hydroxylase, which converts tyrosine to DOPA, direct application of DOPA can bypass this step and increase norepinephrine synthesis.

Inhibition of norepinephrine synthesis is best achieved by blockade of the rate-limiting step, tyrosine hydrox-

TABLE 2. *Drug effects on adrenergic neurotransmission*

Process	Drug	Effect
Norepinephrine synthesis	DOPA	Enhance
	Alpha-methyl-*para*-tyrosine	Inhibit
Norepinephrine storage	Reserpine	Deplete
Norepinephrine release	Tyramine	Increase
	Guanethidine	Inhibit
Actions on adrenergic receptors		
α_1(postsynaptic)	Methoxamine	Agonist
	Prazocin	Antagonist
α_2(presynaptic)	Clonidine	Agonist
	Yohimbine	Antagonist
β_1	Dobutamine	Agonist
	Metoprolol	Antagonist
β_2	Terbutaline	Agonist
	Butoxamine	Antagonist
Norepinephrine neuronal uptake	Desmethylimipramine	Inhibit
MAO activity	Tranylcypromine	Inhibit
COMT activity	4-Methyltropolone	Inhibit

ylase activity. Tyrosine hydroxylase is sensitive to α-methyl-*para*-tyrosinc, which, ovcr a pcriod of hours or days, can deplete adrenergic nerves of norepinephrine content. The cytotoxic agent, 6-hydroxydopamine, is taken up fairly selectively by adrenergic neurons, which are damaged owing to intraneuronal formation of hydrogen peroxide (144). The effect may not be totally selective in that other neurons which possess monoamine transport systems, such as those which release 5-HT, can also be affected (36). After treatment with 6-hydroxydopamine, adrenergic function is disrupted within a few hours and norepinephrine levels are diminished for several days (73), depending on exact experimental conditions and age of the animals. In young animals or after high dosages, the terminals of many adrenergic neurons are destroyed by 6-hydroxydopamine treatment. Neuronal storage of norepinephrine can be inhibited by a variety of rauwolfia alkaloids, such as reserpine. These drugs block the amine transport system of the intraneuronal storage granule membranes, thus allowing escape into the cytoplasm of the granule content of norepinephrine. Once released into the cytoplasm, the adrenergic amine is quickly deaminated by mitochondrial monoamine oxidase. The inactive deaminated metabolites diffuse out of the neuron. The norepinephrine content of tissue is depleted within a few hours after reserpine treatment and levels remain depressed for several days. A special caution is required for investigators choosing to employ drugs that deplete tissues of adrenergic amines. As mentioned above, these treatments are not totally selective. Reserpine, for example, depletes tissues not only of norepinephrine, but also of dopamine and 5-HT and, to a lesser extent, of histamine and peptide hormones. The second caution concerns the relative resistance of gas-

trointestinal tissues to amine depletion. Dosages of α-methyl-*para*-tyrosine, 6-hydroxydopamine, or reserpine that deplete brain, heart, or blood vessels of norepinephrine may have considerably less effect on gastrointestinal concentrations of the adrenergic amine (73). Depletion of gastrointestinal norepinephrine is often achieved only after vigorous pharmacological treatment, and, even then, the success of the treatment cannot be ascertained unless norepinephrine levels are actually measured. Finally, one must be concerned with interpretation of negative results. In some tissues, even 90% depletion of norepinephrine may not markedly impair adrenergic neurotransmission processes. Thus, failure of depletion to block a response may not provide conclusive evidence that noradrenergic transmission is not involved.

Release of norepinephrine from its neuronal stores can be achieved by use of the indirectly acting sympathomimetic agent, tyramine. Tyramine is transported into adrenergic nerves and displaces norepinephrine from readily releasable pools into the synaptic cleft (150). Tyramine has virtually no direct effect on adrenergic receptors. Its effects are due almost entirely to the norepinephrine it releases and its actions in gastrointestinal tissues are virtually identical to those of exogenously applied norepinephrine. Tyramine can be used as an indirect test for the integrity of noradrenergic nerves in a tissue. For example, complete depletion of norepinephrine by α-methyl-*para*-tyrosine, 6-hydroxydopamine, or reserpine should totally prevent responses to tyramine. Persistence of tyramine effects indicates lack of norepinephrine depletion. Again, however, absence of tyramine effects does not prove that amines are depleted.

Guanethidine is a useful drug for preventing release

of norepinephrine. The norepinephrine antirelease effect of guanethidine requires that the drug be transported by the neuronal membrane amine transport system into the nerve. Guanethidine competes with norepinephrine for the neuronal membrane transport mechanism and thus exerts a norepinephrine antiuptake effect. Once inside the neuron, guanethidine prevents exocytotic release of norepinephrine, probably by interference with the influx of calcium required for the release process. Over a period of days or weeks, guanethidine in high doses can cause depletion of neuronal norepinephrine by promoting slow release of the amine from its storage granules into the nerve cytoplasm, where it undergoes oxidative deamination in the mitochondria. The acute effects of guanethidine are limited to its norepinephrine antiuptake and antirelease effects. Guanethidine may exert similar effects on neural and nonneural elements that contain 5-HT.

There are four recognized types of adrenergic receptors, which can be differentiated pharmacologically. Prototype drugs that act on these receptors are listed in Table 3. α_1-Adrenergic receptors are located postsynaptically and mediate effects of adrenergic amines on nerves, glands, and smooth muscle. α_2-Adrenergic receptors are located presynaptically on adrenergic nerve terminals and serve to inhibit norepinephrine release from the neuron. Thus, activation of α_1-adrenergic re-

ceptors causes a typical sympathomimetic effect, whereas activation of α_2-adrenergic receptors inhibits adrenergic neurotransmission. Two types of β-adrenergic receptors can be identified in various tissues on the basis of their sensitivity to agonist and antagonist drugs. There is some evidence for the existence of a presynaptic β-adrenergic receptor on adrenergic nerve terminals which serves to facilitate release of norepinephrine (29). Generally, β-adrenergic receptors are thought to occur postsynaptically on neurons, glands, and particularly on smooth muscle. Intestinal smooth muscle β-adrenergic receptors were tentatively identified as belonging to the β_1 category, but this identification requires reinvestigation with the newer, more selective agents presently available. It is more likely that both β_1- and β_2-adrenergic receptors exist in gastrointestinal tissues (125).

Norepinephrine is an agonist at α_1-, α_2-, and β_1-adrenergic receptors. Phenylephrine and particularly methoxamine are agonists primarily at α_1-adrenergic receptors. Clonidine is a relatively selective agonist at the presynaptic α_2-adrenergic receptors. If it were perfectly selective, clonidine would act exclusively to inhibit neuronal release of norepinephrine. In many tissues, clonidine also acts as an agonist on postsynaptic α_1-adrenergic receptors and thus possesses modest sympathomimetic activity. Phentolamine and phenoxybenzamine are the classic α-adrenergic receptor antag-

TABLE 3. Receptor actions of common adrenergic agents

Drugs	Receptors				
	α_1	α_2	β_1	β_2	Dopamine
Agonists					
Norepinephrine	+	+	+		
Epinephrine	+	+	+	+	
Isoproterenol			+	+	
Dopamine	+[a]		+[b]		+
Phenylephrine	+				
Methoxamine	+				
Clonidine		+			
Dobutamine			+		
Terbutaline				+	
Metaproterenol				+	
Carbuterol				+	
Salbutamol				+	
Antagonists					
Phentolamine	+	+			
Phenoxybenzamine	+	+			
Propranolol			+	+	
Metoprolol			+		
Butoxamine				+	
Prazocin	+				
Yohimbine		+			
Haloperidol					+
Domperidone					+

[a]High doses.
[b]Probably indirect.

onists. Phentolamine, the more selective, is a competitive antagonist at both α_1- and α_2-adrenergic receptors. Phenoxybenzamine functions as a noncompetitive antagonist at both types of α-adrenergic receptors by forming covalent chemical bonds with functional groups that are part of the α-adrenergic receptor. Thus, phentolamine displays kinetics characteristic of competitive antagonism, whereas phenoxybenzamine displays noncompetitive kinetics as an α-adrenergic receptor antagonist. Phentolamine can antagonize 5-HT in certain tissues, implying either drug nonspecificity or receptor similarity. Tolazoline, a chemically related drug, is also an agonist at H_2 histamine receptors (168). Phenoxybenzamine is notoriously nonspecific and can inhibit responses not only to norepinephrine but also to histamine and acetylcholine (Fig. 8). Insofar as effects upon adrenergic receptors are concerned, prazosin is relatively selective as an α_1-adrenergic receptor competitive antagonist, but the drug is also an inhibitor of cyclic nucleotide phosphodiesterase and probably has other actions as well (31). Yohimbine can act as an antagonist on both α_1- and α_2-adrenergic receptors, but it is more selective for α_2-adrenergic receptors than phentolamine, phenoxybenzamine, or prazosin. The α_1-adrenergic receptor antagonists inhibit postsynaptic actions of norepinephrine attributable to its α_1-adrenergic receptor agonist activity. α_2-Adrenergic receptor antagonists tend to promote excessive release of norepinephrine from adrenergic neurons. By blocking norepinephrine postsynaptic effects on α_1-adrenergic receptors while simultaneously

promoting norepinephrine release, phentolamine may intensify actions of norepinephrine on β-adrenergic receptors.

Isoproterenol is a pan-β-adrenergic receptor agonist that activates both β_1- and β_2-adrenergic receptors. Dobutamine, developed for its effects on the heart, is relatively selective as an agonist on β_1-adrenergic receptors. Several relatively selective β_2-adrenergic receptor agonists are available: terbutaline, metaproterenol, carbuterol, and salbutamol. Investigators are cautioned that neither the β_1- nor the β_2-adrenergic receptor agonists are perfectly selective. They simply have relatively greater effects on one type of β-adrenergic receptor or the other. As noted earlier, stimulation of β-adrenergic receptors almost invariably results in activation of adenylyl cyclase with subsequent increases in intracellular concentrations of cAMP. The physiological effects of β-adrenergic receptor activation in a particular cell can be attributed to second messenger functions of cAMP. Consequently, effects of β-adrenergic receptor stimulation are generally mimicked by exogenously applied cAMP or its lipid-soluble derivatives. It follows that the effects of β-adrenergic receptor activation are generally enhanced by inhibitors of cyclic nucleotide phosphodiesterase, such as theophylline.

β-Adrenergic receptor antagonists presently available all act by competitive inhibition. Propranolol, alprenolol, and others are pan-β-adrenergic receptor antagonists that block both β_1- and β_2-adrenergic receptors. Somewhat more selective agents are also available. Practolol and metoprolol are relatively selective antagonists at β_1-adrenergic receptors. Butoxamine, related chemically to methoxamine, is relatively selective as a β_2-adrenergic receptor antagonist. As with the β-adrenergic receptor agonists, the receptor selectivity of the antagonists is not absolute.

The functional significance of dopamine in relation to gastrointestinal motility has barely been explored. In many tissues, dopamine acts on distinct dopamine receptors on nerves or smooth muscle. In higher dosages, dopamine also acts on vascular α_1-adrenergic receptors and on cardiac β_1-adrenergic receptors. The cardiac effect may be largely indirect, resulting from dopamine-induced release of neural norepinephrine. Haloperidol and pimozide have been employed as prototype dopamine receptor antagonists in a variety of preparations (115,147). Metoclopramide and domperidone are effective dopamine receptor antagonists in gastrointestinal tissues (83,109,147), although metoclopramide may have other additional actions (98). The striking pharmacological effects of metoclopromide and domperidone suggest important physiological functions of dopamine in control of gastrointestinal motility (8,33,148).

Present evidence indicates that intestinal α-adrenergic receptors are localized primarily in cholinergic neurons

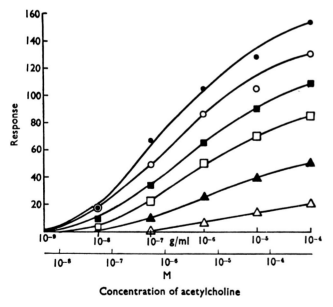

FIG. 8. Anticholinergic effects of the "adrenergic" antagonist phenoxybenzamine. Contractions of guinea pig ileum elicited by acetylcholine were antagonized noncompetitively by phenoxybenzamine in a concentration-dependent manner from 10^{-6} g/ml (O—O) to 10^{-4} g/ml d($\triangle$—$\triangle$). (From Cook, ref. 35, with permission.)

and, when activated by agonists, the α-adrenergic receptors inhibit release of acetylcholine from the intramural neurons (9,160). β-Adrenergic receptors are located on smooth muscle cells and also on cholinergic and other intramural neurons (160). Both α- and β-adrenergic receptors cause inhibition of contractions of the wall of the intestine, but α-adrenergic receptors stimulate contractions of sphincteric smooth muscle (72, 118,122). Phenylephrine causes inhibition of intestinal wall by decreasing release of acetylcholine, isoproterenol by direct inhibitory effects on smooth muscle and by neural inhibition, and epinephrine by both smooth muscle and neural effects (9,160).

Other pharmacological modalities can be used to alter adrenergic neurotransmission processes. In many tissues, including the gastrointestinal system, the major mechanism by which the actions of norepinephrine are terminated is by active uptake into adrenergic neurons. Several drugs can inhibit the uptake process and thereby preserve synaptic norepinephrine. The classic drug that blocks norepinephrine neural uptake is cocaine. However, the strong local anesthetic properties of cocaine often prevent its effective use in gastrointestinal preparations (104). Several of the tricyclic antidepressant drugs are potent inhibitors of norepinephrine uptake. The most selective of these drugs for noradrenergic neurons is desmethylimipramine (61). By preserving synaptic norepinephrine, desmethylimipramine can enhance responses to adrenergic nerve stimulation and to exogenously administered norepinephrine. As in most tissues, enzymatic inactivation of norepinephrine in gastrointestinal smooth muscle is relatively unimportant. Nevertheless, drugs are available that inhibit MAO and COMT activity. MAO exists in at least two forms, A and B (70). Norepinephrine (as well as 5-HT) is acted upon largely by form A. Clorgyline is a relatively selective inhibitor of MAO-type A. Tranylcypromine inhibits both forms A and B. For selectivity of drug action, particularly *in vivo*, clorgyline would be preferred. *In vitro*, use of tranylcypromine would foster inhibition of both forms of the enzyme. The most effective inhibitors of COMT are the tropolones, the most potent of which is 4-methyl tropolone. Theoretically at least, inhibition

of COMT activity should lead to enhancement of responses to norepinephrine; in fact, inhibition of the enzyme generally has relatively little physiological consequence. As neuronal uptake is the major inactivating mechanism for norepinephrine, inhibition of norepinephrine uptake generally produces the most dramatic enhancement of responses to norepinephrine.

DRUG EFFECTS ON 5-HYDROXYTRYPTAMINE

Whether or not 5-HT is a neurotransmitter in the gastrointestinal tract (36), it is present in high concentrations and, when applied exogenously, produces striking effects upon motility. 5-HT is biosynthesized from tryptophan, which is hydroxylated by tryptophan 5-hydroxylase to 5-hydroxytryptophan. 5-Hydroxytryptophan is decarboxylated by means of 5-hydroxytryptophan decarboxylase (probably similar or identical to aromatic 1-amino acid decarboxylase, also known as DOPA decarboxylase) to 5-HT. The presence of the decarboxylase in several types of nerves cautions against use of 5-hydroxytryptophan as a pharmacological tool to increase synthesis of 5-HT. 5-HT is stored in granules in enterochromaffin cells and in nerves. The biological actions of 5-HT are terminated by neural uptake and by oxidative deamination by MAO. Despite exhaustive studies, a physiological role for 5-HT in the gastrointestinal tract is still speculative. 5-HT may function as a nerve transmitter of interneurons in the myenteric plexus (37,165) and can be released from intestinal stores by drugs and by vagal stimulation (24–27,143,145).

The rate-limiting step in 5-HT formation is the hydroxylation of tryptophan. In the brain and probably in the gastrointestinal tract, tryptophan hydroxylation depends primarily on the concentration of substrate, tryptophan. Thus, treatment with tryptophan (Table 4) can increase the rate of synthesis of 5-HT (49,166). Conversely, blockade of 5-HT synthesis is best achieved by inhibition of tryptophan 5-hydroxylase. The drug used most extensively for this purpose is *para*-chlorophenylalanine or its methyl ester (154). In brain, *para*-chlorophenylalanine is relatively selective in pro-

TABLE 4. *Drug effects on 5-HT*

Process	Drug	Effect
5-HT synthesis	Tryptophan	Enhance
	Para-chlorophenylalanine	Inhibit
5-HT storage	Reserpine	Deplete
Actions on 5-HT receptors		
Muscle	Mescaline	Agonist
	Methysergide	Antagonist
Neural	5-Methoxy-*N,N*-dimethyltryptam	Antagonist
5-HT neuronal uptake	Chlorimipramine	Inhibit
MAO activity	Chlorgyline	Inhibit

ducing a long-lasting depletion of 5-HT with only temporary diminution of norepinephrine levels (91). Two major groups of 5-HT neurotoxins are presently available: halogenated amphetamine derivatives, such as *para*-chloroamphetamine, and the hydroxy derivatives of 5-HT, particularly 5,6- and 5,7-dihydroxytryptamine (55). These agents have been studied primarily in brain, where they cause destruction of 5-HT neurons. Gastrointestinal effects of these agents have received little attention (36). As mentioned above, reserpine effectively depletes the intestine of 5-HT as well as norepinephrine.

Traditionally, stimulatory effects of 5-HT in mammalian intestine have been considered to consist of two components: stimulation of intramural cholinergic neurons and a direct smooth muscle action (15,16,58,120). More recently, evidence has been presented that 5-HT stimulates two classes of excitatory intramural neurons, one releasing acetylcholine and the other releasing an unknown neurotransmitter (37,63). There appear to be at least two types of 5-HT receptors, one possibly located on intramural neurons and the other located on smooth muscle cells. In the older literature, the neural receptors for 5-HT were termed M receptors because they were thought to be blocked by morphine (65). Smooth muscle receptors were termed D receptors, as they were inhibited by phenoxybenzamine (Dibenzyline). It is now known that morphine does not block 5-HT receptors in intestinal tissue, it inhibits acetylcholine release from cholinergic nerves (102,129). Likewise, phenoxybenzamine inhibits intestinal responses to a wide variety of substances (163). The M and D receptor terminology should be abandoned. However, the concept of different 5-HT receptors in gastrointestinal organs of some species (124) is still valid. Unfortunately, pressures of the marketplace have stimulated considerably more research on 5-HT inhibitors in the central nervous system than in the gut. In many cases, therefore, more is known about the central nervous system action of 5-HT antagonists than their gastrointestinal effects. In the central nervous system, the drugs unquestionably affect neural 5-HT receptors. The relevance of central nervous system 5-HT receptors to gastrointestinal neural and nonneural 5-HT receptors is questionable (54). Some drugs that are known to affect mainly smooth muscle receptors in the gastrointestinal tract, such as methysergide, are effective 5-HT inhibitors in the brain.

The best-characterized 5-HT antagonists in the gastrointestinal system are the derivatives of LSD. LSD itself is a weak 5-HT antagonist. A halogenated derivative of LSD, 2-bromo-lysergic acid diethylamide (BOL), is a relatively potent antagonist of 5-HT at smooth muscle receptors (65,137). A related compound, methysergide, is even more effective (65) and is generally considered the prototype of 5-HT antagonists.

Cyproheptadine has considerable antihistaminic as well as anti-5-HT activity, but it is relatively selective in some preparations (18). Cinanserin is slightly less potent than methysergide as a 5-HT antagonist but may be more or less selective, depending on the particular preparation (90). In human and rat gastrointestinal tissues, methysergide has been found to be more selective than cinanserin; in dog intestine, cinanserin is more selective than methysergide as a 5-HT antagonist (18,19,90). Methergoline (57) has not been studied in a sufficiently wide variety of gastrointestinal preparations to determine its usefulness and selectivity.

The gastrointestinal neural receptors for 5-HT have been difficult to define. Phenyldiguanide has been suggested as an effective antagonist of 5-HT at intestinal neural receptors in the mouse, but it is nonselective in guinea pig intestine (37). Several hallucinogens and closely related substances are thought to block gastrointestinal neural 5-HT receptors: 5-methoxy-*N,N*-dimethyltryptamine, *N,N*-dimethy-5-hydroxytryptamine, and *N,N*-dimethyltryptamine (116). These substances may interact with neural 5-HT receptors to cause initial stimulation, then blockade (7,53). Methiothepin has 5-HT antagonist properties in the brain but is not totally selective for 5-HT receptors (93). Its actions in gastrointestinal preparations have not been adequately characterized. A number of substances, including metoclopramide and propranolol, have been shown to antagonize neural effects of 5-HT in nongastrointestinal preparations (51,52,87,157).

Often the best antagonist of 5-HT is 5-HT itself. Extended exposure of many tissues, including gastrointestinal tissues, to 5-HT results in rapid desensitization (autoinhibition) of 5-HT receptors to further stimulation by 5-HT. The inhibition produced by 5-HT desensitization is often quite specific for 5-HT (97). The antagonism of 5-HT receptors induced by 5-methoxy-*N,N*-dimethyltryptamine may result from a similar desensitization of 5-HT receptors (7).

In addition to 5-HT itself, other drugs may act as agonists on 5-HT receptors, including 5-methoxy-*N,N*-dimethyltryptamine, which has both agonist and antagonist properties. In some tissues, mescaline is an effective 5-HT agonist (47). Quipazine may also act as a 5-HT agonist in gastrointestinal tissues (56,69).

Neuronal uptake of 5-HT is inhibited by many of the tricyclic antidepressant drugs which also inhibit neural uptake of norepinephrine. Among the tricyclic agents, chlorimipramine is generally considered the most selective for blocking 5-HT uptake (61). A newer drug, fluoxetine, is highly selective for inhibition of 5-HT uptake in the brain (164), but it has not been tested extensively in gastrointestinal preparations. As 5-HT and norepinephrine are substrates for the same type of MAO (type A), chlorgyline effectively inhibits oxidative deamination of either of these monoamines.

DRUG EFFECTS ON HISTAMINE

Histamine is formed *in vivo* from the decarboxylation of histidine and is stored in three types of cells in the gastrointestinal tract; mast cells, APUD (amine precursor uptake and decarboxylase) cells, and a third type of cell, which has not been characterized. In the brain, histamine can exist in neurons. Two different enzyme systems are capable of decarboxylating histidine to histamine. For this reason, attempts to block formation of histamine with drugs, such as semicarbazide, have generally not succeeded in producing specific depletion. Several types of chemical compounds promote release of stored histamine. These include enzymes and venoms, such as phospholipase A and cobra venom, macromolecular compounds, such as dextran, and basic compounds, such as compound 48/80 and *d*-tubocurarine. These substances, especially compound 48/80, have been used experimentally to promote endogenous release of histamine, but they may also release peptides from mast cells (40). The degree of histamine release is rarely sufficient to produce tissue depletion.

In the gastrointestinal tract, histamine can alter motility by actions on smooth muscle and nerves. Its effects are exerted upon two types of receptors: H_1 and H_2 histamine receptors. In aqueous solution, histamine is a mixture of various ionic species, tautomers, and conformers which exist in dynamic equilibrium (59). For H_1 receptor agonist activity, imidazole tautomerism is not required, but the imidazole ring must be able to rotate to achieve coplanarity with the side chain. For H_2 receptor agonist activity, the tautomeric property of the imidazole ring of histamine appears to be of considerable importance. Several histamine analogs exert relatively selective agonist actions on H_1 or H_2 histamine receptors. The standard H_1 histamine receptor agonist is 2-methylhistamine. Several relatively selective H_2 receptor agonists have been developed. These include 5-methylhistamine, N-methylhistamine, N-methyl,5-methylhistamine, 4-methylhistamine, dimaprit, and impromidine. As with other transmitter and autacoid receptor agonists and antagonists, specificity of histamine receptor agonists and antagonists must be established in the particular experimental preparation employed. For example, the H_2 receptor agonist impromidine can antagonize the agonist effects of histamine on H_1 receptors and inhibit the effects of carbachol on cholinergic receptors (46).

H_1 histamine receptor antagonists, the classic antihistamines, include pyrilamine, tripelennamine, chlorpheniramine, and diphenhydramine. In addition to H_1 receptor antagonism, these drugs produce variable degrees of anticholinergic and antiserotonin actions. Many H_1 receptor antagonists are also potent local anesthetics. The established H_2 receptor antagonists are metiamide and cimetidine. Neither of these substances possesses the pharmacological potency required for great selectivity of action. Two more recently developed drugs with greater potency are ranitidine (14) and ICI 125,211 (Tiotidine) (167). The two newer substances may have considerable application as experimental tools.

Histamine exerts direct excitatory effects on most gastrointestinal smooth muscle by direct agonist actions on smooth muscle H_1 histamine receptors. In the lower esophageal sphincter (LES), activation of H_2 receptors may produce excitation or inhibition, depending on the animal species involved (32,34,43). Interestingly, the opossum LES can also be relaxed by activation of histamine H_1 receptors on intramural inhibitory neurons (117).

Metabolic biotransformation of histamine occurs primarily by two pathways. One pathway involves ring N-methylation by imidazole-N-methyltransferase followed by oxidative deamination by MAO to form 1-methylimidazole-4-acetic acid. Conventional MAO inhibitors, such as tranylcypromine, inhibit this pathway. The second catabolic route involves oxidative deamination by diamine oxidase to form imidazole acetic acid. This pathway is inhibited by aminoguanidine. Mammalian tissues, however, have a tremendous capacity to inactivate histamine. Blockade of one metabolic pathway shifts histamine catabolism to an alternate route. As mentioned above, reserpine can release histamine, but the degree of depletion is considerably less than that of norepinephrine or 5-HT (158).

DRUG EFFECTS ON PURINE NUCLEOTIDES

Administered exogenously, adenosine triphosphate (ATP) and related purine derivatives can cause relaxation or contraction of gastrointestinal smooth muscle. The contractions may be mediated by stimulatory effects upon intramural cholinergic neurons or result from direct excitatory effects upon gastrointestinal smooth muscle. ATP and related purine derivatives can also inhibit release of acetylcholine from intramural cholinergic nerves and can act directly upon smooth muscle cells to cause inhibition (127). Owing to interest in the noncholinergic, nonadrenergic inhibitory neurons in gastrointestinal tissues, considerable attention has focused upon the inhibitory effects of purine nucleotides as possible mediators of this mysterious inhibitory neural system (30,99). After treatment with guanethidine, to block norepinephrine release, and with muscarinic cholinergic receptor antagonists, such as atropine or scopolamine, transmural electrical stimulation often induces relaxation of gastrointestinal tissues. The relaxation response to electrical stimulation is frequently blocked by tetrodotoxin, indicating neural mediation. The inhibitory effects of the transmitter released from these inhibitory neurons is apparently exerted directly on smooth muscle cells (2,99).

Several drugs have been tested for selective inhibitory actions against ATP and related purine derivatives. The most widely tested have been theophylline and 2-2'-pyridylisatogen (PIT). Theophylline is a methylxanthine inhibitor of cyclic nucleotide phosphodiesterase, which can itself induce relaxation of intestinal smooth muscle. Likewise, PIT usually induces relaxation of intestinal smooth muscle apparently by blocking influx of extracellular calcium ions (138). Although theophylline and PIT may function as antagonists at purinergic receptors, these additional direct effects on contractile activity in gastrointestinal smooth muscle have complicated their use as tools to probe the validity of the "purinergic nerve" hypothesis (6). One of the most specific methods for blocking ATP receptors is by continued exposure of the tissue to relatively high concentrations of ATP, inducing receptor desensitization or autoinhibition to ATP. Recent studies utilizing theophylline, PIT, and ATP desensitization indicate that the neurotransmitter released by the gastrointestinal noncholinergic, nonadrenergic inhibitory neurons is not ATP or adenosine (6,135). However, theophylline and PIT may be useful tools, when used carefully, to explore gastrointestinal effects of purine nucleotides (6,135,138). The search for the transmitter(s) released by the intramural inhibitory nerves, which could be a peptide (28), will continue.

DRUG EFFECTS ON PROSTAGLANDINS

Unlike other autacoids such as 5-HT and histamine, prostaglandins are not stored in specialized structures. They are released immediately after synthesis depending upon availability of precursor chemicals. Formation of prostaglandins, prostacyclin, and thromboxane show considerable regional variation in gastrointestinal tissues (82). Their many effects upon gastrointestinal motility, which have been reviewed extensively (62,68, 155,162), will not be repeated here. The physiological, pathophysiological, and pharmacological effects of prostaglandins on gastrointestinal smooth muscle can be studied by direct application of these substances, by inhibition of their synthesis, or by blockade of their receptors. In addition to their direct effects on smooth muscle, prostaglandins also exert important actions on neural elements of the intestine, an effect that is often overlooked by investigators. Prostaglandins may decrease neural secretion of norepinephrine and serve to maintain release of neural acetylcholine (11).

The most selective method of inhibiting prostaglandin-mediated responses is by inhibition of their synthesis. This can be accomplished by application of nonsteroidal antiinflammatory drugs, such as indomethacin, or analogs of arachidonic acid, such as 5,8,11,14-eicosatetraynoic acid (ETA) (161). As with other synthesis inhibitors, the investigator must ascertain that these treatments produce the desired effects. This can be de-

termined by testing conversion of arachidonic acid to active prostaglandins before and after application of the synthesis inhibitors. At the same time, other control substances with similar effects (stimulation or inhibition) should be tested in parallel to avoid conclusions based upon nonspecific effects. Indomethacin, in particular, can produce nonspecfic inhibition of smooth muscle *in vitro*. For this reason, it is sometimes necessary to administer indomethacin to the experimental animal before test tissues are removed. Indomethacin and ETA inhibit the cyclo-oxygenase (prostaglandin synthetase) required for conversion of arachidonic acid to cyclic endoperoxides. Other inhibitors will undoubtedly be developed to block conversion of cyclic endoperoxides to prostacyclin, prostaglandins, and thromboxanes.

Prostaglandins act upon at least two types of smooth muscle receptors. The most selective receptor antagonist of prostaglandins available, SC-19,220, does not differentiate well between these receptors and can inhibit responses to a variety of other agonists (126). Ample control experiments are required to demonstrate selectivity of its actions.

DRUG EFFECTS ON PEPTIDES

With the exception of the endorphins, the mechanisms of action of the neuropeptides and hormones of the gastrointestinal tract on motility have not been studied exhaustively because of lack of adequate pharmacological tools. Nonavailability of receptor antagonists has especially hampered research in this important area. For those peptides, such as cholecystokinin, which produce contractions of gastrointestinal smooth muscle by actions on intramural cholinergic neurons, cholinergic involvement can be determined by the methods outlined above (50,139,149). For most of the peptides, however, mechanisms of action have not been established.

Present evidence indicates that substance P, vasoactive intestinal peptide (VIP), and one or more endorphins are contained within neurons of the gastrointestinal tract and may serve as neurotransmitter substances (92,100,146). All three peptides can both affect intramural nerve activity and exert direct effects on smooth muscle (10,76,123). No compelling evidence for physiological functions of these substances has been elucidated.

By the time of their discovery in gastrointestinal tissues, a great deal was known about the actions of the endorphins, owing to the availability of receptor agonists, such as morphine, and antagonists, such as naloxone. Specific opioid receptor binding sites were discovered simultaneously in brain and intestine (106). The existence of specific opioid receptors led to the deliberate search for endogenous ligands; peptide substances with morphine-like actions were discovered in 1975 (71).

Morphine-like activity on guinea pig intestine was an important pharmacological feature of the endogenous substances (38).

The endogenous morphine-like peptides are known generically as endorphins. They correspond to fragments of β-lipotropin, although the actual precursor molecule may be a much larger peptide known as pro-opiocortin (64,85). β-Endorphin (β-LPH 61-91) and met-enkephalin (β-LPH 61-65) probably exist in separate neuronal systems (153). Enkephalins occur in the intestine, probably in nerve fibers (48,136), and can be released *in vitro* by electrical stimulation (113,132). Present evidence suggests the existence of multiple types of opioid receptors, including the opioid receptors in intestine (39,81,134).

The pharmacological effects of opioid alkaloids and peptides depend on the species and the specific preparation tested. Opioid substances exert modest direct effects on some gastrointestinal smooth muscle, but their effects are usually determined by actions on neural control systems. These drugs depress contractions of guinea pig intestine by inhibition of release of acetylcholine from intramural cholinergic neurons (102,128,129). In guinea pig ileum, morphine and enkephalins act directly on myenteric neurons, probably at nerve terminals, to inhibit release of acetylcholine (44,95,96). Workers in the field of opioid pharmacology often ignore the fact that inhibition of intestinal contractions by opioid substances is peculiar to the guinea pig and some other rodents. Intestinal contractile activity is increased by these substances in humans, dogs, cats, rabbits, rats, and monkeys (110,111,119). In the dog, intestinal stimulatory actions of morphine and related substances are apparently mediated in part by release of endogenous 5-HT, which stimulates the intestine through cholinergic and noncholinergic pathways (18,97). The increase in intestinal tone and motility induced by morphine retards propulsion through the bowel, increases resistance to flow of bile through the choledochoduodenal junction, and contributes to a delay in gastric emptying (20,105). Morphine characteristically produces disorganized patterns of contractions in large and small bowel, increases resistance to flow, and thus retards intestinal transit (159). Recently developed synthetic antidiarrheal drugs, diphenoxylate and loperamide, apparently act in the same manner (41,86,108). Although opioid substances can exert direct effects on neural elements of the bowel, a portion of their constipating effect *in vivo* may result from actions on the central nervous system (21,140).

With repeated exposure, tolerance to the intestinal effects of opioid drugs develops readily (22,23,88). Cross-tolerance between morphine and enkephalin has been demonstrated (152). The cross-tolerance extends to the opioid substance released from the intestine by electrical stimulation (114). Intestinal dependence also occurs after prolonged exposure to morphine. Strips of ileum taken from tolerant-dependent guinea pigs dis-play a contracture upon naloxone challenge (131). Contracture is prevented by continuing exposure to morphine or enkephalins (130). After naloxone-precipated withdrawal, intestinal strips exhibit supersensitivity to 5-HT (131).

Treatment of guinea pigs with *para*-chlorophenylalanine, which decreased intestinal 5-HT levels by 40%, enhanced the abstinence-like effects of naloxone in the morphine tolerant-dependent ileum (121). Treatment of guinea pigs with 5,6-dihydroxytryptamine did not alter responses to morphine or 5-HT; however, whether the treatment affected 5-HT levels in the intestine was not determined (151).

Relatively little is known at this time about the mechanisms that control synthesis, storage, or release of endorphins in the gastrointestinal tract. The detailed studies of opioid action in the intestine have been made possible by the availability of the relatively pure opioid antagonist, naloxone. Naltrexone, which has a longer duration of action, is also considered a relatively pure antagonist. Opioid receptor agonists frequently employed in pharmacological studies include morphine, normorphine (which has a shorter duration of action than morphine), met-enkephalin, leu-enkephalin, human β-endorphin, D-ala^2-met^5-enkephalin (which is relatively resistent to catabolism), and a large number of other synthetic peptides (92).

It has not been established whether β-endorphin secreted from the pituitary gland affects motility by actions on gastrointestinal opioid receptors (64). If so, gastrointestinal motility could be modulated by enkephalins released from intramural neurons and by circulating β-endorphin from the pituitary.

ACKNOWLEDGMENT

This work was supported by U.S. Public Health Service Grant DA02163.

REFERENCES

1. Adler-Graschinsky, E., and Langer, S. Z. (1975): Possible role of a beta-adrenoceptor in the regulation of noradrenalin release by nerve stimulation through a positive feed-back mechanism. *Br. J. Pharmacol.*, 53:43–50.
2. Ally, A. I., and Nakatsu, K. (1976): Adenosine inhibition of isolated rabbit ileum and antagonism by theophylline. *J. Pharmacol. Exp. Ther.*, 199:208–215.
3. Andersson, K.-E., Andersson, R. G. G., Hedner, P., and Persson, C. G. A. (1977): Interrelations between cyclic AMP, cyclic GMP and contraction in guinea pig gallbladder stimulated by cholecystokinin. *Life Sci.*, 20:73–78.
4. Andersson, R. (1972): Role of cyclic AMP and Ca^{++} in the metabolic and relaxing effects of catecholamines in intestinal smooth muscle. *Acta Physiol. Scand.*, 85:312–322.
5. Andersson, R., and Nilsson, K. (1972): Cyclic AMP and calcium in relaxation in intestinal smooth muscle. *Nature New Biol.*, 238:119–120.
6. Baer, H. P., and Frew, R. (1979): Relaxation of guinea-pig fundic strip by adenosine, adenosine triphosphate and electrical stimulation: lack of antagonism by theophylline or ATP treatment. *Br. J. Pharmacol.*, 67:293–299.

7. Barlow, R. B., and Kahn, I. (1959): Actions of some analogues of 5-hydroxytryptamine on the isolated rat uterus and the rat fundic strip preparations. *Br. J. Pharmacol.*, 14:265–274.

8. Baumann, H. W., Sturdevant, R. A. L., and McCallum, R. W. (1979): L-Dopa inhibits metoclopramide stimulation of the lower esophageal sphincter in man. *Dig. Dis. Sci.*, 24:289–295.

9. Beani, L., Bianchi, C., and Crema, A. (1969): The effect of catecholamines and sympathetic stimulation on the release of acetylcholine from the guinea-pig colon. *Br. J. Pharmacol.*, 36:1–17.

10. Behar, J., Field, S., and Marin, C. (1979): Effect of glucagon, secretin, and vasoactive intestinal polypeptide on the feline lower esophageal sphincter: mechanisms of action. *Gastroenterology*, 77:1001–1007.

11. Bennett, A., Eley, K. G., and Stockley, H. L. (1976): Inhibition of peristalsis in guinea-pig isolated ileum and colon by drugs that block prostaglandin snythesis. *Br. J. Pharmacol.*, 57:335–340.

12. Berridge, M. G. (1975): The interaction of cyclic nucleotides and calcium in the control of cellular activity. *Adv. Cyclic Nucleotide Res.*, 6:1–98.

13. Birks, R. I., and MacIntosh, F. C. (1957): Acetylcholine metabolism at nerve-endings. *Br. Med. Bull.*, 13:157–161.

14. Bradshaw, J., Brittain, R. T., Clitherow, J. W., Daly, M. H., Jack, D., Price, B. J., and Stables, R. (1979): Ranitidine (AH 19065): a new potent, selective histamine H_2-receptor antagonist. *Br. J. Pharmacol.*, 66:464P.

15. Brownlee, G., and Johnson, E. S. (1963): The site of the 5-hydroxytryptamine receptor on the intramural nervous plexus of the guinea-pig isolated ileum. *Br. J. Pharmacol.*, 21:306–322.

16. Brownlee, G., and Johnson, E. S. (1965): The release of acetylcholine from the isolated ileum of the guinea-pig induced by 5-hydroxytryptamine and dimethylphenylpiperazinium. *Br. J. Pharmacol.*, 24:689–700.

17. Burgen, A. S. V. (1979): Drug receptors. *Br. Med. Bull.*, 35:269–273.

18. Burks, T. F. (1973): Mediation by 5-hydroxytryptamine of morphine stimulant actions in dog intestine. *J. Pharmacol. Exp. Ther.*, 185:530–539.

19. Burks, T. F. (1976): Acute effects of morphine on rat intestinal motility. *Eur. J. Pharmacol.*, 40:279–283.

20. Burks, T. F. (1976): Gastrointestinal pharmacology. *Annu. Rev. Pharmacol. Toxicol.*, 16:15–31.

21. Burks, T. F. (1978): Central sites of action of gastrointestinal drugs. *Gastroenterology*, 74:322–324.

22. Burks, T. F., Castro, G. A., and Weisbrodt, N. W. (1976): Tolerance to intestinal stimulatory actions of morphine. In: *Opiates and Endogenous Opioid Peptides*, edited by H. W. Kosterlitz, pp. 369–376. North-Holland, Amsterdam.

23. Burks, T. F., Jaquette, D. L., and Grubb, M. N. (1974): Development of tolerance to the stimulatory effect of morphine in dog intestine. *Eur. J. Pharmacol.*, 25:302–307.

24. Burks, T. F., and Long, J. P. (1966): 5-Hydroxytryptamine release into dog intestinal vasculature. *Am. J. Physiol.*, 211:619–625.

25. Burks, T. F., and Long, J. P. (1966): Catecholamine-induced release of 5-hydroxytryptamine (5-HT) from perfused vasculature of isolated dog intestine. *J. Pharm. Sci.*, 55:1383–1386.

26. Burks, T. F., and Long, J. P. (1967): Release of 5-hydroxytryptamine from isolated dog intestine by nicotine. *Br. J. Pharmacol.*, 30:229–239.

27. Burks, T. F., and Long, J. P. (1967): Release of intestinal 5-hydroxytryptamine by morphine and related agents. *J. Pharmacol. Exp. Ther.*, 156:267–276.

28. Burleigh, D. E., D'Mello, A., and Parks, A. G. (1979): Responses of isolated human internal anal sphincter to drugs and electrical field stimulation. *Gastroenterology*, 77:484–490.

29. Burnstock, G. (1979): Autonomic innervation and transmission. *Br. Med. Bull.*, 35:255–262.

30. Burnstock, G., Campbell, G., Satchell, D., and Smythe, A. (1970): Evidence that adenosine triphosphate or a related nucleotide is the transmitter substance released by non-adrenergic inhibitory nerves in the gut. *Br. J. Pharmacol.*, 40:668–688.

31. Cavero, I., Fenard, S., Gomeni, R., Lefevre, R., and Roach, A. G. (1978): Studies on the mechanism of the vasodilator effects of prazocin in dogs and rabbits. *Eur. J. Pharmacol.*, 49:259–270.

32. Cohen, S., Kravitz, J. J., and Snape, W. J. (1979): Esophageal histamine receptors. In: *Histamine Receptors*, edited by T. O. Yellin, pp. 69–78. S P Medical and Scientific Books, New York.

33. Cohen, S., Morris, D. W., Schoen, H. J., and DiMarino, A. J. (1976): The effect of oral and intravenous metoclopramide on human lower esophageal sphincter pressure. *Gastroenterology*, 70:484–487.

34. Cohen, S., and Snape, W. J. (1975): Action of metiamide on the lower esophageal sphincter. *Gastroenterology*, 69:911–919.

35. Cook, D. A. (1971): Blockade by phenoxybenzamine of the contractor response produced by agonists in the isolated ileum of the guinea-pig. *Br. J. Pharmacol.*, 43:197–209.

36. Costa, M., and Furness, J. B. (1979): On the possibility that an indoleamine is a neurotransmitter in the gastrointestinal tract. *Biochem. Pharmacol.*, 28:565–571.

37. Costa, M., and Furness, J. B., (1979): The sites of action of 5-hydroxytryptamine in nerve-muscle preparations from the guinea-pig small intestine and colon. *Br. J. Pharmacol.*, 65:237–248.

38. Cox, B. M., Opheim, K. E., Teschemacher, H., and Goldstein, A. (1975): A peptide-like substance from pituitary that acts like morphine. 2. Purification and properties. *Life Sci.*, 16:1777–1782.

39. Creese, I., and Snyder, S. H. (1975): Receptor binding and pharmacological activity of opiates in the guinea-pig intestine. *J. Pharmacol. Exp. Ther.*, 194:205–219.

40. Cutz, E., Chan, W., Track, N. S., Goth, A., and Said, S. I. (1978): Release of vasoactive intestinal polypeptide in mast cells by histamine liberators. *Nature*, 275:661–662.

41. Dajani, E. Z., Roge, E. A. W., and Bertermann, R. E. (1975): Effects of E prostaglandins, diphenoxylate and morphine on intestinal motility in vivo. *Eur. J. Pharmacol.*, 34:105–113.

42. Daniel, E. E. (1975): Peptidergic nerves in the gut. *Gastroenterology*, 75:142–145.

43. De Carle, D. J., Brody, M. J., and Christensen, J. (1976): Histamine receptors in esophageal smooth muscle of the opossum. *Gastroenterology*, 70:1071–1075.

44. Dingledine, R., and Goldstein, A. (1976): Effect of synaptic transmission blockade on morphine action in the guinea-pig myenteric plexus. *J. Pharmacol. Exp. Ther.*, 196:97–106.

45. Drew, G. M. (1978): Pharmacological characterization of the presynaptic α-adrenoceptors regulating cholinergic activity in the guinea-pig ileum. *Br. J. Pharmacol.*, 64:293–300.

46. Durant, G. J., Duncan, W. A. M., Ganellin, C. R., Parsons, M. E., Blakemore, R. C., and Rasmussen, A. C. (1978): Impromidine (SK&F 92676) is a very potent and specific agonist for histamine H_2 receptors. *Nature*, 276:403–405.

47. Dyer, D. C., and Gant, D. W. (1973): Vasoconstriction produced by hallucinogens on isolated human and sheep unbilical vasculature. *J. Pharmacol. Exp. Ther.*, 184:366–375.

48. Elde, R., Hökfelt, T., Johansson, O., and Terenius, L. (1976): Immunohistochemical studies using antibodies to leucine-enkephalin: initial observations on the nervous system of the rat. *Neuroscience*, 1:349–351.

49. Fernstrom, J. D., and Jacoby, J. H. (1975): The interaction of diet and drugs in modifying brain serotonin metabolism. *Gen. Pharmacol.*, 6:253–258.

50. Fisher, R. S., DiMarino, A. J., and Cohen, S. (1975): Mechanism of cholecystokinin inhibition of lower esophageal sphincter pressure. *Am. J. Physiol.*, 228:1469–1473.

51. Fozard, J. R., and Mobarok Ali, A. T. M. (1978): Blockade of neuronal tryptamine receptors by metoclopramide. *Eur. J. Pharmacol.*, 49:109–112.

52. Fozard, J. R., and Mobarok Ali, A. T. M. (1978): Receptors for 5-hydroxytryptamine on the sympathetic nerves of the rabbit heart. *Naunyn-Schmiedebergs Arch. Pharmacol.*, 301:223–235.

53. Fozard, J. R., and Mobarok Ali, A. T. M. (1978): Dual mechanism of the stimulant action of N,N-dimethyl-5-hydroxytryptamine (bufotenine) on cardiac sympathetic nerves. *Eur. J. Pharmacol.*, 49:25–30.

54. Frankhuyzen, A. L., and Bonta, I. L. (1974): Effect of mianserin, a potent anti-serotonin agent, on the isolated rat stomach fundus preparation. *Eur. J. Pharmacol.*, 25:40–50.

55. Fuller, R. W. (1978): Neurochemical effects of serotonin neurotoxins: an introduction. *Ann. NY Acad. Sci.,* 305:178–181.
56. Fuller, R. W., Snoddy, H. D., Perry, K. W., Roush, B. W., Molloy, B. B., Bymaster, F. P., and Wong, D. T. (1976): The effects of quipazine on serotonin metabolism in rat brain. *Life Sci.,* 18:925–934.
57. Fuxe, K., Agnati, L., and Everitt, B. (1975): Effects of methergoline on central monoamine neurons. Evidence for a selective blockade of central 5-HT receptors. *Neurosci. Lett.,* 1:283–290.
58. Gaddum, J. H., and Hameed, K. A. (1954): Drugs which antagonize 5-hydroxytryptamine. *Br. J. Pharmacol.,* 9:240–248.
59. Ganellin, C. R. (1979): Chemical development and properties of histamine H_2-receptor agonists and antagonists. In: *Histamine Receptors,* edited by T. O. Yellin, pp. 377–413. S P Medical and Scientific Books, New York.
60. Gershon, M. D. (1967): Effects of tetrodotoxin on innervated smooth muscle preparations. *Br. J. Pharmacol.,* 29:259–279.
61. Gershon, M. D., Robinson, R. G., and Ross, L. L. (1976): Serotonin accumulation in the guinea-pig myenteric plexus: ion dependence, structure-activity relationship and the effect of drugs. *J. Pharmacol. Exp. Ther.,* 198:548–561.
62. Gorman, R. R. (1976): Prostaglandin endoperoxides: possible new regulators of cyclic nucleotide metabolism. *J. Cyclic Nucleotide Res.,* 1:1–19.
63. Grubb, M. N., and Burks, T. F. (1974): Modification of intestinal stimulatory effects of 5-hydroxytryptamine by adrenergic amines, prostaglandin E_1 and theophylline. *J. Pharmacol. Exp. Ther.,* 189:476–483.
64. Guillemin, R., Vargo, T., Rossier, J., Minick, S., Ling, N., Rivier, C., Vale, W., and Bloom, F. (1977): β-Endorphin and adrenocorticotropin are secreted concomitantly by the pituitary gland. *Science,* 197:1367–1369.
65. Gyermek, L. (1961): 5-Hydroxytryptamine antagonists. *Pharmacol. Rev.,* 13:399–439.
66. Haubrich, D. R., Wang, P. F. L., and Wedeking, P. W. (1975): Distribution and metabolism of intravenously administered choline (methyl-^{3}H) and synthesis of acetylcholine in various tissues of guinea pigs. *J. Pharmacol. Exp. Ther.,* 193:246–255.
67. Hedqvst, P. (1977): Basic mechanisms of prostaglandin action on autonomic neurotransmission. *Annu. Rev. Pharmacol. Toxicol.,* 17:259–279.
68. Hinman, J. W. (1972): Prostaglandins. *Annu. Rev. Biochem.,* 41:161–178.
69. Hong, E., Sancilio, L. F., Vargas, R., and Pardo, E. G. (1969): Similarities between the pharmacological actions of quipazine and serotonin. *Eur. J. Pharmacol.,* 6:274–280.
70. Houslay, M. D., and Tipton, K. F. (1976): Multiple forms of monoamine oxidase: fact and artefact. *Life Sci.,* 19:467–478.
71. Hughes, J. (1975): Isolation of an endogenous compound from the brain with pharmacological properties similar to morphine. *Brain Res.,* 88:295–308.
72. Jenkinson, D. H., and Morton, I. K. M. (1967): The role of α- and β-adrenergic receptors in some actions of catecholamines on intestinal smooth muscle. *J. Physiol. (Lond.),* 188:387–402.
73. Juorio, A. V., and Gabella, G. (1974): Noradrenaline in the guinea pig alimentary canal: regional distribution and sensitivity to denervation and reserpine. *J. Neurochem.,* 22:851–858.
74. Kalix, P., McAfee, D. A., Schorderet, M., and Greengard, P. (1974): Pharmacological analysis of synaptically mediated increase in cyclic adenosine monophosphate in rabbit superior cervical ganglion. *J. Pharmacol. Exp. Ther.,* 188:676–687.
75. Kao, I., Drachman, D. B., and Price, D. L. (1976): Botulinum toxin: mechanism of presynaptic blockade. *Science,* 193:1256–1258.
76. Katayama, Y., and North, R. A. (1978): Does substance P mediate slow synaptic excitation within the myenteric plexus? *Nature,* 274:387–388.
77. Kebabian, J. W., and Greengard, P. (1971): Dopamine-sensitive adenyl cyclase: possible role in synaptic transmission. *Science,* 174:1346–1349.
78. Kebabian, J. W., Steiner, A. L., and Greengard, P. (1975): Muscarinic cholinergic regulation of cyclic guanosine 3′,5′-monophosphate in autonomic ganglia: possible role in synaptic transmission. *J. Pharmacol. Exp. Ther.,* 193:474–488.

79. Kilbinger, H., and Wagner, P. (1975): Inhibition by oxotremorine of acetylcholine resting release from guinea pig-ileum longitudinal muscle strips. *Naunyn-Schmiedebergs Arch. Pharmacol.,* 287:47–60.
80. Kimberg, D. V. (1974): Cyclic nucleotides and their role in gastrointestinal secretion. *Gastroenterology,* 67:1023–1064.
81. Kosterlitz, H. W., and Leslie, F. M, (1978): Comparisons of the receptor binding characteristics of opiate agonists interacting with μ- or κ-receptors. *Br. J. Pharmacol.,* 64:607–614.
82. LeDuc, L. E., and Needleman, P. (1979): Regional localization of prostacyclin and thromboxane synthesis in dog stomach and intestinal tract. *J. Pharmacol. Exp. Ther.,* 211:181–188.
83. Lefebvre, R. A., and Willems, J. L. (1978): Measurement of gastric relaxation in the experimental animal: influence of domperidone. *Arch. Int. Pharmacodyn. Ther.,* 234:342–343.
84. Levine, R. A. (1970): The role of cyclic AMP in hepatic and gastrointestinal function. *Gastroenterology,* 59:280–300.
85. Lewis, R. V., Stein, S., Gerber, L. D., Rubinstein, J., and Udenfriend, S. (1978): High molecular weight opioid-containing proteins in striatum. *Proc. Natl. Acad. Sci.,* 75:4021–4023.
86. Mackerer, C. R., Clay, G. A., and Dajani, E. Z. (1976): Loperamide binding to opiate receptor sites of brain and myenteric plexus. *J. Pharmacol. Exp. Ther.,* 199:131–140.
87. Maj, J., Palider, W., and Baran, L. (1976): The effects of serotonergic and antiserotonergic drugs on the flexor reflex of spinal rat: a proposed model to evaluate the action on the central serotonin receptor. *J. Neural Trans.,* 38:141–147.
88. Mattila, M. (1962): The effects of morphine and nalorphine on the small intestine of normal and morphine-tolerant rat and guinea-pig. *Acta Pharmacol. Toxicol.,* 19:47–52.
89. McAfee, D. A., and Greengard, P. (1972): Adenosine 3′,5′-monophosphate: electrophysiological evidence for a role in synaptic transmission. *Science,* 178:310–312.
90. Metcalfe, H. L., and Turner, P. (1969): Pharmacological studies of cinanserin in human isolated smooth muscle. *Br. J. Pharmacol.,* 37:519P–521P.
91. Miller, F. P., Cox, R. H., Snodgrass, W. R., and Maickel, R. P. (1970): Comparative effects of p-chlorophenylalanine, p-chloroamphetamine and p-chloro-N-methylamphetamine on rat brain norepinephrine, serotonin and 5-hydroxyindole-3-acetic acid. *Biochem. Pharmacol.,* 19:435–552.
92. Miller, R. J., and Cuatrecasas, P. (1979): Neurobiology and neuropharmacology of the enkephalins. In: *Neurochemical Mechanisms of Opiates and Endorphins,* edited by H. H. Loh and D. H. Ross, pp. 187–225. Raven Press, New York.
93. Monachon, M. A., Burkard, W. P., Jalfre, M., and Haefely, W. (1972): Blockade of central 5-hydroxytryptamine receptors by methiothepin. *Naunyn-Schmiedebergs Arch. Pharmacol.,* 274:192–197.
94. Nilsson, K. B., and Andersson, R. G. G. (1977): Effects of carbachol and calcium on the cyclic guanosine-3′,5′-monophosphate (cyclic GMP) metabolism in intestinal smooth muscle. *Acta Physiol. Scand.,* 99:246–253.
95. North, R. A. (1979): Opiates, opioid peptides and single neurones. *Life Sci.,* 24:1527–1546.
96. North, R. A., and Williams, J. T. (1976): Enkephalin inhibits firing of myenteric neurons. *Nature,* 264:460–461.
97. Northway, M. G., and Burks, T. F. (1979): Indirect intestinal stimulatory effects of heroin: direct action on opiate receptors. *Eur. J. Pharmacol.,* 59:237–243.
98. Okwuasaba, F. K., and Hamilton; J. T. (1975): The effect of metoclopramide on inhibition induced by purine nucleotides, noradrenaline, and theophylline ethylenediamine on intestinal muscle and on peristalsis *in vitro. Can. J. Physiol. Pharmacol.,* 53:972–977.
99. Okwuasaba, F. K,, Hamilton, J. T., and Cook, M. A. (1977): Relaxations of guinea-pig fundic strip by adenosine, adenine nucleotides and electrical stimulation; antagonism by theophylline and desensitization to adenosine and its derivatives. *Eur. J. Pharmacol.* 46:181–198.
100. Otsuka, M., and Takahashi, T. (1977): Putative peptide neurotransmitters. *Annu. Rev. Pharmacol. Toxicol.,* 17:425–439.
101. Paiva, T. B., Mendes, G. B., Aboulafia, J., and Paiva, A. C. M. (1976): Evidence against cholinergic mediation of the effect of

angiotensin II on the guinea pig ileum. *Pflügers Arch.*, 365:129–133.

102. Paton, W. D. M. (1957): The action of morphine and related substances on contraction and on acetylcholine output of coaxially stimulated guinea-pig ileum. *Br. J. Pharmacol.*, 11:119–127.

103. Paton, W. D. M., and Vizi, E, S. (1969): The inhibitory action of noradrenaline and adrenaline on acetylcholine output by guinea-pig ileum longitudinal muscle strip. *Br. J. Pharmacol.*, 35:10–28.

104. Paton, W. D. M., and Zar, M. A. (1968): The origin of acetylcholine released from guinea-pig intestine and longitudinal muscle strips. *J. Physiol, (Lond.)*, 194:13–33.

105. Persson, C. G. A. (1971): The action of morphine on the cat choledochoduodenal tract. *Acta Pharmacol. Toxicol.*, 30:321–329.

106. Pert, C. B., and Synder, S. H. (1973): Opiate receptor: demonstration in nervous tissue. *Science*, 179:1011–1014.

107. Pert, C. B., and Snyder, S. H. (1974): High affinity transport of choline into the myenteric plexus of guinea-pig intestine. *J. Pharmacol. Exp. Ther.*, 191:102–108.

108. Piercey, M. F., and Ruwart, M. J. (1979): Naloxone inhibits the antidiarrheal activity of loperamide. *Br. J. Pharmacol.*, 66:373–375.

109. Pinder, R. M., Brogden, R. N., Sawyer, P. R., Speight, T. M., and Avery, G. S. (1976): Metoclopramide: a review of its pharmacological properties and clinical use. *Drugs*, 12:81–131.

110, Plant, O. H., and Miller, G. H. (1926): Effects of morphine and some other opium alkaloids on the muscular activity of the alimentary canal. I. Actions on the small intestine in unanesthetized dogs and man. *J. Pharmacol. Exp. Ther.*, 27:361–383.

111. Pruitt, D. B., Grubb, M. N., Jaquette, D. L., and Burks, T. F. (1974): Intestinal effects of 5-hydroxytryptamine and morphine in guinea pigs, dogs, cats and monkeys. *Eur. J. Pharmacol.* 26: 298–305.

112. Puglisi, L., Berti, D., and Folco, G. C. (1972): Cyclic-GMP interaction with the parasympathetic system of isolated rat stomach. *Pharmacol. Res. Commun.*, 4:227–235.

113. Puig, M. M., Gascon, P., Craviso, G. L', and Musacchio, J. M. (1977): Endogenous opiate receptor ligand: electrically induced release in the guinea pig ileum. *Science*, 195:419–420.

114. Puig, M. M., Gascon, P., and Musacchio, J. (1978): Electrically induced opiate-like inhibition of the guinea-pig ileum: crosstolerance to morphine. *J. Pharmacol. Exp. Ther.*, 206:289–302.

115. Rattan, S., and Goyal, R. K. (1976): Effect of dopamine on the esophageal smooth muscle in vivo. *Gastroenterology*, 70:377–381.

116. Rattan, S., and Goyal, R. K. (1977): Effects of 5-hydroxytryptamine on the lower esophageal sphincter—evidence for multiple sites of action. *J. Clin. Invest.*, 59:125–133.

117. Rattan, S., and Goyal, R. K. (1978): Effects of histamine on the lower esophageal sphincter *in vivo*: evidence for actions at three different sites. *J. Pharmacol. Exp. Ther.*, 204:334–342.

118. Reddy, V., and Moran, N. C. (1968): An evaluation of the adrenergic receptor types in isolated segments of the small intestine of the rabbit. *Arch Int. Pharmacodyn. Ther.*, 176:326–336.

119. Reynolds, A. K., and Randall, L. O. (1957): *Morphine and Allied Drugs*. University of Toronto Press, Toronto.

120. Rocha, E., Silva, M., Valle, J. R., and Picarelli, Z. P. (1953): A pharmacological analysis of the mode of action of serotonin (5-hydroxytryptamine) upon the guinea-pig ileum. *Br. J. Pharmacol.*, 8:378–388.

121. Rodríguez, R., Luján, Campos, A. E., and Chorné, R. (1978): Morphine dependence in the isolated guinea-pig ileum and its modification by p-chlorophenylalanine. *Life Sci.*, 23:913–920.

122. Rubin, M. C., Fournet, J., Snape, W. J., and Cohen, S. (1980): Adrenergic regulation of ileocecal sphincter function in the cat. *Gastroenterology*, 78:15–21.

123. Sakai, K. (1979): Effects of intra-arterial bradykinin and substance P on isolated, blood-perfused small intestine of the rat. *Jpn, J. Pharmacol.*, 29:597–603.

124. Sakai, K., Shiraki, Y., Tatsumi, T., and Tsuju, K. (1979): The actions of 5-hydroxytryptamine and histamine on the isolated ileum of the tree shrew *(Tupaia glis)*. *Br. J. Pharmacol.*, 66:405–408.

125. Salimi, M. (1975): Comparison of β-adrenoceptor blocking properties of sotalol, oxprenolol, propranolol and pindolol on rabbit intestinal smooth muscle. *Pharmacology*, 13:441–447.

126. Sanner, J. H. (1974): Substances that inhibit the actions of prostaglandins. *Arch. Int. Med.*, 133:133–146.

127. Sawynok, J., and Jhamandas, K. H. (1976): Inhibition of acetylcholine release from cholinergic nerves by adenosine, adenine nucleotides and morphine: antagonism by theophylline. *J. Pharmacol. Exp. Ther.*, 197:379–390.

128. Schaumann, W. (1955): The paralysing action of morphine on the guinea pig ileum. *Br. J. Pharmacol.*, 10:456–461.

129. Schaumann, W. (1957): Inhibition by morphine of the release of acetylcholine from the intestine of the guinea-pig. *Br. J. Pharmacol.*, 12:115–118.

130. Schulz, R., and Herz, A. (1976): Dependence liability of enkephalin in the myenteric plexus of the guinea pig. *Eur. J. Pharmacol.*, 39:429–432.

131. Schulz, R., and Herz, A. (1976): Aspects of opiate dependence in the myenteric plexus of the guinea-pig. *Life Sci.*, 19:1117–1128.

132. Schultz, R., Wüster, M., Simantov, R., Snyder, S., and Herz, A. (1977): Electrically stimulated release of opiate-like material from the myenteric plexus of the guinea pig ileum. *Eur. J. Pharmacol.*, 41:347–348.

133. Seno, N., Nakazato, Y., and Ohga, A. (1978): Presynaptic inhibitory effects of catecholamines on cholinergic transmission in the smooth muscle of the chick stomach. *Eur. J. Pharmacol.*, 51:229–237.

134. Simon, E. J. (1976): The opiate receptors. *Neurochem. Res.*, 1:3–28.

135. Small, R. C., and Weston, A. H. (1979): Theophylline antagonizes some effects of purines in the intestine but not those of intramural inhibitory nerve stimulation, *Br. J. Pharmacol.*, 67:301–308.

136. Smith, T. W., Hughes, J., Kosterlitz, H. W., and Sosa, R. P. (1976): Enkephalins: isolation, distribution and function. In: *Opiates and Endogenous Opioid Peptides*, edited by H. W. Kosterlitz, pp. 57–62, North-Holland, Amsterdam.

137. Sollero, L., Page, I. H., and Salmoiraghi, G. C. (1956): Bromlysergic acid diethylamide: a highly potent serotonin antagonist. *J. Pharmacol. Exp. Ther.*, 117:10–15.

138. Spedding, M., and Weetman, D. F. (1978): The mechanism of the relaxant effect of 2-2'-pyridylisatogen on the isolated taenia of the guinea-pig caecum. *Br. J. Pharmacol.*, 63:659–664.

139. Stewart, J. J., and Burks, T. F. (1977): Actions of cholecystokinin octapeptide on smooth muscle of isolated dog intestine. *Am. J. Physiol.*, 232:E306–E310.

140. Stewart, J. J., Weisbrodt, N. W., and Burks, T. F. (1978): Central and peripheral actions of morphine on intestinal transit. *J. Pharmacol. Exp. Ther.*, 205:547–555.

141. Stjarne, L., and Brundin, J. (1976): Beta$_2$-adrenoceptors facilitating noradrenalin secretion from human vasoconstrictor nerves. *Acta Physiol. Scand.*, 97:88–93.

142. Takayanagi, I., Ohkubo, H., and Takagi, K. (1976): Drug-induced smooth muscle contraction with no change in the level of cyclic GMP. *Jpn. J. Pharmacol.*, 26:501–504.

143. Tansy, M. F., Rothman, G., Bartlett, J., Farber, P., and Hohenleitner, F. J. (1971): Vagal adrenergic degranulation of enterochromaffin cell system in guinea pig duodenum. *J. Pharm. Sci.*, 60:81–84.

144. Thoenen, H., and Tranzer, J. P. (1973): The pharmacology of 6-hydroxydopamine. *Annu. Rev. Pharmacol. Toxicol.*, 13:169–180.

145. Thompson, J. H., Spezia, C. A., and Angulo, M. (1969): The release of intestinal serotonin in rats by nicotine, *JAMA*, 207:1883–1886.

146. Uddman, R., Alumets, J;, Edvinsson, L., Hakånson, R., and Sundler, F. (1978): Peptidergic (VIP) innervation of the esophagus. *Gastroenterology*, 75:5–8.

147. Valenzuela, J. E. (1976): Dopamine as a possible neurotransmitter in gastric relaxation. *Gastroenterology*, 71:1019–1022.

148. Van Neuten, J. M., and Janssen, P. A. (1978): Is dopamine an endogenous inhibitor of gastric emptying? In: *Gastrointestinal Motility in Health and Disease*, edited by H. L. Duthie, pp. 173–180. MTP Press, Ltd., Lancaster.

149. Vizi, S. E. (1973): Acetylcholine release from guinea pig ileum by parasympathetic ganglion stimulants and gastrin-like polypeptides. *Br. J. Pharmacol.*, 47:765–777.

150. Wagner, L. A. (1975): Subcellular storage of biogenic amines. *Life Sci.*, 17:1755–1762.

151. Ward, A., and Takemori, A. E. (1976): Effect of 6-hydroxydopamine and 5,6-dihydroxytryptamine on the of the coaxially stimulated guinea-pig ileum to morphine. *J. Pharmacol. Exp. Ther.*, 199:124–130.

152. Waterfield, A. A., Hughes, J., and Kosterlitz, H. W. (1976): Cross tolerance between morphine and methionine-enkephalin. *Nature*, 260:624–625.

153. Watson, S. J., Akil, H., Richard, C. W., and Barchas, J. D. (1978): Evidence for two separate opiate peptide neuronal systems. *Nature*, 275:266–228.

154. Weber, L. J. (1970): p-Chlorophenylalanine depletion of gastrointestinal 5-hydroxytryptamine. *Biochem, Pharmacol.*, 19:2169–2172.

155. Weeks, J. R. (1972): Prostaglandins. *Annu. Rev. Pharmacol. Toxicol.*, 12:317–336.

156. Weiner, N. (1979): Multiple factors regulating the release of norepinephrine consequent to nerve stimulation. *Fed. Proc.*, 38:2193–2202.

157. Weinstock, M., and Schecter, Y. (1975): Antagonism by propranolol of the ganglion stimulant action of 5-hydroxytryptamine. *Eur. J. Pharmacol.*, 32:293–301.

158. White, T. (1973): Effects of drugs on brain histamine. In: *Histamine and Antihistamines (International Encyclopedia of Pharmacology and Therapeutics)*, edited by M. Schacter, Sect. 74, pp. 101–107, Pergamon Press, New York.

159. Wienbeck, M. (1972): The electrical activity of the cat colon *in vivo*. II. The effects of bethanechol and morphine. *Res. Exp. Med.*, 158:280–287.

160. Wikberg, J. (1977): Localization of adrenergic receptors in guinea pig ileum and rabbit jejunum to cholinergic neurons and to smooth muscle cells. *Acta Physiol. Scand.*, 99:190–207.

161. Willis, A. L., Davison, P., and Ramwell, P. W. (1974): Inhibition of intestinal tone, motility and prostaglandin biosynthesis by 5,8,11,14-eicosatetraynoic acid (TYA). *Prostaglandins*, 5:355–368.

162. Wilson, D. E. (1972): Prostaglandins and the gastrointestinal tract. *Prostaglandins*, 4:281–293.

163. Winter, J. C., and Gessner, P. K. (1968): Phenoxybenzamine antagonism of tryptamines, their indene isosteres and 5-hydroxytryptamine in the rat stomach fundus preparation. *J. Pharmacol. Exp. Ther.*, 162:286–293.

164. Wong, D. T., Bymaster, F. P., Horng, J. S., and Molloy, B. B. (1975): A new selective inhibitor for uptake of serotonin into synaptosomes of rat brain: 3-(p-trifluoromethylphenoxy)-N-methyl-3-phenylpropylamine. *J. Pharmacol. Exp. Ther.*, 193:804–811.

165. Wood, J. D., and Mayer, C. J. (1979): Serotonergic activation of tonic-type enteric neurons in guinea pig small bowel. *J. Neurophysiol.*, 42:582–593.

166. Wurtman, R. J., and Fernstrom, J. D. (1976): Control of brain neurotransmitter synthesis by precursor availability and nutritional state. *Biochem. Pharmacol.*, 25:1691–1696.

167. Yellin, T. O., Buck, S. H., Gilman, D. J., Jones, D. F., and Wardleworth, J. M. (1979): ICI 125,211: a new gastric antisecretory agent acting on histamine H_2-receptors. *Life Sci.*, 25:2001–2009.

168. Yellin, T. O., Buck, S. H., and Johnson, E. M. (1979): Imidazoline stimulants of gastric secretion. In: *Histamine Receptors*, edited by T. O. Yellin, pp. 79–98. S P Medical and Scientific Books, New York.

Physiology of the Gastrointestinal Tract, edited by
Leonard R. Johnson. Raven Press, New York © 1981.

Chapter 17

Functional Gastric Morphology

Susumu Ito

The stomach is an enlarged, specialized segment of the digestive tract between the esophagus and small intestine that serves to store as well as process food for absorption by the intestine. Although the stomachs of vertebrates share common structural features, their gross morphology varies remarkably. It is related to species differences in body size and shape, need for food storage, nature of diet, and frequency of food intake. A feature synonomous with function of the stomach is the ability to secrete acid and pepsin. Absorption is not a major function of the stomach, and water-soluble substances are absorbed in limited quantities, although some fat-soluble compounds, such as ethanol, are absorbed readily and quickly (27).

SPECIES VARIATIONS AND SPECIALIZATIONS OF THE STOMACH

Most vertebrates have a glandular stomach, which may be a simple sac or complex with many compartments. Some animals, such as the duckbill platypus and echidna, do not have a glandular stomach, and the esophageal mucosa is joined directly to the small intestine (54). A similar condition exists in the "stomachless fishes," which also lack glandular stomachs and do not secrete acid or pepsin (5). The am-

phioxus and cyclostomes, which are primitive vertebrates, also do not have true stomachs. Comparative studies indicate that absence of the stomach in certain species is the result of specialized adaptation rather than a pattern of evolutionary development.

The large range of variation in the size and shape of stomachs in various animals appears to be related to the evolved size and shape of the animal (181). In species with elongated bodies, the stomach lies in the long axis; in wider bodied animals, it is oriented more transversely. Some stomachs are straight tubular enlargements, whereas others have saccular compartments. The most complex form is found in the ruminants, which have four discrete compartments.

In fishes, the stomach is generally folded, and the cardiac region or initial portion may form a blind pouch which is distensible and allows some fish to swallow prey as large as themselves. Except for the stomachless fishes, the majority have stomachs whose principal glands secrete acid and pepsin and are known as fundic or chief glands. These glands have two main cell types; (a) the oxynticopeptic cells, which form much of the body of the glands and are responsible for both HCl and pepsinogen secretion, and (b) the surface mucous cells, which line the luminal surface and gastric pits (1,128). In the region adjacent to the esophagus are cardiac glands; the region near the duodenum consists of pyloric glands. Both of these gland types contain mucous cells and lack oxynticopeptic cells. In addition, there are endocrine cells in the glands of the piscine stomach, but their role is still poorly understood.

All the amphibians and reptilians that have been studied have stomachs whose histological structure is similar to that found in fishes (128). The mucus-secreting and oxynticopeptic cells are similar to those in the principal gastric glands of fish. Cardiac and pyloric glands resembling those in fish are also present.

The stomach of the bird reflects the special adaptation of its ability to fly and its lack of teeth to grind food. A unique feature in many birds is the presence of the crop, which is a specialized esophageal structure for food storage and some predigestive activity. The stratified squamous epithelium lining of the crop resembles that of the esophagus. The enzymatic content of the crop is provided by the esophageal and oral salivary glands. The glandular stomach of birds is called the proventriculus, which lies between the esophagus and the gizzard. The mucosa of the proventriculus is similar to that of the amphibian and fish stomach, with mucous cells on the free surface and in the gastric pits and oxynticopeptic cells in the glands. Another unique specialization of the avian stomach system is the gizzard or ventriculus. This muscular organ is formed by a thick layer of smooth muscle, an epithelium with tubular glands, and a tough noncellular lining material known as koilin. This lining is apparently secreted by the underlying glandular epithelium of the gizzard (1,128) and is similar to keratin but is distinctive in its composition.

Among the great variety of specialized structures found in the nonmammalian, vertebrate gastric mucosa, some basic similarities persist. Mucus is secreted by the superficial cells, while a single cell type, the oxynticopeptic cell, is responsible for HCl and pepsinogen secretion. Relatively little work has been done to identify the endocrine cell types in the nonmammalian gastric mucosa, but their presence has been documented, and comparison with mammalian endocrine cells has been made (35).

THE MAMMALIAN STOMACH

From the absence of gastric glands in the monotreme stomach to the complex multichambered stomachs of the ruminants, there are wide structural variations in mammalian stomachs. It is the intent of this chapter to provide a general description of the stomach of commonly encountered mammals and to correlate the histology and ultrastructure of the mucosa with its secretory activity.

In primates, most carnivores, and many insectivores, the stomach is a single-chambered organ of relatively simple form. In some species, these simple stomachs are partially subdivided to form bilocular or even trilocular chambers. Further modifications are present in the form of multichambered stomachs with two, three, or four discrete compartments. The most complex form of stomach is found in the ruminant with four chambers: the rumen, reticulum, omasum, and abomasum. The capacious multichambered stomach stores food and provides sites for the fermentation of cellulose and other plant polymers (119). Much of the luminal surface of these large organs is lined with stratified squamous, nonglandular epithelium. Specific chambers consist of gastric glands containing mucous, oxyntic, peptic, and endocrine cells. These are present as typical mucosal glands separated from the submucosa by the muscularis mucosae. In a few species, such as the grasshopper mouse (77), beaver (123), wombat (73), and manatee, additional gastric glands are present as a saccular or nodular thickening on the lesser curvature near the esophageal opening. The functional significance of these glands, the "cardiogastric glands," is not known; they may serve to concentrate gastric secretory activity at focal sites in the stomach.

MAMMALIAN GASTRIC MUCOSA

The mammalian glandular gastric mucosa has been the subject of much investigation because of its clinical as well as biological interest. Much work has been directed toward a better understanding of its unique ability to secrete high concentrations of HCl. It should be noted, however, that the secretions of gastric mucus, pepsinogen, intrinsic factor, and hormones are significant contributions of the stomach. Furthermore, the presence of a nonglandular gastric epithelium, which is not involved in significant secretory activity but lines the chambers for storage and digestion of food, should not be ignored. The objective of this chapter is to describe the morphology of the typical mammalian gastric mucosa in some detail and to relate the structure of the stomach to its function. Attention is directed toward the specialized epithelial cells, since all other aspects, such as nerves, growth, cell renewal, motility, circulation, and regulation, are comprehensively covered in separate chapters of this volume.

Glandular Mucosa

The glandular epithelium of the stomach contains specialized cells which are distinct from cells of other organs (9,11). The entire surface of the glandular stomach is lined by a simple columnar epithelium of surface mucous cells. This same type of cell also lines the numerous tubular invaginations, the gastric pits (also called foveolae or crypts) (Figs. 1–4). Opening into the base of the gastric pits are one or more simple or branched tubular gastric glands. A delicate basement

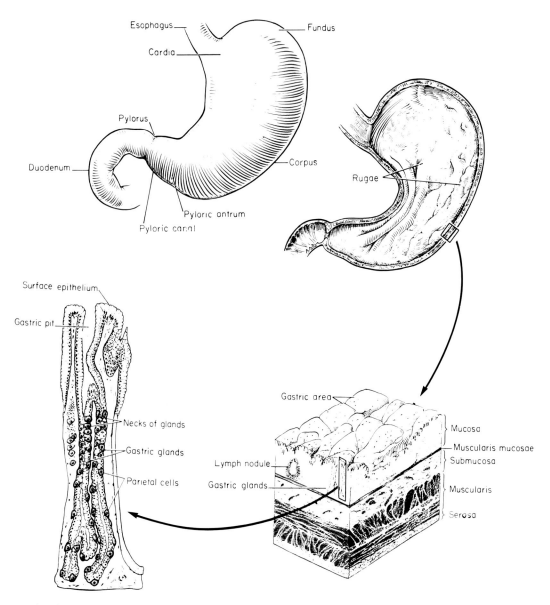

FIG. 1. Diagram of a simple glandular stomach. **Upper,** outer and interior surfaces; **lower,** part of the entire wall from the corpus and a gastric pit with gastric glands. (Modified from ref. 83 and after Braus.)

membrane underlies the epithelium, and the intervening loose connective tissue of the lamina propria contains blood vessels, nerves, smooth muscle cells, and various connective tissue cells (plasma cells, lymphocytes, polymorphonuclear leukocytes, eosinophils, mast cells). The lymphatics in the stomach are generally similar to the system in the small intestine, with blind projections in the lamina propria and plexuses in the muscularis mucosa and submucosa (144). In many routine preparations of normal stomachs, however, the lymphatics are not prominent. Some believe that the stomach contains considerably fewer lymphatics than reported in the early literature (139) (see ref. 185 for a general discussion).

The muscularis mucosa, a thin layer of smooth muscle cells arranged as two or three sublayers, separates the gastric mucosa from the submucosa. In some mammals, a tough layer of dense connective tissue, the stratum compactum, intervenes between the lamina propria and the muscularis mucosae.

The next layer is the submucosa (Fig. 1), which consists of relatively dense connective tissue in which larger blood vessels and nerves, including Meissner plexus, are located. More peripherally, the muscularis or muscular coat of the stomach consists of smooth muscle cells arranged as oblique, circular, and longitudinal layers. The muscle layers in the stomach are not as distinct and discernable as in the muscularis of the intestine. Between the outer two layers of smooth muscle, a parasympathetic nerve plexus (Auerbach plexus) is present. The outermost layer is the serosa, which is a thin layer of loose connective tissue covered by a layer of

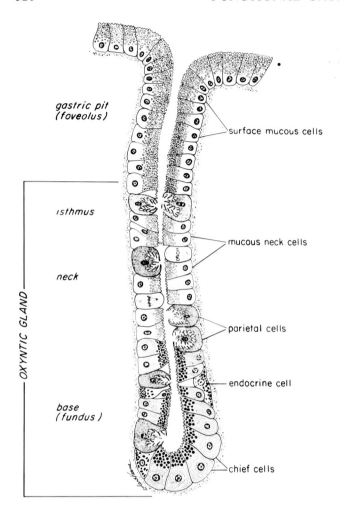

FIG. 2. Diagramatically simplified tubular oxyntic gland from the corpus of a mammalian stomach. Regional designations are after Stevens and Leblond (159). (Modified from ref. 83.)

stratified squamous epithelium to the simple columnar cells of the glandular gastric mucosa. Since the glandular stomach is lined by uniformly similar surface mucous cells, the surface and gastric pit cells of the cardiac glands are indistinguishable from those glands in other regions in the stomach. The cardiac glands, however, are distinct from the oxyntic glands by the absence of the parietal or oxyntic cells and chief cells. Only mucous, undifferentiated, and endocrine cells are present. The zone occupied by cardiac glands varies from a narrow rim of a few millimeters in the cat or human stomach to as much as one-third of the glandular stomach in the pig (10). The gastric pits in these glands are relatively short and are joined by branched tubular glands which are tortuous and coiled. The predominant cells are mucous cells, which are histologically similar to mucous neck cells of the oxyntic glands and to the pyloric gland cells. The functional significance of the cardiac glands is incompletely defined. Its secretion of mucus is generally acknowledged, and the presence of endocrine cells is recognized. The hog cardiac gland has yielded extractable gastrin (52), indicating that this endocrine cell type must be present in these glands.

Pyloric Glands

The pyloric gland area of the stomach generally occupies a region much larger than the cardiac gland area and may be one-fifth or more of the gastric mucosal surface area (96,118). The pyloric antrum (Fig. 1) is adjacent to the oxyntic gland area of the corpus and is continuous with the pyloric canal, which joins the duodenum. The pyloric glands contain mucus-secreting cells, which are similar to mucous neck cells in the oxyntic glands. The characteristic, deep gastric pits penetrate about one-half the thickness of the mucosa and are joined by relatively straight tubular pyloric glands. At the junction with the duodenum is the pyloric sphincter, formed by a thickened circular muscle layer.

Although the major exocrine secretion of these glands is mucus, Grossman and Marks (57) have shown that there is some pepsinogen secretion from dog pyloric pouches. Since their preparations did not contain chief cells, pyloric pepsinogen in the dog is attributed to pyloric gland mucous cells. In a clearly documented study using immunofluorescence, Samloff (147) has shown that human pyloric glands do not contain group I pepsinogens. The basis for these apparent species differences is unclear. A limited number of parietal cells are found in the antral mucosa (12,166). The major source of gastrin is the G cells in the pyloric glands. Since the functional and morphological aspects of gastrin are considered in detail in separate chapters, the G cell is described and discussed only briefly in this chapter. G cell distribution in the pyloric glands has been established by immunolabeling (114). Further-

squamous cells, the mesothelium. These outer layers of the stomach are essentially similar to those in the intestine and are not considered in detail in this chapter.

The mammalian gastric mucosa contains three distinct types of gastric glands: the cardiac, pyloric, and oxyntic glands. Both cardiac and pyloric glands produce a secretion rich in mucus. The cardiac glands are present in a narrow zone near the esophageal orifice; the pyloric glands occupy a sizable region adjacent to the duodenum. The most distinctive gastric gland in the stomach is the oxyntic gland. This gland is also known as the fundic gland, gastric gland, proper gastric gland, or principal gastric gland. To clarify some of the confusion regarding the terminology of this gland, Grossman (55) suggested "oxyntic gland" as an appropriate compromise.

Cardiac Glands

The cardiac glands occupy the zone adjacent to the esophagus where there is an abrupt transition from the

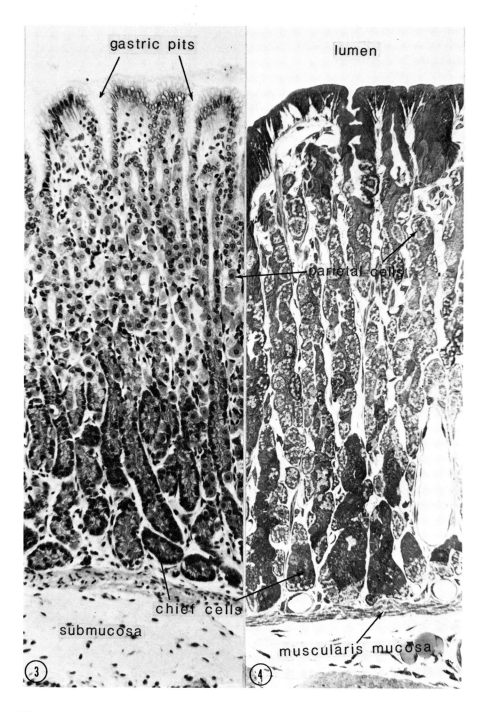

FIG. 3. Photomicrograph of a paraffin section of a monkey stomach stained with hematoxylin and eosin. The surface and gastric pits are lined with surface mucous cells. The parietal cells, which are strongly eosinophylic, appear pale. Chief cells located in the basal portion of the oxyntic glands are stained more intensely. A distinct muscularis mucosae underlies the glands and separates it from the submucosa. × 235.

FIG. 4. A 1 μm-thick section of mouse glandular mucosa from a stomach fixed by vascular perfusion, embedded in plastic, and stained with toluidine blue. The magnification is higher than Fig. 3, but it is readily apparent that much greater cytological detail is preserved in this preparation. Parietal cell mitochondria are seen as fine granules, and the intracellular canaliculi appear as clear channels. Note also scattered smooth muscle cells and expanded vascular spaces. × 380.

more, immunolocalization of gastrin-containing cells has been extended to the electron microscopic level. The definitive ultrastructural identity of the G cell has been made by Greider et al. (53).

Oxyntic Glands

General Consideration

The oxyntic glands are the distinguishing feature of the stomach, occupying most of the fundus and corpus (or body) of the stomach (Fig. 1). The precise area occupied by the oxyntic glands in mammals varies greatly in different species (12,20,76,118,132). As implied by its name, glands containing more than an occasional number of oxyntic or parietal cells, which appear to be the most probable site of gastric HCl secretion, are called oxyntic glands. The second cell type, which is also characteristic of this gland, is the chief cell; it is the acknowledged site of gastric pepsinogen synthesis and secretion. In addition, there are mucous neck cells, undifferentiated cells, and endocrine cells.

As many as seven oxyntic glands may open into a single gastric pit or foveola, but a single gland may join a gastric pit, as depicted in the diagram in Fig. 2. The tubular glands are usually fairly straight but may branch and appear tortuous. The gland is usually divided into three regions: (a) the isthmus, containing parietal and surface mucous cells, (b) the neck, with mainly parietal and mucous neck cells, and (c) the base, which characteristically contains chief cells in addition to some parietal and mucous neck cells. Also present are the endocrine cells, which are scattered throughout the gland. A population of epithelial lymphocytes located between the epithelial cells is a common feature of these glands.

The oxyntic glands are usually not strictly located within distinct boundaries but merge with cardiac and pyloric glands. Furthermore, the distribution of the cell types in the oxyntic gland is variable. In the stomach of humans, dogs, and cats (76,133), parietal cells are more numerous nearer the pylorus than toward the cardia, whereas chief cells have the opposite distribution. Parietal cells comprise about 32% (40% in rats) of the corpus mucosa, whereas chief cells make up about 20 to 26% of the mucosa. The remainder of the gastric mucosal composition is about 18% surface mucous cells, 8% mucous neck cells, and 18% lamina propria. In some glands, parietal cells occupy the basal part of the gland when chief cells are absent. A typical oxyntic gland contains chief cells as the major cell type in the base of the gland; parietal cells predominate in the isthmus and neck regions, intermingled with mucous neck cells, undifferentiated cells, and a few chief cells. The endocrine cells occur as single cells sequestered between the other cell types.

STRUCTURE AND FUNCTIONAL CORRELATES OF THE GASTRIC EPITHELIUM

Although the morphology of the gastric mucosa has been described in detail, much remains to be established regarding the precise functional correlates of gastric secretions. The difficulty is immediately apparent because of the complex intermingling of different cell types and the mixing of secretory products. Thus it is difficult to collect a pure secretory product from one cell type. To study the functions of specific cell types (17,24, 87,137,161), viable stomach cells have been isolated and separated into different populations. This aspect is not considered here, since it is the subject of a separate chapter in this volume. In addition, a promising approach using isolated glands (13,14,31) has been reported.

Despite the incomplete evidence for the direct, positive correlation of gastric secretions with specific cell types, much circumstantial and indirect observations have provided compelling evidence to suggest specific cellular origins of gastric secretory products.

Surface Mucous Cell

The ubiquitous surface mucous cell forms the free surface of the glandular stomach, lines the gastric pits, and intermingles with parietal cells in the isthmus of the gastric glands. These cells resemble intestinal goblet cells but are distinctively different. The role of the stomach is to receive, store, and initiate digestion of all the solid and fluid foodstuffs. In this process, the stomach itself must be protected from detrimental effects, including damage from the wide range of ingested substances as well as from HCl, digestive enzymes, and refluxed contents of the duodenum; this formidable task is relegated to the gastric surface mucous cell.

A few examples illustrate the great diversity and almost unbelievable heterogeneity of mammalian dietary adaptations and preferences. Ingested fluid ranges from water to salt solutions of high osmolar strength and varied alkalinity and acidity; temperatures range from below freezing to near boiling. Solid food intake includes virtually every degree of compactness and fluidity. Furthermore, agents such as ethanol (34), drugs (6,60,74,110,184), and substances like bile salts (33), which can damage or destroy the gastric epithelium, are commonly swallowed. The primary barrier and protective layer of the stomach is the layer of surface mucous cells and its associated gastric mucus.

The stomach is generally lined with a viscous mucus layer overlying the epithelial cells. This tenacious layer is a physical barrier preventing direct contact of particulate matter with the plasma membrane of the surface mucous cells. The ultrastructural features of this cell type are shown in a drawing (Fig. 6) reconstructed from micrographs of various species (human, monkey, mouse, and rat) (see also Figs. 5 and 7–10).

Light microscope preparations of routine paraffin-embedded stomachs show surface mucous cells as a columnar epithelium of cells with lightly staining apical cytoplasm. The mucous granules are not apparent. These cells are often called surface epithelial or columnar cells. When selective stains to demonstrate carbohydrates, such as the periodic acid-Schiff reaction (PAS), are used, the apical cytoplasm is stained intensely.

Recently, Spicer et al. (163) reported a comprehensive ultrastructural histochemical analysis of mucus and carbohydrates in the rat gastric epithelium. The surface mucous cell granules in the interfoveolar cells stained as a hexose-rich neutral mucosubstance. Both the diphasic droplets and monophasic mucous granules in these cells contained a neutral mucosubstance, but the cores of the biphasic granules were not characterized. In the gastric pits, the surface mucous cells contained neutral mucosubstance, but some granules stained for glycoconjugate as well as sulfomucin. Deep in the foveolae, mucous granules were all monophasic and stained for acidic carbohydrates. Thus, although the surface mucous cells are all of one type, varying only in their age and maturation, the characteristics of the mucus varies with location. Furthermore, there is a range of heterogeneity of granules within a single cell.

The amount of mucus stored in these cells is variable and depends on the stage of secretion or synthesis of mucus by the cell. Those cells on the surface usually contain more mucous granules than cells deeper in the gastric pits or isthmus of the glands. In the bat (85), stimulation by feeding after fasting causes a marked reduction in contained mucus, but these changes are not pronounced in the mouse or many other species. Furthermore, there appears to be no effective stimulating agent which will exhaustively deplete cells of their stored mucus. The lack of a selective secretagogue has been a limiting factor in the elucidation of the precise role of these cells in gastric physiology and pathology.

A number of studies (67,83–85,104,140,157) have reported the ultrastructure of the surface mucous cells (Figs. 5–10). The apical part of the cells is packed with mucous granules, and a layer of cytoplasm rich in filaments resembling the terminal web is found in a narrow zone beneath the microvilli and along the lateral cell membrane. This investing layer may appear as a theca around the stored mucus. The mucous granules may be

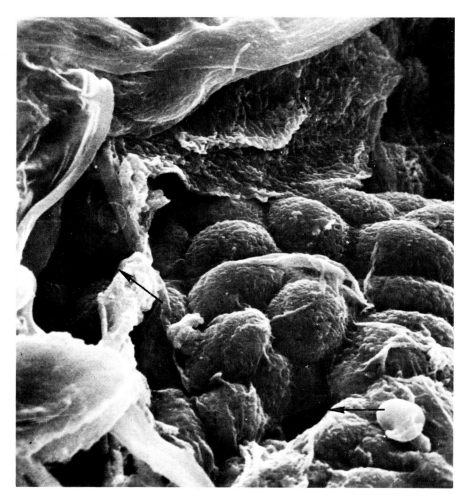

FIG. 5. Scanning electron micrograph of the gastric mucosal surface of a mouse stomach. The surface mucous cells appear as a cobblestone surface mostly covered with a blanket of mucus. At intervals, there are the openings of gastric pits (*arrows*). The mucous coating is preserved as three distinct layers, each with its individual texture and appearance. × 13,825.

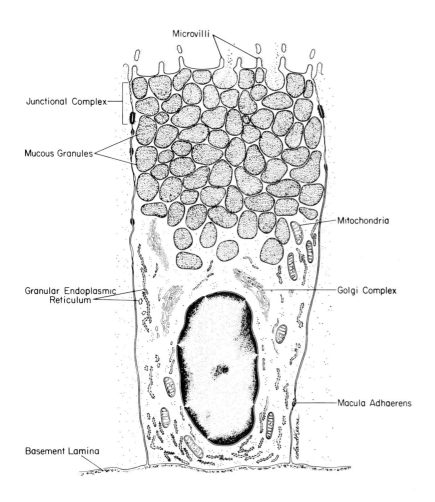

FIG. 6. Surface mucous cell, illustrating some of its salient features.

aggregated and packed together, with little intervening cytoplasm. They are variable in shape, ranging from spherical to ovoid or discoid, but relatively consistent from cell to cell in any one species. When tightly packed, the granules may be deformed and arranged in rouleau-like stacks.

The mucous granules appear as structures of greatly varying density and organization. Some are almost without appreciable density, whereas others are completely opaque. Granules of intermediate density may also be present in the same cell. In some species, the granules may be biphasic, with dense cores and a halo of lower density. In others, the content appears to be preserved as a heterogeneous precipitate-like substance. These variations are presumably due to the preparative process but may represent differences in composition, maturation, or secretory state.

All mucous granules are enclosed in a typical membrane, which appears trilaminar at high magnification. The mucous granule membrane originates from the Golgi complex, where the granules are formed. As in other exocrine secretory cells, the Golgi complex is the site for the terminal stages of synthesizing mucus, including the incorporation of carbohydrates and the formation of granules. In cells where the mucous granule

appear dense, a similar substance is found in the inner or concave lamellae of the Golgi cisternae. Small vesicles containing this substance may be seen fusing with larger granules to form the full or mature mucous granule. Spicer et al. (163) have demonstrated that all Golgi cisternae in surface mucous cells stained positively for hexoses, and increased reactivity was seen in the maturing face. Recognizable mucus in the cytoplasm is confined within membrane-bound compartments and not free in the cytoplasmic matrix.

In many species, the surface mucous cell granules appear as electron-dense granules with no internal structure. Methods used in the preparation of the tissue influence the appearance of the granules. This does not explain why the identical procedure produces different appearances within mucous granules within a single cell. Since it seems likely that granules are similar within a single cell, the varied appearance may be attributable to differences in content due to the formative state of the granules. In the human surface mucous cell, Lillibridge (105) and Rubin et al. (140) found that the mucous granules of both mucous cell types in human stomachs were finely stippled. We previously noted (83,84) that most of the surface mucous cells were dense in some preparations; in other preparations (Fig. 8), the finely stippled

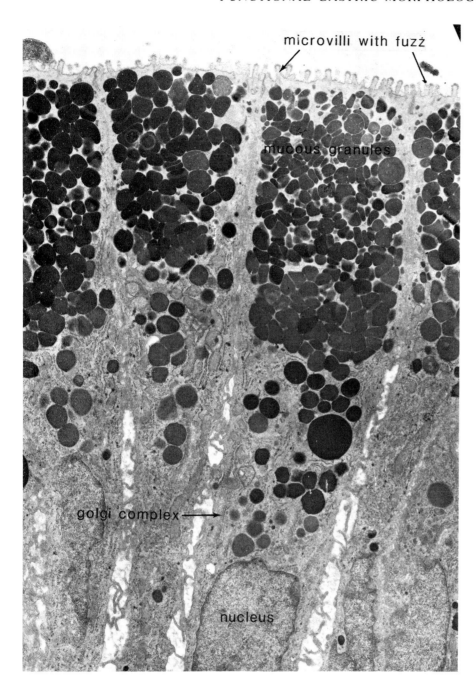

microvilli with fuzz

mucous granules

golgi complex →

nucleus

FIG. 7. Electron micrograph of several surface mucous cells from a human stomach biopsy fixed with osmium tetroxide. The mucous granules are packed densely in the apical cytoplasm. Note that many granules are deformed and appear stacked. The luminal surface has many stubby microvilli coated with fuzz or glycocalyx. Part of a gastric spirillum is seen at the upper left. × 8,075.

appearance was noted. These differences are attributable to methods of preparation, although the effects caused by other factors have not been fully investigated.

The luminal surface of the surface mucous cell has short microvilli with a fuzzy surface coat or glycocalyx of fine filaments. The number and density of microvilli are variable. They may be numerous and closely packed, widely separate, or almost absent. The abundance of microvilli often appears to be inversely proportional to the amount of stored mucus, but other factors, such as the age of the cell and its imminent exfoliation, may determine the number of microvilli present.

Demonstrable near the apex or luminal border of ad-

jacent surface mucous cells is a typical terminal bar, as seen by light microscopy, or a junctional complex, as revealed by electron microscopy and described in all epithelia (36). The zonula occludens or tight junction is a prominent structure with multiple strands of fused outer leaflets. An intermediate junction, or zonula adherens, is present just beneath the tight junction. In addition, desmosomes are distributed periodically along the lateral cell borders. Gap junctions, or nexuses, are also present between surface mucous cells. These are the closely opposed junctions believed to be the sites of electrical coupling between adjacent cells. As far as it is known, all these junctional specializations are present

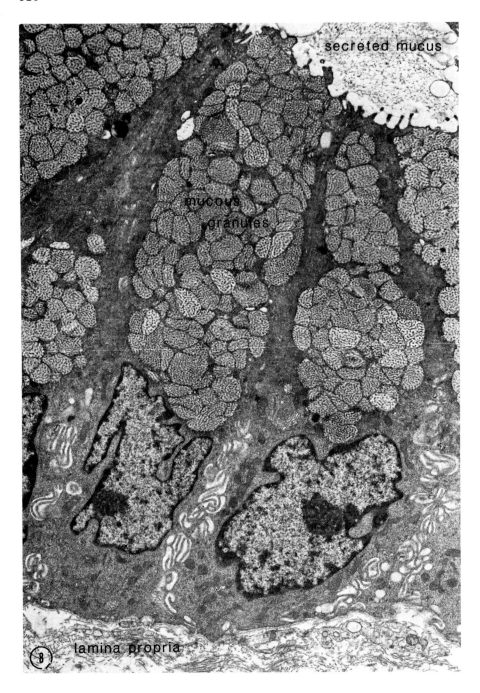

FIG. 8. Human gastric surface mucous cells from the upper part of a gastric pit. The specimen was fixed with aldehydes and then osmicated. Note that the densely packed mucous granules appear mottled and quite different from the granules in Fig. 7. Some profiles in the apical cell border resemble late stages of exocytosis. × 18,500.

between all gastric epithelial cells that have a free luminal border.

The lateral cell membranes are usually parallel to each other, with a minimum space of about 20 nm. Adjacent cells often interdigitate, while still maintaining their intercellular space. Particularly between cells on the luminal surface, however, the intercellular space may be greatly distended, with occasional bridges of adjacent cell folds joining the cells. The functional significance of these spaces is not known but may represent a physiologically important third fluid compartment responsible for the transport of electrolytes and movement of water, as suggested by Kaye et al. (92) in the gall bladder epithelium.

The nucleus of the surface mucous cell is not distinctive; it is located in the basal cytoplasm, may be infolded, and contains a centrally located nucleolus. The cytoplasmic matrix has a moderate amount of rough surfaced endoplasmic reticulum and free ribosomes. The mitochondria are smaller and not as numerous as in parietal cells. Relatively few lysosomes or little evidence of endocytotic activity by these epithelial cells have been noted. Microtubules and filaments are present in the surface mucous cells, but their possible role in mucus secretion has not been investigated. Occasional cells may have relatively large intracellular vacuole-like structures that are lined with microvilli. These appear to be formed by apparent internalization of the apical

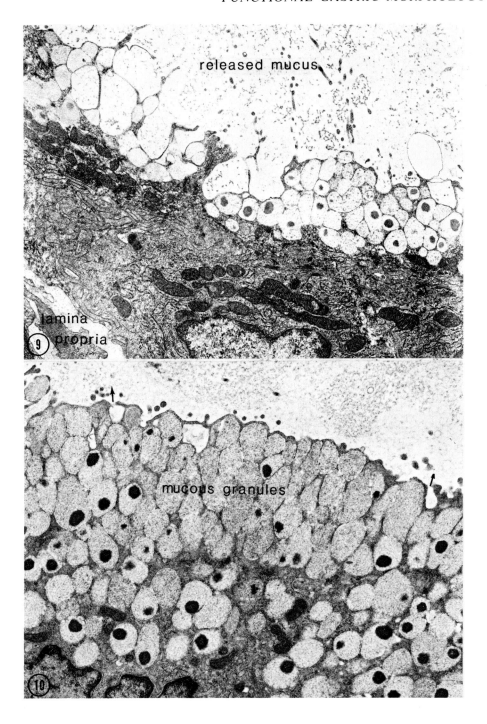

FIG. 9. Rat stomach surface mucous cell from a gastric pit showing the process of massive sudden release of stored mucus by successive exocytosis. Among the secreted mucus in the lumen are slender elements of cytoplasmic processes, which represent residual mucous granule membrane. The remaining granules appear to be smaller than those from the unstimulated gastric mucosa in Fig. 10. × 8,075.

FIG. 10. Rat gastric pit surface mucous cell with many stored granules. A few images representing exocytosis are found in apparently nonsecreting cells and probably represent a constant low level of mucus release. Note the dense cores of the biphasic granules. × 8,075.

plasma membrane. The significance of this structure is not known.

MUCUS SYNTHESIS AND SECRETION

Comprehensive studies on the structural correlates of gastric synthesis of mucus are lacking. Available information and some ongoing studies indicate that the surface mucous cells behave similarly to other mucus-secreting cells, such as intestinal goblet cells (125), in their uptake of labeled carbohydrate precursors into the cell. When tritiated glucose, galactose, or fucose was in-

cubated with pieces of human or mouse gastric mucosae *in vitro* or injected in the submucosa of intact mouse stomachs, the surface mucous cells absorbed the labeled sugar rapidly and avidly. In an early autoradiographic study, Jennings and Florey (89) reported that radioactive sulfur was incorporated into gastric mucous granules in the rat and rabbit stomach. Sulfur uptake by these cells appears to be less evident in other species, such as rat, mouse, and guinea pig.

In a comprehensive autoradiographic study of glycoprotein transport in surface mucous cells of rat stomach incubated with tritiated leucine and galactose, Kramer and Geuze (94) reported that the pathway of glycoprotein synthesis is similar to that in other organs. The Golgi complex was maximally labeled at 40 min and mucous granules after 2 hr. Galactose was incorporated to the glycoprotein in the Golgi complex. Analysis for secreted glycoprotein in the incubation medium was negative after 2 hr, but labeled secreted mucus still attached to the apical part of the cells was observed.

The actual mechanism by which mucous granules are released is incompletely understood. A recent report by Zalewsky et al. (188) undertook a comprehensive ultrastructural analysis of dog gastric mucus and cell release to extend previous studies (65,102,120). On the basis of scanning electron microscopy, it was found that exocytosis, apical expulsion, and cell exfoliation appear to be the three methods of gastric mucus release. Exocytosis of mucous granules was interpreted to be a slow, continuous process in contrast to the sudden release of all the stored mucus during apical expulsion, which was followed by the *in vitro* degeneration of the cell. The final method of release, in which whole cells exfoliate, was observed only rarely. In the gastric pits, only the exocytotic release of mucus was observed, while the exfoliation of cells and expulsive release of the mucus content was restricted to the interfoveolar or free surface of the stomach.

An alternative method for mucus secretion was suggested for human stomachs (83), by exocrine secretion or diffusion through the apparent intact granule and cell membrane. Such a possibility was also suggested as the means for secretion of sulfated glycoprotein from the surface mucous cells in the gastric pits of dogs (163).

Although detailed studies have not been reported, the role of microfilaments and microtubules in the release of mucous granules may be important. Baudin et al. (7) found good evidence to suggest that exocrine pancreatic secretions were associated with microfilaments during the secretory process. It was also found that inhibitory concentrations of secretagogues caused changes in the microtubule and microfilament system that could account for inhibition of pancreatic enzyme secretion. Contractile protein filaments and microtubules may play an important role in the release of secretory granules from surface mucous cells.

The mechanism of stimulation for the release of mucus from the cell is not well known. The normal digestive process and such factors as the uptake, digestion, and absorption of food must be involved with gastric mucus secretion. Morphological studies using, for example, aspirin (47,74), ethanol (34), or stress (65) generally indicate increased mucus release as well as exfoliation of the surface mucous cells. The effect of various cytoprotective agents, such as prostaglandins (135), on the secretion of mucus is unclear; the effects of antiulcer drugs, such as cimetidine and atropine, which are antisecretory, on the surface mucous cells are also unknown.

MORPHOLOGY AND ROLE OF GASTRIC MUCUS

The structure of mucus is discussed in detail in the chapter by Allen elsewhere in this volume. This chapter is concerned only with the microscopic appearance of mucus in the stomach. The morphology of the mucus coat is different from intracellular mucus in secretory granules. As shown in Figs. 8-10 and by a number of published illustrations (65,83,84,106,188), the process of exocytosis results in a sharp decrease in density of the mucus. The released mucus may be preserved as a relatively compact layer (Fig. 5) or as a scattered array of fine, filamentous, or flocculent material. The appearance of mucus in microscope preparations is different from the fresh mucus, which does not lend itself favorably to microscopic study.

In many preparations, much of the mucus is lost during tissue processing, and the exposed microvilli-lined interfoveolar surface mucous cells appear as a naked free surface. When adequately preserved, the mucous coat is present as a thick blanket over the entire epithelium. Some of its characteristics in the dried state can be seen in scanning electron micrographs (Fig.5).

Morphological assessment of the role played by the gastric mucus has not been investigated in detail. In some preliminary studies, we have noted that particulate tracers, such as carbon particles and thorium dioxide, are effectively trapped and do not penetrate the intact coating of mucus. Similarly, most of the ferritin, colloidal iron, and horseradish peroxidase exposed to the stomach surface is prevented from direct contact with surface cells. These tracer localizations indicate that gastric mucus has the ability to protect the underlying cells by providing a physical barrier for the gastric epithelium.

A related but distinct component on the lining of the surface mucous cells is the glycocalyx or fuzzy coat (82). This coat of glycoprotein is attached to the plasma membrane and is a product of the cell on which it is located; it is different from the secreted mucus. Although the gastric glycocalyx has not been studied extensively, it is reasonable to predict that its biology will be similar to that of other cells. Its synthesis, transport, secretion, and turnover from the plasma membrane must allow the surface mucous cells to possess its specific surface properties, such as permeability characteristics, surface antigens, receptors, transport proteins, and digestive enzymes.

The role played by the surface mucous cell of the stomach is remarkable. It must be prepared and be able to accept all the food and fluid intake in a chamber lined with a delicate-appearing, simple columnar epithelium. This appearance is misleading; it can withstand diverse chemical and physical assaults as well as great osmotic variations.

In studies with ethanol damage to the epithelium

(34,50), recovery from the experimental damage occurs within a few hours, indicating an exceptional healing capacity. Although the mechanism by which the epithelium is reestablished is not clear, the migration and differentiation of mucous cells must play an essential role. Another interesting aspect of the gastric mucosa is the cytoprotection provided by prostaglandins to alcohol, boiling water, hypertonic salt (135), or aspirin (60). It is not known whether gastric mucus is concerned with this cytoprotection, but its possible role has been suggested.

Another aspect of the gastric mucosal surface epithelium is the formation of stress ulcers caused by various treatments, such as restraint or surgery. Ultrastructural studies (65) show increased extrusion of cells when animals are stressed; with prolonged stress, surface mucous cells were observed to degenerate *in situ*.

Mucous Neck Cell

In addition to the surface mucous cell, a second type of mucus-secreting cell is present in the gastric mucosa. The mucous neck cells are numerous in the neck and isthmus region where there is a transition in population from surface mucous cells to mucous neck cells. Parietal cells are almost always found in close apposition to mucous neck cells. In the fundus of the oxyntic glands, a few of these cells are scattered among chief cells and parietal cells.

The mucous neck cells in the oxyntic glands and the mucous cells in the cardiac and pyloric glands are similar in appearance; no distinct morphological or histochemical distinction has been demonstrated. Again, the inability of obtaining a pure secretory product of one cell type from a mucosa containing several different secretory cell types makes it difficult to assign precise cellular functions. Some differences among the population of cells classified as mucous neck cells must exist.

Mucous neck cells deep in the oxyntic glands are not always distinguishable from chief cells in routine histological preparations. However, the positive staining for carbohydrates by the PAS reaction of mucous granules readily distinguishes them from chief cell zymogen granules, which do not show significant carbohydrate staining. Both surface mucous cells and the mucous neck cells in the gastric glands stain with PAS reaction, but Alcian Blue staining at low pH for mucous neck cells is more intense than for the surface mucous cells (162,163), indicating the presence of more acidic staining sites in these cells. A possible explanation for this staining capability is suggested by the uptake of radioactive sulfur as shown by autoradiography, which indicates the presence of sulfated glycoproteins. Comparative studies have shown that the mucous neck cells of rabbits and cats are positive for sulfur uptake,

whereas the same cells in the mouse, rat, and guinea pig gastric mucosa do not take up this tracer. More recently, Zalewsky and Moody (187) reported the uptake of sulfur by dog mucous neck cells.

Mucous neck cells are frequently found adjacent to parietal cells, which tend to deform these mucous cells so that they have narrow or broad luminal surfaces and a slender central region. The cytoplasm is not particularly different from that of the surface mucous cell but contains an abundance of free ribosomes and moderate amounts of granular endoplasmic reticulum. In this respect, it is more like the cytoplasm of undifferentiated cells.

The mucous granules in the mucous neck cells differ in their fine structure from those in the surface mucous cells. The granules are larger and often found in the paranuclear region. Often, the granules appear to have a peripheral material of lower or higher density than the core. These differences are in part due to species differences and perhaps also to preparation techniques. Helander and Ekholm (67,68) have described both cell types in the mouse stomach under a single heading, the "mucoid cell," because they could not be distinguished clearly. In a study of the human stomach, Lillibridge (105) noted that there seemed to be transition forms between the two types of mucous cells; he attributed both cells to a common cellular origin.

Included among the mucous neck cell population are the undifferentiated or stem cells of the gastric mucosa. These cells are responsible for the constant replacement of the gastric epithelium by proliferation and differentiation. The surface mucous cells and mucous neck cells are the most rapidly replaced cell types, but the parietal, chief, and endocrine cells are also replaced. This aspect is considered in detail in a separate chapter and has been the subject of a number of early reports (79,109,118, 164).

Appropriate description of the undifferentiated cells has been made by Rubin et al. (140) in human oxyntic glands and by Ferguson (37) in pyloric glands of dogs. These cells are found in the isthmus and neck region of the gland but are present in relatively small numbers. They characteristically have few mucous granules, many free ribosomes and polysomes, and relatively little rough endoplasmic reticula. The nucleus and other cell organelles resemble those of the mucous neck cell. Occasional undifferentiated cells are observed in mitosis. In histological preparations of the stomach, mitotic figures are seen less frequently than in the crypts of the small intestine.

Cell renewal studies indicate that the stomach turns over its epithelial cells similarly to the intestine. Stevens and Leblond (164), as well as Lipkin et al. (109) and others (15,79,100,111,116,164), have documented the kinetics of gastric epithelial cell renewal. The surface mucous cells are renewed more rapidly (about 3 days), whereas mucous neck cells are renewed in about 1 week. Parietal cells and probably chief cells are also replaced (79).

Experimental regeneration studies (50,78,169,184) indicate that the damaged or excised areas are regenerated by rapid migration and proliferation of mucous or undifferentiated cells from the margin of the wound. This new epithelium resembles the differentiation of the stomach in embryonic development (30,146). In human embryos, gastric pits were found in 6- to 9-week-old embryos (30). This was followed by differentiated parietal and chief cells. In adult rats with resected small bowels, a hyperplasia of glandular cells in the stomach was observed (179), similar to the functional adaptation of the remaining intestine after partial intestinal resection.

Parietal or Oxyntic Cell

The most distinctive and characteristic gastric cell of the stomach is the parietal cell, so named because it often bulges outward from the walls of gastric glands. A synonomous term, which is more appropriate but used less commonly, is oxyntic cell, which refers to its ability to secrete acid. There is strong evidence that the gastric parietal cell is the actual source of HCl in the stomach. Among the compelling reasons are the observations that acid is found only in stomachs that contain parietal cells, and that larger numbers of parietal cells result in more acid produced. Also, the presence of acid in the fetal stomach coincides with the differentiation of parietal cells (146,175).

As indicated by their designation, oxyntic glands are those containing oxyntic or parietal cells. Their distribution in various regions of the normal human stomach has been determined (118,124). These cells are found only rarely in the gastric pits or on the luminal surface among the surface mucous cells. In the transition zone adjacent to the cardiac and pyloric glands, some parietal cells are present among the mucous cells, and occasional single cells or clusters of parietal cells have been noted in the pyloric gland area (12,166). Parietal cells are most numerous in the neck or isthmus of the oxyntic glands and are also present in the base or fundus of the glands, particularly in glands where chief cells are absent or scarce.

Histological preparations of the oxyntic glands reveal parietal cells as large oval to pyramidal cells measuring up to 25 μm in diameter with their bases bulging into the lamina propria. These cells stain characteristically with acidic dyes, such as eosin; they are not truly "acidophylic" (51), however, and this staining is not directly indicative of acid secretory activity. Since microscopic observations show an unusual number of mitochondria in parietal cells, this feature must be responsible for the staining with acid dyes.

A structural specialization of parietal cells which was recognized very early (8,107,130,189) is their intracellular canaliculi. These are a network of canals or clefts which are continuous with the gland lumen and may extend into the basal cytoplasm and encircle the nucleus. The canaliculi stain heavily with certain osmium tetroxide and silver stains (8,189).

Since the early electron microscopic studies demonstrated that the intracellular canaliculi were not truly "intracellular" but always open to the lumen, we suggested the term "secretory canaliculus" (85). Our recent studies (88,148), however, have shown that these canaliculi may become internalized in the nonsecreting stage, as described in detail below. The term intracellular canaliculi, therefore, seems appropriate.

With the development of electron microscopic techniques, Dalton (26) first observed microvilli lining the intracellular canaliculi and free surface of parietal cells. This study was followed by publications on the ultrastructure of the parietal cell of mammals and its equivalent oxyntopeptic cells of other nonmammalian vertebrates. Some earlier studies include those by Arevalo (2), Challice et al. (23), Gusek (59), Sedar (149-156), Hally (61-63), Helander (66-72), Ito (81,83,84), Ito and Winchester (85), Kurosumi et al. (95), Lawn (99), Lillibridge (104), Vial and Orrego (170-172), Rohrer et al. (136), Rosa (138), Rubin et al. (140), Shibasaki (157), and others (117,162,180,187). More recently, the studies on parietal cells have been devoted to describing structural changes related to the secretory states (22,45,46,72,86,88,148,171,186) and the steriological analysis of membrane components in these cells (48,71,72,86,88,186).

There is general agreement on the ultrastructure of the parietal cell. The salient features are illustrated in Figs. 11-13 and 16. The most conspicuous structures in parietal cells are the intracellular canaliculi and the abundant, large mitochondria. The microvilli in the secreting parietal cell are long and numerous. They are present on the luminal surface as well as on the canalicular walls and when tightly packed may almost occlude the canalicular lumen. The surface area provided by these microvilli is very large. The shape and extent of the intracellular canaliculi vary somewhat between parietal cells among different species. Even within one stomach, however, there are marked differences in different cells in the amount of microvillar surface between cells presumed to be in the secreting or nonsecreting states.

In parietal cells from gastric mucosae of animals secreting acid at high rates, there are consistent observations among several independent investigators (45,71, 72,86,88,148,186) that the microvillar surface increases rapidly after stimulation of acid secretion. In mice (148), we found that stereological measurements indicated at least a fourfold increase in microvillar surface, as well as a 50% increase in lateral and basal cell

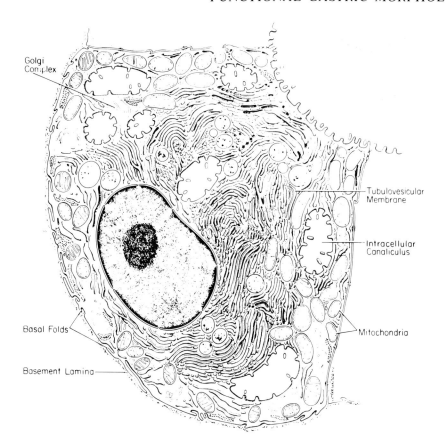

FIG. 11. Nonsecreting parietal cell. The cytoplasm is replete with tubulovesicular membranes, and the intracellular canaliculus has become internalized, distended, and devoid of microvilli.

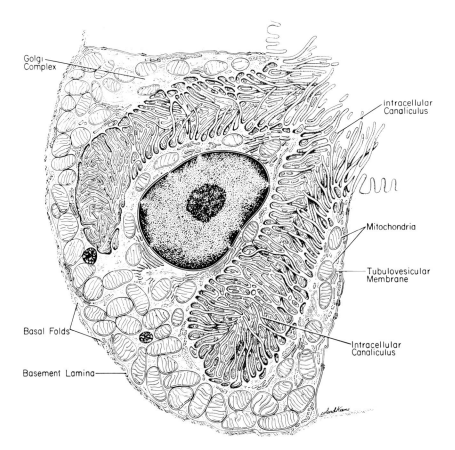

FIG. 12. Acid-secreting parietal cell. The most striking difference is the abundance of long microvilli and the paucity of the tubulovesicular system, which makes the mitochondria appear relatively numerous.

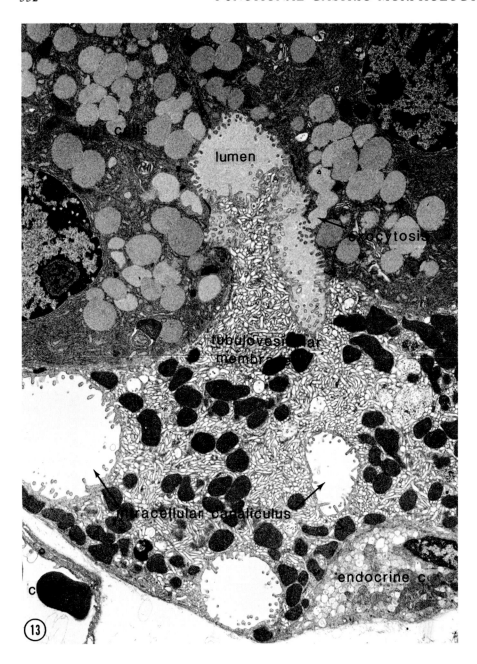

FIG. 13. Low-power electron micrograph of a mouse oxyntic gland with chief cells and a parietal and endocrine cell. The parietal cell contains an abundance of tubulovesicular membranes and numerous dense mitochondria and many multivesicular bodies. The chief cells bordering the gland lumen contain numerous pepsinogen granules and an example of successively fused granules undergoing exocytosis. Note that the granule content density is identical to the luminal content, but the parietal cell intracellular canaliculi is clear. This indicates that the canalicular lumen is no longer in continuity with the gland lumen. × 6,160.

membrane. Concomitantly, there was a 90% reduction in the tubulovesicular membranes of the cytoplasm. Other workers have found even greater increases in the microvillar membrane surface (71,72,186) of secreting parietal cells.

In a recent study using immunolocalization techniques, Saccomani et al. (145) reported that the antibody to the major membrane fractions of hog stomachs with the K^+ ATPase-containing H^+ transport fraction was localized on the apical and canalicular microvilli of parietal cells. Only weak reactions were evident on the zymogenic cells or on the basal and lateral cell surfaces. This study shows that the proton translocation ATPase is in the regions of parietal cells, which are the presumed sites of acid secretion. The histochemical localization of ATPase activity on mammalian parietal cell microvillous membrane has been reported (141), but the tubulovesicular system did not react for this enzyme.

Extensive studies on the antitropic effects of autoantibodies to parietal cells have been reported (see ref. 49 for a recent review). Antibodies to parietal cells and also to intrinsic factor have been localized in parietal cells by immunofluorescence staining. By electron microscopy, the immunolocalization of peroxidase-coupled parietal cell antibody from the sera of pernicious anemia patients revealed that the antigenic sites were restricted to the microvillar membrane of human parietal cells. Interspecies cross reaction with parietal cells of rat, mouse, guinea pig, and hog was observed. This antibody appears to be selective for the outer surface of the microvilli and did not react with the cytoplasmic tubulovesicular membrane (75).

The membrane of parietal cell microvilli lacks the prominent morphological coating or glycocalyx present on the other cells in gastric glands. Further evidence suggesting that the parietal cell plasma membrane is different is the positive staining for neutral carbohydrates on rat parietal cell microvilli after "inert dehydration" in ethylene glycol and staining with acid phosphotungstic acid, as shown by Sedar (154) and in an extensive histochemical study by Forte and Forte (42). More recently, Spicer and Sun (162) confirmed this finding by staining for neutral glycoconjugate, a neutral mucosubstance, on parietal cell microvilli. This is an unusual neutral carbohydrate cell coating, which has not been found on any other cell type. It has been suggested that this feature of parietal cell microvilli may be related to the proton transport believed to take place at this site.

Within the microvilli are numerous thin filaments, which have been shown (172) to be actin by the characteristic binding of heavy meromyosin. Some microtubules have also been observed in the apical cytoplasm (46) and have been suggested as the possible means of withdrawing the microvillar membrane from the surface and into the cytoplasm to reconstitute the tubulovesicular membrane.

The basal and lateral cell membranes of the parietal cell are slightly thinner than the apical plasmalemma. The lateral apical surface of the cell has a typical junctional complex with a prominent tight junction and a zonula adherens. Some desmosomes and gap junctions have also been observed on the lateral borders, which are moderately interdigitated with adjacent cells. The basal border may be smooth but more often has uniform basal folds approximately as thick as the diameter of microvilli (~ 100 nm). These plications are most prominent on parietal cells and are not a regular feature of other gastric epithelial cells. The functional significance of this basal specialization is not known but may represent amplification of surface area associated with the release of bicarbonate into the circulatory system.

The abundant and conspicuous cytoplasmic membrane component of parietal cells in the nonsecreting stomach are the tubulovesicular membranes. These have been variously designated as the agranular endoplasmic reticulum, vacuoles, vesicles, vesicotubules, or bulbotubules. During the early period of electron microscopic study, there were questions regarding the true morphology of this system. Was it vesicular or vacuolar, or was it tubular? This question still remains unresolved. Certain methods of preparation (fixation and embedding) favored the presence of vesicles, whereas others resulted in the apparent preservation of predominantly tubular profiles. Since the tubular system may be more representative of the living state, and because there always are some vesicles and focal regions of some tubules which are enlarged, we prefer the term tubulovesicular system or tubulovesicular membranes for this component. Further evidence that these cytoplasmic membranes are normally of tubular configuration is indicated in ongoing studies by rapid freezing of living tissue and fixation by freeze-substitution. As shown in Fig. 15b, the tubulovesicular system in mouse parietal cells are mainly tubular in shape in these preparations.

In most gastric mucosae, whether the animal was fasting or feeding, considerable variation in the abundance of the tubulovesicular system in different parietal cells has been noted. When maximum gastric secretion is stimulated by secretagogues, such as histamine, carbachol, gastrin, insulin, or reserpine (45,71,72,86,148, 186), there is a rapid depletion of these membranes. A concomitant increase in the number and size of microvilli has been observed and measured stereologically.

The morphology of the secreting parietal cell contrasted with the inactive parietal cell is clear, but we know relatively little of the mechanism or process by which the cell reverts from one morphological state (Figs. 11 and 13) to the other (Fig. 12 and 14). An obvious process that could explain the rapid loss of tubulovesicular membrane and the increase in microvillar membrane is by direct continuity, so that the membrane is exteriorized by membrane flow or exchange, as suggested by a number of investigators (81,101,102,152). This process has not been demonstrated with tracers, however, and there is no evidence that this transposition occurs in mammalian parietal cells (86). If it does take place, our failure to reveal the mechanism may be due to presently inadequate techniques or to the extreme rapidity of the process. On the other hand, some morphological observations suggest the possibility of direct transfer of membranes. These are the occasional very close appositions of tubulovesicular membranes to the plasmalemma (86,148) and extensions of tubular membrane profiles into microvillous cores. In addition, the appearance of the freeze-fracture replicas of microvillar and tubulovesicular membranes (43,44,86,101) (Fig. 16) are similar.

Parietal cell microvillar membranes in freeze-fracture replicas consistently have a dense packing of intramembrane particles on the convex P face, with corresponding pits in the concave E face (Fig. 16). The tubulovesicular membranes have a similar dense packing of particles and pits and are indistinguishable from the microvilli, except for the presence of particles on the concave or cytoplasmic face of the tubulovesicular membrane. Thus the luminal surface of the tubulovesicular system corresponds with the E face of the

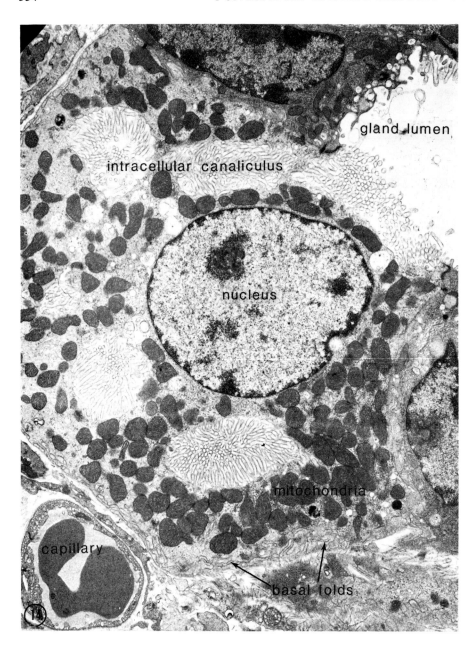

FIG. 14. Mouse parietal cell from a stomach which was secreting acid at a high rate. In contrast to the cell in Fig. 13, there are many long microvilli, an extensive intracellular canalicular system, and almost no tubulovesicular membranes. Numerous mitochondria occupy much of the cytoplasm. There is some increase in the basal plasma membrane in the folds, but this is less apparent than the microvillus membrane. Many parietal cells in this configuration are found only when animals are stimulated maximally. An undifferentiated cell is seen at the upper margin. × 5,950.

microvillous membrane. On the basis of membrane morphology, simple translocation between the two membrane compartments would be the obvious means of changing parietal structure to conform with secretory activity. As indicated above, however, this has been suggested (101) but not demonstrated.

A recent freeze-fracture study (16) has shown a change in the distribution of membrane associated granules in the apical surface plasma membrane between the resting and secreting parietal cells. These changes lend further support to the hypothesis that the tubulovesicular membranes fuse with surface membrane during the onset of acid secretion.

There are some distinct differences between the microvilli and the tubulovesicular system: (a) the histochemical reactions for adenosine triphosphatase and *p*-nitrophenylphosphatase are positive for the microvilli but not the tubulovesicular system (141); and (b) the localization of carbonic anhydrase in the parietal cell appears to be in the microvilli cores and on the cytoplasmic surface of the plasma membrane and is not consistently associated with the tubulovesicular system (165). We have attempted to show the possible continuity between the tubulovesicular system and the plasma membrane of parietal cells (86) but have never found any indication of such connections. There are reported observations (42,152) of frog oxynticopeptic cells in which peroxidase tracer from the lumen was found in the tubulovesicular system, suggesting continuity of the membranes.

When active secretion ceases, parietal cells somehow revert back to the nonsecreting stage and reconstitute

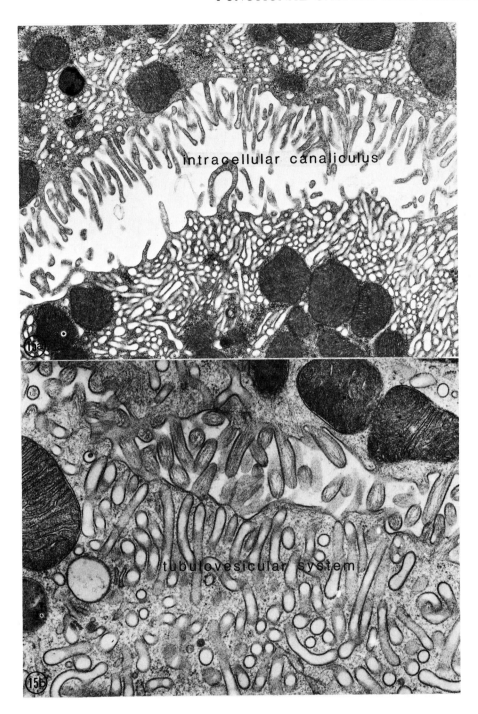

intracellular canaliculus

tubulovesicular system

FIG. 15. a: Part of a mouse parietal cell with cell morphology suggesting intermediate acid secretory activity. Microvilli are moderately abundant, but many tubulovesicular membranes are still present. Note the close approximation of the cytoplasmic membranes to the plasma membrane. × 26,000. **b:** Part of a mouse parietal cell rapidly frozen in the living state on a liquid nitrogen cooled copper block and fixed by freeze substitution at −79° C in OsO_4 and acetone. Note that the tubulovesicular system is predominantly tubular in shape and that the tubules are not open to the intracellular canalicular lumen. × 38,000. (Micrograph courtesy of N. Sugai and A. Ichikawa.)

their tubulovesicular compartment. This process is poorly understood. We recently reported (148) that after intense stimulation and secretory activity, a variety of vesicular elements, such as flattened vesicles, concentric membrane profiles, coated vesicles, and multivesicular bodies, may be involved in the movement of microvillar membrane to the tubulovesicular system in the mouse parietal cell.

In dog gastric parietal cells after stimulation with histamine, Helander and Hirschowitz (71) observed the apparent invagination of microvilli and the merging of their membranes to form a five-layered structure after

acid secretion had ceased. Studies with pig stomachs by Forte et al. (45) revealed the presence of numerous microfilaments and microtubules beneath parietal cell microvilli. These cytoplasmic structures were postulated to be responsible for membrane translocation to form the microvillar membranes during stimulated acid secretion. Upon cessation of histamine stimulation, the microfilaments became disoriented and the microvillar membranes folded upon one another and formed pentalaminar structures, which were endocytosed. This process was also interpreted to involve the microfilaments

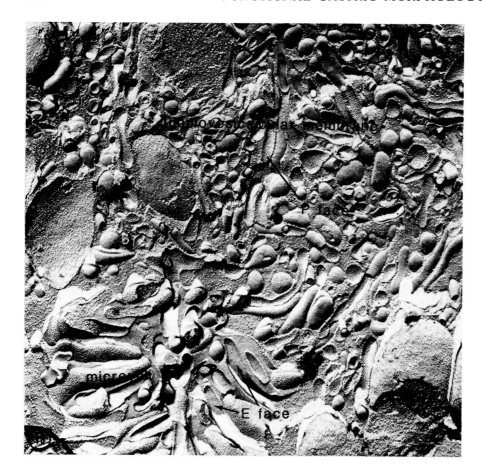

FIG. 16. Freeze-fracture replica of a mouse parietal cell in a secretory state similar to Fig. 15. The microvilli of the intracellular canaliculi have a dense packing of intramembrane granules on the P face and few particles on the E face. The tubulovesicular membranes have a similar density of particles on their respective membrane faces. Note, however, that the concave and convex faces are reversed in the two membrane compartments. × 34,000.

and microtubules. After the endocytic uptake of the pentalaminar structures, the membrane components were believed to be recycled back into the tubulovesicular membranes. Further support for the possible role of the filaments in movement of membranes is the finding by Vial and Garrido (172) that the rat parietal cell microvilli were associated with actin-like filaments demonstrated by heavy meromyosin labeling.

During the course of our morphological studies on the parietal cell, we noted (87,148) that the intracellular canaliculus may become completely internalized and close off its opening to the lumen of the gastric gland. Although this was not a constant feature of all parietal cells in the nonsecreting configuration, some of these cells with distended canaliculi lined with a few stubby microvilli and numerous tubulovesicular membranes exhibited clear evidence of this feature. In some glands, the lumen was filled with a dense product, which appeared to be secreted pepsinogen from chief cells. In nearby parietal cells, the intracellular canaliculi were clear and void of the dense luminal material. This indicates that these parietal cell canaliculi must be truly internalized and intracellular in these inactive cells (Fig. 13).

Further evidence that these canaliculi may become internalized is related to the observation that a bacterium (the gastric spirilla) present in gastric glands and in-

tracellular canaliculi of many apparently normal dogs, cats, and occasional human stomachs (87,107,170) may be phagocytized and destroyed in parietal cell phagosomes (87). This process occurs by the closing off of the canaliculi into which the bacteria had entered and the conversion of the canal into a phagosome; it presumably takes place many times during the lifespan of the cell and may result in the accumulation of dense bodies in parietal cells.

The cytoplasm of parietal cells contains an abundance of large mitochondria which occupy 30 to 40% of the cytoplasmic volume (71,86) and are the major component of the cytoplasm. The mitochondrial cristae are transversely oriented and may have distinct angular configurations. Small, dense intramitochondrial granules are common in the matrix. Most recent studies do not indicate mitochondrial changes associated with active secretion, but an early light microscope study (108) suggested visible changes. The gastric mucosa has long been known to be a tissue with exceptionally high oxidative activity. Studies on isolated enriched parietal cell fractions (137,161) reveal an oxygen consumption rate about five times higher than the mucous cells. Similar findings were reported for the amphibian oxynticopeptic cells (17).

The Golgi complex of the parietal cell is small and easily overlooked. It is formed by smooth surfaced cisternae which are stacked in close array and have associated smooth and coated vesicles. The Golgi complex may be located almost anywhere in the cytoplasm, and several small Golgi complexes may be found in the peripheral or basal cytoplasm of a single parietal cell. Varying numbers of lysosomes, multivesicular bodies (62,148), and scattered glycogen particles are common features of parietal cells.

The remaining cytoplasm of parietal cells contains many free ribosomes and polysomes, as well as a limited amount of rough endoplasmic reticula. The role of these ribosomes is not known, but it is possible that some are involved in the production of intrinsic factor which has been localized in the parietal cells of the human and most mammals. In the rat gastric mucosa, there is evidence that the intrinsic factor is present in chief cells (18).

The parietal cell is the most logical candidate for secretion of HCl. Assuming that our observations on parietal cell morphology are correct, the secretion of HCl must occur across the parietal cell microvillar membrane. The acid then flows out from the intracellular canaliculus, into the gastric gland lumen, and into the stomach. How do the parietal cells and the other epithelial cells protect themselves from secreted 0.1 N HCl? The mucus secreted by the mucous neck and surface mucous cells do not form an impermeable shield over the epithelium. Therefore, the plasma membrane with its glycocalyx must be the effective barrier to withstand the acid environment. Resistance to damage is complicated further by the outpouring of pepsinogen from the chief cells and the resulting potent proteolytic effect of pepsin.

To define the cellular source of gastric HCl, a number of studies and many theories have been proposed; the work up to 1950 was reviewed by Babkin (3). Subsequent work has confirmed and extended the earlier studies, but the accepted role of parietal cells as the source of gastric acid is still based on indirect evidence. An extensive study using 26 indicator dyes on isolated frog and cat gastric mucosa by Bradford and Davies (21) supports the contention that parietal cells are the source of acid, and that the site of acid secretion is the wall of the oxyntic cell canaliculus. It was found that the parietal cell secretion pH was <6.8 with neutral red, <4.85 with acridine in UV light, and <1.4 using toluene-azoamine toluene 2:1:1:4′:3′. Kominick (93) devised a method using silver to precipitate chloride in the lumen and vesicles of parietal cells and interpreted these findings to support the view that parietal cells are the source of gastric hydrochloric acid.

Recent studies by DiBona et al. (31) and Berglindh et al. (14) using isolated rabbit gastric glands examined by interference, electron, and fluorescence microscopy show the formation of intracellular vacuoles in parietal cells. These intracellular compartments were found to be intracellular canaliculi which were internalized and not freely open to the gland lumen. Histamine stimulation greatly enhanced the formation of these vacuoles, which were acidic as shown by the pH-dependent, red metachromasia of acridine orange fluorescence. These studies also indicated that the intracellular vacuoles accumulated aminopyrine when stimulated by histamine of high-K^+ medium. It is assumed that aminopyrine uptake is coincident with acid secretion into parietal cell vacuoles.

OXYNTICOPEPTIC CELL

In place of chief and parietal cells in mammalian gastric glands, nonmammalian vertebrates have a single cell type, the oxynticopeptic cell, which serves a dual function, secreting both acid and pepsinogen (1,128). Because this cell in the amphibian is a useful experimental system, it has been used extensively in physiological and morphological experiments (22,42,43,149,150, 152,167,172). Various aspects of this cell (which is also called the oxyntic or parietal cell) have been included in various parts of this chapter; a brief consideration of its morphology is presented here.

The salient feature of the oxynticopeptic cell from nonsecreting and secreting frog stomach preparation is shown in Figs. 17 and 18. In the inactive state, the luminal plasma membrane is relatively smooth, and there are few microvilli or surface plications. The cytoplasm of such cells is replete with a packed array of tubulovesicular membranes. In contrast, during stimulated secretory activity, the surface plasma membrane is increased greatly by the elaboration of numerous, long, surface plications. Concurrent with the surface amplification, there is a sharp depletion of the tubulovesicular system. It has been suggested (42,81,150) that these membrane compartments are interchangable.

In addition to the acid secretory mechanism, granules of pepsinogen are stored in the cytoplasm, and a moderate amount of rough endoplasmic reticulum is present. In most of these cells, the structures associated with the presumed acid secretory mechanism predominate over the pepsinogenic apparatus.

Relatively little work has been done with the stomach of other vertebrate classes. Toner (167,168) and Vial et al. (173) have studied the ultrastructure of avian oxynticopeptic cells in the proventriculus; and a recent study has reported on the fine structure of an elasmobranch (134). Except for minor differences, these cells closely resemble the oxynticopeptic cells of the frog.

CHIEF CELL

The chief or peptic cell is a typical protein-secreting exocrine cell similar in morphology to the pancreatic

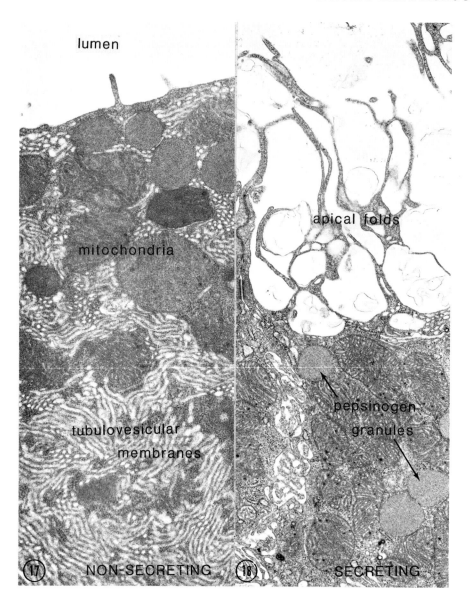

lumen

mitochondria

tubulovesicular membranes

apical folds

pepsinogen granules

⑰ NON-SECRETING   ⑱   SECRETING

FIGS. 17 and 18. Examples of bullfrog oxynticopeptic cells in different secretory states. In Fig. 17, the nonsecretory state, the cell has a relatively smooth luminal surface with few microvilli or surface undulations. The cytoplasm is rich in tubulovesicular membranes. In contrast, the oxynticopeptic cell in Fig. 18 from an active acid-secreting gastric mucosa has a large amplification of the apical plasma membrane arrayed as folds and plications. Only limited amounts of tubulovesicular membrane are found in these cells. The cytoplasm of both cells have numerous mitochondria and some pepsinogen granules. × 17,000.

acinar cell, but it synthesizes, stores, and secretes pepsinogen instead of pancreatic enzymes. Relatively little attention or study has been directed to gastric pepsinogen production. This in part because these cells reside in a gland with several other cell types, and it is difficult to study the sites of secretion in chief cells without influence and contamination by other secretory cells.

As shown in Figs. 2 to 4, chief cells are found predominantly in the base or fundus of the oxyntic gland. Their distribution varies in different parts of the glandular mucosa, but they are most abundant in the corpus of the stomach (20). Chief cells are absent in the cardiac glands and are usually not numerous in the adjacent oxyntic glands of the fundus. These peptic cells are rare or absent in the pyoric glands. In routine histological preparations, chief cell granules are not colored but stain well with Biebrich Scarlet by the method of Bowie (19) and as modified for plastic sections by

Moxey and Yeomans (121). The basal cytoplasm of these cells stains strongly with basic dyes, indicating the presence of abundant ergastoplasm or cytoplasm rich in ribosome-studded endoplasmic reticulum.

A diagram of a typical chief cell is shown in Fig. 19 and illustrated in Fig. 20, where its ultrastructural features are seen. The luminal surface has a few stubby microvilli, and the membrane has a thin glycocalyx or fuzzy coating of glycoprotein. The lateral cell membrane is relatively smooth and is joined to its adjacent cell at the apex by a typical junctional complex of a tight junction and zonula adherens. Desmosomes and gap junctions are also present. As with all epithelial cells, a thin basement lamina underlies the cell.

The zymogen granules, which contain pepsinogen, are usually numerous in the apical cytoplasm. These granules range from about 1 to 3 μm in diameter and are round. Some methods of preservation for electron microscopy do not retain the granule content, so that

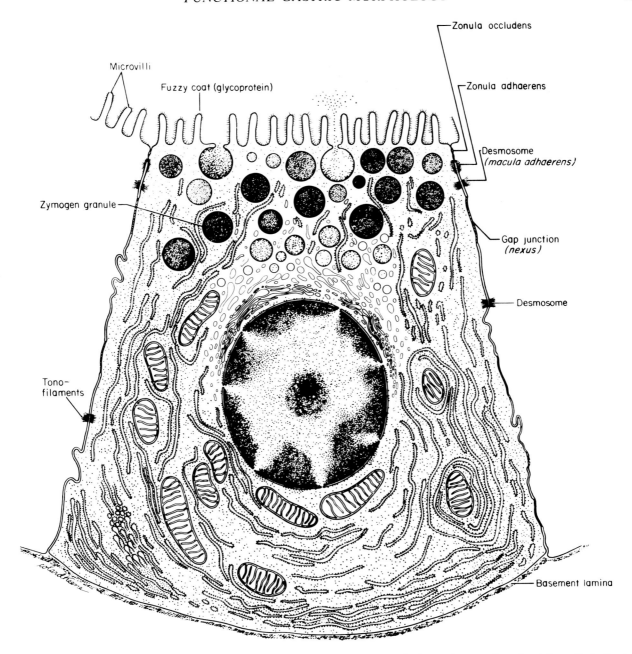

FIG. 19. Gastric chief cell illustrating its ultrastructural features. The cell is a typical protein-secreting glandular cell similar to a pancreatic acinar cell. It contains an abundance of granular endoplasmic reticulum and stored pepsinogen or zymogen granules in addition to the nucleus and other cell organelles. Typical junctional complexes are also present.

they appear empty or filled only with a small amount of fine precipitate. Some of our current techniques (148), however, preserve these granules with a uniformly dense matrix. The granules are enclosed within a trilaminar membrane in favorably fixed material. The presence of pepsinogen granules with enclosing membranes reported to be a single dense line (104) may be due to autolytic changes or differences in preparation techniques. Shibasaki (158) reported unit membranes in deep granules and a single dense line on more apical granules in the same cell. This unusual appearance of pepsinogen granule membranes may have some functional significance.

The abundant studded endoplasmic reticulum is in the basal cytoplasm and extends well into the apical cytoplasm between the secretory granules. Although cisternal arrays are most common, tubular configurations of the reticulum are also present. For reasons that are not apparent, human chief cells (83,105,140) frequently have dense lysosome-like structures among and often adjacent to the zymogen granule. There may be residual components of autophagic activity, but they are not found in abundance in other species, and their significance is unknown.

Pepsinogen release by exocytosis or merocrine secretion (85,95) is similar to pancreatic zymogen secretion.

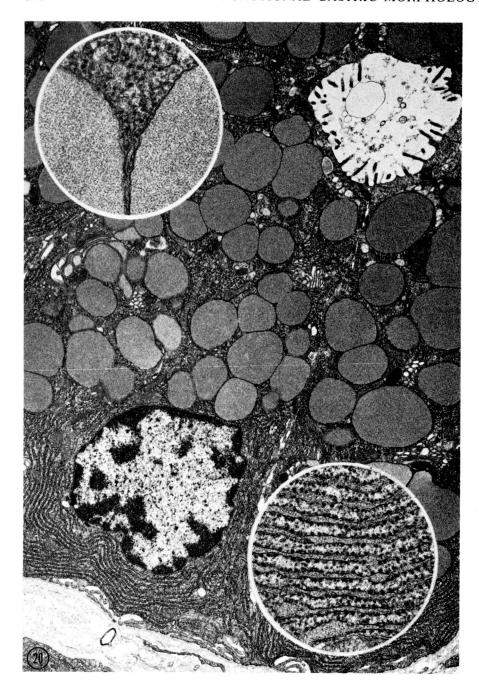

FIG. 20. Chief cells from the fundus of an oxyntic gland from a monkey stomach. These cells contain numerous large secretory granules containing pepsinogen. The basal cytoplasm has an abundance of granular endoplasmic reticulum, which also fills in much of the intergranule cytoplasm. × 12,750. *Upper inset,* higher magnification illustrating the trilaminar membrane surrounding the secretory granules; *lower inset,* ribosome-rich endoplasmic reticulum. × 63,750.

Studies on zymogen granule release in response to feeding or fasting have been investigated (115), but a thorough quantitative analysis with selective secretagogues has not been done. The chief cell, which is an important although not essential gastric cell, has been neglected when compared to the parietal studies.

Although it had long been assumed that gastric chief cells are the source of pepsinogen, the evidence was not definitive until the past decade. The strong immunofluorescent localization of immunolabeled antibodies to pepsinogen has been demonstrated convincingly in human chief cells by Samloff (147). In addition, the mucous neck cells in the same preparation were stained for pepsinogen, suggesting that this mor-

phologically distinct cell type also produces pepsinogen. An unexpected aspect of this immunofluorescence study was that the mucous cells in the pylorus, which closely resemble mucous neck cells, did not react for pepsinogen. An earlier study (57) showed that pyloric glands of the dog, devoid of peptic cells, secrete a pepsinogen-like protease. The cellular source of pepsinogens is considered in greater detail elsewhere in this volume.

ENTEROENDOCRINE CELLS

Although the endocrine cells of the stomach are less conspicuous and comprise only a small part of the glands, they are of great importance as the source of important polypeptide hormones and biogenic amines (113). The enteroendocrine cells are the subject of the chapter by Solcia; his recent comprehensive review of gastric endocrine cells (159), in addition to other recent reviews (41,58,129,132), obviates the need for a detailed description here. The salient features of the endocrine cells that have been identified in the gastric mucosa are considered briefly, and the gastrin cell, found mainly in the pyloric glands, is described in some detail.

Since their first description more than 100 years ago, the enteroendocrine cells were given dozens of names, depending on how they were tinted by various staining procedures (112). A commonly used term for these cells was enterochromaffin cells, because some cells in this group were colored when treated with chromic acid-containing fixatives. Another distinction observed in the granules of certain endocrine cells was that they reduced silver salts; this was the basis for considering them as argentaffin cells (28). Still another distinctive cell is the argyrophile cell, which reacts with silver only after exposure to a reducing substance. In addition, there were cells in this group that did not stain by any of these techniques. It was recently estimated (58) that there are more than 100 staining methods described for these cells, but none provides conclusive identification of the specific cell types. Factors that make the study of these cells difficult include their small numbers, mixed populations, species differences, functional variations, and production of several hormones by the same cell.

In the past two decades, the biochemical purification and synthesis of some of the hormones (52) from these cells allowed the raising of specific antibodies to the individual hormones. The simultaneous development of radioimmunoassay and immunocytochemical techniques (see ref. 56 for a short historic review) provides the technical basis for the current rapid advances in this area. These techniques provided a means to distinguish between the different types of endocrine cells.

According to recent summaries (49,56,129,159,160), there are nine or more different enteroendocrine cell types in the mammalian stomach. Most of these cells have corresponding cells in other organs which secrete the same hormone. The accepted basis for their identification is by specific immunofluorescence of polypeptide hormones correlated with ultrastructural immunolocalization. This evidence has been compared with the electron microscopy studies of the endocrine cells, so that the size and texture of the granules have become another means to identify specific cell types (58,159). The population of cells containing monoamines is identified by specific fluorescence characteristics using specific histochemical methods.

A system to encompass all the common cytological characteristics of cells producing polypeptide hormones has been proposed by Pearse and Takor (129) as the "APUD concept." In this proposal, the common cytochemical properties of the endocrine cells are attributed to their neuroectodermal origin from the neural crest. APUD refers to "amine content and *A*mine *P*recursor *U*ptake and *D*ecarboxylation cells." With respect to the stomach, the actual origin of the gastric APUD cells is yet unproven, and evidence suggests endodermal as well as neuroectodermal origin.

In the gastric mucosa, enterochromaffin cells, which are also argentaffin by their staining reaction, are found in the oxyntic and pyloric glands. These cells are also positive for the APUD reaction and have characteristic granule ultrastructure. The two cell types are the EC cell bound in the stomach and small intestine, and the ECL cell found only in the gastric mucosa. The EC cell contains granules that are about 300 nm in diameter and are flat, oval, or crescent-shaped with little or no clear halo around the dense core (Table 1 and Fig. 23d). The EC cells have a narrow apical cytoplasmic extention to the gastric gland lumen. The ECL cell contains larger granules of up to about 450 nm (Fig. 23b). It is the only enteroendocrine cell found exclusively in the gastric mucosa and was shown by Rubin and Schwartz (143) to synthesize histamine. In the rat, the ECL cell is also an APUD (142).

An endocrine cell with the appropriate appearance and immunoreactivity to pancreatic glucagon has been designated the A cell. These cells contain dense granules about 250 nm diameter with a narrow clear halo within the enclosing granule membrane (Fig. 23c). The A cells are the source of gastric glucagon, as shown by immunolabeling (4). Including the gastrin cells (described below), there are currently nine gastric endocrine cell types. These are summarized in Table 1, as compiled by Grube and Forssmann (58), and are not discussed individually here. The nine cell types found in the stomach are reproduced in Table 1. As indicated by the incompleteness and uncertainty of their contents, much remains to be done to fully understand these cells. Exploration of the structure and identification of non-mammalian endocrine cells has been relatively limited (35), but the avian endocrine cells have been examined in some detail (97,131,168,182,183).

Gastrin Cell

The gastrin or G cell was among the earliest to be identified immunocytochemically (114). Because of its importance in stimulation of gastric acid secretion, it has been studied extensively. Furthermore, gastrin or pentagastrin appears to stimulate gastric mucosal cell proliferation (90,178). Selective staining studies for G cells by various histochemical methods have been used. Some of these methods no doubt stain these cells. However, McGuigan et al. (114) found no precise staining for G cells with six of the widely used methods

TABLE 1. Enteroendocrine cells[a]

CELLTYPE	LOCALIZATION	SECRETION GRANULES (size in nm)	AMINES	PEPTIDES
EC_n	Stomach (Small intestine)	200	Serotonin	?
ECL	Stomach	450	Histamine Serotonin?	?
G	Stomach (Duodenum) (Pancreas)	300	Tryptamine? Dopamine?	Gastrin ACTH-and Lipotropin-related peptides ?
D	Stomach Small intestine Pancreas	350		Somatostatin Met-Enkephalin ? Gastrin (Pancreas) ?
D1 (H)	Stomach Small intestine Large intestine Pancreas	160		VIP
A	Pancreas (Stomach) (Small intestine?)	250		Glucagon, Glicentin Pancreas Glucagon, GLI-1 CCK-PZ?(Endorphin)
X (AL)	Stomach (Small intestine) (Large intestine) (Pancreas)	300		?
PP (F)	Pancreas (Stomach) (Small intestine) (Large intestine)	180		Pancreatic Polypeptide Met-Enkephalin ?
P	Stomach Small intestine (Pancreas)	120	?	Bombesin ?

[a]Compiled by Grube and Forssmann (58). Only those cell types found in the gastric mucosa (and elsewhere) have been selected. The cell type nomenclature is the currently accepted terminology. Secretion granule size and ultrastructural characteristics, as well as their content of amines and peptides, are also indicated.

believed to reveal G cells when compared with the immunolabeling method.

Several investigators (25,29) have quantitated the number of G cells and have estimated that there are about 5×10^5 cells per cm^2 in the dog, cat, and rat gastric mucosa. In another study (40), the relative number of G cells in rat pyloric glands was found to be about 2% of the total glandular cells, as determined by cell counts of isolated rat pyloric gland cells, which do not have attached gastric pits. G cells were found to proliferate when the antrum was chronically stimulated (103).

The G cell was identified immunocytochemically at the ultrastructural level by Greider et al. in 1972 (53), but the ultrastructure of the cell and its tentative identification, which has been confirmed as the source of gastrin, was made earlier (38,39). Many studies (40,159,160) have confirmed and extended the identification and functional parameters of this cell. Gastrin appears to retain its antigenic labeling characteristic after the routine fixation of stomachs in formalin, while Bouin's fixed tissues result in greater intensity of fluorescence. A recent report (177) has shown that conventionally fixed, paraffin-embedded tissues already stained with hematoxylin and eosin can be labeled subsequently with fluorescein-labeled antibodies. The ability of gastrin to retain its immunoreactivity after histological processing is a feature that greatly favors its study.

The G cell is the predominant cell type in the pyloric antrum; an idealized G cell is shown in Fig. 21, and an electron micrograph is shown in Fig. 22. It is a medium-sized cell and shares features common to other enteroendocrine cells. A typical basement lamina underlies the cell, and most if not all of them have a narrow apical cell border with long microvilli. A typical junctional complex joins G cells to the neighboring pyloric gland cells.

Granules in G cells are the storage sites and the distinguishing feature of these cells. The granules have been reported to be from 150 to 400 nm in diameter (53,58), and their content varies from a dense core to an intermediate density, or to granules that appear clear or empty. Granules are most numerous in the basal

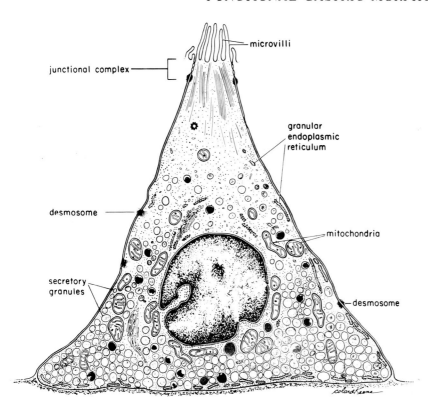

FIG. 21. Diagram of a G cell from the pyloric gland. Gastrin endocrine cells have infranuclearly located secretory granules and a wide basal cytoplasm on the lamina propria. Of the many types of endocrine cells in the stomach, only the G cell and EC cell have a luminal border with microvilli.

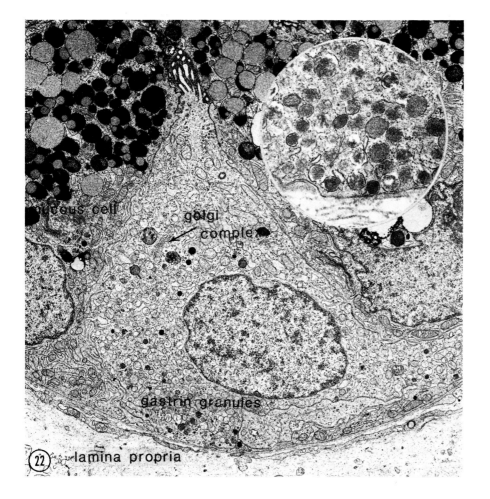

FIG. 22. Low-power electron micrograph of a human G cell from the pyloric antrum. The base of the cell does not lie continuously on the basal lamina but is underlain by processes from neighboring cells. Most of the secretion granules are of low density. The narrow apical border has a few relatively large microvilli. × 6,800. *Circular inset,* a higher magnification of the basal region of a G cell with secretion granules of intermediate density. × 23,800 (Micrograph courtesy of W. G. Forssmann.)

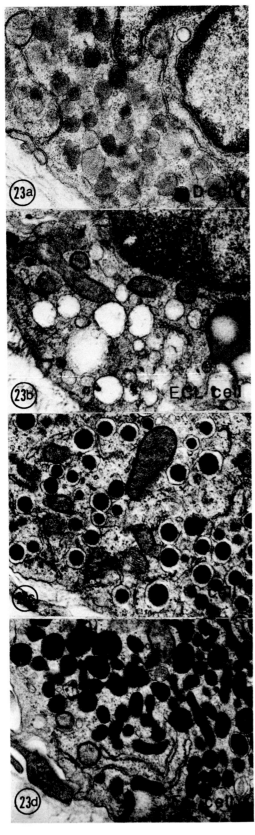

FIG. 23. Electron micrographs of selected parts of *Tupaia* pyloric antral endocrine cells showing their characteristic granule ultrastructure: **a:** D cell with granules of low density. **b:** ECL cell with large clear granules containing eccentrically located dense material. **c:** A cell with characteristic round, dense-cored granules very much like pancreatic A cells. **d:** EC cell with dense, elongated granules. All figures × 28,000. (Micrographs courtesy of W. G. Forssmann.)

cytoplasm where they are crowded. The remaining cytoplasm contains a limited number of mitochondria, some granular endoplasmic reticulum, and free ribosomes. The nucleus and para- or supranuclear Golgi complex are not distinctive.

The release of gastrin, as well as all the peptide hormones, has been shown to be by exocytosis or emiocytosis, where there is initial fusion of the secretory granule membrane with the plasma membrane. This is followed by the opening of the merged membranes and the release of the secretory product into the extracellular space. In contrast to exocrine cells where secretion is at the apical end of the cell into the gland lumen, endocrine cells release their product at the base or lateral cell surfaces. Exocytosis is a process that occurs in many different cell types, and the possible role of contractile filaments and microtubules in this process has been suggested but remains to be substantiated. This process has been described in detail in freeze-fracture replicas (126,127).

OTHER CELL TYPES IN THE GASTRIC EPITHELIUM

The major cell types thus far considered comprise the preponderant majority of the normal gastric mucosa. There are, however, several additional cell types that have been described and are consistent features of this epithelium, including the intraepithelial lymphocytes, globular leukocytes, and caveolate cells. In addition, other cell types may be present as rare residents in the epithelium. As may be expected, the role that these cells play in gastric function is less than clear.

Intraepithelial lymphocytes between gastric mucosal cells are usually much less numerous than in the intestine. These wandering cells, which form no specialized junctional complexes with epithelial cells, resemble other epithelial lymphocytes in various parts of the alimentary tract. Unlike the intestinal lymphocytes, which have been studied extensively (32), there seems to be little work or interest in gastric epithelial lymphocytes. It is reasonable to presume that they play an immunological role similar or related to the intraepithelial lymphocytes in the intestine.

Another enigmatic cell found in the gastric mucosa of certain species is the so-called "globular leukocyte." These are wandering cells between intestinal and gastric epithelial cells that contain numerous large granules staining vividly in routine H and E slides and resembling eosinophils. Globular leukocytes are not found in human stomachs but have been seen in cat, rat, and mouse gastric mucosa.

The final cell type described here is the caveolated or fibrillovesicular cell. The ultrastructure of these cells have been described in detail in the stomach (64,91,122). Similar cells have also been described in the intestine and respiratory tract, and thus caveolated cells are not unique to the gastric mucosa. These cells are scattered throughout the gastric mucosa but appear to be more numerous in the pylorus than in the corpus or fundus regions. Caveolated cells have a narrow apical border and a wide base and share some features in common with undifferentiated and G cells. The apical border has stubby to long microvilli and prominent core filaments that extend deep into the cytoplasm. From the intermicrovillar spaces, caveolae or channels course for some distance into the cytoplasm. The role of this cell is entirely speculative; caveolated cells may secrete some product, absorb material from the lumen, serve as a sensory receptor to sample the luminal environment, or play an entirely unknown role in gastric physiology.

CYTOLOGY OF THE NONGLANDULAR GASTRIC MUCOSA AND THE OUTER LAYERS

Nonglandular Gastric Mucosa

As mentioned above, the gross structure of the stomach varies remarkably in different species, and these differences have been the subject of many comparative studies (1,128). In animals with a simple or single-chambered stomach, the mucosa is usually of the glandular type, even though certain primates, rodents, and undulates may have some areas of the stomach which do not contain any gastric glands. On the other hand, most of the multichambered stomachs of mammals are lined with nonglandular or stratified squamous epithelium, and only one chamber is the glandular stomach.

The nonglandular gastric mucosa is a typically keratinized stratified squamous epithelium and is similar to the esophageal mucosa. Developmental studies (176) indicate that the origin of nonglandular mucosa is not by the modification of the esophagus but from the same tissue that forms the glandular mucosa.

The relative area occupied by the nonglandular mucosa is variable. In the mouse and rat (1), the single-chambered stomach is subdivided; the upper half, which corresponds to the fundus and adjacent corpus of the stomach, is lined with stratified squamous epithelium. In the grasshopper mouse (77), the whole stomach is lined almost completely with stratified squamous cells, and the gastric glands are restricted to the specialized cardioesophageal glands. In ruminants and other herbivores, only the last chamber (abomasum), which is adjacent to the duodenum, contains the usual gastric glands. All the remaining chambers are lined with nonglandular mucosa (98).

The gastric stratified squamous epithelium is similar to other keratinized stratified squamous epithelium. A typical basal layer rests on a basement lamina; superficially, there is a stratum spinosum, stratum granulo-

sum, and a stratum corneum. Some electron microscopy of this nonglandular epithelium has been reported for the mucosa of the bovine rumen (80,98).

Lamina Propria and Outer Layers

The lamina propria, which is a loose connective tissue, serves the overlying epithelium and must be of vital importance for the normal functions of the mucosa. The outermost limit of the lamina propria is the basement membrane or lamina. This structure is found beneath all epithelia; evidence in other organ systems indicates that it is a product of the epithelial cells rather than a connective tissue derivative.

Beneath the basement lamina are varying amounts of collagen and small reticular fibers. Some elastic fibers are also present. The vascular supply in the lamina propria consists primarily of capillaries and small arterioles from plexuses in the submucosa. The capillaries are of the fenestrated type and form a rich network in the lamina propria. In certain regions, they form venous plexuses or lakes. The outflow is via venules to the submucosa.

Lymphatic vessels have been described in the lamina propria. They are not prominent in preparation of normal gastric mucosa, and it has been suggested (144) that the frequency of lymphatics in the lamina propria may be less abundant than generally assumed. The cell types in the lamina propria are numerous, but their numbers vary. There are scattered smooth muscle cells extending from and oriented perpendicular to the muscularis mucosae. Other cells that are commonly found include lymphocytes, plasma cells, eosinophils, polymorphonuclear leukocytes, mast cells, and fibroblasts. Occasional endocrine-like cells and globular leukocytes have also been observed.

The distribution of nerve fibers from the vagus nerve, as well as the autonomic ganglia and intrinsic enteric ganglia, is not entirely clear but is presumed to be similar to nerves of the small intestine. Fine structure studies reveal small unmyelinated nerve fibers and varicosites, but none has been found in direct apposition with the plasma membrane of gastric epithelial cells. The muscularis mucosa is a band of smooth muscle made up of several layers oriented in different directions to form a distinct boundary between the lamina propria and the submucosa.

External to the muscularis mucosa is the submucosa, through which are distributed the vascular elements and nerves to the mucosa and muscularis. This dense connective tissue layer has a compact accumulation of collagen fibers and some elastic fibers. In this meshwork, arterioles and vessels are prominent. Some lymphatic vessels are also obvious. Relatively few connective tissue cells are present in the submucosa.

CLOSING REMARKS

This chapter provides a relatively simple and only moderately detailed review of gastric mucosal structure and function. During this undertaking, however, it became increasingly apparent that a chapter of limited size could not cover the intended material adequately. The field is so active that there are many new papers and obvious omissions of relevant publications and perhaps inclusions of material that may not be as pertinent. Furthermore, there is unavoidable incorporation of personal opinion and interpretation of presumed gastric functions in relation to mucosal structure. Some of my views may be less than appropriate or even erroneous. Finally, it is the presumption of most morphologists that all functions have morphological correlates. This may be correct, but we should realize that with currently available technology, most of the physiological and biochemical processes in cells and tissues cannot be visualized and are, therefore, amicroscopic. There is before us a challenge of a dimension which seems almost insurmountable but will someday be overcome. Our present knowledge may seem archaic and totally superficial in the very near future. For the present, however, it is hoped that this attempt will serve some useful purpose.

ACKNOWLEDGMENTS

This work was supported in part by USPHS grant RO1 Am17255.

The invaluable assistance of Ms. Louise M. Aulenbach and Ms. Dorothy J. Rowe in the preparation of this chapter is gratefully acknowledged.

REFERENCES

1. Andrew, W. (1959): *Textbook of Comparative Histology.* Oxford University Press, New York.
2. Arevalo, F. R. (1962): Ultrastructure of the parietal cell of the human gastric mucosa in the resting state and after stimulation with histalog. *GEN,* 17:51–65.
3. Babkin, B. D. (1950): *Secretory Mechanisms of the Digestive Glands.* Hoeber, New York.
4. Baetens, D., Rufener, C., Srikant, B. C., Dobbs, R., Unger, R., and Orci, L. (1976): Identification of glucagon-producing cells (A cells) in dog gastric mucosa. *J. Cell Biol.,* 69:455–464.
5. Barrington, E. J. W. (1957): The alimentary canal and digestion. In: *The Physiology of Fishes,* edited by M. E. Brown, pp. 109–161. Academic Press, New York.
6. Baskin, W. N., Ivey, K. J., Krause, W. J., Jeffrey, G. E., and Gemmell, R. T. (1976): Aspirin-induced ultrastructural changes in human gastric mucosa. *Ann. Intern. Med.,* 85:299–303.
7. Baudin, H., Stock, C., Vincent, D., and Grenier, J. F. (1975): Microfilamentous system and secretion of enzymes in the exocrine pancreas. *J. Cell Biol.,* 66:165–181.
8. Beams, H. W., and King, R. L. (1932): Notes on the cytology of the parietal cells of the stomach of the rat. *Anat. Rec.,* 53:31–41.
9. Bensley, R. R. (1898): The structure of the mammalian gastric glands. *Q. J. Microscop. Sci.,* 41:361–389.
10. Bensley, R. R. (1902): The cardiac glands of animals. *Am. J. Anat.,* 2:105–156.
11. Bensley, R. R. (1932): The gastric glands. In: *Special Cytology,* edited by E. V. Cowdry, vol. 1, pp. 198–230. Hoeber, New York.
12. Berger, E. H. (1934): The distribution of parietal cells in the stomach: a histotopographic study. *Am. J. Anat.,* 54:87–114.
13. Berglindh, T., and Obrink, K. J. (1976): A method for preparing isolated glands from the rabbit gastric mucosa. *Acta Physiol. Scand.,* 96:150–159.
14. Berglindh, T., Dibona, R., Ito, S., and Sachs, G. (1980): Probes of parietal cell function.
15. Bertalanffy, F. D. (1963): Cell renewal in the gastrointestinal tract of man. *Gastroenterology,* 43:472–475.
16. Black, J. A., Forte, T. M., and Forte, J. G. (1980): Structure of oxyntic cell membranes during conditions of rest and secretion of HCl as revealed by freeze-fracture. *Anat. Rec.,* 196:163–172.
17. Blum, A. L., Shah, G. T., Wiebelhaus, V. D., Brennan, F. T., Helander, H. F., Ceballos, R., and Sachs, G. (1971): Pronase method for isolation of viable cells from necturus gastric mucosa. *Gastroenterology,* 61:189–200.
18. Boas, A., and Wilson, T. H. (1963): Cellular localization of gastric intrinsic factor in the rat. *Am. J. Physiol.,* 206:783–786.
19. Bowie, D. J. (1935): A method for staining the pepsinogen granules in gastric glands. *Anat. Rec.,* 64:357–362.
20. Bowie, D. J. (1940): The distribution of the chief or pepsin-forming cells in the gastric mucosa of the cat. *Anat. Rec.,* 78:9–18.
21. Bradford, N. M., and Davies, R. E. (1950): The site of hydrochloric acid production in the stomach as determined by indicators. *Biochem. J.,* 46:414–420.
22. Carlisle, K. S., Chew, C. S., and Hersey, S. J. (1978): Ultrastructural changes and cyclic AMP in frog oxyntic cells. *J. Cell Biol.,* 76:31–42.
23. Challice, C. E., Bullivant, S., and Scott, D. B. (1957): The fine structure of some cytoplasmic inclusions of oxyntic cells. *Exp. Cell Res.,* 13:488–492.
24. Croft, D. N., and Ingelfinger, F. J. (1969): Isolated gastric parietal cells: Oxygen consumption, electrolyte content, and intracellular pH. *Clin. Sci.,* 37:491–501.
25. Crowley, D. J., Ganguli, D. C., Dolak, J. M., Elder, J. B., and Pearse, A. G. E. (1975): The G cell population of the pyloric antrum of the cat. *Digestion,* 12:25–31.
26. Dalton, A. J. (1951): Electron micrography of the epithelial cells of the gastro-intestinal tract and pancreas. *Am. J. Anat.,* 89:109–134.
27. Davenport, H. W. (1977): *Physiology of the Digestive Tract,* 4th edition. Yearbook, Chicago.
28. Dawson, A. B. (1948): Argentaffin cells in the gastric mucosa of the rat. *Anat. Rec.,* 100:319–327.
29. Delaney, J. P., Michel, H. M., Eisenberg, M. M., and Bonsack, M. (1978): Quantitation of antral gastric cell populations in the dog. *Gastroenterology,* 74:708–712.
30. DeLemos, C. (1977): The ultrastructure of endocrine cells in the corpus of the stomach of human fetuses. *Am. J. Anat.,* 148:359–384.
31. DiBona, R., Ito, S., Berglindh, T., and Sachs, G. (1979): Cellular site of gastric acid secretion. *Proc. Natl. Acad. Sci. U.S.A.,* 76:6689–6693.
32. Douglas, A. P., and Weetman, A. P. (1975): Lymphocytes and the gut. *Digestion,* 13:344–371.
33. Eastwood, G. L. (1975): Effect of pH on bile salt injury to mouse gastric mucosa. A light- and electron-microscope study. *Gastroenterology,* 68:1456–1465.
34. Eastwood, G. L., and Kirchner, J. P. (1974): Changes in the fine structure of mouse gastric epithelium produced by ethanol and urea. *Gastroenterology,* 67:71–84.
35. Falkmer, S., and Ostberg, Y. (1976): Phylogeny and ontogeny of endocrine cells of the gastrointestinal tract. In: *Endocrinology Vol. 2,* edited by V. H. T. James, pp. 443–447. Exerpta-Medica, Amsterdam.
36. Farquhar, M. G., and Palade, G. E. (1963): Junctional complexes in various epithelia. *J. Cell Biol.,* 17:375–414.

37. Ferguson, D. J. (1969): Structure of antral gastric mucosa. *Surgery,* 65:280–291.

38. Forssmann, W. G., and Orci, L. (1969): Ultrastructure and secretory cycle of the gastrin-producing cell. *Z. Zellforsch.,* 101:419–432.

39. Forssmann, W. G., Orci, L., Pictet, R., Renald, A. E., and Rouiller, C. (1969): The endocrine cells in the epithelium of the gastrointestinal mucosa of the rat: An electron microscope study. *J. Cell Biol.,* 40:692–715.

40. Forssmann, W. G., Lichtenberger, L. M., Helmstaedter, and Ito, S. (1979): Studies of isolated and enriched rat antral mucosa gastrin cells. *Cell Tissue res.,* 200:163–178.

41. Forssmann, W. G., and Helmstaedter, V. (1979): Intestinal hormone. In: *Die ultrastructor der endokrinen Zellen des GEP-Systems. I. Intestinale Hormone,* edited by G. A. Martini, pp. 15–39. George Thieme Verlag, Stuttgart.

42. Forte, T. M., and Forte, J. G. (1970): Histochemical staining characterization of glycoproteins in acid-secreting cells of frog stomach. *J. Cell Biol.,* 47:437–453.

43. Forte, T., and Forte, J. G. (1971): A freeze-fracture study of bullfrog gastric oxyntic cells. *J. Ultrastruct. Res.,* 37:322–334.

44. Forte, J. G., Forte, T. M., and Ray, T. K. (1972): Membranes of the oxyntic cell: Their structure, composition, and genesis. In: *Gastric Secretion,* edited by G. Sachs, E. Heinz, and K. J. Ulrich, pp. 37–68. Academic Press, New York.

45. Forte, T. M., Machen, T. E., and Forte, J. G. (1975): Ultrastructure and physiological changes in piglet oxyntic cells during histamine stimulation and metabolic inhibition. *Gastroenterology,* 69:1208–1222.

46. Forte, T. M., Machen, T. E., and Forte, J. G. (1977): Ultrastructural changes in oxyntic cells associated with secretory function: A membrane-recycling hypothesis. *Gastroenterology,* 73:941–955.

47. Frenning, B., and Obrink, K. J. (1971): The effects of acetic acid and acetylsalicylic acids on the appearance of the gastric mucosal surface epithelium in the scanning electron microscope. *Scand. J. Gastroenterol.,* 6:605–612.

48. Frexinos, J., Carballido, M., Louis, A., and Kibet, A. (1971): Effect of pentagastrin on human parietal cells: an electron microscopic study with quantitative evaluation of cytoplasmic structures. *Dig. Dis.,* 16:1065–1074.

49. Glass, G. B. J. (1977): Antitrophic effects of gastric autoantibodies on parietal and peptic cells. In: *Progress in Gastroenterology,* edited by G. B. Jerzy Glass, pp. 73–106. Grune & Stratton, New York.

50. Grant, R. (1945): Rate of replacement of the surface of the epithelial cells of the gastric mucosa. *Anat. Rec.,* 91:175–186.

51. Graumann, W. (1965): Uber die angebbiche der Acidophilie der Belegzellen. *Histochemie,* 5:437–440.

52. Gregory, R. A., and Tracy, H. J. (1961): The preparation and properties of gastrin. *J. Physiol. (Lond.),* 156:523–543.

53. Greider, M. H., Steinberg, V., and McGuigan, J. E. (1972): Electron microscopic identification of the gastrin cell of the human antral mucosa by means immunocytochemistry. *Gastroenterology,* 63:572–583.

54. Griffiths, M. (1965): Digestion, growth and nitrogen balance in an egg-laying mammal, *Tachyglossus aculeatus* (Shaw). *Comp. Biochem. Physiol.,* 14:357–375.

55. Grossman, M. I. (1958): The names of the parts of the stomach. *Gastroenterology,* 34:1159–1162.

56. Grossman, M. I. (1977): A short history of digestive endocrinology. In: *Advances in Experimental Medicine and Biology, 106,* edited by M. I. Grossman, V. Speranza, N. Basso, and E. Lezoche, pp. 5–10. Plenum Press, New York.

57. Grossman, M. I., and Marks, I. N. (1960): Secretion of pepsinogen by the pyloric glands of the dog, with some observations on the histology of the gastric mucosa. *Gastroenterology,* 38:343–352.

58. Grube, D., and Forssmann, W. G. (1979): Morphology and function of the entero-endocrine cells. *Horm. Metab. Res.,* 11:603–620.

59. Gusek, W. (1961): Zur ultramikroskopischen cytologie der Belegzellen in dem Magenscheimbaut des menschen. *Z. Zellforsch.,* 55:790–809.

60. Guth, P. H., Aures, D., and Paulsen, G. (1979): Topical aspirin plus HCl gastric lesions in the rat. Cytoprotective effect of prostaglandin, cimetidine, and probanthine. *Gastroenterology,* 76:88–93.

61. Hally, A. D. (1959): The fine structure of the gastric parietal cell of the mouse. *J. Anat.,* 93:217–225.

62. Hally, A. D. (1959): Functional changes in the vacuole-containing bodies of the gastric parietal cell. *Nature,* 183:408.

63. Hally, A. D. (1960): The electron microscopy of the unusual "Golgi apparatus" of the gastric parietal cell. *J. Anat.,* 94:425–431.

64. Hammond, J. B. and LaDeur, L. (1968): Fibrillovesicular cells in the fundic glands of the canine stomach: evidence for a new cell type. *Anat. Rec.,* 161:393–412.

65. Harding, R. K., and Morris, G. P. (1977): Cell loss from normal and stressed gastric mucosae of the rat. An ultrastructural analysis. *Gastroenterology,* 72:857–863.

66. Helander, H. F. (1961): A preliminary note on the ultrastructure of the argyrophile cells of the mouse gastric mucosa. *J. Ultrastruct. Res.,* 5:257–262.

67. Helander, H. F. (1962): Ultrastructure of fundus glands of the mouse gastric mucosa. *J. Ultrastruct. Res. [suppl.],* 4:1–123.

68. Helander, H., and Ekholm, R. (1959): Ultrastructure of epithelial cells in fundus glands of the mouse gastric mucosa. *J. Ultrastruct. Res.,* 3:74–83.

69. Helander, H. F., and Olivecrona, T. (1970): Lipolysis and lipid absorption in the stomach of the suckling rat. *Gastroenterology,* 59:22–35.

70. Helander, H. F., Sanders, W. S., Rehm, W. S., and Hirschowitz. (1972): Quantitative aspects of gastric morphology. In: *Gastric Secretion,* edited by G. Sachs, E. Heinz, and K. J. Ullrich, pp. 69–90. Academic Press, New York.

71. Helander, H., and Hirschowitz, B. I. (1972): Quantitative ultrastructural studies on gastric parietal cells. *Gastroenterology,* 63:951–961.

72. Helander, H. F., and Hirschowitz, B. I. (1974): Quantitative ultrastructural studies on inhibited and on partly stimulated gastric parietal cells. *Gastroenterology,* 67:447–452.

73. Hingson, D. J., and Milton, G. W. (1968): The mucosa of the stomach of the wombat (*Vombatus hirsutus*) with special reference to the cardio-gastric gland. *Proc. Linnean Soc.,* 93:69–75.

74. Hingson, D. J., and Ito, S. (1971): Effect of aspirin and related compounds on the fine structure of mouse gastric mucosa. *Gastroenterology,* 61:156–177.

75. Hoedemaeker, P. J., and Ito, S. (1970): Ultrastructural localization of gastric parietal cell antigen with peroxidase-coupled antibody. *Lab. Invest.,* 22:184–188.

76. Hogben, C. A. M., Kent, T. H., Woodward, P. A., and Sill, A. J. (1974): Quantitative histology of the gastric mucosa: man, dog, cat, guinea pig, and frog. *Gastroenterology,* 67:1143–1154.

77. Horner, B. E., Taylor, J. M., and Padykula, H. A. (1965): Food habits and gastric morphology of the grasshopper mouse. *J. Mammal.,* 45:513–535.

78. Hunt, T. E. (1958): Regeneration of the gastric mucosa in the rat. *Anat. Rec.,* 131:193–212.

79. Hunt, T. E., and Hunt, E. A. (1962): Radioautographic study of proliferation in the stomach of the rat using thymidine-H^3 and compound 48/80. *Anat. Rec.,* 142:505–517.

80. Hyden, S., and Sperber, I. (1965): Electron microscopy of the ruminant fore-stomach. In: *Physiology of Digestion in the Ruminant,* edited by R. W. Dougherty, R. S. Allen, W. Burroughs, N. L. Jacobson, and A. D. McGilliard, pp. 51–67.

81. Ito, S. (1961): The endoplasmic reticulum of gastric parietal cells. *J. Biophys. Biochem. Cytol.,* 11:333–347.

82. Ito, S. (1965): The enteric surface coat on cat intestinal microvilli. *J. Cell Biol.,* 27:475–491.

83. Ito, S. (1966): Fine structure of the gastric mucosa. In: *Gastric Secretions: Mechanisms and Control,* edited by T. K. Shnitka, J. A. L. Gilbert, and R. C. Harrison, pp. 3–24. Pergamon Press, Oxford.

84. Ito, S. (1968): Anatomic structure of the gastric mucosa. In: *Handbook of Physiology, Section 6, Alimentary Canal,* edited

by C. F. Code, pp. 705–741. American Physiological Society, Washington, D.C.

85. Ito, S., and Winchester, R. J. (1963): The fine structure of the gastric mucosa in the bat. *J. Cell Biol.,* 16:541–578.
86. Ito, S., and Schofield, G. C. (1974): Studies on the depletion and accumulation of microvilli and changes in the tubulovesicular compartment of mouse parietal cells in relation to gastric acid secretion. *J. Cell Biol.,* 63:364–382.
87. Ito, S., Munro, D. R., and Schofield, G. C. (1977): Morphology of the isolated mouse oxyntic cell and some physiological parameters. *Gastroenterology,* 73:887–898.
88. Ito, S., and Schofield, G. S. (1977): Ultrastructural changes in mouse parietal cells after high H$^+$ secretion. *Acta Physiol. Scand. [Special Suppl.],* 1978:25–34.
89. Jennings, M. A., and Florey, H. F. (1956): Autoradiographic observations on the mucous cells of the stomach and intestine. *Q. J. Exp. Physiol.,* 41:131–152.
90. Johnson, L. R., Aures, D., and Hakanson, R. (1969): Effect of gastrin on the in vivo incorporation of ^{14}C-leucine into protein of the digestive tract. *Proc. Soc. Exp. Biol. Med.,* 132:996–998.
91. Johnson, F. R., and Young, B. A. (1968): Undifferentiated cells in gastric mucosa. *J. Anat.,* 102:541–551.
92. Kaye, G., Nathan, I., Wheeler, H. O., and Whitlock, R. T. (1965): Fluid transport in the rabbit gall bladder: A combined physiological and electron microscopic study. *Anat. Rec.,* 151:369.
93. Kominick, H. (1963): Zur funktionellen Morphologie der Salzsaureproduktion in der Magenschleimhaut. *Histochemie,* 3:354–378.
94. Kramer, M. F., and Geuze, J. J. (1977): Glycoprotein transport in the surface mucous cells of the rat stomach. *J. Cell Biol.,* 73:533–547.
95. Kurosumi, K. Shibasaki, S., Uchida, G., and Y. Tanaka. (1956): Electron microscope studies on the gastric mucosa of normal rats. *Arch. Histol. Jpn.,* 15:587–624.
96. Landboe-Christensen, E. (1944): Extent of the pylorus zone in the human stomach. *Acta Pathol. Microbiol. Scand. [Suppl.],* 54:671–692.
97. Larsson, L. I., Sundler, F., Hakanson, R., Refeld, J. F., and Stadil, F. (1974): Distribution and properties of gastrin cells in the gastrointestinal tract of chicken. *Cell Tissue Res.,* 154:209–421.
98. Lavker, R., Chalupa, W., and Dickey, J. F. (1969): An electron microscopic investigation of rumen mucosa. *J. Ultrastruct. Res.,* 28:1–15.
99. Lawn, A. M. (1960): Observations on the fine structure of the gastric parietal cell of the rat. *J. Biophys. Biochem. Cytol.,* 7:161–166.
100. Leblond, C. P., and Lee, E. R. (1979): Renewal of the pyloric epithelium. In: *Cell Lineage, Stem Cells, and Cell Determination,* edited by N. Le Dovarin, pp. 325–334. Elsevier, Amsterdam.
101. Leeson, T. S. (1971): Parietal cell canaliculi: a freeze-etch study. *Cytobiologie,* 5:352–362.
102. Leeson, T. S. (1973): Canaliculi and tubulovesicles of rat parietal cells. *Am. J. Anat.,* 136:541–547.
103. Lehy, T., Voillemot, N., Dubrasquet, M., and Dufougeray, F. (1975): Gastrin cell hyperplasia in rats with chronic antral stimulation. *Gastroenterology,* 68:71–82.
104. Lillibridge, C. B. (1961): Membranes of the human pepsinogen granule. *J. Biophys. Biochem. Cytol.,* 10:145–149.
105. Lillibridge, C. B. (1964): The fine structure of normal human gastric mucosa. *Gastroenterology,* 47:269–296.
106. Lillibridge, C. B., Brown, M. R., and Hall, J. G. (1974): The electron microscopic appearance of presecreted gastric mucus in cystic fibrosis. *Pediatrics,* 53:913–919.
107. Lim, R. K. S. (1922): The gastric mucosa. *Q. J. Microscop. Sci.,* 66:187–212.
108. Lim, R. K. S., and Ma, W. C. (1926): Mitochondrial changes in the cell of the gastric glands in relation to activity. *Q. J. Exp. Physiol.,* 16:87–110.
109. Lipkin, M., Shenock, P., and Bell, B. (1963): Cell proliferation kinetics in the gastrointestinal tract of man. II. Cell renewal in the stomach, ileum, colon, and rectum. *Gastroenterology,* 45:721–729.
110. MacDonald, W. C. (1973): Correlation of mucosal histology and aspirin intake in chronic gastric ulcer. *Gastroenterology,* 65:381–389.
111. MacDonald, W. C., Trier, J. S., and Everett, N. B. (1964): Cell proliferation and migration in the stomach, duodenum, and rectum of man: Radioautographic studies. *Gastroenterology,* 46:405–417.
112. Macklin, C. C., and Macklin, M. T. (1932): The intestinal epithelium. In: *Special Cytology,* edited by E. V. Cowdry, p. 233. Hoeber, New York.
113. Makhlouf, G. M. (1974): The neuroendocrine design of the gut. The play of chemicals in a chemical playground. *Gastroenterology,* 67:159–184.
114. McGuigan, J. E., Greider, M. H., and Grawe, L. (1972): Staining characteristics of the gastrin cell. *Gastroenterology,* 62:959–969.
115. Menzies, G. (1962): The effects of starvation and of feeding following starvation on the pepsinogen granules of the rat's stomach. *J. Pathol. Bacteriol.,* 83:475–481.
116. Messier, B., and Leblond, C. P. (1960): Cell proliferation and migration as revealed by radioautography after injection of thymidine-H^3 into male rats and mice. *Am. J. Anat.,* 106:247–285.
117. Michaels, J. E. (1979): Formation of concentric saccules in murine parietal cells after injection of diazo-oxo-norleucine. *Anat. Rec.,* 193:775–790.
118. Miyagawa, J. (1921): The exact distribution of the gastric glands in man and in certain animals. *J. Anat.,* 55:56–67.
119. Moir, R. J. (1965): The comparative physiology of ruminant-like animals. In: *Physiology of Digestion in the Ruminant,* edited by R. W. Dougherty, R. S. Allen, W. Burroughs, N. L. Jacobson, and A. D. McGilliard, pp. 1–14. Butterworths, Washington.
120. Morris, G. P., and Harding, K. (1974): Topography and fine structure of acute fundic mucosal erosions in the rat. *Lab. Invest.,* 30:639–646.
121. Moxey, P. C., and Yeomans, N. D. (1976): Identification of cell types in thin epoxy sections of gastric fundic mucosa. *J. Histochem. Cytochem.* 24:755–756.
122. Nabeyama, A., and Leblond, C. P. (1974): "Caveolated cells" characterized by deep surface invaginations and abundant filaments in mouse gastro-intestinal epithelia. *Am. J. Anat.,* 140:147–166.
123. Nasset, E. S. (1953): Gastric secretion in the beaver (*Castor canactensis*). *J. Mammal.,* 34:204–209.
124. Neuburger, P. H., Lewin, M., deRecherche, C., and Bonfils, S. (1972): Parietal and chief cell populations in four cases of the Zollinger-Ellison syndrome. *Gastroenterology,* 63:937–942.
125. Neutra, M. R., Grand, R. J., and Trier, J. S. (1977): Glycoprotein synthesis, transport, and secretion by epithelial cells of human rectal mucosa. *Lab. Invest.,* 36:535–546.
126. Orci, L., Amherdt, F., Malaisse-Lagae, Rouiller, C., and Renold, A. E. (1973): Insulin release by emiocytosis: Demonstration with freeze-etching technique. *Science,* 179:82–83.
127. Orci, L. (1977): Morphologic events underlying the secretion of peptide hormones. In: *Endocrinology, Vol. 2,* edited by V. H. T. James. Exerpta Medica, Amsterdam.
128. Patt, D. I., and Patt, G. R. (1969): *Comparative Vertebrate Histology.* Harper & Rowe, New York.
129. Pearse, A. G. E., and Takor, T. (1976): Neuroendocrine embryology and the APUD concept. *Clin. Endocrinol. [Suppl.],* 5:229–244.
130. Plenk, H. (1932): Der Magen. In: *Handbuch der Mikroskopische Anatomie des Menschen, Vol. 5,* edited by W. v. Mollendorff. pp. 1–234. Springer, Berlin.
131. Polak, J. M., Pearse, A. G. E., Adams, C., and Garaud, J. C. (1974): Immunohistochemical and ultrastructural studies on the endocrine polypeptide (APUD) cells of the avian gastrointestinal tract. *Experientia,* 30:564–567.
132. Polak, J. M., and Bloom, S. R. (1977): Peptidergic innervation of the gastrointestinal tract. In: *Advances in Experimental Medicine and Biology, 106,* edited by M. I. Grossman, V. Speranza, N. Basso, and E. Lezoche, pp. 27–49. Plenum Press, New York.
133. Read, G. M., and Johnstone, F. R. C. (1961): The distribution of parietal cells in the gastric mucosa of the cat. *Anat. Rec.,* 139:525–530.
134. Rebolledo, I. M., and Vial, J. D. (1979): Fine structure of the

oxynticopeptic cell in the gastric glands of an elasmobranch species (*Halaeburus chilensis*). *Anat. Rec.,* 193:805–822.

135. Robert, A., Nezamis, J. E., Lancaster, C., and Hanchar, A. J. (1979): Cytoprotection by prostaglandins in rats. Prevention of gastric necrosis produced by alcohol, HCl, NaOH, Hypertonic NaCl, and thermal injury. *Gastroenterology,* 77:433–443.

136. Rohrer, G. V., Scott, J. R., Joel, W., and Wolf, S. (1965): The fine structure of human gastric parietal cells. *Am. J. Dig. Dis.,* 10:13–21.

137. Romrell, L. J., Coppe, M. R., Munro, D. R., and Ito, S. (1975): Isolation and separation of highly enriched fractions of viable mouse gastric parietal cells by velocity sedimentation. *J. Cell Biol.,* 65:428–438.

138. Rosa, F. (1963): Ultrastructure of the parietal cell of the human gastric mucosa in the resting state and after stimulation with histalog. *Gastroenterology,* 45:354–363.

139. Rubin, W. (1972): An unusual intimate relationship between endocrine cells and other types of epithelial cells in the human stomach. *J. Cell Biol.,* 52:219–227.

140. Rubin, W., Ross, L. L., Sleisenger, M. H., and Jeffries, G. H. (1968): The normal human gastric epithelia. A fine structural study. *Lab. Invest.,* 19:598–626.

141. Rubin W., and Allasgharpour, A. A. (1970): Demonstration of a cytochemical difference between the tubulovesicles and plasmalemma of gastric parietal cells by ATPase and NPPase reactions. *Anat. Rec.,* 184:251–264.

142. Rubin, W., and Schwartz, B. (1979): An electron microscopic radioautographic identification of the "enterochromaffin-like" APUD cells in murine oxyntic glands. Demonstration of a metabolic difference between rat and mouse gastric A-like cells. *Gastroenterology,* 76:437–449.

143. Rubin, W., and Schwartz, B. (1979): Electron microscopic radioautographic identification of the ECL cell as the histamine-synthesizing endocrine cell in the rat stomach. *Gastroenterology,* 77:458–467.

144. Rusznyak, I. (1967): The gastro-intestinal tract. In: *Lymphatics and Lymph Circulation: Physiology and Pathology,* edited by L. Youlten, pp. 92–97. Pergamon Press, Oxford.

145. Saccomani, G., Helander, H. F., Crago, S., Chang, H. H., Dailey, D. W., and Sachs, G. (1979): Characterization of gastric mucosal membranes. X. Immunological studies of gastric (H$^+$ + K$^+$) ATPase *J. Cell Biol.,* 83:271–283.

146. Salenius, P. (1962): On the ontogenesis of the gastric epithelial cells. *Acta Anat. [Suppl.],* 46:1–76.

147. Samloff, M. (1971): Cellular localization of group pepsinogens in human gastric mucosa by immunofluorescence. *Gastroenterology,* 61:188–188.

148. Schofield, G. C., Ito, S., and Bolander, R. P. (1979): Changes in membrane surface areas in mouse parietal cells in relation to high levels of acid secretion. *J. Anat.,* 128:669–692.

149. Sedar, A. W. (1961): Electron microscopy of the oxyntic cells in the gastric glands of the bullfrog (Rana catesbiana). I. The non-acid-secreting gastric mucosa. *J. Biophys. Biochem. Cytol.,* 9:1–18.

150. Sedar, A. W. (1961): Electron microscopy of the oxyntic cells in the gastric glands of the bullfrog (Rana catesbiana). II. The acid-secreting gastric mucosa. *J. Biophys. Biochem. Cytol.,* 10: 47–57.

151. Sedar, A. W. (1962): The fine structure of the oxyntic cell in relation to functional activity of the stomach. *Ann. N.Y. Acad. Sci.,* 99:9–29.

152. Sedar, A. W. (1962): Electron microscopy of the oxyntic cell in the gastric glands of the bullfrog (Rana catesbiana). III. Permanganate fixation of the endoplasmic reticulum. *J. Cell Biol.,* 14:152–156.

153. Sedar, A. W. (1965): Fine structure of the stimulated oxyntic cell. *Fed. Proc.,* 24:1360–1367.

154. Sedar, A. W. (1969): Electron microscopic demonstration of polysaccharides associated with acid-secreting cells of the stomach after "inert dehydration." *J. Ultrastruct. Res.,* 28:112–124.

155. Sedar, A. W., and Friedman, M. H. F. (1961): Correlation of fine structure of the gastric parietal cell (dog) with functional activity of the stomach. *J. Biophys. Biochem. Cytol.,* 11:349–363.

156. Sedar, A. W., and Forte, J. C. (1964): Effects of calcium deple-

tion on the junctional complex between oxyntic cells of gastric glands. *J. Cell Biol.,* 22:173–188.

157. Shibasaki, S. (1961): Experimental cytological and electron microscopic study on the rat gastric mucosa. *Arch. Histol. Jpn.,* 21:251–288.

158. Shibasaki, S., Lobayashi, K., and Umahara, Y. (1966): Electron microscope studies on the gastric chief cells of hibernating bats (Rhinolopus ferrum-equinum nippon). *Arch. Histol. Jpn.,* 26: 389–412.

159. Solcia, E., Capella, C., Vassallo, G., and Butta, R. (1975): Endocrine cells in the gastric mucosa. *Int. Rev. Cytol.,* 42:223–286.

160. Solcia, E., Capella, C., Buffa, R., Usellini, L., Fontana, P., and Frigerio, B. (1977): Endocrine cells of the gastrointestinal tract: general aspects, ultrastructure and tumor pathology. In: *Advances in Experimental Medicine and Biology,* edited by M. Grossman, V. Speranza, N. Basso, and E. Lezoche, pp. 11–22. Plenum Press, New York.

161. Soll, A. H. (1978): The action of secretagogues on oxygen uptake by isolated mammalian parietal cells. *J. Clin. Invest.,* 61: 370–380.

162. Spicer, S. S., and Sun, D. C. H. (1967): Part II: The role of the mucous barrier in the defense of the stomach vs. peptic ulceration. Carbohydrate histochemistry of gastric epithelial secretions in dog. *Ann. N.Y. Acad. Sci.,* 140:762–783.

163. Spicer, S. S., Katsuyama, T., and Sannes, P. L. (1978): Ultrastructural carbohydrate cytochemistry of gastric epithelium. *Histochem. J.,* 10:309–331.

164. Stevens, C. E., and Leblond, C. P. (1953): Renewal of the mucous cells in the gastric mucosa of the rat. *Anat. Rec.,* 115: 231–245.

165. Sugai, N., and Ito, S. (1980): Carbonic anhydrase, ultrastructural localization in the mouse gastric mucosa and improvements in the technique. *J. Histochem. Cytochem. (in press).*

166. Tominaga, K. (1975): Distribution of parietal cells in the antral mucosa of human stomachs. *Gastroenterology,* 69:1201–1207.

167. Toner, P. G. (1963): The fine structures of resting and active cells in the submucosal glands of the fowl proventriculus. *J. Anat.,* 97:575–583.

168. Toner, P. G. (1964): Fine structure of argyrophic and argentaffin cells in the gastro-intestinal tract of the fowl. *Z. Zellforsch.,* 63:830–839.

169. Townsend, S. F. (1961): Regeneration of gastric mucosa in rats. *Am. J. Anat.,* 109:133–141.

170. Vial, J. D., and Orrego, H. (1960): Electron microscope observations of the fine structure of parietal cells. *J. Biophys. Biochem. Cytol.,* 7:367–372.

171. Vial, J. D., and Orrego, H. (1963): Action of 2,4-dinitrophenol and iodoacetate on the ultrastructure of the oxyntic cells. *Exp. Cell Res.,* 30:232–235.

172. Vial, J. D., and Orrego, H. (1976): Actin-like filaments and membrane rearrangements in oxyntic cells. *Proc. Natl. Acad. Sci. USA,* 73:4032–4036.

173. Vial, J. D., Garrido, J., Dabike, M., and Koenig, C. (1979): Muscle proteins and the changes in shape of avian oxynticopeptic cells in relation to secretion. *Anat. Rec.,* 194:293–310.

174. Voillemot, N., Potet, F., Mary, J. Y., and Lewin, M. J. M. (1978): Gastrin cell distribution in normal human stomachs and in patients with Zollinger-Ellison syndrome. *Gastroenterology,* 75:61–65.

175. Vollrath, L. (1959): Uber entwicklung und function der Belegzellen der Magendrussen. *Z. Zellforsch.,* 50:36–60.

176. Warner, R. G., and Flatt, W. P. (1965): Anatomical development in the ruminant stomach. In: *Physiology of Digestion in the Ruminant,* edited by R. W. Dougherty, R. S. Allen, W. Burroughs, N. L. Jacobson, and A. D. McGilliard. pp. 24–38. Butterworths, Washington.

177. Weinstein, W. M., and Lechago, J. (1977): Gastrin cell immunofluorescence in conventionally fixed and stained tissue sections. *Gastroenterology,* 73:765–767.

178. Willems, G., and Lehy, T. (1975): Radioautographic and quantitative studies on parietal and peptic cell kinetics in the mouse. A selective effect of gastrin on parietal cell proliferation. *Gastroenterology,* 69:416–426.

179. Winborn, W. B., Seelig, L. L., Nakayama, H., and Weser, E.

(1974): Hyperplasia of the gastric glands after small bowel resection in the rat. *Gastroenterology,* 66:384–395.

180. Winborn, W. B., and Seelig, Jr., L. L. (1974): Pattern of osmium deposition in the parietal cells of the stomach. *J. Cell Biol.,* 63:99–108.

181. Wolf, S. (1965): *The Stomach.* Oxford University Press, New York.

182. Yamada, J., Iwanaga, T. Okamoto, T., Yamashita, T., Misui, M., and Yanahara, N. (1980): Ultrastructure of avian gastrin cell granules. *Arch. Histol. Jpn.,* 43:57–63.

183. Yamada, J., Yoshina, M., Yamashita, T., Misu, M., and Yanaihara, N. (1979): Distribution and frequency of gastrin cells in the digestive tract of the Japanese quail. *Arch. Histol. Jpn.,* 42:33–39.

184. Yeomans, N. D., St. John, D. J. B., and deBoer, W. G. R. M. (1973): Regeneration of gastric mucosa after aspirin-induced injury in the rat. *Dig. Dis.,* 18:773–780.

185. Yoffey, J. M., and Courtice, F. C. (1956): *Lymphatics, Lymph, and Lymphoid Tissue.* pp. 126–127. Edward Arnold Ltd., London.

186. Zalewsky, C., and Moody, F. G. (1977): Stereological analysis of the parietal cell during acid secretion and inhibiton. *Gastroenterology,* 73:66–74.

187. Zalewsky, C. A., and Moody, F. G. (1979): Mechanisms of mucus release in exposed canine gastric mucosa. *Gastroenterology,* 77:719–729.

188. Zalewsky, C. G., Moody, F. G., and Simons, M. A. (1975): Effects of p-chloromercuribenzene sulfonate upon ultrastructure of canine gastric surface cells. *Gastroenterology,* 69:427–438.

189. Zimmerman, K. W. (1889): Beitrage zur Kenntnis einiger Driissen und Epithelien. *Arch. Mikroskop. Anat.,* 52:522–706.

Physiology of the Gastrointestinal Tract, edited by
Leonard R. Johnson. Raven Press, New York © 1981.

Chapter 18

Electrolyte Composition of Gastric Secretion

G. M. Makhlouf

This chapter deals with the ionic composition of nascent parietal acid secretion and the changes it undergoes as a result of admixture with other secretions and of passive movements of ions and water across the mucosa. It pays special attention to the passive properties of the mucosa and stresses the importance of mucosal structure in determining the permeability to H$^+$ and water.

METHODS

Gastric secretion in humans can be collected only by suction with a tube. The main drawbacks to this technique are the uncertainties regarding adequacy of collection and freedom from contamination with extragastric secretions, chiefly saliva. The only effective way to prevent contamination with saliva is to place cotton rolls in the sulci of the cheeks and under the tongue and to change them frequently (80).

In animals, secretion can be collected from the whole stomach or from innervated or denervated pouches equipped with cannulae. Because denervated pouches secrete poorly, collection of secretion at low flow rates may be incomplete. Also, the pouches deteriorate with time, and their permeability to ions and water increases.

An acute preparation, first introduced by Thull and Rehm (114), consists of an isolated segment of canine fundic mucosa with intact blood supply and with the lumen enclosed in one or more chambers (7,90). The chief advantages of this technique are ease of sampling, good recovery of secretion or instillates, and a fixed mucosal surface area. The disadvantage is a lower secretory rate than that observed in the stomach of the conscious animal.

A technique introduced by Makhlouf (78,79) permits the study of nascent secretion *in vitro* and has thus far been used in amphibians only (Fig. 1). The stomach is stripped of external muscle layers and maintained as a tube equipped with a microdrainage system. Only the serosal side is exposed to a bathing solution. The unilateral preparation maintains a high transmucosal potential difference for several hours and secretes a fluid that parallels in ionic composition the secretion of the intact mammalian stomach.

FUNCTION AND STRUCTURE OF GASTRIC MUCOSA

The luminal surface of the gastric mucosa is extensively infolded into pits and tubules. This arrangement considerably enlarges the transporting surface, but it also creates a long diffusion path between the main lumen and the site of active transport and engenders high velocities of tubular flow during active secretion (99,100).

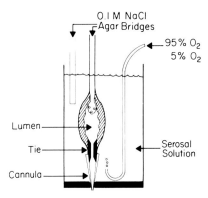

FIG. 1. Unilateral mucosal preparation. Frog mucosa is stripped of external muscle layers and maintained as a tube equipped with a drainage system. Only the serosal side is exposed to a bathing solution. The preparation maintains a high potential difference and secretes for at least 6 hr. Saline bridges are used to avoid contamination of secretion with K^+. Appropriate corrections are made for junction potentials.

The location, dimensions, and cellular properties of the pits and tubules contribute to the apparent luminal impermeability of the mucosa to ions and water.

The mucosa of the adult human has a surface area of 800 cm², a volume of 50 cm³, and a thickness of 0.06 cm (23). Eighty percent of mucosal volume and surface area is located in the fundus. The parietal cells (10^9 cells) comprise one-third of the cell mass and are capable of secreting maximally 35 mEq acid/hr in a volume of 250 ml (19,72,74). The parietal cell mass and secretory capacity of a 20-kg dog are similar to those of a human adult (84).

There are 10^4 pits/cm² of gross surface area in the dog (18). The average diameter of the pits is 25 μm; their total cross-sectional area is 0.05 cm²/cm² or 5% of gross surface area. The surface area of the tubules (5 tubules per pit; average diameter, 10 μm; average length, 300 μm) is 5 cm²/cm² of gross surface area. Thus 80% of the luminal surface is embedded in the tubules. The apical (i.e., canalicular) surface of the parietal cells is 50 cm²/cm² of gross surface area in the resting state and 500 cm²/cm² in the secreting state (52,53,57). The tubules expand the area of the lumen by a factor of 5; the parietal cells expand it further by a factor of 10 in the resting state and by a factor of 100 in the secreting state.

THEORIES OF SECRETION: A BRIEF SURVEY

A number of theories have been advanced to account for the variations in the composition of gastric secretion. Pavlov (98) claimed that nascent gastric secretion had a constant acidity which was modified by admixture with alkaline mucus. Hollander (58–61) expanded this view and concluded that gastric secretion consisted of a variable mixture of an isotonic solution of HCl secreted by the parietal cells and an alkaline secretion(s) of constant composition containing all the other ele-

ments of the juice. Rosemann (102) claimed that gastric secretion had a constant total chloride and that variations of acidity were due to conversion of variable proportions of "neutral" chloride to "acid" chloride by the parietal cells. This view was revived recently by Hirschowitz (54), who proposed that gastric juice arose in the blind end of the tubules as a secretion of NaCl, which was partly exchanged for HCl on its way to the gastric lumen. The Rosemann-Hirschowitz view has found little experimental support and few adherents.

Teorell (110,111) proposed that a primary acidity, which may or may not be constant, was altered by diffusion of H^+ from the lumen of the stomach. Teorell and later Obrink (95,96) provided formal statements of this hypothesis, emphasizing the importance of analyzing secretion in the steady state, and presented supporting evidence based on model instillation experiments. Makhlouf et al. (80) provided a formal statement of the Pavlov-Hollander two-component hypothesis: As a result of this treatment and the revised version given in this review, it was recognized that the two hypotheses, long thought to be at odds, could be stated in identical formal terms. Although somewhat primitive in concept, the hypotheses provide adequate descriptions of the composition of gastric secretion and the changes it undergoes in the lumen of the stomach.

ACID SECRETION

Postulates of the Two-Component Hypothesis

According to the two-component hypothesis (80), the flow rate of secretion in the steady state (v) consists of a nonparietal component of fixed volume (k) and a parietal component (v-k) which varies with the intensity of stimulation. The amount of secreted acid is represented by:

$$[H] \, v = H_o \, (v - k) \qquad [1]$$
$$= H_o v - H_o k$$

and the concentration of acid by:

$$[H] = H_o \, (1 - k/v) \qquad [2]$$

From Eq. 1, the relationship between acid output ([H]v), and flow rate (v) is linear with a slope equal to H_0, the initial or primary acid concentration, and an intercept equal to k at [H] = 0 (Fig. 2). From Eq. 2, the relationship between [H] and flow rate is hyperbolic with an asymptote equal to H_o and an intercept equal to k at [H] = 0 (Figs. 3 and 4). The relationship between [H] and 1/v is both linear and inverse, with intercepts equal to H_o and 1/k.

It should be noted that if only the fit of data is considered, there is no reason to invoke the existence of a neutralizing constituent in the nonparietal component.

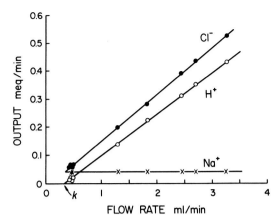

FIG. 2. Relationship between Cl, H, and Na output and flow rate. Note the constancy of Na output despite increasing flow rate. Intercept = k or flow rate of nonparietal component. Data from one human subject (80).

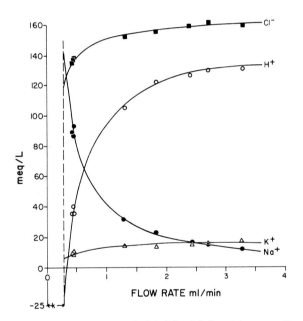

FIG. 3. Relationship between [Cl], [H], [Na], [K], and flow rate. Data from one human subject (see Fig. 2 and ref. 80); k may be read at [H] = 0 or at [H] = −b (see Eqs. 2 and 6 in text).

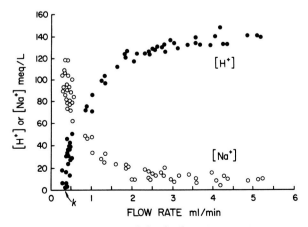

FIG. 4. Relationship between [H] or [Na] and flow rate in two human subjects. Data obtained in the basal state and during infusion of gastrin II (80).

This component would then act as a neutral diluent, which may be recovered in pure form in the absence of parietal acid secretion.

Postulates of the Diffusion Hypothesis

According to the diffusion hypothesis (51,95,111), the observed flow rate, v, and the parietal flow rate are the same. The amount of acid recovered, [H]v, differs from the amount of acid initially secreted, $H_o v$, by the amount of acid that has diffused across the mucosa. Teorell assumed that the secreted volume was instantly and thoroughly mixed with the volume previously secreted and claimed that the decrement due to diffusion was proportional to the gradient between the concentration of acid in the main lumen and the interstitial fluid, i.e., ([H] − 0). Obrink (95) pointed out that instantaneous mixing may not occur, in which case the appropriate gradient would be the difference between the primary acidity and the interstitial fluid, i.e., $(H_o − 0)$. The decrement due to diffusion would then be $(k_H H_o)$. Since the permeability coefficient for acid, k_H, and the primary acidity, H_o, are constant quantities, the loss of acid by diffusion would be constant. A constant loss of acid, is, in fact, probable, since the locus of diffusion appears to be the tubules (see below). These permeable structures represent a constant surface area (80% of total area), which is continuously exposed to nascent acid secretion flowing at high velocities on its way to the main gastric lumen.

The amount of acid recovered may be expressed by:

$$[H] \, v = H_o v − H_o \, k_H \qquad [3]$$

and the concentration of acid by:

$$[H] = H_o \, (1 − k_H / v) \qquad [4]$$

The formal similarity between Eqs. 3 and 4 of the diffusion hypothesis and Eqs. 1 and 2 of the two-component hypothesis is evident. The dimensions of k_H, like those of k in Eqs. 1 and 2, are volume/unit time for a given area and thickness of mucosa. k_H is related to the apparent diffusion coefficient of acid in the mucosa (D_H) by the function $k_H = D_H \, (A/d)$, where A and d are the surface area and thickness of the mucosa, respectively.

In addition to the formal similarity of the two hypotheses, there is an intuitive conceptual similarity. Equation 3 states that a fixed amount of acid is lost from the parietal secretion and replaced by NaCl with little or no change in volume. Equation 1 states that a fixed amount of saline mixes with a greater amount of parietal secretion. In either case, when no acid is present, a neutral solution of NaCl is recovered with a volume equal to k or k_H (intercepts in Figs. 3 and 4).

The fit of data obtained in human subjects to Eqs. 1 and 3 is shown in Fig. 2; the fit of data to Eqs. 2 and

4 is shown in Figs. 3 and 4. In all instances, a clear-cut intercept on the flow rate axis is seen equal to k or k_H (80,93). A good fit of data to Teorell's original formulation has been reported in some studies using canine denervated pouches (69,95). According to that formulation ([H] = $(H_o v)/(v + k_H)$), the hyperbolic curve relating [H] and flow rate, v, passes through the origin. However, low flow rates in denervated pouches can be easily underestimated; this would lead to a spurious shift of the curve to the origin that would mask the intercept.

Neutralization by Bicarbonate

It is probable that the nonparietal component reduces acidity further by neutralization. The main neutralizing constituent appears to be bicarbonate, as discussed in detail later; the contributions of mucus and partly digested protein are minor (81,95). Equations 1 and 2 can be expanded to take into account the effect of neutralization:

$$[H]\ v = H_o\ (v - k) - bk \qquad [5]$$
$$= H_o v - k(H_o + b)$$
$$[H] = H_o - (k/v)(H_o + b) \qquad [6]$$

The predictions of Eqs. 5 and 6 are similar to those of Eqs. 1 and 2 except that estimates of k are obtained at [H] = −b, where b is an assumed (32,47,48,80) or measured (1,10,17,61,72) value for bicarbonate concentration in the nonparietal component (see Table 3). The estimates of k obtained from Eqs. 5 and 6 are only marginally smaller than those obtained from Eqs. 1 and 2 (Fig. 3).

Neutralization must also be considered in the formulation of the diffusion hypothesis. Since the diffusional movement of Na from the interstitial fluid involves both its companion anions Cl and HCO_3, the appropriate gradient for the "disappearance" of acid should include the concentration of bicarbonate in the interstitial fluid, i.e., $(H_o + b)$. Equations 3 and 4 can be expanded to take this into account:

$$[H]\ v = H_o v - k_H(H_o + b) \qquad [7]$$
$$[H] = H_o - (k_H/v)(H_o + b) \qquad [8]$$

Here again, the formal similarity between Eqs. 7 and 8 of the diffusion hypothesis and Eqs. 5 and 6 of the two-component hypothesis is evident.

Estimates of H⁺ Permeability and Nonparietal Flow Rate

Values of k_H (the permeability coefficient for H⁺) or of k (the flow rate of the nonparietal component) cal-

culated from the fit of human secretory data are identical (0.35 ± 0.04 and 0.35 ± 0.03 ml/min, respectively; mean ± SEM) (80,93). These values represent 6 to 8% of maximal secretory flow rate. Individual values depend on the functional size of the stomach, particularly on the mucosal surface area (92). Expressed per cm^2 of human gastric mucosa, the mean value of k or k_H is 4.5 × 10^{-4} ml/cm^2-min. Values for canine denervated pouches of indeterminate area are probably of the same order (0.1 ml/min) (93,95).

SODIUM SECRETION

Postulates of the Two-Component Hypothesis

According to the two-component hypothesis, Na derives solely from the nonparietal component. The amount of Na in secretion, [Na] v, is equal to the amount of Na initially present in the nonparietal component, Na_o k:

$$[Na]\ v = Na_o\ k \qquad [9]$$
$$[Na] = Na_o\ k/v \qquad [10]$$

Equation 9 states that Na output during steady-state secretion remains constant. Equation 10 states that [Na] tends to zero at high flow rates and to its initial level, Na_0, at v = k.

The constancy of Na output leads to the conclusion that the nonparietal component is produced in fixed quantities during steady-state secretion. This phenomenon has been described in the human (80), dog (47), cat (12,85), and rabbit (10). Figure 2 and Table 1 show that Na output in humans remains constant, despite a sevenfold increase in flow rate and a hundredfold increase in the dose of gastrin (80). Detailed data from five individuals (kindly made available by Dr B. Nordgren; for other details, see ref. 93) show that Na output in the basal state (30 μEq/min) does not change with weak, moderate, or intense stimulation with histamine (30 to 33 μEq/min). During prolonged infusions of histamine in dogs (4 hr), the integrated Na output increases with the dose of stimulant; these results cannot be usefully interpreted since the flow rate and acid secretion declined drastically within 90 min of the start of infusion (55).

Postulates of the Diffusion Hypothesis

According to the diffusion hypothesis, Na enters the lumen of the stomach by diffusion down its concentration gradient. Teorell (111) assumed the gradient to be the difference between the concentration of Na in the interstitial fluid and the concentration of Na in the luminal contents, i.e., $(Na_o − [Na])$. From this, he de-

TABLE 1. *Flow rate and ionic secretion in response to infusion of gastrin II in a human subject*[a]

Gastrin II (pmoles/kg-hr)	Flow rate (ml/min)	[H]	[Na]	[K]	[Cl]	Na output	H output
		(mEq/liter)				(μEq/min)	
Basal	0.48	30.7	86.7	9.7	126.5	41.6	14.8
1.1	0.43	35.5	88.7	9.0	135.1	38.3	15.3
2.7	0.45	40.0	86.5	8.5	137.5	38.9	18.0
5.4	0.47	35.6	93.1	10.6	139.1	43.8	16.8
11.0	1.31	105.7	31.8	14.2	153.3	41.7	138.3
14.6	1.83	122.7	23.1	13.6	156.2	42.3	224.6
18.2	2.44	127.1	16.9	15.4	159.7	41.2	310.2
36.4	2.70	131.1	15.7	15.5	162.3	42.4	354.0
109.1	3.28	131.8	12.5	17.1	160.5	41.0	431.6

[a] From ref. 80.

rived the following equation to describe the relationship between [Na] and flow rate:

$$[Na] = (Na_o\, k_{Na})/(v + k_{Na}) \qquad [11]$$

where k_{Na} is the permeability coefficient for Na.

There is no convincing evidence from the fit of secretory data that Eq. 11 describes adequately the state of Na in secretion (69). According to this equation, at $v = k_{Na}$, $[Na] = Na_o/2$ or approximately 75 mEq/liter. At this flow rate, which is equal to or less than the intercepts in Figs. 3 and 4, the concentration of acid should be zero; yet Figs. 3 and 4 show concentrations of Na between 90 and 120 mEq/liter in the presence of appreciable concentrations of acid (5 to 40 mEq/liter). Similar considerations apply to data from canine denervated pouches (69).

For the same reasons adduced above in deriving the true gradient for acid, the gradient for Na is more correctly stated as $(Na_o - 0)$, because Na diffuses across the tubular cell layer into nascent secretion, which is Na-free. Since the gradient for Na is constant (i.e., Na_o), the diffusional flux of Na into nascent secretion is also constant:

$$[Na]\, v = Na_o\, k_{Na} \qquad [12]$$

Equation 12 is formally similar to Eq. 9 derived on the basis of the two-component hypothesis and leads to the same predictions. Because Na^+ is less mobile than H^+, k_{Na} should, in theory, be less than k_H. Estimates from secretory studies (95) show the ratio of k_H to k_{Na} to be about 1.5. Estimates from instillation experiments (4,5,11,20,31,34,77,103,111,112) show ratios ranging from 1 to 2.2, the theoretical maximum for diffusion of HCl and NaCl as ion pairs in aqueous solutions. The meaning and variability of k_H and k_{Na} are discussed below.

Relationship Between [H] and [Na]

Combining Eqs. 6 and 10 of the two-component hypothesis (or Eqs. 8 and 12 of the diffusion hypothesis)

to eliminate the volume function k/v (or v in the diffusion hypothesis) yields a linear relationship between [H] and [Na]:

$$[Na] = Na_o(H_o - [H])/(H_o + b) \qquad [13]$$

It is clear from Eq. 13 that the relationship between [H] and [Na] is independent of flow rate and, therefore, should hold during steady- and nonsteady-state secretion. H_o and Na_o correspond to the intercepts at [Na] = 0 and at [H] = $-b$, respectively (Figs. 5 to 7). Estimates of H_o and Na_o are listed in Tables 2 and 3.

Much has been made of a linear or curvilinear relationship between [H] and [Na] as a test of the validity of the two-component or diffusion hypothesis. Since the two hypotheses can be stated in similar formal terms,

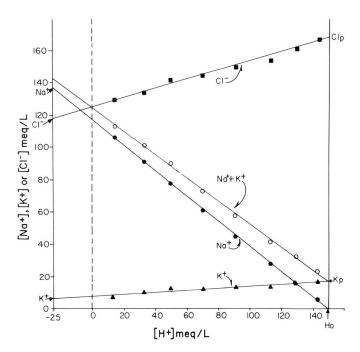

FIG. 5. Linear relationship between [H] and [Na], [K] or [Cl] in human gastric secretion. Data from one human subject (see Figs. 2 and 3 and ref. 80). The intercepts on the right and left vertical axes (*arrows*) correspond to the concentrations in the parietal and nonparietal components, respectively (Tables 2 and 3).

TABLE 2. *Composition of parietal secretion*

Reference	Species	Origin	[H]	[Na]	[K]	[Cl]	All cations
					(mEq/liter)		
Nordgren (93)	Human	Whole stomach	144.1	3.4	16.4	164.1	163.9
Makhlouf et al. (80)	Human	Whole stomach	148.9	—	16.9	166.3	165.8
Moody (87)	Dog	Segment	164.1	4.8	6.4	173.6	175.3
Gray and Bucher (47)	Dog	Pouch	158.6	—	7.4	166.0	166.0
Milton et al. (85)	Cat	Whole stomach	146.0	22.0	9.5	180.4	177.5
Beauville et al. (10)	Rabbit	Pouch	152.3	1.8	19.6	176.3	173.9

TABLE 3. *Composition of nonparietal component*

Reference	Species	Origin	[Na]	[K]	All cations	[HCO₃]	[Cl]	All anions
					(mEq/liter)			
Makhlouf et al. (80)	Human	Whole stomach	136.7	6.4	143.1	25.0[b]	117.8	142.8
Makhlouf (72)	Human[a]	Whole stomach	134	12	146	14	125	139
Gray and Bucher (47)	Dog	Pouch fundus	135.4	7.4	142.8	25.0[b]	117.8	142.8
Bugajski et al. (17)	Dog	Pouch fundus	136.0	6.2	142.2	10.0	141.5	151.5
Grossman (49)	Dog	Pouch antrum	151.0	9.2	160.2	8.0	145.3	153.3
Beauville et al. (10)	Rabbit	Pouch						
		Fundus	143.3	6.7	150.0	17.7	126.1	143.8
		Antrum	147.7	5.6	153.3	19.6	127.8	147.4

[a]Patient with pernicious anemia.
[b]Assumed values.

the relationship loses its discriminant value. Curvilinearity accompanied by wide scatter of data is usually an artifact of salivary contamination in humans and animals (42,56,62–64,66,67), as the instructive analysis of Hobsley and Silen shows (56). Where special care is taken to avoid salivary contamination (73,80,81,93), linearity between [H] and [Na] is maintained (Figs. 5 and 6). A departure from linearity is sometimes seen at high acid concentrations in data obtained from canine denervated pouches where extragastric contamination is not possible (Fig. 8) (62,69). The phenomenon may be peculiar to canine denervated pouches and could result from an increase in the permeability to H⁺ and Na⁺ during intense stimulation.

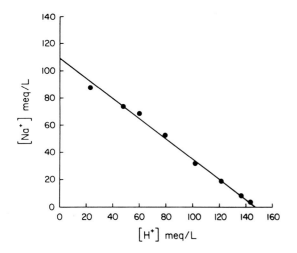

FIG. 6. Inverse linear relationship between [H] and [Na]. Mean data from five human subjects in the basal state and during histamine stimulation. (Courtesy of Bengt Nordgren.)

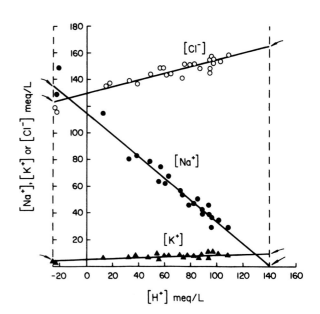

FIG. 7. Linear relationship between [H] and [Cl], [Na] or [K] in gastric secretion from rabbits in the basal state and during stimulation with gastrin. Note the fit of the lines to [Cl], [Na], and [K] obtained in alkaline secretion. Vertical intercepts designate parietal (*right*) and nonparietal (*left*) concentrations. [Redrawn from Beauville et al. (10).]

Linearity is evident in data obtained from denervated pouches in the rabbit (Fig. 7) (10). These data are unique in that they span the entire spectrum of acid and alkaline concentrations. The intercepts for Na, K, and Cl at the observed alkaline concentrations (i.e., at [H] = −b) are of special interest. They are listed in column 7 of Table 3, which also provides estimates of the nonparietal component in several species (10,17, 47,49,72,80).

Analysis of secretion obtained from a unilateral mucosal preparation in the frog (Fig. 1) discloses striking similarities to mammalian secretion (79). The Na concentration and osmolarity in the serosal medium were altered by addition or withdrawal of NaCl. The maneuver yielded hypertonic, isotonic, or hypotonic secretions in which the relationship between [H] and [Na] was invariably linear (Fig. 9) (G. M. Makhlouf, *unpublished observations*).

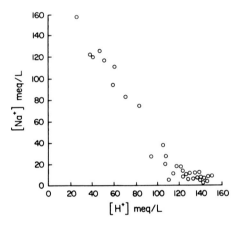

FIG. 8. Inverse relationship between [H] and [Na] in gastric secretion obtained from canine denervated pouches. [Data of Linde and Obrink (69) redrawn from Hung and Wan (62).] A departure from linearity is noted at high acid concentrations.

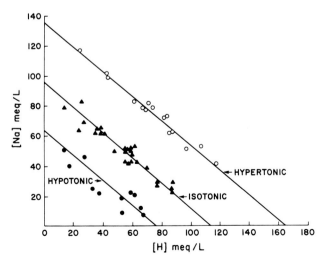

FIG. 9. Inverse linear relationship between [H] and [Na] in gastric secretion obtained from a unilateral mucosal preparation in the frog. Hypertonic and hypotonic secretions were generated by addition or withdrawal of NaCl from the serosal bathing medium. (G. M. Makhlouf, *unpublished data*.)

POTASSIUM SECRETION

Potassium is present in both parietal and nonparietal components. At high flow rates, secretion consists solely of HCl and KCl; at these rates, the limiting concentration of K is 17 mEq/liter in humans and about 10 mEq/liter in dogs (Table 2 and Fig. 3). At low flow rates, [K] tends to a level slightly higher than that in plasma (Table 3, Fig. 3). A positive relationship exists between K output and H output and between [K] and [H], which suggests a link between the secretion of the two cations (Figs. 5 and 7) (10,60,62,73,80,82).

The link was examined recently in a unilateral mucosal preparation bathed on the serosal side with variable concentrations of K (78). Secretory [K] was found to be linearly related to serosal [K] (Fig. 10). The slope of the relationship indicated that K was concentrated threefold in the water of secretion. Despite its higher concentration in secretion, K was distributed at or near electrochemical equilibrium. Since the water of secretion is osmotically coupled to the active transport of the major ions, H and Cl, an inevitable correlation should develop between K and H secretion. Thus a stoichiometric relationship between K and H flux and between [K] and [H] (Fig. 11) probably derives from the inde-

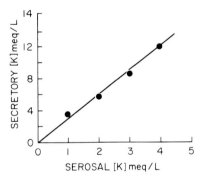

FIG. 10. Linear relationship between secretory [K] and serosal [K]. Slope = 3. Data obtained from a unilateral mucosal preparation in the frog exposed on the serosal side to various concentrations of K.

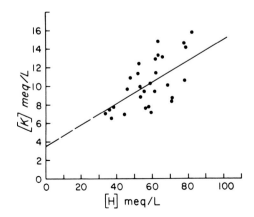

FIG. 11. Linear relationship between [H] and [K] in gastric secretion obtained from a unilateral mucosal preparation in the frog (79).

pendent link of each cation to the water of secretion (78,118). The coupling between the movements of K and water is further supported by experiments in which the secretions of H and K were dissociated. This was accomplished by progressively raising the osmolarity of the serosal medium. The maneuver produced an increase in [H] and osmolarity of the secreted fluid and a decrease in flow rate and [K].

There are two possible pathways for the movement of K into the lumen of the stomach: intercellular and transcellular. In the latter case, K would originate in a labile intracellular compartment, traverse the luminal membrane of the cell, and distribute in the secreted fluid at or near electrochemical equilibrium. This sequence would identify the parietal cell, the main site of active ionic transport and osmotic equilibration, as also the main site of passive K transport (118). The sweep of water through the labile compartment could generate [K] transients, such as that usually seen at the start of secretion before a steady state is established (73,80,97).

CALCIUM SECRETION

The pattern of Ca secretion is similar in most respects to the pattern of Na secretion (46,91,116). At low flow rates, the concentration of Ca in secretion approaches the concentration of ionized Ca in plasma. At high flow rates, the concentration of Ca tends to low levels in dogs (0.1 to 0.4 mEq/liter) but to somewhat higher levels in humans (about 1 mEq/liter). The difference is probably attributable to the binding of Ca to pepsin (91); the latter is strongly stimulated by histamine in humans but not in dogs. Calcium also binds to mucus and can be readily displaced from it by acid, a probable factor in the neutralizing capacity of mucus (46,95).

CHLORIDE SECRETION

Chloride is the sole anion in parietal secretion and the main anion in nonparietal secretion. At high flow rates, [Cl] increases to its limiting level in parietal secretion (Fig. 3); the level is somewhat higher in animals than in humans (Table 2). At low flow rates, [Cl] decreases to its level in the nonparietal component. In terms of the diffusion hypothesis, the decrease in [Cl] at low flow rates results from the greater mobility of HCl relative to NaCl.

On the basis of similar considerations as those used to derive Eq. 13, expressions can be derived to show that the relationship between [H] and [Cl] or [K] is linear (for details, see ref. 80) (Figs. 5,7 and 11).

OSMOLARITY OF SECRETION

The osmolarity of acid secretion parallels the concentration of Cl and can be calculated from the following

expression: Osmolarity of secretion = 2 × [Cl] × osmotic coefficient (0.944).

The osmolarity of histamine-stimulated acid secretion is about 6% higher than the osmolarity of arterial plasma and can be made to increase or decrease in parallel with it by oral or intravenous administration of saline or water (44,45,87,114). The osmolarity of gastric venous plasma is higher than that of arterial plasma because of the clearance of water with H⁺ formed de novo in the mucosa (6). When compared with the osmolarity of gastric venous plasma, gastric secretion appears to be isoosmotic (6).

Experiments in vitro support the view that secretion is isoosmotic with the solution immediately bathing the mucosa (28,29). Samples obtained from a unilateral mucosal preparation show that if all secreted ions are considered, including NaCl and KCl, the calculated osmolarity equals that of the serosal bathing solution (79). When the flow rate is low and acid concentration declines, however, secretion becomes distinctly hypotonic (Fig. 12). A nadir is reached, which is about 20% less than the osmolarity of highly acid secretion. The same phenomenon has been observed repeatedly in mammalian secretion (63,64,68,80,95). The factors that determine the development of hypotonicity are neutralization by bicarbonate, which dissipates osmotically active H⁺, and the lower mobility of NaCl diffusing into the lumen relative to the mobility of HCl diffusing out of the lumen (110).

WATER TRANSPORT

Water flows across the gastric mucosa in response to osmotic gradients created within the tissue by the active transport of solutes, chiefly HCl (87). Water flow can be maintained against hydrostatic as well as external osmotic gradients of 100 mOsmoles/liter (26,29). The relationship between water and solute flow is illustrated in Fig. 2 by the linear relationship between Cl output (an index of total ionic flow) and volume flow rate. A similar relationship exists for secretion obtained from

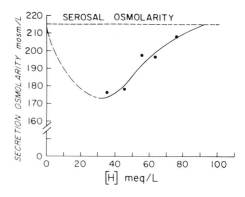

FIG. 12. Relationship between secretory osmolarity and [H]. Data obtained from a unilateral mucosal preparation in the frog (79).

a unilateral mucosal preparation (Fig. 13) (79). The slope of the relationship for mammalian secretion corresponds to 166 mEq/liter Cl or 314 mOsmoles/liter which is slightly hypertonic to arterial plasma but probably isotonic to gastric venous plasma (see above). The slope of the relationship for amphibian secretion is identical to the osmolarity of the bathing serosal solution (200 mOsmoles/liter) (Fig. 13).

The obligatory dependence of water flow on solute flow is best demonstrated *in vitro*, where changes in the osmolarity of a solution bathing the serosal side of a unilateral mucosal preparation can be induced by addition or withdrawl of NaCl or by substitution of glucose for NaCl (75,82). Secretory osmolarity increases or decreases with serosal osmolarity (Fig. 14). The osmotic

difference brought about by addition of glucose to the serosal solution is matched by the secretion of ions. A deviation from isoosmolarity occurs, however, when the serosal solution is rendered hypotonic. This is probably due to swelling of the cells wsith partial obliteration of paracellular, tubular, or canalicular channels (H. Helander, *personal communication*), thus rendering osmotic equilibration more difficult to achieve (105).

The osmotic transport of water can also be studied by modifying the endogenous osmotic gradient from the luminal side. Using a technique introduced by Teorell and co-workers (51, 70), Moody and Durbin (89) instilled isotonic solutions of the buffer glycine or of various impermeable electrolytes or nonelectrolytes on the luminal surface of a histamine-stimulated canine mucosa and calculated that the concentration of secreted acid increased beyond its limiting value in normal secretion (H_0). The increase was due primarily to a reduction in the rate of net water flow toward the lumen. The results indicate that the osmotic gradient created by the secretion of H and Cl into the canaliculi could be diluted by the diffusion of impermeable solutes to these sites of osmotic equilibration. Glycine acted also to reduce the osmotic gradient by buffering H^+. The effect was most prominent at the lowest secretory rates, when the velocity of secreted fluid in the tubules and canaliculi is minimal and the diffusion of instilled solutes into the tubules optimal (Fig. 15).

Durbin (28) confirmed these results in unilateral amphibian mucosa and showed further that hypotonic instillates (10% of normal) abolish net water flow. From the difference in net secretory water flow into isotonic and hypotonic instillates, Durbin calculated the osmotic permeability to be about 45 nl/cm²- hr-mOsm differ-

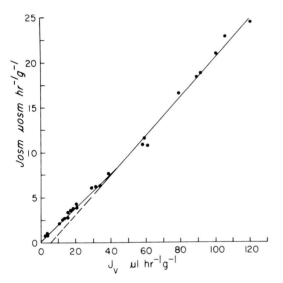

FIG. 13. Relationship between solute flow and water flow. Data obtained from a unilateral mucosal preparation in the frog (79). The linear component of the slope is equal to serosal osmolarity.

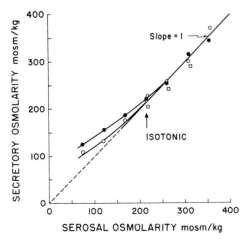

FIG. 14. Relationship between secretory osmolarity and serosal osmolarity in data obtained from a unilateral mucosal preparation in the frog (75). *Closed circles*, first 3 hr; *open circles*, last 3 hr; *open squares*, substitution of glucose for NaCl. Note deviation from isoosmotic secretion when the serosal bathing solution is rendered hypotonic.

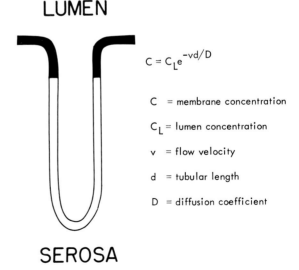

FIG. 15. Schematic representation of the pits (*blacked area*) and tubules. Equation describes the concentration profile of a solute diffusing from the lumen and the effect of tubular secretion flowing toward the lumen (see text for details). The pits are considered impermeable and the tubules permeable to H ions and water.

ence. This value is similar to that measured by application of exogenous osmotic gradients (see below). These values are probably underestimates of the osmotic permeability. The infolding of the mucosa into tubules and the parietal cells into canaliculi increases the velocity of secretory flow and hampers the access of instilled solutes to the sites of osmotic equilibration. This makes it likely that only a fraction of the applied osmotic gradient reaches the luminal surface of the parietal cells (99).

BICARBONATE SECRETION

Bicarbonate secretion is discussed in greater detail by Flemström elsewhere in this volume. Only those aspects of bicarbonate transport pertinent to the regulation of acidity are discussed here. Bicarbonate enters the lumen of the stomach by active secretion, by diffusion, and, in some instances, by bulk flow of interstitial fluid. The amounts of bicarbonate that can be recovered from the lumen of the stomach are as follows: 40 $\mu Eq/hr$ from the canine antrum (5,49); 15 to 45 $\mu Eq/hr$ from canine denervated fundic pouches of various sizes (17,65); 40 $\mu Eq/hr$ from a chambered canine fundic segment (surface area, about 100 cm^2) (2–4); 40 $\mu Eq/hr$ from the whole stomach of the guinea pig (41); and about 350 $\mu Eq/hr$ from the stomach of patients with pernicious anemia (42,66,72). Expressed per cm^2 mucosa, bicarbonate production in humans (0.4 $\mu Eq/cm^2$-hr) and dogs (0.4 $\mu Eq/cm^2$-hr) is similar to bicarbonate production by the amphibian antrum (0.3 $\mu Eq/cm^2$-hr) or fundus (0.25 to 0.55 $\mu Eq/cm^2$-hr) in vitro (33,36,43). These amounts are small compared to acid secretion, rarely exceeding 5%. Nonetheless, the flow rate and Na content of the fluid in which bicarbonate is found (0.4 ml/min and 54 $\mu Eq/min$ Na for the whole stomach in man or 5 × 10^{-4} ml/cm^2-min and 7 × 10^{-2} $\mu Eq/cm^2$-min Na) correspond to the flow rate and Na content of the nonparietal component, as calculated from Eqs. 5 and 6 and from the fit of secretory data in Figs. 3 and 4.

It is not known to what extent the amount of bicarbonate recovered from the mammalian stomach is the result of active secretion rather than diffusion or bulk flow of interstitial fluid. Active secretion of bicarbonate has been conclusively shown in amphibian fundic and antral mucosa only (33,36). The evidence points to active secretion of bicarbonate by the mammalian antral and fundic mucosa also (13,39,65). Early attempts to determine whether fundic mucosa could secrete bicarbonate were hampered by the problem of residual acid secretion (9,14,39,40,107,115). This problem has now been resolved by the combined use of inhibitors of acid secretion (cholinergic and histamine-H^2 receptor antagonists or prostaglandins) and/or stimulants of alkaline secretion (prostaglandins). The electrolyte composition of fundic alkaline secretion is similar to that of antral

secretion (Table 3). The stomachs of patients with pernicious anemia yield an alkaline fluid, which also resembles the secretion of antral and resting fundic mucosa (Table 3). Characteristically, these fluids contain higher [K] and [Cl] and lower [HCO$_3$] than interstitial fluid. A higher [K] is consistent with passive movement of this ion down a favorable electrical gradient. A high [Cl] indicates the presence of an active Cl mechanism in the surface epithelial and mucous cells of the antrum and fundus (33,36). A Cl carrier subserves active Cl transport as well as exchange diffusion of Cl (82); the carrier may also be capable of transporting other monovalent anions, such as HCO$_3$, but with lesser affinity than Cl. The exchange diffusion process could involve Cl as well as HCO$_3$; the latter can be made readily available by the action of carbonic anhydrase in the surface epithelial and mucous cells (94,106). In the presence of acid, a luminal HCO$_3$/Cl exchange diffusion process could lead to a considerable influx of bicarbonate into the lumen, resulting in greater loss of acid than accountable for by the actual bicarbonate content of alkaline secretion.

Bicarbonate can also enter the lumen as part of the bulk flow of interstitial fluid. Bulk flow occurs if arterial pressure exceeds 200 mm Hg or if mucosal capillary pressure is raised mechanically or by close intra-arterial injection of acetylcholine (1,7,8). The flow occurs predominantly through a small set of large pores, 60 to 90Å in radius, which occupy 10 to 12% of the effective pore area of the gastric mucosa. Topical application of acetylcholine (61) or detergents (24,25,107) and exposure of the mucosa to excessive osmotic gradients (greater than 600 mOsm) (37,38) disrupt the mucosa, causing leakage of interstitial fluid. Altamirano (3) has pointed out that the mucosa is occasionally exposed to high osmotic gradients in the form of soup, juice, or syrup (0.5 to 2 OsM)

Bicarbonate and other ions accumulate in small, constant amounts in isotonic or hypotonic instillates (2,3,86,88). The entry of bicarbonate in these instances could represent diffusion of bicarbonate into the lumen and/or secretion of bicarbonate by the mucous and surface epithelial cells.

MUCOSAL PERMEABILITY TO ACID AND SODIUM

Structural Determinants of Permeability

The gastric mucosa is a tight epithelium (27) characterized by a high transmucosal potential difference, high transmucosal resistance, low osmotic permeability, and steep solutes gradients resulting from the active transport of ions (82). These properties are largely determined by the relative permeabilities of the paracellular (i.e., between cells) and transcellular (i.e., across both the luminal and basolateral membranes of the cell) pathways to ions and water. The permeability of the paracellular pathway in antral mucosa is 10 times greater than that in fundic mucosa (109).

The geometry of the tubules adds considerably to the impermeability of the mucosa. The tubules, which contain 80% of the cell mass and include 80% of the surface area, are relatively inaccessible to the solutes present in the main lumen. At rest, they constitute a long and narrow diffusion pathway. During secretion, the high velocity of water flow sweeps away solutes that had diffused from the main lumen.

The permeability of the luminal side to cations is low (15,16,21,22,82,101). H+ disappear from the lumen of the stomach more rapidly than Na+ or K+, in this order (21). The rate of diffusion of Na from the lumen of the resting fundus is less than 0.5%/min; diffusion of Na from the lumen stops during active secretion (21,22). The rate of diffusion of Na in the antrum is higher than in the fundus and is not affected by acid secretion. This points to the tubules as the main sites of Na diffusion.

Rehm et al. (16,99,100,114) were the first to focus attention on the tubules as the main sites of H+ diffusion and osmotic water transport. Rehm considered the surface epithelial and mucous cells which line the pits (average depth, 100 μm) to be impermeable to H+ and water, in contrast to the parietal cells which line the tubules. Because tubular cells are separated from the main lumen by a long, narrow, unstirred pathway, they are exposed to only a fraction of H+ and osmotic gradients present in the main lumen. When acid solutions are instilled in the stomach, H+ diffuse toward the tubules and from there cross the mucosal cell layer; Na+ enter the tubular lumen at the same site. Because the mobilities of the H+ and Na+ are unequal, a Na/H profile is established in the pits and tubules, which renders the blind tubular end transiently hypertonic and obligates the entry of water. The entry of water in turn renders the instillate in the main lumen transiently hypotonic. In accordance with the predictions of Rehm's model (Fig. 15) (99), studies in which recovery of volume is adequate show a net increase in the volume of acid in-

stillates coincidentally with the disappearance of acid and the development of hypotonicity (see also Figs. 17 and 18).

The effect of acid secretion on the permeability of the mucosa to instilled solutes is described in terms of Rehm's model by the following expression:

$$C = C_L e^{-vd/D} \qquad [14]$$

where C_L is the initial concentration of solute in the main lumen; C, the concentration of the solute at a distance, d, in the pits and tubules; D, the diffusion coefficient of the solute; and v, the velocity of flow in the tubules calculated from the secretory flow rate and mean cross-sectional area of the tubules (Fig. 15).

When the rate of secretion is high, the concentration profile within the tubules and pits is rapidly dissipated and the solute (or H+, if the instillate is acid) is swept back to the main lumen. H+ derived from secretion occupy the tubules, and the gradient for back-diffusion now becomes (H_0 + b), as noted earlier (Eqs. 7 and 8).

Permeability to Instilled Acid

Although the conditions that prevail during instillation of exogenous acid differ from those that prevail during active secretion, the permeability coefficients for H (k_H) determined in both states should be similar, provided the appropriate gradients are defined and the stimulus to secretion does not alter the permeability of the mucosa.

There are numerous studies in which acid was instilled in the stomach (4,50,71,95,96,104,110,119); only a few are amenable to comparative analysis of fluxes or to calculation of the permeability coefficients. Estimates of the permeability coefficients for H (k_H) and Na (k_{Na}) expressed in ml/cm²-min or cm-min are listed in Table 4. The coefficients were derived from the ratio of the normalized H or Na fluxes in μEq/cm²-min and the H or Na gradients in μEq/ml (flux in μEq/cm²-min = permeability coefficient in ml/cm²-min × gradient in μEq/ml). The estimates were obtained from studies on dener-

TABLE 4. *Fluxes and permeability coefficients of H+ and Na+*

Reference	Species	Origin	H+ flux (μEq/cm²-min)	k_H (μl/cm²-min)	Na+ flux (μEq/cm²-min)	k_{Na} (μl/cm²-min)
Chung et al. (20)	Dog	Fundus	0.13	0.78	0.14	0.96
Dyck et al. (31)	Dog	Fundus	0.10	0.64	0.09	0.62
Berkowitz and Janowitz (11)	Dog	Fundus	0.15	0.97	0.10	0.66
Rudick et al. (103)	Dog	Fundus	0.18	1.11	0.16	1.08
		Mean	0.14 ± 0.02	0.88 ± 0.10	0.12 ± 0.02	0.83 ± 1.1
Dyck et al. (31)	Dog	Antrum	0.20	1.30	0.34	2.36
Rudick et al. (103)	Dog	Antrum	0.23	1.46	0.45	3.08
		Mean	0.22 ± 0.02	1.38 ± 0.08	0.40 ± 0.06	2.72 ± 0.36
Terner (112)	Frog	Fundus	0.06	0.70	—	—
Makhlouf (77)	Frog	Fundus	0.09	0.90	—	—

vated canine fundic and antral pouches (11,20,31,103) and from chambered amphibian fundic mucosa *in vitro* (77,83,112). The approximate surface area of the pouches was calculated from the volume of their contents in the absence of distension, assuming the pouches to be spheres of the same capacity. The following conclusions may be drawn from the data presented in Table 4:

a. H loss (0.14 ± 0.02 μEq/cm²-min) equaled Na gain (0.12 ± 0.02 μEq/cm²-min) in canine fundic pouches. This was reflected in similar values for k_H and k_{Na} (0.88 ± 0.10 and 0.83 ± 0.11 μliter/cm²-min, respectively).

b. Na gain (0.40 ± 0.06 μEq/cm²-min) exceeded H loss (0.22 ± 0.02 μEq/cm²-min) in the antrum. The values for k_H (1.38 ± 0.08 μliter/cm²-min) and k_{Na} (2.72 ± 0.36 μliter/cm²-min) were 1.5 and 3 times greater than the corresponding values in the fundus. Values reported by Altamirano (4) for the chambered canine mucosal segment are one-half those reported by other investigators, probably because the surface area of the stretched mucosa was used in the calculation.

c. Permeability coefficients for H calculated for non-secreting frog mucosa were similar to those calculated for canine mucosa, probably because the cellular barrier in both species is one cell thick.

d. an apparent diffusion coefficient for HCl (D_{HCl}) in gastric mucosa may be calculated if an approximate value is assigned to the thickness of the overall diffusion barrier (e.g., 0.02 cm). D_{HCl} (= k_H × thickness) in canine gastric mucosa is 1.76 × 10⁻⁵ cm²/min or 100 times less than D_{HCl} in aqueous solutions; the difference is an indication of the restriction to H movement in the mucosa.

Variability of the Permeability Coefficients for H⁺ and Na⁺

The values calculated for k_H and k_{Na} depend on the secretory status of the fundic mucosa. A residual acid secretion manifests itself as a decrease in k_H. Conversely, bicarbonate secretion leads to an overestimate of k_H. Altamirano (4) measured the extent of neutralization by bicarbonate from the slope relating H flux and H gradient: a loss of acid was detected in the form of an intercept in the absence of a H gradient. The extent of loss due to neutralization was independently confirmed by measuring the accumulation of bicarbonate in neutral instillates (see above). Neutralization appears to account for only 10% of the total loss of H from instillates and for a corresponding increase in the value of k_H.

A substantial overestimate of k_{Na} could result from bicarbonate secretion. The Na content of this secretion is at least 10 times the bicarbonate content. A combination of Na diffusion and Na secretion could thus account for the apparent equality of k_{Na} and k_H. When Na

secretion is minimized, the ratio of k_H to k_{Na} approaches that expected from the mobilities of the two cations. This is illustrated in Fig. 16 for data obtained from frog mucosa *in vitro* (77). The analysis is based on the assumption that the independent movements of HCl and NaCl obey first order kinetics (111). The approximations based on luminal concentrations of H and Na are adequate if sufficient time is allowed to pass.

At time t, [H] in an acid instillate is related to initial concentration, H_o, by the following function:

$$[H] = H_o e^{-k_H t/p} \qquad [15]$$

[Na] is related to Na concentration on the serosal side, Na_o, by the function:

$$[Na] = Na_o(1 - e^{-k_{Na} t/p}) \qquad [16]$$

Combining Eqs. 15 and 16 to eliminate t/p (where p is the volume of instillate) yields a linear relationship between log [H] and log (Na_o − [Na]) with a slope equal to k_H/k_{Na}. The ratio of k_H to k_{Na} in frog gastric mucosa (2.2) was similar to the ratio of the diffusion coefficients of HCl and NaCl in free solution (D_{HCl}/D_{NaCl} = 2.1). The ratio in canine pouches [calculated from the data of Berkowitz and Janowitz (11)] was slightly less (1.8). The closeness of the observed ratios to the theoretically predictable ratio suggests that the movements of Na and H across gastric mucosa, although severely restricted, occur in aqueous channels. Because the true ratio of k_H to k_{Na} is probably greater than 1, it seems unlikely that the movements of H and

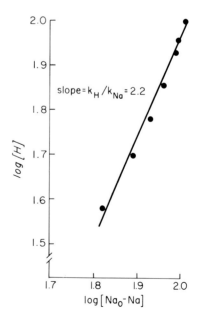

FIG. 16. Linear relationship between log [H] and log (Na_o − [Na]). The slope of the relationship is equal to the ratio of the permeability coefficients for H and Na. Data obtained from frog mucosa exposed to 100 mM HCl on the luminal side and unbuffered nutrient solution on the serosal side (77).

Na are coupled in a unitary exchange mechanism. This conclusion is supported by the fact that Na accumulates at the same rate in neutral and acid instillates (2–4,88).

Permeability and Mucosal Integrity

The permeability of the gastric mucosa to H$^+$ depends, of course, on its integrity (24,108,113). A variety of weak acids [e.g., acetic, acetylsalicylic, and taurocholic acids (23,34,35)] and steroids (20) can damage the mucosa and produce an increase in permeability to acid. Other agents, such as the secretory inhibitor thiocyanate, can increase the permeability of the mucosa to acid and water. In the presence of thiocyanate, k_H increases threefold (Fig. 17); consistent with the predictions of Rehm's model (99), the greater loss of acid is accompanied by more rapid entry of water into the instillate and by development of hypotonicity (Fig. 18) (83).

Diffusion Versus Neutralization by Bicarbonate

The estimates of k_H derived from instillation experiments are sufficiently close to those derived from the fit of secretory data for diffusion to be considered as a mechanism of acidity regulation (see above). On the other hand, the amounts of bicarbonate (and Na) that are known to enter the stomach by a combination of secretion and diffusion are sufficient to account for regulation of secreted acidity by a process of dilution and neutralization (see above). The same amounts of bicarbonate account for only a small fraction of the acid that disappears from instillates. It is possible, however, that in this case also the residual acid is neutralized by bicarbonate, recycled at the surface of the cell via a Cl/HCO$_3$ exchange mechanism (see above).

Thus the experimental evidence as well as the formal considerations presented in the first part of this chapter suggest that the two-component hypothesis is merely a contraction or "clearance" of the diffusion hypothesis and that the disappearance of acid, apparently by diffusion, may be accomplished at the cellular level by one or more processes involving neutralization by bicarbonate.

MUCOSAL PERMEABILITY TO WATER

In the dog, 88% of the effective pore area of the gastric mucosa is occupied by pores with radii of 2.5 Å and 12% with radii of 90 Å. In the frog, the mucosa is occupied by a similar set of pores (117). In both species, the distribution is highly skewed in favor of the smaller pores but is probably continuous between the two extremes. The larger pores may represent transient defects resulting from cell turnover or from experimental damage.

The flow of water in response to hydrostatic gradients occurs predominantly via the small set of large pores [flow proportional to (radius)^4 in accordance with Poiseuille's law]. Flow in response to osmotic gradients occurs predominantly via the large set of small pores. This difference in pathways only partly explains why hydrostatic permeability is 100 times greater than osmotic permeability (30,90).

The gastric mucosa responds to external osmotic gradients by net water flow in the expected direction. The flow is symmetric (i.e., independent of the direction in which it occurs) when gradients ranging from 0 to 200 mOsm are applied from the luminal side (Fig. 19) (7,76). Gradients created by addition of solutes to the serosal side, however, elicit a lesser flow.

Water flow is near linear for gradients up to 200 mOsM (Fig. 19) (29,76). Beyond that level, water flow

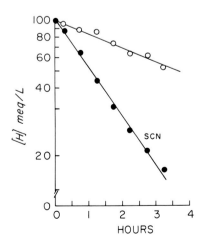

FIG. 17. Disappearance of H$^+$ from the luminal surface of frog mucosa with and without thiocyanate (83).

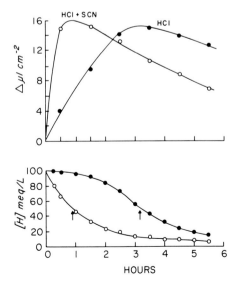

FIG. 18. Accumulation of water in the acid instillate coincidentally with the loss of H ions. Same data as in Fig. 20. *Arrows,* time for [H] decrease to H$_0$/2.

diminishes progressively (16,29,76). The deviation from linearity, also seen in canine mucosa (7,16), is probably due to polarization of solutes within the tubules. The entry and exit of water from these restricted spaces alters the composition of the solutions within the spaces before the change becomes manifest in the bulk solutions. The net effect is to reduce the osmotic gradient to which the tubular cells are exposed. Because of this, values of osmotic permeability based on gradients in the bulk solutions may be gross underestimates and further magnify the difference between osmotic and hydrostatic permeability.

Values for osmotic permeability range from 68 to 81 nl/cm²-hr-mOsm in amphibian mucosa *in vitro* (28,29,76,118) and from 53 to 77 nl/cm²-hr-mOsm in canine mucosa *in vivo* (7,90,100) (Fig. 19). The values depend to some extent on the nature of the solute used to impose a gradient and on the secretory state of the mucosa. From Eq. 14 of Rehm's model, which describes the concentration profile of solutes in the tubule, the gradient within the tubules depends on the balance between the rate of diffusion of the solute down the tubule and the velocity of secretory flow up the tubule. Solutes with low diffusion coefficients are least effective osmotically, particulary during active secretion, when they are rapidly swept away from the tubules into the main lumen. This phenomenon, together with the nonlinearity of osmotic flow, and the accumulation of water in isotonic acid instillates with ensuing hypotonicity, establish the tubules as the main sites of osmotic water flow.

CONCLUSION

It may be a truism worth repeating that the stomach is designed to secrete. Its exposed surface, a small frac-

tion of the total, is impermeable to cations, including H+, and water. The remaining surface is infolded into tubules and canaliculi, which are permeable to water and ions. The infolding of the surface endows the mucosa with long, narrow channels, which are unstirred at rest but vigorously stirred during secretion, conditions that enhance the secretory effectiveness of the mucosa and diminish its absorptive potential. During secretion, the permeable loci of the mucosa (i.e., the tubules) are exposed to constant Na and H gradients arising from a nascent isotonic secretion of fixed composition. Consequently, the diffusional loss of H and gain of Na remain constant despite large variations in secretory activity and can be expressed in the form of a nonparietal component. At the cellular level, the apparent loss of H by diffusion may be mediated by a combination of bicarbonate secretion and diffusion.

REFERENCES

1. Altamirano, M. (1963): Alkaline secretion produced by intra-arterial acetylcholine. *J. Physiol. (Lond.)*, 168:787–803.
2. Altamirano, M. (1969): Action of solutions of reduced osmotic concentration on the dog gastric mucosa. *Am. J. Physiol.*, 216:25–32.
3. Altamirano, M. (1969): Action of concentrated solutions of non-electrolytes on the dog gastric mucosa. *Am. J. Physiol.*, 216:33–40.
4. Altamirano, M. (1970): Backdiffusion of H+ during gastric secretion. *Am. J. Physiol.*, 218:1–6.
5. Altamirano, M., and Cruz, L. (1974): Ionic permeability of canine antrum. *Am. J. Physiol.*, 227:256–263.
6. Altamirano, M., Izaquirre, E., and Milgram, E. (1969): Osmotic concentration of the gastric juice of dogs. *J. Physiol. (Lond.)*, 202:283–296.
7. Altamirano, M., and Martinoya, C. (1966): The permeability of the gastric mucosa of the dog. *J. Physiol.*, 184:771–790.
8. Altamirano, M., Requena, M., and Durbin, R. P. (1974): Effects of gastric arterial and venous pressures on gastric secretion in the dog. *Am. J. Physiol.*, 227:152–260.
9. Baxter, S. G. (1934-5): Sympathetic secretory innervation of the gastric mucosa. *Am. J. Dig. Dis.*, 1:36–39.
10. Beauville, M., Raynaud, P., and Bernay, M. (1974): Secretion gastrique du lapin et théorie des deux composants. *Biol. Gastroenterol. (Paris)*, 7:215–219.
11. Berkowitz, J. M., and Janowitz, H. D. (1966): Alteration in composition of hydrochloric acid solutions by gastric mucosa. *Am. J. Physiol.*, 210:216–220.
12. Blair, E. L., and Yassin, A. K. (1961): The electrolyte content of histamine-stimulated gastric secretion in the cat. *J. Physiol. (Lond.)*, 159:82–83.
13. Bolton, J. P., and Cohen, M. M. (1978): Stimulation of non-parietal cell secretion in canine Heidenhain pouches by 16, 16-dimethyl prostaglandin E₂. *Digestion*, 17:291–299.
14. Bolton, C., and Goodhart, G. W. (1931): The variations in the acidity of the gastric juice during secretion. *J. Physiol. (Lond.)*, 73:115–135.
15. Bond, A. M., and Hunt, J. N. (1956): The effect of sodium fluoride on the output of some electrolytes from the gastric mucosa of cats. *J. Physiol. (Lond.)*, 133:317.
16. Bornstein, A. M., Dennis, W. H., and Rehm, W. S. (1959): Movement of water, sodium, chloride and hydrogen ions across the resting stomach. *Am. J. Physiol.*, 197:333–336.
17. Bugajski, J., Code, C. F., and Schlegel, J. F. (1972): Sodium-hydrogen ion exchange across canine resting gastric mucosa. *Am. J. Physiol.*, 222:858–863.
18. Canosa, C., and Rehm, W. S. (1958): Microscopical dimensions of the pit region of the dog's gastric mucosa. *Gastroenterology*, 35:292–297.

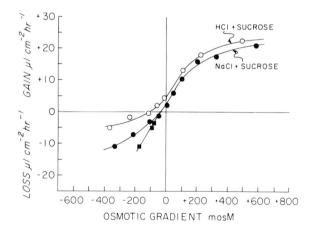

FIG. 19. Water movement in response to osmotic gradients in frog gastric mucosal sacs. (Gain = accumulation in sac). Note symmetric linear flow for gradients up to ± 200 mOsM imposed from the luminal side. *Closed squares,* luminal hypotonic solutions. Deviation from linearity occurs at higher gradients. Gradients imposed in the presence of HCl produce greater accumulation of water in the lumen (see Fig. 18 and text) (76,83).

19. Card, W. I., and Marks, I. N. (1960): The relationship between acid output of the stomach and the parietal cell mass. *Clin. Sci.,* 19:147–163.

20. Chung, R. S. K., Field, M., and Silen, W. (1978): Effects of methylprednisolone on hydrogen ion absorption in the canine stomach. *J. Clin. Invest.,* 62:262–270.

21. Code, C. F., Higgins, J. A., Moll, J. C., Orvis, A. L., and Scholer, J. F. (1963): The influence of acid on the gastric absorption of water, sodium and potassium. *J. Physiol. (Lond.),* 16:110–119.

22. Cope, O., Cohn, W. E., and Brenizer, A. G. (1943): Gastric secretion. II. Absorption of radioactive sodium from pouches of the body and antrum of the stomach of the dog. *J. Clin. Invest.,* 22:102–110.

23. Cox, A. J. (1952): Stomach size and its relation to chronic peptic ulcer. *Arch. Pathol.,* 54:407–422.

24. Davenport, H. W. (1972): The gastric mucosal barrier. *Digestion,* 5:162–165.

25. Davenport, H. W., Warner, H. A., and Code, C. F. (1964): Functional significance of gastric mucosal barrier to sodium. *Gastroenterology,* 47:142–152.

26. Davies, R. E., and Terner, C. (1949): The effects of applied pressure on secretion by isolated amphibian gastric mucosa. *Biochem. J.,* 44:377–384.

27. Diamond, J. M. (1978): Channels in epithelial cell membranes and junctions. *Fed. Proc.,* 37:2639–2644.

28. Durbin, R. P. (1979): Osmotic flow of water in isolated frog gastric mucosa. *Am. J. Physiol.,* 236:E63–E69.

29. Durbin, R. P., Frank, H., and Solomon, A. K. (1956): Water flow through frog gastric mucosa. *J. Gen. Physiol.,* 39:535–551.

30. Durbin, R. P., and Helander, H. F. (1978): Distribution of osmotic flow in stomach and gallbladder. *Biochem. Biophys. Acta,* 513:179–181.

31. Dyck, W. P., Werther, J. L., and Rudick, J., and Janowitz, H. D. (1969): Electrolyte movement across canine antral and fundic gastric mucosa. *Gastroenterology,* 56:488–495.

32. Fisher, R. B., and Hunt, J. N. (1950): The inorganic components of gastric secretion. *J. Physiol. (Lond.),* 111:138–149.

33. Flemström, G. (1977): Active alkalinization by amphibian gastric fundic mucosa in vitro. *Am. J. Physiol.,* 233:E1–E12.

34. Flemström, G., Frenning, B., and Obrink, K. J. (1964): The disappearance of acetic acid and acetate from the cat's stomach and its influence on the permeability for hydrochloric acid. *Acta Physiol. Scand.,* 62:422–428.

35. Flemström, G., and Frenning, B. (1968): Migration of acetic acid and sodium acetate and their effects on the gastric transmucosal ion exchange. *Acta Physiol. Scand.,* 74:521–532.

36. Flemström, G., and Sachs, G. (1975): Ion transport by amphibian antrum in vitro. I. General characteristics. *Am. J. Physiol.,* 228:1188–1198.

37. Frenning, B. (1973): The effects of large osmolality variations on the gastric mucosal surface ultrastructure. *Scand. J. Gastroenterol.,* 8:185–192.

38. Frenning, B. (1974): The effects of large osmolality variations on the gastric mucosal ion permeability. *Acta Physiol. Scand.,* 90:1–13.

39. Fromm, D., and Fuhro, R. (1976): Active bicarbonate secretion by mammalian antrum. *Surg. Forum,* 27:437–440.

40. Gamble, J. L., and McIver, M. R. (1928): The acid-base composition of gastric secretions. *J. Exp. Med.,* 48:837–847.

41. Garner, A., and Flemström, G. (1978): Gastric HCO_3 secretion in the guinea pig. *Am. J. Physiol.,* 234:E535–E541.

42. Gardham, J. R. C., and Hobsley, M. (1970): The electrolytes of alkaline human gastric juice. *Clin. Sci.,* 39:77–87.

43. Garner, A., and Heylings, J. R. (1979): Stimulation of alkaline secretion in amphibian-isolated gastric mucosa by 16,16-dimethyl PGE_2 and PGF_2. *Gastroenterology,* 76:497–508.

44. Gilman, A., and Cowgill, G. R. (1931-2): Osmotic relations of blood and glandular secretions. 1. The regulatory action of total blood electrolytes on the concentration of gastric chlorides. *Am. J. Physiol.,* 99:172–178.

45. Gilman, A., and Cowgill, G. R. (1933): Osmotic relationship of blood and gastric juice. *Am. J. Physiol.,* 103:143–152.

46. Grant, R. (1941): The relation of calcium content to acidity and buffer value of gastric secretions. *Am. J. Physiol.,* 132:467–473.

47. Gray, J. S., and Bucher, G. R. (1941): The composition of gastric juice as a function of the rate of secretion. *Am. J. Physiol.,* 133:542–550.

48. Gray, J. S., Bucher, G. R., and Harman, H. H. (1941): The relationship between total acid and neutral chloride of gastric juice. *Am. J. Physiol.,* 132:504–516.

49. Grossman, M. I. (1960): The pyloric gland area of the stomach: A brief survey. *Gastroenterology,* 38:1–6.

50. Harmon, J. W., and Woods, M., and Gurll, N. J. (1978): Different mechanisms of hydrogen ion removal in stomach and duodenum. *Am. J. Physiol.,* 235:E692–E698.

51. Heinz, E., and Obrink, K. J. (1954): Acid formation and acidity control in the stomach. *Physiol. Rev.,* 34:643–673.

52. Helander, H. F. (1972): Quantitative aspects of gastric morphology. In: *Gastric Secretion,* edited by G. Sachs, E. Heinz, and K. Ullrich, pp. 69–82. Academic Press, New York.

53. Helander, H. F. (1977): An attempt to correlate functional and morphological data for the gastric parietal cells. *Gastroenterology,* 73:956–957.

54. Hirschowitz, B. I. (1960): Gastric osmolar clearance and ionic barter. Two mechanisms of electrolyte secretions by the human stomach. *J. Appl. Physiol.,* 15:933–938.

55. Hirschowitz, B. I. (1968): Apparent kinetics of histamine dose-responsive gastric water and electrolyte secretion in the dog. *Gastroenterology,* 54:514–522.

56. Hobsley, M., and Silen, W. (1970): The relation between the rate of production of gastric juice and its electrolyte concentrations. *Clin. Sci.,* 39:61–75.

57. Hogben, C. A. M., Kent, T. H., Woodward, P. A., and Sill, A. J. (1974): Quantitative histology of the gastric mucosa: man, dog, cat, guinea pig, and frog. *Gastroenterology,* 67:1143–1154.

58. Hollander, F. (1934): Studies in gastric secretion. V. The composition of gastric juice as a function of its acidity. *J. Biol. Chem.,* 104:33–42.

59. Hollander, F. (1934-5): The composition of pure gastric juice. *Am. J. Dig. Dis.,* 1:319–329.

60. Hollander, F. (1952): Gastric secretion of electrolytes. *Fed. Proc.,* 11:706–714.

61. Hollander, F. (1963): The electrolyte patterns of gastric mucinous secretions: its implications for cystic fibrosis. *Ann. N.Y. Acad. Sci.,* 106:757–766.

62. Hunt, J. N., and Wan, B. (1967): Electrolytes of mammalian gastric juice. In: *Handbook of Physiology, Section 6: Alimentary Canal, Volume II. Secretion,* edited by C. F. Code, pp. 781–804. American Physiological Society, Washington, D.C.

63. Ihre, B. (1938): Human gastric secretion. A quantitative study of gastric secretion in normal and pathological conditions. *Acta Med. Scand. [Suppl.],* 95:1–226.

64. James, A. H. (1957): *The Physiology of Gastric Digestion.* Edward Arnold Ltd., London.

65. Kauffman, G. I., and Grossman, M. I. (1976): Gastric alkaline secretion: Effect of topical and intravenous 16-16 dimethyl prostaglandin E_2. *Gastroenterology,* 76:1165.

66. Lambling, A., Bernier, J. J., Majean, Y., and Badoz-Lambling, J. (1961): Gastric juice in pernicious anaemia. Physico-chemical composition of gastric juice in complete achlorhydria and composition of primary alkaline secretion of the stomach. *Am. J. Dig. Dis.,* 6:629–645.

67. Lee, Y. H., and Thompson, J. H. (1969): Gastric electrolyte secretion during nonsteady-state secretion in gastric fistula rats. *Am. J. Physiol.,* 216:1481–1485.

68. Lifson, N., Varco, R. L., and Visscher, M. B. (1943): Relation between osmotic pressure of gastric juice and its acidity. *Gastroenterology,* 1:784–802.

69. Linde, S., and Obrink, K. J. (1950): On behaviour of electrolytes in gastric juice induced by histamine. *Acta Physiol. Scand.,* 21:54–60.

70. Linde, S., Teorell, T., and Obrink, K. J. (1947): Experiments on the primary acidity of the gastric juice. *Acta Physiol. Scand.,* 14:220–231.

71. Lindner, A. E., Cohen, N., Dreiling, D. A., and Janowitz, H. D. (1963): Electrolyte changes in the human stomach following instillation of acid solutions. *Clin. Sci.,* 25:195–205.

72. Makhlouf, G. M. (1965): The action of gastrin II on gastric secretion in man. Doctoral dissertation, University of Edinburgh.

73. Makhlouf, G. M. (1968): The relationship between secretory rate, acid and potassium concentration in gastric secretion. In: *The Physiology of Gastric Secretion,* edited by L. S. Semb and J. S. Myren, pp. 546–551. Universitetsforlaget, Oslo.

74. Makhlouf, G. M. (1968): Measures of gastric acid secretion in man. *Gastroenterology,* 55:423–429.

75. Makhlouf, G. M. (1971): Direct evidence of isoosmotic gastric secretion. *Gastroenterology,* 60:784.

76. Makhlouf, G. M. (1972): Osmotic volume flow in isolated frog gastric mucosa. *Fed. Proc.,* 31:964.

77. Makhlouf, G. M. (1973): Determinants of the permeability to acid of gastric mucosa in vitro. *Gastroenterology,* 64:866.

78. Makhlouf, G. M. (1974): A model for the passive transport of potassium by the stomach: evidence from in vitro studies. *Am. J. Physiol.,* 227:1285–1288.

79. Makhlouf, G. M., and Duckworth, G. R. (1973): Secretion and electrical activity of a unilateral in vitro gastric mucosa. *Gastroenterology,* 65:907–911.

80. Makhlouf, G. M., McManus, J. P. A., and Card, W. I. (1966): A quantitative statement of the two-component hypothesis of gastric secretion. *Gastroenterology,* 51:149–171.

81. Makhlouf, G. M., Moore, E. W., and Blum, A. L. (1970): Undissociated acidity of human gastric juice: Measurement and relationship to protein buffers. *Gastroenterology,* 58:345–351.

82. Makhlouf, G. M., and Rehm, W. S. (1974): Gastric secretion in amphibia. In: *Chemical Zoology, Vol. IX,* edited by Marcel Florkin and Bradley T. Scheer, Academic Press, New York.

83. Makhlouf, G. M., and Yau, W. M. (1973): Osmotic flow into and out of acid gastric solutions. *Fed. Proc.,* 32:907.

84. Marks, I. N., Komarov, S. A., and Shay, H. (1960): Maximal acid secretory response to histamine and its relation to the parietal cell mass in the dog. *Am. J. Physiol.,* 199:579–588.

85. Milton, G. W., Skyring, A. K., and George, G. P. (1963): Histamine secretory tests in cats: an evaluation of results based upon Hollander's two-component theory. *Gastroenterology,* 44:642–653.

86. Moody, F. G. (1971): Waster movement through canine stomach during thiocyanate inhibition of gastric acid secretion. *Am. J. Physiol.,* 220:467–471.

87. Moody, F. G. (1972): Water flow through gastric secretory mucosa. In: *Gastric Secretion,* edited by G. Sachs, E. Heinz, and K. Ulbrich, pp. 432–452. Academic Press, New York.

88. Moody, F. G., and Davis, W. L. (1970): Hydrogen and sodium permeation of canine gastric mucosa during histamine and sodium thiocyanate administration. *Gastroenterology,* 59:350–357.

89. Moody, F. G., and Durbin, R. P. (1965): Effect of glycine and other instillates on concentrations of gastric acid. *Am. J. Physiol.,* 209:122–126.

90. Moody, F. G., and Durbin, R. P. (1969): Water flow induced by osmotic and hydrostatic pressure in the stomach. *Am. J. Physiol.,* 217:255–261.

91. Moore, E. W., and Makhlouf, G. M. (1968): Calcium in normal human gastric juice: A 4-component model with speculation on the relation of calcium to pepsin secretion. *Gastroenterology,* 55:465–481.

92. Nordgren, B. (1958): Aspects of gastric acid secretion in man. *Acta Med. Scand.,* 161:221–231.

93. Nordgren, B. (1963): The rate of secretion and electrolyte content of normal gastric juice. *Acta Physiol. Scand. [Suppl. 202],* 58:1–83.

94. O'Brien, P., Rosen, L., Trencis-Buck, L., and Silen, W. (1977): Distribution of carbonic anhydrase within the gastric mucosa. *Gastroenterology,* 72:870–874.

95. Obrink, K. J. (1948): Studies on the kinetics of the parietal secretion of the stomach. *Acta Physiol. Scand. [Suppl. 51],* 15:1–106.

96. Obrink, K. J., and Waller, M. (1965): The transmucosal migration of water and hydrogen ions in the stomach. *Acta Physiol. Scand.,* 63:175–185.

97. Obrink, K. J., and Waller, M. (1967): Potassium in gastric juice under non-steady-state conditions. *Scand. J. Gastroenterol.,* 2:44–48.

98. Pavlov, I. P. (1902): *The Work of the Digestive Glands,* translated by W. H. Thompson. Charles Griffin, London.

99. Rehm, W. S., Butler, C. F., Spangler, S. G., and Sanders, S. S. (1970): A model to explain uphill water transport in the mammalian stomach. *J. Theor. Biol.,* 27:433–453.

100. Rehm, W. S., Schlesinger, H., and Dennis, W. H. (1953): Effect of osmotic gradients on water transport, hydrogen ion and chloride ion production in the resting and secreting stomach. *Am. J. Physiol.,* 175:473–486.

101. Reitemeier, R. J., Code, C. F., and Orvis, A. L. (1957): Barrier offered by gastric mucosa of healthy persons to absorption of sodium. *J. Appl. Physiol.,* 10:261.

102. Rosemann, R. (1907): Contributions to the physiology of digestion. The properties and composition of the dog's gastric juice obtained by sham-feeding. *Pflegers Arch. Ges. Physiol.,* 118:467–524.

103. Rudick, J., Werther, J. L., Chapman, M. L., and Janowitz, H. D. (1970): Ionic flux across the gastric mucosa: effects of atropine on the permeability of fundus and antrum. *Proc. Soc. Exp. Biol. Med.,* 135:605–608.

104. Rune, S. J., and Henriksen, F. W. (1969): Carbon dioxide tensions in the proximal part of the canine gastrointestinal tract. *Gastroenterology,* 56:758–762.

105. Sanders, S. S., Shanbour, L. L., and Rehm, W. S. (1970): Resistance changes of in vitro frog gastric mucosa bathed in very hyptonic fluids. *Biophys. Soc. Abstr.,* 10:32a.

106. Schiessel, R. (1980): Prostaglandin stimulated gastric chloride transport: Possible key to cytoprotection. *Nature (in press).*

107. Shay, H., Komarov, S. A., Siplet, H., and Fels, S. S. (1946): A gastric mucigogue action of the alkyl sulfates. *Science,* 103(2663):50–52.

108. Skillman, J. J., and Silen, W. (1972): Gastric mucosal barrier. *Surg. Annu.,* 4:213–237.

109. Spenney, K. G., Flemström, G., Shoemaker, R. L., and Sachs, G. (1974): The antral "barrier." *Gastroenterology,* 66:781A.

110. Teorell, T. (1939): On the permeability of the stomach mucosa for acids and some other substances. *J. Gen. Physiol.,* 23:263–274.

111. Teorell, T. (1947): Electrolyte diffusion in relation to the acidity regulation of the gastric juice. *Gastroenterology,* 9:425–443.

112. Terner, C. (1949): The reduction of gastric acidity by back-diffusion of hydrogen ions through the mucosa. *Biochem. J.,* 45:150–158.

113. Thjodleifsson, B., and Wormsley, K. G. (1977): Back-diffusion—fact or fiction? *Digestion,* 15:53–72.

114. Thull, N. B., and Rehm, W. S. (1956): Composition and osmolarity of gastric juice as a function of plasma osmolarity. *Am. J. Physiol.,* 185:317–324.

115. Toby, C. G. (1936): Effect of different types of stimuli on the composition of gastric juice. *Q. J. Exp. Physiol.,* 26:45–57.

116. Van Geertruyden, J., and Dejardin, N. (1964): Les lois de la secretion des ions Ca^{++} et Mg^{++} par la muqueuse gastrique. *Acta Gastroenterol. Belg.,* 27:409–415.

117. Villegas, L. (1963): Equivalent pore radius in the frog gastric mucosa. *Biochim. Biophys. Acta,* 75:131–134.

118. Villegas, L. (1963): Action of histamine on the permeability of the frog gastric mucosa to potassium and water. *Biochim. Biophys. Acta,* 75:377–386.

119. Winship, D. H., and Robinson, J. E. (1974): Acid loss in the human duodenum. *Gastroenterology,* 66:181–188.

Physiology of the Gastrointestinal Tract, edited by
Leonard R. Johnson. Raven Press, New York © 1981.

Chapter 19

Physiology of the Parietal Cell

G. Sachs and T. Berglindh

In recent years, the establishment of the chemiosmotic mechanism as central to biological energy conservation (113) and the key role of proton gradients in the theory has resulted in a resurgence of interest in the H^+ secretory process in the gastric mucosa. This chapter is not intended to be an exhaustive review of the extensive literature on gastric acid secretion but rather attempts to explain the known tissue characteristics by means of a series of hypotheses for an understanding of the basis for current trends in gastric research. It should be understandable to the general biologist or student; where possible, electrical and mathematical models have been avoided and the original literature references used instead.

Detailed descriptions of gastric phenomena are not presented; instead wider, general biological principles are included. The general approach is selective and depends on the prejudices of the authors; it should not be viewed as always true but as one alternative. In terms of the phenomenology of gastric acid secretion, we describe the cell types present in the tissue, histology and ultrastructure of the parietal cell, stimuli of acid secretion, products of the gastric mucosa associated with acid secretion, and electrical characteristics of the mucosa. Some of these topics are described in more detail elsewhere in this volume but with different emphases.

STRUCTURE OF THE GASTRIC MUCOSA

The stomach is divided into two general functional portions: the fundus and the antrum. The former has been shown to secrete acid, the latter to be involved in the secretion of hormones. (We refer to the antrum only occasionally, since our major emphasis is on acid secretion.)

The epithelium in the gastric fundus is a single layer of various cell types that is highly infolded, forming glands buried in the stomach wall. These glands communicate with the gastric lumen through pits that open onto the luminal surface. More than one gastric gland is associated with a single pit; thus, when viewed from the lumen, the pit with its associated glands has the appearance of a tree, with three to five main branches. This infolding effectively increases the surface area of the stomach about 20-fold. A macroscopic mucosal area of 1 cm^2 would have an actual cellular area of 20 cm^2. The actual membrane area producing acid is even greater due to the further infolding of the apical surface of the parietal cells of the gastric gland.

The cells in the gastric fundus also vary in terms of their location. The gastric surface is composed of a uniform layer of mucus-secreting cells named surface epithelial cells. The gastric pits are partially lined by these cells, which are then gradually replaced by a larger cell type, mucous neck cells. Little is known of the function of mucous neck cells except that they are considered to be the stem cells of the epithelium, i.e., the dividing cell which differentiates into the other major cell types in the gastric lining (87).

The gastric glands are composed of two major cell types: the pepsinogen-secreting chief cells and the parietal cells. The parietal cell, as indicated by its name, is placed peripherally and is conical to allow insertion into the core of the gland and to communicate with the lumen of the gland. The gland is inserted into a network of capillaries, thus assuring the blood supply to this area of the tissue. There is also complex innervation of the gastric glands where nerve fibers arising from the intramural plexus contact both the parietal and peptic cells. There is evidence that several neurotransmitters, such as acetylcholine (ACh) and epinephrine, modulate the function of the cells, and paracrine cells are also present.

The questions raised by this tissue structure are multiple. Which cell type is responsible for HCl secretion? Which cell is responsible for transepithelial Cl$^-$ or Na$^+$ transport? What forces determine the movement of solvent from gland lumen to gastric surface? These must be answered, and most are discussed herein.

ULTRASTRUCTURE OF THE PARIETAL CELL

The histological and ultrastructural appearance of the parietal cell undergoes large changes from rest to acid secretion (164). This finding alone has classified it as the cell in the gastric mucosa responsible for secreting acid.

The cell is shaped like a cone or pyramid and is inserted into the gastric gland so that the basolateral surface extends out from the wall of the cylindrical gland. Ultrastructurally, it contains large numbers of mitochondria, which account for about 34% of the cell volume (73). Since gastric secretion requires considerable energy input, the parietal cell is likely involved in the elaboration of acid.

Evident at the light microscope level is the presence of an infolding of the apical plasma membrane, termed the intracellular or secretory canaliculus. The special nature of this structure and the large H$^+$ gradient generated by the stomach clearly suggest an association between the canaliculus and transport.

Electron microscopy shows that at rest, the cytoplasm is filled with smooth membrane structures named tubulovesicles. During secretion, these structures decrease in number and are replaced by an expansion of the secretory canaliculus in the form of microvilli (73). It is important to establish the mechanism whereby this morphological transformation occurs and what it represents. The occurrence of this transformation has been interpreted to indicate that secretory canaliculus plays a vital role in acid secretion. In its active form, the structural appearance of the parietal cell is not unique. The KCl-secreting cell of insect malpighian tubule or midgut (3,20) and the Cl$^-$ cell of the fish gill (121) resemble the parietal cell, although the morphological changes between rest and secretion have not been shown to occur in those cells.

The massive infolding of the apical membranes of the parietal cell has an additional multiplying effect on the effective surface area of the gastric mucosa. In addition to the infolding due to the gastric glands, the amplification factor by the apical membranes is about 10. The change that occurs between rest and secretion also affects the electrical resistance of the mucosa. For example, if the gastric secretion were due to an electrogenic process with its associated conductance, there would be a fall in resistance when such a pump was activated. If, on the other hand, there were an increase in surface area (assuming constant resistance per unit), this would also result in a fall of resistance. A decrease in resistance associated with the onset of acid secretion is not evidence for electrogenicity of the acid secretory process. To support an electrogenic concept, one must know the resistance of the unit area of the secretory canalicular membrane and the numerical value of the area expansion term and show that the resistance decrease exceeds the theoretically expected fall by a significant margin. If the resistance decrease corresponds exactly to the predicted value on the basis of area, this may be interpreted as evidence against an electrogenic mechanism for acid secretion on the assumption that the apical membrane of the resting gastric parietal cell does not contain inactive pump units that are turned in upon stimulation.

STIMULATION OF ACID SECRETION

Three main groups of secretagogues have been studied: histamine, peptides (e.g, gastrin), and ACh or more stable cholinergic compounds. They differ from species to species in terms of the composition of the secretion elicited. In man but not in dog, for example, histamine induces pepsin secretion, whereas gastrin and cholinergic substances stimulate both acid and pepsin secretion in all species studied (68,78).

In recent years, an insight into the complexity of parietal cell receptors has been provided by the use of the newly developed histamine H_2 receptor antagonists. It had been recognized for many years that the classic antihistamines had no effect on histamine or other secretagogue-mediated secretion *in vivo* (94). The H_2 antagonists, however, have been shown to be effective as acid secretory inhibitors (25). These compounds inhibit secretion *in vivo* regardless of origin, supporting the idea that the histamine pathway is common to all acid secretory stimulation.

Another common event resulting from secretory stimulation is the increase of gastric blood flow. The anatomy of the gastric circulation allows blood flow across the gastric wall without significant supply to the gastric glands. Stimulation not only increments the total blood perfusing the stomach but also results in a redistribution of the flow so that the gland cells are supplied (85).

The intact stomach is subject to neural control as well as to direct secretagogue stimulation. The effectiveness of antimuscarinic agents in reducing stimulation elicited by insulin (81) or 2-deoxyglucose (80) has provided evidence that one of the neurogenic stimuli is cholinergic in nature and is vagally mediated.

On the other hand, recent evidence on isolated rabbit gastric glands demonstrates that a major mediator of peptic secretion is cyclic AMP (cAMP). The level of this second messenger is augmented by β-agonists, and pepsin secretion thus induced is blocked by β-antagonists (94).

GASTRIC SECRETION

From the time of Beaumont, the acid component of gastric secretion has been of central interest. Under a variety of conditions, the HCl content approximates 160 mM, being essentially isotonic to plasma. The composition of gastric juice during brisk secretion as compared to the resting secretion shows that there is an increase in HCl at the expense of NaCl, with KCl remaining fairly constant. At full secretion, the only major cation present in addition to H^+ is K^+. In the absence of secretion of acid, there also appears to be active secretion of alkali, in the form of HCO_3^-. In addition to these inorganic contents, the secreted juice is rich in organic solutes, such as mucus and pepsin.

Based solely on the concentration of acid found in gastric juice, this must be due to active transport. The pH gradient from blood to lumen is 6.6. In electrical terms, this can be translated to a potential across the membrane of 400 mV, a potential not found anywhere in mammalian biology. In contrast, the concentration of other cations does not require the presence of active pumps oriented transepithelially. The transport of Cl^- determines the orientation of the transepithelial potential difference (PD). In the intact mucosa, the PD is between 30 and 60 mV lumen negative. This implies an active transport for Cl^-; however, the transport of this ion may not be active but secondary to other active processes. The reason for this cautious conclusion is that the epithelial cells of this tissue are polarized with different properties in the apical and basolateral surfaces. Such differences can result in secondary active transport of a given solute across the whole epithelium.

ELECTRICAL CHARACTERISTICS

The presence of a transepithelial PD is mentioned above. The orientation, lumen negative, must be due to active secretion of an anion or active reabsorption of a cation. The PD drops upon stimulation of acid. It was recognized that this drop is most likely due to the appearance of HCl secretion and the considerable diffusion potential between isotonic saline and 0.16 M HCl (135). When this diffusion potential is taken into account, there are no changes in PD; at first analysis, this finding argues against the induction of an electrogenic H^+ pump. The lack of change of PD, however, could be due to the simultaneous and equal stimulation of an electrogenic H^+ and electrogenic Cl^- pump (or an inward electrogenic cation pump).

The existence of cell junctions affects the properties of an epithelium in predictable fashion. Originally these were labeled by anatomists as tight junctions. It is now recognized that in several epithelia, these junctions are not tight but are leaky to ions (59). Often this leak, now termed the paracellular pathway, is the major route for ion movement across the tissue. In the gastric fundus, however, it has been shown that only 20% of tissue conductance originates from the tight junctions (174). This value rises to 80% in the antrum (173). Accordingly, the fundic mucosa can be classified as a tight epithelium, the antrum as moderately leaky.

As in other epithelia, gap junctions (desmosomes) exist, allowing both electrical and chemical communication between cells (106). Such communication exists between surface epithelial cells and between glandular cells; intercommunication between these two cell classes in the stomach has not yet been established.

Changes in electrical resistance of an epithelium can provide information about ion pathways (i.e., whether ion flow is cellular or paracellular) and can determine whether onset of secretion is associated with activation of an electrogenic pump. Such a pump must be reversible with respect not only to ion gradients but also to the electrical PD across the pump-containing membrane. Hence with onset of secretion, resistance should fall, as in fact it does. The change in surface area occurring with onset of secretion makes suspect the conclusion, derived from resistive changes, that the H^+ pump is electrogenic.

Given that an epithelium is ohmic (that is, that the voltage current curve is linear), the measurements of PD and resistance are sufficient to calculate the current generated. The origin of the current can be assigned by measuring ion fluxes in the absence of external driving forces for the ions (184). This is done by clamping the transepithelial voltage at zero and measuring the current necessary to achieve this. This current, termed the short-circuit current, must exactly balance the ion current generated by the tissue. The unidirectional flux of one or more ions must be greater in one direction than in the other, resulting in net flux. In the case of the stomach, two ions show net fluxes when short-circuited: Cl^- toward the lumen, Na^+ toward the blood or serosal side (82). The latter net flux is absent in some species. By definition, therefore, transport of these two ions is active. Based simply on this fact, we cannot define the active transport as primary or secondary; more information is needed.

The secreting stomach has an additional flux of HCl not eliminated by short-circuiting. Thus the equation relating short-circuit current and ion fluxes can be written as:

$$I_{SC} = [J_{Cl_{S-M}} - J_{Cl_{M-S}}] - J_{H_{S-M}} + [J_{Na_{M-S}} - J_{Na_{S-M}}]$$

The current or flux terms must be in equivalent units; 1 μmole net flux of a monovalent ion is equivalent to 26.8 μAmps current.

The measurement of ion fluxes also allows assessment of the nature of the ion pathways across the tissue. Thus if the ion flux is exactly equivalent to that predicted from the electrical resistance, it can be concluded that ion flow is conductive. If, on the other hand, the ion flux exceeds the predicted amount, then a proportion of the ion flow is through electrically silent pathways, such as electroneutral cotransport or exchange. In the stomach, Cl^- flux exceeds the predicted amount considerably (47), showing that much of the flux of this ion is electrically silent.

ENERGETICS

Historically, two primary energy sources have been considered for ion transport in mammalian cells, namely, ATP and oriented redox systems (75), leading to the dual suggestion for the energy source for H^+ secretion, an ATPase or a redox pump. One of the earliest observations was the absolute O_2 dependence of acid secretion (42). This observation has led to a reluctance to accept a completely ATP-dependent H^+ pump, although redox processes occurring across the plasma membranes of mammalian cells have not yet been established.

SUMMARY

Many facets of the gastric epithelium must be developed beyond the descriptive; fortunately, the field has progressed to the point that satisfying explanations can be given for many of the phenomena outlined above. These explanations rest mostly on the development of mammalian *in vitro* gastric models. It is appropriate, therefore, to begin our more detailed description by discussing the models available and their advantages and limitations.

MODELS FOR THE STUDY OF GASTRIC PHYSIOLOGY

To understand the mechanism of any of the complex processes outlined above, simplification is essential.

Intact Tissue

The first effort made many decades ago was to depart from the standard procedure of measuring acid secretion in the living animal by gastric fistulas or gastric suction and to exteriorize the stomach with the circulation intact, providing the dog flap preparation (132). This allows direct measurement of PD. Since the serosal side still cannot be controlled, the short-circuit technique can be applied only with difficulty. This technique was followed by the use of amphibian mucosa in Ussing chambers. Here the muscle layer is removed and the epithelium with its associated connective tissue is used to separate two solutions of defined composition. In this preparation, not only are acid secretion, ion flux, PD, and resistance directly accessible, but short-circuiting is straightforward (67,184). The trade-off in the increased precision of both the dog flap and Ussing chamber methods is the loss of the ability to study the neurogenic component of acid secretion. The problem of easy access to the nutrient surface of many cell types also remains. For example, many ionophores of proven effectiveness are apparently ineffective in the frog gastric mucosa (91). Since there is no reduction in the cell types present, the secretory and electrical contributions of each individual cell type cannot be discriminated. On the other hand, although the development of chamber techniques for mammalian mucosae has been slow, guinea pig (116), piglet (57), and, to a lesser degree, mature rats (119) provide relatively viable preparations. In some instances, the data provided from a given model raise questions as to techniques used or uniqueness of species. A case in point is the claim that rabbit mucosa actively secretes Na^+ when short-circuited (59). This is different from the other preparations studied and is difficult to explain based on known pump properties.

More sophisticated use of either the dog flap or the Ussing chamber preparation is provided by microelectrodes (29,173,174). This allows measurements independently of the electrical properties of different cell types and of the apical and basolateral membranes of these cell types. With the development of ion-specific electrodes (i.e., Na^+, K^+, Cl^-, Ca^{2+}, and H^+), the activity of these ions in the cells can also be measured (4,117). Less easy are measurements of the more deeply located cells, such as parietal cells. In fact, one is forced to resort to dye marking techniques where the dye is electrophoresed into the cell during electrically defined puncture in order to label the cell type being studied. Since the marked cell must be found subsequently in frozen section, this increases significantly the difficulty of measurement and reduces the number of measurements that can be made. Another problem often encountered is the poor visualization due to the presence of secreted mucus. Nevertheless, microelectrode technique has provided some insights into the electrical structure of the stomach when applied to the intact tissue (173,174).

As an example, the use of microelectrodes has shown that the relative resistance of the apical and basal surfaces of the surface epithelial cell are about equal, that the basal surface is selectively permeable to K^+ and Cl^-, and that paracellular conductance makes only a minor contribution to the conductance of the epithelium.

Isolated Cells

Even in a well-functioning *in vitro* gastric mucosa, there are many difficult problems. In the mammal and perhaps even in the amphibian, the effectiveness of gas exchange is a vital question, namely, to provide adequate access of O_2 to avoid the presence of an anaerobic core, and the exchange of CO_2/HCO_3 to avoid excessive pH changes in the cell which may produce unrecognized artifacts. Biochemical experiments on the entire mucosa restrict the number of samples that can be taken; dose response curves require a large number of animals; allocation of membrane properties to a given cell type requires purification of that cell and its membranes, which is difficult if the starting material is the heterocellular intact tissue. For these and other reasons, the development of cell and gland isolation techniques has occupied investigators more and more. For stomach, the choice of techniques has been reduced to the use of enzymes, such as pronase or collagenase (12). The latter permits the production of gastric glands or, when used in conjunction with Ca^{2+} chelating agents, such as EGTA, isolated cells. Pronase alone (27) or subsequent to collagenase will also yield isolated cells.

If the starting material is the intact mucosa, a mixture of all cells present will be obtained, whereas a partial purification with mainly parietal and peptic cells is obtained using isolated gastric glands. In the choice between working with a gland preparation or a cell preparation, one must consider the problems to be studied and the tools that can be provided. As explained below, there are means of studying acid formation in cells even in a mixed preparation. The glands represent a more intact system with tight junctions, maintained polarization of the cells, normal shape of the cells, and cell-to-cell communication. Since the glands have been prepared with less abuse, this preparation is sturdy, with minimal cell death even after long incubations. The glands in themselves represent an enrichment in parietal cells from 20% in the intact mucosa to 50% by volume; they are the preparation of choice when studying specific cell functions that can be discriminated in a mixed cell population.

For such studies as amino acid uptake, ion fluxes, biochemical constituents in one particular cell type, and cell specific receptors, we must turn to purified isolated cells.

To separate single cell types from a mixed cell population, either different mass of the cells (138,170) or different electric charge or variation of antigenic structure have been used or proposed. Currently, there appear to be three accepted methods for enrichment of a given cell type in adequate yield: (a) The production of gastric glands automatically enriches the parietal cell population from 20 to 50%. (b) The step gradient purification of rat cells using Percoll produces the highest purity of viable parietal cells yet published (138). (c) The use of the elutriator rotor where solvent flow is used to fix the position of a cell type in a centrifugal field has been useful in dissecting some vexing problems, such as the cell response to prostaglandins (188).

A major drawback in isolated tissue and cell techniques is the maintenance of function. In the chambered preparation, measurement of acid secretion in response to hormones is convenient. In cell or gland suspensions, the measurement of pH changes in the medium is generally not useful, since the H^+ produced results in the equivalent production of OH^- or HCO_3^-. Thus any net change of medium pH must be due to an unequal rate of release of one of these, which can only be transient, or to compartment storage of either H^+ or OH^-. Clearly, without a measure of the generation of H^+ gradients, isolated gland or cell technology would be of limited value. Since we have excluded medium pH changes as a reasonable method, measurement of a low pH compartment is the only alternative. In isolated glands, the canaliculus of the parietal cell and the lumen of the gland would be expected to be the site of such compartments.

Theoretically, weak bases with a suitable pK_a could be used to monitor low pH comparments. Ideally, we should use a base that is unprotonated and uncharged at pH 7; furthermore, it should be lipid soluble at that pH so that it can cross biological membranes. Finally, if it enters a compartment where the pH is lower than the pK_a, the subsequently formed protonated species of the base should be lipid impermeable and thus trapped in the compartment. A weak base that comes reasonably close to these specifications is aminopyrine (12). The pH of the trapping compartment can be calculated, provided its volume is known. The distribution of weak base between compartment and medium must be determined. Hence a radioactive weak base is the most convenient for multiple sample handling, or a weak base that changes optical properties upon concentration would be convenient for continuous recording. Optical probes that have been used in vesicle studies include 9-aminoacridine (142) and acridine orange (43).

In gastric cells or glands, we expect a large pH gradient. Therefore, a weak base with a low pK_a would be particularly useful, avoiding excessive accumulation. For example, a weak base of pK_a 9 added to cells incubated in a pH 7 medium, if the cells contained an acid compartment of pH 1, would be concentrated 1 million-fold; on the other hand, a weak base, such as aminopyrine, would be concentrated only 10,000-fold since its pK_a is 5. No accumulation of aminopyrine would take place in a compartment with a pH greater than 5. Probes with a higher pK_a occasionally must be used at low rates of acid secretion to determine the acidity of a compartment with pH between 5 and 7.4.

Isolated parietal cells also accumulate weak bases, showing that the acid compartment cannot solely be the gland lumen (although this may be partially responsible), but that an intracellular compartment also is involved. Isolated cells often show a closed apical membrane, thereby making an intracellular space where acid can accumulate. These weak base probes are the single most important criterion of gastric parietal cell viability, both qualitatively (i.e., is there any weak base ac-

cumulation.[2]) and quantitatively (i.e., what accumulation ratio is actually achieved?). The weak base accumulation should also be sensitive to hormones at physiological levels, thereby providing a secondary criterion of viability. In addition, an increase in oxygen consumption associated with stimulation is a valuable criterion in that it will increase in proportion to increased acid secretory rates. Finally, the morphological status of the preparation provides an index of the quality of the preparation at the light and especially at the electron microscopic level. It must be emphasized that without these criteria, isolated cell or gland preparations may provide anomalous data. The accumulation of weak base in an acid compartment does not necessarily provide a direct index of the rate of acid secretion but rather is a measure of the concentration of sequestered acid in a specific space.

Isolated Glands as a Morphological Tool

Isolated glands or cells lend themselves to observation by nondestructive microscopic techniques. Of particular use is differential interference contrast microscopy (Nomarski optics). This gives an apparent three-dimensional image with a narrow focal plane permitting optical sectioning of a living cell.

The morphological transformation from rest to secretion in parietal cells in glands has been observed (9). From displaying a fairly featureless image in the resting state, the addition of histamine induces formation of vacuoles in the cytoplasm of the parietal cell within 10 min. However, the morphological transformation either seen as an increase in the secretory membrane surface as in the electron microscope or in vacuoles under Nomarski is not proof of the presence of HCl. In fact, no one has ever shown that the parietal cell is the source of acid secretion. We have tried to approach that question, i.e., the source of the acid, in two different ways: (a) If aminopyrine in the millimolar range were added to glands, it might accumulate in a low pH space to an extent exceeding isoosmolarity, provided acid formation continued. This would induce a swelling of that space, which might be observed with Nomarski techniques. In the presence of high extracellular aminopyrine concentration, vacuoles appeared in unstimulated parietal cells, much like the histamine condition. These artificially induced vacuoles did not appear in the presence of SCN^-, thereby indicating that the presence of acid was essential for the induced swelling. (b) The fluorescent probe acridine orange has weak base properties and will accumulate on the acid side of a pH gradient. When accumulated in sufficiently high concentrations, the dye changes its emission spectrum from green to red. The addition of acridine orange to unstimulated glands resulted in a homogenous green fluorescence of the parietal cells as viewed by fluorescent microscopy. Following stimulation of the glands, deep red areas appeared, always starting at the base of the cell. Combination of fluorescence and Nomarski optics showed that the red areas totally coincided with the vacuoles seen in strict Nomarski. The red acridine orange fluorescence did not appear under SCN⁻ conditions or disappeared upon addition of SCN⁻.

From these *in vitro* morphological studies, we can conclude that the parietal cell and more specifically the secretory cannaliculus is the origin of acid production. The astonishing morphological changes induced by aminopyrine raises questions as to the mechanism of morphological transformation. The prevailing hypothesis suggests a recycling of membranes where tubulovesicles fuse and form an enlarged secretory surface. An alternative possibility is that the resting parietal cell contains a network of collapsed canaliculi which, upon stimulation, would swell and fill most of the cytoplasmic space (9). The parietal localization of the parietal cell might thus be explained by its need to expand upon stimulation. In the isolated gland, the parietal cell can expand freely without counteracting forces, permitting the intracellular channels to swell and form vacuoles. In the intact mucosa, the general structure and supporting tissue would prevent any extensive swelling of the cell, thereby forcing the canalicular content into the lumen of the gland. This hypothetical train of events could not take place if the acid-secreting cell were embedded as a rigid structure in the glandular body. These aspects are outlined in Fig. 1.

Isolated Membranes

Despite the many advantages of isolated cell systems, the cell internal environment is in general self regulating. Thus, for example, to attempt to establish the energetic basis of acid secretion using ATP measurements may be futile since the ATP level is maintained constant despite large variations in energy demand. It is an advantage at times to be able to study isolated membranes, especially if duality of function can be preserved. This duality of function implies an enzyme, such as an ATPase, and a transport activity in response to the addition of ATP, as well as a receptor activity in terms of ligand binding coupled to a function in terms of production or flux of second messenger. Understanding of the molecular mechanism of any process requires purification beyond the cell level and must begin by purification of the membrane of interest.

The presence of a given activity can usually be followed. Transport activity is amenable to direct measurement in terms of gradients generated. In general, the electrical events in conjunction with transport in membrane vesicles can also be established. Measurement of either ΔpH or ΔPD rests on either the distribution of weak base or weak acid consistent with the principles outlined above or on the distribution of lipid-permeable ions based on electrophoretic movement of the ion dependent on the PD across the vesicle membrane. Vesicular potentials can either be spontaneous or created by ionophores.

It is often possible to purify membrane vesicles containing essentially only pump protein, but the protein or activity of interest is usually only a minor constituent of the isolated membrane. To advance further in our understanding of the mechanism at the protein level, it is necessary to go beyond membrane purification and to isolate a particular protein or group of proteins from the membrane. This necessitates eventual solubilization of the protein with consequent loss of an identifiable function that depends on the presence of a membrane-limited boundary. To restore the transport function, we

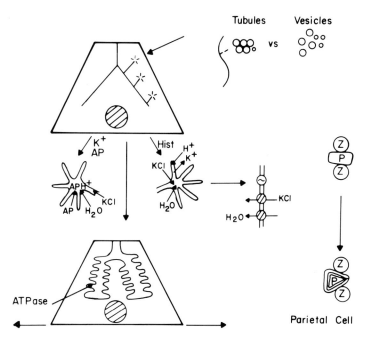

FIG. 1. Conceptual model of the transformation of the resting to the secreting parietal cell. The resting intracellular membranes are visualized as collapsed tubules, and stimulation results in expansion due perhaps to KCl influx and communication with the medium.

must reinsert the protein not only into a lipid bilayer but into a bilayer that separates two solutions. This technique is known as reconstitution and can be performed either in artificial vesicles (liposomes) or planar films separating two bulk solutions (black lipid films). In the former case, net transport is measured, as in the case of natural membrane vesicles; in the latter, basically the same electrical measurements can be carried out as are performed in Ussing chambers, namely PD, resistance, and current. In addition, the high resistance of black lipid membranes allows the detection of electrical events that are too small to be detected in intact epithelia, where the background resistance is much lower, and changes of conductance due to opening and closing of channels are not measurable without sophisticated noise analysis techniques (177).

SUMMARY

Some of the techniques that have been applied in studies of the stomach are outlined. Increasingly simplified models facilitate our ability to explain the phenomena found. On the other hand, we often lose sight of the subtle regulatory processes present in the intact animal and may be misled as to the prominence of a process by its ease of study in isolated form.

It is essential to refer back to the intact animal or at least to intact tissue data to see whether or not the information obtained in isolated cells or organelles makes both mechanistic and physiological sense. The development of a consistent picture at all levels of analysis is a major goal of current research.

STIMULUS SECRETION COUPLING IN THE PARIETAL CELL

Receptors

Gastric acid secretion is hormonally regulated and can be evoked in a number of ways. It is now well established that the initial action of a hormone on its target cell is binding to a receptor on or in the cell. This binding reaction initiates a complex series of events increasing cAMP or cGMP levels or changing Ca^{2+} pools in the cell.

Receptors and the complexes in which they reside are probably multimeric proteins with considerable hydrophobic interaction with the membrane. For this reason, receptors, catalytic or conductance units, or coupling factors have not yet been purified to homogeneity.

The types of studies that must be performed to define a system, short of purification of the components, involve binding measurements, cyclase activation, Ca^{2+} and other electrolyte fluxes and correlation of these events quantitatively and temporally with the physio-

logical response. Many such studies in the field of gastric secretion have only partially fulfilled these criteria. Based on other tissues, some general statements can be made in relation to either cyclase activation or Ca^{2+} permeability modulation.

Studies of hormone-receptor interaction should be conducted with agonists of proven biological activity; the radioligand should have unmodified biological activity. Also, binding studies should always relate membrane and intact cell or system data. The technique used in binding studies is to incubate the labeled ligand with increasing amounts of nonlabeled ligand with the receptor preparation and then to separate bound from unbound hormone. To determine nonspecific binding of the radioligand, an excess of unlabeled ligand (approximately 1,000-fold) is added; the remaining bound activity is denoted as nonspecific binding. The technique used for separation depends on the dissociation constant that applies. High affinity binding is stable for a sufficient time so that filtration, columns, or other techniques are applicable. Lower affinity binding requires centrifugation or dialysis since the half-life of the complex is too short to remain stable during other techniques. The correlation between binding and effect can be performed determining activation of adenylate cyclase or enhancement of Ca^{2+} permeability, preferably in parallel runs. The data obtained in membrane fractions or membrane containing fractions should correlate in terms of effects of binding and requirements for binding to data obtained in intact cells or organs. The data are usually analyzed in terms of binding constants where the affinity is obtained either from equilibrium methods or by measuring the rate of binding and rate of dissociation of the hormone where the affinity is expressed in terms of the ratio of the two rates.

Binding constants have more than physiological importance. If, for example, an antagonist of one activity has an apparent pA_2 of about 9 (i.e., an effective affinity of 10^{-9}) and the same antagonist blocks another activity at a pA_2 of 3, it can be concluded that the receptors to which the antagonist binds in the two systems are not identical. These distinctions are particularly relevant in complex receptor systems with multiple interactions, as appears to be the case with the parietal cell.

There are a large number of hormones that affect acid secretion in terms of either stimulation or inhibition. These may be classified as peptide or nonpeptide, stimulatory or inhibitory; the stimulatory hormones can be identified as histaminic, cholinergic, and peptide types. We discuss those in turn in terms of receptor studies.

Histamine

The role of histamine in acid secretion has been long disputed; because the presence of histamine is universal, its occurrence in the stomach does not instantly classify it as a physiological secretagogue. Destructive enzymes are present in all tissues; hence circulating levels of histamine may bear little relation to its hormonal status. Thus the stated role of histamine as a gastric hormone has oscillated between no role at all or the central role in parietal cell stimulation. The latter attitude is now becoming more prevalent, largely because of the development of a new group of antagonists.

Histamine interacts with many organs in the body, such as the central nervous system (CNS), capillaries, heart, uterus, and stomach. The original antihistamines developed several decades ago were effective in blocking vasodilatory effects of histamine and also had CNS effects (28). Antisecretory activity at acceptable blood levels was minimal. Either the histamine-induced secretion was not a true physiological response, the antihistamine did not reach the receptors, or the histamine receptor in the stomach was different in terms of structural requirements from the histamine receptor in blood vessels (98).

The structure of histamine suggests that there are two sites that may be modified singly or separately, the imidazole ring and the ethylamine side chain. The antihistamines effective against histamine action on smooth muscle show only minimal modification of the side chain, whereas the other components do not have to bear any resemblances to the imidazole ring. If the gastric receptors were indeed different, the gastric antagonist would have as its major modification an alteration in the ethyl amine side chain. Although not this straightforward, this proved to be the case. A series of histamine antagonists is now available which has considerable selectivity in blocking gastric acid secretion and uterine motility and has cardiac effects. These drugs have been classified as H_2 antagonists. Their actions on the stomach have revised attitudes about the gastric receptor and its interaction. The definition of the H_2 receptor to date has involved few binding studies and relied largely on cellular or tissue responses. With this screening method, the synthesis of a variety of histamine analogs and determination of their actions and affinities has given the following generalizations: The

stomach contains an activating receptor which recognizes specific structural features of the imidazole ring. Modification of the latter, for example, by methylation of the 4 position, results in increased selectivity for the gastric as opposed to the ileal receptor. With imidazole or the methylated imidazole, appropriate modification of the side chain results in an antagonist of the histamine action on gastric secretion. The compound now used therapeutically to inhibit acid secretion is cimetidine (Tagamet). Various compounds can be compared in cellular models as well as in intact animals, and some are listed in Table 1. Here the effect of both H_1 and H_2 agonists and antagonists are listed in terms of relative effect on acid secretion in isolated rabbit gastric glands. It can be seen that there is a considerable range of effectiveness either as a stimulus of acid secretion or as an antagonist of histamine-induced acid secretion. Noteworthy also is the finding that there is some antagonism of acid secretion by the H_1 antagonists, contrary to what is found *in vivo;* but this inhibition is not competitive.

These compounds then allow studies to be performed on the histamine receptor itself in gastric cells or gastric membranes. Considerable problems have been experienced in using histamine as the radioligand. The expected affinity would be of the order of 10^{-6}. With such a low affinity, we would have problems in measuring binding. Thus far, however, the major problem is a large nonreceptor-associated background; that is, radioactivity that is not displaced by excess cold histamine represents the major fraction of the total counts found in cells or membrane fractions. In isolated rabbit gastric glands, a histamine uptake system has been detected, which is of such a magnitude that receptor binding studies using histamine as a radioligand are impossible. This uptake system features characteristics resembling those of an amino acid uptake pathway; thus the uptake is energy dependent and Na^+ driven. Addition of an H_2 antagonist in large excess will inhibit further uptake but will not displace any radioactivity associated with the glands (13,14). The uptake seems selective in terms of H_2 agonists; i.e., there is a good correlation between

TABLE 1. *Effect of histamine and analogs on secretory parameters of rabbit gastric glands*[a]

Compound	AP acc[b]	O_2 consumption	cAMP content	Adenylcyclase activity
Cimetidine	6.7	6.7	6.9	6.9
Histamine	5.6	5.6	5.4	5.5
N^α-methylhistamine	5.3	5.3	5.3	5.4
Dimaprit	4.6	4.9	4.8	5.0
4-Methylhistamine	4.5	4.8	4.7	4.5
D,L-tetrahydrozoline	4.4	4.4	4.4	4.3

[a] Values taken from ref. 36.
[b] AP acc, aminopyrine accumulation.
pA2 or pED50 for histamine-like compounds.

acid stimulatory potency and ability to inhibit histamine uptake. H_1 agonists, such as 2-pyridyl-ethylamine (2-PEA), are weak secretagogues and weak inhibitors of histamine uptake (36). On the antagonistic side, the correlation is not as strict, and H_1 antagonists show a high affinity for the uptake pathway.

The radioactive histamine taken up at 10^{-6} M is not readily exchangeable. In fact, if we homogenize glands and subsequently perform a velocity centrifugation, we find an enrichment of radioactive substance in the microsomal pellet obtained at $100,000 \times g$ (60 min). Thin layer chromatography (TLC) shows that less than 10% of this radioactivity is associated with histamine. Thus, at least at low extracellular histamine concentrations, the histamine taken up is to a major extent converted, which would explain why excess of histamine cannot displace accumulated product. In contrast, the uptake of H^3-metiamide (H_2 blocker), which shows the same kinetics as the histamine uptake, can be reversed by excess cold metiamide and is not enriched in the microsomal pellet.

As our knowledge of the uptake system stands today, we cannot define a specific role for it. We know that it cannot be involved in the direct activation of the parietal cell, based on the relatively low affinity of the H_2 antagonists. Two other possibilities emerge: (a) The uptake system is there to remove and inactivate histamine, perhaps via a telemethylation of the imidazole ring. (b) The system is used by the cells to store histamine or converted histamine. It is known that isolated gastric glands do contain a considerable amount of histamine, despite the absence of mast cells. Release of histamine from the glands can be of utmost importance for the stimulatory pattern overall. Finally, a high histamine-forming capacity has been found only in the mucosa of rats, hamsters, and mice, making a histamine-conserving uptake system a speculative but attractive alternative in other species.

Binding of histamine to its receptor must result in activity of the parietal cell. Binding defines only the initial essential step. It is classic to assume that the receptor is on the external face of the membrane for most but not all hormones. The effect of the binding reaction, therefore, must affect membrane properties and subsequently lead to an intracellular reaction. It is presumed that the receptor, by binding the hormone, alters quaternary structure so that a change occurs in a membrane channel or in a regulatory subunit of a membrane bound enzyme, such as adenylate cyclase. This initial conformational change has eluded investigators in any system.

Gastrin Receptor

The demonstration of the existence of gastrin—its isolation, sequence, radioimmunoassay, and description of physiological effects—was the major event in gastric physiology of the 1960s (67). Although radioiodinated gastrin has been available for more than a decade, only recently has an iodinated form with defined biological activity served as a ligand for receptor studies. As before, the methodology is to correlate binding studies with physiological action, using gastrin and gastrin analogs. This has allowed novel studies of this hormone so that its action can be directly related to its binding reaction (181, 182).

Cholinergic Receptors

ACh, which is released from parasympathetic nerve terminals, activates two types of receptors. One, prevalent in the nervous system, is nicotinic in nature and is not involved in acid secretion. The other is classified as muscarinic and is sensitive to atropine with a pA_2 of 9. Since atropine blocks neural and cholinergic agonist activation of acid secretion, the receptor in the stomach is muscarinic (6, 68, 170).

Studies of this receptor type require the use of a specific muscarinic antagonist with sufficient affinity to give significant relative binding. Two compounds have become available with the necessary characteristics: quinuclidinyl [phenyl-4(n)-^{3}H] benzilate (QNB) (190) and N-methyl scopolamine (22). The usual method for detecting specific muscarinic binding is to use the atropine inhibition of binding as assay and then, using various agonists and antagonists, to identify the receptor and compare the ligand binding properties with the properties implied by intact cell or tissue studies. Only recently have such studies been initiated using isolated rat cells as the functional model (51). A problem using QNB has been noted in pancreatic acini. Binding of QNB inactivates the muscarinic receptor; after continued incubation, the quantity of QNB bound remains constant, but the cholinergic reponse returns. This finding suggests that QNB binding data should be viewed with caution.

The binding of ACh should result in a change in membrane properties to facilitate the cell response. What we know about its mechanism sets this receptor apart from the histamine receptor in terms of not only binding of ligand but of secondary effects as well.

Stimulus Transduction

The effect of hormone binding to its receptor is eventually to change the concentration of second messenger in the target cell. The three types of second messenger considered here are the cyclic nucleotides, Ca^{2+}, and prostaglandins.

cAMP and cGMP

There are necessary criteria for establishing cAMP as a second messenger in a hormonal response: (a) cAMP levels should increase in the target cell prior to the response; (b) an adenylate cyclase should be present and activated by the hormone; and (c) cAMP or its permeable derivatives should mimic or potentiate the hormone response (180). It should be emphasized that these criteria are minimal, and their establishment does not necessarily prove the role of cAMP as second messenger or as exclusive second messenger. In some instances, the requirements might be obscured; for example, *in vivo*, secondary factors may obscure the response of a tissue to exogenous cAMP or to phosphodiesterase inhibition. It is also vital that in a heterocellular tissue, the cAMP levels measured are those of the target cell in question; otherwise, misleading data may be obtained.

The number of species in which cAMP involvement in gastric acid secretion has been established is growing. Initially, the frog gastric mucosa *in vitro* showed that theophylline resulted in an increase in acid secretion (1). Necturus gastric mucosa was shown to contain a histamine-sensitive adenylate cyclase (115). This species, often nonsecreting when prepared *in vitro*, responded to the addition of cAMP by onset of acid secretion, as well as to the addition of aminophylline (116). Cyclic nucleotide levels were shown to increase in dog gastric mucosa with onset of secretion (21). Guinea pig (120) and rabbit (180) were the first mammalian species to be shown to contain an histamine-sensitive adenylate cyclase. The data for adenylate cyclase stimulation in the rabbit at the time correlated well with acid secretory responses in the better-studied secretory models of rat and dog for a variety of agonists (179). The adenylate cyclase from rabbit stomach did not discriminate between H_1 and H_2 antagonists as well as expected. More recent data on steady-state cAMP levels in intact frog gastric mucosa did not show correlation between secretion and cAMP levels (35).

At least two major cell types in the intact mucosa may have opposite changes in cAMP in response to secretagogues. In rabbit gastric glands, a study of acid secretion by the aminopyrine uptake method, oxygen consumption, adenylate cyclase activity, and cAMP levels showed for both agonists and antagonists (Table 1) a remarkable linear correlation between any two of the parameters. This is convincing evidence for the role of cAMP as the second messenger for acid secretion in this species (36). Similar conclusions have been made for isolated dog gastric mucosal cells (171). It is probable that with increasing sophistication of measurement, similar data will be obtained for all species.

Further analysis of some of the data relating cAMP levels and acid secretory response show some peculiarities. When the dose response curve for changes in acid secretion and cAMP levels are compared in the presence of the phosphodiesterase inhibitor isobutyl methylxanthine, (IMX), the cAMP level in the presence of inhibitor changed by a greater amount than expected based on acid secretion rates (34).

There are few detailed studies on gastric adenylate cyclase. Our knowledge of the regulation of adenylate cyclase has considerably increased in recent years based on investigation in other tissues. The hormone-sensitive enzyme consists of at least three subunits: the receptor, the enzyme itself, and a regulatory subunit (23). In some instances, the intact system has been solubilized. A diagram of the postulated arrangement of the system is shown in Fig. 2. Of particular interest is the regulatory subunit. This subunit acts as a GTPase and GTP, or analogs, such as GDP-N-P, interact with this subunit and activate the cyclase. It has been suggested that dissociation of bound GDP is required for hormonal stimulation (30). The subunit that is activated by GTP also hydrolyzes its activator, thus being autoinhibitory. Most of these steps have not yet been shown to be present in the gastric mucosa, but the gastric adenylate cyclase has been shown to be activated by GPP-N-P (183).

The histamine-activated cyclase has not yet resulted in definition of the hormone receptor (141). It has been our experience that attempted purification of the crude 3,000 × g precipitate results in loss of histamine-activated cyclase. This could be due to a loss of receptor activity, since the fluoride-stimulated adenylate cyclase remains; or it could be due to a loss of other essential factors involved in the activation. Similar purification of the gastrin receptor allows maintenance of gastrin binding, although whether or not the membrane effect attributable to this binding still persists remains to be elucidated (181,182).

Many details of the regulation of cAMP in the parietal cell are unknown. A similar complex control system may be expected, however, since the major regulatory enzymes, namely, adenylate cyclase and phosphodiesterase, are present in the cell.

Cyclic GMP may also play a role in the hormone response of various cells. Although a guanyl cyclase has been shown to occur in the gastric mucosa (179), cGMP does not seem to influence acid secretion. Rather, there is evidence that this cyclic nucleotide is related to the process of alkali secretion, largely a surface cell property (54). This alkali secretion may be an important defense mechanism for this cell type in the stomach for resisting acid damage.

Neither ACh nor gastrin has been shown to activate gastric adenylate cyclase or to directly affect cAMP

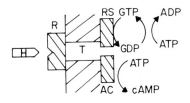

FIG. 2. Model for the H2 receptor in the parietal cell showing the four putative subunits, including the adenylate cyclase (AC) and the GTP regulatory subunit (RS). H, histamine; R, receptor; T, transducer.

levels in the tissue (179). Their second messengers must be other than cAMP.

Ca²⁺

Elevation of cytosolic Ca²⁺ levels is thought to be an alternative means of hormone transduction. Initially, evidence on the role of Ca²⁺ in the gastrointestinal tract was obtained by measurements of the effect on the response of pancreatic amylase release at different medium Ca²⁺ levels (83).

Removal of Ca²⁺ from the medium in gastric glands from rabbit or dog mucosal cells has little effect on the histamine stimulation of acid secretion. In contrast, the response to gastrin or ACh is largely reduced, suggesting that the response of the parietal cell to these hormones involves Ca²⁺.

Definition of the mechanism of Ca²⁺-dependent activation of enzyme secretion in another gastrointestinal tissue, the pancreas, has relied on measurement of changes in Ca²⁺ permeability using ^{45}Ca²⁺ (97). Various workers have shown that with cholinergic or other stimulus, bidirectional fluxes of Ca²⁺ are enhanced, indicating general increase of membrane permeability to this ion. Since the intracellular Ca²⁺ level is about three to four orders of magnitude less than normal extracellular Ca²⁺, enhanced Ca²⁺ permeability would result in increase in cell Ca²⁺. The changes in Ca²⁺, however, are more complex. Addition of hormone to cells in apparent equilibrium with isotope results in a transient efflux of radioactivity, showing that there is a Ca²⁺ pool that is higher than medium Ca²⁺, allowing efflux against the apparent gradient, or that there is activation of a membrane-located Ca²⁺ pump (96). Studies on the stomach as detailed as these have not been published, but it has been shown in the frog that stimuli do result in Ca²⁺ efflux from cells; this was not done under equilibrium conditions (90).

Strict regulation of the low Ca²⁺ level in the cytosol is essential for a role for this ion as a second messenger. Ca²⁺ homeostasis in the environment is maintained by various hormones and the low solubility product of $Ca_3(PO_4)_2$. In the cell, there must be organelles that are capable of removing free Ca²⁺ as well as a plasma membrane pump active at low levels of cytosolic Ca²⁺.

The mitochondrion has been universally shown to be able to accumulate Ca²⁺ against a concentration gradient in a reversible fashion in that there is release of Ca²⁺ in response to decreases in the driving force for accumulation. The pathway for Ca²⁺ involves either electroneutral Ca²⁺:H⁺ or electrogenic Ca²⁺ or Ca²⁺:Na⁺ porters. An alternative Ca²⁺ pool is the endoplasmatic reticulum of epithelial cells. Both the stimulus pathway and the regulatory system could be mediated by regulation of this system. The mitochondrial pathway is probably too slow acting to play a role as fast regulator and

can act only as a Ca²⁺ buffer rather than as a hormonally modulated component of the Ca²⁺ pathway. The Ca²⁺-ATPase system of the endoplasmic reticulum could play such a role, releasing Ca²⁺ with stimulation and also being able to take up Ca²⁺ when the stimulus is removed. Such a system may account for the initial transient Ca²⁺ efflux seen in pancreatic cells, defined as the Ca²⁺ trigger pool (96).

In addition to a trigger pool (perhaps contained in specialized vesicles) and plasma membrane permeability changes, the plasma membrane must also contain mechanisms able to extrude Ca²⁺. Many cells are able to do this by virtue of a Ca²⁺ + Mg²⁺ ATPase with properties similar to the better known sarcoplasmic reticulum (SR) Ca²⁺-ATPase. In the stomach, none of these Ca²⁺ systems has yet been defined, but that such systems must be involved is certain. The interactions of Ca²⁺ mechanisms are shown in Fig. 3.

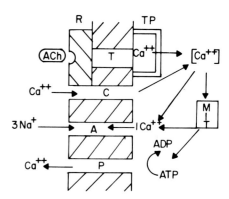

FIG. 3. Model for Ca²⁺ as a second messenger. Acetylcholine (ACh) activates trigger pool (TP) for Ca²⁺ and a Ca²⁺ permease. In addition, a Ca²⁺ pump is present and an electrogenic Na⁺:Ca²⁺ antiport (A), as well as mitochondria to maintain cell [Ca²⁺]. R, receptor; C, Ca²⁺ channel; P, Ca²⁺ ATPase.

Prostaglandins

These derivatives of arachidonic acid are ubiquitous and have been shown to have strong inhibitory actions on gastric secretion (139). Other similar compounds, such as thromboxane, have been shown to enhance histamine-induced secretion (128). Illustrating the complexity of data from intact heterocellular organs, prostaglandins increase cAMP levels in gastric mucosa, which is anomalous for a secretory inhibitor. When the effect of prostaglandins is measured as a function of the number of parietal cells present in an isolated cell preparation, however, it is clear that parietal cell cAMP levels are not affected, whereas other cells respond by increases in cAMP. The latter response probably is a pharmacological effect seen only at higher concentrations of PGE_2. At low (physiological) concentrations, prostaglandins will inhibit histamine-induced cAMP production in parietal cells; this is the reason for the inhibitory effect of certain prostaglandins on acid secretion (188).

The origin of prostaglandin is from arachidonic acid, which is usually present in the 2' position in phospholipids, notably phosphatidyl inositol. Release of the precursor is dependent on the activation of appropriately located Ca^{2+} dependent phospholipase A_2. Thus prostaglandins may act as third messengers in Ca^{2+}-dependent hormone pathways (111). In the parietal cell, where Ca^{2+} is involved in the positive pathway, prostaglandins may provide the regulatory system interacting with the cAMP system allowing interaction between the two second messengers (Fig.4).

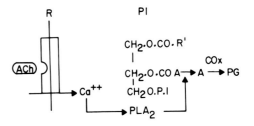

FIG. 4. Model for prostaglandin-dependent exocytosis where a change in cell $[Ca^{2+}]$ activates phospholipase A_2 (PLA_2) with release of arachidonic acid (A) and thus cycloxygenase-dependent synthesis of prostaglandins (PG). R, receptor; PI, phosphatidyl inositol; CO_x, cyclooxygenase; R^1, fatty acid.

Acid Secretory Responses to Individual Stimuli

In vivo

The *in vivo* stimulatory pattern of acid secretion is complex. Since this aspect is covered in other chapters of this volume, we only tabulate the major secretory effects *in vivo*.

Cholinergic influence. Vagal stimulation or stable muscarinic agonists will evoke high rates of acid secretion. Secretion is inhibited by atropine, histamine H_2 antagonists, and prostaglandins.

Gastrin. Gastrin stimulates potently and dose dependently and will give maximal secretion. It is inhibited by atropine, H_2 antagonists, and prostaglandins.

Histamine. Histamine stimulates potently and dose dependently and will give maximal secretion. It is inhibited by atropine only in high concentrations and is strongly inhibited by H_2 antagonists and prostaglandins.

In Vivo Interactions. In vagally denervated fundic mucosa, the efficacy (ED_{50}) but not the potency (V_{max}) of histamine is decreased. With a small dose of cholinergic agonist, the efficacy is restored to normal values (80).

In vitro

The effects of the different secretagogues on isolated mammalian cell systems are covered more extensively elsewhere. Here we list the major responses with special emphasis on the most intact system, the gastric glands.

Histamine. Histamine will dose dependently increase both oxygen consumption and aminopyrine accumulation with ED_{50} of $3 \cdot 10^{-6}$ and 10^{-6} M, respectively. Maximal and sustained response for both parameters is reached within 25 to 30 min (5,7,12), which corresponds to the *in vivo* responses. The histamine response is potentiated by phosphodiesterase inhibitors, such as aminophylline, theophylline, or IMX. Histamine response is inhibited by H_2 antagonists in a competitive fashion. Atropine will inhibit only at high concentrations and then in an apparently nonspecific way.

ACh. An isolated cell system is totally denervated, whereas in an inervated stomach there is always a cholinergic background. Addition of ACh or the more stable analog carbamylcholine (carbachol) to glands induces a transient response in terms of both respiration and aminopyrine accumulation, with a peak within 10 to 15 min (6,13). These transients have not been reported to appear in isolated gastric cells. The transients are true responses, however, since they are not seen on a small background of histamine or IMX, as discussed below. Thus these rapid transient responses might be seen as "clean" cholinergic activation of muscarinic receptors on the parietal cell. All cholinergic responses are blocked by low concentrations of atropine, whereas H_2 receptor antagonists are without effect (171). If the $[Ca^{2+}]$ is lowered from 1 mM to 10 μM, the response to ACh is significantly inhibited, and no transient response is observed (18).

Gastrin. Since gastrin is such a potent secretagogue *in vivo*, one would anticipate such a response also in isolated cell systems. In the rabbit gastric glands, however, we fruitlessly sought gastrin responses and were able to show that the nonresponsiveness was not due to damage by the isolation procedure; mucosal pieces did not respond to pentagastrin either. In contrast, some stimulation in canine gastric cells was observed; however, it amounted to only a 10 to 15% increase in oxygen consumption (170,171). We found that 15-leucine human gastrin I (HGI) would increase the aminopyrine accumulation ratio 1 to 2%, which is far from impressive for an acid secretagogue; however, there are means of strongly potentiating this response. If HGI is added to glands against a background of 10^{-5}M IMX, we obtain dose-dependent increase in aminopyrine accumulation with an apparent K_m of $2 \cdot 10^{-9}$ M for gastrin. IMX, a potent phosphodiesterase inhibitor, will in itself stimulate AP accumulation. Part of that stimulation is inhibited by cimetidine, indicating that endogenously released histamine plays a part in the IMX stimulation. Cimetidine will dose dependently inhibit the gastrin part of the gastrin + IMX stimulation ($K_i \approx 3 \cdot 10^{-7}$ M). Thus a histaminic compound released from gastric glands seems to play a major role in the gastrin response. This was confirmed by the inhibitory effect of diamine oxidase (histaminase) on gastrin-induced AP accumulation (15,18).

Finally, the gastrin + IMX response is totally dependent on extracellular Ca^{2+} (18). Histamine release from rabbit gastric glands has been detected following pentagastrin treatment (19). With normal amounts of glands (≈ 3 mg dry wt/ml), endogenously released histamine will not reach a high enough concentration to stimulate by itself. With the presence of IMX, even a minute histamine-induced respone will be amplified to a point where it can be detected. Thus one aspect of the gastrin response can be explained by histamine release.

If histamine is added at around K_m concentration for its stimulation and gastrin added subsequently, no significant increase above the histamine response is obtained. Gastrin but not histamine needs extracellular Ca^{2+} for secretagogue activity. This might be explained by a Ca^{2+} requirement for gastrin-induced histamine release but is also indicative of a gastrin-mediated Ca^{2+} pathway in the parietal cell.

All these effects bring us to the complicated question of how the individual secretagogues work in concert to establish the final result. With a multiplicity of stimuli affecting a single target process, there are interactions between the individual pathways.

It is certain that histamine and ACh receptors are present on the parietal cell. Although not as well established, it appears as if we might also have a gastrin receptor. As outlined above, gastrin does not stimulate gastric glands on its own, which makes receptor identification more difficult.

Histamine is the only secretagogue that can induce all the secretory responses expected of the parietal cell, when ACh and gastrin activation is impaired. ACh response is normalized if a threshold concentration of histamine is present, i.e., still a fast increase but up to a stable steady-state level. ACh and histamine do potentiate each other, as was the case *in vivo*. This potentiation must originate beyond a simple receptor interaction, since dibutryl-cAMP (db-cAMP)-induced secretion is potentiated by cholinergic compounds (6). Also, a response similar to that between gastrin and IMX can be obtained with ACh + IMX, i.e., normalization and strong potentiation of the ACh effect with a K_m for ACh of $2 \cdot 10^{-7}$ M. This combined effect is inhibited by cimetidine, with the same pA_2 as in the case of gastrin, and is also sensitive to histaminase treatment. Again, the presence of a small amount of histamine or histaminic substance is essential for the ACh response, at least under IMX conditions (15).

Even in a simplified system, events are complicated.

The effect of IMX strongly indicates the necessity of cAMP for a normal response. However only small changes in cAMP levels would therefore be required, since 10^{-5} M IMX gives only a marginal increase in cAMP (34). Since the gastrin response is not equally supported by similar cAMP levels induced by histamine or db-cAMP, it is possible that IMX has an additional, unknown effect.

Based on present facts, histamine still seems to be the key substance, without which no acid secretion will take place; this is indicated by the effects of H_2 antagonists. Histamine might be necessary only as an activator of the parietal cell and not necessarily be the control device for acid secretory rate. That role would be left to ACh and gastrin, which both would release histamine and, simultaneously via a Ca^{2+} pathway, activate the parietal cell. A model for hormonal stimulation of acid secretion is shown in Fig. 5. The final stage of hormone action requires a cell system interacting with the second messenger, the intracellular target.

Second Messenger Target

Several changes occur during acid secretion in the parietal cell: changes in cell morphology, changes in metabolism, and activation of the proton pump. This section defines the site of action within the cell that may induce all or part of the cell response.

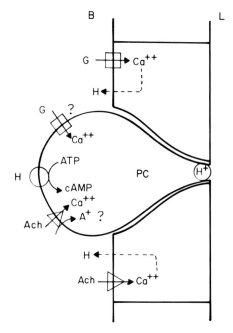

FIG. 5. Model of stimulus-secretion coupling events in the parietal cell (PC) and associated endocrine cells. Definitive evidence exists for histamine (H) and cholinergic (muscarinic) receptors on parietal cells. It is also postulated that acetylcholine (ACh) and gastrin (G) release histamine by a Ca^{2+}-mediated mechanism. L, lumen; B, blood.

cAMP

The discovery of cAMP resulted from the discovery that alterations in glycogen metabolism in muscles were hormonally dependent. The basis of cyclic nucleotide action was eventually discovered to be conversion of the inactive phosphorylase b to the active phosphorylase a (140). The activation was dependent on the addition of ATP and another protein factor, phosphorylase b kinase, with consequent phosphorylation of the target enzyme. Cyclic AMP activated the kinase responsible for the phosphorylation event. This principle protein phosphorylation, dependent on the presence of cAMP, has been generalized to the overall mechanism of action of this nucleotide (86). Cells responding to this nucleotide have been shown to contain both soluble and membrane-bound protein kinases, which phosphorylate a variety of proteins ranging from histones to membrane-bound peptides.

The soluble kinase exists as a tetramer consisting of what is called the catalytic subunit, the component responsible for the phosphorylation reaction and the regulatory subunit, which when bound to the catalytic subunit inhibits its activity (188). The binding of cAMP to the regulatory subunit results in dissociation with consequent activation of the catalytic subunit. The soluble kinase is thus present as an R_2C_2 complex; in the presence of cAMP, it is then dissociated into the active C_2 complex.

This complex may be responsible for the phosphorylation of cell proteins associated with the acid secretion. Usually a variety of proteins are phosphorylated, some soluble and some membrane-bound. The gastric mucosa contains soluble kinase, which has been partially purified in rabbit gastric mucosa (137) and purified to homogeneity from rabbit gastric glands (84). There has also been a report of a membrane-bound kinase in the stomach with cAMP-dependent phosphorylation of membrane (129). Although protein kinase is present in this tissue, the site and mechanism of action have not been defined.

Ca²⁺

The cellular free Ca^{2+} levels are maintained between 0.1 and 1.0 μM. Ca^{2+}-dependent stimulation demands the opening of Ca^{2+} channels in either the plasma membrane or in membrane-bound cellular compartments. This Ca^{2+} increase allows the binding of Ca^{2+} to a Ca^{2+} binding protein, calmodulin (33). This protein was initially discovered as an activator of phosphodiesterase; it has been purified and sequenced, and its quaternary structure is under investigation. There are four Ca^{2+} binding sites with dissociation constants of 4 to 18 nM. This protein in its Ca^{2+} loaded form regulates the activity of several enzymes, such as adenylate cyclase, phosphodiesterase, myosin light chain kinase, NAD

kinase, phospholipase A_2, phosphorylase kinase, and membrane phosphorylation. Thus with this protein there can be interaction with the cAMP-dependent kinase, which also phosphorylates membrane proteins, and with prostaglandins, which require the activation of phospholipase A_2 for their synthesis.

Calmodulin thus could regulate both the synthesis and breakdown of cAMP and the synthesis of prostaglandins, thereby having a pivotal function in second messenger interaction. For this protein to play a role in parietal cell function, it must be present in this cell in adequate amounts; removal or inhibition should reduce cell activity; and the addition of Ca^{2+} in its presence should alter cell enzymes or other features. It has been claimed that Ca^{2+} enhances the KCl permeability of gastric vesicles (112), but whether calmodulin has a part in this is not known (Fig. 6).

METABOLISM AND SECRETION

The high mitochondrial content of the gastric parietal cell indicates an important contribution of oxidative metabolism to the energy economy of the cell. Since mitochondria oxidize substrates and generate ATP, the finding that H^+ secretion is absolutely dependent on the presence of O_2 does not discriminate between the ATP or redox hypotheses of acid secretion. Before discussing the known metabolic events, these hypotheses are considered since they provide a conceptual framework for an understanding of the major reasons for studying parietal cell metabolism.

The earliest suggestion for the basis of H^+ secretion was the vectorial orientation of a redox reaction separating protons and electrons. As illustrated in Fig. 7, a proton donor, AH_2, is oxidized by a membrane-bound redox system so that H^+ is transported across the membrane and the electrons are donated to an acceptor located on the cytoplasmic surface. This concept antedated the discovery of ATP and the germinal suggestions of Mitchell in the chemiosmotic hypothesis (113). In fact, this could represent a redox loop in the mito-

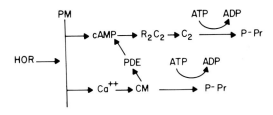

FIG. 6. Model illustrating putative targets for cAMP and Ca^{2+} as second messengers, the former activating protein kinase (C_2) by dissociation of the regulatory R_2 from the catalytic C_2 subunits, the latter via calmodulin (CM). HOR, hormone; R_2C_2, inactive kinase; PDE, phosphodiesterase; P-Pr, phosphoprotein.

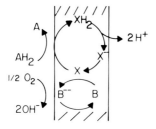

FIG. 7. Illustration of a redox pump generating 2 H$^+$/O and using an electron acceptor to shuttle the electrons to oxygen.

chondrial respiratory chain. There are significant restrictions on the nature of the redox loop. The necessary difference in redox potential between donor and acceptor, if this is the sole H$^+$ pumping mechanism, is set by the pH gradient. With the cytosolic pH corresponding to 7.7 during secretion, the voltage drop must be of the order of 420 mV. It is necessary to have this drop across a single loop; otherwise, reversal would occur before the final pH gradient was generated. To date, neither the redox reaction nor its components are known.

The alternative hypothesis followed the discovery of the Na$^+$K$^+$ATPase (166). It was suggested that ATP also provided the energy for acid secretion. The mechanism has been defined only recently. Much of the early work in acid secretion was dedicated to attempts to prove one or the other mechanism. The first type of experiment measured the stoichiometry between O$_2$ consumption and acid secretion. Many variations were tried with this general protocol. Most experiments were carried out in the *in vitro* frog mucosa mounted in an Ussing chamber. Changes in acid rate were correlated with changes in O$_2$ consumption. The changes in acid rate were induced either by stimulation or by the use of inhibitors, such as thiocyanate. In the former, even in the dog flap, H/O ratios never exceeded 2. This demonstrated the possibility of the presence of a redox pump; for a single redox loop, this would be the predicted ratio. Evidently, as the overall span between NADH and O$_2$ was 1,100 mV, almost three loops would be possible; hence, these data are not decisive. Moreover, the ΔG of ATP hydrolysis under physiological conditions would dictate a maximal H/ATP ratio of 1. With a P/O ratio of 2, the maximal ratio even for the ATP hypothesis is also not more than 2. Ratios much larger than this can be obtained using SCN (56). However, since this inhibitor changes O$_2$ consumption rather little, indicating an uncoupling action, these data have little meaning.

The early work discussed above was concerned with the primary energy source for acid secretion. The difficulties of determining this by the techniques applied have been discussed. Subsequent work can be divided into three areas: (a) the determination of whether ATP is involved in acid secretion, (b) the role of redox components other than ATP synthesis, and (c) the role of substrate metabolism.

ATP as an Energy Source for Acid Secretion

It might be predicted that as ATP turnover is stimulated due to the onset of acid secretion, there would be a fall in the high energy phosphate pool. The creatine phosphate/creatine (PCr/Cr) ratio would be the first to fall; this might be followed by a fall in the phosphorylation potential, the ATP/(ADP + Pi) value. Measurements in the frog gastric mucosa *in vitro* (50) and in parietal cell-enriched biopsies from dog gastric mucosa *in vivo* (160) show little if any change of the values expected, except for a rise in the inorganic phosphate values in the dog. It is only this change that alters the phosphorylation potential. The source of the Pi is not clear. There may be significant utilization of phospholipid or phosphorylcholine. [The data in isolated rabbit glands do show a significant fall in the ATP/ADP ratio, with certain substrates consonant with the utilization of ATP by the acid secretory process (76).] An alternative is to measure ATP turnover either by measurement of ^{32}Pi incorporation at rest and during secretion or by measuring the incorporation of ^{18}O from H$_2$^{18}O under the same conditions. Data on frog gastric mucosa show that there is an increased ATP turnover (46).

In the dog gastric mucosa, the PCr/Cr ratio actually tends to increase. This can be used to calculate the change in pH during acid secretion, due to the equilibrium

$$H^+ + PCr \rightleftharpoons Cr + Pi$$

so that an increase in pH will result in a rise in the PCr/Cr ratio. We conclude from the increase and the equilibrium constant of the reaction that the pH of the secreting oxyntic cell increases by at least 0.3 units (52).

The development of isolated cell models, such as the rabbit gastric glands, and the use of probes of acid accumulation within the secretory canaliculus (either aminopyrine or acridine orange) have provided a direct test of the ATP dependence of acid secretion. Using high voltage dielectric discharge over a gland or cell suspension results in an increase in the permeability of the cell, notably to molecules, such as ATP. Shocked permeable glands no longer are able to accumulate aminopyrine or acridine orange, either following shocking alone or in the additional presence of CN$^-$, N$_3$$^-$, or amytal, which are inhibitors of the mitochondrial respiratory chain. In the presence of elevated medium K (108 mM), the addition of ATP restores the property of acid secretion. This is illustrated in terms of AP accumulation in Fig. 8. Similar conclusions were derived from AO accumulation when measured optically. The data are complementary. The former gives the overall efficiency of the

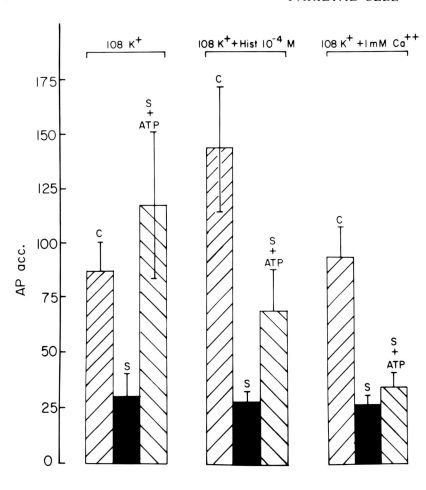

FIG. 8. Aminopyrine accumulation ratio (pH gradient) in control (C), shocked (S), and shocked rabbit gastric glands + ATP added (S + ATP) in the absence of Ca^{2+} and in the presence of EGTA and in the presence of Ca^{2+} where noted. The restoration of aminopyrine accumulation by ATP is noteworthy, as is the inhibition of the process by added Ca^{2+}.

readdition of ATP, whereas the latter not only allows a cell-by-cell evaluation of the response to ATP but also confirms that the restimulation occurs within the same glandular structure as normal secretagogue-induced stimulation, namely, the secretory canaliculi of the parietal cell (10).

From this approach, it may be concluded that ATP can indeed serve as an energy source for acid secretion. The data do not allow the conclusion that ATP is the sole energy source required for the process of acid secretion by the parietal cell. At least ATP must be involved in the terminal step; otherwise, no pH gradient would be generated.

Redox Components

The alternative to ATP driven acid secretion that has been widely considered is the redox pump hypothesis. The major components of the redox chain give a characteristic signal when changes occur between oxidation and reduction. For observation of scattering samples, either a split beam spectrophotometer is used, where one-half of the tissue serves as a control so that changes due to altered secretory status of the other half can be detected, or a dual or multiple wavelength spectropho-

tometer can be used, so that the optical density at the reference wavelength of any redox component can be compared to the optical density at the peak absorbance change (31).

With this technique, pyridine nucleotides, flavins, and cytochromes can be measured. The experimental protocol is usually to measure a change in redox state and to quantitate the change by comparison to the optical changes in the fully oxidized and fully reduced state.

With this approach in the frog gastric mucosa, even at resting conditions, there is considerable reduction of the cytochromes, including cytochrome oxidase (74). This finding has been interpreted to mean that there is some special feature of the redox chain in the gastric mucosa. The alternative explanation, that there is limitation of the access of O_2 to the oxyntic cell region of the tissue, has been considered but dismissed based on the similarity of data obtained under hyperbaric conditions (92).

With stimulation of secretion, the redox components that are readily observed undergo reduction (74). In general, with a fall in phosphorylation potential, as might occur with onset of acid secretion, one would predict an oxidation of the respiratory chain if the limitation on oxidation were the availability of ADP or Pi. If the limitation were access of oxidizable substrate, then the alteration toward reduction would not be unexpected.

Analysis of the quantity of components that are spectrally observable does not provide any evidence for abnormalities of ratios of the redox components, as might be expected if there were nonmitochondrial location of segments of the respiratory chain. Thus observations of either ATP levels or redox state of the frog gastric mucosa do not provide decisive evidence as to the nature of the primary energy source (75).

In the isolated rabbit glands, with changes in secretion, only transient changes in the redox components are observed. The overall oxidation state of the cytochromes appears to be about 75% oxidized (16), in contrast to the frog gastric mucosa. This might suggest better oxygenation of cell suspensions as the reason for the higher oxidation level. It also suggests that the reduced state in the frog gastric mucosa, as well as the change toward reduction with secretory onset, is attributable to inadequate or increasingly inadequate oxygenation.

Inhibitors of phosphorylation or oxidation invariably inhibit acid secretion (154). Since the oxidation and phosphorylation activities of mitochondria are tightly coupled, the use of inhibitors does not discriminate between the two postulated energy sources. If there were purely a redox source for acid secretion, with no utilization of ATP, it might be expected that acid secretion would not be sensitive to uncouplers of phosphorylation, since oxidation continues, despite lack of ATP synthesis. Since the action of uncouplers is to inhibit acid secretion, along with an increase in tissue electrical resistance, acid secretion is not solely dependent on redox reactions.

Evidently, the permeable isolated gastric glands provide the best model in which to establish not only the utilization of ATP, as has already been done, but also whether there is any additional redox component required for HCl elaboration.

Substrate Metabolism

Two interconnected aspects have been studied: the alterations in substrate turnover observed with onset of acid secretion, and the substrate(s) specifically involved in support of the energy source for acid secretion.

In amphibian gastric mucosa, the effect of substrate addition to the bathing solutions, along with measurements of respiratory quotient, has shown that in general fatty acids are better substrates in terms of both CO_2 production and support of acid rate (2). In contrast, in both rabbit glands and the piglet mucosa (55), glucose is an adequate substrate for acid secretion. Thus the support of acid secretion in amphibia may be dependent on fatty acid oxidation, whereas in mammals, glycolysis with consequent oxidation of pyruvate may suffice; in rabbit glands, however, substrates, such as β-OH butyrate, are clearly adequate (77).

An alternative approach is to measure the level of a series of metabolites in nonsecreting and secreting gastric mucosa. This has been done in some detail in biopsies from dog gastric mucosa *in vivo*. Using parietal cell-enriched sections, the data of Figs. 9 and 10 were

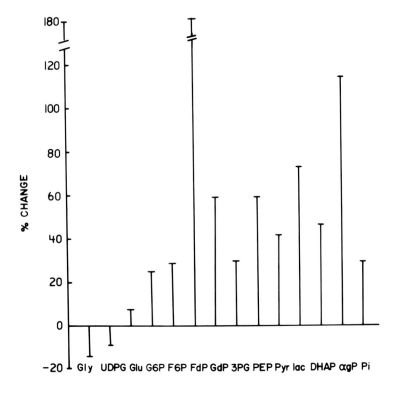

FIG. 9. Percent change in living dog parietal cells of the intermediates of glycolysis following stimulation of acid secretion.

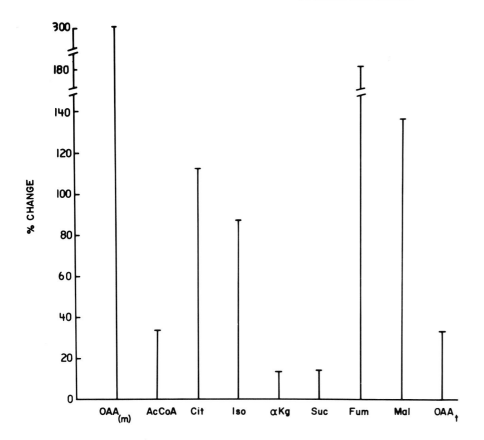

FIG. 10. Percent change in living dog parietal cells of the intermediates of the Krebs cycle following stimulation of acid secretion.

obtained (161). There is a large increase in tricarboxylic acid intermediates, and the relative changes in glycolysis show that there is also an increment in carbohydrate metabolism. This may be due entirely to a pH increase in the cytosol (152,160). In this particular series of studies, no evidence was sought for an increase in fatty acid oxidation.

The measurement of metabolites by the Lowry cycling technique also allows compartmental analysis of the ratio of oxidized and reduced pyridine nucleotides. The demonstrated increase in reduction can be due to changes in metabolite flux or to pH changes, as discussed for the creatine kinase equilibrium. The reaction $A + NADH + H^+ \rightarrow NAD^+ + AH_2$ shows that alkalinization would drive the reaction to the left. From the changes found, it can be calculated that there is a ΔpH of about 0.3 pH units with onset of acid secretion (160).

From metabolite measurement, it is not clear which are the control points in parietal cell metabolism. The general increase in Krebs cycle intermediates suggests that the entry of the tri- or dicarboxylic acids into mitochondria may be the regulated portion of parietal cell metabolism. The onset of secretion would then depend on increased quantities of cytosolic intermediates, on adequate mitochondrial transport of cytosolic intermediates, and on activity of the redox chain.

There is little evidence for a special role of any par-

ticular enzyme step in regulation of parietal cell metabolism. Nevertheless, the 16-fold increase of O_2 consumption found in dog gastric mucosa *in vivo* with onset of acid secretion (114) and the more than twofold increase found in rabbit gastric glands associated with secretagogue activation (5) strongly implies the presence of one or more reaction steps that are regulated.

The net result of all the metabolic studies performed on the gastric mucosa may be summarized as showing that ATP is required for acid secretion and that the source of ATP is probably mitochondrial metabolism. The more modern techniques of ^{31}P and ^{13}C NMR spectroscopy may provide the insights necessary for resolution of many of the vexing questions still unanswered in this cell.

ENZYMIC CORRELATES OF SECRETION

Certain enzymes have been studied intensively with respect to their role in acid secretion. These can be classified into two groups: those concerned primarily with the process of H^+ transport and secondarily with supply of ions to the primary pump, or those involved with buffering of the OH^- produced. The gastric $H^+ K^+$ ATPase is discussed in a separate section; here we consider the role of carbonic anhydrase, cytochrome b5, and the $Na^+ K^+$ ATPase.

Carbonic Anhydrase

Carbonic anhydrase, a Zn-containing enzyme, occurs in high concentrations in the gastric parietal cell (110). Chemically, the enzyme corresponds to a type C carbonic anhydrase. Histochemical staining shows intimate association with the microvilli of the secretory canaliculus (39).

The reason for interest in the role of this enzyme is that associated with export of protons from the gastric parietal cell, there must be accumulation of OH^- on the cytosolic surface of the proton pump (Fig. 11a). Since substantial amounts of HCO_3^- are produced by the stomach, the presence of carbonic anhydrase indicates that the base formed is rapidly converted to HCO_3^-. Accordingly, inhibition of this enzyme reduces the rate of acid secretion because of an increase in pH (77). The strict location of the enzyme to the site of acid secretion would suggest an even more specific role.

Thiocyanate ion has long interested gastric physiologists because of its inhibition of acid secretion at concentrations of 1 to 10 mM. At these concentrations, the chaotropic properties of this lipid-permeable anion cannot account for the inhibition. Also intriguing is the lack of any substantial inhibition of oxygen consumption; SCN^- acts like an uncoupler of acid secretion. The earliest hypothesis was that the action of this ion was due to the inhibition of carbonic anhydrase (40) but, with the discovery that more potent inhibitors of the enzyme had lesser effects on acid secretion, this theory fell into disfavor. Perhaps the demise of this theory was premature, if one considers the different mechanisms of inhibition exerted by compounds, such as diamox and SCN^-. The active site of the enzyme contains Zn and catalyzes the interaction of OH^- and CO_2. The enzyme also presumably contains an anion channel selective for OH^- to allow approach of the two reactants from either side of the catalytic center. Inhibition of the reaction center would not result in any marked slowing of diffusion of OH^- to the center. However, a pseudohalide, such as SCN^-, would result in blockade of the channel and restriction of OH^- diffusion. Accordingly, with an activated proton pump producing OH^-, the presence of SCN^- would result in significant alkalinization of the

cytoplasmic face of the ATPase to which carbonic anhydrase is bound. This in turn could lead to leak of OH^- into the acid compartment generated by the pump, with consequent uncoupling of acid secretion. A neutralization process in the form of a reunion of OH^- and H^+ was suggested, based on the effect of SCN^- in gastric glands (7). The addition of SCN^- to prestimulated glands rapidly dissipated the accumulated aminopyrine gradient, an effect that must be explained by an active neutralization process and not merely a diffusion process following a shutdown of the H^+ pump.

A neutralization process is also supported by the finding that weak bases, such as imidazole or aminopyrine, when added to the nutrient side of a frog gastric mucosa, could prevent the SCN^- effect (159). If the weak base combines with the acid, it would prevent a neutralization by making the OH^- gradient less steep. If the pH on the secretory side of the mucosa is kept above the pK_a of the base, the proton will leave the base and thus become titratable. A hypothetical model for an SCN^- interaction with the carbonic anhydrase is given in Fig. 11 (*right*), where the H^+ pump and carbonic anhydrase are tightly associated.

Cytochrome b5

The presence of cytochrome b5 has been established in membrane fractions of rat gastric mucosa (102). Also in fractions derived from hog gastric mucosa apparently free of mitochondrial contamination, the presence of a cytochrome absorbing at 561 nm has been described (151). The occurrence of these redox components in a cell type devoid of smooth membrane structures other than the secretory tubulovesicles might indicate its presence in these structures. In chromaffin granule membranes where it has been established that there is an ATP-dependent H^+ pump process (88) apparently similar to the mitochondrial type, the presence of a similar type of cytochrome has also been observed (53). In neither case has there been any convincing demonstration of its function. Until a plausible role for redox reactions has been found, the presence of these cytochromes remains an interesting mystery.

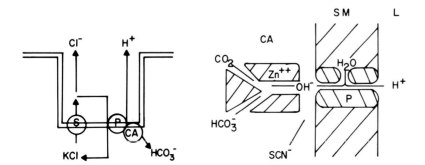

FIG. 11. Left: Model of acid secretion by the parietal cell, involving a $K^+:H^+$ exchange pump (P) in parallel with a KCl entry into the lumen of the cell (S). SCN^- is postulated to inhibit translocation of OH^- from the pump by carbonic anhydrase (CA). **Right:** Detailing of the role of carbonic anhydrase (CA) in gastric acid secretion showing the possible location of the site of action of SCN^-. SM, secretory membrane; P, acid pump.

Na⁺ K⁺ ATPase

This enzyme, located in the basolateral membrane, will translocate three Na⁺ outward and two K⁺ inward for each ATP molecule utilized (63). This makes the overall reaction electrogenic, inside negative. Since K⁺ is essential for HCl secretion, especially in the parietal cell, Na⁺ must be supplied for the accumulation of K⁺. It has been suggested that Na⁺ enters the cell as NaCl through cotransport or symport (11,108). Since there is current flow through the pump, we must complete the circuit with net transport of charge across the apical or basal membrane. We can now use this current to model how active Cl⁻ transport would occur across the apical membrane. From a neutral NaCl entry, it can be predicted (and has in fact been found) that intracellular Cl⁻ is not in electrochemical equilibrium with the extracellular Cl⁻ (44). This Cl⁻ disequilibrium is generated by the Na⁺, K⁺ ATPase. Therefore, the Cl⁻ exiting across the apical membrane would in fact be driven by the ATPase; i.e., net Cl⁻ flux is due to secondary active transport. Evidence favoring this interpretation is that the Cl⁻ transport is absolutely Na⁺ dependent (157) and is inhibited by ouabain (57).

Figure 12 illustrates a model of the resting parietal cell showing the presence of the Na⁺, K⁺ ATPase associated with an Na⁺ and K⁺ cycle in the basal membrane. This model results in the secretion of Cl⁻. Na⁺ absorption can be modeled similarly as also illustrated, but now the requirements of the pump are met by the apical entry of Na⁺. The role of this pump in mediating acid secretion is discussed in more detail when the properties of the H⁺: K⁺ ATPase are presented. Direct evidence for the nature of the NaCl flux pathways across the basolateral membrane has not yet been obtained. For example, it is not possible to exclude a coupled Na⁺:H⁺ and Cl⁻:OH⁻ (HCO₃⁻) antiport as the mechanism of NaCl symport. Both pathways appear to be present in intestinal but not renal brush-border membranes (105).

ACTIVE TRANSPORT OF SOLUTE OTHER THAN HCl

In all gastric mucosae studied, there appears to be active transport of Cl⁻ in the direction serosa to mucosa. In some but not all species, there is also Na⁺ absorption. Both transport processes are inhibited by the specific inhibitor of the Na⁺ K⁺ ATPase, ouabain (57). In addition, inhibition of HCl secretion can be reversed by increasing medium K⁺ (41).

These data have not been ascribed to any specific cell type in the tissue but are discussed in relation to the parietal cell in terms of Cl⁻ transport; Na⁺ is discussed in relation to the nonparietal cells of the stomach.

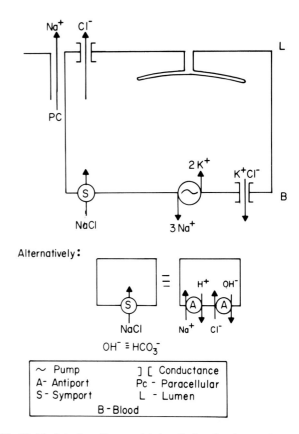

FIG. 12. Model of resting parietal cell showing ion pathways present. Notable is the coupling between NaCl symport, Na⁺K⁺ ATPase and active Cl⁻ pumping on the opposite membrane. An NaCl symport could also be a Na⁺:H⁺ Cl⁻:OH⁻ exchanger.

ELECTRICAL PROPERTIES

In Cl⁻ solutions, the gastric mucosa generates a PD, lumen negative. This potential persists whether or not acid secretion is present. In the case of the surface cell, measurement of cell membrane potentials using microelectrodes shows that there is a negative well with the apical membrane less polarized than the basal (174). Changes of K⁺ or Cl⁻ concentration on the basal surface show that this membrane is selectively permeable to these two ions (158). Moreover, the change in PD across the basolateral surface is almost exactly reflected by a change across the apical membrane (174), showing that the paracellular pathway contributes little to the tissue conductance. There appears to be little conductance for either Na⁺ or HCO₃⁻ (134).

When Cl⁻ is removed (in the frog) and replaced by sulfate in resting tissue, the PD drops to low values and tissue resistance rises (72). In the presence of acid secretion, the PD actually inverts and is then linearly related to the rate of acid secretion. This is strong evidence for the electrogenicity of acid secretion (134). Alternative hypotheses can also explain this, based on the K$^+$ exchange theory of acid secretion (38).

The presence of an electrogenic pump in a tissue would be expected to decrease its resistance if the pump were reversible with respect to both ion gradient and electrical potential. In fact, one of the earliest pieces of evidence that H$^+$ pumping was electrogenic was that application of voltage resulted in the alteration of H$^+$ rate, depending on the direction of applied current (134). Again, this can be explained not only by an electrogenic pump concept but also by the K$^+$ exchange mechanism.

A decrease in tissue resistance is indeed found with onset of acid secretion. This is consistent with insertion of electrogenic pump subunits into the parietal cell apical membrane. In addition, cell apical surface area increases with stimulation of secretion. Capacitance measurements show that the drop in resistance can be accounted for by increase in area by addition of constant subunits (109) (Fig. 13). The electrical properties of the parietal cell membranes have not been well defined. In the case of isolated oxyntic cells from Necturus, the cell membrane appears also to have K$^+$ and Cl$^-$ conductance pathways, as does the surface cell (26,158).

Overall, the electrical properties of the gastric mucosa have not provided definite information on the mechanism of acid secretion. Concepts of electrogenic transport have their historic origins in this tissue and have had considerable influence on the development of thought in other epithelia.

Microelectrode approaches are of little use in defining potentials in intracellular compartments, such as the mitochondria or secretory canaliculus. To measure these, lipid permeable ions, whose distribution can be measured optically or radioactively, may be used. This approach has been used successfully in the case of neuroblastoma cells (104). Radiolabeled ions that have been used in different systems are thallium, tetraphenylphosphonium (TPP$^+$), and triphenylmethylphosphonium (TPMP$^+$) (72,167,168).

In gastric cells, the problem is that the potential of an intracellular compartment, which may be at a high voltage (about 180 mV) in series with a plasma membrane voltage of about 60 mV, may be the major determinant of ion distribution. The plasma membrane voltage can be measured directly using microelectrodes; the additional accumulation of, for example, TPP$^+$, may be accounted for by the presence of an intracellular high voltage compartment. Alternatively, depolarization of the mitochondrial membrane by intracellular lipid permeable cation can be detected using carbocyanine dyes. If the dye response can be calibrated using K$^+$ in the presence of valinomycin, the mitochondrial potential can be calculated, provided total mitochondrial volume is known. A third way is to take advantage of the finding that whereas Tl$^+$ distributes across the mitochondrial volume membrane according to voltage, its distribution across the plasma membrane is due to the function of the Na$^+$K$^+$ATPase (97). Hence, knowing the cytosolic concentration of this ion (approximately a 16-fold distribution, as for K$^+$ or Rb$^+$), the distribution ratio for mitochondria can be calculated. With this, the mitochondrial potential in gastric glands is between 140 and 160 mV. In neuroblastoma cells, the calculated potential appears to be considerably lower (104).

IONIC BASIS OF SECRETION

The four ions that are clearly implicated in parietal cell HCl transport are Cl$^-$, HCO$_3^-$, Na$^+$, and K$^+$. Although the mechanism whereby any of these ions are involved is not completely understood, the general areas of interaction with the secretory system have been recently defined.

Cl$^-$

Removal of Cl$^-$ in some species of amphibian gastric mucosa results in detectable acid secretion and a positive lumen potential. (The interpretation of this is discussed above.) In the presence of sulfate, the K$^+$ conductance of the apical surface of the gastric mucosa equals the K$^+$ conductance of the basal surface

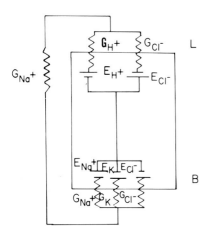

L :   Lumen
B :   Blood
E_{H^+} G_{H^+}: H$^+$ pump

E_{Cl^-}, G_{Cl^-}: Cl$^-$ diffusion potential, conductance
E_{Na^+} G_{Na^+}: Na$^+$ pump
E_{K^+} G_{K^+}: K$^+$ diffusion potential, conductance
G_{Na^+} : Na$^+$ conductance paracellular

FIG. 13. Equivalent current model of the parietal cell modeled as an electrogenic H$^+$ pump in parallel with an electrogenic Cl$^-$ pump on luminal membrane and Na$^+$, K$^+$, and Cl$^-$ diffusion potentials basally.

(133,158). This would be expected from a cell where the apical and basal surfaces contain both a K^+ conductance and a Cl^- conductance but where the Cl^- conductance of the apical membrane masks the K^+ conductance.

In piglet gastric mucosa (57) and in isolated rabbit gastric glands (8), there is no detectable constant secretion in sulfate solutions. Preincubating glands at low temperature, however, will give rise to a rapid transient acid production when put into 37° C. This phenomena could be due to initial K^+ accumulation at the apical surface, which subsequently could be used for H^+ secretion (17). There is also a secretagogue-induced increase in O_2 consumption without a corresponding increase in aminopyrine accumulation in the rabbit (11). This uncoupling between metabolism and acid secretion in Cl^--free medium could be caused by either an increased amount of available substrate or protons actually forming but subsequently being neutralized. The effect of Cl^- removal cannot be bypassed by high medium K^+ or by lipid permeable ions, even in the presence of high medium K^+ concentrations (17). Other halides and other monovalent cations can substitute for Cl^- in the sequence $Br^- > NO_3^- > I^- > ClO_3^-$ (49). Fluoride inhibits acid secretion.

The anion sequence and lack of reversal by lipid permeable ions even in the presence of K^+ suggests strict coupling between cation and anion as a requirement for acid secretion in the mammalian system.

HCO_3^-

The presence of HCO_3^- buffer in the bathing medium increases the rate of acid secretion in the *in vitro* frog gastric mucosa but is not an absolute requirement, other buffers being able to substitute (136). The endogenous CO_2 production from mitochondria can suffice. As discussed above, there is no HCO_3^- conductance in the plasma membrane but rather electroneutral exchange systems. Studies on the *in vitro* requirements for HCO_3^- have not been performed in the chambered mammalian mucosa.

Na^+

The regulation of Na^+ level in the cell depends on the activity of the basal Na^+, K^+ ATPase. The reduction of acid secretion that occurs with K^+ removal, e.g., in rabbit glands, is partially reversed by the additional removal of the Na^+. This implies that not only is K^+ required for acid secretion, but also that Na^+ levels might be inhibitory. The further finding that removal of Na^+ does not block acid secretion in frog gastric mucosa shows that Na^+ is not essential for all Cl^- entry into the parietal cell (158).

K^+

It was shown more than three decades ago that K^+ removal from the solutions bathing frog gastric mucosa blocked acid secretion (70). Replacement of K^+ on either side of the tissue restored the acid rate. Thus *in vitro* acid secretion shows dependence on K^+ in the bathing medium.

In rabbit gastric glands, the measurement of K^+ levels following changes in bathing medium are shown in Table 2. The removal of K^+ alone results in a fall in intercellular K^+ to about 60 mM. The removal of Na^+ or the addition of ouabain at 5.4 mM K^+ in the medium results in a fall of K^+ to 35 and 45 mM, respectively. That acid secretion is inhibited by K^+ removal but not by Na^+ removal does not correlate with the measured cellular K^+ levels. The simultaneous removal of Na^+ and K^+ produces a similar fall in cell K^+, but now there is a finite acid rate. This shows that K^+ is required for acid secretion, and that Na^+ inhibits proton transport. The K^+ level, even in the absence of medium cations other than choline, does not fall much below 25mM, indicating that there may be a membrane-bounded compartment of K^+. To correlate medium K^+ levels precisely with cellular levels at the secretory site, this compartment must also be depleted of K^+.

Without depletion of all cellular K^+, some information about the electrolyte interactions can be obtained. In the absence of ouabain, 0.9 mM extracellular K^+ is enough to drive aminopyrine accumulation to half-maximum value. Since these experiments were performed in the presence of 30 mM Na^+, K^+ will naturally accumulate because of the Na^+ K^+ ATPase. In the presence of ouabain, extracellular K^+ will more closely reflect the intracellular values. Again in the presence of 30 mM Na^+, unstimulated glands showed an ED_{50} of 60 mM, whereas the apparent K^+ affinity in the presence of histamine dropped to 30 mM (9). These figures are only relative and depend on the amount of Na^+ present.

When the medium is made Na^+ free and acid secretion is monitored as a function of medium K^+ with or without histamine, acid secretion is higher at low K^+

TABLE 2. *Cation levels in rabbit gastric glands*

Control	K^+ (mM)	Na^+ (mM)
[5K$^+$ 142.4 Na$^+$]	134	25
$-K^+$	64	90
$-Na^+$	38	5
$-K^+$, $-Na^+$	25	5
C + ouabain	45	100
C + amphotericin B	10	145
$-Na^+$, $-K^+$ + amphotericin B	5	2

levels than in the presence of Na$^+$ but is still sensitive to medium K$^+$ and histamine. The presence of cell Na$^+$ thus has large effects on the rate of acid secretion at low K$^+$ levels, but removal of Na$^+$ does not alter the maximal secretory capacity of the system.

Under the above conditions, namely, with no Na$^+$ present, evidently small changes in medium K$^+$ levels have large effects on acid secretion. It is necessary for a quantitative correlation between cell K$^+$ levels and acid secretion to eliminate the K$^+$ compartment, since neither its location nor volume occupancy are known. To achieve this, we have used a neutral ionophore amphotericin (95). Nigericin, an exchange ionophore, will also deplete the intracellular K$^+$ compartment but, in contrast to amphotericin, will inhibit acid secretion. Thus a direct correlation between intracellular K$^+$ and H$^+$ secretion can be obtained in an intact cell. The apparent intracellular ED$_{50}$ is now of the order of 18 mM and, in the presence of histamine, is reduced to 12 mM. This shows that, as above, histamine does increase the affinity of the system and that the K$^+$ requirement corresponds to what has been determined for isolated gastric vesicles for measureable H$^+$ transport.

THE GASTRIC H$^+$, K$^+$ ATPase

The discovery that the gastric mucosa of various species, such as frog (60), dog (149), hog (150), rabbit (11,63), and man (145) contains an ATPase that is activated by cations in the sequence in terms of affinities Tl$^+$ > K$^+$ > Rb$^+$ $\gg$ Cs$^+$ > Na$^+$, Li$^+$ that does not require Na$^+$ and is not inhibited by ouabain indicates the presence of a plasma membrane transport ATPase different from the Ca^{2+} or Na$^+$, K$^+$ ATPase described in other tissue. The further demonstration that this enzyme activity in vesicular form is stimulated by K$^+$ ionophores implies that K$^+$ transport may occur in these vesicles (61). Finally, the demonstration that the addition of ATP resulted in H$^+$ transport into these gastric vesicles provided compelling evidence for the role of this enzyme in acid secretion (101). In this section, we explore the detailed properties of the system and correlate these with properties of the intact parietal cell.

In most species where the enzyme has been sought, there is no difficulty in demonstrating its presence. A notable exception is the rat, where there is a high level of Mg^{2+}-activated ATPase but little if any K$^+$ stimulation in purified membrane fractions (148); the significance of this is not yet known. A considerable amount of work has been done on the so-called HCO$_3^-$ ATPase (176). Most workers agree that the presence of this enzyme is due to mitochondrial contamination (172); in our view, this position has not been proved. It is difficult in many species to separate the K$^+$-stimulated

from the HCO$_3^-$-stimulated activities. The highest purity fraction thus far has been derived from hog gastric mucosa, where no HCO$_3^-$ activation has been detected (150).

Purification of ATPase

The gastric mucosa contains several cell types. Partial enrichment of the parietal cell population can be obtained either by removal of surface cells with salt solution or by preparing gastric glands. In membrane fractions obtained by differential and density gradient fractionation, although essentially free of mitochondrial contamination, there are at least three other enzyme activities that copurify with the gastric K$^+$-activated ATPase and K$^+$ pNPPase activities: (a) 5'-nucleotidase, (b) Mg^{2+}ATPase, and (c) cytochrome b561. These are separated from the K$^+$-activated ATPase and pNPPase by the free flow electrophoretic fractionation procedure. The fraction enriched in K$^+$ATPase activity still contains some Mg^{2+}ATPase activity, but this activity in this fraction is a property of the K$^+$ATPase. The Na$^+$, K$^+$-activated ATPase, as measured by ouabain binding, occurs in a denser membrane fraction. The only known enzymes associated with the anodic group of vesicles are K$^+$ATPase and pNPPase. The fraction consists of vesicles. SDS gel electrophoresis shows that one group of peptides present, MW 105,000, accounts for 90% of the protein. Carbohydrate staining and analysis shows that glycoprotein is present in this band, free of sialic acid. The amino acid composition is similar to that of Na$^+$, K$^+$ATPases, and there is considerable peptide homology (R. L. Post, *personal communication*).

SDS gel characterization is not sufficient to determine whether only a single peptide is involved. In fact, tryptic digestion in the absence or presence of ATP provides evidence for heterogeneity of this single molecular weight region on the gel, since ATP will protect only part of the 105,000 moiety from digestion (146). Either two or three peptides appear to be present. One is a trypsin-resistant glycoprotein. The subunit that is protected by the presence of ATP provides labeled fragments when digestion follows incubation with γ^{32}-P-ATP: Mg^{2+} is evidently the catalytic subunit. The other fragment that does not label and is not protected against fragmentation by trypsin may be either the catalytic subunit oriented in the membrane so that ATP cannot bind or a different subunit altogether.

The molecular weight of the functioning enzyme is 280,000 (144). Cross-linking studies also gave evidence that there may indeed be a trimer associated with ATPase activity. The data suggesting polymeric functional units for this type of ATPase are characteristic of the plasma membrane type of transport ATPase.

Orientation of the ATPase

When membranes are isolated, the fragments resulting from homogenization may be inverted, right-side out vesicles or open pieces. Several methods determine sidedness. Electron microscopy using tannic acid glutaraldehyde fixation gives the density of protein on either surface. Since the protein is asymmetrically distributed, a quantitative statement can be made about orientation. If the vesicles are broken and the ATPase activity increases, then it might be concluded that some vesicles have the ATP site on the inside face. In the case of gastric vesicles, it is important to do this type of experiment under unrestricted K^+ entry conditions, for example, in the presence of ionophores, such as nigericin or gramicidin. Using either type of approach, the data indicate that there is essentially only an external ATP side (rim side out) orientation of the gastric vesicles as isolated. Freeze fracture of the vesicles can also show the orientation of the protein, provided it is not evenly distributed between the fracture faces of the membranes (100). There are particles of about 80 Å diameter, largely on the concave face of the membranes. The diameter of the particles suggests a 200,000 MW.

Localization of the ATPase

Although the ATPase is present in membrane fractions derived from gastric glands, which contain essentially only parietal and peptic cells, it is important to determine the exact localization within the tissue, as well as to examine the distribution of the enzyme in different organs. Antibodies were generated against the purified enzyme and further purified by precipitation and absorption to the antigen (the ATPase). Tests of monospecificity, such as rocket immunoelectrophoresis or crossed immunoelectrophoresis, are essential for exact interpretation of the data. Using monospecific antibody, staining of the gastric mucosa showed the presence of the ATPase only in the parietal cell and within the cell only on the microvilli of the secretory canaliculus; therefore, the location is appropriate for an acid-generating enzyme (147). Figure 14 illustrates these results. Of 15 tissues surveyed for the presence of the K^+ ATPase using this antibody, only the thyroid and even more weakly the thymus cross reacted using immunodiffusion. Specialized regions of other organs may contain the enzyme.

With respect to the H^+K^+ ATPase, two classes of antibody are produced in rabbit: those that bind and inhibit enzyme activity, and those that bind but do not inhibit enzyme activity (147).

The antibody can be used to study membrane flow in isolated cells. When cells are freshly isolated, the antibody reacts only with the apical surface, thereby yielding polar staining, if fluorescent coupling methods are used. After about 60 min, however, there is a uniform halo of fluorescence around the cell, showing lateral diffusion of the marker, the ATPase. The data reflecting a unique localization of antibody are en-

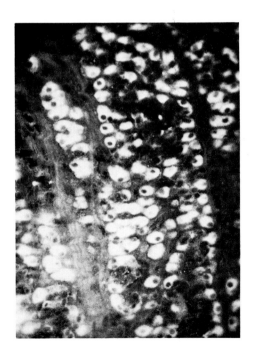
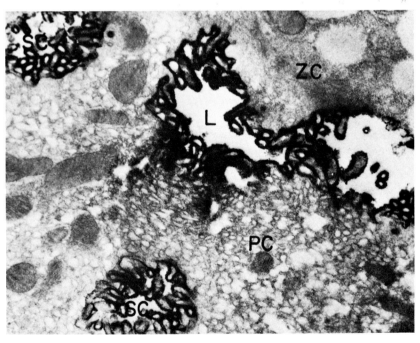

FIG. 14. Left: Immunofluorescence micrograph of a gastric section following treatment with anti-ATPase antibody showing parietal cell localization of the ATPase **Right:** Electron micrograph showing localization of the ATPase to the microvilli of the secretory canaliculus (SC) and the apical surface of the parietal cell (PC).

couraging in terms of a role for this enzyme in acid secretion. The K⁺ ATPase antibody does not affect the Mg^{2+} ATPase in the second peak after free flow separation, showing that the enzyme in this fraction is not part of the K⁺ ATPase.

Reaction Pathway

To date, two types of transport ATPases have been well characterized. The mitochondrial ATPase, which transports 2 H⁺ per ATP hydrolyzed and is reversible with respect to the electrical or H⁺ gradient generated, belongs to the category of enzymes that apparently do not form covalent intermediates during the reaction. F_1 is composed of five subunits, some (α and β) necessary for substrate binding and others (γ, δ, and ϵ) necessary for the interaction with the true membrane-bound portion of the complex, the F_0 portion. The F_1 and F_0 together form the proton translocating portion. The F_0 is also composed of more than one peptide. One is the proton translocating potion, and others are the DCCD and oligomycin binding proteins. The result of action of this type of enzyme is to produce an electrochemical gradient of H⁺ across mitochondrial, chloroplast, or bacterial membranes (127). The understanding of this process is based on the chemiosmotic hypothesis of oxidative phosphorylation. The mechanism of translocation of H⁺ through the F_1 complex with generation of ATP is not understood.

The other class of transport ATPases that has been described is exemplified by the Na^+-, K^+-, or Ca^{2+} ATPases (64,107). Here the protein is phosphorylated by the terminal phosphate of ATP during the reaction. Usually one ionic ligand, Na^+, is essential for phosphorylation, and the other, K^+, accelerates the dephosphorylation. The general scheme is:

$$ENZ' + Na^+_i + ATP \rightarrow ENZ - P \cdot Na_i$$

$$ENZ - P_i \cdot Na_0 \cdot \rightarrow ENZ - P \cdot Na_0$$

$$ENZ - P \cdot Na_0 + K_0 \rightarrow ENZ - P \cdot K_0 + Na_0$$

$$ENZ - P \cdot K^+_0 \rightarrow ENZ + P_i + K_i + P_i$$

It is important to define this pathway in the gastric ATPase, not only in terms of the role of the phosphoenzyme but also in terms of the reactions with ionic ligands involved in the reaction.

The Presence of Phosphorylation

When the gastric ATPase is incubated with $\gamma - {}^{32}P - ATP$, ^{32}P is incorporated into the enzyme (130). In the presence of K⁺, this phosphorylation is reduced (63,130,149). It is clear from these data that the gastric ATPase is a member of the class of enzymes occupied by the Na^+, K^+ and Ca^{2+} ATPases. Two classes of enzymes may be distinguished by the requirements for loss of phosphoenzyme (covalent or electrovalent binding). In the case of the F_1 type, although breakdown of ATP to form enzyme phosphate (EP) requires H⁺, as does the $H^+:K^+$ ATPase to form EP, the rate of loss of P from the enzyme is not affected by ions on the *trans* side of the enzyme (the ATP binding site being on the *cis* side). Hence H⁺ transport through the enzyme complex is not accompanied by counterion flow. This may be true of the Neurospora ATPase (C. Slayman, *personal communication*). In the case of the mammalian plasma membrane ATPases, K⁺ (or its equivalent) is necessary for loss of Pi by binding to a site *trans* to the ATP or initial cation site (Fig. 15). Depending on the stoichiometry of the two ionic ligands, such pumps may be electroneutral or partially electrogenic (e.g., with the Na^+, K^+ ATPase with three Na^+ for two K^+ stoichiometry, activity results in one charge transported per three ions translocated). Such pumps also show several modes of operation, such as (a) normal transport, (b) $Na^+:Na^+$ exchange, (c) $K^+:K^+$ exchange, (d) uncoupled Na^+ flux, and (e) reverse flux, indicating that the state of the enzymes are separable (64). It is pertinent to discuss the possible role of the EP form in the enzyme reaction.

Formation of EP

Kinetic studies of reaction intermediates usually require rapid methods of formation and quenching of the reaction. Hence the studies to be described utilize a rapid reaction machine, where reactants are rapidly mixed in a given sequence, aged for a predetermined time, the reaction stopped, and the products analyzed.

The sequence of reaction can be determined by the addition of Mg^{2+} to the enzyme after first mixing with

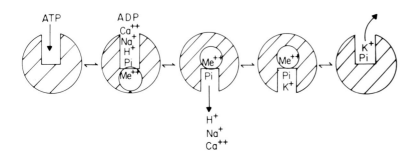

FIG. 15. Conceptual model illustrating an antiport pump operating via a phosphorylated intermediate pumping H⁺, Na⁺, or Ca^{2+} in one direction and K⁺ in the other. The uniport does not require K⁺. Me⁺⁺ represents Mg^{2+}.

ATP, or by mixing enzyme with Mg^{2+}ATP. The reactions are:

$$ENZ \quad ATP + Mg^{2+} \rightarrow ENZ - P$$

$$or \quad ENZ + Mg^{2+} \quad ATP \rightarrow ENZ - P$$

If the enzyme is premixed with ATP before the addition of Mg^{2+}, the rate of formation of EP is faster than if free enzyme is reacted simultaneously with Mg^{2+}ATP. The rate constants are 4,400 and 1,200 per min. In either case, the formation of enzyme phosphate is faster than the overall reaction rate of ~ 210 min^{-1}. The sequence of reaction is:

$$ENZ + ATP \rightarrow ENZ \cdot ATP$$

$$ENZ \cdot ATP + Mg^{2+} \rightarrow ENZ - P + ADP$$

The reversibility of this reaction can also be investigated kinetically. Thus if the enzyme and labeled ATP mixture is mixed with Mg^{2+} and unlabeled ATP, the labeling of enzyme will be reduced, because of the dissociation of the enzyme-ATP complex. Since there is inhibition of EP formation, ATP binding is reversible. Reversibility of the second step can be determined by the addition of ADP. However, the addition of ADP does not reduce the formation of phosphoenzyme any more than does unlabeled ATP. This implies poor reversibility of the second step of the reaction as shown.

The rate of formation of the EP increases with decreasing extravesicular pH. It can be shown that the rate of phosphorylation is essentially independent of the concentration of H^+ inside the vesicles. Thus the H^+ ion may act in a manner similar to the Na^+ ion in the Na^+, K^+ ATPase reaction. The overall reaction may be written:

$$ENZ \cdot H_0 + ATP <-> ENZ \cdot ATP \cdot H_0$$

$$ENZ \cdot H_0 \cdot ATP + Mg \rightarrow ENZ - Pi \cdot H_0 + ADP$$

The H_0 in this reaction is on the cystolic face of the enzyme (177,185,186).

Breakdown of EP

Enzyme phosphate can be formed in the rapid reaction apparatus, further formation stopped by the addition of the Mg^{2+} chelator CDTA, and the level of EP measured as a function of time. This gives the spontaneous rate of breakdown of EP. Increasing the internal pH accelerates the rate of breakdown of EP. This is also reflected in the steady-state measurement of the Mg^{2+}ATPase activity, which increases with increasing pH. Moreover, the spontaneous rate of breakdown of the EP complex increases in the presence of K^+, but this reaches maximal rate at low K^+ concentrations. This can be interpreted according to the equation:

$$ENZ - Pi_I \rightarrow ENZ - Pi_{II}$$

$$ENZ - Pi_{II} + K^+ \rightarrow ENZ + Pi + K^+$$

where ENZ-Pi_I and ENZ-Pi_{II} are two different conformations of the intermediate. As the pH increases on the luminal face of the enzyme, the rate of breakdown of the EP is increasingly accelerated by the addition of K^+. Accordingly, the rate of the enzyme reaction would be maximal with low pH external and high pH internal to the vesicles. The rate of breakdown of the intermediate is always accelerated by the addition of K^+. The interaction of K^+ with the enzyme is more complex than simply catalyzing EP breakdown.

Sidedness of K^+ Interaction

When the steady-state rate of the K^+ATPase is investigated as a function of K^+ concentration in lyophilized vesicles, K^+ activates the enzyme at low concentrations and inhibits the enzyme at higher concentrations (186). The reactions discussed above do not provide an explanation for the inhibition by K^+. When the EP complex is formed in tight vesicles and K^+ added, only a slow dephosphorylation is seen. In contrast, if K^+ is added to the vesicles prior to the addition of ATP, there is large reduction in the rate of phosphoenzyme formation. Hence external K^+ inhibits the enzyme reaction. Na^+ is even more potent than K^+ as an inhibitor of phosphorylation. The reaction scheme must now be expanded to:

$$ENZ - Pi \cdot K_i \rightarrow ENZ - Pi - K_0$$

$$ENZ - Pi \cdot K_0 \rightarrow ENZ \cdot K_0 + Pi$$

$$ENZ \cdot K_0 + ATP \rightarrow ENZ \cdot ATP + K_0$$

Thus there are two K^+ sites: an internal activating site of high affinity (~ 200 μM) and an external site of lower affinity (15 mM at 2 mM ATP). The affinity change is one of the necessary conditions for K^+ transport out of the vesicles. When the interaction of H^+ with the phosphorylation reaction is considered, there is again a high affinity site external to the vesicles, as shown by the increasing rate of phosphorylation with increasing H^+ concentration. From the kinetics, therefore, it can be predicted that the vesicles should transport H^+ inward and K^+ outward. The reaction scheme thus far determined is shown in Fig. 16.

The K^+ Site

Kinetic investigations are most readily interpreted as being due to the presence of two K^+ sites, one internal and one external to the vesicles when the ATP binding site is external to the vesicles.

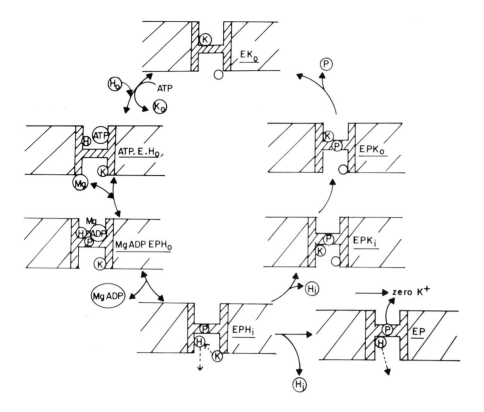

FIG. 16. Possible catalytic sequence for the H+:K+ ATPase. The reaction starts by displacement of K+ from the cytosolic face of the pump by ATP or H+. Mg^{2+}-dependent phosphorylation follows; with dissociation of Mg ADP, H+ is translocated across the barrier (much thinner than the biomembrane). K+ displaces H+, with movement of H+ into the lumen; K+ is then transported in the opposite direction with loss of bound phosphate.

Better definition of these K+ sites can be obtained by using a carboxyl group-activating reagent, ethoxy carbonyl ethoxy dihydroquinoline (EEDQ). Its mechanism is activation of carboxyl groups with reaction with NH$_2$-R groups on the protein. This reagent inhibits the ATPase, and the enzyme is protected by low K+ concentrations (143). When the K+ is present only external to the vesicles, no protection is exerted; when it is present on the vesicle interior, there is complete protection as before. Hence the activating K+ site, which is internal to the vesicles, is a carboxyl group that interacts with EEDQ. The pK of this group as defined by interaction with EEDQ is about 7, showing that it is hydrophobic. Evidence for the hydrophobicity of the group is also obtained by considering the possible reason for the high affinity of Tl+ for the activiting site (10-fold that of K+) (124). This is due to the higher polarizability of this large group III cation as opposed to K+. In contrast to the high affinity of Tl+ for the internal activating site, the affinity of Tl+ for the external inhibitory K+ site is about the same order of magnitude as that for K+, showing that it is a less hydrophobic group that is responsible for the K+ binding external to the vesicles.

The action of EEDQ also elicits another property of the enzyme. The pNPPase activity, which is clearly a partial reaction of the ATPase, is also inhibited by EEDQ. K+ present on both sides of the vesicles also protects the pNPPase activity. However, if K+ is present only on the vesicle interior, only 50% protection is obtained; if K is present externally, again only 50% pro-

tection is provided. This suggests that the enzyme may be at least a dimer, where both halves of the dimer are required for ATPase activity, but either monomer can hydrolyze pNPP (143).

The H+ Site

Although the K+ site has been demonstrated to be a carboxyl group, the H+ site is not as well defined. The use of site-specific reagents, such as diethyl pyrocarbonate, which interacts with histidine groups and inhibits gastric ATPase activity, may show that external H+ site is a histidine group (143). However, the difficulty of changing H+ concentration without additional complications is such that it is more difficult to define the site of interaction of H+ with the enzyme. NH$_2$ groups are also essential for enzyme function.

Role of Phospholipids

The ATPase is a membrane-bound enzyme intrinsic to the membrane. Accordingly, the phospholipids may play a vital role in the function of this enzyme. Removal of phospholipids to the extent of 50% of the hydrolyzable components by phospholipase A2 inhibits the ATPase but not the pNPPase, provided the products are removed by defatted serum albumin. ATPase activity is restored by the addition of either phosphatidylcholine or ethanolamine. It should also be noted that there is an increase of Mg^{2+}ATPase activity with removal of phospholipids, and that this activity falls with readdition of the lipids. The lipid requirement is not very specific in terms of ATP turnover. The finding that ATPase activity can be inhibited without an effect on pNPPase activity is consistent with a requirement for dimer for ATPase activity but monomer function in pNPPase activity (143).

The kinetic analysis provides evidence that the gastric ATPase belongs to the class of transport ATPases that form phosphorylated intermediates. Also, H^+ and K^+ are the interactive cations for the activity of this enzyme. Based on the analogy with the Na^+, K^+ and Ca^{2+}ATPases, it can be suggested that the gastric ATPase functions as an H^+:K^+ antiport pump as the Na^+, K^+ and Ca^{2+}ATPases function as Na^+:K^+ and Ca^{2+}: K^+ pumps. The presence of a phosphorylated intermediate alters pump function from an uniport mechanism. This in turn is based on the requirements for phosphate cycling by the enzyme. In the case of an uniport pump, the enzyme does not form a covalent Pi intermediate, and the noncovalent-bound phosphate can dissociate from the enzyme without the entrainment of another cation. In the case of the antiporter pumps, a covalent phosphate is formed that required destabilization by the countertransported cation, thus far universally K^+. These schemes are illustrated in Fig. 15.

Transport by Gastric Vesicles

The seminal observation in this area was the uptake of H^+ by dog or hog gastric microsomes upon the addition of ATP in the presence of K^+ (101,152,155). Before describing the details of the process, it is necessary to discuss some of the experimental methods available for measuring ion transport in vesicular systems (153). The size of the vesicles (average diameter 0.15 μm) precludes direct electrode measurements.

The vesicle membrane defines an intravesicular space. Since the vesicle space is not accessible to electrodes, ion-selective electrodes allow measurement of uptake into or efflux from vesicles from medium changes. The most sensitive ion electrode is the pH electrode, but K^+, Na^+, and Cl^- electrodes are also available. Since, functional H^+ concentrations are about 10^{-7}M, whereas the other ions usually must be present in the millimolar range, uptake of H^+ into a relatively small volume is measured with greater sensitivity.

Uptake or release of radioactive ions into or from the vesicle space can be measured, provided there are rapid means of separating vesicles from medium without leak of ions. This often can be done by filtration, centrifugation, or column separations.

In some instances, separation is not necessary, provided uptake into vesicle space makes a significant concentration difference in the medium, since the rate of

dialysis across a dialysis membrane is a function of the concentration of material in the extravesicular space. Alternatively, probes are available that are sensitive to gradients of H^+ or potential across the vesicle membrane. Thus weak bases, such as aminopyrine, acridine orange, and 9-aminoacridine are trapped in intravesicular water as a function of low pH internally. Lipid permeable cations, such as diethyloxocabodicyanine, are trapped as a function of a negative potential internally, and anilinonapthosulfonic acid shows a change in fluorescence as a function of an internal positive potential; the lipid permeable anion SCN is also trapped. Thus both optical and radioactive probes of pH and potential gradients are available (123). The resonance signal of ^{31}P is also a function of the environmental pH; hence NMR spectroscopy can be used to define the pH gradient generated by vesicles. Thus far, no probes define K^+, Na^+, or Cl^- concentration gradients.

Permeability of vesicles to water and solutes can also be measured by using light scattering to monitor vesicle volume. Addition of an osmotic gradient results in loss of water, the rate of which depends on the osmotic water permeability of the vesicle membrane. The reswelling of the vesicles in turn depends on the entry rate of the solute used to generate the osmotic gradient (125). Thus several techniques are available to measure permeabilities and active transport by gastric vesicles.

Compounds are also available that selectively modify the permeability of the vesicle membrane to ions. These are known as ionophores and differ in allowing net charge flow (protonophores, such as tetrachlorsalicylanilide, the K^+ ionophore valinomycin, and the K^+:H^+ exchange channel gramicidin) or only functioning as electroneutral antiporters (nigericin, which is a K^+, Na^+, or H^+ exchanger, monensin, which is more selective for Na^+ than K^+, and tributyltin, which is a Cl^-:OH^- antiporter).

There can be no violation of electroneutrality using any of these ionophores; hence they allow a simple determination of the nature of the electrical pathways available for ions across membranes. For example, if TCS does not dissipate a proton gradient, no associated conductances are present; otherwise, the H^+ could flux through the electrogenic TCS pathway with associated flow of the other conductive ion through the other conductance. Equally, if there is a potential gradient generated by pump activity, electroneutral exchange ionophores may dissipate the ion gradient but will then increase the potential difference across the vesicle membrane.

Active H^+ Transport

The addition of ATP to gastric vesicles results in uptake of H^+ into the vesicle space only if there is intravesicular K^+. This is shown in Fig. 17, where ATP is added to gastric vesicles loaded with varying K^+ by varying times of preincubation. The loss of H^+ from the medium is monitored by a pH electrode at pH 6.1. Back-titration allows an exact measure of the rate of transport of H^+, provided there is an exact return to baseline with the addition of an appropriate ionophore, such as nigericin or valinomycin with protonophore. When 150 mM KCl is equilibrated across the vesicle membrane, there is loss of about 100 nmoles H^+/mg vesicle protein (32,152); this depends on the quantity of K^+ in the vesicles.

Similar data are obtained using acridine orange or 9-amino acridine, in that K^+ is required in the vesicle interior for H^+ uptake (100,123). These probes can be used to measure the intravesicular pH in a quantitative manner (Table 3). There is a considerable discrepancy in the loss of H^+ from the medium and the appearance of free protons in the vesicle interior. This shows the presence of buffering in the vesicle space. The expected Δ pH of more than 6 is not achieved, but this cannot be accounted for only by vesicle buffering (123,152).

The effect of K^+ on the exterior of the vesicle as opposed to the interior can be determined by fixing internal K^+ and varying external K^+ by dilution into a choline medium or Na^+ medium with the Cl^- held constant. The data show that both external K^+ and external Na^+ are inhibitory to the transport reaction. The effect is on the rate of transport but not on the maximal gradient. These data are expected from the kinetic data discussed above (186). The H^+ transport data are consistent with the ATPase kinetics that have been described and with the presence of a H^+:K^+ exchange mechanism.

Passive H^+ Transport

Passive H^+ transport can be determined by using probes of ΔpH following the application of a pH pulse to induce H^+ gradient across the vesicle membrane and then measuring the rate of decay of the H^+ gradient as monitored by the probe. In the absence of cations, the H^+ permeability of the gastric vesicles is quite low. The addition of Cl^- or K^+ increases the rate of dissipation of the pH gradient, showing the presence of H^+Cl^- or K^+:H^+ pathways in the vesicle membrane. Although the calculated H^+ permeability is low, it is at least an order of magnitude higher than the passive permeability to K^+. The ratio of H^+ to K^+ permeability limits the size of the H^+ gradient that can be generated by the gastric vesicles at a given initial K^+ internal concentration (156) following ATP addition.

Active K^+ Transport

The simplest means of measuring active K^+ transport is to load the vesicles with radioactive cation, such as Rb^+ or Tl^+, and to add ATP directly to the equilibrated vesicles. Any efflux of cation must be active, and both Rb^+ and Tl^+ are transported (124,162). This K^+ efflux is linked to H^+ influx in the vesicles.

Both the uptake of H^+ or the efflux of K^+ can be secondary to the development of a vesicle potential gradient, with consequent electrophoresis of the counter ion. Ionophores can exclude this possibility. Thus if H^+ uptake were attributable to the development of an internal negative potential, the addition of TCS should increase the rate and probably magnitude of H^+ uptake, as well as ATPase activity. Since this does not occur, uptake of H^+ is not secondary to a K^+ pump-induced potential. If K^+ efflux were attributable to the generation of a positive interior potential due to an electrogenic H^+ pump, the addition of valinomycin should increase the H^+ rate, even in equilibrated vesicles, and increase the magnitude and rate of cation efflux. Since this does not happen, it excludes cation movement as being secondary to an H^+ pump potential. The potential generated by the gastric vesicle can be measured directly.

Passive K^+ Transport

Radioactive cations can be used in the absence of ATP to measure the passive flux rate across the gastric vesicle membrane. Passive cation and anion uptake are slow, the half-time being about 40 min at room temperature (162). Osmotic shrink swell experiments

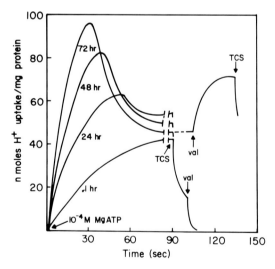

FIG. 17. H^+ uptake by gastric vesicles at 22° C following addition of ATP after exposure to KCl (150 mM) for the times indicated (at 4° C) showing increasing H^+ uptake with increased intravesicular K^+ and dissipation of the ion gradient by the protonophore tetrachlorsalicylanilide (TCS) followed by the K^+ ionophore valinomycin. Valinomycin added first enhances the gradient due to increased rate of reentry of KCl.

TABLE 3. *ΔpH in gastric vesicles (hog) following ATP*

Probe	pH 6.1	pH 7.4
Electrode	4.92	—[a]
Bromcresol green	4.92	—[a]
9-Amino acridine	2.2	2.8
Aminopyrine	3.37	4.41
Acridine orange	3.2	4.6
DOCC + TCS	3.7	5.9

[a] Not measurable due to ATP hydrolysis.

also show that there is low permeability to KCl (126). Both radioactive and light scattering measurements show that Cl^- or other monovalent anions give the maximal flux of K^+. Sulfate severely restricts K^+ movement; hence longer preincubation times are required for demonstrating H^+ transport in the presence of this anion. Nevertheless, in contrast to the intact tissue, H^+ transport is found in gastric vesicles in the presence of sulfate, provided lengthy incubation is used.

In intact gastric vesicles, the rate-limiting step in ATP turnover and H^+ transport is the entry of KCl into the vesicle. Knowing the rate of proton transport per square micron *in vivo* and the surface area of the vesicles, it is possible to compare directly the maximum proton rate *in vivo* and *in vitro*. Under KCl equilibrated conditions, the initial velocity of H^+ uptake by gastric vesicles is comparable to the *in vivo* rate. However, the rate of penetration of KCl is more than one order of magnitude too slow to account for the continuous *in vivo* acid rate. Physiological regulation of the KCl permeability or K^+ interaction with the enzyme must occur if the gastric ATPase is to serve as the primary proton pump.

It has been claimed that Ca^{2+} levels in the medium do affect KCl permeability. This would account for the Ca^{2+}-dependent hormone activation of acid secretion but does not explain the requirement for cAMP changes described earlier (122).

Electrogenicity of Transport

As discussed above, the transport data in gastric vesicles are due to an ATP-activated H^+:K^+ exchange; the process was probably electroneutral. To establish the electroneutrality of the transport process, it is necessary to measure the potential across the vesicle membrane during the transport reaction.

The presence of an interior negative potential can be established by using lipid-permeable cations, such as DOCC, Tl^+, or TPP^+ and by measuring distribution of the cation following ATP addition to gastric vesicles. In the absence of ionophore, there is no change in the optical signal due to DOCC with the addition of ATP (123). Since a H^+ gradient is developed, it is possible to

induce a diffusion potential due to H^+ by the addition of the protonophore, TCS. Accordingly, no negative interior potential is developed during H^+ transport by gastric vesicles.

Similarly, the presence of a positive interior potential can be established by measuring the uptake of SCN^- (162) or the fluorescence of ANS^- (103). Again, in the absence of ionophore, the addition of ATP does not result in any change of distribution of the lipid permeable anions used. Since a K^+ gradient is formed, the addition of valinomycin results in the development of an interior positive potential and a change in ANS fluorescence.

Based on the use of potential probes in these gastric vesicles, there is no evidence for the electrogenicity of the gastric ATPase under the conditions in which it has been studied. If these data are applied to the intact tissue, the data relating to electrogenicity derived from the intact tissue must be interpreted differently. For example, the effect of current application to the intact tissue in activating or inhibiting acid secretion can be reinterpreted on the basis of electrophoresis of K^+ to or from the secretory surface of the ATPase.

Ion Movement in Intact Cell

With the model that has been developed for the gastric vesicles—a KCl entry step and then an active K^+:H^+ exchange—the K^+ is cycled across the secretory membrane. The earlier model for the basolateral membranes, where both K^+ and Na^+ cycles across this membrane were postulated, can readily be combined with the model developed for H^+ transport by adding the K^+ cycle on the secretory canalicular surface, as shown in Fig. 18. The modification that occurs with secretion is the export of Cl^- across the secretory surface and the transport of HCO_3^- across the basal surface.

A major point of ignorance is the means whereby KCl enters the transport site of the enzyme. It is predicted that a pump inhibitor in the presence of stimulus will result in loss of KCl from the tissue. This is borne out by data using a benzimidazole derivative, an inhibitor of the ATPase, in the intact guinea pig (118). There is suppression of HCl secretion and stimulation of KCl secretion. Similarly, a relationship between K^+ and H^+ transport has been elucidated in the frog gastric mucosa by using a nonpermeant sulfhydryl inhibitor, *p*-chloromercuribenzoate (131).

The action of SCN^- in blocking acid secretion at 10 mM is not reproduced by the isolated gastric vesicles (152). The addition of SCN^- to the permeable gastric glands, where acid secretion is stimulated by ATP, does inhibit weak base accumulation. When these vesicles are isolated, the action of SCN^- disappears. Thus upon removal of the membrane from the cell, a factor is lost

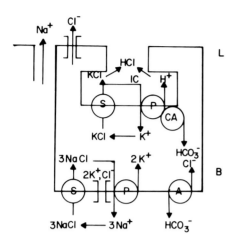

FIG. 18. Model of a secreting parietal cell showing the various ion pathways present on apical, canalicular, and basolateral surface. IC: intracellular canaliculus, L: lumen, B: blood, S: symport, A: antiport, P: pump,][: conductance.

that is essential for SCN⁻ action; it is suggested that this factor is carbonic anhydrase. In isolated frog gastric vesicles, SCN⁻ does inhibit H⁺ but not K⁺ transport (125), which may mean that in this species association of carbonic anhydrase with the gastric ATPase is retained during purification, in contrast to the mammalian system.

PERSPECTIVES

Much has been achieved in the first five decades of research into modern gastric physiology: (a) The function of the major cell types of the gastric epithelium is known; (b) the hormones that regulate this function have in large part been defined; (c) the second messengers responsible for activation of the parietal cell are known; (d) the intracellular target of these second messengers is suspected and perhaps one (Cl⁻ permeability) established; (e) metabolism and its regulation in the parietal cell has had its boundries determined; (f) the site of acid secretion is known; and (g) the H⁺ pump and many of its properties have been investigated.

Nevertheless, at all levels of integration, much remains to be learned. From what has come, understanding of gastric digestion and methods of treatment have evolved. For example, blockade of secretion is now possible without surgical intervention; it is likely that inhibitors of the H⁺ pump will be developed soon. On the other hand, functions that require integration of many parameters, such as resistance to ulceration, the preneoplastic state, and the level of acid secretion in an individual, remain mysteries and require biological approaches, many of which are undeveloped or in their infancy. Tissue culture of gastric cells (24) and of the epithelium itself will contribute significantly in the future to the solution of clinical problems.

ACKNOWLEDGMENTS

This work was supported in part by NIH grants AM15878, AM21588, and AM25520 and by NSF grants PCM 78-09208 and PCM 80-08625.

REFERENCES

1. Alonso, D., and Harris, J. B. (1965): Effect of xanthines and histamine on ion transport and respiration by frog gastric mucosa. *Am. J. Physiol.,* 208:18–23.
2. Alonso, D., Nigon, K., Donr, T., and Harris, J. D. (1967): Energy sources for gastric secretion substrates. *Am. J. Physiol.,* 212:992–1000.
3. Anderson, E., and Harvey, W. R. (1966): Active transport by the cecropia midgut. II. Fine structure of the midgut epithelium. *J. Cell. Biol.,* 31:107–134.
4. Armstrong, W. M., Bixenman, W. R., Frey, K. F., Garcia-Diaz, J. F., O'Regan, M. G., and Owens, J. L. (1979): Energetics of coupled Na⁺ and Cl⁻ entry into epithelial cells of bullfrog small intestine. *Biochim. Biophys. Acta,* 551:207–219.
5. Berglindh, T., Helander, H. F., and Obrink, K. J. (1976): Effects of secretagogues on oxygen consumption, aminopyrine accumulation and morphology in isolated gastric glands. *Acta Physiol. Scand.,* 97:401–414.
6. Berglindh, T. (1977): Potentiation by carbachol and aminophylline of histamine and db-cAMP induced parietal cell activity in isolated gastric glands. *Acta Physiol. Scand.,* 99:75–84.
7. Berglindh, T. (1977): Effects of common inhibitors of gastric acid secretion on secretagogue-induced respiration and aminopyrine accumulation in isolated gastric glands. *Biochim. Biophys. Acta,* 464:217–233.
8. Berglindh, T. (1977): Absolute dependence on chloride for acid secretion in isolated gastric glands. *Gastroenterology,* 73:874–880.
9. Berglindh, T., DiBona, D. R., Ito, S., and Sachs, G. (1980): Probes of parietal cell function. *Am. J. Physiol.,* 238:G165–G176.
10. Berglindh, T., DiBona, D. R., Pace, C. S., and Sachs, G. (1980): ATP dependence of H⁺ secretion. *J. Cell Biol.,* 85:392–401.
11. Berglindh, T., Helander, H. F., and Sachs, G. (1979): Secretion at the parietal cell level: A look at rabbit gastric glands. *Scand. J. Gastroenterol. [Suppl.],* 55:7–14.
12. Berglindh, T., and Obrink, K. J. (1976): A method for preparing isolated glands from the rabbit gastric mucosa. *Acta Physiol. Scand.,* 96:150–159.
13. Berglindh, T., and Obrink, K. J. (1979): Histamine as a physiological stimulant of gastric parietal cells. In: *Histamine Receptors,* edited by T. Yellin, pp. 35–56. S. P. Medical and Scientific Books, New York.
14. Berglindh, T., and Sachs, G. (1979): Histamine uptake and release from isolated gastric glands. In: *Hormone Receptors in digestion and Nutrition,* edited by G. Rosselin, P. Fromageot, and S. Bonfils, pp. 373–381. Elsevier, New York.
15. Berglindh, T., and Sachs, G. (1980): 3-Isobutyl-l-methylxanthine will normalize the response to gastrin and acetycholine in isolated gastric glands. *Fed. Proc.,* 39:376 (Abstr.).
16. Berglindh, T., and Sachs, G. (1980): (*Unpublished observations*).
17. Berglindh, T., and Sachs, G. (1980): (*Unpublished observations*).
18. Berglindh, T., Takeguchi, N., and Sachs, G. (1980): Ca⁺⁺ dependent secretagogue stimulation in isolated rabbit gastric glands. *Am. J. Physiol,* 2:690–694.
19. Bergqvist, E., and Obrink, K. J. (1979): Gastrin-histamine as a normal sequence in gastric acid stimulation in the rabbit. *Ups. J. Med. Sci.,* 84:145–154.
20. Berridge, M. J. (1966): Metabolic pathways of isolated Malpighian tubules of blowfly functioning in an artificial medium. *J. Insect Physiol.,* 12:1523–1538.
21. Bieck, P. R., Oates, J. A., Robison, G. A., and Adkins, R. B.

(1973): Cyclic AMP in the regulation of gastric secretion in dogs and humans. *Am. J. Physiol.,* 224:158–164.

22. Birdsall, N. J. M., Berrie, C. P., Burgen, A. V. S., and Holme, A. C. (1980): Modulation of binding properties of muscarinic receptors. Evidence for receptor effector coupling. *Adv. Biochem. Pharmacol.,* 21:107–116.

23. Birnbaumer, L., Swartz, T. L., Abramowitz, J., Mintz, P. W., and Iyengar, R. (1980): Transient and steady state kinetics of the interaction of guanyl nucleotides with the adenylyl cyclase system from rat liver plasma membranes. *J. Biol. Chem.,* 255:3542–3551.

24. Bisbee, C. A., Rutten, M. J., Logsdon, C. D., and Machen, T. E. (1980): Stomach epithelial cells in monolayer culture: Ultrastructure and electrophysiology. *Fed. Proc.,* 39:714 (Abstr.).

25. Black, J. W., Duncan, W. A. M., Durant, C. J., Ganellin, C. R., and Parsons, E. M. (1972): Definition and antagonism of histamine H_2 receptors. *Nature,* 236:385–390.

26. Blum, A. L., Hirschowitz, B. I., Helander, H. F., and Sachs, G. (1971): Electrical properties of isolated cells of Necturus gastric mucosa. *Biochim. Biophys. Acta,* 241:261–272.

27. Blum, A. L., Shah, G. T., Wiebelhaus, V. D., Brennan, F. T., Helander, H. F., Ceballos, R., and Sachs, G. (1971): Pronase method for isolation of viable cells from Necturus gastric mucosa. *Gastroenterology,* 61:189–200.

28. Bovet, D. (1950): Introduction to antihistamine agents and antergan derivatives. *Ann. N.Y. Acad. Sci.,* 50:1089–1126.

29. Canosa, C. A., and Rehm, W. S. (1968): Microelectrode studies of dog's gastric musoca. *Biophys. J.,* 8:415–420.

30. Cassel, D., and Selinger, Z. (1978): Mechanism of adenylate cyclase activation through the β-adrenergic receptor: Catecholamine-induced displacement of bound GDP by GTP. *Proc. Natl. Acad. Sci. USA,* 75:4155–4159.

31. Chance, B., and Williams, G. R. (1955): Respiratory enzymes in oxidative phosphorylation. II. Difference spectra. *J. Biol. Chem.,* 217:395–407.

32. Chang, H., Saccomani, G., Rabon, E., Schackmann, R., and Sachs, G. (1977): Proton transport by gastric membrane vesicles. *Biochim. Biophys. Acta,* 464:313–327.

33. Cheung, W. Y. (1980): Calmodulin plays a pivotal role in cellular regulation. *Science,* 207:19–27.

34. Chew, C. S., and Hersey, S. J. (1979): Characteristics of histamine receptor in isolated gastric glands. In: *Hormone Receptors in Digestion and Nutrition,* edited by G. Rosselin, P. Fromageot, and S. Bonfils, pp. 361–372. Elsevier, New York.

35. Chew, C. S., and Hersey, S. J. (1978): Dissociation between xoyntic cell cAMP formation and HCl secretion in bullfrog gastric mucosa. *Am. J. Physiol.,* 235:E140–E149.

36. Chew, C. S., Hersey, S. J., Sachs, G., and Berglindh, T. (1980): Histamine responsiveness of isolated gastric glands. *Am. J. Physiol.,* 238:G312–G320.

37. Code, C. F. (1965): Histamine and gastric secretion: A later look. 1955–1965. *Fed. Proc.,* 24:1311–1321.

38. Conway E. J. (1953): *Biochemistry of Gastric Acid Secretion.* Charles C. Thomas. Springfield, Illinois.

39. Cross, S. A. M. (1970): Ultrastructural localization of carbonic anhydrase in rat stomach parietal cells. *Histochemie,* 22:219–225.

40. Davenport, H. W. (1940): The inhibition of carbonic anhydrase and of gastric acid secretion by thiocyanate. *Am. J. Physiol.,* 129:505–514.

41. Davenport, H. W. (1962): Effect of ouabain on acid secretion and electrolyte content of frog gastric mucosa. *Proc. Soc. Exp. Biol. Med.,* 110:613–615.

42. Davenport, H. W., and Chavre, V. J. (1950): Conditions affecting acid secretion by mouse stomachs in vitro. *Gastroenterology,* 15:467–480.

43. Dell'Antone, P., Caolonna, R., and Azzone, G. F. (1971): Metachromatic effects and binding of organic cations to energized submitochondrial particles. *Biochim. Biophys. Acta,* 234:541–544.

44. DiBona, D. R., Ito, S., Berglindh, T., and Sachs, G. (1979): The cellular site of gastric acid secretion. *Proc. Natl. Acad. Sci. USA,* 76:6689–6693.

45. Durant, G. J., Emmett, J. C., and Ganellin, C. R. (1977): pp. 1–12. *Excerpta Medica.*

46. Durbin, R. P. and Hanzel, D. (1980): Uptake and incorporation of phosphate by frog gastric mucosa. *Am. J. Physiol. (in press).*

47. Durbin, R. P., and Heinz, E. (1958): Electromotive chloride transport and gastric acid secretion in the frog. *J. Gen. Physiol.,* 41:1035–1047.

48. Durbin, R. P., and Kasbekar, D. K. (1965): Adenosine triphosphate and active transport by the stomach. *Fed. Proc.,* 24:1327–1381.

49. Durbin, R. P., Kitahana, S., Stahlmann, K., and Heinz, E. (1964): Exchange diffusion of chloride in frog gastric mucosa. *Am. J. Physiol.,* 207:1177–1180.

50. Durbin, R. P., Michelangeli, F., and Nickel, A. (1974): Active transport and ATP in frog gastric mucosa. *Biochim. Biophys. Acta,* 367:177–189.

51. Ecknauer, R., Thompson, W. J., Johnson, L. R., and Rosenfeld, G. C. (1980): Isolated pariental cells: QNB binding to putative cholinergic receptors. *Am. J. Physiol. (in press).*

52. Ekblad, M. (1980): Increase of intracellular pH in secreting frog mucosa. *Biochim. Biophys. Acta,* 632:335–375.

53. Flatmark, T., and Terland, O. (1971): Cytochrome b561 of the bovine adrenal chromaffin granules. A high potential b-type cytochrome. *Biochim. Biophys. Acta,* 253:487–491.

54. Flemstrom, G. (1977): Active alkalinization by amphibian gastric fundic mucosa in vitro. *Am. J. Physiol.,* 233:E1–E12.

55. Forte, J. G. (1980): *Am. J. Physiol. (in press).*

56. Forte, J. G., and Davies, R. E. (1964): Relation between hydrogen ion secretion and oxygen uptake by gastric mucosa. *Am. J. Physiol.,* 206:218–222.

57. Forte, J. G., Forte, T. M., and Machen, T. E. (1975): Histamine-stimulated hydrogen ion secretion by in vitro piglet gastric mucosa. *J. Physiol.,* 244:15–31.

58. Fromm, D., Schwartz, J. H., Robertson, R., and Fuhra, R. (1976): Ion transport across isolated antral mucosa of the rabbit. *Am. J. Physiol.,* 231:1783–1789.

59. Fromter, E. M., and Diamond, J. M. (1972): Route of passive ion permeation in epithelia. *Nature,* 235:9–13.

60. Ganser, A. L., and Forte, J. G. (1973): K^+ stimulated ATPase in purified microsomes of bullfrog oxyntic cells. *Biochim. Biophys. Acta,* 307:169–180.

61. Ganser, A. L., and Forte, J. G. (1973): Ionophoretic stimulation of K^+-ATPase of oxyntic cell microsomes. *Biochem. Biophys. Res. Commun.,* 54:690–696.

62. Forte, J. G., Ganser, A. L., and Tanisawa, A. S. (1974): The K^+-stimulated ATPase system of microsomal membranes from gastric oxyntic cells. *Ann. N.Y. Acad. Sci.,* 242:255–267.

63. Garrahan, P. J., and Glynn, I. M. (1967): The stoichiometry of the sodium pump. *J. Physiol.,* 192:217–235.

64. Glynn, I. M., and Karlish, S. J. D. (1975): The sodium pump. *Ann. Rev. Physiol.,* 37:13–55.

65. Goodall, M. C., and Sachs, G. (1977): Resonstitution of a proton pump from gastric mucosa. *J. Membr. Biol.,* 35:285–301.

66. Gray, J. S., and Adkinson, J. L. (1941): The effect of inorganic ions on gastric secretion in vitro. *Am. J. Physiol.,* 134:27–31.

67. Gregory, R. A., and Tracy, H. J. (1961): The preparation and properties of gastrin. *J. Physiol.,* 156:523–543.

68. Grossman, M. I. (1967): Neural and hormonal stimulation of gastric secretion. *Handbook of Physiology, Vol. 2, Secretion,* edited by C. F. Code and W. Heidel, pp. 835–862. Am. Physiol. Soc., Washington, D.C.

69. Grossman, M. I. (1970): Gastrin and its activities. *Nature,* 228:1147–1150.

70. Harris, J. B., and Edelman, I. S. (1960): Transport of potassium by the gastric mucosa of the frog. *Am. J. Physiol.,* 198:280–284.

71. Heinz, E., and Durbin, R. (1959): Evidence for an independent hydrogen-ion pump in the stomach. *Biochim. Biophys. Acta.,* 31:246–247.

72. Heinz, E., Geck, P., and Pietrzyk, C. (1975): Driving forces of amino acid transport in animal cells. *Ann. N.Y. Acad. Sci.,* 264:428–441.

73. Helander, H. F., and Hirschowitz, B. I. (1972): Quantitative ultrastructural studies on gastric parietal cells. *Gastroenterology,* 63:951–961.

74. Hersey, S. J. (1971): The energetic coupling of acid secretion in gastric mucosa. *Philos. Trans. R. Soc. Lond. [Biol.]*, 262: 261–275.

75. Hersey, S. J. (1974): Interactions between oxidative metabolism and acid secretion in gastric mucosa. *Biochim. Biophys. Acta*, 344:157–203.

76. Hersey, S. J. (1980): ATP metabolism in isolated gastric glands. *Fed. Proc. (in press)*.

77. Hersey, S. J., and High, W. L. (1971): On the mechanism of acid secretory inhibition by acetozolamide. *Biochim. Biophys. Acta*, 233:604–609.

78. Hirschowitz, B. I. (1967): Secretion of pepsinogen. In: *Handbook of Physiology, Vol. 2, Secretion*, edited by C. F. Code and W. Heidel, pp. 889–918. Am. Physiol. Soc., Washington, D.C.

79. Hirschowitz, B. I., and Hutchinson, G. A. (1975): Effects of vagotomy on urecholine-modified histamine dose responses in dogs. *Am. J. Physiol.*, 228:1313–1318.

80. Hirschowitz, B. I., and Sachs, G. (1965): Vagal gastric secretory stimulation by 2-deoxy-D-glucose. *Am. J. Physiol.*, 209:452–460.

81. Hirschowitz, B. I., and Sachs, G. (1969): Atropine inhibition of insulin; histamine and pentagastrin-stimulated gastric electrolyte and pepsin secretion in the dog. *Gastroenterology*, 56:693–702.

82. Hogben, C. A. M. (1955): Active transport of chloride by isolated frog gastric epithelium; origin of the gastric mucosal potential. *Am. J. Physiol.*, 180:641–649.

83. Hokin, L. E. (1966): Effects of calcium omission on acetylcholine-stimulated amylase secretion and phospholipid synthesis in pigeon pancreas slices. *Biochim. Biophys. Acta*, 115: 219–221.

84. Jackson, R. J. *(Unpublished observations)*.

85. Jacobson, E. D., Swan, K. G., and Grossman, M. I. (1967): Blood flow and secretion in the stomach. *Gastroenterology*, 52:414–420.

86. Johnson, E. M., Ueda, T., Maena, H., and Greengard, P. (1972): Adenosine 3,5 monophosphate dependent phosphorylation of a specific protein in synaptic membrane fractions from rat cerebrum. *J. Biol. Chem.*, 247:5650–5652.

87. Johnson, L. R. (1977): Gastrointestinal hormones and their functions. *Ann. Rev. Physiol.*, 39:135–158.

88. Johnson, R. G., Pfisten, D., Carty, S. E., and Scarpa, A. (1979): Biological amine transport in chromaffin ghosts. Coupling to the transmembrane proton and potential gradients. *J. Biol. Chem.*, 254:10963–10972.

89. Kagawa, Y., Kandnach, A., and Racker, E. (1973): Partial resolution of the enzymes catalyzing oxidative phosphorylation. XXVI. Specificity of phospholipids required for energy transfer reactions. *J. Biol. Chem.*, 248:676–684.

90. Kasbekar, D. K. (1974): Calcium-secretagogue interaction in the stimulation of gastric acid secretion. *Proc. Soc. Exp. Biol. Med.*, 145:234–239.

91. Kasbekar, D. K. (1980): *(Unpublished observations)*.

92. Kidder, G. W. (1980): *Am. J. Physiol.* Further studies on the sudden potential drop in gastric mucosa, with a model for its production. *(in press)*.

93. Kier, L. B. (1968): Molecular orbital calculations of the preferred conformations of histamine and a theory on its dual activity. *J. Med. Chem.*, 11:441–445.

94. Koelz, H., Berglindh, T., and Sachs, G. (1981): Properties of pepsin secretion in the isolated rabbit gastric glands. *Am. J. Physiol. (submitted)*.

95. Koelz, H. R., Sachs, G., and Berglindh, T. (1981): Interaction of intracellular K^+ and Na^+ on acid formation in isolated gastric glands. *Am. J. Physiol. (submitted)*.

96. Kondo, S., and Schulz, I. (1976): Ca^{++} fluxes in isolated cells of rat pancreas. Effect of secretagogues and different Ca^{++} concentrations. *J. Membr. Biol.*, 29:185–203.

97. Landowne, D. (1975): A comparison of radioactive thallium and potassium fluxes in the giant axon of the squid. *J. Physiol.*, 252: 79–96.

98. Larose, L., Lanoe, J., Morisset, J., Geoffrion, L., Dumont, Y., Lord, A., and Poirier, G. G. (1979): Rat pancreatic muscarinic cholinergic receptors. In: *Hormone Receptors in Digestion and Nutrition*, edited by G. Rosselin, P. Fromageot, and S. Bonfils, pp. 229–238. Elsevier, New York.

99. Lee, H. C., Breitbart, H., Berman, M., and Forte, J. G. (1979):

100. Lee, H. C., Breitbart, H., Forte, J. G. (1980): Functional role of K^+ ATPase in proton transport. *N. Y. Acad. Sci.*, 341:297–310.

101. Lee, J., Simpson, G., and Scholes, P. (1974): An ATPase from dog gastric mucosa: Changes of outer pH in suspensions of membrane vesicles accompanying ATP hydrolysis. *Biochem. Biophys. Res. Commun.* 60:825–834.

102. Lewin, M. J. M., Ghesquier, D., Soumarmon, A., Cheret, A. M., Grelac, F., and Guesnon, J. (1978): Cytochrome b_5 and K^+-pNPPase: specific characterization in the isolated rat gastric parietal cell. *Acta Physiol. Scand.* [Suppl.], 267–282.

103. Lewin, M. J. M., Saccomani, G., Schackmann, R., and Sachs, G. (1977): The use of ANS as a probe of gastric vesicle transport. *J. Membr. Biol.*, 32:301–318.

104. Lichtstein, D., Kaback, H. R., and Blum, A. J. (1979): Use of a lipophilic cation for determination of membrane potential in neuroblastoma-glioma hybrid cell suspensions. *Proc. Natl. Acad. Sci. USA*, 76:650–654.

105. Liedtke, C. M., and Hopfer, U. (1980): Chloride-sodium symport versus chloride/hydroxide or chloride uniport as mechanisms for chloride transport across rat intestinal brush border membrane. *Fed. Proc.*, 39:734 (Abstr.).

106. Loewenstein, W. R. (1973): Cell coupling. In: *Transport Mechanisms in Epithelia*, edited by H. H. Ussing, and N. A. Thorn, pp. 20–27. Munksgaard, Copenhagen.

107. MacLennan, D. H., and Holland, P. C. (1975): Calcium transport in sarcoplasmic reticulm. *Annu. Rev. Biophys. Bioeng.*, 4:377–404.

108. Machen, T. E., and Logsdon, C. D. (1980): Involvement of Extracellular Calcium in Gastric Stimulation. *Am. J. Physiol. (in press)*.

109. Machen, T. E., Clausen, C., and Diamond, J. M. (1977): Electrical events during stimulation of HCl secretion by frog gastric mucosa in vitro. *Gastroenterology*, 73:970.

110. Maren, T. H. (1967): Carbonic anhydrase: chemistry, physiology and inhibition. *Physiol. Rev.*, 47:595–781.

111. Marshall, P., Dixon, J. F., and Hokin, L. E. (1980): Evidence for a role in stimulus-secretion coupling of prostaglandins derived from release of arachidonyl residues as a result of phosphatidylinositol breakdown. *Proc. Natl. Acad. Sci. USA*, 77(6):3292–3296.

112. Michelangeli, F., and Proverbio, F. (1978): Effect of calcium on the H^+/K^+ ATPase of hog gastric microsomes. *J. Membr. Biol.*, 42:301–315.

113. Mitchell, P. (1966): Chemiosmotic coupling in oxidative and photosynthetic phosphorylation. *Biol. Rev.*, 41:445–502.

114. Moody, F. G. (1968): Oxygen consumption during thiocyanate inhibition of gastric acid secretion in dogs. *Am. J. Physiol.*, 215:127–131.

115. Nakajima, S., Hirschowitz, B. I., and Sachs, G. (1971): Studies on adenyl cyclase in Necturus gastric mucosa. *Arch. Biochem. Biophys.*, 143:123–126.

116. Nakajima, S., Shoemaker, R. L., Hirschowitz, B. I., and Sachs, G. (1970): Comparison of actions of aminophylline and pentagastrin on Necturus gastric mucosa. *Am. J. Physiol.*, 219: 1259–1262.

117. O'Doherty, J., Garcia-Diaz, J. F., and Armstrong, W. M. (1979): Sodium selective liquid ion-exchanger microelectrodes for intracellular measurements. *Science*, 203:1349–1351.

118. Olbe, L., Berglindh, T., Elander, B., Helander, H., Fellenius, E., Sjostrand, S. E., Sundell, G., and Wallmark, B. (1979): Properties of a new class of gastric acid inhibitors. *Scand. J. Gastroenterol. [Suppl.]*, 55:131–132.

119. Parsons, M. E., and Bunce, K. T. (1978): Gastric H^+ secretion in isolated whole rat stomach. *Acta Physiol. Scand.* [Suppl.], 141–142.

120. Perrier, C. V., and Laster, L. (1970): Adenyl cyclase activity of guinea pig gastric mucosa: Stimulation by histamine and prostaglandins. *J. Clin. Invest.*, 49:73a (Abstr.).

121. Philpott, C. W. (1980): Tubular system membranes of teleost chloride cells: Osmotic response and transport sites. *Am. J. Physiol.*, 238: R171–R184.

122. Proverbio, F., and Michelangeli, F. (1978): Effect of calcium on

the H^+/K^+ ATPase of hog gastric microsomes. *J. Membr. Biol.,* 42:301–315.

123. Rabon, E., Chang, H. H., and Sachs, G. (1978): Quantitation of hydrogen ion and potential gradients in gastric plasma membrane vesicles. *Biochemistry,* 17:3345–3353.

124. Rabon, E., and Sachs, G. (1981): The interaction of TL with gastric ATPase vesicles. *J. Membr. Biol. (submitted).*

125. Rabon, E., Saccomani, G., Kasbekar, D. K., and Sachs, G. (1979): Transport characteristics of frog gastric membranes. *Biochim. Biophys. Acta,* 551:432–447.

126. Rabon, E., Takeguchi, N., and Sachs, G. (1980): Water and salt permeability of gastric vesicles. *J. Membr. Biol.,* 53:109–117.

127. Racker, E. (1979): Mechanisms of ion transport and ATP formation. In: *Membrane Transport in Biology,* edited by G. Giebisch, D. C. Tosteson, and H. H. Ussing, Vol. 1, pp. 259–290. Springer Verlag, New York.

128. Ramswell, P., Crane, B. H. (1976): Arachidonic acid and facilitation of acid secretion in stimulus secretion coupling in GI tract. In: edited by R. H. Case and H. Cioebell, pp. 107–116. MTP Press.

129. Ray, T. K., and Forte, J. G. (1974): Soluble and bound protein kinases of rabbit gastric secretory cells. *Biochem. Biophys. Res. Commun.,* 61:1199–1206.

130. Ray, T. K., and Forte, J. G. (1976): Studies on the phosphorylated intermediates of a K^+-stimulated ATPase from rabbit gastric mucosa. *Biochim. Biphys. Acta,* 443:451–467.

131. Ray, T. K., and Tague, L. L. (1978): Role of K^+ ATPase in H^+ and K^+ transport by bullfrog gastric mucosa in vitro. *Acta Physiol. Scand. [Suppl.],* 283–292.

132. Rehm, W. S. (1945): The effect of electric current on gastric secretion and potential. *Am. J. Physiol.,* 144:115–125.

133. Rehm, W. S. (1965): Electrophysiology of the gastric mucosa in chloride-free solutions. *Fed. Proc.,* 24:1387–1395.

134. Rehm, W. S. (1972): Proton transport. In: *Metabolic Pathways,* 3rd edition, edited by L. E. Hokin, Vol. 6, pp. 187–241. Academic Press, New York.

135. Rehm, W. S., Davis, T. L., Chandler, C., and Gohmann, E. (1963): Frog gastric mucosae bathed in chloride-free solutions. *Am. J. Physiol.,* 204:233–242.

136. Rehm, W. S., and Sanders, S. S. (1975): Implications of the neutral carrier $Cl\text{-}HCO_3$ exchange mechanism in gastric mucosa. *Ann. N.Y. Acad. Sci.,* 264:442–455.

137. Reimann, E. M., and Rapino, N. G. (1974): Partial purification and characterization of an adenosine 3,5 monophosphate dependent protein kinase from rabbit gastric mucosa. *Biochim. Biophys. Acta,* 350:201–204.

138. Reyl, F., Silve, C., and Lewin, M. J. M. (1979): Somatostatin receptors on isolated gastric cells. In: *Hormonal Receptors in Digestion and Nutrition,* edited by G. Rosselin, P., Fromageot, and S. Bonfils, pp. 391–400, Elsevier, New York.

139. Robert, A. (1976): Antisecretory, antiulcer, cytoprotective and diarrheogenic properties of prostaglandins. *Adv. Prostaglandin Thromboxane Res.,* 2:507–520.

140. Robison, G. A., Butcher, R. W., and Sutherland, E. W. (1971): *Cyclic AMP.* Academic Press, New York.

141. Rosenfeld, G. C., Jacobson, E. D., and Thompson, W. J.: (1976): Re-evaluation of the role of cyclic AMP in histamine-induced gastric acid secretion. *Gastroenterology,* 70:832–835.

142. Rottenberg, H., and Lee, C. P. (1975): Energy dependent hydrogen ion accumulation in submitochondrial particles. *Biochemistry,* 14:2675–2680.

143. Saccomani, G., Barcellona, M., and Sachs, G. (1981): Reactivity of gastric $(H^+ + K^+)$ ATPase to N-ethoxycarbonyl-2-ethoxyl-1, 2-dihydro quinoline. *J. Biol. Chem. (submitted).*

144. Saccomani, G., Capuletti, J., Chung, J., and Sachs, G. *In preparation.*

145. Saccomani, G., Chang, H. H., Mihas, A. A., Crago, S., and Sachs, G. (1979): An acid transporting enzyme in human gastric mucosa. *J. Clin. Invest.,* 64:627–635.

146. Saccomani, G., Dailey, D., and Sachs, G. (1979): The action of trypsin on the gastric (H^+/K^+) ATPase. *J. Biol. Chem.,* 254:2821–2827.

147. Saccomani, G., Helander, H. F., Crago, S., Chang, H. H., and Sachs, G. (1979): Characterization of gastric mucosal membranes. X. Immunological studies of gastric (H^+/K^+) ATPase. *J. Cell Biol.,* 83:271–282.

148. Saccomani, G., Lewin, M. J. M., and Sachs, G. (1980) (unpublished observations).

149. Saccomani, G., Shah, G., Spenney, J. G., and Sachs, G. (1975): Characterization of gastric mucosal membranes. VIII. The localization of peptides by iodination and phosphorylation. *J. Biol. Chem.,* 250:4802–4809.

150. Saccomani, G., Stewart, H. B., Shaw, D., Lewin, M., and Sachs, G. (1977): Characterization of gastric mucosal membranes. IX. Fractionation and purification of K^+-ATPase containing vesicles by zonal centrifugation and free flow electrophoresis technique. *Biochim. Biophys. Acta,* 465:311–330.

151. Sachs, G., Chang, H., Rabon, E., Schackmann, R., Sarau, H. M., and Saccomani, G. (1977): Metabolic and membrane aspects of gastric H^+ transport. *Gastroenterology,* 73:931–940.

152. Sachs, G., Chang, H., Rabon, E., Schackmann, R., Lewin, M., and Saccomani, G. (1976): A non-electrogenic H^+ pump in plasma membranes of hog stomach. *J. Biol. Chem.,* 251: 7690–7698.

153. Sachs, G., Jackson, R. J., and Rabon, E. C. (1980): The use of plasma membrane vesicles. *Am. J. Physiol.,* 238:G151–G164.

154. Sachs, G., Collier, R. H., Shoemaker, R. L., and Hirschowitz, B. I. (1968): Energy source for gastric H^+ secretion. *Biochim. Biophys. Acta,* 162:210–219.

155. Sachs, G., Rabon, E., Saccomani, G., and Sarau, H. M. (1975): Redox and ATP in acid secretion. *Ann. N.Y. Acad. Sci.,* 264:456–475.

156. Sachs, G., Rabon, E., and Saccomani, G. (1979): Active and passive ion transport by gastric vesicles. In: *Cation Flux Across Biomembranes,* edited by Y. Mukohata and L. Packer, pp. 53–66. Academic Press, New York.

157. Sachs, G., Shoemaker, R. L., and Hirschowitz, B. I. (1966): Effect of sodium removal on acid secretion by the frog gastric mucosa. *Proc. Soc. Exp. Biol. Med.,* 123:47–52.

158. Sachs, G., Shoemaker, R. L., Blum, A. L., Helander, H. F., Makhlouf, G. M., and Hirschowitz, B. I. (1971): Microelectrode studies of gastric mucosa and isolated gastric cells. *Electrophysiology of Epithelial Cells,* pp. 257–279.

159. Sanders, S. S., Pirkle, J. A., Shoemaker, R. L., and Rehm, W. S. (1978): Effect of weak bases on secreting acid inhibited in vitro frog gastric mucosa. *Acta Physiol. Scand. [Suppl.],* 155–164.

160. Sarau, H. M., Foley, J., Moonsamy, G., Wiebelhaus, V. D., and Sachs, G. (1975): Metabolism of dog gastric mucosa. I. Nucleotide levels in parietal cells. *J. Biol. Chem.,* 250: 8321–8329.

161. Sarau, H. M., Foley, J. J., Moonsamy, G., and Sachs, G. (1977): Metabolism of dog gastric mucosa. II. Levels of glycolytic citric acid cycle and other intermediates. *J. Biol. Chem.,* 252:8572–8581.

162. Schackmann, R., Schwartz, A., Saccomani, G., and Sachs, G. (1977): Cation transport by gastric $H^+{:}K^+$ ATPase. *J. Membr. Biol.,* 32:361–381.

163. Schatzmann, H. J. (1973): Dependence on calcium concentration and stoichiometry of the calcium pump in human red cells. *J. Physiol.,* 235:551–559.

164. Sedar, A. W., and Friedman, M. H. F. (1961): Correlation of the fine structure of the gastric parietal cell (dog) with functional activity of the stomach. *J. Biophys. Biochem. Cytol.,* 11: 349–363.

165. Shoemaker, R. L., Sachs, G., and Hirschowitz, B. I. (1966): Secretion by guinea pig gastric mucosa in vitro. *Proc. Soc. Exp. Biol. Med.,* 123:824–827.

166. Skou, J. C. (1965): Enzymatic basis for active transport of Na^+ and K^+ across cell membrane. *Physiol. Rev.,* 45:596–617.

167. Skulachev, V. P. (1971): Energy transformations in the respiratory chain. *Curr. Top. Bioenerg.,* 4:127–190.

168. Skulskii, I. A., Savina, M. V., Glasunov, V. V., and Saris, N. L. (1978): Electrophoretic transport of Tl^+ in mitochondria. *J. Membr. Biol.,* 44:187–194.

169. Soll, A. H. (1978): The actions of secretagogues on oxygen uptake by isolated mammalian parietal cells. *J. Clin. Invest.,* 61:370–380.

170. Soll, A. H. (1980): Secretagogue stimulation of [^{14}C] aminopyrine accumulation by isolated canine parietal cells. *Am. J. Physiol.*, 238:G366–G375.

171. Soll, A. H., and Wollin, A. (1979): Histamine and cyclic AMP in isolated canine parietal cells. *Am. J. Physiol.*, 237:E444–E450.

172. Soumarmon, A., Lewin, M., Cheret, A. M., and Bonfils, S. (1974): Gastric HCO_3^- stimulated ATPase: Evidence against its microsomal localization in rat fundus mucosa. *Biochim. Biophys. Acta*, 339:403–414.

173. Spenney, J. G., Flemstrom, G., Shoemaker, R. L., and Sachs, G. (1975): Quantitation of conductance pathways in antral gastric mucosa. *J. Gen. Physiol.*, 65:645–662.

174. Spenney, J. G., Saccomani, G., Spitzer, H. L., and Sachs, G. (1974): Composition of gastric cell membranes and polypeptide fractionation using ionic and non-ionic detergents. *Arch. Biochem. Biophys.*, 161:456–471.

175. Spenney, J. G., Shoemaker, R. L., and Sachs, G. (1974): Microelectrode studies of fundic gastric mucosa: cellular coupling and shunt conductance. *J. Membr. Biol.*, 19:105–128.

176. Spenney, J. G., Strych, A., Price, A. H., Helander, H. F., and Sachs, G. (1973): Properties of ATPase of gastric mucosa. V. Preparation of membranes and mitochondria by zonal centrifugation. *Biochim. Biophys. Acta*, 311:545–564.

177. Stewart, H. B., Wallmark, B., and Sachs, G. (1981): The interaction of H^+ and K^+ with the partial reactions of gastric (H^+/K^+) ATPase. *J. Biol. Chem. (submitted)*.

178. Rosenfeld, G. C., Thompson, W. J., and Jacobson, E. D. (1976): Gastric mucosal binding of ^{3}H-metiamide to putative histamine H_2-receptors. *Gastroenterology*, 70:963 (Abstr.).

179. Sung, C. P., Jenkins, B. C., Burns, L. R., Hackney, V., Spenney, J. G., Sachs, G., and Wiebelhaus, V. D. (1973): Adenyl and guanyl cyclase in rabbit gastric mucosa. *Am. J. Physiol.*, 225:1359–1363.

180. Sutherland, E. W., and Rall, T. W. (1958): Fractionation and characterization of a cyclic adenine ribonucleotide formed by tissue particles. *J. Biol. Chem.*, 232:1077–1091.

181. Takeuchi, K., Speir, G. R., and Johnson, L. R. (1979): Mucosal gastrin receptor. I. Assay standardization and fulfillment of receptor criteria. *Am. J. Physiol.*, 237:E284–E294.

182. Takeuchi, K., Speir, G. R., and Johnson, L. R. (1979): Mucosal gastrin receptor. II. Physical characteristics of binding. *Am. J. Physiol.*, 237:E295–E300.

183. Thompson, W. J., Change, L. K., and Rosenfeld, G. C. (1981): Histamine regulation of adenyl cyclase of enriched rat gastric parietal cells. *Am. J. Physiol.*, 240:G76–684.

184. Ussing, H. H. (1978): Interpretation of tracer fluxes. In: *Membrane Transport in Biology*, edited by G. Giebisch, D. C. Tosteson, and H. H. Ussing, Vol. 1, pp. 115–140. Springer, New York.

185. Wallmark, B., and Mardh, S. (1979): Phosphorylation and dephosphorylation kinetics of potassium stimulated ATP phosphohydrolase from hog gastric mucosa. *J. Biol. Chem.*, 254:11899–11902.

186. Wallmark, B., Stewart, H. B., Rabon, E., Saccomani, G., and Sachs, G. (1980): The catalytic cycle of gastric ATPase. *J. Biol. Chem. (in press)*.

187. Witt, J. J., and Roskoski, R., Jr. (1975): Bovine brain adenosine 3,5 monophosphate dependent protein kinase. Mechanism of regulatory subunit inhibition of the catalytic subunit. *Biochemistry*, 14:4503–4507.

188. Wollin, A., Soll, A. H., and Samloff, I. M. (1979): Actions of histamine, secretin, and PGE_2 on cyclic AMP production by isolated canine fundic mucosal cells. *Am. J. Physiol.*, 237:E437–E443.

189. Yamamura, H. I., and Snyder, S. H. (1974): Muscarinic cholinergic binding in rat brain. *Proc. Natl. Acad. Sci. USA*, 71:1725–1729.

Physiology of the Gastrointestinal Tract, edited by
Leonard R. Johnson. Raven Press, New York © 1981.

Chapter 20

Gastric Secretion of Bicarbonate

Gunnar Flemström

Full understanding of the electrolyte composition of gastric juice requires detailed knowledge of the mechanism for transport of ions by the gastric mucosal cells and the permeability characteristics of the gastric epithelium. Many studies in this field have provided information about the mechanism for transport of HCl into the gastric lumen and about stimulatory and inhibitory pathways of acid secretion. Transport of other ions and water by the gastric mucosa and its ion permeability characteristics are also important in this context but have received somewhat less attention.

The existence of a nonacid HCO_3 –containing secretion into the gastric lumen was proposed as early as 1892 by Danish physiologist Schierbeck (73). In carefully controlled experiments in dogs, he observed that the pCO_2 in gastric contents reached values up to 150 mm Hg, i.e., considerably higher than in blood. He also observed that a sham-feeding procedure increased the gastric output not only of acid but also of CO_2. Gastric transport of HCO_3^- has since been considered by several authors and is fundamental to the two-component hypothesis for gastric acidity regulation put forward by Hollander (42) and others. The presence of HCO_3^- in (nonacid) gastric secretions from humans and some animal species has been reported earlier, but only recently has gastric HCO_3^- transport been demonstrated to be an active process which can be stimulated and inhibited by various means. It is proposed that active HCO_3^- transport protects the gastric epithelium from damage by alkalinization of the surface boundary of the mucosal membrane (16,17,24,33). This concept has gained support from findings that several potential ulcerogens, including antiinflammatory drugs (35) and alpha-adren-

ergic agonists (18), inhibit gastric HCO_3 secretion. Furthermore, some prostaglandins with known antiulcer activity stimulate active HCO_3 transport in isolated mucosa (34,35) and increase the output of HCO_3 –containing secretion in the dog fundic pouch (7,51), suggesting that use of stimulants of HCO_3^- transport may provide a new approach to ulcer therapy.

Studies of HCO_3^- transport, however, must consider the experimental difficulty that under most conditions, HCO_3^- transport is masked by the larger simultaneous transport of H^+. This chapter describes the various methods employed to overcome this problem, and some of the difficulties involved in evaluation of the source of gastric HCO_3^-, and the nature of the transport process.

Some possible mechanisms leading to the appearance of HCO_3^- in the gastric lumen, namely, active transport of HCO_3, passive diffusion of HCO_3, ultrafiltration of HCO_3, permeation of CO_2 combined with neutralization of H^+, and contamination by salivary or duodenal HCO_3^-, are considered. A summary of some recent studies of the characteristics of active gastric HCO_3^- transport is made, and its possible role in regulation of gastric acidity and mucosal protection against acid is discussed. Some experiments on HCO_3^- transport by duodenal surface epithelium are also described.

METHODS OF STUDY

In vitro Studies of Antrum and H^+-inhibited Fundus

Antral or fundic mucosa from amphibia (17,24,36) or rabbit (28) is mounted as a membrane in *in vitro* chambers. This technique permits control of ion concentrations on both sides of the epithelium and allows characterization of some electrical properties of the mucosa (41,66).

The antrum has no, or very few, H$^+$-secreting (parietal) cells and is composed mainly of surface epithelial and mucous cells. These are morphologically indistinguishable from those in the fundic area; antrum was used as a model for studies of gastric nonparietal ion transport (37).

In most species *in vitro*, fundus secretes acid spontaneously, probably because of continuous release of histamine from endogenous sources (50,65). Neither histamine H$_2$ receptor antagonists nor SCN$^-$ have any effect on alkalinization in the antrum (17,34) and have been used to inhibit fundic H$^+$ secretion for investigations of HCO$_3^-$ transport. Studies in several amphibian species showed that inhibition of H$^+$ transport disclosed a net alkaline transport. The basal rate (0.25 to 0.50 μEq/cm^2/hr) amounts to 5 to 10% of the maximal H$^+$ secretion in the same species. Its characteristics are independent of the type of agent used to counteract H$^+$ secretion (17). The results of studies with stimulants and inhibitors (see below) indicate that HCO$_3$ transport is an active transport process that shows similar properties in H$^+$-inhibited fundus and spontaneously alkalinizing antrum.

Most studies on the isolated gastric mucosa are performed with an unbuffered solution gassed with 100% O$_2$ on the luminal side, and a HCO$_3^-$-containing solution gassed with 95% O$_2$ and 5% CO$_2$ on the nutrient (submucosal) side. The rate of luminal alkalinization is determined by continuous titration with HCl to a predetermined level of pH. The reason for using HCO$_3^-$/CO$_2$ is that gastric mucosal cells *in vivo* face interstitial HCO$_3^-$/CO$_2$. An external supply of CO$_2$ is also essential for maintenance of normal acid secretory rates by gastric mucosa both *in vitro* (52,72) and *in vivo* (71).

The presence of HCO$_3^-$/CO$_2$ in the nutrient solutions makes it necessary to consider the effects of possible passive permeation of these agents on luminal alkalinization. Passive leakage of HCO$_3^-$ would increase luminal alkalinization. This is not likely to occur in amphibian fundus since removal of nutrient HCO$_3^-$/CO$_2$ (with hepes$^-$/O$_2$ replacement) has no effect on the measured rates of HCO$_3^-$ transport (17). In the amphibian antrum, however, this procedure results in a 20 to 40% decrease in alkalinization (17,24,36); in the rabbit antrum, complete cessation of luminal alkalinization has been observed (28). Some of the antral luminal alkalinization may thus reflect passive permeation of HCO$_3^-$. This part of the stomach also has a considerably higher shunt conductance (78) than has the "tight" fundic epithelium (72,77). The sensitivity of amphibian and rabbit antral HCO$_3$ transport to inhibitors and stimulants indicates that active transport is responsible in part for luminal alkalinization by this tissue. The probable

presence in the antrum of both active and passive components of HCO$_3$ transport may explain the qualitatively similar but quantitatively weaker response of antral compared with fundic alkalinization to some inhibitors, including indomethacin (35).

Some agents, by effects on paracellular or other pathways of the mucosa, may induce passive permeation of HCO$_3$ ions and thereby increase luminal alkalinization. This phenomenon is illustrated (Figs. 1 and 2) in the alkalinizing frog fundic mucosa in studies with ethanol, which has previously been proposed to increase mucosal pathways for permeation of ions and molecules (11). Experiments were performed with a HCO$_3^-$-containing (17.8 mM) nutrient side solution gassed with O$_2$/CO$_2$ (95/5) and an unbuffered solution gassed with 100% O$_2$ on the luminal side. The pH on the nutrient side was 7.20; on the luminal side, it was kept at 7.40. At nutrient side concentrations of 3.5 and 7% (vol/vol), ethanol inhibited HCO$_3$ transport (Fig. 1). This was associated by some rise in transepithelial electrical resistance.

At the higher concentration of 14% (nutrient side), there was an initial decline in luminal alkalinization followed by an increase to a level above that preceding ethanol treatment (Fig. 2). The electrical resistance showed a transient increase followed by a marked decrease. The luminal alkalinization did not increase until the electrical resistance had begun to decline. The effects of ethanol were also tested in experiments in which a nonvolatile buffer, hepes$^-$, gassed with 100% O$_2$, was used instead of HCO$_3^-$/CO$_2$ on the nutrient side (Fig. 2). In this case, there was no increase in luminal alkalinization, although the electrical resistance decreased to a low level. Nutrient HCO$_3$ and hepes probably both permeate the low resistance (high conductance) ethanol-treated mucosa. Only HCO$_3^-$ is titrated on the luminal side, since gassing of a luminal solution containing permeated HCO$_3^-$ with 100% O$_2$, by the removal of CO$_2$ and formation of CO$_3^-$ (or OH$^-$), increases its pH. Hepes$^-$ is a nonvolatile buffer; gassing with O$_2$ should not affect the pH of a solution containing this agent. Although ethanol is an inhibitor of active HCO$_3^-$ transport, at high concentrations it may induce transmucosal, passive permeation of HCO$_3$ (and other ions) and thereby increase luminal alkalinization. H$^+$ secretion exhibited much smaller sensitivity to nutrient ethanol than did active HCO$_3^-$ transport; 14% ethanol caused only 7% inhibition, and 3.5 and 7% ethanol had no effect on H$^+$ transport.

Drug-induced passive permeation of HCO$_3^-$ has been demonstrated with acetylsalicylic acid. At low concentrations (1 to 3 mM), this drug inhibits active gastric HCO$_3^-$ transport *in vitro* and *in vivo* (31,32); at higher concentrations (10 to 20 mM), it induces mucosal permeation of HCO$_3^-$. The nonsteroidal, antiinflammatory drug fenclofenac has a similar effect (35).

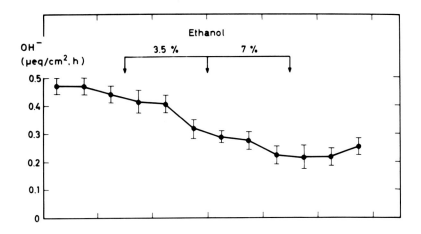

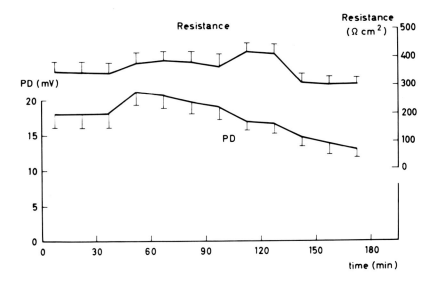

FIG. 1. Ethanol (nutrient side) was added, as indicated, to the alkaline-secreting isolated frog (Rana temporaria) fundic mucosa. Metiamide (10^{-3}M) was present in the nutrient solution throughout the experiments to counteract H^+ secretion. Mean values $\pm$ SE of the rate of HCO_3^- transport (OH^-), transepithelial electrical potential difference (PD), and resistance are presented, N = 10.

Use of a titration endpoint above 7 is advantageous in determining rates of HCO_3 transport. At lower pH values, it is difficult to exclude the possibility that diffusion of H^+ from the luminal solution into the mucosa contributes to the alkalinization of the luminal side.

The disadvantage with use of a nonacid luminal pH for titration is that CO_2 permeating from the nutrient side may acidify the luminal side (72,76), resulting in an underestimate of the rate of HCO_3^- transport. Permeation of CO_2 across the H^+-secreting fundic mucosa *in vitro* is probably slow, since luminal and nutrient side application of CO_2 has different effects on mucosal ion transport (48) and since the external supply of CO_2 is rate-limiting for H^+ secretion (52). Inhibition of H^+ secretion per se, however, may favor permeation of CO_2, since H^+-secreting cells normally consume CO_2 for use in the H^+ secretory process (52,71,72). The problem of CO_2 permeation can probably be minimized by careful gassing of the luminal side with non-CO_2-containing gas and by the use of steady-state conditions (17).

Even if potent inhibitors of H^+ secretion are used to disclose alkalinization, there may be a residual small, and therefore masked, H^+ transport. An increase in this

transport induced, for instance, by cyclic AMP (cAMP) or a high concentration of another stimulator of H^+ secretion, may appear as an inhibitor of the net alkaline (HCO_3^- minus H^+) transport. Comparison between antral and fundic epithelium, determination of electrical properties of the mucosa, or measurement of the output of some electrolyte, at least in part associated with H^+ transport, such as Cl^-, can provide information on the likelihood of this occurrence. Stimulation of H^+ secretion is associated with much greater changes in the transepithelial electrical potential difference and resistance than is stimulation of HCO_3^- transport (Fig. 3).

In Vivo Studies of Antrum and H+-Inhibited Fundus

Antral and fundic pouch secretion in dogs contain 8 to 15 mM HCO_3^- (Table 1). Antrum has no H^+ secretion, and HCO_3^- transport can be studied directly (37). Fundic HCO_3^- transport, on the other hand, has been studied in vagotomized pouches of antrectomized animals (7,42) or during administration of histamine H_2 receptor antagonists (51).

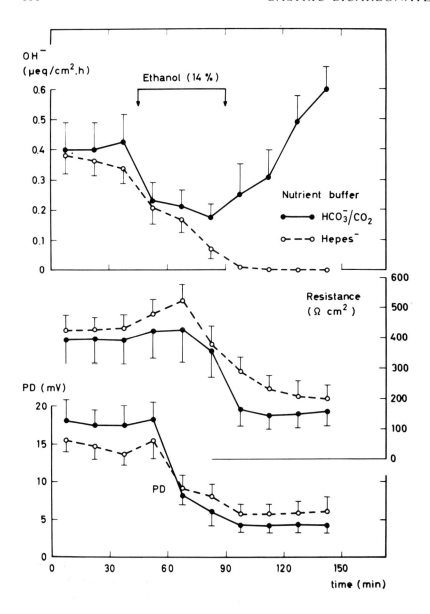

FIG. 2. Ethanol, at a higher concentration (14%, vol/vol) than before (Fig. 1), was added to the nutrient side of the metiamide-treated alkaline-secreting frog (Rana temporaria) fundic mucosa. An unbuffered solution gassed with 100% O_2 was always used on the luminal side. The pH on this side was kept at 7.40 by titration with HCl. Either 5 mM Hepes$^-$ gassed with 100% O_2 or 17.8 mM HCO_3^- gassed with 95% and 5% O_2/CO_2 was used as the nutrient side buffer (pH 7.20). Note that active HCO_3^- transport alone is titrated with hepes$^-$/O_2 on the nutrient side. With HCO_3^-/CO_2 on this side, both active transport of HCO_3^- and passively permeating nutrient HCO_3^- contribute to luminal alkalinization. Means ± SE; N = 9 with both types of experiment.

Passive permeation of HCO_3^- induced by drugs and low (masked) rates of H^+ secretion, despite the use of inhibitors, present similar problems in evaluation of experimental results *in vivo* and *in vitro*. The output of glucose and serum proteins (33) or gastric absorption of macromolecules (23, 24) may be used as an index of drug-induced increased mucosal permeability. Under *in vivo* conditions, changes in mucosal blood flow and capillary permeability may affect mucosal permeation of HCO_3^- and CO_2.

Gastric arterial injection of acetylcholine (5 to 50 µg/kg) or an artificially applied gastric arterial pressure of 200 mm Hg increases the mucosal interstitial pressure and causes ultrafiltration of HCO_3^- into the gastric fundus (2–4). This ultrafiltrate, however, also contains glucose and 10 to 20 g/liter protein and bears a marked resemblance to the fluid appearing in the gastric lumen when the permeability of the mucosa is increased by exposure to high concentrations of un-ionized acetyl-

salicylic acid (9). Induction of ultrafiltration or an increase of a normally occurring ultrafiltration at a low degree may thus result in an increase in intragastric HCO_3^-.

The dog stomach *in vivo* has been reported to extract CO_2 from arterial blood under basal (nonstimulated) conditions (71). Stimulation of H^+ secretion decreases pCO_2 in gastric venous blood to about 30 mm Hg (14), i.e., to levels below that in the arterial blood. Inhibition of H^+ secretion by histamine H_2 receptor antagonists may favor permeation of tissue CO_2 into the gastric lumen, since less CO_2 would be used in the H^+ secretory process. H_2 antagonists, due to the decrease in mucosal blood flow (8), may also decrease the amount of CO_2 available for diffusion. Gastric mucosal permeation of CO_2 was slow in the guinea pig (33) during inhibition of H^+ secretion by H_2 antagonists.

The nature of an intragastrically instilled solution may affect transmucosal exchange of CO_2. In alkaline

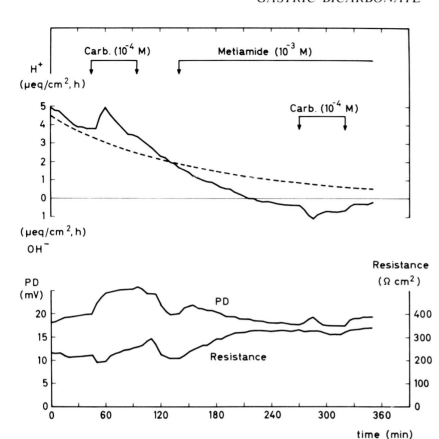

FIG. 3. This experiment illustrates that in the same (isolated frog) fundic mucosa, carbachol stimulates both H^+ and HCO_3^- transports. Interrupted line shows continuous decline of H^+ secretion occurring in an untreated mucosa. [From Flemström (17).]

buffer solutions (76), H^+ formed from CO_2 and water would be neutralized and HCO_3^- would be trapped. Trapping of HCO_3^- would also be associated with low values of intragastric pCO_2. High levels (70 to 80 mM) of intragastric HCO_3^- have been reported after intragastric instillation in humans of hypertonic solutions containing 500 mM glycine at pH 9.4 (5). Solutions containing glycine or some other relatively impermeable solutes may also reduce mucosal transport of water (61),

and hypertonic solutions may increase mucosal passive permeation of ions (27), including HCO_3^-.

Gastric secretions contain mucous glycoproteins with some, probably low (1,39,53,63), buffering capacity. By the neutralization of H^+ formed from CO_2 and water, these might contribute to the appearance of HCO_3^- in gastric contents. The findings of pCO_2 values in gastric contents in the dog (70,73) and guinea pig (33) above those reported for gastric arterial and venous blood

TABLE 1. *Measured mean concentrations of gastric electrolytes at low rates or in the absence of acid secretion*

Ref.	Na^+	K^+	Cl^-	HCO_3^-
Human (parietal cell atrophy)				
Lambling et al. (55)	94	20	83	18
Gardham and Hobsley (29)	80	17	92	8
Okosdinossian and El Munshid (64)	58	14	93	8
Human (normal subjects)				
Kristensen (53)[a]	132	11	117	13
Dog fundus				
Hollander (42)	133	4	120	13
Dog antrum				
Grossman (37)	151	9	145	8

[a]Similar but incomplete data are presented by Ihre (47). Note that variations in Na^+ and Cl^- concentrations may reflect some passive permeation of these ions through the mucosa, not associated with HCO_3^- transport (33), or in the case of fundic Cl^-, residual HCl secretion.

(14,71) suggest that this is of little importance under normal conditions. High pCO_2 per se indicates that permeation of CO_2 through the gastric mucosa is probably slow. High levels of pCO_2 have also been observed in the proximal tubule of the kidney and are probably the result of an intratubular H^+/HCO_3^- neutralization reaction (49,75).

Concomitant Measurement of Gastric H^+ and HCO_3^- Transport

Intragastric determination of pCO_2 and pH have been used to make simultaneous measurements of the gastric transport of HCO_3^- and H^+ into instilled isotonic mannitol or NaCl solutions (33). Prerequisites for this technique are that intragastric CO_2 is formed mainly during the reaction between secreted H^+ and HCO_3^- and that diffusion of CO_2 out of or into the stomach is slow. These seemed to be satisfied under the experimental conditions employed. The total amount of alkali (measured as CO_2 plus HCO_3^-) appearing in the gastric lumen was approximately the same during spontaneous H^+ secretion (when almost only CO_2 appeared), partial inhibition of H^+ secretion by histamine H_2 receptor antagonists (when CO_2 plus HCO_3^- appeared), and potent inhibition of H^+ secretion (when almost exclusively HCO_3^- appeared). There was also quantitative agreement between CO_2 released and the reduction of HCO_3^- when exogenous HCl was instilled. In the guinea pig, HCO_3^- transport occurred at a steady basal rate and was sensitive to some inhibitors and stimulants. It amounted to approximately 10% of the maximum H^+ transport in this species.

High rates of H^+ secretion, however, may be associated with removal of luminal CO_2 by the H^+-secreting cells for use in the H^+ secretory process. Feeding procedures increased intragastric pCO_2 in dogs (70,73). Stimulation of H^+ secretion by histamine in the same species has been reported to decrease the gastric ouput of CO_2 (54), or no CO_2 has been found (56). Cholinergic stimuli (17,33) but not histamine (17,24) increases gastric HCO_3^- transport. A simultaneous rise in HCO_3^- output may mask removal of luminal CO_2 by the mucosa after stimulation of H^+ secretion by feeding.

Indirect Methods

Gastric secretion of a HCO_3^- containing fluid was proposed by Hollander (42) to be the main mechanism for regulation of gastric acidity. Most but not all his evidence supporting the two-component hypothesis was indirect and derived from experiments in which only the net acid (H^+ minus HCO_3^-) was measured. In their mathematical analysis of this hypothesis, Makhlouf et al. (58) used Na^+ transport into the gastric lumen as an index of the nonparietal secretion. The secretion was

assumed to have a fixed concentration of HCO_3^-, to occur at a constant rate, and to have a defined volume. Published data (29,40,58) indicate that their approach is a satisfactory approximation for many experimental conditions. As discussed previously (33,46), however, there may be some permeation of Na^+ that is not associated with HCO_3^-. HCO_3^- transport both *in vitro* and *in vivo* can also be stimulated (and inhibited) by various means, including cholinergic agents. Reaction between H^+ and HCO_3^- would result in a decrease in the osmolarity of the combined secretion. This excess water would diffuse along its chemical gradient into the mucosa (13). Thus, even if transport of HCO_3^- into the gastric lumen is associated with water flux, an increase in intragastric volume may give an incorrect estimate of the amount of HCO_3^- transported.

Measurement of HCO_3^- in Human Gastric Juice

The occurrence of free HCO_3^- in human secretions has been reported by several authors. Two types of experimental conditions have been used. HCO_3^- has been measured in secretions obtained at spontaneously low rates of H^+ transport in apparently normal subjects (47,53) or in patients with pernicious anemia and some other diseases associated with parietal cell malfunction (29,55,64). As discussed earlier (46,53), with both categories there may be a residual but small and therefore masked H^+ secretion, giving falsely low values of gastric HCO_3^-. Parietal cell malfunction might also be associated with impairment of other ion transport characteristics of the gastric mucosa. Nevertheless, there is good agreement between figures published by most authors (Table 1). Thus human gastric secretion has been reported to contain between 8 and 20 mM HCO_3^- under basal conditions.

Values of pH in gastric nonacid secretions provide little information unless determined at a fixed pCO_2. At pCO_2 40 mm Hg (53), the pH has been reported to vary between 6.5 and 7.3. Various methods have been used to estimate contamination by salivary or duodenal HCO_3^- in humans. Salivary contamination has been excluded by use of dental pledgets in trained subjects (58) or the amount of such contamination estimated from the K^+ content of the gastric juice (29,53,64). Contamination by pancreatic HCO_3^- and bile has been excluded from the absence of bile staining (53), estimated by indirect methods, including dilution techniques (74) and measurement of Na^+ in the gastric juice (64), or prevented by intraduodenal aspiration (74).

CHARACTERISTICS OF ACTIVE GASTRIC HCO_3^- TRANSPORT

Fundic and antral mucosa *in vitro* have been used to study effects of stimulants and inhibitors of gastric

HCO$_3^-$ transport. It has been found that gastric HCO$_3^-$ transport can be affected by various agents (Table 2). The combined data strongly suggest that fundic HCO$_3^-$ transport *in vitro* is an active process. In the antrum, there is both active transport and passive permeation of HCO$_3^-$.

Stimulants *In Vitro*

In amphibian fundic and antral mucosa, stimulation of HCO$_3^-$ transport has been found with carbachol (Fig. 3), dibutyryl cGMP (17), Ca^{2+} ions (18), and the prostaglandins 16,16-dimethyl E$_2$ and F$_{2\alpha}$ (32). Some effective stimulants of gastric H$^+$ secretion (histamine, gastrin, pentagastrin, and dibutyryl cAMP) had no effect (17,18). Cholecystokinin (10^{-8} M) increased HCO$_3^-$ transport in fundic epithelium, whereas secretin (10^{-8}M) had no effect (G. Flemström, J. R. Heylings, and A. Garner, *unpublished*).

Further studies are required to elucidate the stimulatory pathway for gastric HCO$_3^-$ transport. Cholinergic stimuli (but not histamine) have been reported to increase the cGMP content of the gastric mucosa (15). It is not known whether the stimulatory effect of an increase in nutrient Ca^{2+} from 1.8 to 7.2 mM reflects a direct effect on HCO$_3^-$ transporting cells, sensitization of these cells, or local release of acetylcholine. Atropine abolishes the Ca^{2+} effect, which may favor the latter hypothesis (G. Flemström and A. Garner, *unpublished*).

Robert and others (69) have established that some prostaglandins protect against gastric ulcerations in several species, including man. PGE$_2$ and PGI$_2$ probably exert this effect by inhibition of H$^+$ secretion, while 16,16 dimethyl-PGE$_2$ possesses antiulcer activity at concentrations too low to affect H$^+$ secretion, and PGF$_{2\alpha}$ has no effect on gastric H$^+$ secretion. The two latter prostaglandins stimulate active HCO$_3$ transport, which may contribute to their antiulcer activity (34,35).

Inhibitors *In Vitro*

HCO$_3$ transport *in vitro* is sensitive to anoxia and CN$^-$, which inhibit tissue metabolism, and to 2:4-dinitrophenol, which uncouples oxidative phosphorylation (17,24). Diamox is a more effective inhibitor of gastric HCO$_3^-$ than H$^+$ secretion and more potent if administered on the luminal side (17). HCO$_3^-$ transport has also been found to be inhibited by alpha-adrenergic receptor agonists (18) while beta-agonists had no effect (Fig. 4). This inhibition was prevented by pretreatment of the mucosa with the alpha-antagonist phentolamine (Fig. 5). Administration of this antagonist (60) or splanchnic sympathectomy (45) prevents gastric stress ulceration *in vivo*.

Some nonsteroidal, antiinflammatory drugs inhibit HCO$_3^-$ transport alone or have a much greater effect on gastric HCO$_3^-$ than on H$^+$ transport. This has been found with acetylsalicylate (31,32), indomethacin, and fenclofenac (35). The latter is a new antiinflammatory drug which caused a large increase in the rate of exfoliation of gastric mucosal cells in the guinea pig (30). Inhibition of HCO$_3^-$ transport by indomethacin was prevented by pretreatment with 16,16-dimethyl PGE$_2$ (35). Hydrocortisone had no effect on gastric HCO$_3^-$ (and H$^+$) secretion, even in very high concentrations

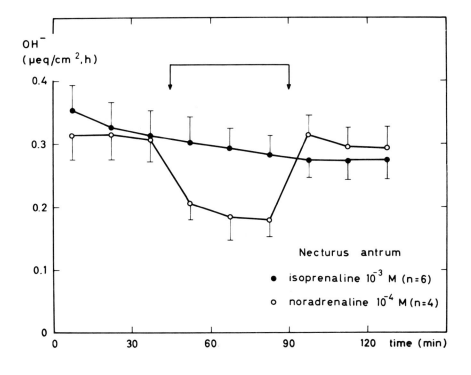

FIG. 4. Norepinephrine but not isoprenaline inhibited HCO$_3^-$ transport by Necturus antrum. The catecholamine was present in the nutrient side solution, as indicated. Means ± SE. [From Flemström (18).]

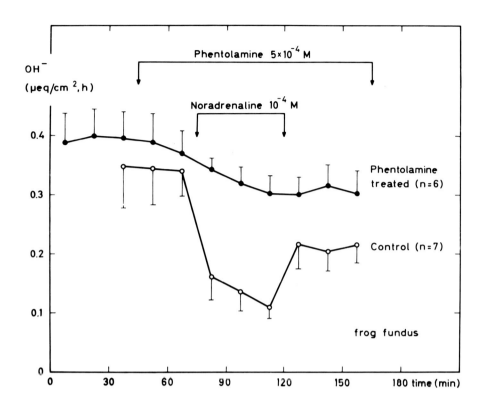

FIG. 5. Pretreatment with phentolamine prevented inhibition of HCO_3^- transport by norepinephrine. Norepinephrine alone was used in the control experiments. Results obtained in isolated frog fundus are shown. [From Flemström (18).]

(35). Ethanol (nutrient side) inhibited HCO_3^- transport at a concentration as low as 3.5% (Fig. 1), while 14% ethanol was required from some reduction of H^+ transport.

In Vivo Studies

Relatively few attempts have been made to stimulate or inhibit HCO_3 transport *in vivo*. Bethanechol had no effect on HCO_3^- output in the dog antral pouch (32),

TABLE 2. *Properties of active HCO_3^- transport by amphibian fundus and antrum in vitro[a]*

Basal rate
    5 to 10% of maximal H^+ transport (both measured in fundus, per cm^2 surface area)
Stimulants
    $Ca^{a,b}$ carbachol[b], cholecystokinin[c], dibutyryl-cGMP, 16,16-dimethyl PGE_2[b], PGF_{2a}, glucagon[c]
Inhibitors
    Alpha-adrenergic agonist, anoxia, acetazolamide, acetylsalicylate[b], CN^-, 2:4-dinitrophenol, ethanol, fenclofenac, indomethacin, parathyroid hormone[c]
No effect
    Beta-adrenergic agonists, dibutyryl cAMP, gastrin, histamine, hydrocortisone, PGE_2, ouabain, secretin[c]

[a] From refs. 16–18, 24, 31–36.
[b] Tested and shown effective *in vivo* (7,32,33,51).
[c] G. Flemström and A. Garner, *unpublished results.*
Atropine prevents cholinergic stimulation of HCO_3^- transport but does not affect the basal output (33).

while vagal stimulation increased the volume of nonacid secretion in the antral pouch of sheep (59).

In the guinea pig, intravenously administered carbachol (Fig. 6) increased the output of HCO_3^- and H^+. Both responses were inhibited by atropine, while H_2 receptor antagonists only inhibited the rise in H^+ secretion (33). Ca^{2+} stimulated both HCO_3^- and H^+ transport (G. Flemström and A. Garner, *unpublished*); and acetylsalicylate (5 mg/kg i.v.) inhibited HCO_3^- transport in the guinea pig (32). 16,16-Dimethyl PGE_2 has been tested in dog fundic pouches (7,51). It caused significant increases in the HCO_3^- output; administration into the pouch seemed more effective than the intravenous route. Some stimulants of active HCO_3^- transport *in vitro* have been shown to increase the HCO_3 output in mammals *in vivo*.

Secretin has been reported to stimulate gastric HCO_3^- transport in patients with antritis (74). Cholinergic stimuli are known to increase Na^+ output in the human stomach, an effect not obtained with histamine or gastrin (58). Na^+ output increased together with HCO_3^- in the guinea pig (33) and dog (7).

ORIGIN OF GASTRIC HCO_3^-

HCO_3^- transport in amphibian fundus *in vitro* was found to be independent of the presence of HCO_3^-/CO_2 on the nutrient side and was inhibited or stimulated by various agents, indicating that it is an active process. Antral alkalinization probably in part reflects transmucosal permeation of HCO_3, but its sensitivity to

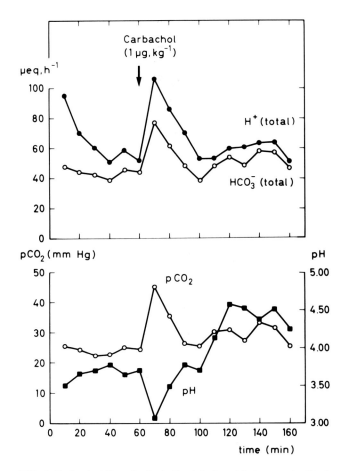

FIG. 6. Carbachol (1 µ g/kg i.v.) stimulated gastric transport of both H + and HCO₃⁻ in the guinea pig. [From Garner and Flemström (33).]

stimulants and inhibitors indicates that an active transport mechanism is also involved in luminal alkalinization in this part of the stomach.

The occurrence of active HCO_3^- transport with similar properties in the antrum and fundus indicates that is is nonparietal in origin. The surface epithelial cells contain most of the gastric mucosal carbonic anhydrase (6,57) and cGMP diesterase (79). The sensitivity of alkalinization to the carbonic anhydrase inhibitor acetazolamide and to dibutyryl cGMP suggests that it originates from surface epithelial cells in fundus and antrum.

Experiments were performed to study the mechanism for HCO_3^- transport (Table 3). All Cl^- (91.4 mM) in solutions bathing both sides of metiamide-inhibited, net alkalinizing, frog fundic mucosae was replaced by SO_4^{2-} or isethionate (2-hydroxyethylsulfonate). To ensure removal of Cl^-, the mucosa was washed repeatedly during a 15-min period with the Cl^--free solutions. Removal of Cl^- resulted in a decrease of luminal alkalinization to values too low to be titrated at a luminal side pH of 7.40. Readdition of Cl^- to the luminal side alone resulted in reestablishment of HCO_3^- transport, while readdition of Cl^- to only the nutrient side had no effect.

Immediately after a change to non-Cl^- solutions, the pH on the luminal side was 7.00. A rise in luminal pH above 7.00 was used as a further test for residual HCO_3^- transport. With isethionate on both sides of the mucosa, there was practically no pH increase (< 0.02 pH U/30 min). With SO_4^{2-} on both sides, or with Cl^- on the nutrient side and SO_4^{2-} on the luminal side, the luminal pH increased somewhat (0.10 ± 0.02 pH U/30 min, mean ± SE, N = 12). This increase was much smaller than that observed with Cl^- on the luminal side alone (0.39 ± 0.05, N = 6) or in controls with Cl^- on both sides (0.44 ± 0.07, N = 7).

Fundic HCO_3^- transport *in vitro* thus depends on the presence of Cl^- on the luminal side. This suggests that HCO_3^- transport involves a HCO_3^-/Cl^- exchange mechanism. SO_4^{2-} may substitute for Cl^- to a small extent. Removal of Cl^- resulted in an increase in tissue resistance; the presence of Cl^- on only one side changed the transmucosal electrical potential difference, the opposite side becoming more negative (nutrient Cl^-) or less positive (luminal Cl^-). This is in accordance with previous findings (26,41) of some passive diffusion of Cl^- across the fundic mucosa.

Stimulation of HCO_3^- transport *in vitro* by carbachol, dibutyryl cGMP (17), or Ca^{2+} (18) was associated with only a slight rise in the transmucosal electric potential difference. Upon stimulation by prostaglandin 16,16-dimethyl E_2 or $F_{2\alpha}$ (34), no changes in the electrical potential difference were observed. This is further support for HCO_3^- transport taking place by an (electroneutral) ion exchange mechanism. In view of the greater sensitivity to acetazolamide placed on the luminal side (17), the process may be located at the luminal cell membrane.

Replacement of nutrient (tissue) HCO_3^-/CO_2 or Cl^- is not possible *in vivo,* and measurement of electrical characteristics is more difficult *in vivo* than *in vitro.* The similar sensitivity of alkalinization *in vitro* and *in vivo* to carbachol, 16,16-dimethyl PGE_2, and low concentrations of acetylsalicylate, however, suggest that luminal alkalinization in the mammalian stomach *in vivo* at least partly reflects active transport of HCO_3^-.

Some ultrafiltration of HCO_3^- into the gastric lumen may also take place *in vivo.* Altamirano and collaborators (2–4) observed that gastric intra-arterial injection of acetylcholine caused output of HCO_3^- and large amounts of protein into the gastric lumen. The latter indicates that the mucosal permeability was increased. Albumin, although in much smaller amounts, does appear in secretions from normal subjects (83). It is thus possible that some ultrafiltration of HCO_3^- contributes to the appearance of HCO_3^- in the gastric lumen *in vivo.*

Cardiac epithelium covers a large part (30 to 40%) of the gastric surface area in the pig. Secretions from innervated cardiac pouches in this species contain ap-

TABLE 3. *Effects of replacement of Cl⁻ on HCO₃⁻ transport and electrical properties of frog fundic mucosa*

Luminal/nutrient	PD (mV)	Resistance (Ω cm²)	OH⁻ (μEq/cm²-hr)
Cl⁻/Cl⁻	18.3 ± 1.3	348 ± 35	0.33 ± 0.04
SO₄²⁻/SO₄²⁻	13.4 ± 0.8	497 ± 50	0
Cl⁻/SO₄²⁻	0.9 ± 0.8	433 ± 57	0.28 ± 0.05
Cl⁻/Cl⁻	22.2 ± 1.6	406 ± 82	0.43 ± 0.13
SO₄²⁻/SO₄²⁻	20.3 ± 1.7	579 ± 98	0
SO₄²⁻/Cl⁻	29.7 ± 1.8	392 ± 75	0
Cl⁻/Cl⁻	22.3 ± 1.1	438 ± 53	0.27 ± 0.05
Isethionate⁻/isethionate⁻	13.4 ± 1.4	690 ± 71	0
Cl⁻/isethionate⁻	−0.3 ± 1.5	530 ± 64	0.34 ± 0.08

Net alkaline secretion was induced in *Rana temporaria* fundus by pretreatment with the histamine H_2 receptor antagonist metiamide (10^{-3}M). The bathing solutions were changed, as indicated, to solutions containing SO_4^{2-} or isethionate⁻ instead of Cl⁻. The mean values ± SE of transmucosal electrical potential difference (PD), electrical resistance, and rate of luminal alkalinization (OH⁻) during the last 30 min in each consecutive 90-min experimental period are given. The latter was determined by titration with H_2SO_4 at pH 7.40 under automatic control by a pH-stat instrument. With each type of ion replacement, N = 6.

proximately 80 mM HCO_3^- (43). HCO_3^- transport is inhibited by gastrin tetrapeptide amide, norepinephrine, acetylcholine, feeding, or gastric instillation of various fluids (44). Most other species have much smaller cardiac areas, whether cardiac epithelium transports HCO_3^- in other species is not known.

Several agents, including dithiothreitol (62), ethanol, and high concentrations of un-ionized acetylsalicylic acid (9,10), increase the rate of disappearance from the gastric lumen of instilled or secreted acid. Un-ionized acetylsalicylic acid, however, has been reported to increase mucosal permeation of serum proteins (9), large uncharged saccharide molecules (22,25), and this drug per se (21). Under conditions of increased permeability, which might be the result of gastric disease (62,74), pathways for transport along the chemical gradient of H^+ out of and HCO_3^- into the gastric lumen might also occur. The latter was found here *in vitro* after ethanol treatment (Fig. 2). In the dog *in vivo,* however, instillation of sodium acetylsalicylate did not increase the intragastric pCO_2 (38). This may reflect the use by these authors of the anion, which has much smaller permeability effects than the un-ionized acid (10).

SUGGESTED PROTECTIVE ROLE OF ACTIVE GASTRIC HCO₃⁻ TRANSPORT

Active transport of HCO_3^- would increase the pH at the mucosal surface and may thus protect the mucosa from damage by intraluminal acid. This proposed protective role (16,17,24) is supported by the inhibitory effect on HCO_3^- transport by several potential ulcerogens and the stimulation of HCO_3^- transport by ulceroprotective prostaglandins. It has been observed in dogs that intravenous injection of high doses of acetazolamide rapidly decreases the ability of fundic mucosa to resist a low luminal pH. Damage occurred only when H^+ concentration of the luminal solution was higher than 30 mM; changes appeared primarily in the surface epithelial cells (82).

In view of the differences in magnitude between the normally large H^+ secretion and the smaller HCO_3^- transport, the HCO_3^- would be ineffective if secreted directly into the intragastric bulk solution, the rise in pH would be very small. Active transport of HCO_3^- into a surface boundary zone with low turbulence (18) would be more effective. H^+/HCO_3^- counterdiffusion in a membrane model has been examined by Teorell (80). The viscoelastic mucous gel at the mucosal surface has physical properties (1,29) appropriate for supporting HCO_3^- and H^+ gradients. The concentration profiles within the surface boundary (Fig. 7) would depend on the amounts of H^+ and HCO_3^- available for diffusion, the presence of other ions, and the structure and electrical charge of the mucus. Recent measurements with pH-sensitive microelectrodes (84), showing a pH gradient across the rabbit gastric mucous layer, with the cell-facing side slightly alkaline (mean pH, 7.59) and lumen-facing side acid (mean pH, 2.36), support this hypothesis.

HCO₃⁻ IN REGULATION OF GASTRIC ACIDITY

Regulation of the acidity of the gastric contents has more than theoretical interest since it underlies interpretation of secretory data obtained clinically or exper-

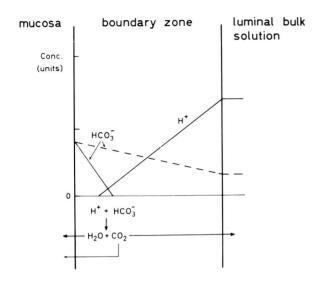

mucosa   boundary zone   luminal bulk solution

Conc. (units)

0

FIG. 7. Model for neutralization of H^+ by HCO_3^- in a boundary zone at the luminal surface of the gastric epithelium. With acid gastric contents (solid lines), all HCO_3^- appearing in the luminal bulk solution should be in the form of CO_2. At high rates of H^+ secretion, some of the CO_2 may be reabsorbed by the mucosa for utilization by the parietal cells in the H^+ secretory process. Free HCO_3^- should appear only in nonacid bulk solutions (*dashed line*). [From Flemström (18).]

imentally. Gastric juice concentrations and outputs of H^+, Na^+, K^+, and Cl^- have been frequently analyzed to obtain information about the secretory process. Hollander (42), in the two-component hypothesis, proposed that a HCO_3^--containing fluid, originating from unstimulated parietal cells, another cell type in the mucosa, or leaking from the interstitial space, diluted and neutralized acid gastric contents. Teorell (81) proposed that from the kinetic point of view, H^+ could be considered to diffuse into the mucosa in exchange for Na^+.

HCO_3^- transport in amphibian fundic mucosa *in vitro* and in the guinea pig *in vivo* takes place at a steady basal rate amounting to 5 to 10% of maximal H^+ output in the same species. An output of HCO_3^- amounting to 1 to 2% of maximal H^+ output would be sufficient to account for acidity regulation in humans, and 5% would account for acid disappearance from the stomach in dogs. These ratios are calculated from the experimental data and mathematical analyses of acidity regulation published by Makhlouf and collaborators (58) and by Öbrink (63). The amount of HCO_3^- necessary to account for acid disappearance has been calculated as the product of "volume of alkaline secretion and HCO_3^- concentration" and of "primary acidity and permeability coefficient for H^+ ions," respectively. The amount of HCO_3^- transported by the mucosa is probably quantitatively sufficient to account for the well-known continuous loss of H^+ ions from acid gastric contents.

This is in accordance with the hypothesis of Hollander. Because of the higher mobility and usual excess of H^+ ions, the process of neutralization occurs in the

immediate vicinity of the luminal cell membranes. Na^+ may be transported together with HCO_3^- or diffuse into the lumen when H^+ is neutralized. The net result of HCO_3^- transport might then appear as an interdiffusion between H^+ and Na^+. Also, reaction between HCO_3^- and H^+ should reduce the osmolarity of the combined secretion, and excess water may diffuse along its chemical gradient into the mucosa. A diluting effect of a HCO_3^--containing secretion would thus be difficult to detect at the normally low values of intragastric pH; HCO_3^- transport may then appear as surface neutralization of H^+ ions rather than as a secretion with a defined volume.

DUODENAL SURFACE EPITHELIAL TRANSPORT OF HCO_3^-

Gastric contents pass into the duodenum, where the acid disappears and neutrality is restored. Until recently, restoration of neutrality in the duodenum was attributed solely to the HCO_3^--containing secretions of the pancreas, glands of Brunner, and liver. Various investigators (12,38,85) have demonstrated that duodenal mucosa per se has the ability to dispose of acid. The mechanism by which this occurs has been the subject of some controversy. Proposed mechanisms include diffusion of acid and ultrafiltration or diffusion of HCO_3^- into the duodenal lumen.

It has also been reported that PGE_2 and 16,16-dimethyl PGE_2 protect against duodenal ulceration in rats caused by administration of cysteamine (69) or stimulants of H^+ secretion (68). The mechanism for this protection is not clear, although antiulcer activity may reflect the inhibitory action of these prostaglandins on H^+ secretion (67). The finding that active HCO_3^- transport by gastric epithelium is stimulated by 16,16-dimethyl PGE_2 and $PGF_{2\alpha}$ (34) led to the examination of whether a similar HCO_3^- transport occurred in duodenal epithelium. Isolated proximal duodenum from the bullfrog, a preparation devoid of glands of Brunner, was chosen for this purpose (19,20). The duodenum alkalinized the mucosal surface at a rate of approximately $1 \mu Eq/cm^2/hr$, and transport was inhibited by CN^-, indomethacin, and acetazolamide. The rate of alkalinization increased 100% on nutrient side administration of PGE_2 (Fig. 8) or 16,16-dimethyl PGE_2 and 60% after administration of $PGF_{2\alpha}$. The minimal effective concentrations were 10^{-8} to 10^{-9} M with PGE_2 and 16,16-dimethyl PGE_2 and 10^{-6} M with $PGF_{2\alpha}$. Stimulation of HCO_3^- transport was always associated with an increase in the transmucosal electrical potential difference (Fig. 9). The results suggest that duodenal surface epithelial HCO_3^- transport is, at least in part, an active process. It may contribute to the ability of duodenal epithelium to resist acid.

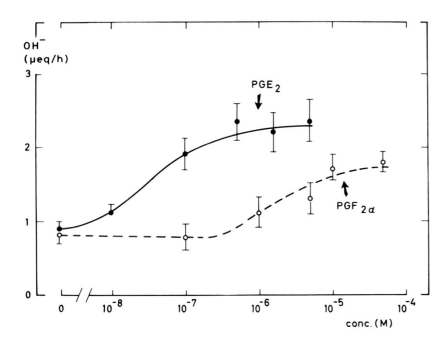

FIG. 8. Effects of PGE_2 and $PGF_{2\alpha}$ on the rate of luminal alkalinization by bullfrog isolated proximal duodenum. The prostaglandin was added only to the nutrient (submucosal) side. Each value is the mean ± SE of eight or more experiments.

PGE_2, which had no effect on gastric alkalinization, stimulated duodenal alkalinization. A prostaglandin-induced increase in alkalinization was associated with an increase in the transepithelial electrical potential difference in duodenum but not in gastric fundus or antrum. In the same species (bullfrog), the basal rate of alkalinization in duodenum ($\sim$1 $\mu Eq/cm^2/hr$) was somewhat larger than that occurring in H^+-inhibited fundus ($\sim$0.55 $\mu Eq/cm^2/hr$) or antrum ($\sim$0.45 $\mu Eq/cm^2/hr$).

Further studies are necessary to determine whether gastric and duodenal epithelial HCO_3^- transport also differ in other aspects. Knowledge about stimulants of

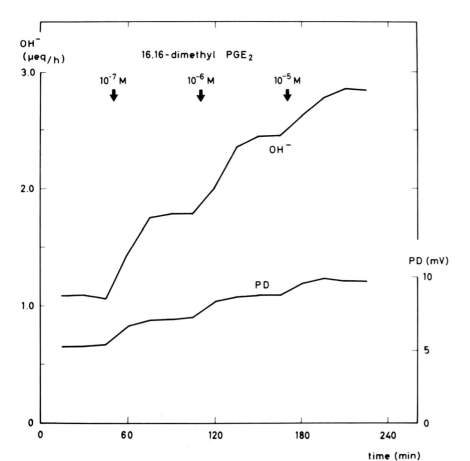

FIG. 9. This experiment illustrates the simultaneous rise in the transepithelial electrical difference (PD) occurring when HCO_3^- transport by bullfrog isolated proximal duodenum was stimulated by prostaglandins; 16,16-Dimethyl PGE_2 was added to the nutrient side, as indicated.

duodenal epithelial HCO_3^- transport may permit experimental evaluation of its possible role in protection against duodenal ulceration.

ACKNOWLEDGMENTS

I wish to thank Ms. Carin Hulth for excellent technical assistance and Dr. A. Garner and Prof. K. J. Öbrink for invaluable discussions of the manuscript. The prostaglandins used for studies of duodenal HCO_3^- transport was a kind gift from Dr. E. R. Walker, I.C.I. Ltd., Macclesfield, England. Financial support was given by the Swedish Medical Research Council (04X-3515).

REFERENCES

1. Allen, A. (1978): Structure of gastrointestinal mucus glycoproteins and the viscous and gel-forming properties of mucus. *Br. Med. Bull.*, 34:29–33.

2. Altamirano, M. (1963): Alkaline secretion produced by intraarterial acetylcholine. *J. Physiol. (Lond.)*, 168:787–803.

3. Altamirano, M., Requena, M., and Durbin, R. P. (1974): Effects of gastric arterial and venous pressures on gastric secretion in the dog. *Am. J. Physiol.*, 227:152–160.

4. Altamirano, M., Requena, M., and Perez, T. C. (1975): Interstitial fluid pressure and alkaline gastric secretion. *Am. J. Physiol.*, 229:1421–1426.

5. Andre, C., Bruhiere, J., Vagne, M., and Lambert, R. (1973): Bicarbonate secretion in the human stomach. *Acta Hepatogastroenterol.*, 20:62–69.

6. Boass; A., and Wilson, T. C. (1964): Cellular localization of gastric instrinsic factor in the rat. *Am. J. Physiol.*, 206:783–786.

7. Bolton, J. P., and Cohen, M. M. (1978): Stimulation of nonparietal secretion in canine Heidenhain pouches by 16,16-dimethyl prostaglandin E_2. *Digestion*, 17:291–299.

8. Cheung, L. Y., and Lowry, S. F. (1976): Canine gastric blood flow and oxygen consumption during cimetidine inhibition of acid secretion. *Surg. Forum*, 27:390–392.

9. Davenport, H. W. (1966): Fluid produced by the gastric mucosa during damage by acetic and salicylic acids. *Gastroenterology*, 50:487–499.

10. Davenport, H. W. (1967): Salicylate damage to the gastric mucosal barrier. *N. Engl. J. Med.*, 276:1307–1312.

11. Dawson, D. C., and Cooke, A. R. (1978): Parallel pathways for ion transport across rat gastric mucosa: Effect of ethanol. *Am. J. Physiol.*, 235: E7–E15.

12. Dorricott, N. J., Fiddian-Green, R. G., and Silen, W. (1975): Mechanisms of acid disposal in canine duodenum. *Am. J. Physiol.*, 228:269–275.

13. Durbin, R. P. (1976): Coupling of water to solute movement in isolated gastric mucosa. In: *Ciba Foundation Symposium 38: Lung Liquids*, pp. 161–177. Elsevier, New York.

14. Eichenholz, A., McQuarrie, D., Blumentals, A. S., and Vennes, J. A. (1967): Unique acid-base parameters of gastric venous blood during secretory activity. *J. Appl. Physiol.*, 22:580–583.

15. Eichhorn, J. H., Salzman, E. W., and Silen, W. (1973): Cyclic GMP in stimulated gastric mucosa. *Surg. Forum*, 24:363–365.

16. Flemstrom, G. (1976): Properties of isolated gastric antral and SCN^- inhibited fundic mucosa. In: *Gastric Hydrogen Ion Secretion*, edited by D. K. Kasbekar, G. Sachs, and W. S. Rehm, pp. 102–116. Dekker, New York.

17. Flemström, G. (1977): Active alkalinization by amphibian gastric fundic mucosa in vitro. *Am. J. Physiol.*, 233: E1–E12.

18. Flemström, G. (1978): Effect of catecholamines, Ca^{++} and gastrin on gastric HCO_3^- secretion. *Acta Physiol. Scand. [Suppl.]*, *Gastr. Ion Transp.*, 81–90.

19. Flemström, G. (1978): HCO_3^- transport by bullfrog duodenum. *Acta Physiol. Scand.*, 105:13A–14A.

20. Flemström, G. (1980): Stimulation of HCO_3 transport in isolated proximal bullfrog duodenum by prostaglandins. *Am. J. Physiol.*, 239:6198–6203.

21. Flemström, G. (1979): Kinetics of acetylsalicylate and D-lactate transport across isolated frog gastric mucosa. *Ups. J. Med. Sci.*, 84:137–144.

22. Flemström, G., and Marsden, N. V. B. (1973): Dextran permeability, electrical properties, and H^+ secretion in isolated frog gastric mucosa after acetylsalicylic acid. *Gastroenterology*, 64:278–284.

23. Flemström, G., and Marsden, N. V. B. (1974): Increased inulin absorption from the cat stomach exposed to acetylsalicylic acid. *Acta Physiol. Scand.*, 92:517–525.

24. Flemström; G., and Sachs, G. (1975): Ion transport by amphibian antrum in vitro. I. General characteristics. *Am. J. Physiol.*, 228:1188–1198.

25. Flemström, G., Marsden, N. V. B., and Richter, W. (1976): Passive cutaneous anaphylaxis in guinea pigs elicited by gastric absorption of dextran induced by acetylsalicylic acid. *Int. Arch. Allergy Appl. Immunol.*, 51:627–636,

26. Forte, J. G. (1969): Three components of Cl^- flux across the isolated bullfrog gastric mucosa. *Am. J. Physiol.*, 216:167–174.

27. Frenning, B. (1974): The effects of large osmolality variations on the gastric mucosal ion permeability. *Acta Physiol. Scand.*, 90:1–13.

28. Fromm, D., Schwartz, J. H., Robertson, R., and Fuhro, R. (1976): Ion transport across isolated antral mucosa in the rabbit. *Am. J. Physiol.*, 231:1783–1789.

29. Gardham, J. R., and Hobsley, M. (1970): The electrolytes of alkaline human gastric juice. *Clin. Sci.*, 39:77–87.

30. Garner, A. (1977): Assessment of gastric mucosal damage: Comparative effects of aspirin and fenclofenac on the gastric mucosa of the guinea pig. *Toxicol. Appl. Pharmacol.*, 42:477–486.

31. Garner, A. (1977): Effects of acetylsalicylate on alkalinization, acid secretion and electrogenic properties in the isolated gastric mucosa. *Acta Physiol. Scand.*, 99:281–289.

32. Garner, A. (1978): Mechanisms of action of aspirin on the gastric mucosa of the guinea pig. *Acta Physiol. Scand. [Suppl.]*, *Gastr. Ion Transp.* 101–110.

33. Garner, A., and Flemström, G. (1978): Gastric HCO_3 secretion in the guinea pig. *Am. J. Physiol.*, 234:E535–E542.

34. Garner, A., and Heylings, J. R. (1979): Stimulation of alkaline secretion in amphibian isolated gastric mucosa by 16,16-dimethyl PGE_2 and $PGF_{2\alpha}$: A proposed explanation for some of the cytoprotective actions of prostaglandins. *Gastroenterology*, 76:497–503.

35. Garner, A., Flemström, G.; and Heylings, J. R. (1979): Effects of antiinflammatory agents and prostaglandins on acid and bicarbonate secretions in the amphibian-isolated gastric mucosa. *Gastroenterology*, 77:451–457.

36. Graper, W. P., Crass, R. A., Halpern, N. B., Fromm, D., and Silen, W. (1976): Secretion of base by the in vitro amphibian antrum. *Surg. Forum*, 27:435–437.

37. Grossman, M. I. (1959): The secretion of the pyloric glands of the dog. *21st Int. Congr. Physiol. Sci., Buenos Aires*, pp. 226–228. (abstr.)

38. Harmon, J. W., Woods, M., and Gurll, N. J. (1978): Different mechanisms of hydrogen ion removal in stomach and duodenum. *Am. J. Physiol.*, 235:E692–E698.

39. Heatly, N. G. (1959): Mucosubstance as a barrier to diffusion. *Gastroenterology*, 37:313–317.

40. Hobsley, M., and Silen, W. (1970): The relation between the rate of production of gastric juice and its electrolyte concentrations. *Clin. Sci.*, 39:69–75.

41. Hogben, C. A. M. (1955): Active transport of chloride by isolated frog gastric epithelium. Origin of the gastric mucosal potential. *Am. J. Physiol.*, 180:641–649.

42. Hollander, F. (1954): The two-component mucous barrier. *Arch. Int. Med.*, 94:107–120.

43. Höller, H. (1970): Untersuchungen über Sekret und Sekretion der Cardiadrüsenzone im Magen des Schweines. I. *Zentralbl. Veterinaermed. [A]*, 17:685–711.

44. Höller, H. (1970): Untersuchungen über Sekret und Sekretion der cardiadrusenzone im Magen des Schweines. II. *Zentralbl. Veterinaermed. [A]*,17:857–873.

45. Hottenrott, C., Seufert, R. M., Kühne, F. W., and Büsing, M. (1977): Experimental gastric sympathectomy: An effective prophylaxis of gastric stress lesions. *Ann. Surg.,* 762–765.

46. Hunt, J. N., and Wan, B. (1967): Electrolytes of human gastric juice. In: *Handbook of Physiology, Section 6: Alimentary Canal, Vol. II. Secretion,* edited by C. F. Code, pp. 781–804. American Physiological Society, Washington, D.C.

47. Ihre, B. (1938): Human gastric secretion. *Acta Med. Scand.[Suppl.],* 95:1–226.

48. Imamura, A. (1970): The effects of carbon dioxide and bicarbonate on chloride fluxes across frog gastric mucosa. *Biochim. Biophys. Acta,* 196:245–253.

49. Karlmark, B., and Danielson, B. G. (1974): Titrable acid, bicarbonate and ammonium ions along the rat proximal tubule. *Acta Physiol. Scand.,* 91:243–258.

50. Kasbekar, D. K. (1967): Studies of resting isolated frog gastric mucosa. *Proc. Soc. Exp. Biol. Med.,* 125:267–271.

51. Kauffman, G. L., J. J. Reeve, and Grossman, M. I. (1980): Gastric bicarbonate secretion: Effect of topical and intravenous 16, 16-dimethyl prostaglandin E_2. *Am. J. Physiol.,* 239:G44–G48.

52. Kidder, G. W., III, and Montgomery, C. W. (1974): CO_2 diffusion into frog gastric mucosa as rate-limiting factor in acid secretion. *Am. J. Physiol.,* 227:300–304.

53. Kristensen, M. (1975): Titration curves for gastric secretion. *Scand. J. Gastroenterol. [Supp. 32],* 10:1–149.

54. Kurtz, L. D., and Clark, B. B. (1947): The inverse relationship of the secretion of hydrochloric acid to the tension of carbon oxide in the stomach, *Gastroenterology,* 9:594–602.

55. Lambling, A., Bernier, J.-J., Najean, Y., and Badoz-Lambling, J. (1959): Le suc gastrique dans l'anémie pernicieuse. *Rev. Fr. Etudes Clin. Biol.,* 4:582–592.

56. Linde, R., Teorell, R., and Öbrink, K. I. (1947): Experiments on the primary acidity of the gastric juice. *Acta Physiol. Scand.,* 14:220–232.

57. Lönnerholm, G. (1977): Carbonic anhydrase in the intestinal tract of the guinea pig. *Acta Physiol. Scand.,* 99:53–61.

58. Makhlouf, G. M., McManus, M. B., and Card, W. I. (1966): A quantitative statement of the two-component hypothesis of gastric secretion. *Gastroenterology,* 51:149–171.

59. McLeay, L. M., and Titchen, D. A. (1975): Gastric, antral and fundic pouch secretion in sheep. *J. Physiol. (Lond.),* 248:595–612.

60. Menguy, R., and Masters, Y. F. (1978): Mechanism of stress ulcer. Influence of alpha-adrenergic blockade on stress ulceration and gastric mucosal energy metabolism. *Am. J. Dig. Dis.,* 23:493–497.

61. Moody, F. G., and Durbin, R. P, (1965): Effects of glycine and other instillates on concentration of gastric acid. *Am. J. Physiol.,* 209:122–126.

62. Munro, D. R. (1974): Route of protein loss during a model protein-losing gastropathy in dogs. *Gastroenterology,* 66:960–972.

63. Öbrink, K. J. (1948): Studies on the kinetics of the parietal secretion of the stomach. *Acta Physiol. Scand. [Suppl. 51],* 15:1–106.

64. Okosdinossian, E. T., and El Munshid, H. A. (1977): Composition of the alkaline component of human gastric juice: Effect of swallowed saliva and duodeno-gastric reflux. *Scand. J. Gastroenterol.,* 12:945–950.

65. Rangachari, P. K. (1975): Histamine release by gastric stimulants. *Nature,* 253:53–55.

66. Rehm, W. S., and Sanders, S. S. (1977): Electrical events during activation and inhibition of gastric HCl secretion. *Gastroenterology,* 73:959–969.

67. Robert, A. (1976): Antisecretory, antiulcer, cytoprotective and diarrheogenic properties of prostaglandins. In *Advances in Prostaglandin and Thromboxane Research, Vol. 2,* edited by B. Samuelsson and R. Poaletti, pp. 507–520. Raven Press, New York.

68. Robert, A., Stowe, D. F., and Nezamis, J. E. (1971): Prevention of duodenal ulcers by administration of prostaglandin E_2 (PGE_2). *Scand. J. Gastroenterol.,* 6:303–305.

69. Robert, A., Nezamis, J. E., Lancaster, C., and Badalamenti, J. N. (1974): Cysteamine-induced duodenal ulcers: A new model to test antiulcer agents. *Digestion,* 11:199–214.

70. Rune, S. J., and Henriksen, F. W. (1969): Carbon dioxide tensions in the proximal part of the canine gastrointestinal tract. *Gastroenterology,* 56:758–762.

71. Russel, J. C., and Kowalewski, K. (1974): The acid-base balance in gastric H^+ secretion. *Physiol. Chem. Phys.,* 6:269–274.

72. Sanders, S. S., Hayne, V. B., and Rehm, W. S. (1973): Normal H^+ rates in the stomach in the absence of exogenous CO_2 and a note on pH stat method. *Am. J. Physiol.,* 225:1311–1321.

73. Schierbeck, N. P. (1892): Ueber Kohlensäure im Ventrikel. *Scand. Arch. Physiol.,* 3:437–474.

74. Silvis, S. E., and Doscherholmen, A. (1972): Production of HCO_3^- by the human stomach. *Am. J. Gastroenterol.,* 58:138–144.

75. Sothell, M. (1979): P_{CO_2} of the proximal tubular fluid and the efferent arteriolar blood in the rat kidney. *Acta Physiol. Scand.,* 105:137–145.

76. Spenney, J. G. (1979): Physical chemical and technical limitations to intragastric titration. *Gastroenterology,* 76:1025–1034.

77. Spenney, J. G., Shoemaker, R. L., and Sachs, G. (1974): Conductance properties of gastric fundic mucosa. *J. Membr. Biol.,* 19:105–128.

78. Spenney, J. G., Flemström, G., Shoemaker, R. L., and Sachs, G. (1975): Quantitation of conductance pathways in antral gastric mucosa. *J. Gen. Physiol.,* 65:645–662.

79. Sung, C. P., Wiebelhaus V. D., Jenkins, B. C., Adlercreutz, P., Hirschowitz, B. I., and Sachs, G. (1972): Heterogeneity of 3', 5'-phosphodiesterase of gastric mucosa. *Am. J. Physiol.,* 223:648–650.

80. Teorell, T. (1936): A method of studying conditions within diffusion layers. *J. Biol. Chem.,* 113:735–748.

81. Teorell, T. (1947): Electrolyte diffusion in relation to the acidity regulation of the gastric juice. *Gastroenterology,* 9:425–443.

82. Werther, J. L., Hollander, F., and Altamirano, M. (1965): Effect of acetazolamide on gastric mucosa in canine vivo-vitro preparations. *Am. J. Physiol.,* 209:127–133.

83. Wetterfors, J., Gullberg, R., Liljedahl, S., Platin, L., Birke, G., and Olhagen, G. (1960): Role of the stomach and small intestine in albumin breakdown. *Acta Med. Scand.,* 168:347–363.

84. Williams, S. E., and Turnberg, L. A. (1980): Studies of the ''protective'' properties of gastric mucus: Evidence for a mucus-bicarbonate barrier. *Gut,* 20:A922–A923.

85. Winship, D. H., and Robinson, J. E. (1974): Acid loss in human duodenum. *Gastroenterology,* 66:181–188.

Physiology of the Gastrointestinal Tract, edited by
Leonard R. Johnson, Raven Press, New York © 1981.

Chapter 21

Structure and Function of Gastrointestinal Mucus

Adrian Allen

Mucus is secreted as a viscoelastic gel that provides a flexible protective cover that adheres to the mucosal surface. It contrasts with other gastrointestinal secretions which are water soluble. Because of its gelatinous nature and structure of complex glycoprotein molecules, mucus is difficult to study and, therefore, despite the ubiquity of mucus throughout the gastrointestinal tract, its physiology and pathology are poorly defined. Until now, much of the work in this field has concentrated on unraveling mucus structure as a necessary prerequisite to a better understanding of its biology; such a bias is reflected in this chapter.

FUNCTION OF MUCUS

A clear function of gastrointestinal mucus is to protect the delicate mucosal epithelium from mechanical damage by the passage of food, fecal material, and the vigorous forces that attend digestion (39,40,71). Mucus provides a slimy lubricant for the passing of solid material, yet its strongly adhesive properties ensure that much of the gel still remains firmly stuck to the mucosa to protect it from the next round of mechanical abuse. Another important feature of the mucous gel is its ability to retain water (154) and provide a perpetual aqueous environment for the mucosal surface; at the same time, the gel resists excessive swelling and solubilization by the luminal solutions.

Since immunity of the gastric-duodenal mucosa from autodigestion and its breakdown in ulceration was first recognized, mucus has been implicated as part of the protective barrier. Hollander (71) developed this concept in his proposal of a two-component barrier consisting of the mucous gel on one hand and the underlying rapidly regenerating mucosal cell layer on the other. However, it is still a matter of debate as to what constitutes the barrier to autodigestion (see Chapter 27 by Fromm) and in particular the role in this of the mucus itself (4). There is circumstantial evidence that mucus may protect against ulceration; for example, gastric production is inhibited by various ulcerogenic agents (57,118), such as the antiinflammatory drug salicylate (88,120). In contrast, the antiulcer agents prostaglandins (19,33) and carbenoxolone (129,164) are reported to increase mucus production. Isolated gastric mucus-secreting cells are sensitive to low pH and cease to synthesize mucus or even to respire in an environment below pH 5.0 (158). *In vivo,* only the mucous gel separates these cells from the luminal acid.

The gastric mucous gel does not provide an impenetrable barrier to acid, since it is permeable to H^+. Heatley (68) proposed that mucus protects the mucosa by acting as a barrier to gross mixing and by ensuring that a mucosal alkaline secretion within the gel was restricted to the luminal surface and so neutralized the acid diffusing in from the lumen. The recent demonstration of HCO_3^- secretion by the gastric mucosa (see Chapter 27) has provided considerable support for this hypothesis. If mucus and its contained HCO_3^- is to prove an effective first line of defense against acid, the mucous gel should fulfill two conditions (4). First, it should provide an unstirred layer and thus maintain the secreted HCO_3^- secretion on the mucosal surface at a high concentration and prevent mixing with the bulk of the luminal HCl. The relatively dense molecular structure of the mucous gel (7) makes it well suited to provide such an unstirred layer. Second, the flux of H^+ from the lumen through the unstirred layer of the mucous gel must not exceed the flux of HCO_3^- from the mucosal surface. Calculations suggest that free diffusion of H^+ through an unstirred layer is a rapid process (26). Even under conditions of maximal stimulation, gastric HCO_3^- secretion is unlikely to be more than one-tenth of the HCl output. Much of the secreted acid, however, will be buffered by food and lost from the stomach by gastric emptying. In practice, therefore, the amount of acid penetrating the gel *in vivo* may not, under normal conditions, exceed the output of HCO_3^-. It remains to be determined whether the rate of H^+ flux through the gel matrix *in vivo* is such that it could be neutralized by the HCO_3^- it contains. If there is such surface neutralization, one would expect a pH gradient across the mucous gel from pH 1 to 2 on the luminal side to approximately pH 7 on the serosal side. This is supported by a recent report in which microelectrodes showed a gradient from pH 2.36 to 7.59 across the mucus on isolated rabbit gastric mucosa (179). The buffering capacity of gastric mucus, in the absence of HCO_3^-, is small and not a major factor in protection of the mucosa from acid.

It has been suggested that mucus protects the underlying mucosal cells from the proteolytic enzymes of the gastrointestinal tract, but many mucous gel secretions are solubilized and degraded by proteolysis. Thus pepsin is not inhibited by gastric mucus, and in fact pepsin continually solubilizes and degrades the luminal surface of the mucous gel layer (2,143). The result is a dynamic balance *in vivo* between peptic erosion of the mucus and its secretion by the mucosa. Mucous secretions from lower down the tract are also susceptible to enzymic degradation (43,66,76). The diffusion of these large molecular weight degradative enzymes through the unstirred layer of the thick mucous gel matrix, however, may be severely restricted. This would be particularly pertinent to the stomach, where, despite persistent peptic erosion of its luminal surface, the mucous gel would provide a relatively impenetrable barrier to pepsin in the gastric juice and prevent it from reaching the susceptible mucosal cells. Such a hypothesis raises the question of how pepsin secreted by the chief cells in the gastric pits gains access through the mucous coat to the lumen. There is probably no mucus covering the surface of the gastric glands below the level of the mucous neck cells. Presumably, the membranes of these cells must be resistant to their own secretions. Mucus, however, does cover the neck cells of the gastric glands. It would be surprising if it did not at times block the neck at this

point. The pressure of flow from the secretion of an active gastric gland may be sufficient to force this secretion into the gastric lumen. The mucous plug would reform and thus reseal the gastric gland from the lumen once secretion of acid and pepsin is finished.

A variety of other functions have been attributed to gastrointestinal mucus but have not yet been investigated in detail. One such function proposed for mucus is that of an antibacterial and antiviral agent (39,43). The mucus could provide a barrier between the pathogenic organism and the mucosa or alternatively combine directly with the organism or its toxin and thereby inactivate it. Pig gastric mucus, for example, binds to cholera toxin and prevents its attachment to the cell surface (166). On the other hand, mucus is important to the maintenance of gastrointestinal flora. This is evident from the interactions of salivary mucus and oral streptococci (52,103) and the demonstration that soluble mucus is a nutrient source for endogenous bacteria in the gut (76). Other functions shown for gastrointestinal mucus include the binding of cations, such as iron (17) and calcium (44), but the physiological significance of this is uncertain. Mucus can also facilitate digestion; thus rat small intestinal mucus stimulated the hydrolysis of casein and brush border membranes by trypsin and chymotrypsin (153).

STRUCTURE OF MUCUS

Constituents

The molecules responsible for the viscous and gel-forming properties of mucus are the glycoproteins or mucins (71), which constitute between 1 and 10% by weight of the gel. The bulk of mucus consists of water, up to 95% by weight, with about 1.0% by weight of dialyzable salts, with an electrolyte composition close to plasma (72); the remainder is nondialyzable glycoproteins, proteins, and nucleic acids (2,24,73,73a). Isolated mucus is heterogeneous and contains material from sloughed epithelial cells, bacteria, digested food, plasma proteins, digestive enzymes, secretory IgA, bile, and virtually all other constituents found in gastrointestinal juice (43,53). Mucous glycoproteins have been isolated in varying degrees of purity and integrity from gastrointestinal mucous secretions. They are molecules of high molecular weight, from 2×10^5 to 15×10^6 daltons, and consist of protein cores with carbohydrate side chains (Fig. 1). An analogy is sometimes made between this structure and a bottle brush, where the bristles are the carbohydrate chains and the wire supports the protein core. The sugar constituents are *N*-acetylglucosamine, *N*-acetylgalactosamine, galactose, fucose, and various forms of neuraminic acid (sialic acids). Mucous glycoproteins are distinct from membrane-bound glycoproteins or glycolipids on the surfaces of

Over 70% by weight carbohydrate.

Carbohydrate chains contain: N-acetylgalactosamine, N-acetylglucosamine, galactose, fucose and sialic acids*.

Do not contain: uronic acid, mannose or glucose

Carbohydrate chains often branched with 2—22 sugars per chain.

Negatively charged due primarily to sialic acid and ester sulphate

High molecular weight: $2 \times 10^5 \longrightarrow 15 \times 10^6$ daltons

Viscous and form gels

Possess 'bottle brush structure' of protein core with carbohydrate side chains attached.

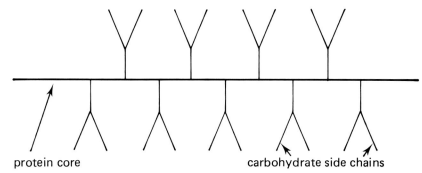

protein core   carbohydrate side chains

FIG. 1. Some characteristics of gastrointestinal mucous glycoproteins.

For more details of the structure of glycoproteins and the constituent sugars the reader is referred to a short review by Clamp (23) and books edited by Gottschalk (61) and Horowitz & Pigman (75),

* Sialic acid is a generic name for the various neuraminic acids which differ from each other in whether they are substituted with an acetyl or glycollyl residue on their amino group and the number of 0-acetyl substitutions on the hydroxyl groups,

cells and from the constituents of intercellular connective tissue, the proteoglycans (acidic mucopolysaccharides). Mucous glycoproteins do not contain either uronic acid, which is a sugar characteristic of the proteoglycans of connective tissue, or mannose, which is found in serum glycoproteins and some membrane glycoproteins.

Mucus can be obtained by the collection of gastrointestinal juice from fistulas and pouches, by intubation and aspiration of the secretions, or by scraping the mucous gel from the surface of isolated mucosa or in small amounts by biopsy. Mucus in gastrointestinal juice is partially degraded (2) and is contaminated with nonmucous secretions, as well as mucus from other regions of the tract (97,98). When mucous gel is obtained by scraping the mucosal surface, heavy contamination often results from simultaneous removal of the mucosal cells. This accounts for the low glycoprotein content of 15 and 5% by weight found in pig small intestinal (113) and pig colonic (115) mucous scrapings, respectively, which consist principally of protein (between 70 and 80% by weight) with small amounts of nucleic acid. Pig gastric mucous scrapings contain more than 50% by weight glycoprotein (163) due to less tissue damage on removal. Relatively pure preparations of gastric mucus

can be obtained from canine stomach pouches after stimulation by acetylcholine (74), although even this preparation contains substantial amounts of free protein, particularly serum albumin.

A number of specific proteins have been identified in mucous secretions. Some of these are plasma proteins, such as serum albumin, which are considered to arise by passive transudation across the mucosa (24). In contrast, IgA in mucous secretions is actively secreted, combined with an extra protein of about 70,000 MW, the secretory component (168). Secretory IgA is a glycoprotein, but it differs in structure from mucous glycoproteins by possessing less than 10% by weight carbohydrate, of which mannose is a constituent (14). Some of this IgA may be strongly bound to mucous glycoproteins (22), possibly through disulfide bridges, which are important in the structure of both these molecules. The traces of mannose in purified mucous glycoproteins may reflect the presence of bound secretory IgA, but contamination by free serum glycoproteins usually accounts for the significant amounts of mannose sometimes found in analyses of gastric juice (93,147).

Other nonmucous gastric glycoprotein secretions are the vitamin B_{12}-binding proteins: intrinsic factor (17.5%

by weight carbohydrate) and a glycoprotein (35.5% by weight carbohydrate) that binds B_{12} but does not possess the transport and assimilative properties of the former (11). These molecules, like IgA, differ from mucous glycoproteins by containing substantially less carbohydrate. Two other glycoprotein secretions are the poorly defined gastrones, which inhibit acid secretion (54,55), and the iron-binding gastric glycoprotein gastroferrin (27). Gastric mucous glycoprotein binds iron as strongly as gastroferrin (17). Since both molecules have a similar analysis (142), they are probably the same molecular entity.

A rather different class of polysaccharide-containing molecules frequently found in isolated mucous secretions, particularly those derived by proteolysis of mucosal preparations, are the acidic proteoglycans of connective tissue (56,73,73a,121,127,172). These proteoglycans, which can be identified by the presence of uronic acid, are specifically absent in several purified gastrointestinal mucous preparations (2,61,73,73a). When proteoglycans are found in mucous secretions, their presence probably reflects loss of connective tissue associated with the continual shedding of mucosal cells. Excessive amounts could be an indication of mucosal damage. In cat and dog gastric mucosa, acid polysaccharides are found in the chief cells (100) and can be a component of gastric juice preparations (172). Recently, glycolipids have been found in gastric mucus from perfusates of rat stomach (156). They were predominantly glycerolipids and distinct from the glycosphingolipids and phospholipids of the gastric mucosal membranes.

Solubilization of Mucous Gel

Most of the mucous gel scraped from the mucosal surface, or the visible mucus in gastric washouts, dissolves only slowly in salt solutions and can be separated by centrifugation or filtration. Before the glycoprotein constituents are purified and studied, therefore, the gel must be solubilized. The viscous and gel-forming properties of these mucous glycoproteins, however, are easily lost upon chemical manipulation (24), and the strength and efficiency of the solubilization procedure must be balanced against this potential loss of rheological properties in the glycoproteins. The two most effective methods for solubilizing many mucous gels are: (a) reductive cleavage of disulfide bridges with thiol reagents, or (b) proteolysis with either endogenous (e.g., pepsin) or added proteolytic enzymes (Table 1). The success of both these methods depends on the splitting of covalent disulfide bridges and peptide bonds, respectively. As a result, chemically degraded glycoproteins of lower molecular weight are produced, which have lost much of their viscous and gel-forming properties (35,143,152,159). If the carbohydrate side chains alone are the subject for study, then proteolysis is a rapid and efficient way to obtain relatively pure mucous

glycoprotein. Autolysis by pepsin has long been an established method for the isolation of blood group substances from gastric mucosa (85). Reductive cleavage of the disulfide bridges has the advantage over proteolysis in that the soluble glycoprotein possesses a more intact protein core, albeit without inter- and intrachain disulfide bridges.

Noncovalent bond-breaking solvents must be used if the rheological properties of the glycoprotein are to be preserved. Complete solubilization of the mucous gel can be achieved in isotonic saline if physical shear is applied. For example, pig gastric mucous gel is completely dissolved in 0.2 M NaCl by brief homogenization for 30 to 60 sec to yield a glycoprotein possessing the full gel-forming properties (1). Solutions of strong denaturants, e.g., 6 M urea (74,176) and 4 M guanidinium chloride, will dissolve the gel when stirred (Table 1). Strong denaturants, however, can cause conformational changes in the glycoprotein. This is seen in pig gastric mucous glycoprotein, which retains its molecular weight of 2×10^6 daltons in 4 M guanidinium chloride but, when the denaturant was removed by dialysis against isotonic saline, aggregated to give a soluble component of about 8×10^6 daltons (161). It is essential with all nondegradative isolation methods to avoid proteolytic degradation during the procedure; the mucous preparations should always be kept cool (4°C); and, where possible, other means of inhibiting endogenous proteolytic enzymes should be used. This can be done with gastric mucus by raising the pH to above 5 when pepsin activity is abolished, or by collecting mucus from a nonacid-secreting stomach pouch (74). As a matter of routine, 0.02% sodium azide, or some other antibacterial agent, should be added to the mucous preparations to eliminate bacterial growth.

Purification of Mucous Glycoproteins

An understanding of the extent of purity of the isolated material is essential for the elucidation of the physiological and rheological aspects of mucus. The many methods that have been used to purify and fractionate mucous glycoproteins could occupy a chapter on their own; specific books, reviews, or papers (see refs. 24,36,61,75 and Table 1) should be consulted for details.

One method used at some point in many purification procedures is gel filtration with large pore size gels (45,49,146,157). Because of their large molecular size, the mucous glycoproteins are excluded by such gels and well separated from the lower molecular weight contaminant proteins and other constituents. The strong negative charge of mucous glycoproteins is the basis for several separation methods, including electrophoresis (90,127,176), ion exchange (16,127), and selective precipitation with cationic detergents (16,62,127) or solutions of low pH (62,126). A particular drawback with

TABLE 1. *Methods for isolating glycoproteins from gastrointestinal mucous gels*

Method	Source	Form of glycoprotein	
Degradative: covalent bond breaking			
Proteolysis (e.g., pepsin, trypsin, pronase, papain)	Gastric mucus: human (78,148), canine (127), pig (85,155)	Carbohydrate chains intact; protein partly degraded	Loss of viscous and gel-forming properties
	Colonic mucus: sheep (89), pig (79)		
Reductive cleavage of disulfide bridges (e.g., 2-mercapthethanol, dithiothreitol, Na_2SO_3.	Gastric mucus: human (150), canine (90)	Carbohydrate chains and protein intact, except for disulfide bridges	
Nondegradative: noncovalent bond breaking			
Denaturants (e.g., urea, guanidinium chloride, phenol/ H_2O)	Gastric mucus: human (74,78,176), pig (141)	Primary structure intact; viscous and gel-forming properties retained although some loss can occur, especially with denaturants; physical shear, e.g., homogenization, necessary to dissolve gel in salt solutions	
	Colonic mucus: human (58), rat (123)		
Salt solutions, etc. (e.g., 0.2 M NaCl, 3.5 M CsCl, EDTA, H_2O)	Salivary mucus: human (111,126), sheep, cow, pig (62)		
	Gastric mucus: human (13,131,146), pig (157,163)		
	Small intestinal mucus: human (82), rat (16,45), pig (113), rabbit (124)		
	Colonic mucus: pig (115), rat (123)		

For further details of methods for gastrointestinal mucous glycoproteins as well as for respiratory, cervical, and ovarian cyst mucus, see refs. 24,36,61,75.

these methods is the complete removal of nonglycoprotein material, which binds strongly although noncovalently to the glycoprotein and separates with it during the isolation procedure (24,163). For example, all the contaminant protein in the mucus, because of its much lower molecular weight, should be easily separable from the glycoprotein by gel filtration. However, mucous glycoproteins isolated by gel filtration in 0.2 M NaCl still contain up to 20% contaminant, nonglycoprotein protein, which is attached to it by strong noncovalent interactions and excluded with it by the sepharose gel (163).

Coprecipitation of contaminant protein with the glycoprotein has been shown to account for the varying protein contents of submaxillary gland mucous glycoprotein preparations (132). Stronger noncovalent bond-breaking solvents, e.g., sodium dodecylsulfate, must be used if the glycoprotein and protein are to be completely separated by these methods. Preparative equilibrium centrifugation in a density gradient of CsCl or a similar salt is probably the only satisfactory way to obtain quantitatively undegraded mucous glycoprotein free of

noncovalently bound protein (25,163). This method separates the glycoprotein on the basis of its density from the lower density protein and higher density nucleic acid, respectively. At the same time, the high ionic strength of the cesium salt (e.g., 3.5 M CsCl) counteracts the strong noncovalent interactions between the macromolecules, in particular protein-glycoprotein interactions. In practice, purification procedures for glycoproteins involve several steps; an example for human or pig gastric mucous glycoprotein is outlined in Fig. 2. Examples of the isolation of mucous glycoproteins by other methods, including ion exchange chromatography and selective precipitation, are exemplified in the purification of glycoproteins from dog gastric mucus (90,127) and the various submaxillary gland mucous secretions (62).

Assessment of the purity of the isolated mucous glycoprotein includes not only whether it is free of nonglycoprotein constituents but also to what extent it is a single homogeneous species of glycoprotein. The question of homogeneity of mucous glycoproteins is complicated by the fact that these molecules are polydisperse

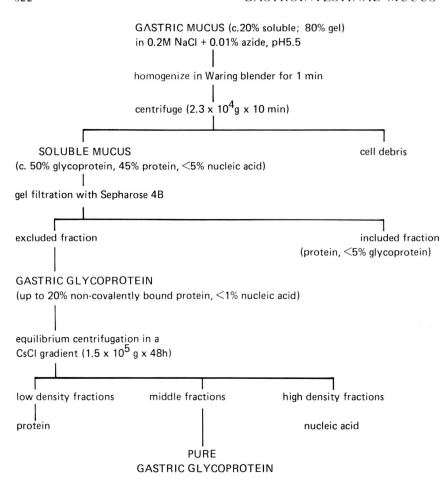

FIG. 2. Procedure for the isolation and purification of undergraded human or pig gastric mucous glycoprotein.

in size, primarily because of differences in the number of carbohydrate residues per chain and the number of these chains per molecule (25,49). This results in variation about a mean of such properties as molecular weight, density, and charge of glycoprotein molecules from a single secretion of an individual. Thus a pure, homogeneous glycoprotein fractionated by gel filtration or ion exchange chromatography will elute as a broad peak from the column and on ultracentrifugation sediment under a broad envelope, in contrast to the sharp profiles obtained by these methods with a single species of protein.

Gibbons (49) proposed that a homogeneous glycoprotein preparation could be distinguished from a heterogeneous preparation in that for the former, the variations of all the molecular parameters throughout the sample should be unimodal. No single method is sufficient for demonstrating homogeneity of a mucous glycoprotein preparation; as many different methods as possible should be used to check this (73,73a). Such

methods may include sedimentation velocity and equilibrium ultracentrifugation analysis (24,49,81), column chromatography by gel filtration, ion exchange, electrophoretic methods, and identification of the components by immunological analysis (61,90). Gel electrophoresis in sodium dodecyl sulfate is a particularly good method for checking whether the glycoprotein is free of all noncovalently bound, lower molecular weight proteins (45). The carbohydrate and amino acid analysis of the glycoprotein should be consistent from preparation to preparation. No uronic acid should be present, for this indicates the absence of connective tissue-type proteoglycans. The removal of nucleic acid contaminants can be monitored by analysis for phosphate or the sugars ribose and deoxyribose. Finally, the isolated mucous glycoprotein should be shown to be the major high molecular weight polysaccharide-containing constituent of the mucous secretion; this has seldom been achieved. In fact, the successful isolaton of pure mucous glycoproteins, which at the same time possess full rheological properties, has been an obstacle to progress in the mucus field.

Carbohydrate Side Chains of Mucous Glycoproteins

There are considerable variations in the structure of the carbohydrate chains in glycoproteins from different regions of the gastrointestinal tract in the same species as well as between species. This is apparent from the sugar composition of different mucous glycoproteins (Table 2), where the molar ratios of the five different sugars characteristic of these molecules (Figs. 1 and 3) vary considerably. In some glycoproteins, one or more of these sugars may be absent. The size of the carbohydrate chains attached to the protein core varies from a relatively simple two sugars to a complex structure of up to 19 sugars (Fig. 3). The sequence of the sugars and the conformation of the glycosidic linkages between them, however, is always the same for a given glycoprotein.

Sheep submaxillary mucous glycoprotein has simple chains of N-acetylgalactosamine linked to N-acetylneuraminic acid and contains approximately 800 of these chains in a molecule of more than 1×10^6 MW (62). Pig submaxillary mucous glycoprotein is more complicated, containing a maximum of five sugar residues per chain and about 500 such chains per molecule of 1×10^6 MW (20). In contrast, the glycoproteins from human (150) or pig gastric mucus (155) have branched chains that are up to 19 sugars in length joined by 10 or so different glycosidic linkages (Fig. 3) and about 600 of these chains on molecule of 2×10^6 MW. The largest

carbohydrate side chain known is that from rat colonic mucus, which is branched, with an average of 22 sugars per chain (123). Too few complete sequences of these sugar chains have been elucidated to know what special structural features are associated with mucous glycoproteins from different regions of the gastrointestinal tract. In the one gastrointestinal tract, namely, the pig, where the structure of the carbohydrate side chains of both submaxillary mucous and gastric mucous glycoproteins have been determined, that found in the former is much simpler than in the latter. Recent work shows that the pig small intestinal mucous glycoprotein has a simple carbohydrate chain similar to that from pig submaxillary mucus and unlike that from pig gastric mucus (113).

There are certain common structural patterns that can be discerned by comparing the known carbohydrate chain structures. For example, N-acetylgalactosamine is always found at the reducing end, joining the chain to the serine or threonine residues of the protein core (21). The only other position where N-acetylgalactosamine occurs is at the other, nonreducing, end of the carbohydrate chains in some mucous glycoproteins (Fig. 3). Sialic acid and fucose are also always found in terminal positions at the nonreducing ends of main or branch chains.

Another feature common to many of these mucous glycoproteins is that they are ABH antigens for the ABO blood group system; the structure of the terminal portions of their carbohydrate side chains are the same as those of the blood group antigens on the surface of the red cell (177). Therefore, when included in an agglutination assay, they compete with the antibody and

TABLE 2. *Composition of some gastrointestinal mucous glycoproteins*

Source	GlcNAc	Carbohydrate GalNAc	(molar ratios)[a] Gal	Fuc	NeuNAc/ NeuNGl	Ester sulfate (% by wt.)	Protein (% by wt.)	Ref.
Saliva								
Human	1.2	1	1.5	0.9	0.6	+	34	126
Pig	0	1	0.5	0.4	0.4	0	34	61
Sheep	0	1	0	0	1.0	0	46	61
Stomach								
Human	2.4	1	3.1	2.1	0.2	7.0	17	148
Pig	2.8	1	2.9	1.9	0.2	3.1	13	9
Small intestine								
Human	1	1	2	0.6	0.2	0	12	82
Pig	0.6	1	0.7	0.3	0.5	2.6	18	113
Rat	1	1	3	1	0.8	0.03	12-16	45
Colon								
Human[b]	1	1	1.1	0.5	0.7	1.6	33	58
Pig	2.9	1	2.5	1.5	0.2	3.0	13	115

[a]Abbreviations: Fuc; fucose; Gal; galactose; GalNAc, N-acetylgalactosamine; GlcNAc, N-acetylglucosamine; NeuNAc, N-acetylneuraminic acid; NeuNGl, N-glycollylneuraminic acid.
[b]Mucoprotein antigen from human colonic mucosa.
With human glycoproteins, the sugar composition will depend on the blood-group secretor status; all examples given are for A secretors.

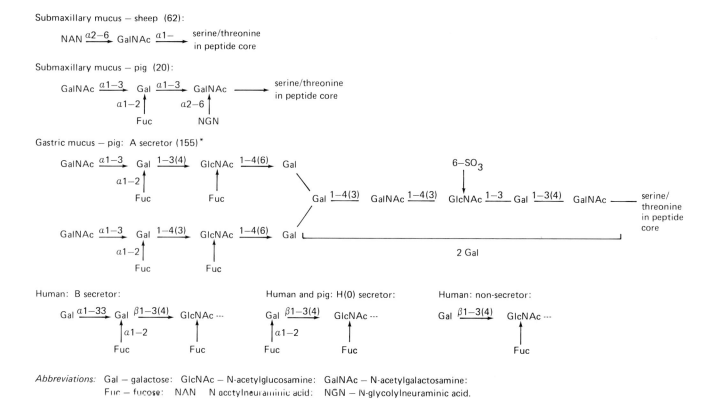

FIG. 3. Structure of carbohydrate side chains of some glycoproteins from gastrointestinal mucus.

thereby inhibit the agglutination of the red cells. The ABH antigenic activity of human mucous glycoproteins from all regions of the gastrointestinal tract is reflected in the structure of their carbohydrate chains, which end in either N-acetylgalactosamine (A secretor) or galactose (B secretor), or with just the terminal fucose α-2 galactose (H secretor) (Fig. 3). About 20% of people are nonsecretors (recessive form of the Se gene). In this case, the secretions possess neither A, B, nor H activity, and the carbohydrate chains of the glycoproteins end in a single galactose without the terminal fucose residue (178). In pig mucous secretions, the glycoproteins from all regions of the gut have either A or H antigenic activity, again showing common structural features in the carbohydrate side chains of these different mucous glycoproteins.

While the sequence, type of linkage, and maximum number of possible sugar residues per chain are genetically specified, the number of sugars per chain, together with the number of chains per glycoprotein molecule, varies between molecules from the same secretion. In pig submaxillary mucous glycoprotein from A secretors, five different sizes of carbohydrate chains are found from a single N-acetylgalactosamine residue to completed chains with all five residues (20). This microheterogeneity in size and number of the carbohydrate chains per mucous glycoprotein molecule is considered

to be the reason for the polydispersity in their molecular parameters, such as molecular weight, density, and charge (discussed above). The polydispersity in charge per molecule is attributable to differences in the number of sialic acid and ester sulfate residues which are located on the carbohydrate chains. While microheterogeneity results at the level of biosynthesis of the carbohydrate chains, it can also be caused by modification of the secreted mucous glycoprotein by endogenous hydrolytic glycosidase enzymes in the gut (77). An example of this is the removal of the terminal sialic acid residues from gastric mucous glycoprotein by the hydrolytic enzyme neuraminidase produced by bacteria in the mucus (10). Proteolytic enzymes in the gut can hydrolyze parts of the protein of the mucous glycoproteins; this could result in microheterogeneity in the amino acid composition of the isolated material (143).

Gastrointestinal glycoproteins are strongly negatively charged, primarily because of the presence of carbohydrate bound ester sulfate and sialic acid residues, each of which has a single negative charge. Sialic acid is the family name for a series of sugars based on N-acetyl- or N-glycolylneuraminic acid (61). The neuraminic acids always possess a free negatively charged carboxyl group; often, hydroxyl positions on the sugars are substituted further with O-acetyl groups. In bovine salivary mucous glycoproteins, 10 forms of N-acetyl- and glycolylneuraminic acid with different acetyl substitutions have been isolated (133). The sialic acid residues are found in terminal positions on the carbohydrate chains, while ester sulfate residues are located internally, for example, as N-acetylglucosamine-6-sulfate in pig gastric mucus (155), or as N-acetylglucosamine-3- or 4-sulfate in dog submaxillary mucus (108). Sialic acid and ester sulfate often are together in the same glycoprotein preparations; in dog submaxillary mucus, however, there is evidence that they are on different carbohydrate chains (108). The content of sialic acid and sulfate varies considerably from one mucous glycoprotein secretion to another (Table 2) and between glycoprotein molecules from the same secretion. Fractionation of dog gastric mucous glycoprotein by ion exchange chromatography produces fractions that vary considerably in their content of ester sulfate and sialic acid (127). Until more detailed analysis has been performed on glycoprotein preparations from a given source, it is not possible to say to what extent such preparations consist of distinct classes of sulfated and sialic acid-containing glycoproteins.

Protein of Mucous Glycoproteins

Mucous glycoproteins have an amino acid composition with a characteristically high serine, threonine, and proline content when compared to a typical globular protein (Table 3). Threonine and serine are the amino acids involved in the linkage of the carbohydrate side chains to the protein core by N-acetylgalactosamine (21). The carbohydrate side chains can be packed very closely together; for example, in pig gastric mucus, one in three or four amino acids on the protein core must carry a chain on the average of 15 sugar residues in length. In the ovarian cyst mucous glycoprotein, which has a similar carbohydrate chain structure, peptides (e.g., Pro-Thr-Thr-Thr-Pro-Ser and Ala-Pro-Thr-Thr-Ser-Gly-Ser) have been isolated with all the serine and threonine residues glycosylated (60). The high proline content may reflect a role for this amino acid in maintaining a particular conformation in the protein core that will enable the close packing of these large carbohydrate side chains. With such a protective sheath of carbohydrate (80% by weight of the glycoprotein), the protein core buried inside is protected from attack by proteolytic enzymes. It was on this basis that the original preparation of blood group active glycoproteins from the gastric mucosa by autodigestion through pepsin was successful (85). Blood group active glycoproteins isolated from pig gastric mucus by this method are still large molecules of 5×10^5 daltons, yet they are resistant to further proteolysis by pepsin, trypsin, and even the less specific proteases, such as papain and pronase (143).

Several gastrointestinal mucous glycoproteins isolated by nondegradative methods and purified free of noncovalently bound protein (see above) have an extra portion of protein not found in the same glycoprotein isolated by proteolysis (Table 3). This has resulted in the concept of two regions of protein in these glycoproteins, a glycosylated region rich in serine, threonine, proline, and a nonglycosylated (or "naked") region, which is not covered by a sheath of carbohydrate and therefore is accessible to proteolytic attack. Nonglycosylated protein is lost when undegraded pig gastric mucous glycoprotein is incubated with proteolytic enzymes, e.g., pepsin or papain, and represents about 35% by weight of the total protein content or about 4 to 5% by weight of the molecule (143,163). This is equivalent to approximately 750 amino acid residues, larger than the average

TABLE 3. *Amino acid composition of some gastrointestinal mucous glycoproteins*

| Source | Amino acid composition (moles/100 moles protein) | | | | | | | | | | Ref. |
	Thr	Ser	Pro	Glu	Asp	Ala	Gly	Arg	Lys	Cys	
Saliva											
Pig	13.6	23.3	5.4	5.7	1.9	14.5	19.7	2.7	1.0	—	62
Sheep	12.7	15.2	8.2	7.1	4.9	10.9	14.9	4.0	2.1	0.8	62
Stomach											
Human	25.3	14.2	17.8	4.7	2.4	10.8	6.7	2.1	4.8	—	148
Pig native	18.1	15.8	15.3	7.7	4.8	4.7	5.8	3.2	3.9	3.1	143
Pig pronase digested	26.3	24.0	18.5	5.0	2.0	4.0	4.3	0.9	1.8	0.4	143
Small intestine											
Human	16.8	10.5	9.8	8.7	8.1	6.5	7.4	3.1	3.3	1.5	82
Pig	26.5	10.4	15.4	4.2	4.6	3.8	5.6	2.2	2.2	4.3	113
Rat	23.5	10.2	11.8	8.6	6.4	5.2	6.1	2.7	4.5	2.0	45
Colon											
Pig native	24.1	12.2	14.8	5.3	4.8	5.2	5.5	3.5	2.6		115
Pig pronase/mercaptoethanol treated	36.8	17.4	19.8	7.6	2.0	5.0	5.3	—	—		115

The aromatic and long chain aliphatic amino acids are present only in small amounts.

globular protein, and its removal has a drastic effect on the polymeric structure of the glycoprotein, as discussed in the next section. Comparison of the amino acid composition of the proteolytically degraded pig gastric mucous glycoprotein with the purified undegraded material shows that the amino acid composition of the nonglycosylated protein is close to that of an average globular protein; in particular, it is low in serine, threonine, and proline, which predominate in the glycosylated region of the protein core (Table 3). There is evidence for similar naked, nonglycosylated regions of the protein in glycoproteins from other gastrointestinal mucous secretions, including those from human gastric mucus (131), pig small intestinal mucus (113), pig colonic mucus (115), and the related ovarian cyst mucous glycoproteins (34,35).

Polymeric Structure of Mucous Glycoproteins

The molecular weight of the undegraded glycoprotein from pig gastric mucus, which is 2×10^6 daltons, is markedly decreased in size to 5×10^5 daltons following proteolysis by pepsin and other proteases (9,143). Furthermore, the undegraded glycoprotein is dissociated on reductive cleavage of the disulfide bridges with mercaptoethanol into four equal sized subunits of MW 5×10^5 daltons (159), the same size as those obtained by proteolysis. From detailed studies on pig gastric mucus, a model has been proposed for its structure (1), which explains these results (Fig. 4). The undegraded glycoprotein consists of four subunits of equal size. The protein of each subunit is composed of two parts, a glycosylated region and a nonglycosylated region which is naked and susceptible to proteolytic attack. The four subunits are joined together by disulfide bridges, about 39 per molecule, most of which are located in the nonglycosylated region. Recently, it has been shown that a separate protein of 70,000 MW joined to the glycoprotein subunits by disulfide bridges is the main component of the naked protein of each glycoprotein molecule (130).

The importance of naked protein and disulfide bridges to the gel-forming structures of glycoproteins from a wide variety of mucous secretions is clear from the ready solubilization of these secretions by proteolytic enzymes and thiol reagents (e.g., Table 1). To demonstrate a polymeric structure, as described above for pig gastric mucous glycoprotein, it is essential to isolate the undegraded glycoprotein free of all noncovalently bound protein. Degradative methods of preparation, which use proteolytic enzymes or reducing agents to isolate water-soluble glycoproteins from the gelatinous mucus, inevitably destroy the polymeric structure of the glycoprotein and produce degraded subunits (Table 1). In constrast, nondegradative agents, which break only noncovalent bonds, e.g., 2 M NaCl, 3.5 M CsCl, 6 M guanidinium chloride, or sodium dodecyl sulfate, do not dissociate the glycoprotein polymer but dissociate glycoprotein from contaminant, noncovalently bound protein.

Other undegraded glycoproteins have been isolated by methods similar to those developed for pig gastric

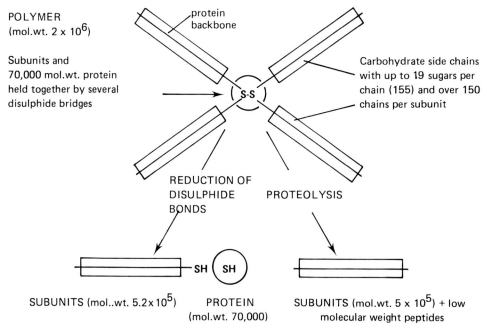

FIG. 4. Diagrammatic representation of the proposed structure for pig gastric mucous glycoprotein (MW 2×10^6). [Data from Allen (1,2) and Pearson and Allen (130).] The arrangement in space of the subunits and protein is not known. Human gastric mucous glycoprotein has the same overall structure (131).

mucous glycoprotein, namely, a combination of equilibrium density gradient centrifugation and gel filtration (Fig. 2). Human gastric mucus, pig small intestinal mucus, and pig colonic mucus have all been shown to possess a polymeric structure composed of subunits joined by interchain disulfide bridges and dependent on regions of naked protein which is accessible to proteolytic attack (Table 4). Human gastric mucous glycoprotein, MW 2×10^6, has a polymeric structure like that found in pig gastric mucus and which is broken down into glycoprotein subunits of about MW 5×10^5 by pepsin, papain, pronase, or reduction with mercaptoethanol (131). Since the carbohydrate side chains of human and pig gastric mucus are also very close in their structure (150,155), pig gastric mucus, which can be obtained in plentiful supply, is a good model for human secretion (8). The glycoprotein from pig small intestinal mucus (MW 1.8×10^6 daltons) has a different polymeric structure from that of pig gastric mucus in that it consists of subunits (MW 2.3×10^5 daltons) about one-eighth the size of the polymeric glycoprotein (5). The glycoprotein from pig colonic mucus was found to have a large molecular weight of 15×10^6 (115). The glycoprotein is broken down by proteolysis and mercaptoethanol treatment to relatively small glycoprotein units, the smallest of which has a molecular weight of 7.6×10^5 daltons; however, the relative contributions of covalent and noncovalent linkages in the structure of the original glycoprotein are not yet clearly defined. There is evidence from gel electrophoresis for a polymeric structure in pig and dog submaxillary mucous glycoproteins (70). It is becoming evident that such polymeric structures occur widely in glycoproteins of mucous secretions from nongastrointestinal sources,

namely, cervical (50), respiratory (138), and ovarian cyst mucus (35).

There are some well-documented examples of mucous glycoproteins that are not broken down by reductive cleavage of disulfide bridges (Table 4); these are sheep and cow submaxillary mucous glycoproteins (69,70), rat small intestinal glycoprotein (45), and human small intestinal glycoprotein (46). In the case of the rat and human small intestinal glycoproteins, the effect of proteolysis on molecular size has yet to be investigated. Sheep submaxillary glycoprotein possesses a polymeric structure, but one involving particularly strong noncovalent interactions between subunits of MW 154,000 daltons and which are reversibly dissociated at high salt concentrations, namely, 2.0 M NaCl (69).

VISCOUS AND GEL-FORMING PROPERTIES OF MUCUS

Properties of the Mucous Glycoprotein Gel

The viscoelastic mucous gel has properties intermediate between those of a solid gel and a liquid (51,106,125,154). It is not merely a viscous liquid, since once fully hydrated, it can remain in an aqueous medium without swelling. It will anneal if sectioned, yet it is resistant to flow and has a yield point, i.e., an externally applied force below which it will not flow. These properties arise at the molecular level from a balance of the polymer-polymer interactions between the glycoprotein molecules themselves and the polymer-solvent interactions of the hydrophilic glycoprotein interacting with its aqueous environment (122). Mucous glycoproteins are "sticky" molecules, with respect not only

TABLE 4. *Molecular size and structure of mucous glycoproteins*

Source	Molecular weight		Ref.
	Polymer	Subunit	
Dissociated by reduction of			
Disulfide bridges			
Pig gastric	2×10^6	5×10^5	2,9,159
Human gastric	2×10^6	5×10^5	8,131
Pig small intestinal	1.8×10^6	2.4×10^5	5
Pig colonic	15×10^6	7.2×10^5	115
Pig submaxillary	1×10^6	lower MW	70
Canine submaxillary	—		70
Cervical	1.6 to 4×10^6	3 to 6×10^5	50
Respiratory	1 to 3×10^6	lower MW	138
Ovarian cyst	1 to 2×10^6		35
Dissociated by 2 M NaCl			
Ovine submaxillary	1×10^6	1.5×10^5	69
No detectable subunit structure			
Rat small intestinal	2×10^6		45
Human small intestinal			46

to each other, but also to other molecules; they will bind to cell surfaces (6). This stickiness ensures that mucus adheres to the mucosal surface and provides a slimy coat to facilitate the passage of solid material through the gut.

Nondegradative solvents (Table 1) will dissolve the mucous gel completely to give the soluble glycoproteins because noncovalent interactions between these molecules are responsible for gel formation. Furthermore, isolated undegraded glycoproteins will reversibly gel at concentrations similar to that found in the native mucous gel in vivo (7,113). The gel-forming potential of the soluble glycoprotein is reflected in its intrinsic viscosity (viscosity extrapolated to infinite dilution), which is high for the undegraded glycoprotein, e.g., 320 ml g^{-1} for pig gastric mucous glycoprotein in 0.2 M NaCl and about 400 ml g^{-1} for rat small intestinal mucous glycoprotein in 0.01 M tris, respectively (45,160). As the concentration of the glycoprotein increases, the viscosity rises, not linearly, but asymptotically (Fig. 5), until the solution assumes viscoelastic gel-like properties, and gel formation occurs.

A model for gel formation in pig gastric mucus has been proposed (7) based on physical studies that show in dilute solution that the glycoprotein is a highly expanded, hydrated, roughly spherical molecule. At a concentration of approximately 20 mg/ml, the glycoprotein molecules fill the entire solution volume. This (Fig. 5) is the point at which the viscosity begins to rise sharply. As the concentration of glycoprotein molecules increases further, so does the overlap of their domains; the noncovalent intermolecular interactions increase; and the viscoelastic properties of the system develop with the formation of a gel. The higher the glycoprotein concentration becomes, the greater will be the degree of interpenetration of the molecules within the gel, the stronger will be their interactions, and the thicker and

more stable the gel will become. The mucous gel has a relatively high molecular density, with the glycoprotein molecules completely filling the gel volume and where much of the solvent is intramolecular. Such an arrangement within the mucous gel matrix undoubtedly provides an excellent unstirred layer and prevents HCO_3^- secreted at the gastric mucosal surface from mixing with the major part of the HCl in the lumen.

The permeability properties of gastrointestinal mucous gels have yet to be clearly defined. Gastric mucus in vitro and in vivo is permeable to ions, e.g., H^+, HCO_3^-, and small molecules (26,68,179), but the upper limit on the size molecule that can permeate the gel has not been determined. The glycoprotein gel matrix, with its unstirred solution within, is likely to be a considerable barrier to the passage of larger molecules, such as pepsin. However, the mucous gel is still more than 90% by volume water. While this is contained within the unstirred layer of the gel matrix, less than 1% will be physically bound to the glycoprotein. Therefore, the rate of diffusion of small ions, such as H^+, through the mucous gel would be the same as that through an unstirred layer. Calculation shows that this is a rapid process, taking only a few minutes (26). It remains to be shown experimentally whether the rate diffusion of H^+ through gastric mucous gel is the same as that theoretically expected for an unstirred layer and how this is affected by neutralization with HCO_3^-.

Relationship Between the Viscous and Gel-Forming Properties of Mucus and the Glycoprotein Structure

If the pig or human gastric mucous glycoprotein polymer (MW 2×10^6) is dissociated into its subunits (MW 5×10^5), the viscous and gel-forming properties of the native mucus are lost (2,9,131) (Fig. 4). This explains at the molecular level the solubilization of the gastric

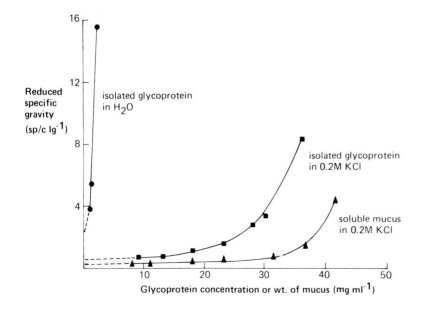

FIG. 5. Viscosity of pig gastric mucous glycoprotein. [Data from Allen (1,2).]

mucous gel by proteolysis or by reduction of the disulfide bridges (Table 1). It is reflected in the isolated glycoprotein by the large decrease in viscosity when it is dissociated into its component subunits by either of the above procedures. The solubilization of dog gastric mucus by proteolysis (66,127) or reduction (90) and of cat gastric mucus (86) indicates a dependence on an analogous covalent polymeric structure in the glycoprotein for the gel-forming properties of these secretions. In the pig, in addition to gastric mucus, mucus from the colon (115), small intestine (113), and submaxillary gland (70) depends on the polymeric structures of the glycoproteins for its viscous and gel-forming properties. A similar dependence on glycoprotein polymeric structure for rheological properties has been demonstrated for respiratory, cervical, and ovarian cyst mucus from humans (Table 4). The glycoproteins of sheep submaxillary mucus and rat small intestinal mucus do not possess a polymeric structure dependent on interchain disulfide bridges. In these secretions, gel formation is considered to take place by the interlinking of negatively charged, long chain, random coil polymers (45,62).

The role in gel formation of the polysaccharide, which comprises at least 70% of the weight of the glycoprotein, is not yet clearly defined. The hydrophilic carbohydrate side chains ensure strong interaction of the mucus with its aqueous environment. Since most of the surface of the glycoprotein consists of sugar residues, it is also likely that the noncovalent interactions involved in gel formation are between the polysaccharide chains. There are many different polysaccharides, e.g., agar, that interact noncovalently to form gels. In these instances, the interactions are specific, form cooperatively, and are stronger than those found in mucus (137). The precise chemical structure of the carbohydrate chains in mucous glycoproteins does not determine whether these molecules can form a gel. Within the same tissue from the same species, the composition of the terminal sugars in these mucous glycoproteins can vary according to secretor status (177); in nonsecretors, the chains can be deficient by three sugars; in all cases, an effective gel is produced. Furthermore, the size of the polysaccharide chain in glycoproteins from different secretions can differ between two and 22 sugars, although all these mucous glycoproteins form gels. The considerable differences in carbohydrate chain structure between these glycoproteins may be reflected in as-yet unrecognized properties of the gel matrix which influence the physiological functions of the mucus *in vivo*.

Mucous glycoproteins are negatively charged, for which the functional significance is not fully understood. It may be a matter of physiological importance that the presence of negative charges can hinder enzymic degradation of the glycoproteins in the gut; the tryptic digestion of sheep submaxillary mucous glycoprotein, for example, may only occur after the sialic acid residues have been removed from the carbohydrate chains (62). The nature of the charge on the glycoprotein does influence the viscosity of mucus; but such changes occur only at very low ionic strengths. Thus the viscosity of pig gastric mucus (160) (Fig. 5), rat small intestinal mucus (45), and sheep submaxillary mucus (62) increases markedly if the total ionic concentration falls below about 10 mM. This increase in viscosity can be attributed to a polyelectrolyte effect caused by repulsion between the negatively charged groups on the glycoprotein, which causes expansion of the molecule. This repulsion between the negative charges is significant only at very low ionic strengths, when there are insufficient cations in solution to act as a shield between them. As a result, the expanded glycoprotein will influence a larger volume of solution and show more intermolecular interactions and greater viscosity at a given concentration (1). The negative charges responsible for this effect are presumed to be the ester sulfate and sialic acid residues on the carbohydrate chains. This is confirmed in rat small intestinal mucous glycoprotein, in which the rise in viscosity at low salt concentrations is abolished by removal of the sialic acid with the enzyme neuraminidase (45). These changes in viscosity caused by repulsion between negatively charged residues in the glycoprotein are at such low ionic strengths that they are unlikely to be of significance *in vivo*. The negatively charged residues may be the site of cation bonding by the glycoprotein, for example, Ca^{2+}. Addition of Ca^{2+} to rat small intestinal mucus produces a reduction in viscosity and the formation of clumps of material (44). This may be important in the formation of mucous plugs in the Ca^{2+}-rich secretions of cystic fibrosis patients (41).

The effect of H^+ concentration on the physical properties of mucus is uncertain. Visual observations by several workers have pointed to solubilization of the visible gastric mucous gel at low pH (67,74,151), although it has not been determined whether this is a direct result of the pH change or the indirect result of stimulation of pepsinolysis. The viscosity of dilute solutions of isolated pig gastric mucous glycoprotein is the same over a pH range of 1 to 8 (3), but more detailed investigations on pH and mucus rheology, preferably on the gel itself, are needed.

Another area of uncertainty surrounding the control of the viscous and gel-forming properties of mucus are the effects of free protein and other nonglycoprotein constituents. The presence of protein impurities in the solubilized mucus is responsible for its lowered viscosity relative to the viscosity of a comparable concentration of purified glycoprotein (Fig. 5). In some instances, however, noncovalently bound protein can interact with the glycoprotein and increase its viscosity, possibly by functioning as a link between the glycoprotein molecules (24,105,138). This hypothesis is difficult to substantiate. At present, there is no definitive evidence that noncovalently bound protein is a factor in raising the viscosity of mucous secretions *in vivo*. Bovine serum albumin has been shown to increase the viscosity of pig gastric mucous glycoprotein (105). This was not under physiological conditions, however, since a high ratio of protein to glycoprotein (2:1) was investigated; the glycoprotein, which was from a commercial source, is enzymatically degraded and possesses an intrinsic viscosity less than half that of the undegraded material. Bile is another factor that may affect the properties of mucus *in vivo*. It has been reported that bile salts decrease the gel strength of respiratory mucus *in vitro* (117). Respiratory mucus is particularly heterogeneous (24); this effect of bile may not be applicable to other mucous secretions.

TURNOVER OF MUCUS

The effectiveness of mucus *in vivo* depends on the depth of its layer covering the mucosal surface and on the structure of its gel. The depth of the mucous gel on the mucosal surface is not static; it is the result of a dynamic balance between its secretion and erosion (Fig. 6). Proteolytic enzymes, e.g., pepsin in the stomach, solubilize the mucous gel to produce degraded subunits in the lumen. This erosion depends on the extent of luminal proteolysis and is augmented by mechanical forces during the process of digestion. Balancing this erosion of the mucus is its secretion by the mucosal cells, with their high biosynthetic activity and turnover rate. The greater the depth of mucous gel covering the surface epithelium, the better the protection against mechanical damage and, in the stomach and duodenum,

the better the containment of mucosal HCO_3^- secretion. The structure of the secreted glycoprotein molecules determines whether a gel is formed, the strength of the gel, and the tenacity with which it adheres to the mucosal surface. The concentration of glycoprotein secreted must be at a certain threshold before a gel can be formed; then, the greater the concentration, the denser the molecular matrix of the gel, and the greater its strength.

The intracellular biosynthetic pathways for mucous glycoproteins are known in some detail (61,144,145,178). Briefly, the protein core is made by translation of messenger RNA (mRNA) at the membrane-bound ribosomes. The attachment of *N*-acetylgalactosamine to serine and threonine residues, which is the starting point for the biosynthesis of the carbohydrate side chains, occurs next in the rough endoplasmic reticulum. It is during the passage of the precursor glycoprotein through the smooth endoplasmic reticular system and in the Golgi apparatus that most of the carbohydrate chain is formed by the stepwise addition of one sugar after another. In the Golgi apparatus, the glycoprotein is packed into secretory vesicles, and the new mucus is secreted by these vesicles fusing with the plasma membrane and disgorging their contents into the lumen (see Ito, Chapter 17). An intriguing and as yet unanswered question relates to the timing of the stage at which the glycoprotein ceases to exist in the soluble phase and becomes a gel; presumably, this occurs during or after it is contained within the membrane-bound vesicles.

The enzymes that catalyze the stepwise addition of sugars to the growing carbohydrate chain are called glycosyltransferases. As substrates, they require the precursor glycoprotein together with an activated nucleo-

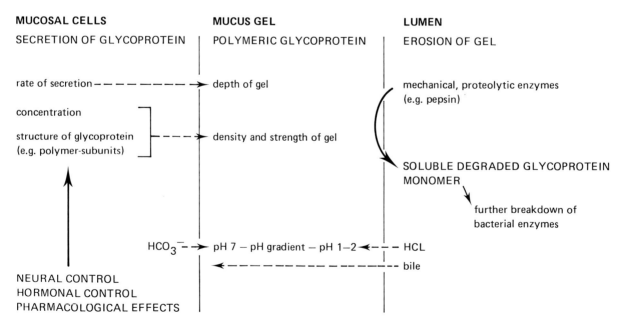

FIG. 6. Factors influencing the nature of the gastric mucus gel on the surface mucosa.

tide sugar derivative (145,178). These glycosyltransferases are highly specific; there is a separate enzyme for every sugar linkage. For example, 16 different enzymes can be involved in the biosynthesis of a carbohydrate side chain of human or pig gastric mucous glycoprotein (Fig. 3). Thus the final biosynthetic step in the formation of a glycoprotein with A blood group activity is the transfer of UDP-*N*-acetylgalactosamine by the relevant glycosyltransferase, which is found only in the mucosa of A and AB secretors. Similarly, for B and AB secretors, there is a glycosyltransferase in the mucosa that transfers UDP-galactose to the penultimate galactose residue. Both enzymes are absent from the mucosa of H secretors and from nonsecretors (Fig. 3).

The pathways for degradation of the mucous glycoproteins can be conveniently considered in two stages: (a) proteolysis of the glycoprotein with solubilization of the gel, and (b) subsequent breakdown of the soluble glycoprotein into low molecular weight sugars and amino acids that can be reutilized by either the body or the enteric flora. The enzymic solubilization of mucus from the stomach and lower gut has been reported (66,71,76,83). From studies on the hydrolysis of gastric mucous glycoprotein by pepsin, this can be explained by the proteolytic dissociation of the glycoprotein polymer into degraded soluble glycoprotein monomers and their release into the lumen (2,143). There may be inhibition of pepsin by mucus, possibly attributable to sulfated glycoproteins (97,116). Pig gastric mucus, which is well sulfated, is readily attacked by pepsin (143). When present in a thousandfold excess by weight, the isolated glycoprotein does not inhibit pepsin activity (3). Similar proteolytic degradation of the glycoproteins into lower molecular weight units and concomitant solubilization of the gel probably occurs with mucous secretions further down the gastrointestinal tract by the action of enzymes, such as trypsin, or bacterial proteases. The remaining protein core of the soluble proteolytically degraded glycoprotein is resistant to further proteolysis, unless the carbohydrate chains are first removed. There are glycosidase enzymes which hydrolyze the bonds between the sugar residues, one sugar at a time, from the free ends of the carbohydrate chains. Such enzymes, which are specific to the type of sugar and the conformation of the sugar linkage, originate almost entirely from the gut flora and are particularly plentiful in the oropharyngeal cavity and colon (76,77).

MUCUS *IN VIVO*

Analysis

Studies on isolated mucous secretions have yielded considerable information about the structure and bulk properties of mucus, but it remains to be considered how far this knowledge helps elucidate the physiological role of the surface mucous gel *in vivo* and how this is influenced by pharmacological and pathological factors. (See refs. 36,38, and 100 for detailed studies on mucus *in vivo,* particularly on its histochemistry.)

It is necessary to consider the major limitations of the available methods for analysis of mucus (Table 5). In no instance do these methods provide a comprehensive picture of the structure and quantity of mucus on the mucosal surface *in vivo.*

Mucous secretions can be classified into three groups on the basis of their histochemical staining: (a) neutral mucins, which stain only with the PAS technique, (b) sialic acid-containing mucins, and (c) ester sulfate-containing mucins. The acidic mucins stain with the basophilic dyes Alcian blue or high iron diamine; the distinction between sialic acid and sulfate groups is achieved by varying the salt concentration or pH of the staining solutions (38,101). The specificity of these techniques is increased by the use of enzymes to remove sugar residues; neuraminidase, for example, selectively removes sialic acid. It is often difficult to correlate histochemical results with the detailed chemical structure of the mucous glycoprotein. Therefore, there is uncertainty about whether or not sulfated glycoproteins are always present in normal human gastric mucous secretions. Mucous glycoproteins isolated from gastric juice (56,64,148) contain sulfate; fluorescent antibodies to these glycoproteins show their presence in the gastric mucosa (64,65). Histochemical staining shows only traces of sulfated glycoproteins in the normal human gastric mucosa. Their presence in gastric juice has been explained by contamination with saliva (96,97).

Biochemical studies and histochemical staining both show the presence of sulfated glycoproteins in the gastric mucous secretions of other mammals, e.g., rat and dog. Several workers (100,173,180), by staining or autoradiography using $^{35}SO_4^{2-}$, have shown that in the rat and dog, mucous glycoprotein produced by the cells of the gastric pits is much richer in ester sulfate residues than the mucous glycoprotein produced by the same cells once they attain the mucosal surface. Such differences in the sulfation of the mucous glycoproteins secreted by individual cells of the same tissue partially explain the microheterogeneity in the ester sulfate content found in bulk preparations of isolated mucous glycoproteins. An example of the degree of specificity that can be achieved with histochemical methods is seen by the distinction between mucus produced by the acinar cells and that produced by the serous cells in the bovine submandibular glands (174). This method picks out differences in the position of *O*-acetyl groups on the sialic acids by altering the conditions for periodate oxidation. It must be remembered, however, that biochemical studies have so far failed to provide a general role for sialic acid and ester sulfate in glycoproteins. Until this is achieved, the interpretation of these histochemical

TABLE 5. *Methods used for quantitating the content of mucus in secretions*

Method	Ref.

Carbohydrate composition
    Individual sugars by colorimetric methods
        Sialic acid
        Fucose
        Galactose
        Hexosamines
	12,18,29,31—33,
	84,98,104,118,119,167,
	170–172

Total sugar composition by colorimetric methods
    Periodic acid Schiff
    Alcian blue
	81,112,
	19

Total spectrum of sugars Gas liquid chromatography	92–94,98,110, 116,140,146–152

Incorporation of radioactively labeled glycoprotein precursors
in vivo or *in vitro* with isolated cells or tissue
    Radioactive precursor
        $^{14}C/^3H$ glucose, galactose, glucosamine
        $^{35}SO_4$
        $^{14}C^3H$ threonine, serine, and other amino acids
	42,88,95,99,109,
	128,129,173,175

Histochemical
    Stains for periodate oxidizable and acidic groups in the glycoprotein
    Autoradiography
    Antibodies
	30,37–39,48,
	63–65,100–102,
	162,164,174,180

Radioimmunoassay	47,135
Viscosity	66,86,134
Precipitation and turbidity	56

studies in terms of mucus physiology must remain in doubt.

The most common method for quantitating mucus *in vivo* is the analysis of the quantity and spectrum of sugars from mucous glycoproteins in gastric juice (Table 5). Such an approach has serious shortcomings, however; it does not distinguish between polymeric undegraded glycoprotein characteristic of the gel and degraded glycoprotein produced by peptic erosion (2,3). Although a rise in the glycoprotein content of gastric juice could be caused by secretion, it could also be caused by increased erosion of the surface gel with or without a concomitant increased secretion. The gel on the surface could be either thicker or thinner, or unaltered in depth. These results are also subject to misinterpretation if the method used to measure mucous glycoprotein is interfered with by other molecules; for example, the different acidic proteoglycans of connective tissue between them contain all the sugars found in the mucous glycoproteins. In these analyses, the presence or absence of uronic acid in mucous secretions can provide a useful indication of proteoglycan contamination, because it is absent from mucous glycoproteins. Colorimetric estimations, particularly those involving concentrated sulfic acid for galactose or fucose, are notorious for interference from other sugars and protein. The most informative method for estimating the sugars of mucous

glycoproteins is by gas-liquid chromatography, where the entire spectrum of sugars is unambiguously obtained; but this method is time-consuming for a large number of samples. Two colorimetric methods for rapid estimation of glycoprotein are modifications of the PAS (112) and the Alcian blue (19) staining assays, which rely on the number of periodate oxidizable hydroxyl groups and the charge of the carbohydrate, respectively. With both these methods, it is necessary to use the purified glycoprotein as a standard and to eliminate interference from other periodate oxidizable or negatively charged molecules. Finally, when quantifying mucus, it is preferable to estimate more than one sugar, particularly with respect to sialic acid and fucose. These are found in the terminal position of the carbohydrate chains. The content of both can vary with the secretory state of the tissue (31), while sialic acid in particular can be readily removed by endogenous degradative enzymes (10).

The development of radioimmunoassays for mucous glycoproteins (47) provides a new and sensitive technique for estimating mucus. The use of antibodies offers a sensitive and specific method for both quantitative estimation and cellular localization (48,65,162). An antibody against human goblet cell mucin was found to cross-react with colonic mucus but only weakly with gastric mucous glycoproteins (135). The results show that there are fundamental similarities in the structure of glycoproteins from mucous secretions throughout the gastrointestinal tract and support the evidence from structural analysis and histological studies showing that gastric and small intestinal glycoproteins are different. The human goblet cell mucin antibody cross-reacts with intestinal glycoproteins from other species, namely, dog, monkey, and rabbit, but not with those from pig or rat. It is not yet clear what the antigenic determinants are on these glycoproteins, but they are independent of blood group activity; therefore, the antibodies are directed against other parts of the molecule than the terminal sugar residues. It is important to use pure glycoprotein to raise the antibody; if strongly noncovalently bound protein is present, this will also be antigenic.

Incorporation of radioactively labeled glycoprotein precursor has been used widely in biosynthetic studies on mucus *in vitro* and sometimes *in vivo*. Suitable precursors are radioactive sugars, $^{35}SO_4^{2-}$, or amino acids. Changes in the incorporation of such radioactivity should be measured in the isolated mucous glycoprotein and not the total within the mucosa where the radioactivity may be incorporated into proteoglycan, membrane glycoproteins, or glycolipids. An illustration of this pitfall relates to the interpretation of the increased incorporation of radioactive glucosamine into rat small intestinal mucosal tissue when treated with cortisol. This incorporation was found to be into certain membrane glycoproteins only, and incorporation into other glycoproteins was inhibited (42). Another pitfall with radioactive labeling of mucus is contamination by bacteria, which avidly incorporate the radioactive mucous precursors. Unless a strong antibiotic cocktail is included, most of the radioactivity incorporated into high molecular weight products by mucosal cells *in vitro* can be into bacterial products and not mucus (10).

A physical method for investigating changes in mucus is the measurement of its viscosity. Mucous viscosity is related to the gel-forming potential of the glycoprotein and is dependent on the concentration of undegraded glycoprotein present. Viscosity measurement has its difficulties; it is essential that it be related to the glycoprotein concentration because of the nonlinear relationship between viscosity and concentration (Fig. 5). A difference in viscosity between two samples may be due simply to a difference in glycoprotein concentration and not to a structural change. For example, an alteration to the rate of flow of any nonglycoprotein secretion would be sufficient to change the viscosity without any change in mucus content or structure. Viscosity should be expressed in terms of the concentration of the pure glycoprotein; this is illustrated in Fig. 5, where the viscosity at a given concentration of the soluble mucus, which contains 30 to 40% free protein, is much lower than for purified mucus, which contains about 5% free protein.

In the following sections, much of the work reviewed must be interpreted with caution in view of the limitations on the above methods. It is particularly important to remember that a change in the content of mucous glycoprotein in luminal juice could reflect secretion or erosion and on its own cannot be extrapolated to provide information about the mucous gel on the mucosal surface. For a more complete picture of the origin of mucous glycoprotein present in gastric juice, it is desirable to measure viscosity, glycoprotein concentration, and the ratio of undegraded to degraded glycoprotein present (86).

Physiological and Pharmacological Effects on Mucus Production

Mucus is produced throughout the length of the gastrointestinal tract by a variety of cell types: esophageal mucous glands, cardiac, fundic, and pyloric glands of the stomach, Brunner's glands of the duodenum, goblet cells of the small and large intestines, and superficial mucous cells found all through the tract (38,100). The control of mucus production by these cells can occur at two levels: (a) secretion of preformed mucus, and (b) mucus biosynthesis. In a normal mucus-secreting cell, one might expect these two processes to be interdependent, since an increase in secretion alone would soon exhaust the cell of mucus unless there was also an increase in its biosynthesis. However, stimulation of mucus secretion by excessive mechanical or chemical irritation might exceed the rate of biosynthesis and exhaust the mucus within the cells. This ultimately would cause a breakdown of the mucosal barrier (see Chapter 27 by Fromm). The production of a thick mucous secretion in response to acid was first observed by Ivy and Oyama (80) and has since been observed with a number of other chemical irritants, e.g., mustard oil and ethanol (30,39,43,57). Recent scanning electron microscopy studies of the anesthetized dog gastric mucosa by Zalewsky and Moody (180) have shown three mechanisms by which mucus is released: (a) a continuous exocytosis of a few granules at a time; (b) an explosive release of mucus by apical expulsion of the older cells in the interfoveolar area; and (c) the relatively rare event of cell exfoliation. The explosive release of mucus from mucosal cells in contact with irritants is in keeping with apical expulsion (87,180), which is maximal on gastric mucosa away from the foveolae; this is the site of maximal damage in gastric mucosal injury.

There is a large body of evidence that the output of mucus can be increased in the luminal juice by neural or hormonal stimulation. Stimulation of the splanchnic or vagus nerves or topical application of acetylcholine produces a copious gastric mucous gel in dogs (39,71, 74,83). Acetylcholine stimulated radioactive mucus release from rabbit and human colonic biopsies *in vitro* but did not affect the rate of glycoprotein biosynthesis

(109). Salivary mucus is stimulated by either sympathetic or parasympathetic stimulation. Two different glycoproteins or groups of related glycoproteins are formed, depending on which nerve is stimulated to evoke submaxillary secretion. Thus the ratio of sialic acid to fucose or hexosamines was higher and the size of the salivary glycoproteins smaller in secretion evoked by sympathetic than parasympathetic stimulation (31).

The two best documented hormonal stimulants of gastric mucus production are secretin and the prostaglandins. Secretin increases the sugars of mucous glycoproteins in gastric juice from humans (12), cats (169–171), and dogs (92) and also in Brunner canine pouch secretions (165). Secretin infusion produces a sharp rise in the viscosity of cat gastric juice. Recently, this has been shown to be associated with an increase in the native glycoprotein characteristic of the gel rather than its pepsin degraded subunit (86). Prostaglandins, which as judged visually cause an increased production of viscous mucus (19,33), produce a rise in the glycoprotein-bound sialic acid content of gastric washouts in man when given with pentagastrin (33,84). Prostaglandins also increase the soluble mucus in rat gastric juice, although no change in the glycoprotein content of the surface mucous gel was observed (19). A prostaglandin endoperoxide analog was shown to be more effective than the prostaglandin E_2 in stimulating an increase in glycoprotein-bound sialic acid from Heidenhain pouch dogs (167). These results, which suggest an increased mucus production by prostaglandins, are particularly interesting in view of their known cytoprotective effect and their stimulatory effect on bicarbonate secretion (see Chapter 20 by Flemström). Various other gastrointestinal hormones, including gastrin, CCK-PZ, and histamine, have been shown to increase the fucose and galactose content of gastric juice from cats prepared with fistulas or pouches (171,172), although there was no information on viscosity or on whether the glycoprotein was degraded and therefore the result of peptic erosion. Both 5-HT and carbachol increased mucus production by the rat colon, as measured by increased hexose content of the perfused lumen *in vivo* (18). Atropine abolished the action of carbachol, and application of either histamine or isoprenaline alone had no effect on the hexose content.

Several factors that decrease mucus production have been described. Any cytotoxic agents that reach the mucosal cells are to be expected to decrease mucus production. Decreased biosynthesis of mucus is caused by a number of antiinflammatory drugs (57,118,128). Salicylates decreased the amount of mucus produced in rat stomachs and in dog gastric pouches (120), as determined by staining and estimation of glycoprotein sugars in washouts. Salicylates also decreased glycoprotein biosynthesis *in vitro* in sheep colonic and human gastric mucosa measured by the incorporation of radioactive

precursors into the isolated mucous glycoproteins (88). Similar observations have been made by others (57,136) and include an *in vivo* study on explanted canine antrum (175) in which salicylate caused an initial loss of the adherent mucus followed by an increase in cell metabolism above normal to compensate for the original damage. Corticosteroids and ACTH decrease the amount of both stainable mucus in the mucosa and glycoprotein sugars in gastric juice (29,57,119). Glass and co-workers (57,102) have shown that there can be a biphasic response to corticosteroids in the dog stomach: an initial hyperplastic response and increased glycoprotein production, as measured by $^{35}SO_4^{2-}$ incorporation, followed by its impairment.

The antiulcer drug carbenoxolone, which increases the lifespan of epithelial cells in the mucosa (see Chapter 4 by Lipkin), increases the stainable gastric mucus present in human biopsies (164). Carbenoxolone has also been shown to increase the incorporation of bound radioactive glycoprotein sugars into whole rat gastric mucosa (129) and to raise the glycoprotein-bound sialic acid content of gastric washouts in humans (32). Other factors that stimulate mucus production include immunological effects where bovine serum albumin stimulated the release of intestinal goblet cell mucus in rats that have been previously immunized by oral administration of bovine albumin (95). The production of mucus can also be dependent on the nutritional state of the animal. Thus incorporation of radioactive precursors into isolated mucus-type glycoproteins is reduced in the intestines from vitamin A-deficient rats (28). Dibutyryl cyclic AMP and theophylline stimulate the production of radioactive colonic glycoprotein in mucosal organ cultures of rabbit colon (99).

Mucus in Pathological Conditions

Despite the possible importance of disorder of mucus in the etiology of gastrointestinal disease, particularly ulceration, little is known about how it is affected in disease states. Visible breakdown of the mucous gel layer clearly has taken place when erosion of the mucosal surface has occurred; it is not established, however, whether this was associated with an intrinsic weakness in the protective mucus in the first place. Comparisons have been made of the ratios of the glycoprotein sugars in gastric washouts from ulcer patients and control subjects (57,139,151). Although the results have been conflicting and often negative, in one investigation there was less glycoprotein-bound sialic acid in the gastric juice from ulcer patients compared with controls (32). In contrast, a study of gastric washouts, where the glycoprotein was purified by equilibrium density gradient centrifugation (140), showed an increase compared with control subjects in total mucous glycoprotein in the gastric juice from patients with gastric ulcer but not in gastric juice from those with duodenal ulcers. In both groups of patients, the ratio of the sugars compared with control subjects was the same.

A rise in the luminal glycoprotein sugars has been found with the development of erosions when experimental animals or humans are placed under stress (57). This rise has been explained by a breakdown of the mucosal barrier with a concomitant shedding of mucus and cells. For reasons that are discussed above, it is not apparent that much useful information about the role of mucus in ulceration will come from a study of the composition of the carbohydrate chains; it is more likely to come from a study of the polymeric structure and gel-forming potential of the mucus. A rise in the viscosity of mucus in the gastric washouts of patients with duodenal ulcer has been reported (134); but as the viscosity was not related to glycoprotein concentration, the results are not readily interpretable and could be due to differences in the volume of secretion affecting the concentration of glycoprotein or to changes in the concentration of protein contaminants.

There is histochemical and biochemical evidence for changes in the mucous glycoproteins associated with malignant mucosa or intestinalized gastric mucosa (57,91,100). Hakkinen and colleagues (64,65) have demonstrated antigenic differences between normal and carcinomatous tissues. Of the three antigens isolated from gastric juice, all of which were sulfated mucus-type glycoproteins, one (No) was present in gastric mucosa at all ages, while the other two (I and FSA) were characteristic of fetal, aging, and diseased mucosa only (63). A sulfated glycoprotein antigen with a high N-acetylgalactosamine ratio to other sugars has been isolated from gastric tumors (15). This high N-acetylgalactosamine content is indicative of short carbohydrate side chains, since this sugar is found only at either end of the chains in mucous glycoproteins. The antigen is associated with intestinal metaplasia in human gastric tissue and is also present in the normal goblet cells of the small and large intestine. Glycoproteins isolated from gastric juice of patients with intestinal metaplasia also show a rise in the molar ratio of N-acetylgalactosamine to other sugars (151). An increase in the sulfate and sialic acid content has been shown in the mucus glycoproteins isolated from neoplastic mucosa compared with those isolated from normal gastric mucosa (149). An apparent change in secretor status of patients with gastric carcinoma is further evidence for changes in the structure of the sugar chains of their mucous glycoproteins. In some cases where the host red cells were O, the gastric mucus indicated an A secretor, thus pointing to the expression of a new enzymic activity in the tumor cells (151). Histological studies show that a switch from sulfated mucins to sialomucins may be associated with colonic malignancy; this is accompanied by an increase in

the sialic acid content of the isolated mucus (37,38). The mucoprotein antigen isolated from the human colon, which is probably the major mucus secretory component of the large bowel, changes its chemical and immunological properties with neoplasia (58,59). There is a 40% by weight increase in aspartic acid and a corresponding decrease in threonine content of the glycoprotein from the neoplastic tissue, together with a lower density of carbohydrate chains per molecule.

THE FUTURE

A knowledge of the structure and properties of the soluble glycoproteins from mucus secretions is gradually being accumulated. Although the structure of the protein component of these glycoproteins and how this is related to the polymeric structure remains to be elucidated, the recent demonstration that pig gastric mucous glycoprotein contains a 70,000 MW protein joined by disulfide bridges to the glycoprotein subunits (130) is particularly interesting. Studies are now focusing on the properties of the intact mucous gels, which at present can only be explained in general terms. It is important to know the detailed chemical basis for the interactions involved in gel formation in order to interpret how gel structure may change under different conditions. Comparison of the properties of mucus secretions from different parts of the gastrointestinal tract may reveal changes in gel structure correlated with the changes in the constituent glycoproteins and how these are related to their different physiological functions. Accumulation of accurate data on the permeability of mucus to ions and other molecules is clearly important for elucidating its function and, in the case of the stomach and duodenum, for assessing the contribution of mucus in mucosal protection.

A most important requirement in the study of the physiology and pathophysiological significance of mucus is to bridge the gap that exists between the studies on isolated mucus and the studies on the surface mucous gel *in vivo*. There is no doubt about the importance of the dynamic balance *in vivo* between secretion of the mucous gel and its erosion by enzymic degradation, especially with respect to pepsin action in the stomach. Measurement of glycoprotein content alone in gastric juice has been shown to be insufficient for the study of changes in mucus secretion. Such studies should include some estimation of the extent of degradation of the glycoprotein. Increased mucus degradation could be as important as decreased secretion in the etiology of gastrointestinal disease. It is only when we can qualitate and quantitate the dynamic changes in the mucous gel covering defined areas of the mucosal surface *in vivo* and know the factors that control these that we will understand the physiology of gastrointestinal mucus.

REFERENCES

1. Allen, A. (1977): Structure and function in gastric mucus. In: *Mucus in Health and Disease,* edited by M. Elstein and D. V. Parke, pp. 275-299. Plenum Press, New York.
2. Allen, A. (1978): Structure of gastrointestinal mucus glycoproteins and the viscous and gel-forming properties of mucus. *Br. Med. Bull.,* 34:28-33.
3. Allen, A. (1979): Mucus and mucosal defence. In: *Peptic Ulcer Disease: An Update,* pp. 63-76. Biomedical Information Corporation, New York.
4. Allen, A., and Garner, A. (1980): Gastric mucus and bicarbonate secretion and their possible role in mucosal protection. *Gut,* 21:249-262.
5. Allen, A., Mantle, M., and Pearson, J. P. (1980): The polymeric structure and properties of mucus glycoproteins. In: *Perspectives in Cystic Fibrosis,* edited by J. Sturgess, pp. 102-112. Canadian Cystic Fibrosis Foundation, Toronto.
6. Allen, A., and Minnikin, S. M. (1975): The binding of the mucoprotein from gastric mucus to cells in tissue culture and the inhibition of cell adhesion. *J. Cell Sci.,* 17:617-631.
7. Allen, A., Pain, R. H., and Robson, T. (1976): Model for the structure of the gastric mucus gel. *Nature,* 264:88-89.
8. Allen, A., Pearson, J. P., and Venables, C. W. (1979): The glycoprotein from human gastric mucus gel and its breakdown by pepsin. *J. Physiol.,* 293:30P.
9. Allen, A., and Snary, D. (1972): The structure and function of gastric mucus. *Gut,* 13:666-672.
10. Allen, A., and Starkey, B. J. (1974): Neuraminidase in pig gastric mucus. *Biochim. Biophys. Acta,* 338:364-368.
11. Allen, R. H., and Mehlman, C. S. (1973): Isolation of gastric vitamin B_{12} binding proteins using affinity chromatography. Purification of properties of hog intrinsic factor and hog nonintrinsic factor. *J. Biol. Chem.,* 248:3660-3680.
12. Andre, C., Lambert, R., and Descos, F. (1972): Stimulation of gastric mucous secretions in man by secretin. *Digestion,* 7:284-293.
13. Andre, F., and Descos, F. (1975): Purification of human gastric glycoprotein and study of its carbohydrate components. *Biochim. Biophys. Acta,* 386:129-137.
14. Baenziger, J., and Kornfeld, S. (1974): Structure of the carbohydrate units of IgA immunoglobulin. *J. Biol. Chem.,* 249:7260-7269, 7270-7281.
15. Bara, J., Paul-Gardais, A., Loisillier, F., and Burton, P. (1978): Isolation of a sulphated glycopeptide antigen from human gastric tumors: its localisation in normal and cancerous gastrointestinal tissue. *Int. J. Can.,* 21:133-139.
16. Bella, A., and Kim, Y. S. (1972): Rat small intestinal mucin: isolation and characterisation of a water soluble mucin fraction. *Arch. Biochem. Biophys.,* 150:679-689.
17. Bella, A., and Kim, Y. S. (1973): Iron binding of gastric mucins. *Biochim. Biophys. Acta,* 304:580-585.
18. Black, J. W., Bradbury, J. E., and Wyllie, J. H. (1979): Stimulation of colonic mucus output in rat. *Br. J. Pharmacol.,* 66:456P.
19. Bolton, J. P., Palmer, D., and Cohen, M. M. (1978): Stimulation of mucus and nonparietal cell secretion by the E_2 prostaglandins. *Am. J. Dig. Dis.,* 23:359-364.
20. Carlson, D. M. (1968): Structures and immunochemical properties of oligosaccharides isolated from pig submaxillary mucus. *J. Biol. Chem.,* 243:616-626.
21. Carlson, D. M. (1977): Chemistry and biosynthesis of mucin glycoproteins. In: *Mucus in Health and Disease,* edited by M. Elstein and D. V. Parke, pp. 251-273. Plenum Press, New York.
22. Clamp, J. R. (1977): The relationship between secretory immunoglobulin A and mucus. *Trans. Biochem. Soc.,* 5:1579-1581.
23. Clamp, J. R. (1978): Chemical aspects of mucus. *Br. Med. Bull.,* 34:25-27.
24. Creeth, J. M. (1978): Constituents of mucus and their separation. *Br. Med. Bull.,* 34:17-24.
25. Creeth, J. M., and Denborough, M. A. (1970): The use of equilibrium density methods for the preparation and characterization of blood group specific glycoproteins. *Biochem. J.,* 117:879-891.
26. Davenport, H. W. (1967): Physiological structure of the gastric mucosa. In: *Handbook of Physiology, Alimentary Canal, Vol. II,* edited by C. F. Code, pp. 759-779. American Physiological Society, Washington, D.C.
27. Davis, P. S., Luke, C. G., and Deller, D. G. (1967): Gastric iron binding protein in iron chelation by gastric juice. *Nature (Lond.),* 214:1126.
28. DeLuca, L., Schumacher, M., and Wolf, G. (1970): Biosynthesis of a fucose-containing glycopeptide from rat small intestine in normal and vitamin A deficient conditions. *J. Biol. Chem.,* 245:4551-4558.
29. Desbaillets, L., and Menguy, R. (1967): Inhibition of gastric mucous secretion by ACTH. *Am. J. Dig. Dis.,* 12:583-588.
30. Dinoso, V. P., Ming, S., and Meniff, J. (1976): Ultrastructural changes of the canine gastric mucosa after topical application of graded concentrations of ethanol. *Dig. Dis.,* 21:626-632.
31. Dische, Z., Kahn, N., Rothschild, C., Danilchenko, A., Liebling, J., and Wang, S. C. (1970): Glycoproteins of submaxillary saliva of the cat: differences in composition produced by sympathetic and parasympathetic nerve stimulation. *J. Neurochem.,* 17:649-658.
32. Domschke, W., Domschke, S., Classen, M., and Demling, L. (1972): Some properties of mucus in patients with gastric ulcer. Effect of treatment with carbenoxolone sodium. *Scand. J. Gastroenterol.,* 7:647-651.
33. Domschke, W., Domschke, S., Hornig, D., and Demling, L. (1978): Prostaglandin-stimulated gastric mucus secretion in man. *Acta Hepatogastroenterol.,* 25:292-294.
34. Donald, A. S. R. (1973): The products of pronase digestion of purified blood group-specific glycoproteins. *Biochim. Biophys. Acta,* 317:420-436.
35. Dunstone, J. R., and Morgan, W. T. (1965): Further observations on the glycoproteins in human ovarian cyst fluids. *Biochim. Biophys. Acta,* 101:300-314.
36. Elstein, M., and Parke, D. V. (eds.) (1977): *Mucus in Health and Disease.* Plenum Press, New York.
37. Filipe, M. I. (1977): Mucin histochemistry in the detection of early malignancy in the colonic epithelium. In: *Mucus in Health and Disease,* edited by M. Elstein and D. V. Parke, pp. 413-422. Plenum Press, New York.
38. Filipe, M. I. (1979): Mucins in the human gastrointestinal epithelium: A review. *Invest. Cell Pathol.,* 2:195-216.
39. Florey, H. (1955): Mucin and the protection of the body. *Proc. R. Soc. Lond. [B],* 143:144-158.
40. Florey, H. (1962): The secretion and function of intestinal mucus. *Gastroenterology,* 42:326-329.
41. Forstner, G. G. (editor) (1977): *Mucus secretions and cystic fibrosis. Mod. Probl. Paediatr.,* 19:1-207.
42. Forstner, G., and Garland, G. (1975): The influence of hydrocortisone on the synthesis and turnover of microvillous membrane glycoproteins in suckling rat intestine. *Can. J. Biochem.,* 54:224-232.
43. Forstner, J. F. (1978): Intestinal mucins in health and disease. *Digestion,* 17:234-263.
44. Forstner, J. F., and Forstner, G. G. (1975): Calcium binding to intestinal goblet cell mucin. *Biochim. Biophys. Acta,* 386:283-292.
45. Forstner, J. F., Jabbal, I., and Forstner, G. G. (1973): Goblet cell mucin of rat small intestine. Chemical and physical characterization. *Can. J. Biochem.,* 51:1154-1166.
46. Forstner, J. F., Jabbal, I., Qureshi, R., Kells, D. I. C., and Forstner, G. G. (1979): Role of disulphide bonds in human intestinal mucin. *Biochem. J.,* 181:725-732.
47. Forstner, J. F., Ofosu, F., and Forstner, G. G. (1977): Radioimmunoassay of intestinal goblet cell mucin. *Anal. Biochem.,* 83:657-665.
48. Forstner, J., Taichman, N., Kalnins, V., and Forstner, G. G. (1973): Intestinal goblet cell mucus: isolation and identification by immunofluorescence of a goblet cell glycoprotein. *J. Cell Sci.,* 12:585-597.
49. Gibbons, R. A. (1972): Physico-chemical methods for determination of purity, molecular size and shape of glycoproteins. In: *Glycoproteins,* edited by A. Gottschalk, pp. 31-109. Elsevier, Amsterdam.

50. Gibbons, R. A. (1978): Mucus of the mammalian genital tract. *Br. Med. Bull.,* 34:34–38.

51. Gibbons, R. A., and Sellwood, R. (1972): The macromolecular biochemistry of cervical secretions. In: *Biology of the Cervix,* edited by R. J. Blandau and Moghissi, pp. 251–265. Chicago University Press, Chicago.

52. Gibbons, R. J., and Qureshi, J. V. (1978): Selective binding of blood group reactive salivary mucins by Streptococcus mutans and other oral organisms. *Infec. Immun.,* 22:665–671.

53. Glass, G. B. J. (1964): Proteins, mucosubstances and biologically active components of gastric secretion. *Clin. Chem.,* 7:235–322.

54. Glass, G. B. J. (1974): Gastrone. *Gastroenterology,* 67:740–741.

55. Glass, G. B. J., and Code, C. F. (1968): Gastrone, endogenous inhibitor of gastric secretion. *Prog. Gastroenterol.,* 1:221–247.

56. Glass, G. B. J., Mori, H., and Pamer, T. (1969): Measurement of sulphated and non-sulphated glycoproteins in human gastric juice under fasting conditions and following stimulation with histamine, pentagastrin and insulin. *Digestion,*

57. Glass, G. B. J., and Slomiany, B. L. (1977): Derangements in gastrointestinal injury and disease. In: *Mucus in Health and Disease,* edited by M. Elstein and D. V. Parke, pp. 311–347. Plenum Press, New York.

58. Gold, D. V., and Miller, F. (1974): Characterisation of human colonic mucoprotein antigen. *Immunochemistry,* 11:369–375.

59. Gold, D. V., and Miller, F. (1978): Comparison of human colonic mucoprotein antigen from normal and neoplastic mucosa. *Can. Res.,* 38:3204–3211.

60. Goodwin, S., and Watkins, W. M. (1974): The peptide moiety of blood group specific glycoproteins. *Eur. J. Biochem.,* 47:371–382.

61. Gottschalk, A. (editor) (1972): *Glycoproteins: Their Composition, Structure, and Function,* 2nd edition. Elsevier, Amsterdam.

62. Gottschalk, A., Bhargava, A. S., and Murty, V. L. N. (1972): Submaxillary gland glycoproteins. In: *Glycoproteins: Their Composition, Structure and Function,* 2nd edition, pp. 810–829. Elsevier, Amsterdam.

63. Hakkinen, I. P. T. (1974): FSA—Foetal sulphoglycoprotein antigen associated with gastric cancer. *Transplant. Rev.,* 20:61–76.

64. Hakkinen, I., Hartiala, H., and Tesho, T. (1965): The fractionation and characterization of the acid polysaccharides in human gastric juice. *Acta Chem. Scand.,* 19:797–806.

65. Hakkinen, I., Jarvi, O., and Gronroos, J. (1968): Sulphoglycoprotein antigens in the human alimentary canal and gastric cancer. An immunohistological study. *Int. J. Can.,* 3:582–592.

66. Hantiala, K., and Grossman, M. I. (1952): Studies on chemical and physical changes in duodenal mucus. *J. Biol. Chem.,* 195:251–256.

67. Heatley, N. G. (1959): Some experiments on partially purified gastrointestinal mucosubstance. *Gastroenterology,* 37:304–312.

68. Heatley, N. G. (1959): Mucosubstance as a barrier to diffusion. *Gastroenterology,* 37:313–318.

69. Hill, M. D., Reynolds, R. J., and Hill, R. L. (1977): Purification, composition, molecular weight, and subunit structure of ovine submaxillary mucin. *J. Biol. Chem.,* 252:3791–3795.

70. Holden, K. G., Yim, N. C. F., Griggs, L. J., and Weisback, J. A. (1971): Electrophoresis of mucous glycoproteins. II. Effect of physical disaggregation and disulphide bond cleavage. *Biochemistry,* 10:3110–3113.

71. Hollander, F. (1954): The two-component mucus barrier. *Arch. Intern. Med.,* 93:107–120.

72. Hollander, F. (1963): The electrolyte patterns of gastric secretions: its implication for cystic fibrosis. *Ann. N.Y. Acad. Sci.,* 106:298–310.

73. Horowitz, M. I. (1977): Purification of glycoproteins and criteria of purity. In: *The Glycoconjugates, Vol. I,* edited by M. I. Horowitz and W. Pigman, pp. 15–34. Academic Press, New York.

73a. Horowitz, M. I. (1977): Gastrointestinal glycoproteins: In: *The Glycoconjugates, Vol. I,* edited by M. I. Horowitz and W. Pigman, pp. 189–213. Academic Press, New York.

74. Horowitz, M. I., and Hollander, F. (1961): Evidence regarding the chemical complexity of acetylcholine stimulated gastric mucus. *Gastroenterology,* 40:785–793.

75. Horowitz, M. I., and Pigman, W. (eds.) (1977): *The Glycoconjugates, Vol. I.* Academic Press, New York.

76. Hoskins, L. C. (1978): Degradation of mucus glycoproteins in the gastrointestinal tract. In: *The Glycoconjugates, Vol. II,* edited by M. I. Horowitz and W. Pigman, pp. 235–250. Academic Press, New York.

77. Hoskins, L. C., and Boulding, E. T. (1976): Degradation of blood group antigens in human colon ecosystems. I. *In vitro* production of ABH blood group-degrading enzymes by enteric bacteria. *J. Clin. Invest.,* 57:63–73.

78. Hough, L., and Jones, J. V. S. (1972): Human gastric mucosa. Part I. The preparation of a glycopolypeptide and some aspects of its structure. *Carbohydr. Res.,* 23:1–16.

79. Inoue, S., and Yosizawa, Z. (1966): Purification and properties of sulphated sialopolysaccharides isolated from pig colonic mucosa. *Arch. Biochem. Biophys.,* 117:257–265.

80. Ivy, A. C., and Oyama, Y. (1921): Studies on the secretion of the pars pylorica gastri. *Am. J. Physiol.,* 57:51–60.

81. Jabbal, I., Forstner, G., Forstner, J. F., and Kells, D. I. C. (1975): Sedimentation velocity studies on microgram quantities of rat intestinal goblet cell mucin. *Anal. Biochem.,* 69:558–571.

82. Jabbal, I., Kells, D. I. C., Forstner, G., and Forstner, J. F. (1976): Human intestinal goblet cell mucin. *Can. J. Biochem.,* 54:707–716.

83. Jarowitz, H. D., and Hollander, F. (1954): Viscosity of cell-free canine gastric mucus. *Gastroenterology,* 26:582–594.

84. Johansson, C., and Kollberg, B. (1979): Stimulation by intragastrically administered E_2 prostaglandins of human gastric mucus output. *Eur. J. Clin. Invest.,* 9:229–232.

85. Kabat, A. (1956): *Blood Group Substances.* Academic Press, New York.

86. Kaura, R., Allen, A., and Hirst, B. H. (1980): Mucus in the gastric juice of cats during pentagastrin and secretin infusions. The viscosity in relation to glycoprotein structure and concentration. *Biochem. Soc. Trans.,* 8:52–53.

87. Kelly, D. G., Code, C. F., Lechago, J., Bugajski, J., and Schelgel, J. F. (1979): Physiological and morphological characteristics of progressive disruption of the canine gastric mucosal barrier. *Am. J. Dig. Dis.,* 24:424–441.

88. Kent, P. W., and Allen, A. (1967): The biosynthesis of intestinal mucins: Effect of salicylate on glycoprotein biosynthesis by sheep colonic and human gastric mucosal tissues *in vitro.* *Biochem. J.,* 106:645–658.

89. Kent, P. W., and Marsden, J. C. (1963): A sulphated sialoprotein from sheep colonic mucin. *Biochem. J.,* 87:38–39P.

90. Kim, Y. S., and Horowitz, M. I. (1971): Solubilisation and chemical and immunological characterisation of sparingly soluble canine gastric mucin. *Biochim. Biophys. Acta,* 234:686–701.

91. Kimoto, E., Kuramari, T., Masuda, H., and Takeughi, M. (1968): Isolation and characterization of a glycopeptide from mucinous carcinoma of human stomach. *Biochem. J.,* 63:542–549.

92. Kowalewski, K., Pachkowski, T., and Kolodej, A. (1979): Effect of secretin on mucinous secretion by the isolated canine stomach perfused extracorporeally. *Pharmacology,* 16:78–82.

93. Kowalewski, K., Pachkowski, T., and Secord, D. C. (1976): Mucinous secretion from canine Heidenhain pouch after stimulation with food, pentagastrin and histamine. *Eur. Surg. Res.,* 8:635–544.

94. Kowalewski, K., Pachkowski, T., and Secord, D. C. (1977): Gastric mucinous secretion under various conditions of stimulation in hypothyroid dogs. *Pharmacology,* 15:348–358.

95. Lake, A. H., Black, K. J., Neutra, M. R., and Walker, A. W. (1979): Intestinal goblet cell mucus release. *In vivo* stimulation by antigen in the immunized rat. *J. Immunol.,* 122:834–837.

96. Lambert, R., and Andre, C. (1972): Sulphated muco-substances and gastric disease. *Digestion,* 5:116–122.

97. Lambert, R., Andre, C., and Bernard, A. (1971): Origin of sulphated glycoproteins in human gastric secretions. *Digestion,* 4:234–249.

98. Lambert, R., Andre, C., Descos, F. M., and Andre, F. (1973): Influence of a gastric tube on salivary and pharyngeal mucous secretions in man. *Digestion,* 8:227–238.

99. LaMont, T., and Ventola, A. (1977): Stimulation of colonic glycoprotein synthesis by dibutyryl cyclic AMP and theophylline. *Gastroenterology,* 72:82–86.

100. Lev, R. (1970): The histochemistry of mucus producing cells in normal and diseased gastrointestinal mucosa. *Prog. Gastroenterol.,* 2:13–41.

101. Lev, R. (1977): Histochemistry. In: *The Glycoconjugates, Vol. I,* edited by M. I. Horowitz and W. Pigman, pp. 35–48. Academic Press, New York.

102. Lev, R., Siegal, H. I., and Glass, G. B. J. (1970): Histochemical studies of the mucosubstances in the canine stomach. III. The effects of corticosteroids. *Gastroenterology,* 58:495–507.

103. Levine, M. J., Herzberg, M. C., Levine, M. S., Ellison, G. A., Stinson, M. W., Li, H. C., and Van Dyke, T. (1978): Specificity of salivary bacterial interactions: Role of terminal sialic acid residues in the interaction of salivary glycoproteins with Streptococcus sanguis and Streptococcus mutans. *Infect. Immun.,* 19:107–115.

104. Ley, R., Bremen, J., Verbustel, S., Woussen-Colle, M. C., and DeGraff, J. (1969): Physiology of the secretion of acid, pepsin sulphated polysaccharides and glycoproteins by the dog fundic mucosa. *Digestion,* 2:113–123.

105. List, S. J., Findlay, B. P., Forstner, G. G., and Forstner, J. F. (1978): Enhancement of the viscosity of mucin by serum albumin. *Biochem. J.,* 175:565–571.

106. Litt, M., Wolf, D. P., and Khan, M. A. (1977): Functional aspects of mucus rheology. In: *Mucus in Health and Disease,* edited by M. Elstein and D. V. Parke, pp. 191–201. Plenum Press, New York.

107. Lloyd, K. O., and Kabat, E. A. (1968): Immunochemical studies on blood groups, XLI. Proposed structures for the carbohydrate portions of blood group ABH, Lewis[a] and Lewis[b] substances. *Proc. Natl. Acad. Sci. USA,* 61:1407–1477.

108. Lombart, C. G., and Winzler, R. J. (1974): Isolation and characterisation of oligosaccharides from canine submaxillary mucin. *Eur. J. Biochem.,* 49:77–86.

109. MacDermott, R. P., Donaldson, R. M., and Trier, J. S. (1974): Glycoprotein synthesis and secretion by mucosal biopsies of rabbit colon and human rectum. *J. Clin. Invest.,* 54:545–554.

110. Machado, G., Clamp, J. R., and Read, A. E. (1977): Carbohydrate content of endoscopic gastric biopsies in carcinoma of the stomach. *Gut,* 18:670–672.

111. Mandel, I. D. (1977): Human submaxillary, sublingual and parotid glycoproteins and enamel pellicle. In: *The Glycoconjugates, Vol. I,* edited by M. I. Horowitz and W. Pigman, pp. 153–179. Academic Press, New York.

112. Mantle, M., and Allen, A. (1978): A colorimetric assay for glycoproteins based on the periodic acid/Schiff stain. *Biochem. Soc. Trans.,* 6:607–609.

113. Mantle, M., and Allen, A. (1981): Isolation and characterisation of the native glycoprotein from pig small intestine. Polymeric structure of pig small intestinal mucus glycoprotein. *Biochem. J. (in press).*

114. Marcus, D. M. (1969): The ABO and Lewis blood-group system. *N. Engl. J. Med.,* 280:994–1006.

115. Marshall, T., and Allen, A. (1978): Isolation and characterisation of the high molecular weight glycoproteins from pig colonic mucus. *Biochem. J.,* 173:569–578.

116. Martin, F., Mathian, R., Berard, A., and Lambert, R. (1969): Sulphated glycoproteins in human salivary and gastric secretions. *Digestion,* 2:103–112.

117. Martin, G. P., Marriott, C., and Kellaway, I. W. (1978): Direct effect of bile salts and phospholipids on the physical properties of mucus. *Gut,* 19:103–107.

118. Menguy, R. (1969): Gastric mucus and the gastric mucous barrier. *Am. J. Surg.,* 117:806–812.

119. Menguy, R., and Masters, Y. F. (1963): Effect of cortisone on mucoprotein secretion by gastric antrum of dogs: pathogenesis of steroid ulcer. *Surgery,* 54:19–28.

120. Menguy, R., and Masters, Y. F. (1965): The effects of aspirin on gastric mucus secretion. *Surg. Gynaecol. Obstet.,* 92:1–7.

121. Meyer, K., Smyth, E. M., and Palmer, J. (1937): On glycoproteins in polysaccharides from pig gastric mucosa. *J. Biol. Chem.,* 119:73–84.

122. Morris, E. R., and Rees, D. A. (1978): Principles of biopolymer gelation. *Br. Med. Bull.,* 34:49–53.

123. Murty, V. L., Downs, F. J., and Pigman, W. (1978): Rat colonic mucus glycoprotein. *Carbohydr. Res.,* 61:139–145.

124. Munabata, H., and Yosizawa, Z. (1978): Isolation and characterization of a sulphated glycoprotein from rabbit small intestine. *J. Biochem. Tokyo,* 24:1587–1592.

125. Odeblad, E. (1977): Physical properties of cervical mucus. In: *Mucus in Health and Disease,* edited by M. Elstein and D. V. Parke, pp. 217–225. Plenum Press, New York.

126. Oemrawsingh, I., and Roukema, P. A. (1974): Isolation, purification and chemical characterisation of mucins from human submandibular glands. *Arch. Oral Biol.,* 19:615–624.

127. Pamer, T., Jerzy-Glass, G. B., and Horowitz, M. I. (1968): Purification and characterisation of sulphate glycoproteins and hyaluronidase resistant mucopolysaccharides from dog gastric mucosa. *Biochemistry,* 7:3812–3829.

128. Parke, D. V. (1978): Pharmacology of mucus. *Br. Med. Bull.,* 34:89–94.

129. Parke, D. V., and Symons, A. M. (1977): The biochemical pharmacology of mucus. In: *Mucus in Health and Disease,* edited by M. Elstein and D. V. Parke, pp. 423–441. Plenum Press, New York.

130. Pearson, J. P., and Allen, A. (1980): A protein, 70,000 molecular weight, is joined by disulphide bridges to pig gastric mucus glycoprotein. *Trans. Biochem. Soc.,* 8:388–389.

131. Pearson, J. P., Allen, A., and Venables, C. W. (1980): Gastric mucus: isolation and polymeric structure of the undegraded glycoprotein: its breakdown by pepsin. *Gastroenterology,* 78:709–715.

132. Pigman, W. (1977): Submandibular and sublingual glycoproteins. In: *The Glycoconjugates, Vol. I,* edited by M. I. Horowitz and W. Pigman, pp. 137–152. Academic Press, New York.

133. Pfeil, R., and Schauer, R. (1979): Isolation of new acyl neuraminic acids from bovine submandibular glands. In: *The Glycoconjugates,* edited by R. Schauer, P. Boer, E. Buddecke, M. F. Kramer, J. F. G. Vliegenthart, and H. Wiegandt, pp. 44–45. Georg Thieme, Stuttgart.

134. Pringle, R. (1977): Gastric mucus, viscosity and peptic ulcer. In: *Mucus in Health and Disease,* edited by M. Elstein and D. V. Parke, pp. 227–238.

135. Qureshi, R., Forstner, G. C., and Forstner, J. F. (1979): Radioimmunoassay of human intestinal goblet cell mucin. *J. Clin. Invest.,* 64:1149–1156.

136. Rainsford, K. D. (1978): The effects of aspirin and other non-steroid anti-inflammatory/analgesic drugs on gastrointestinal mucus glycoprotein biosynthesis *in vivo*: Relationship to ulcerogenic actions. *Biochem. Pharmacol.,* 27:877–885.

137. Rees, D. A. (1972): Shapely polysaccharides. *Biochem. J.,* 126:257–273.

138. Roberts, G. P. (1978): Chemical aspects of respiratory mucus. *Br. Med. Bull.,* 34:39–41.

139. Roberts, S. H., Hefferman, C., and Douglas, A. P. (1975): The sialic acid and carbohydrate content and the synthesis of glycoprotein from radioactive precursors by tissues of the normal and diseased upper intestinal tract. *Clin. Chim. Acta,* 63:121–128.

140. Roberts-Thompson, J. C., Clarke, A. E., Maritz, V. M., and Denborough, M. A. (1975): Gastric glycoproteins in chronic peptic ulcer. *Aust. N.Z. J. Med.,* 5:507–514.

141. Robson, T., Allen, A., and Pain, R. H. (1975): Non-covalent forces hold glycoprotein molecules together in mucus gel. *Biochem. Soc. Trans.,* 3:1105–1107.

142. Rudzki, Z., and Della, D. J. (1973): The iron binding glycoprotein of human gastric juice. *Digestion,* 8:35–52.

143. Scawen, M., and Allen, A. (1977): The action of proteolytic enzymes on the glycoprotein from pig gastric mucus. *Biochem. J.,* 163:363–368.

144. Schacter, H. (1978): Glycoprotein biosynthesis. In: *The Glycoconjugates, Vol. II,* edited by M. I. Horowitz and W. Pigman, pp. 87–181. Academic Press, New York.

145. Schacter, H., and Tilley, C. A. (1978): The biosynthesis of human blood group substances. In: *International Review of Biochemistry, Biochemistry of Carbohydrates II,* edited by D. J. Manners, vol. 16, pp. 210–246. University Park Press, Baltimore.

146. Schrager, J. (1969): The composition and some structural features of the principal gastric glycoprotein. *Digestion,* 2:73–89.

147. Schrager, J., and Oates, M. D. G. (1970): Further observations on the principle glycoprotein of the gastric secretion. *Digestion,* 3:231–242.

148. Schrager, J., and Oates, M. D. G. (1971): The isolation and partial characterisation of the principal gastric glycoprotein of "visible mucus." *Digestion,* 4:1–12.

149. Schrager, J., and Oates, M. D. G. (1973): A comparative study of the major glycoproteins isolated from normal and neoplastic gastric mucosa. *Gut,* 14:324–329.

150. Schrager, J., and Oates, M. D. G. (1974): The isolation and partial characterization of a glycoprotein isolated from human gastric aspirates and from extracts of gastric mucosa. *Biochim. Biophys. Acta,* 372:183–195.

151. Schrager, J., and Oates, M. D. G. (1978): Human gastrointestinal mucus in disease states. *Br. Med. Bull.,* 34:79–82.

152. Sheffner, A. L. (1963): The reduction *in vitro* in viscosity of mucoprotein solutions by a new mucolytic agent, Nacetylcysteine. *Ann. N.Y. Acad. Sci.,* 106:298–309.

153. Shora, W., Forstner, G. G., and Forstner, J. F. (1975): Stimulation of proteolytic digestion by intestinal goblet cell mucus. *Gastroenterology,* 68:470–479.

154. Silberberg, A, Meyer, F. A., Gilboa, A., and Gelman, R. A. (1977): Function and properties of epithelial mucus. In: *Mucus in Health and Disease,* edited by M. Elstein and D. V. Parke, pp. 171–180. Plenum Press, New York.

155. Slomiany, B. L., and Meyer, K. (1972): Isolation and structural studies of sulphated glycoproteins of hog gastric mucosa. *J. Biol. Chem.,* 247:5062–5070.

156. Slomiany, A., Slomiany, B. L., and Glass, G. B. J. (1978): Lipid composition of the gastric mucous barrier in the rat. *J. Biol. Chem.,* 253:3785–3791.

157. Snary, D., and Allen, A. (1971): Studies on gastric mucoproteins. The isolation and characterisation of the mucoprotein of the water soluble mucus from pig cardiac gastric mucosa. *Biochem. J.,* 123:845–853.

158. Snary, D., and Allen, A. (1972): Studies on gastric mucoproteins: The production of radioactive mucoproteins by pig gastric mucosal scrapings *in vitro. Biochem. J.,* 127:577–587.

159. Snary, D., Allen, A., and Pain, R. H. (1970): Structural studies on gastric mucoproteins. Lowering of molecular weight after reduction with 2-mercaptoethanol. *Biochem. Biophys. Res. Commun.,* 40:844–851.

160. Snary, D., Allen, A., and Pain, R. H. (1971): The structure of pig gastric mucus. Conformational transitions induced by salt. *Eur. J. Biochem.,* 24:183–189.

161. Snary, D., Allen, A., and Pain, R. H. (1974): Conformational changes in gastric mucoproteins induced by caesium chloride and guanidinium chloride. *Biochem. J.,* 141:641–646.

162. Spree-Brand, R., Strous, G., and Kramer, M. F. (1979): Immunocytochemical characterisation of mucous glycoproteins in the rat stomach. In: *Glycoconjugates,* edited by R. Schauer, pp. 187–188. George Thieme, Stuttgart.

163. Starkey, B. J., Snary, D., and Allen, A. (1974): Characterisation of gastric mucoproteins isolated by equilibrium density gradient centrifugation in caesium chloride. *Biochem. J.,* 141:633–639.

164. Steer, H. W., and Colin-Jones, D. G. (1975): Mucosal changes in gastric ulceration and their response to carbenoxolone sodium. *Gut,* 16:590–597.

165. Stening, G. F., and Grossman, M. I. (1969): Hormonal control of Brunner's gland. *Gastroenterology,* 56:1047–1052.

166. Strombeck, D. R., and Harrold, D. (1974): Binding of cholera toxin to mucins and inhibition by gastric mucin. *Infect. Immun.,* 10:1266–1272.

167. Tao, P., Scruggs, W., and Wilson, D. E. (1979): The effects of a prostaglandin endoperoxide analogue on canine gastric acid and mucous secretion. *Am. J. Dig. Dis.,* 24:449–454.

168. Tomasi, T. B., and Bienenstock, J. (1968): Secretory immunoglobulins. *Adv. Immunol.,* 9:1–96.

169. Vagne, M. (1974): Dose-response curve to secretin on gastric mucus secretion in conscious cats. *Digestion,* 10:402–412.

170. Vagne, M., and Fargier, M. (1973): Effect of pentagastrin and secretin on gastric mucus secretion in conscious cats. *Gastroenterology,* 65:757–763.

171. Vagne, M., and Perret, G. (1976): Effect of duodenal acidification on gastric mucus and acid secretion in conscious cats. *Digestion,* 14:332–341.

172. Vagne, M., and Perret, G. (1976): Regulation of gastric mucus secretion. *Scand. J. Gastroenterol. [Suppl.],* 42:63–74.

173. Van Huis, G. A., Smits, H. L., and Kramer, M. F. (1979): Glycoprotein synthesis in various mucus cells of rat stomach during vascular perfusion. In: *The Glycoconjugates,* edited by R. Schauer, P. Boer, E. Buddecke, M. F. Kramer, J. F. G. Vliegenthart, and H. Wiegandt, pp. 526–527. Georg Thieme, Stuttgart.

174. Veh, R. W., Cornfeld, A. P., Schauer, R., and Andres, K. H. (1979): The bovine submandibular gland. 1. Morphological and morphometric results. 2. Histochemical and biochemical results. In: *The Glycoconjugates,* edited by R. Schauer, P. Boer, E. Buddecke, M. F. Kramer, J. F. G. Vliegenthart, and H. Wiegandt, pp. 191–194. Georg Thieme, Stuttgart.

175. Waldron-Edward, D. (1977): The turnover of mucin glycoprotein in the stomach. In: *Mucus in Health and Disease,* edited by M. Elstein and D. V. Parke, pp. 301–308. Plenum Press, New York.

176. Waldron-Edward, D., and Skoryna, S. C. (1970): Studies on human gastric gel mucin. *Gastroenterology,* 59:671–682.

177. Watkins, W. M. (1966): Blood group substances. *Science,* 152:172–181.

178. Watkins, W. M. (1974): Genetic regulation of the structure of blood group specific glycoproteins. *Biochem. Soc. Symp.,* 40:125–146.

179. Williams, S. E., and Turnberg, L. A. (1979): Studies of the "protective" properties of gastric mucus. Evidence for mucus bicarbonate barrier. *Gut,* 20:A922–923.

180. Zalewsky, C. A., and Moody, F. G. (1979): Mechanisms of mucus release in exposed canine gastric mucosa. *Gastroenterology,* 77:719–729.

Physiology of the Gastrointestinal Tract, edited by
Leonard R. Johnson. Raven Press, New York © 1981.

Chapter 22

Intrinsic Factor and the Transport of Cobalamin

Robert M. Donaldson, Jr.

HISTORICAL CONSIDERATIONS

Only with precise knowledge of what happens normally can we understand disease. That is what is generally taught, but more often than not the reverse is true: observations about disease lead to the first real insights into normal events. No better example can be found than the physiology of vitamin B_{12} or, as it is now called, cobalamin. As is apparent throughout this chapter, most of what we know about the normal absorption of cobalamin originated from investigations in patients unable to assimilate the vitamin. Indeed, one might justifiably wonder how long it would have taken to discover the existence of cobalamin had it not been for a disease, pernicious anemia.

Although clearly described by Addison in 1855 (2), this usually fatal anemia lacked any effective treatment until 1926 when Minot and Murphy (97) documented striking clinical and hematologic improvement in 45 patients who ate large amounts of liver. Reticulocyte counts regularly and dramatically increased in these patients within 10 days after they began to eat at least 120 to 240 g liver daily; equal amounts of chopped beef had no such effect. This objective demonstration soon led to the preparation of injectable liver extracts capable of inducing reticulocytosis and maintaining patients in hematologic remission. Extracts of increasing purity were subsequently obtained. In 1948, two laboratories (113,128) successfully isolated in crystalline form the active principle in liver known as vitamin B_{12}. The pure substance that was first obtained proved to be cyanocobalamin.

Long before Minot and Murphy reported their cure for pernicious anemia, the stomachs of patients dying with the disease were known to be atrophied and incapable of digesting hard-boiled egg white. Moreover, by 1921, gastric secretory tests had unequivocally confirmed the uniform failure of living patients to secrete hydrochloric acid. This achlorhydria was observed in some patients before actual anemia developed; it persisted long after liver extract had corrected all other manifestations of pernicious anemia. These clinical observations led Castle (27) to suppose that impaired gastric function was somehow responsible for the disease, a concept he systematically tested in 1929. Using patients with untreated pernicious anemia as their own controls, Castle found that neither 200 g beef fed daily nor 150 ml normal human gastric juice administered every day by stomach tube produced a reticulocyte response. Yet simultaneous administration of both beef and gastric juice regularly caused reticulocytosis as brisk as that induced by liver (Fig. 1). Castle explained these results by proposing that an "intrinsic factor" normally present in gastric juice reacted with an "extrinsic factor" in beef to form a "hemopoietic factor" which is stored in the liver. Patients with pernicious anemia, according to this hypothesis, could not form the hemopoietic factor because their atrophied stomachs did not produce the necessary intrinsic factor.

Although this hypothesis explained all previous clinical and experimental observations in patients with pernicious anemia, Castle points out in his detailed historic account (28) that "the natural supposition that the gastric intrinsic factor was an enzyme could not be sub-

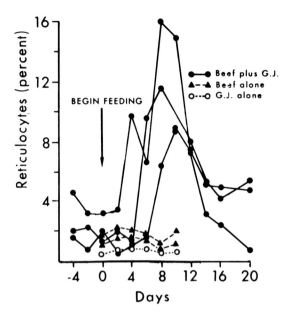

FIG. 1. Reticulocyte response of three pernicious anemia patients fed beef, gastric juice (G.J.) and beef plus gastric juice. [Drawn from tabular data reported by Castle (27).]

stantiated." Moreover, normal human gastric juice was found to potentiate the hemopoietic activity of small amounts of orally administered liver extract itself (111), an observation to which little attention was paid but which made Castle's original formulation seem untenable. Only when isotopically labeled cyanocobalamin became available in 1950 was it possible to understand fully the role of Castle's intrinsic factor. Fecal (60) and urinary (121) excretion tests of the absorption of radioactive cyanocobalamin soon established that patients with pernicious anemia required intrinsic factor to assimilate effectively the tiny quantities of cobalamin present, for example, in chopped beef. How then did Minot and Murphy cure pernicious anemia when they fed 120 to 240 g liver each day without also administering normal gastric juice? The answer lies in the large amount of cobalamin present in liver. Minot and Murphy produced a hematologic response because intrinsic factor is not needed for nonspecific diffusion of the vitamin across mucosal membranes. This process, although inefficient, will nevertheless permit patients with pernicious anemia to assimilate therapeutic amounts (1 to 2 μg) of cobalamin from the 100 to 200 μg present in the quantities of liver Minot and Murphy fed their patients.

Thus it was objective studies in patients with pernicious anemia that first brought to light a substance essential for normal viability of mammalian cells and called attention to a previously unknown normal function of the stomach. Following these germinal observations by Minot and Murphy and by Castle, clinical investigations contributed substantially to the present understanding of normal cobalamin absorption and transport. Studies in patients have not only localized the site of intrinsic factor production but have also substantiated the presence of two distinct functional sites on the intrinsic factor molecule, have led to the discovery of ileal membrane receptors for intrinsic factor-bound cobalamin, have pointed out a role for the pancreas as well as the stomach in normal cobalamin absorption, and have focused attention on the involvement of cobalamin-binding proteins other than intrinsic factor in normal transport of the vitamin (38).

COBALAMIN

Although the hemopoietic factor purified from liver extracts was first identified as cyanocobalamin (113), it is now clear that this compound, although remarkably stable, is in fact an artifact that results from isolation procedures. If present at all in nature, cyanocobalamin occurs only in trace amounts. In mammalian tissues, the vitamin exists largely as hydroxycobalamin, methylcobalamin, and adenosylcobalamin. Since all of these compounds have the biologic activities formerly attributed to vitamin B$_{12}$, it is now recommended (69) that the general term for the vitamin should be cobalamin, except when a specific compound is meant. The term vitamin B$_{12}$, if used at all, should refer only to cyanocobalamin.

Figure 2 illustrates the structure of adenosylcobalamin. A single cobalt atom in the nucleus of the molecule is coordinated in the center of a planar corrin ring by the nitrogens of the four pyrroline rings. The Co-α ligand lies below the planar ring. In the case of all cobalamins, this ligand consists of dimethylbenzimidazole linked to a ribose phosphate, which in turn is linked to the D-pyrroline ring by an amino alcohol. The Co-β ligand, shown in Fig. 2 as 5'-deoxyadenosine, can vary markedly without affecting binding to proteins or biologic activity; but even slight changes in either the corrin ring or the Co-α ligand results in profound changes in biologic properties and in protein binding (52,63,94).

Like the formation of heme, the biosynthesis of cobalamin (49) begins with d-aminolevulinic acid. Unlike heme, however, cobalamin cannot be synthesized by mammalian tissues but only by microorganisms. A wide variety of bacteria and protozoa are capable of *de novo* production of cobalamin, and microbial synthesis of the vitamin serves as the ultimate source for the mammalian organism. In addition to synthesizing cobalamin, these microorganisms produce a large number of related cobalamin analogs which cannot sustain the growth of cobalamin-dependent microbial mutants, substitute for the vitamin in cobalamin-dependent enzyme reactions, or correct the clinical manifestations of cobalamin deficiency. Such inactive analogs include (a) cobinamide, which consists only of the corrin ring with its amide side

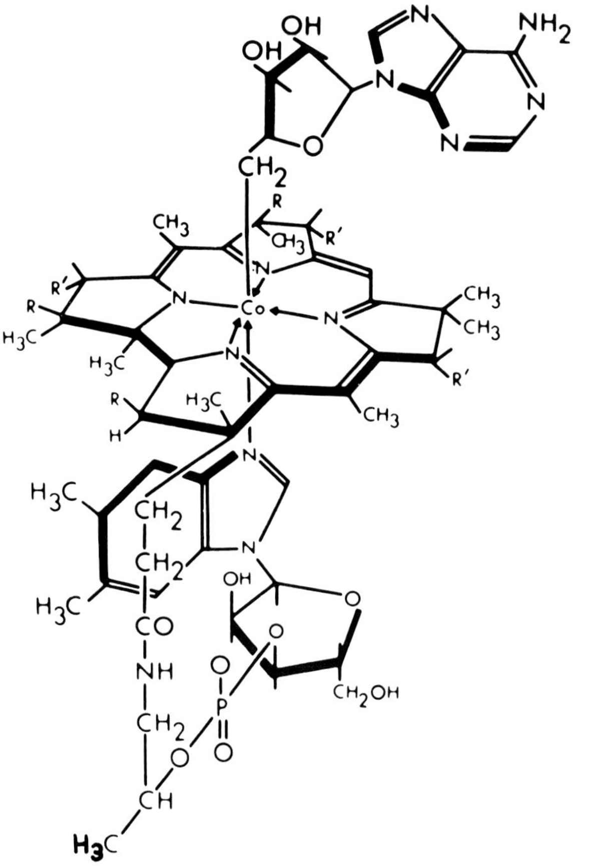

FIG. 2. Adenosylcobalamin. R, CH_2CONH_2; R^1, $CH_2CH_2CONH_2$.

chains but without the Co-α-linked base, (b) cobamides, in which benzimidazole, adenine, or other bases substitute for dimethylbenzimidazole, and (c) a variety of other corrinoids (66). To date, there is no evidence that mammalian cells can synthesize cobalamin or any of its analogs.

Mammalian tissues are capable of efficiently converting hydroxycobalamin to the coenzymes methylcobalamin and adenosylcobalamin. These conversions require sequential reduction of trivalent cobalt, Co(111), to divalent Co(11) and then to monovalent Co(1) by two apparently distinct reductase systems. Although the intracellular site for methylation of hydroxyco(1)balamin remains uncertain, there is some evidence (92,98) that a mitochondrial enzyme system is responsible for adenosylation. In any event, adenosylcobalamin functions as the coenzyme for the mitochondrial apoenzyme methylmalonyl CoA reductase, which is responsible for the cobalamin-dependent conversion of methylmalonate to succinate. Methylcobalamin, on the other hand, serves as the coenzyme for methyltetrahydrofolate homocysteine methyltransferase, a cytoplasmic apoenzyme that transfers a methyl group from N^5-methyltetrahydrofolate to homocysteine and thus converts homocysteine to methionine.

The conversion of methylmalonate to succinate re-

quires adenosylcobalamin, and the formation of methionine from homocysteine requires methylcobalamin. These are the only two unequivocally established cobalamin-dependent reactions in mammalian cell metabolism, although additional cobalamin-mediated events are known to occur in microorganisms. In keeping with these two cobalamin-dependent conversions, methylmalonic and homocysteinuria occur frequently in patients who are deficient in the vitamin or who suffer from an inherited disorder of cobalamin metabolism. Nevertheless, there is no adequate explanation for the absolute dependence of the mammalian organism on the vitamin for normal cellular replication and survival; nor do we understand the basis for the neurologic defects and megaloblastic anemia that characterize clinical cobalamin deficiency (13,104).

Although the vitamin is crucial for tissue viability, the mammalian organism does not effectively assimilate cobalamin by any simple passive process. As is evident from Fig. 2, cobalamin is a relatively large molecule, with a molecular weight of 1,355 daltons and a radius that far exceeds the "effective pore size" of intestinal absorptive membranes (52). Moreover, this large molecule possesses several highly polar groups, including the six amide groups on the side chains of the corrin ring, the phosphate moiety, and the hydroxyl groups of the ribose and amino alcohol constituents. These hydrophilic groups result in a substance that is highly soluble in water and virtually insoluble in most organic solvents. It is not surprising that this bulky, polar, water-soluble, lipid-insoluble molecule does not readily pass through the lipid bilayer of biologic membranes and, therefore, requires highly specialized membrane transport mechanisms if it is to be efficiently assimilated and used by the mammalian host. Moreover, these membrane transport processes not only must be capable of identifying and extracting the tiny quantities (10 to 15 μg/day for humans) of cobalamin available in the diet but also must be sufficiently specific to distinguish cobalamin from structurally similar but inactive and possibly harmful cobalamin analogs.

THE COBALAMIN-BINDING TRANSPORT PROTEINS

To meet these imposing requirements for its efficient absorption and transport, the cobalamin molecule binds with high affinity to three distinct transport proteins: intrinsic factor, transcobalamin II, and the R proteins (Table 1). Intrinsic factor is secreted by the stomach, while transcobalamin II is present in plasma. The R proteins are a family of glycoproteins found in plasma, granulocytes, and several glandular secretions. These binders were originally called R proteins because of their rapid migration during electrophoresis (52). Largely as a consequence of the work of Allen (3) and co-work-

TABLE 1. *Characteristics of human cobalamin binding proteins*[a]

Characteristic	Intrinsic factor	Transcobalamin II	R protein
Location	Gastric juice	Plasma	Multiple
Binding properties			
Cobalamin binding sites	1	1	1
Affinity (K_A)	1.9 pM^{-1}	0.5 pM^{-1}	7.5 pM^{-1}
Specificity	High	Moderate	Low
Molecular weight[b]	45,000	38,000	56,000 to 66,000
Carbohydrate (%)	15	0	33 to 40
Sialic acid residues	2	0	16 to 19
Membrane receptors	Ileum	All cells	Hepatocytes
Function	Ileal absorption	Delivery to cells	Storage, excretion

[a]Summarized from Allen (3) and Kolhouse and Allen (81).
[b]Molecular weights based on ultracentrifugation and on analyses of amino acids and carbohydrates.

ers, these three transport proteins have now been purified to homogeneity and have been sufficiently characterized to permit a reasonable understanding of how they function.

All three proteins tightly bind cobalamin in a macromolecular complex that involves a single cobalamin-binding site per protein molecule. The affinity of cobalamin for its transport proteins is remarkably high, with association constants in the picomolar range. Affinity remains high whether the Co-β ligand of the cobalamin molecule consists of a hydroxyl, cyanide, methyl, or adenosyl residue (3,81,94).

Of the three binding proteins, intrinsic factor is the most selective. For example, among 14 cobalamin analogs tested by Kolhouse and Allen (81), only two cobamides with minor changes in the benzimidazole base had an affinity for intrinsic factor approaching that of cobalamin. The binding requirements of transcobalamin II are somewhat less specific, and this protein binds a few additional cobamides. The R proteins, however, are nonspecific in that they bind with affinity a wide variety of cobamides as well as cobinamide, an analog that lacks the entire nucleotide moiety of cobalamin.

The molecular weights of the three binding proteins range from 38,000 to 66,000 daltons. Transcobalamin II is a polypeptide, whereas intrinsic factor and the R proteins are glycoproteins. Carbohydrate moieties are probably responsible for the falsely high molecular weights obtained when intrinsic factor or R proteins are analyzed by gel filtration or gel electrophoresis (9). The relatively large number of sialic acid residues on the R proteins accounts for the rapid anionic migration of these binders during electrophoresis. The amino acid compositions of the three transport proteins are distinct, and there is no immunologic cross-reactivity among intrinsic factor, transcobalamin II, and the R proteins (4,5). On the other hand, R proteins isolated from different sources cross-react and have similar amino acid compositions (19,20). Variations in carbohydrate composition are responsible for the observed differences in the molecular weight and charge of various R proteins.

Intrinsic factor, transcobalamin II, and the R proteins are also distinctive in that each has specific membrane receptors present on the surface of cells. Receptors for intrinsic factor are found only on microvillous membranes of ileal absorptive cells (41), whereas a wide variety of dividing cells contain receptors for transcobalamin II (3). Receptors specific for R proteins, however, are present only on hepatocytes. Intrinsic factor and its ileal membrane receptors are discussed in detail in subsequent sections of this chapter. Here it is necessary to consider only the transport functions of transcobalamin II and the R proteins.

Transcobalamin II

This plasma globulin accounts for most of the unsaturated cobalamin-binding capacity of plasma (3). The site of formation of circulating transcobalamin II remains uncertain, although there is considerable indirect evidence to suggest its synthesis by the liver (31,110) as well as by other organs, including the kidney, intestine (110) and monocytes (109). Although the amount of transcobalamin II in plasma is minute (25 μg/liter), there is considerable evidence to suggest that this protein is the plasma binder responsible for the delivery of cobalamin to tissues. Only a tiny proportion of circulating transcobalamin II is bound to endogenous cobalamin, and both newly absorbed cobalamin (57) and injected cyanocobalamin (40,58) bind promptly and virtually exclusively to unsaturated apotranscobalamin II.

Although the quantity of transcobalamin circulating at any one time is small, turnover of the protein, whether free or bound to cobalamin, is rapid, with a half-life of about 90 min in rabbits (122). Comparable disappearance rates for [57]Co-labeled cyanocobalamin bound to transcobalamin II have also been described in humans (67). When ^{125}I-labeled transcobalamin II is bound to [57]Co-labeled cyanocobalamin and is then injected into rabbits, both ^{125}I and [57]Co are rapidly cleared from the plasma. Within 30 min, small ^{125}I-labeled peptide fragments of transcobalamin II unaccompanied by [57]Co appear in the urine (122). After 60 min, [57]Co begins to reappear in plasma. Rapid uptake of both ^{125}I and [57]Co occurs in all tissues studied, including liver, spleen, heart, lungs, and intestine. Thus cobalamin bound to transcobalamin II is rapidly taken up by tissues throughout the body, which then degrade the transport protein to small fragments that are excreted by the kidney. Unwanted cobalamin is gradually returned to the circulation for redistribution, storage, or excretion by the liver.

Transcobalamin II greatly facilitates the uptake of cobalamin *in vitro* by a variety of cells, including reticulocytes (112), tumor cells (33), lymphoblasts (117), and fibroblasts (143). Cellular uptake of cobalamin mediated by transcobalamin II can be divided into two phases (47). The initial phase occurs rapidly, requires divalent cations, is not temperature dependent, does not require cellular metabolic energy, and presumably represents uptake of cobalamin-bound transcobalamin II by cell surface receptors. These receptors are specific for transcobalamin II since uptake of cobalamin bound to intrinsic factor or to R protein does not occur. The surface receptor recently has been isolated from human placenta (125). It appears to be a glycoprotein with a molecular weight of 50,000 daltons and an amino acid composition similar to that of transcobalamin II.

The second phase is characterized by continuous uptake of cobalamin for several hours. This phase is temperature dependent, is blocked by metabolic inhibitors, and represents transfer of cobalamin into the cell (33).

The fate of both transcobalamin II and cobalamin during cellular uptake has been examined by cell fractionation studies. These studies have been conducted with liver (107) and kidney (99) after *in vivo* binding of [57]Co-labeled cyanocobalamin and with fibroblasts cultured with transcobalamin II-bound cyanocobalamin (142,143). The results of these investigations are depicted in Fig. 3. The cobalamin-transcobalamin II complex enters the cell intact perhaps by endocytosis. Transcobalamin II then is degraded by lysosomal enzymes after fusion of endocytic vesicles with lysosomes. Finally, the cobalamin is released into the cytosol. Additional studies (82,96) suggest that the released cobalamin binds to the methylmalonyl mutase apoenzyme in the mitochondria. Although this proposed sequence for cellular uptake of cobalamin requires more direct confirmation by morphologic techniques, it is consistent with data obtained by cell fractionation. In addition, the fact that some cobalamin has been found in the cytosol still bound to transcobalamin II raises the possibility that mechanisms other than endocytosis and lysosomal digestion may also be operating to affect cellular transport (101).

It is not clear whether cells take up transcobalamin II that is bound to cobalamin more readily than free transcobalamin II. The affinity of cobalamin-bound transcobalamin II is greater than that of unsaturated transcobalamin II for human placental membranes (50). Moreover, in human subjects, saturation of circulating transcobalamin II results in a prompt and striking decline in plasma levels of transcobalamin II (40), suggesting more rapid tissue uptake of the bound than the unbound protein. In rabbits, however, unsaturated transcobalamin II disappears from plasma somewhat more rapidly than cobalamin-bound transcobalamin II. Direct comparisons of tissue uptake of cobalamin-bound and unbound transcobalamin II are obviously needed.

The rapid turnover of transcobalamin II in plasma is consistent with the concept (3) that changes in the availability of this polypeptide may modulate the delivery of cobalamin to cells that require the vitamin. Moreover, the importance of transcobalamin II is emphasized by observations in patients who lack this protein (56). Patients with constitutional deficiency of transcobalamin

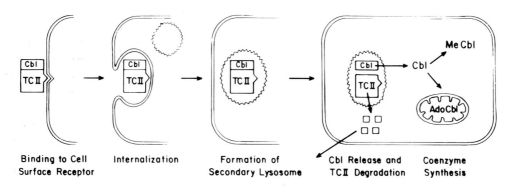

FIG. 3. Transcobalamin II-mediated cellular uptake and transport of cobalamin. TC II, transcobalamin II; Cbl, cobalamin; MeCbl, methylcobalamin; AdoCbl, adenosylcobalamin. [Reproduced with permission from Youngdahl-Turner et al. (143).]

II have severe megaloblastic anemia, despite normal or elevated serum levels of cobalamin.

R proteins

More difficult to establish has been the transport role of the family of cobalamin-binding R proteins that are found in granulocytes and in many body fluids and secretions, including plasma, saliva, gastric juice, bile, milk, tears, and amniotic fluid (127). This difficulty is enhanced by the fact that patients who are deficient in R proteins have no obvious clinical abnormality that can be attributed to impaired utilization of cobalamin (25).

R proteins are present in plasma as transcobalamin I, which carries at least 90% of circulating endogenous cobalamin (58,67), and as transcobalamin III, which is derived from granulocytes (26). In fact, most of the transcobalamin III in normal plasma is probably released from granulocytes after blood has been collected (124). When either ^{125}I-labeled transcobalamin III or ^{131}I-labeled granulocyte R protein, which are similar in their molecular structure (20), is bound to [57]Co-labeled cobalamin and injected intravenously into rabbits, both the ^{125}I and the [57]Co disappear rapidly from the plasma (21). Virtually all the injected radioactivity is taken up by the liver. This organ secretes a portion of the radioactivity labeled R protein-cobalamin complex into the bile intact, degrades the remainder of the complex, and stores some of the cobalamin while returning the rest to the circulation.

The turnover of granulocyte R protein or transcobalamin III in plasma is extremely rapid, with a half-life of about 5 min (21) as compared to the very slow (half-life, 10 days) disappearance rate of transcobalamin I. Uptake of R proteins by hepatic plasma membranes is mediated by the general mechanism for desialylated glycoproteins described by Ashwell and Morell (12). Thus when transcobalamin I, which is relatively rich in sialic acid residues and only slowly removed from circulation, is treated with neuraminidase, the rate of removal by liver cells is increased severalfold (3,21). R protein-mediated uptake of cobalamin by liver cells involves rapid calcium-dependent attachment of cobalamin-bound R protein to saturable cell surface receptors, followed by a slower energy-requiring process, resulting in entry of cobalamin into the hepatocyte (3).

The circulating endogenous cobalamin which is bound to transcobalamin I constitutes a storage form of the vitamin, which is delivered very slowly to tissues for use or excretion. It is uncertain whether or not the cobalamin bound to transcobalamin I in plasma interacts with the rapidly turning over transcobalamin II.

All the R proteins, whether present in granulocytes, plasma, or glandular secretions, bind with high affinity not only to cobalamin but also to a wide variety of bacterially synthesized, potentially harmful cobalamin analogs. Thus, as proposed by Allen (3), the R proteins function to bind unwanted cobalamin analogs or excessive cobalamin for either storage, delivery to the liver, biliary excretion, or removal via glandular secretions. The locations, turnover rates, and binding specifications of intrinsic factor, transcobalamin II, and the R proteins strongly suggest that these transport proteins act in concert to deliver needed cobalamin to cells while simultaneously protecting the body from cobalamin analogs (81). Intrinsic factor selectively recognizes cobalamin and promotes its intestinal absorption but rejects any bacterially produced cobalamin analogs present in the bowel lumen. In the plasma, transcobalamin II binds and delivers cobalamin to cells that need it, but fails to bind or deliver most analogs that may have gained access to the circulation. In contrast, R proteins in granulocytes, plasma, and glandular secretions are capable of binding unwanted cobalamin analogs along with excess cobalamin. The bound substances are stored or excreted.

INTRINSIC FACTOR

Site of Intrinsic Factor Production

Since Castle's original observations (27), many investigations have confirmed that the stomach is the site of intrinsic factor secretion in humans. Total gastrectomy is regularly accompanied by cobalamin malabsorption, which is corrected by human gastric juice (59). Unless the vitamin is administered parenterally, this operation leads to cobalamin deficiency in 3 to 5 years (88). It is the oxyntic mucosa of the body and fundus of the human stomach rather than the gastric antrum that is responsible for intrinsic factor secretion. Atrophy of fundic but not antral mucosa occurs in addisonian pernicious anemia (141), and selective resection of the body of the stomach leads to impaired cobalamin absorption (87). In addition, autoradiographic (65) and immunofluorescent (48) studies have demonstrated localization of intrinsic factor to the parietal cells in human gastric mucosa. Similarly, in the rabbit, monkey, cat, guinea pig, and ox, intrinsic factor is present in parietal cells (65). In human subjects, immunocytochemical studies have clearly demonstrated the presence of intrinsic factor antigen on membranes of the perinuclear envelop, rough endoplasmic reticulum, Golgi apparatus, and tubulovesicular membrane system of the parietal cell (85).

In contrast to these findings, intrinsic factor is found in the chief cell in mouse and rat (65), and hog intrinsic factor appears to be located in mucus cells that populate the duodenum and pyloric area of the stomach (65). Hog intrinsic factor is not found in the fundus of the stomach.

Mechanisms Involved in Intrinsic Factor Secretion

Like acid secretion, intrinsic factor secretion by the human stomach is stimulated by histamine (11,70), pentagastrin (11,137) and cholinergic agents (137) and is inhibited by cimetidine (14). The pattern of intrinsic factor secretion is different from that of acid secretion (23). As illustrated in Fig. 4, intrinsic factor secretion responds rapidly to stimulation and reaches peak levels within 15 to 30 min, a time when acid secretion is still increasing. By the time acid secretion is maximal, intrinsic factor secretion has already returned to levels close to control values. This phenomenon has been attributed to washout of preformed intrinsic factor (23), although repeating the stimulus results in secretion of additional intrinsic factor, and continuous infusion of either betazole or pentagastrin yields reasonably steady intrinsic factor secretion for prolonged periods.

The amounts of intrinsic factor secreted by the stomach greatly exceed what is needed to bind and assimilate dietary cobalamin. In 1 hr, the stimulated human stomach secretes enough intrinsic factor to bind all the cobalamin usually present in the diet for an entire day (70).

The cellular mechanisms responsible for the control of intrinsic factor secretion remain poorly understood. Recent insights, however, have been achieved by investigations with biopsies of rabbit oxyntic mucosa maintained in organ culture. This approach allows direct examination of macromolecular secretion *in vitro* under steady-state conditions for 24 hr (131). Intrinsic factor secretion by cultured biopsies is stimulated by histamine and acetylcholine and is inhibited by cimetidine (73). A role for cyclic nucleotides in the mediation of intrinsic factor secretion is suggested by several observations (74). The phosphodiesterase inhibitor isobutlylmethylxanthine and dibutyryl cyclic AMP (but not dibutyryl cyclic GMP) markedly stimulate intrinsic factor secretion by isolated rabbit gastric mucosa. Moreover,

the intrinsic factor secretion induced by isobutylmethylxanthine is preceded by increased mucosal levels of cyclic nucleotides. In addition, histamine induces an increase in tissue levels of cyclic AMP but not cyclic GMP in cultured gastric mucosa, and cimetidine blocks both the rise in tissue cyclic AMP and the increased intrinsic factor secretion induced by histamine.

In vitro experiments with isolated rabbit gastric mucosa have also demonstrated that the secretory responses of the parietal cells which secrete intrinsic factor are distinctly different from the responses of pepsinogen-secreting chief cells (73). Although the secretion of both pepsinogen and intrinsic factor are stimulated by acetylcholine, dose-response curves are quite different. In addition, atropine inhibits the unstimulated secretion of intrinsic factor, while basal pepsinogen secretion is unaffected. Moreover, histamine stimulates intrinsic factor but not pepsinogen secretion by isolated gastric mucosa, and cimetidine inhibits basal secretion of intrinsic factor but not pepsinogen. Most striking was the difference in response to topical application of 50 mN HCl to the mucosal surface of cultured mucosal biopsies. Topical HCl induced a marked increase in pepsinogen secretion, consistent with the *in vivo* response observed in humans (22) and dogs (71); at the same time, intrinsic factor secretion was virtually abolished. Additional experiments are required to determine whether acidification of the surface of oxyntic mucosa blocks intrinsic factor secretion *in vivo* and whether this phenomenon might account for the pattern of intrinsic factor secretion illustrated in Fig. 5.

The cellular mechanism for secreting intrinsic factor may vary considerably from species to species. In mouse and rat, for example, intrinsic factor appears to be localized to chief cells (65). In this cell, intrinsic factor may be packaged in secretory granules, as has been so carefully documented for pancreatic enzymes (102). The same may hold for hog intrinsic factor, which appears

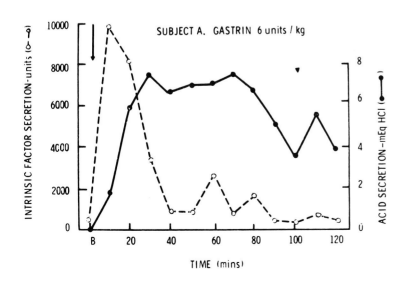

FIG. 4. Pattern of intrinsic factor and acid secretion after injection of pentagastrin given at the time indicated by the arrow. [Reproduced with permission from the review by Callender (23).]

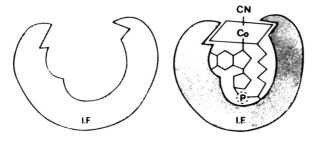

FIG. 5. Binding of cyanocobalamin by intrinsic factor (I.F.). [Reproduced with permission from the review by Callender (23) and as originally proposed by Gräsbeck (52).]

to be secreted by mucus cells (65). A similar mechanism, however, is unlikely for the parietal cell, which secretes human intrinsic factor (23). Localization of intrinsic factor to the membranes of the Golgi apparatus and tubulovesicular system of the parietal cell (85) suggests an important role for membrane translocation in the release of intrinsic factor by this cell.

Gastric oxyntic mucosa has long been identified as the site of intrinsic factor secretion; only recently, however, has it been possible to demonstrate that it also synthesizes intrinsic factor *de novo* (126). When biopsies of rabbit fundic mucosa are cultured for 24 hr, the amount of intrinsic factor recovered from biopsy tissue remains unchanged, while the quantity of intrinsic factor increases steadily and at 24 hr amounts to about 70% of that present in the biopsy. This direct demonstration of the formation of new intrinsic factor *in vitro* is further substantiated by the fact that both ³H-labeled leucine and ³⁵S-labeled methionine are incorporated by cultured biopsies into intrinsic factor isolated by affinity chromatography. The labeled intrinsic factor is homogeneous on polyacrylamide slab gel electrophoresis, reacts with anti-intrinsic factor antibodies, and promotes the uptake of cobalamin by ileal cells. Synthesis of human intrinsic factor almost certainly occurs in the parietal cell of oxyntic mucosa, since immunocytochemical studies have clearly documented intrinsic factor in rough endoplasmic reticulum of that cell (85).

Thus (a) intrinsic factor is synthesized and secreted by parietal cells in most animal species; (b) the amounts of intrinsic factor secreted are far in excess of the quantities needed to promote physiologic absorption of the vitamin; and (c) the processes involved in the control of intrinsic factor secretion probably differ from those responsible for the secretion of acid and pepsinogen. We need a more precise understanding of the fundamental mechanisms involved in the synthesis and secretion of this critical cobalamin-binding transport protein. Further investigations with isolated parietal cell preparations (129) may provide important information about the assembly and secretion of intrinsic factor in the parietal cell.

Physicochemical and Binding Properties of Intrinsic Factor

Investigators have now purified from hog pyloric mucosa (6,52,93) and human gastric juice (5,52) preparations of intrinsic factor that facilitate cobalamin absorption and that appear to be homogenous both by polyacrylamide gel electrophoresis and analytical ultracentrifugation. Intrinsic factor is a globular glycoprotein that contains about 15% carbohydrate. Preparations isolated from human gastric juice (5) contain 340 amino acid residues and 36 sugar residues (Table 2) which combine to yield a molecular weight of 44,000 daltons. This compares closely with a molecular weight of 45,000 to 48,000 daltons obtained by sedimentation equilibrium ultracentrifugation (5). The larger molecular weights (55,000 to 70,000 daltons) estimated for intrinsic factor by gel filtration or electrophoresis probably reflect the falsely high values these techniques often yield for glycoproteins (9).

When intrinsic factor is reduced, alkylated, and analyzed by ultracentrifugation in 6 M guanidine HCl, the observed molecular weight is not altered. Allen (3) has concluded, therefore, that intrinsic factor protein consists of a single polypeptide chain. The quantity of cob-

TABLE 2. *Composition of human intrinsic factor[a]*

Composition	Residues[b]
Amino acid	
Lysine	20
Histidine	5
Arginine	6
Aspartate	38
Threonine	24
Serine	30
Glutamate	35
Proline	22
Glycine	20
Alanine	23
Half-cystine	6
Valine	21
Methionine	10
Isoleucine	21
Leucine	34
Tyrosine	9
Phenylalanine	10
Tryptophan	6
Carbohydrate	
Fucose	7
Galactose	6
Mannose	12
Galactosamine	3
Glucosamine	5
Sialic acid	3

[a]As reported by Allen and Mehlman (5).
[b]Residues per mole bound cobalamin.

alamin bound by homogeneous intrinsic factor (30 μg/mg intrinsic factor protein) indicates that each molecule of intrinsic factor binds one molecule of cobalamin. Although the composition of intrinsic factor has been defined, its amino acid sequence and oligosaccharide structure remain to be elucidated. Until the complete configuration of the molecule is described and the cobalamin-binding site identified, it will not be possible to understand fully how intrinsic factor functions.

Intrinsic factor tightly binds cobalamin in a macromolecular complex. This binding is virtually instantaneous with cobalamin, exhibiting an extremely high affinity for the protein (52,64). Over a wide range of concentrations of cobalamin, a Scatchard plot of binding to intrinsic factor is linear, suggesting that each cobalamin molecule combines at a separate binding site. At very low cobalamin concentrations, however, the Scatchard plot suggests binding cooperativity (94). Although the bond formed between intrinsic factor and cobalamin is extremely strong under physiologic conditions, it is readily disrupted above a pH of 12.6 (52). Below pH 3.0, affinity is markedly reduced; in an acid environment, binding of cobalamin to R protein is greatly favored over binding to intrinsic factor (7). The intrinsic factor molecule undergoes distinct changes as it binds to cobalamin. The molecule becomes more compact, since binding is accompanied by a 10 to 15% decrease in the calculated Stokes radius and apparent molecular weight of intrinsic factor (52). Cobalamin-bound intrinsic factor is also distinctly more resistant to destruction by proteases than is free intrinsic factor (1). In addition, free intrinsic factor exists in dilute solutions only as monomers, while the cobalamin-intrinsic factor complex occurs as monomers, dimers, and larger oligomers (5,52).

As emphasized earlier, intrinsic factor is the most specific of the cobalamin binders. Cyanocobalamin, hydroxycobalamin, methylcobalamin, or adenosylcobalamin all bind to intrinsic factor with approximately the same high affinity (7,52,94). Thus the Co-β ligand can be markedly altered without affecting binding. Both the corrin ring and the dimethylbenzimidazole base are critical for binding, and even slight changes in either of these moieties markedly reduces affinity for intrinsic factor (81,94). Several studies of binding (7,81,94) have provided support for the model for binding first proposed by Gräsbeck (52), who suggested that the cobalamin molecule fits into a pit on the globular IF-molecule with the nucleotide facing inward and the β-substituent facing outward (Fig. 5).

The site on the intrinsic factor molecule that binds cobalamin appears to be separate from that which attaches to the absorptive surface of the ileum. Evidence favoring separation of these two sites has been derived from clinical investigations. Serum samples from at least 70% of patients (54) with pernicious anemia contain an IgG known as "antibody I" or "blocking antibody," which prevents intrinsic factor from combining with cobalamin to form a macromolecular complex (10,119), as illustrated in Fig. 6. Sera from approximately one-third of patients with pernicious anemia contain an additional immunoglobulin, usually IgG but occasionally IgA or IgM, which combines with cobalamin-bound intrinsic factor and is called "antibody II" or "binding antibody" (119). These anti-intrinsic factor antibodies have proved invaluable as reagents for identifying and measuring intrinsic factor. Of some interest is the fact that injecting animals with purified intrinsic factor, whether or not saturated with cobalamin, produces only antibodies of the "blocking" type. Thus the "binding" or "type II" antibody appears to be unique to pernicious anemia. Both type I and type II antibodies combine with the intrinsic factor molecule (119), and their effects support the notion of two separate functional sites on that molecule. Type I or "blocking" antibody keeps cyanocobalamin from binding to intrinsic factor but does not interfere with ileal uptake of intrinsic factor-bound cyanocobalamin once the macromolecular complex has formed (118,119). In contrast, type II or "binding" antibody specifically prevents the intrinsic factor-cobalamin complex from attaching to its ileal membrane receptor (118,120).

Additional support for distinct cobalamin-binding and receptor-attaching sites comes from a patient with cobalamin malabsorption resulting from gastric secretion of an abnormal intrinsic factor (79). This patient's intrinsic factor, although incapable of promoting intestinal absorption of cobalamin, could not be distinguished from normal intrinsic factor on the basis of physicochemical characteristics (80). This abnormal intrinsic factor bound cyanocobalamin with the same high affinity as did normal intrinsic factor and reacted appropriately with anti-intrinsic factor antibody but totally lacked the capacity to attach to the ileal membrane receptor for intrinsic factor.

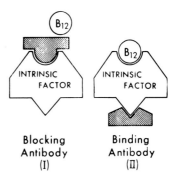

FIG. 6. Anti-intrinsic factor antibodies in sera of some patients with pernicious anemia. B$_{12}$, cyanocobalamin. *Shaded portions,* antibodies.

GENERAL FEATURES OF COBALAMIN ABSORPTION

Some information about the overall process of cobalamin absorption is needed as background for a detailed examination of the sequence of individual events involved in intrinsic factor-mediated assimilation of the vitamin. Although cobalamin is essential for survival, only tiny quantities are required. Human beings, for example, must assimilate only 1 to 2 µg daily to maintain normal stores (35). Most sources of animal protein provide adequate amounts of dietary cobalamin. Liver and kidney are particularly rich in the vitamin, but meat, fish, milk, and eggs all substantially contribute to the average dietary intake of 10 to 20 µg/day. On the other hand, fruits, vegetables, and grains lack cobalamin, and strict vegetarians will slowly develop cobalamin deficiency unless they supplement their diet (62). It should be kept in mind that microbial synthesis constitutes the ultimate source of dietary cobalamin, and that herbivorous animals must depend on rumen bacteria or some other regular access, such as coprophagy, to microbial products.

The vitamin exists in food as adenosyl-, methyl-, or hydroxycobalamin. Although cyanocobalamin is the substance most often used to investigate cobalamin absorption, this compound is actually found in only trace amounts in the diet. Fortunately, the naturally occurring cobalamins apparently use the same mechanisms for absorption as have been documented for cyanocobalamin (86,94). It should also be pointed out that although ingested cobalamin is bound to food proteins (45), investigations into the absorption of the vitamin are almost always conducted with crystalline cyanocobalamin, either free or bound to intrinsic factor.

Ellenbogen (46) has recently reviewed the methods available for quantifying cobalamin absorption in humans. The technique most widely used is the urinary excretion test first described by Schilling (121). A small (0.5 to 2.0 µg) quantity of cyanocobalamin labeled with ^{57}Co or ^{58}Co is fed to the fasting subject. To release absorbed radioactivity from tissues so that it can be excreted in the urine, a "flushing dose" of 1,000 µg nonradioactive cyanocobalamin is administered intramuscularly within 2 hr of the oral dose. Under these conditions, about one-third of the absorbed radioactivity is recovered from the urine (24), and healthy subjects generally excrete 10 to 20% of the administered radioactivity in urine collected for 24 hr. Patients with pernicious anemia, however, excrete much less (0 to 5%) radioactivity, unless the radioactive cyanocobalamin is fed with a biologically active preparation of intrinsic factor. Therefore, if the urinary excretion test indicates impaired absorption of free cyanocobalamin, the test must be repeated by feeding radioactive vitamin together with an excess of intrinsic factor but only under conditions that assure that residual radioactivity from the first test will not be excreted in the urine (46). This procedure can be considerably shortened by feeding a mixture of cyanocobalamin containing two different radioactive isotopes of cobalt, one free and the other bound to intrinsic factor, so that the absorption of free and intrinsic factor-bound cyanocobalamin can be determined simultaneously (76).

The urinary excretion test measures only the amount of cyanocobalamin excreted after absorption, not the amount absorbed. More direct assessment of absorption of the vitamin can be achieved by measuring radioactivity excreted in feces (60) or retained in the body (108) after an oral dose of labeled cyanocobalamin. These tests indicated that healthy subjects absorb 30 to 60% of an oral dose of 1 µg cyanocobalamin. Both procedures, however, may require as long as 10 days before all unabsorbed radioactivity is excreted in feces. Furthermore, prolonged fecal collections are inconvenient, and measurement of total body radioactivity requires equipment that is not always available. Determination of hepatic uptake (140) or plasma levels (16) of radioactivity also provide indirect measures of cobalamin absorption that, like the more widely used urinary excretion test, correlate reasonably well with more direct methods that rely on fecal excretion or total body retention of radioactivity (16,108). Nevertheless, these indirect techniques must be validated by direct methods during investigations into mechanisms of cobalamin absorption.

Assimilation of the vitamin occurs by two fundamentally different processes, depending on the quantity ingested. When the tiny quantities of cobalamin ordinarily present in the diet are administered, absorption is quite efficient: 30 to 60% of a dose less than 10 µg will be retained (24,60). When doses of 100 µg or more are ingested, however, less than 1% is absorbed from the entire alimentary canal by nonspecific diffusion, and peak blood levels are achieved within 1 to 2 hr (43). In contrast, efficient absorption of physiologic amounts of the vitamin is remarkably slow and occurs only from the ileum.

Investigations in several mammalian species indicate that cobalamin is absorbed from distal rather than proximal small bowel (15). In humans, the distal third to half of the ileum is responsible for efficient absorption of the vitamin. Assimilation is markedly impaired following resection of this portion of the ileum but not of the duodenum or jejunum (15,95). Moreover, intrinsic factor-bound cobalamin is readily absorbed when infused directly into the distal ileum (9), whereas the colon is clearly incapable of assimilating the bound vitamin (100).

When labeled cyanocobalamin is ingested by healthy individuals, levels of radioactivity in the plasma are not maximal until 6 to 8 hr after ingestion (43). This slow absorption does not result from delay in the liver since similar curves of plasma radioactivity are observed in patients with surgically created vascular shunts that bypass the liver (44). Similarly, the ileal site for cobalamin absorption does not explain this delay. Plasma levels of conjugated bile salts are maximal within 2 hr of ingestion, even though these compounds are also absorbed by the ileum (84).

From this discussion, it is apparent that absorption of cobalamin by the intestine is unusual in several respects when compared to the absorption of most other nutrients. First, efficient absorption requires that the vitamin form a macromolecular complex with a glycoprotein secreted by the stomach. Second, investigations in patients (95,135) and experimental animals (132) with pancreatic insufficiency indicate that pancreatic proteases are necessary for normal cobalamin absorption; yet these proteases do not appear to digest cobalamin or cobalamin-intrinsic factor complex (7,136). Third, the vitamin is efficiently absorbed only from distal portions of the bowel in all species thus far studied (15,30). Fourth, the capacity of the intestine to absorb cobalamin is remarkably limited. In human subjects, for example, no more than 1 to 2 μg cyanocobalamin can be absorbed from any given dose, even when fed with an excess of intrinsic factor (51). Finally, assimilation of cobalamin occurs extremely slowly, with the delay occurring at the ileal mucosa (44). A complete explanation of how cobalamin is absorbed must ultimately take into account all these distinctive features.

SEQUENTIAL EVENTS INVOLVED IN COBALAMIN ABSORPTION

Twenty years ago, Cooper and Castle (32) proposed the concept now widely accepted that efficient absorption of physiologic quantities of cobalamin results from an orderly sequence of discrete events. These events include: (a) the release of cobalamin from dietary protein, (b) the intragastric binding of cobalamin to R proteins of salivary and gastric origin, (c) digestion of R protein-cobalamin complexes by pancreatic proteases with release of cobalamin, (d) binding of the vitamin by intrinsic factor, (e) attachment of intrinsic factor-bound cobalamin to the absorptive surface of the ileum, (f) absorption of cobalamin by ileal mucosal cells, and (g) release of newly absorbed vitamin into the portal circulation.

Intragastric and Intraduodenal Events

Dietary cobalamin is bound to proteins that consist of either the apoenzymes responsible for cobalamin-dependent reactions (82,96) or the R proteins that function to store the vitamin in tissues or plasma (3). Although interactions between the vitamin and ingested proteins have not been studied extensively, it is clear that the acid environment of the stomach rapidly frees cobalamin from food protein complexes (32). This release does not require pepsin and does not appear to be the rate-limiting step in cobalamin absorption under ordinary circumstances. Nevertheless, some patients with achlorhydria cannot effectively extract and absorb the vitamin from foods, even though these individuals secrete adequate amounts of intrinsic factor and absorb crystalline cobalamin normally (45).

Until recently, it was generally assumed that cobalamin, once freed from food protein, immediately became bound to intrinsic factor in the stomach (51). Recent *in vitro* studies (7), however, suggest that the vitamin may first bind to salivary and gastric R proteins, particularly when the pH of gastric contents is acid. Human salivary R protein binds cobalamin with affinities that are three- and 50-fold greater than those of human intrinsic factor at pH 8 and 2, respectively. At neither pH is the vitamin transferred from R protein to intrinsic factor (7). When a meal is eaten, however, gastric contents may be sufficiently neutralized by food, while intrinsic factor secretion may be sufficiently stimulated to favor the initial binding of cobalamin to intrinsic factor rather than to R proteins. Clearly needed are *in vivo* measurements of the relative binding of labeled cyanocobalamin to intrinsic factor and R proteins not only under the conditions of fasting that usually prevail during clinical tests of cobalamin absorption but also during the ingestion of an ordinary meal. Any cobalamin that is initially bound by R proteins in the stomach is probably released promptly within the proximal small intestine, since pancreatic proteases rapidly degrade R proteins, thereby freeing cobalamin from R protein-cobalamin complexes (7).

In patients with exocrine pancreatic insufficiency, however, one might expect digestion of R protein to be impaired, and it is of considerable interest that cobalamin malabsorption was observed in pancreatic insufficiency as early as 1956 (95). Subsequent systematic investigations (132,138) have documented impaired absorption of the vitamin corrected by pancreatic extract in 40 to 50% of cases of steatorrhea due to pancreatic disease. Cobalamin malabsorption also occurs regularly in rats subjected to partial pancreatectomy (132). In both clinical and experimental settings, however, the extent of cobalamin malabsorption is unrelated to the severity of steatorrhea (133), and the corrective factor in pancreatic extract clearly has the physicochemical properties of pancreatic proteases (134). Indeed, highly purified trypsin corrects cobalamin malabsorption associated with pancreatic insufficiency (136).

Allen and co-workers (7,8) have proposed that cobalamin malabsorption in pancreatic insufficiency results from impaired proteolytic release of cobalamin from its complex with R protein and consequent inability of cobalamin to bind to intrinsic factor. In support of this view is the observation that administration of a large excess of cobinamide, a cobalamin analog that avidly binds R proteins but does not bind to intrinsic factor, regularly increases absorption of labeled cobalamin in patients who lack pancreatic proteases (18). In this situation, the large quantities of cobinamide block the available binding sites on R protein, permitting the test dose of cobalamin to bind initially to intrinsic factor. It should also be pointed out that virtually all the labeled vitamin is bound to intrinsic factor when recovered from the duodenal contents of subjects with normal pancreatic function (72,103), whereas in a patient with exocrine pancreatic insufficiency, most of the recovered radioactivity was bound to R protein (103). Since pancreatic proteases do not demonstrably alter the physicochemical or antigenic properties of intrinsic factor (136) and are not required for the function of ileal membrane receptors for intrinsic factor-bound cobalamin (41,132), impaired intraduodenal release of the vitamin is the most satisfactory explanation for malabsorption of the vitamin in patients with pancreatic insufficiency.

Further studies are needed in which the intraluminal binding of cobalamin to intrinsic factor and to R protein is compared in patients with pancreatic insufficiency who do and do not absorb the vitamin normally.

Figure 7 summarizes the subsequent events involved in absorption of the vitamin. After its release from R proteins within the proximal small bowel, the vitamin combines with intrinsic factor to form a remarkably stable macromolecular complex, as described in detail above. When labeled cyanocobalamin is fed to healthy volunteers, virtually all the radioactivity subsequently recovered from small bowel contents is bound to intrinsic factor (103). Unlike R proteins, the intrinsic factor-cobalamin complex resists digestion by proteolytic enzymes (1,7). In addition, intrinsic factor serves to protect the vitamin from bacterial utilization within the bowel lumen (36,37) while the macromolecular complex is being delivered to the ileum.

Attachment of Intrinsic Factor-Bound Cobalamin to Ileal Membrane Receptors

The next step is absorption of intrinsic factor-bound cobalamin onto the surface of ileal mucosa. This results from the attachment of the complex to specific receptors that have been localized to the outer surface of ileal microvillous membranes (41). Attachment is rapid, with a second order rate constant of $1.3 \times 10^6 M^{-1}/sec$ (94). Binding of the intrinsic factor-cobalamin complex to its receptor is unaffected by temperatures from 4° to 37° C and does not require cellular metabolic energy (41). The ileal membrane receptor has a high affinity (K_D

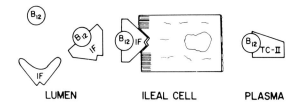

FIG. 7. Sequence of events involved in the intestinal absorption of cyanocobalamin (B_{12}). IF, intrinsic factor; TC-II, transcobalamin II. [Reproduced with permission from the review by Donaldson (39).]

= 0.25 nM) for intrinsic factor-bound cobalamin (41,94), and the receptor site is highly specific in that it does not take up free cobalamin, cobalamin analogs, or cobalamin that is bound to transcobalamin II or to a wide variety of R proteins (41,68,94). The nature of the Co-β ligand of the cobalamin molecule does not alter affinity of the complex for its ileal receptor (81,94). As described earlier, the site on the intrinsic factor molecule that attaches to the receptor appears to be separate from that which binds cobalamin. As illustrated in Fig. 7, the intrinsic factor molecule probably is interposed between the membrane receptor and the cobalamin molecule (52).

Attachment to ileal receptors requires calcium ions and a pH greater than 5.6 (89). Calcium thus may form "salt bridges" between critical anions, and these bridges may either maintain the appropriate configuration of the ileal receptor or actually link the intrinsic factor molecule to the receptor molecule.

The number of receptors for intrinsic factor-bound cobalamin on the surface of ileal absorptive cells is remarkably small in all species thus far examined (42,68,77). In the hamster, for example, there are no more than 300 to 400 receptors per ileal absorptive cell, or approximately one receptor per microvillus (42). This limited number of receptor sites adequately accounts for the limited capacity of the ileum to absorb cobalamin, since in hamster (42) as well as in guinea pig and human (68) ileum, the total binding capacity of membrane receptors approximates the maximal amount of cobalamin that can be absorbed from a single dose. The receptor sites appear to be distributed over human ileum in a patchy fashion that varies considerably from individual to individual (55), an observation that may explain the unexpected results of Schilling tests sometimes obtained after ileal resection.

The number of ileal receptors for intrinsic factor-bound cobalamin appears to increase substantially during pregnancy in mice without a concomitant increase in affinity of the receptor for the complex (114). Absorption of the vitamin is increased in pregnant women (61) as well as in mice (17). In mice, both *in vivo* absorption and the number of ileal receptors approximately double during pregnancy (17,114); this is further evidence that the number of receptors may determine the capacity of the intestine to absorb the vitamin. How the number of receptors increases during pregnancy is far from clear, but it would appear that ileal receptors return to control numbers within 24 hr of hysterectomy in pregnant mice, and that this decrease is prevented by injecting either serum from pregnant mice (17) or as little as 1 μg human placental lactogen (114).

The limited number of receptor sites for intrinsic factor-bound cobalamin or ileal microvillous membranes has made isolation and characterization of the receptor extremely difficult. Workers have solubilized receptors from guinea pig (78,123) and human (77) intestine and have partially purified small amounts by affinity chromatography. In general, however, the quantities isolated have been insufficient for further purification and characterization. Recently, Grasbeck and co-workers (93) have solubilized receptor activity from hog ileum. By serial chromatography on affinity columns (93) or by a simpler procedure using pH adjustments (83), these workers have achieved 70,000- to 84,000-fold purifications of solubilized receptor. Their purified preparation was a glycoprotein which was homogenous by isoelectric focusing and contained two subunits with apparent molecular weight of 70,000 and 130,000 daltons on SDS gel electrophoresis. The smaller subunit reacted with intrinsic factor-bound cobalamin but not with cobalamin bound to an abnormal intrinsic factor (79) that is incapable of promoting cobalamin absorption. Preliminary results with receptor activity isolated from human ileum (83) indicate that the human receptor also consisted of two subunits with apparent molecular weights of 90,000 and 140,000 daltons.

Transcellular Transport of Cobalamin by Ileal Mucosa

In contrast to the detailed information now available concerning the attachment of intrinsic factor-bound cobalamin to ileal microvillus membranes, relatively little is known about how cobalamin is subsequently absorbed into and transported across ileal absorptive cells. Investigations have been greatly hampered by the fact that currently available *in vitro* techniques cannot be used to examine intrinsic factor-mediated transport of cobalamin from mucosal to serosal surface of ileal epithelium. Studies with everted sacs of ileum, for example, have shown that absorption of the vitamin into ileal mucosal cells requires metabolic energy, but transport of labeled cyanocobalamin into fluid bathing the serosal surface of these sacs could not be documented (130). Similarly, strips of mucosa from rabbit ileum that bind intrinsic factor-bound cobalamin and also actively transport sodium were unable to transfer the vitamin from mucosal to serosal fluid in a manner that was potentiated by intrinsic factor (39). Since *in vivo* absorption of cobalamin is remarkably delayed (43), the time

required for transport into or across ileal mucosa may simply be too long to demonstrate transmucosal movement of the vitamin within the time constraints of present *in vitro* techniques.

To circumvent this difficulty, various investigators have fed labeled cyanocobalamin to intact guinea pigs (105) or have instilled intrinsic factor-bound radioactive vitamin into loops of ileum *in vivo* (115) and then measured radioactivity associated with subcellular fractions of ileal mucosal homogenates. Experiments thus performed have demonstrated increasing specific activity of cobalamin recovered from mitochondrial fractions over a 2-hr period, during which time radioactivity associated with brush border fractions declined (105). Subsequent investigations (106) showed that both methylcobalamin and adenosylcobalamin accumulated in mitochondrial fractions during absorption, and that labeled adenosylcobalamin could be recovered from these during intrinsic factor-mediated absorption of [57]Co-labeled cyanocobalamin.

In contrast to what has been observed with transcobalamin II-mediated uptake of cobalamin by liver (107) and fibroblasts (143), association of labeled vitamin with lysosomal fractions was not demonstrated during intrinsic factor-mediated absorption of the vitamin by ileal mucosa (105). Moreover, whether intrinsic factor enters ileal cells along with cobalamin remains unsettled (39,46); some experiments suggest entry of intrinsic factor (115,116), while others have failed to detect intracellular cobalamin bound to intrinsic factor (105). Thus there is little evidence to indicate that ileal cells absorb intrinsic factor-bound cobalamin by a pinocytotic mechanism similar to that described for transcobalamin II-mediated cellular uptake.

These cell fractionation experiments must be interpreted cautiously. First, there is the question of cross-contamination of subcellular fractions, particularly with fragmented membranes. Experiments must be monitored by morphologic localization of cobalamin in the intact cell in order to determine if the observed subcellular distribution of labeled cobalamin occurs during fractionation rather than during transport. Unfortunately, it has not been possible to document the movement of physiologic quantities of cobalamin into and through intact ileal cells by autoradiographic or other morphologic techniques.

With respect to elucidating the fate of intrinsic factor during ileal absorption of cobalamin, experiments must be performed in which intrinsic factor is purified and separately labeled, as has already been accomplished with radioiodinated transcobalamin II (143). Although intrinsic factor can be iodinated (90), such preparations have been unsatisfactory because of rapid separation of the iodine label from the intrinsic factor molecule (90). A preliminary report from our laboratory (75) describes incubation of isolated ileal cells (139) with intrinsic factor biosynthetically labeled with ^{35}S-methionine (126) and bound to ^{57}Co-labeled cyanocobalamin. After incubation at 4° C or at 37° C in the presence of an uncoupler of oxidative phosphorylation, both the ^{57}Co and ^{35}S radioactivity can be completely removed from the surface of ileal cells by washing with EDTA or with a buffer at pH 5.0. On the other hand, after incubations for 30 min at 37° C in the presence of oxygen, approximately half the ^{57}Co and ^{35}S radioactivity taken up by ileal cells is "internalized"; it can no longer be washed from the surface. This internalized radioactivity is associated with a macromolecule that has the same chromatographic, electrophoretic, and immunologic properties as intrinsic factor (75). Although these experiments do not unequivocally document entry of intrinsic factor into ileal cells, they do show that after attachment of intrinsic factor-cobalamin complex to ileal membrane receptors, an energy-dependent process somehow prevents the intrinsic factor molecule as well as the cobalamin molecule from being removed from the cell surface. Further investigations with biosynthetically labeled intrinsic factor are needed to clarify subsequent events during ileal mucosal absorption of cobalamin.

How absorbed cobalamin leaves the ileal cell is also poorly understood. Although some absorbed cyanocobalamin may be converted to cobalamin coenzymes for use within the cell, measurable quantities of cyanocobalamin can also be transported to plasma unchanged (106). It is clear that cobalamin is absorbed into portal blood rather than lymphatics (34), and that it is no longer bound to intrinsic factor when it emerges from the intestine. After labeled cyanocobalamin is fed, newly absorbed radioactivity is bound to transcobalamin II in the plasma (57). Investigations in healthy human subjects (29) and in guinea pigs (116) indirectly suggest that as it leaves the absorptive cell, cobalamin may immediately bind to an ileal pool of transcobalamin II, which is distinct from circulating transcobalamin II. Transcobalamin II may be necessary for normal cobalamin absorption, since impaired absorption of the vitamin has been described in association with transcobalamin II deficiency (56). Still lacking is experimental evidence that directly indicates that transcobalamin II is required for efficient ileal transport of cobalamin. In one study which examined portal rather than systemic plasma, newly absorbed cobalamin appeared to be bound to a macromolecule that differed from both intrinsic factor and transcobalamin II (34).

SUMMARY

Cobalamin is a vitamin that is synthesized by microorganisms and is crucial for normal division and viability of mammalian cells. Yet mammalian tissues cannot synthesize this essential nutrient, and cobalamin does not readily diffuse through biologic membranes because of its large molecular size and hydrophilic properties. We are gradually beginning to understand how the mammalian organism assimilates cobalamin and delivers it to cells that require it while simultaneously rejecting structurally similar but biologically inactive, possibly harmful cobalamin analogs that are also synthesized by microorganisms. Effective absorption and transport of the vitamin depends on its ability to bind avidly and specifically to at least three distinct mammalian transport proteins: intrinsic factor, transcobalamin II, and the R proteins. Each of these transport proteins forms a stable macromolecular complex with cobalamin and then attaches to its specific membrane receptor located on the surface of cells. Attachment to the membrane receptor is immediate; it does not require cellular energy, but it does involve divalent cations. Surface attachment is followed by a slower, energy-dependent process that transfers cobalamin into the cell. In the case of transcobalamin II-mediated transport at least, this process appears to involve endocytosis of the intact protein-cobalamin complex followed by lysosomal degradation of transcobalamin II and release of cobalamin.

Intrinsic factor recognizes and binds cobalamin but rejects virtually all cobalamin analogs. The intrinsic factor-cobalamin complex is delivered to the distal small bowel, where it attaches to specific receptors that are found only on the microvillous membranes of ileal absorptive cells. How cobalamin enters and traverses the ileal cell remains poorly understood, but the newly absorbed vitamin immediately binds to transcobalamin II. This plasma polypeptide turns over rapidly and appears to modulate the delivery of cobalamin to cells that require it. Surface membrane receptors for transcobalamin II are present on all cells thus far examined. Since transcobalamin II binds very few cobalamin analogs, this transport protein prevents cellular uptake of any analogs that may have gained access to the circulation. R proteins, on the other hand, bind a wide variety of cobalamin analogs in addition to cobalamin itself, and receptors for this family of glycoproteins appear to be present only on the surface of liver cells. The R proteins appear to function primarily to bind excessive cobalamin or unwanted cobalamin analogs for storage and ultimate excretion via the liver.

Just as clinical investigations have always played a key role in uncovering fascinating processes responsible for the transport of cobalamin, observations in patients continue to point out aspects still to be clarified. Patients with selective familial cobalamin malabsorption, for example, fail to assimilate the vitamin, although they absorb all other nutrients normally (53). These patients secrete ample amounts of functionally active intrinsic factor, and cobalamin malabsorption is not corrected by pancreatic extract or by antibiotics. Moreover, their ileal mucosal receptors effectively take up intrinsic factor-bound cobalamin, and plasma levels of trans-cobalamin II are normal (91). It is apparent that some crucial step in the transfer of the vitamin into, across, or out of the ileal absorptive cell is defective in these patients. Identification of this specific defect will undoubtedly enhance our understanding of how cobalamin is absorbed normally.

REFERENCES

1. Abels, J., and Schilling, R. F. (1964): Protection of intrinsic factors by vitamin B_{12}. *J. Lab. Clin. Med.*, 60:375–384.
2. Addison, T. (1855): *On the Constitutional and Local Effects of Disease of the Suprarenal Capsules.* Samuel Highley, London.
3. Allen, R. H. (1975): Human vitamin B_{12}-transport proteins. *Prog. Hematol.*, 9:57–84.
4. Allen, R. H., and Majerus, P. W. (1972): Isolation of vitamin B_{12}-binding proteins using affinity chromatography. III. Purification and properties of human plasma transcobalamin II. *J. Biol. Chem.*, 247:7709–7717.
5. Allen, R. H., and Mehlman, C. S. (1973): Isolation of gastric vitamin B_{12}-binding proteins using affinity chromatography. I. Purification and properties of human intrinsic factor. *J. Biol. Chem.*, 248:3660–3669.
6. Allen, R. H., and Mehlman, C. S. (1973): Isolation of gastric vitamin B_{12}-binding proteins using affinity chromatography. II. Purification and properties of hog intrinsic factor and hog nonintrinsic factor. *J. Biol. Chem.*, 248:3670–3680.
7. Allen, R. H., Seetharam, B., Podell, E., and Alpers, D. H. (1978): Effect of proteolytic enzymes on the binding of cobalamin to R protein and intrinsic factor. In vitro evidence that a failure to partially degrade R protein is responsible for cobalamin malabsorption in pancreatic insufficiency. *J. Clin. Invest.*, 61:47–54.
8. Allen, R. H., Seetharam, B., Allen, N. C., Podell, E. R., and Alpers, D. H. (1978): Correction of cobalamin malabsorption in pancreatic insufficiency with a cobalamin analogue that binds with high affinity to R protein but not to intrinsic factor. In vivo evidence that a failure to partially degrade R protein is responsible for cobalamin malabsorption in pancreatic insufficiency. *J. Clin. Invest.*, 61:1628–1634.
9. Andrews, P. (1965): The gel-filtration behavior of proteins related to their molecular weights over a wide range. *Biochem. J.*, 96:595–606.
10. Ardeman, S., and Chanarin, I. (1963): A method of the assay of human gastric intrinsic factor and for the detection of titration of antibodies against intrinsic factor. *Lancet*, 2:1350–1354.
11. Ardeman, S., Chanarin, I., and Doyle, J. C. (1964): Studies on secretion of gastric intrinsic factor in man. *Br. Med. J.*, 2:600–603.
12. Ashwell, G., and Morell, A. G. (1974): The role of surface carbohydrates in the hepatic recognition and transport of circulating glycoproteins. *Adv. Enzymol.*, 41:99–128.
13. Beck, W. S. (1975): Metabolic features of cobalamin deficiency in man. In: *Cobalamin: Biochemistry and Pathophysiology*, edited by B. M. Babior, pp. 403–450. Wiley, New York.
14. Binder, H. J., and Donaldson, R. M. (1978): Effect of cimetidine on intrinsic factor and pepsin secretion in man. *Gastroenterology*, 74:535–539.
15. Booth, C. C. (1967): Sites of absorption in the small intestine. *Fed. Proc.*, 26:1583–1588.
16. Booth, C. C., and Mollin, D. L. (1956): Plasma, tissue and urinary radioactivity after oral administration of ^{58}Co-labeled vitamin B_{12}. *Br. J. Haematol.*, 2:223–236.
17. Brown, J., Robertson, J., and Gallagher, N. (1977): Humoral regulation of vitamin B_{12} absorption by pregnant mouse small intestine. *Gastroenterology*, 72:881–885.
18. Brugge, W. R., Goff, J. S., Podell, E., Allen, N. C., and Allen, R. H. (1980): Development of a dual label Schilling test for pancreatic exocrine function based on the differential absorption of

cobalamin bound to intrinsic factor and R protein. *Gastroenterology*, 78:937–941.
19. Burger, R. L., and Allen, R. H. (1974): Characterization of vitamin B_{12}-binding proteins isolated from human milk and saliva by affinity chromatography. *J. Biol. Chem.*, 249:7220–7227.
20. Burger, R. L., Mehlman, C. S., and Allen, R. H. (1975): Human plasma R-type vitamin B_{12} binding protein. I. Isolation and characterization of transcobalamin I, trancobalamin III and the normal granulocyte vitamin B_{12} binding protein. *J. Biol. Chem.*, 250:7700–7706.
21. Burger, R. L., Schneider, R. J., Mehlman, C. S., and Allen, R. H. (1975): Human plasma R-type vitamin B_{12} binding protein. II. The role of transcobalamin I, transcobalamin III and the normal granulocyte vitamin B_{12}-binding protein in the plasma transport of vitamin B_{12}. *J. Biol. Chem.*, 250:7707–7713.
22. Bynum, T. E., and Johnson, L. R. (1975): Stimulation of human pepsin output by topical hydrochloric acid. *Am. J. Dig. Dis.*, 20:607–612.
23. Callender, S. T. (1972): The parietal cell and intrinsic factor. In: *Recent Advances in Gastroenterology*, edited by J. Badenoch and B. N. Brooke, pp. 162–172. Churchill Livingston, Edinburgh.
24. Callender, S. T., and Evans, J. R. (1955): Observtions on the relationship of intrinsic factor to the absorption of labelled vitamin B_{12} from the intestine. *Clin. Sci.*, 14:387–393.
25. Carmel, R., and Herbert, V. (1969): Deficiency of vitamin B_{12}-binding alpha globulin in two brothers. *Blood*, 33:1–12.
26. Carmel, R., and Herbert, V. (1972): Vitamin B_{12}-binding protein of leukocytes as a possible major source of the third vitamin B_{12}-binding protein of serum. *Blood*, 40:542–549.
27. Castle, W. B. (1929): Observations on the etiologic relationship of achylia gastrica to pernicious anemia. *Am. J. Med. Sci.*, 178:748–764.
28. Castle, W. B. (1975): The history of corrinoids. In: *Cobalamin: Biochemistry and Pathophysiology*, edited by B. M. Babior, pp. 1–17. Wiley, New York.
29. Chanarin, I., Muir, M., Hughes, A., and Hoffbrand, A. V. (1978): Evidence for intestinal origin of transcobalamin II during vitamin B_{12} absorption. *Br. Med. J.*, 1:1453–1455.
30. Citrin, Y., DeRosa, C., and Halsted, J. A. (1957): Sites of absorption of vitamin B_{12}. *J. Lab. Clin. Med.*, 50:667–672.
31. Cooksley, W. G. E., England, J. M., Louis, L., Down, M. C., and Tavill, A. S. (1974): Hepatic vitamin B_{12} release and transcobalamin II synthesis in the rat. *Clin. Sci. Mol. Med.*, 47:531–545.
32. Cooper, B. A., and Castle, W. B. (1960): Sequential mechanisms in the enhanced absorption of vitamin B_{12} by intrinsic factor in the rat. *J. Clin. Invest.*, 39:199–214.
33. Cooper, B. A., and Paranchych, W. (1961): Selective uptake of specifically bound cobalt-58 vitamin B_{12} by human and mouse tumor cells. *Nature*, 191:393–395.
34. Cooper, B. A., and White, J. J. (1968): Absence of intrinsic factor from human portal plasma during 57 Co B_{12} absorption in man. *Br. J. Haematol.*, 14:73–78.
35. Darby, W. J. (1958): Vitamin B_{12} requirement of adult man. *Am. J. Med.*, 25:726–732.
36. Donaldson, R. M. (1962): Malabsorption of labeled cyanocobalamin in rats with intestinal diverticula. I. Evaluation of possible mechanisms. *Gastroenterology*, 43:271–281.
37. Donaldson, R. M., Corrigan, H., and Natsios, G. (1962): Malabsorption of labeled cyanocobalamin in rats with intestinal diverticula. II. Studies on contents of the diverticula. *Gastroenterology*, 43:282–290.
38. Donaldson, R. M. (1975): Mechanisms of malabsorption of cobalamin. In: *Cobalamin: Biochemistry and Pathophysiology*, edited by B. M. Babior, pp. 335–368. Wiley, New York.
39. Donaldson, R. M. (1977): Intestinal transport of cobalamin. In: *Intestinal Permeation*, edited by M. Kramer and F. Lauterbach, pp. 363–376. Excerpta Medica, Amsterdam.
40. Donaldson, R. M., Brand, M., and Serfilippi, D. (1977): Changes in circulating transcobalamin II after injection of cyanocobalamin. *N. Engl. J. Med.*, 296:1427–1430.
41. Donaldson, R. M., Mackenzie, I. L., and Trier, J. S. (1967): Intrinsic factor-mediated attachment of vitamin B_{12} to brush

borders and microvillous membranes of hamster intestine. *J. Clin. Invest.*, 46:1215–1228.

42. Donaldson, R. M., Small, D. M., Robins, S., and Mathan, V. I. (1973): Receptors for vitamin B_{12} related to ileal surface area and absorptive capacity. *Biochim. Biophys. Acta*, 311:477–481.

43. Doscherholmer, A., Hagen, P. S., and Liu, M. (1957): A dual mechanism of vitamin B_{12} plasma absorption. *J. Clin. Invest.*, 36:1551–1557.

44. Doscherholmer, A., Hagen, P. S., and Olin, L. (1959): Delay of absorption of radiolabeled cyanocobalamin in the intestinal wall in the presence of intrinsic factor. *J. Lab. Clin. Med.*, 54:434–439.

45. Doscherholmer, A., and Swain, W. R. (1973): Impaired absorption of egg Co^{57} vitamin B_{12} in patients with hypochlorhydria and achlorhydria and after gastric resection. *Gastroenterology*, 64:913–919.

46. Ellenbogen, L. E. (1979): Uptake and transport of cobalamins. *Int. Rev. Biochem.*, 27:45–96.

47. Finkler, A. E., and Hall, C. A. (1967): Nature of the relationship between vitamin B_{12} binding and cell uptake. *Arch. Biochem. Biophys.*, 120:79–85.

48. Fisher, J. M., and Taylor, K. B. (1969): The intracellular localization of castle's intrinsic factor by immunofluorescent technique using autoantibodies. *Immunology*, 16:779–786.

49. Friedmann, H. C. (1975): Biosynthesis of corrinoids. In: *Cobalamin: Biochemistry and Pathophysiology*, edited by B. M. Babior, pp. 75–109. Wiley, New York.

50. Friedman, P. A., Shia, M. A., and Wallace, J. K. (1977): A saturable high affinity binding site for transcobalamin II-vitamin B_{12} complexes in human placental membrane preparations. *J. Clin. Invest.*, 59:51–58.

51. Glass, G. B. J. (1974): *Gastric Intrinsic Factor and Other Vitamin B_{12} Binders*. Georg Thieme, Stuttgart.

52. Gräsbeck, R. (1969): Intrinsic factor and other vitamin B_{12} transport proteins. *Prog. Hematol.*, 6:233–260.

53. Gräsbeck, R., Gordin, R., Kantero, I., and Kuhlback, (1960): Selective vitamin B_{12} malabsorption and proteinuria in young people, a syndrome. *Acta Med. Scand.*, 167:289–296.

54. Gullberg, R. (1971): Sensitive test for antibody type I to intrinsic factor. *Clin. Exp. Immunol.*, 9:833–840.

55. Hagedorn, C. H., and Alpers, D. H. (1977): Distribution of intrinsic factor-vitamin B_{12} receptors in human intestine. *Gastroenterology*, 73:1010–1022.

56. Hakami, N., Neiman, P. E., Canellos, G. P., and Lagerson, J. (1971): Neonatal megaloblastic anemia due to inherited transcobalamin II deficiency in two siblings. *N. Engl. J. Med.*, 285:1163–1170.

57. Hall, C. A. (1975): Transcobalamins I and II as natural transport proteins of vitamin B_{12}. *J. Clin. Invest.*, 56:1125–1131.

58. Hall, C. A., and Finkler, A. E. (1965): The dynamics of transcobalamin II: A vitamin B_{12} binding substance in plasma. *J. Lab. Clin. Med.*, 65:459–468.

59. Halsted, J. A., Gassten, M., and Drenick, E. J. (1954): Absorption of radioactive vitamin B_{12} after total gastrectomy. *N. Engl. J. Med.*, 251:161–164.

60. Heinle, R. W., Welch, A. D., Scharf, V., Meacham, G. C., and Prusoff, W. H. (1952): Studies of excretion and absorption of Co^{60}-labeled vitamin B_{12} in pernicious anemia. *Trans. Assoc. Am. Phys.*, 65:214–222.

61. Hellegers, A., Okuda, K., Nesbitt, R. E. L., Smith, D. W., and Chow, B. F. (1957): Vitamin B_{12} absorption in pregnancy and in the newborn. *Am. J. Clin. Nutr.*, 5:327–331.

62. Hines, J. D. (1966): Megaloblastic anemia in an adult vegan. *Am. J. Clin. Nutr.*, 19:260–268.

63. Hippe, E., Haber, E., and Olesen, H. (1971): Nature of vitamin B_{12} binding. II. Steric orientation of vitamin B_{12} on binding and number of combining sites of human intrinsic factor and the transcobalamins. *Biochim. Biophys. Acta*, 243:75–82.

64. Hippe, E., and Olesen, H. (1971): Nature of vitamin B_{12} binding. III. Thermodynamics of binding to human intrinsic factor and transcobalamins. *Biochim. Biophys. Acta*, 243:83–89.

65. Hoedemaker, P. J., Abels, J., Wachters, J. J., Arends, A., and Nieweg, H. O. (1966): Investigations about the site of production of Castle's gastric intrinsic factor. *Lab. Invest.*, 15:1163–1171.

66. Hogenkamp, H. P. C. (1975): The chemistry of cobalamins and related compounds. In: *Cobalamin: Biochemistry and Pathophysiology*, edited by B. M. Babior, pp. 21–73. Wiley, New York.

67. Hom, B. L. (1967): Plasma turnover of ^{57}Cobalt-vitamin B_{12} bound to transcobalamin I and II. *Scand. J. Haematol.*, 4:321–332.

68. Hooper, D. C., Alpers, D. H., Mehlman, C. S., and Allen, R. H. (1973): Characterization of ileal vitamin B_{12}-binding using homogeneous human and hog intrinsic factors. *J. Clin. Invest.*, 52:3074–3083.

69. IUPAC-IUB Commission on Biochemical Nomenclature (1974): The nomenclature of corrinoids (1973 recommendations). *Biochemistry*, 13:1555–1560.

70. Jeffries, G. H., and Sleisenger, M. H. (1965): The pharmacology of intrinsic factor secretion in man. *Gastroenterology*, 48:444–448.

71. Johnson, L. R. (1972): Regulation of pepsin secretion by topical acid in the stomach. *Am. J. Physiol.*, 223:847–850.

72. Kapadia, C. R., Bhat, P., Jacob, E., and Baker, S. J. (1975): Vitamin B_{12} absorption—a study of intraluminal events in control subjects and in patients with topical sprue. *Gut*, 16:988–993.

73. Kapadia, C. R., and Donaldson, R. M. (1978): Macromolecular secretion by isolated gastric mucosa. Fundamental differences in pepsinogen and intrinsic factor secretion. *Gastroenterology*, 74:535–539.

74. Kapadia, C. R., Schafer, D. E., Donaldson, R. M., and Ebersole, E. R. (1979): Evidence for involvement of cyclic nucleotides in intrinsic factor secretion by isolated rabbit gastric mucosa. *J. Clin. Invest.*, 63:1044–1049.

75. Kapadia, C. R., Serfilippi, D., and Donaldson, R. M. (1979): Uptake of biosynthetically labeled intrinsic factor by isolated ileal cells. *Clin. Res.*, 27:455A (Abstr.).

76. Katz, J. H., Dimase, J., and Donaldson, R. M. (1963): Simultaneous administration of gastric juice bound and free radioactive cyanocobalamin. *J. Lab. Clin. Med.*, 61:266–271.

77. Katz, M., and Cooper, B. A. (1974): Solubilized receptor for vitamin B_{12}-intrinsic factor complex from human intestine. *Br. J. Haematol.*, 26:569–578.

78. Katz, M., and Cooper, B. A. (1974): Solubilized receptor for intrinsic factor-vitamin B_{12} complex from guinea pig intestinal mucosa. *J. Clin. Invest.*, 54:733–739.

79. Katz, M., Lee, S. K., and Cooper, B. A. (1972): Vitamin B_{12} malabsorption to a biologically inert intrinsic factor. *N. Engl. J. Med.*, 287:425–429.

80. Katz, M., Mehlman, C. S., and Allen, R. H. (1974): Isolation and characterization of an abnormal human intrinsic factor. *J. Clin. Invest.*, 53:1274–1283.

81. Kolhouse, J. F., and Allen, R. H. (1977): Absorption, plasma transport, and cellular transport of cobalamin analogues in the rabbit. *J. Clin. Invest.*, 60:1381–1392.

82. Kolhouse, J. F., and Allen, R. H. (1977): Recognition of two intracellular cobalamin binding proteins and their identification as methylmalonyl-CoA mutase and methionine synthetase. *Proc. Natl. Acad. Sci. USA*, 74:921–925.

83. Kouvonen, I., and Grasbeck, R. (1979): A simplified technique to isolate porcine and human ileal intrinsic factor receptors and studies on their subunit structures. *Biochem. Biophys. Res. Commun.*, 86:358–364.

84. LaRusso, N. F., Korman, M. G., Hoffman, N. E., and Hofmann, A. F. (1974): Dynamics of the enterohepatic circulation of bile acids. *N. Engl. J. Med.*, 291:689–692.

85. Levine, J. S., Nakane, P. K., and Allen, R. H. (1980): Immunocytochemical localization of human intrinsic factor: The nonstimulated stomach. *Gastroenterology*, 79:493–502.

86. Linnell, J. C. (1975): The fate of cobalamin in vivo. In: *Cobalamin: Biochemistry and Pathophysiology*, edited by B. M. Babior, pp. 287–335. Wiley, New York.

87. Lowenstein, F. (1958): Absorption of cobalt ^{60}-labeled vitamin B_{12} after subtotal gastrectomy. *Blood*, 13:339–348.

88. MacDonald, R. M., Ingelfinger, F. J., and Belding, H. W. (1947): Late effects of total gastrectomy in man. *N. Engl. J. Med.*, 237:887–890.

89. Mackenzie, I. L., and Donaldson, R. M. (1972): Effect of divalent cations and pH on intrinsic factor-mediated attachment

of vitamin B_{12} to intestinal microvillons membranes. *J. Clin. Invest.*, 51:2465–2471.

90. Mackenzie, I. L., Donaldson, R. M., and Schilling, R. F. (1968): Radioiodination of human intrinsic factor. *J. Clin. Invest.*, 48:516–524.

91. Mackenzie, I. L., Donaldson, R. M., Trier, J. S., and Mathan, V. I. (1972): Ileal mucosa in familial selective vitamin B_{12} malabsorption. *N. Engl. J. Med.*, 286:1021–1025.

92. Mahoney, M. J., and Rosenberg, L. E. (1975): Inborn errors of cobalamin metabolism. In: *Cobalamin: Biochemistry and Pathophysiology*, edited by B. M. Babior, pp. 369–402. Wiley, New York.

93. Marcoullis, G., and Grasbeck, R. (1977): Solubilized intrinsic factor receptor from pig ileum and its characteristics. *Biochim. Biophys. Acta*, 496:36–51.

94. Mathan, V. I., Babior, B. M., and Donaldson, R. M. (1974): Kinetics of the attachment of intrinsic factor-bound cobamides to ileal receptors. *J. Clin. Invest.*, 54:598–608.

95. McIntyre, P. A., Sachs, M. V., Krevans, J. R., and Conley, C. L. (1956): Pathogenesis and treatment of macrocytic anemia: Information obtained with radioactive vitamin B_{12}. *Arch. Intern. Med.*, 98:541–549.

96. Mellman, I. S., Youngdahl-Turner, P., Willard, H. F., and Rosenberg, L. E. (1977): Intracellular binding of radioactive hydrocobalamin to cobalamin-dependent apoenzymes in rat liver. *Proc. Natl. Acad. Sci. USA*, 74:921–925.

97. Minot, G. R., and Murphy, W. P. (1926): Treatment of pernicious anemia by a special diet. *JAMA*, 87:470–475.

98. Newmark, P. (1971): Metabolism of vitamin B_{12} in the kidney at a subcellular level. In: *The Cobalamins*, edited by H. R. V. Arnstein and R. J. Wrighton, pp. 79–91. Churchill-Livingstone, Edinburgh.

99. Newmark, P., Newman, G. E., and O'Brien, J. R. P. (1970): Vitamin B_{12} in the rat kidney: Evidence for an association with lysosomes. *Arch. Biochem. Biophys.*, 141:121–130.

100. Okuda, K., and Sasayama, K. (1965): Intestinal distribution of intrinsic factor and vitamin B_{12} absorption. *Am. J. Physiol.*, 208:14–17.

101. Ostroy, F., and Gams, R. A. (1977): Cellular fluxes of vitamin B_{12}. *Blood*, 50:877–888.

102. Palade, G. E. (1975): Intracellular aspects of the process of protein synthesis. *Science*, 189:347–358.

103. Parmentier, Y., Marcoulis, G., and Wicolas, J. P. (1979): The intraluminal transport of vitamin B_{12} and the exocrine pancreatic insufficiency. *Proc. Soc. Exp. Biol. Med.*, 160:396–400.

104. Pelliniemi, T., and Beck, W. S. (1980): Biochemical mechanisms in the Killman experiment. *J. Clin. Invest.*, 65:449–460.

105. Peters, T. J., and Hoffbrand, A. V. (1970): Absorption of vitamin B_{12} by the guinea pig. I. Subcellular localization of vitamin B_{12} in the ileal enterocyte during absorption. *Br. J. Haematol.*, 19:369–382.

106. Peters, T., Linnell, J. C., Matthews, D. M., and Hoffbrand, A. V. (1971): Absorption of vitamin B_{12} in the guinea pig. III. The forms of vitamin B_{12} in ileal mucosa and portal plasma in the fasting state and during absorption of cyanocobalamin. *Br. J. Haematol.*, 20:299–305.

107. Pletsch, Q. A., and Coffey, J. W. (1971): Intracellular distribution of radioactive vitamin B_{12} in rat liver. *J. Biol. Chem.*, 246:4619–4629.

108. Pollycove, M., and Apt, L. (1956): Absorption, elimination and excretion of orally administered vitamin B_{12} in normal subjects and in patients with pernicious anemia. *N. Engl. J. Med.*, 255:207–212.

109. Rachmilewitz, B., Rachmilewitz, M., and Chaouat, M. (1978): The production of TC II—the vitamin B_{12} transport protein—by mouse mononuclear phagocytes. *Blood*, 52:1089–1097.

110. Rappazzo, M. E., and Hall, C. A. (1972): Transport function of transcobalamin II. *J. Clin. Invest.*, 51:1915–1918.

111. Reimann, F. (1931): Versuche zur Potenzierung der Wirkuns oral verabreichter Leber. *Med. Klin.*, 27:880–881.

112. Retief, F. P., Gottlieb, C. W., and Herbert, V. (1966): Mechanism of vitamin B_{12} uptake by erythrocytes. *J. Clin. Invest.*, 45:1907–1915.

113. Rickes, E. L., Brink, N. G., Koniuszy, F. R., Wood, T. R., and

Folkers, K. (1948): Crystalline vitamin B_{12}. *Science*, 107:396–397.

114. Robertson, J. A., and Gallagher, N. D. (1979): Effects of placental lactogen on the number of intrinsic factor receptors in the pregnant mouse. *Gastroenterology*, 77:511–517.

115. Rothenberg, S. P. (1968): Identification of a macromolecular factor in ileum which binds intrinsic factor. *J. Clin. Invest.*, 47:913–923.

116. Rothenberg, S. P., Weiss, J. P., and Colter, R. (1978): Formation of transcobalamin II-vitamin B_{12} complex by guinea pig ileal mucosa in organ culture after in vivo incubation with intrinsic factor-vitamin B_{12}. *Br. J. Haematol.*, 40:401–414.

117. Ryel, E. M., Meyer, L. M., and Gama, R. A. (1974): Uptake and subcellular distribution of vitamin B_{12} in mouse L1210 leukemic lymphoblasts. *Blood*, 44:427–433.

118. Samloff, I. M., Kleinman, M. D., Turner, M., Sobel, V., and Jeffries, G. H. (1968): Blocking and binding antibodies to intrinsic factor and parietal cell antibody in pernicious anemia. *Gastroenterology*, 55:575–583.

119. Schade, S. G., Abels, J., and Schilling, R. F. (1967): Studies on antibody to intrinsic factor. *J. Clin. Invest.*, 46:615–620.

120. Schade, S. G., Feick, P., Muckerheide, M., and Schilling, R. F. (1966): Occurrence in gastric juice of antibody to a complex of intrinsic factor and vitamin B_{12}. *N. Engl. J. Med.*, 275:528–531.

121. Schilling, R. F. (1953): Intrinsic factor studies. II. The effect of gastric juice on the urinary excretion of radioactivity after the oral administration of radioactive vitamin B_{12}. *J. Lab Clin. Med.*, 42:860–866.

122. Schneider, R. J., Mehlman, C. S., and Allen, R. H. (1976): The role and fate of rabbit and human transcobalamin II in the plasma transport of vitamin B_{12} in the rabbit. *J. Clin. Invest.*, 57:27–38.

123. Schneider, R. P., Donaldson, R. M., and Babior, B. M. (1974): Evidence for the solubilization of the intestinal intrinsic factor receptor by sonication of ileal brush borders. *Biochym. Biophys. Acta*, 373:58–65.

124. Scott, J. M., Bloomfield, F. J., Stebbins, R., and Herbert, V. (1974): Studies on the derivation of transcobalamin III from granulocytes. *J. Clin. Invest.*, 53:228–239.

125. Seligman, P. A., and Allen, R. H. (1978): Characterization of the receptor for transcobalamin II isolated from human placenta. *J. Biol. Chem.*, 253:1766–1772.

126. Serfilippi, D., and Donaldson, R. M. (1979): Biosynthesis of radiolabeled intrinsic factor by isolated gastric mucosa. *Gastroenterology*, 76:1241 (Abstr.).

127. Simons, K. (1964): Vitamin B_{12} binders in human body fluids and blood cells. *Commentat. Biol. Soc. Sci. Fenn.*, 27:1–94.

128. Smith, E. L. (1948): Purification of anti-pernicious anemia factor from liver. *Nature*, 161:638–639.

129. Soll, A. H. (1978): The actions of secretagogues on oxygen uptake by isolated mammalian parietal cells. *J. Clin. Invest.*, 61:370–380.

130. Strauss, E. W., Wilson, T. H., and Hotchkiss, A. (1960): Factors controlling B_{12} uptake by intestinal sacs *in vitro*. *Am. J. Physiol.*, 198:103–107.

131. Sutton, D., and Donaldson, R. M. (1975): Synthesis and secretion of pepsinogen by rabbit gastric mucosa. *Gastroenterology*, 69:166–174.

132. Toskes, P. P., and Deren, J. J. (1972): The role of the pancreas in vitamin B_{12} absorption: Studies of vitamin B_{12} absorption in partially pancreatectomized rats. *J. Clin. Invest.*, 51:216–223.

133. Toskes, P. P., and Deren, J. J. (1973): Vitamin B_{12} absorption and malabsorption. *Gastroenterology*, 65:662–683.

134. Toskes, P. P., Deren, J. J., and Conrad, M. E. (1972): Trypsin-like nature of the pancreatic factor that corrects vitamin B_{12} malabsorption associated with pancreatic dysfunction. *J. Clin. Invest.*, 52:1660–1672.

135. Toskes, P. P., Hansell, J., Cerda, J., and Deren, J. J. (1971): Vitamin B_{12} malabsorption in chronic pancreatic insufficiency. Studies suggesting the presence of a pancreatic "intrinsic factor." *N. Engl. J. Med.*, 248:627–632.

136. Toskes, P. P., Smith, G. W., Francis, G. M., and Sander, E. G. (1977): Evidence that pancreatic proteases enhance vitamin B_{12} absorption by acting on crude preparations of hog gas-

tric intrinsic factor and human gastric juice. *Gastroenterology,* 72:31–36.

137. Vatn, M. H., Schrumpf, E., and Myren, J. (1975): The effect of carbechol and pentagastrin on the gastric secretion of acid, pepsin and intrinsic factor in man. *Scand. J. Gastroenterol.,* 10:55–58.

138. Vecger, W., Abels, J., Hellemans, N., and Nieweg, H. O. (1962): Effect of sodium bicarbonate and pancreatin on the absorption of vitamin B_{12} and fat in pancreatic insufficiency. *N. Engl. J. Med.,* 267:1341–1344.

139. Weiser, M. M. (1973): Intestinal epithelial cell surface membrane glycoprotein synthesis. I. An indicator of cellular differentiation. *J. Biol. Chem.,* 245:2536–2541.

140. Weissberg, H., and Glass, G. B. J. (1966): A rapid quantitative method for measuring intestinal absorption of vitamin B_{12} in man using a double label hepatic uptake test. *J. Lab. Clin. Med.,* 68:163–172.

141. Witts, L. J. (1966): *The Stomach and Anemia.* Athlone Press, London.

142. Youngdahl-Turner, P., Mellman, I. S., Allen, R. H., and Rosenberg, L. E. (1979): Protein mediated vitamin uptake. Absorptive endocytosis of the transcobalamin II-cobalamin complex by cultured human fibroblasts. *Exp. Cell Res.,* 118:127–134.

143. Youngdahl-Turner, P., Rosenberg, L. E., and Allen, R. H. (1978): Binding and uptake of transcobalamin II by human fibroblasts. *J. Clin. Invest.,* 61:133–141.

Physiology of the Gastrointestinal Tract, edited by
Leonard R. Johnson. Raven Press, New York © 1981.

Chapter 23

Regulation of Gastric Acid Secretion

Morton I. Grossman

The aim of this chapter is to describe the mechanisms that operate to regulate acid secretion by the parietal cells of the gastric mucosa in the resting state and in response to meals. The description includes identification of (a) the agent initiating the change, (b) the site in the body where this initiator acts, (c) the paths by which the effect is conveyed to the parietal cells, and, insofar as they are known, (d) the stimulatory and inhibitory transmitters that are delivered to the parietal cells to produce the observed effect.

The classic division of gastric acid secretion into interdigestive and digestive periods and the further subdivision of the digestive period into cephalic, gastric, and intestinal phases is still useful for descriptive purposes. It must be emphasized, however, that the terms designating the phases refer only to the site at which initiators act and should not be taken to indicate any one mechanism. It was once thought that each phase had only one mechanism; for example, the cephalic phase was thought to be mediated solely by vagal cholinergic effects directly on the parietal cell. It is now known, however, that vagal release of gastrin is also involved. It is probably the rule rather than the exception that each initiator uses more than one mechanism in producing its effect on acid secretion. Thus initiators and sites should not be taken as designators of a single mechanism.

The activity of all cells of the body, including the acid-secreting parietal cells of the stomach, are regulated by chemical messengers. These chemical messengers move from their cells of origin to their targets by one of three modes of delivery, namely, neurocrine, endocrine, or paracrine (40). Three substances found in the body which are capable of acting directly on the parietal cell to stimulate acid secretion have been identified. These are acetylcholine, gastrin, and histamine. Each of these chemical messengers uses one of the three possible modes of delivery. Acetylcholine, released at or near the parietal cells by postganglionic neurons, is an example of neurocrine delivery. Gastrin, released by the G cells of the mucosa of the antrum and the first part of the duodenum into the blood which carries it to the parietal cells, is an example of endocrine delivery. Histamine, released from the mast-like cells of the lamina propria of the oxyntic (acid-secreting) mucosa into the extracellular fluid through which it diffuses to the adjacent parietal cells, is an example of paracrine delivery.

There is convincing evidence that all three of these substances participate in the physiological regulation of gastric acid secretion. In the case of acetylcholine and histamine, specific antagonists are available, namely, muscarinic antagonists, such as atropine, and histamine H_2 antagonists, such as cimetidine. Both atrophine and cimetidine strongly inhibit all physiological mechanisms of gastric acid secretion, including basal secretion and all three phases of the response to a meal (cephalic, gastric and intestinal) (43). Pharmacological antagonists, such as atropine and cimetidine, are specific only within defined dosage ranges. Even within these ranges, atropine and cimetidine inhibit all physiological mechanisms of acid secretion. No specific antagonist of gastrin is available, but its physiological role has been demonstrated by showing that the blood concentration of gastrin increases after ingestion of a meal composed of a mixture of amino acids and that causing a similar increase by infusing exogenous gastrin will stimulate acid secretion to a similar extent (31). Also, removal of the sources of gastrin, the antrum and the first part of the duodenum, decreases basal and meal-stimulated acid secretion (4).

When two of the three direct parietal cell stimulants (acetylcholine, gastrin, and histamine) act simultaneously, the response is greater than the sum of the responses to each of the two agents given separately, a phenomenon called potentiation. Various other definitions of potentiation have been used in the past, but this is the one most widely used at present (32). Potentiation may or may not produce maximal responses that are greater than the maximal responses to the agents given singly; conversely, greater maximal response to combinations than to single agents is not a reliable criterion of potentiation. In Heidenhain pouches in dogs, all three pairs (cholinomimetic-gastrin, cholinomimetic-histamine, and gastrin-histamine) have been shown to produce potentiation (38). In isolated parietal cells of dog, only the pairs involving histamine have been shown to produce potentiation, but potentiation of all three agents acting simultaneously has been found (95).

The mechanism by which potentiation occurs is not known. One proposal was that the occupation of one receptor, for example, the histamine receptor, might change the affinity or efficacy of another receptor, such as the gastrin receptor (43). Studies on isolated parietal cells of the stomach (96) and acinar cells of the pancreas (32), however, have shown that potentiation involves events beyond the receptor, but the exact locus or mechanism of potentiation is not yet known.

In dogs, atropine inhibits the response not only to cholinomimetic stimulants but also to gastrin and histamine (45). Similarly, cimetidine inhibits the response not only to histamine but also to gastrin (43) and cholinomimetics (42). Also, vagotomy decreases the response to both gastrin and histamine (23). These findings suggest that during the basal state, the parietal cells are exposed to a constant background of acetylcholine and histamine, which sensitize them to additional amounts of these agents, or of gastrin. Thus the inhibition by atropine of the responses to exogenous gastrin or histamine could be seen as withdrawal of the sensitizing action of the basal background acetylcholine. Similarly, the inhibition by cimetidine of the responses to exogenous gastrin and cholinomimetics can be viewed as removal of the potentiating action of basal background histamine.

Since acetylcholine and histamine are always present as a potentiating background, counteracting them with atropine or cimetidine would be expected to (and indeed does) interfere with all physiological modes of gastric acid stimulation. Such interference does not tell us whether the antagonist has acted only against the basal background amount of agonist or whether additional amounts of agonist have been released in the situation under study. For example, cimetidine markedly inhibits acid secretion in response to sham feeding. This tells us that histamine is involved in the response. It does not tell us whether the histamine involved is only the basal background histamine or an additional amount of histamine that has been released by the sham feeding. Only in the case of gastrin, in which blood concentrations can be measured by radioimmunoassay, can we determine whether a certain mechanism of stimulation involves additional release of the agent. At present, no methods are available for determining how much of the acetylcholine or histamine that is stored in the gastric mucosa is being released and presented to the parietal at any given moment. We infer from the effects of atropine and cimetidine on exogenous stimulants that acetylcholine and histamine are being constantly released as a basal background, but we do not know how much of additional amounts of these stores have been released and are available to stimulate the parietal cells after any given mode of stimulation.

Two of the three direct parietal cell stimulants, namely, gastrin and acetylcholine, act both as basal background sensitizers of the parietal cell and as phasic stimulants. Gastrin is present in blood in the basal state, and large increases in its concentration in blood occur in response to eating. From the observation that atropine inhibits acid secretion evoked by exogenous gastrin or histamine, we deduce that acetylcholine is delivered continously to the parietal cells. Activation of vagal reflexes during the cephalic and gastric phases of the response to eating is assumed to increase the delivery of acetylcholine to the parietal cells to levels substantially above basal rates. In the case of the third direct stimulant, histamine, there is strong evidence that it is delivered to the parietal cell as a continous basal background, since histamine H_2 antagonists inhibit acid secretion evoked by stimulants, such as exogenous gastrin. There is, however, no convincing evidence that phasic increase in histamine release occurs in most species during stimulation of acid secretion by eating or by exogenous stimulants. Acetylcholine and gastrin release histamine from frog gastric mucosa (86), and gastrin releases histamine from gastric mucosa in rat and a few related species (55); but this has not been seen in humans or dogs. The demonstration that the parietal cell of the dog has receptors for each of the three primary stimulants (96) disposes of the once widely held hypothesis that histamine is the sole final common chemical mediator for all stimulants of acid secretion (10). The question of whether an increase in the rate of histamine release and delivery to the parietal cell is one of the factors involved in the physiological regulation of gastric secretion awaits the application of more refined methods to the problem.

The same line of reasoning applies to the effects of

vagotomy and antrectomy. The finding that a certain mechanism of acid secretion is depressed by vagotomy cannot be taken to mean that the mechanism entails an increase in vagal activity. The depression may be due to removal of basal background activity. The same principle applies to the effect of antrectomy on a mechanism of acid secretion. Only if the mechanism is completely abolished by a procedure such as vagotomy or antrectomy, rather than merely being decreased, can one assume that the structure that was ablated plays more than a permissive role in the mechanism in question.

It is likely that additional direct stimulants of the parietal cell remain to be discovered. In particular, the hypothetical hormone of the intestinal phase, enterooxyntin, has not yet been isolated. A large number of chemical messengers that inhibit acid secretion are known, including norepinephrine, epinephrine, dopamine, serotonin, secretin, vasoactive intestinal peptide, glucagon, somatostatin, and calcitonin. The physiological role of these inhibitors is unknown, and we do not know whether they act directly on the parietal cell.

The mechanisms of gastric acid secretion have been studied more extensively in dog than in any other species. Results obtained from those studies are the basis for most of the descriptions in this chapter. When important species differences are known to exist, they will be pointed out. The stomach in a 20-kg dog is about the same size as that in a 70-kg man and has about the same number of parietal cells (about 1 billion) and about the same maximal capacity to secrete acid (about 22 mmoles hr^{-1}) (72).

PHASES OF GASTRIC SECRETION AND THEIR MECHANISMS

Basal Secretion

Basal or interdigestive secretion is that which occurs in the absence of all intestinal stimulation. It is usually studied at least 6 hr after the stomach has emptied to ensure that the intestinal phase of secretion is over. Recently, there has been reconfirmation (74) of the observation (33) that complete emptying of a meal of solid food from the stomach of dog normally takes about 12 hr, compared with about 4 hr in man (71). Failure to appreciate this slow emptying in dogs has probably led to observations being made under what were assumed to be basal conditions but in fact were not. Despite this error, dogs have usually been found to have a low rate of basal secretion, in comparison with other species. Hirschowitz (44) found that basal acid secretion was detected in only about one in 20 gastric fistula dogs. Most studies report low levels of basal acid secretion in dog (about 0.1 mmoles hr^{-1}, which is less than 1% of maximal capacity). In rat, basal secretion is about 30% of maximal capacity (82), whereas in man, it is about

10% (110). Wyrwicka and Garcia (111) recently found that gastric fistula cats secreted about 0.2% of their maximal capacity when unrestrained in cages but secreted about 3.7% of maximal capacity when restrained in the kind of harness usually used for collecting secretion.

In both dogs (2) and humans (34), basal acid secretion is reduced but not abolished by vagotomy. Addition of antrectomy to the vagotomy further decreases basal secretion to near zero levels in both dogs (49) and humans (5). In some species, such as *Rana catesbiana,* high rates of basal secretion continue, even after the mucosa is isolated in an *in vitro* chamber (58), indicating that it is independent of both hormones and extrinsic nerves. Certain glands and muscles exhibit spontaneous activity of this kind as an inherent property of the particular tissue (41).

Basal secretion in man shows a circadian rhythm characterized by a high rate in the evening and a low rate in the morning. The cause of this circadian variation is unknown; it is not accompanied by a corresponding change in blood gastrin concentration (75).

In dogs with gastric fistulas, the rate of basal acid secretion was about twice as great during the activity front of the interdigestive myoelectric complex as during other times (98), but even this enhanced rate amounted to only about 0.2% of the maximal rate.

Cephalic Phase

The cephalic phase (Table 1) is that gastric secretion evoked by agents acting in the region of the head. It is mediated entirely by the vagus nerves and is eliminated by vagotomy.

Initiators of the Cephalic Phase

The initiators of the cephalic phase include the components that occur during the experimental procedure called sham feeding in which food is chewed but is not allowed to enter the stomach, being either spit out or diverted to the outside by an esophageal fistula. Food must be used as the stimulus; sham drinking of water is ineffective (80). Few studies have been done on the relative effectiveness of various kinds of food. For example, it is not known whether meals consisting only of carbohydrate or only of fat would be effective or whether protein is required. The magnitude of the response increases as the duration of sham feeding increases. In dogs with innervated antral pouches, the response of the main stomach to sham feeding for 100 min was about equal to the maximal response to exogenous gastrin (84). By contrast, the maximal response that has been attained to sham feeding in man is about 40% of the maximal response to exogenous pentagastrin (29).

TABLE 1. *Sites, initiators, paths to parietal cell, and mediators at parietal cell*

Site	Initiator	Path	Mediator at parietal cell
Head	Feeding, sham or real[a]	Direct vagal Vagal-antral gastrin-blood[b]	Acetylcholine Gastrin
	Impairment of supply or utilization of glucose by brain[a]		
Stomach	Distention[a,c]	Vagovagal reflexes (same two efferent paths as for feeding) Local intramural reflexes (same two postganglionic paths as for feeding)	
	Calcium, amino acids, peptides	Release of gastrin into blood by topical action on G cells	Gastrin
Intestine	Distention	At least in part by release into blood of unidentified hormone	Enterooxyntin
	Amino acids and peptides	At least in part by amino acids absorbed into blood	Amino acids

[a] In mechanisms involving both direct neural action on the parietal cell and neural release of gastrin, the relative importance of these two components varies with species, initiators, and conditions of testing.

[b] The mediator for release of gastrin from antral G cells by vagal or local reflexes has not been identified.

[c] See Table 2 for a further analysis of gastric reflexes initiated by distention.

A conditioned reflex can be established by appropriate pairing of an unconditioned stimulus, such as food, with a conditioned stimulus, such as the sound of a bell. The conditioned stimulus will become extinguished unless it is periodically reinforced. Little is known about the minimal requirements for initiating the unconditioned reflex or about the central pathways involved in the response to sham feeding.

Another initiator of cephalic stimulation of gastric secretion of acid is interference with the supply of glucose to the brain. This can be initiated by hypoglycemia induced by exogenous insulin (4) or by release of endogenous insulin by agents such as tolbutamide (108), or by giving analogs of glucose which cannot be metabolized. The most potent of these agents is 2-deoxy-D-glucose (48), which gives a maximal response about equal to that of gastrin in dogs (23) and humans (25).

There is evidence that 2-deoxy-D-glucose may act at more than one site to stimulate acid secretion. Kadekaro et al. (57) have proposed that it acts at hypothalamic, diencephalic, and medullary sites in the brain, as well as at hepatic sites in the periphery, with the vagal outflow as the final common efferent path.

Mechanism of the Cephalic Phase

In dogs, truncal vagotomy permanently abolishes responses to cephalic phase stimuli, such as 2-deoxy-D-glucose. By contrast, cutting only those branches of vagus that go to the acid-secreting part of the stomach (proximal gastric vagotomy) completely abolished the response to 2-deoxy-D-glucose for a few months, but recovery began by 6 months and by 16 months had sta-

bilized at about 60% of the prevagotomy level (46). After all forms of vagotomy in humans, a few patients show a small response to stimuli, such as insulin, in the immediate postoperative period. The number of responders increases during the first 2 years, by which time more than half the patients have some response to insulin (56). Even in those who show some response to insulin, however, it is usually much smaller than the preoperative response. The maximal response to pentagastrin in these insulin-positive subjects is reduced by about 50%, about the same as in the insulin-negative subjects (35). Whether the responses to cephalic phase stimulants that occur in man early after vagotomy are caused by missed vagal fibers or a nonvagal mechanism is not known. The recovery of response with time in dogs after selective vagotomy and in humans after all types of vagotomy may be attributable to regeneration of nerves, possibly by sprouting from uncut fibers, but this has not been established. Because the responses to all forms of cephalic phase stimulation are completely abolished in most subjects in the early period after vagotomy, we assume that the cephalic phase is mediated solely by the vagus nerves.

Uvnas (104) introduced the notion that vagal impulses activate gastric acid secretion by two mechanisms, a direct action on the parietal cells and an indirect action by release of gastrin from antral mucosa. Between 1942 when Uvnas first proposed this hypothesis and 1968 when the first reliable radioimmunoassay for plasma gastrin was introduced by McGuigan and Trudeau (73), the possible release of gastrin by cephalic phase stimuli could be monitored only by its effect on acid secretion. In dog, sham feeding causes an increase in the plasma concentration of gastrin (Fig. 1), as measured by radioimmunoassay (76,103). The increment in response to sham feeding is about half as great as that to a mixed meal. In man, some investigators (30) have found an increase in plasma gastrin concentration in response to sham feeding; others have not (100). (A fuller discussion of this topic is presented in the chapter by Richardson).

Large doses of atropine decrease gastrin release produced by sham feeding in dogs (76,103). Such large doses may produce nonspecific effects, and the effects of smaller doses that could be presumed to be more specific have not yet been reported. In cats (106), release of gastrin by electrical stimulation of the vagi is not inhibited by atropine. In humans, small doses of atropine augment gastrin release in response to sham feeding (30) and to insulin hypoglycemia (26). The failure of small doses of atropine to block vagal release of gastrin suggests that the muscarinic action of acetylcholine is not the mediator of this effect. Bombesin has been proposed as the possible mediator because it is present in antral mucosa (107) and because it releases gastrin by an atropine-resistant mechanism (51).

Sham feeding releases more gastrin in dog than in man; correspondingly, acid secretion in response to sham feeding appears to be more dependent on gastrin in dog than in man. Thus, in dogs, antrectomy does not reduce the response to exogenous gastrin but reduces the acid secretion in response to sham feeding by about 70% (84). In humans, antrectomy reduces the response to exogenous gastrin and to sham feeding by about 50% (60). In dogs, infusing a subthreshold dose of gastrin restores the acid secretion in response to sham feeding to its preantrectomy level (77), whereas in humans, infusion of gastrin does not restore the response (60).

The postganglionic neuroeffector mediator of direct vagal stimulation of the parietal cells is presumed to be a muscarinic action of acetylcholine. Atropine abolished acid secretion in response to sham feeding in dogs (76) and greatly reduces the response in humans (30). The failure of atropine to abolish completely acid secretion in response to sham feeding in man may or may not indicate that a mediator in addition to acetylcholine is involved.

As reviewed above, removal of the main sources of gastrin, the antrum and the first part of the duodenum, reduces but does not abolish acid secretion in response to sham feeding in man and dog. This indicates that neither vagal release of gastrin nor basal background gastrin is essential for direct vagal activation of the parietal cells. Thus the direct vagal-parietal component can operate in the absence of the vagal-gastrin component. Is the converse also true? Can the vagal-gastrin mechanism stimulate acid secretion in the absence of the vagal-parietal component? In man, when the acid-secreting part of the stomach is vagally denervated but the vagal innervation to the antrum is left intact, sham feeding causes a greater release of gastrin than before parietal call vagotomy, but no acid secretory response is seen (28). This may be because the sensitivity of the parietal cells to gastrin is reduced by vagotomy. Studies in dogs, however, indicate that an additional factor may be involved. Physiologists have long been puzzled by the observation that the gastrin released by sham feeding produces little or no stimulation of acid secretion from a Heidenhain pouch. For example, in dogs with vagally innervated antral pouches, sham feeding released substantial amounts of gastrin but failed to stimulate acid secretion from a Heidenhain pouch (103). Based on this

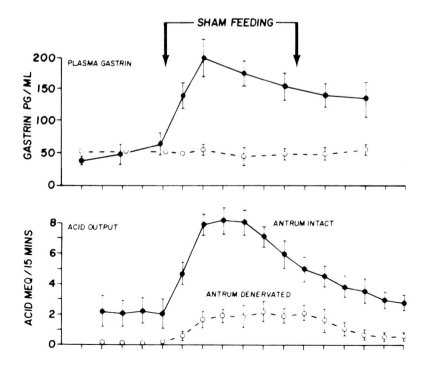

FIG. 1. Effect of sham feeding on plasma gastrin concentration and acid output from a vagally innervated gastric fistula in dogs with vagally innervated antral pouches. Studies were done before and after vagal denervation of the antral pouches. Vagal denervation of the antral pouch abolished gastrin release and greatly decreased but did not abolish acid output, indicating that vagal stimulation can activate the parietal cells without participation of vagal release of gastrin. [Reproduced with permission from Tepperman and co-workers (103).]

finding, Preshaw (85) postulated that sham feeding releases an inhibitor of gastrin-stimulated acid secretion that is effective in vagally denervated but not in vagally innervated oxyntic mucosa. The studies supporting this view are presented in a later section of this chapter.

Gastric Phase

The gastric phase (Table 1) of acid secretion is that which results from stimuli acting in the stomach. There are two classes of initiators of the gastric phase: distention and the chemical constituents of food.

Distention

The introduction of even small amounts of fluid into the stomach of dogs increases the rate of acid secretion. For example, introduction of 50 ml isotonic saline increased acid secretion to about 0.6 mmoles hr^{-1}, measured by intragastric titration, from a basal rate of about 0.1 mmole hr^{-1}, measured by gravity drainage from a gastric fistula, without a detectable increase in serum gastrin concentration (27). In dogs with intact stomachs, graded increases in intragastric pressure, produced by introducing isotonic saline under barostatic control, produced graded increases in acid secretion (101). The response plateaued at 20 cm water pressure, which gave an intragastric volume of about 400 ml and an acid secretion rate of about 13 mmoles hr^{-1}, which represented about 40% of the maximal response to exogenous gastrin. The graded increases in intragastric pressure produced a small and ungraded increase in serum gastrin concentration. Thus distention of the whole stomach of dog stimulates moderate rates of acid secretion by mechanisms that do not primarily involve release of gastrin and are presumed on the basis of indirect evidence, to be mediated by long (vagovagal) and short (intramural) reflexes.

Graded distention of a vagally innervated antral pouch produced graded increases in serum gastrin concentration and graded increases in acid secretion from a vagally innervated gastric fistula (17). Thus distention is a much more effective releaser of gastrin when acting in an antral pouch than when acting in the intact stomach. The reason for this difference is not known. If the distention of the vagally innervated antral pouch is carried out with an acidified solution (100 mM HCl), release of gastrin is completely prevented, but the acid secretory response of the gastric fistula is only moderately decreased (Fig. 2). If the antral pouch is vagally denervated, distension of it with an acidified solution no longer produces a secretory response from the gastric fistula. Thus the stimulation of acid secretion from the gastric fistula produced by distention of the vagally innervated pouch involves at least two mechanisms. One, release of gastrin, can be prevented by acidification. The other is abolished by vagal denervation of the antral pouch and therefore involves a vagovagal reflex from the antral pouch to the gastric fistula. This has been called the pyloro-oxyntic reflex. Since distention of the intact stomach produces moderate stimulation of acid secretion with little increase in serum gastrin concentration, this reflex may play an important role in that response.

In dogs with vagally innervated pouches of both the oxyntic gland area (Pavlov pouch) and the pyloric gland area (antrum), graded distention of the Pavlov pouch while the antral pouch was alkaline produced graded increases in gastrin release and in acid secretion from the Pavlov pouch (19). Acidification of the antral pouch abolished the gastrin response and greatly decreased the acid response. These findings were interpreted as indicating the existence of a vagovagal oxyntopyloric reflex initiated by distention of the oxyntic gland area and leading to release of gastrin from the pyloric gland area. Since distention of the intact stom-

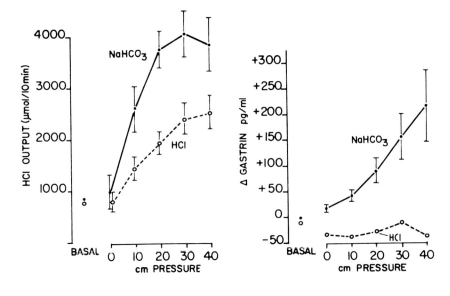

FIG. 2. Effect of distension of a vagally innervated antral pouch with 100 mM NaHCO$_3$ or 100 mM HCl on acid output from vagally innervated gastric fistula and on increment in serum gastrin concentration. Acidification of the antral pouch abolished gastrin release but only moderately reduced acid output, indicating that a pyloro-oxyntic reflex was operating. Vagal denervation of the antral pouch abolished the effect. [Redrawn from Debas and co-workers (17).]

ach produces only small increments in serum gastrin, the large increments seen with distention of antral or oxyntic pouches must be suppressed.

Vagal denervation of an antral pouch greatly decreases the release of gastrin produced by distention (17) or by bathing the pouch with chemical stimulants (103). By contrast, vagal denervation of the whole stomach causes an increase in gastrin release in response to eating. The reason for this discrepancy is not known.

Distention of the vagally innervated antrectomized stomach causes a modest increase in acid secretion presumed to be mediated by a vagovagal reflex (37). Distention of a vagally denervated Heidenhain pouch produces slight stimulation of acid secretion but marked augmentation of acid secretion in response to exogenous stimulants, such as histamine or gastrin (38). This response is presumed to be mediated by a local intramural reflex. Table 2 summarized the reflexes for gastrin and acid secretion that can be elicited by distending dogs' stomachs.

Chemical Agents

The only chemical substances that are regularly ingested and are known to stimulate acid secretion are caffeine, alcohol, calcium ions, and the digestion products of protein.

Caffeine alone stimulates acid secretion in man (8) but not in dog, but it potentiates the response in dog to histamine and to meals (13). The mechanism by which caffeine stimulates acid secretion is not known, but it is hypothesized that it acts by inhibiting breakdown of cyclic AMP by phosphodiesterase (see chapter by Soll). Caffeine is not the main stimulant of acid secretion in coffee; decaffeinated coffee is as strong a stimulant as caffeinated coffee (11).

Hypertonic solutions of ethanol stimulate acid secretion when applied to the mucosa of antral pouches (22), presumably by releasing gastrin; this has not been measured by radioimmunoassay. Also, like other agents that damage gastric mucosa, they produce transient stimulation of acid secretion when applied to oxyntic

mucosa of dogs (14). Intravenous infusion of alcohol stimulates acid secretion in dog (109) and man (47) by unknown mechanisms. Although ethanol was long used as a gastric secretory test meal in man, recent studies show that ethanol solutions in concentrations of 8 to 16% instilled into the human stomach have no greater effect on gastrin release or acid secretion than water (12).

Calcium ions in the human stomach are a strong stimulus for gastrin release and for acid secretion (70); this effect is not seen in the dog (3).

Although food in general stimulates acid secretion through distention of the stomach, the only macronutrient known to act as a chemical stimulant of acid secretion is protein. Instillation of undigested albumin solution into a vagally denervated antral pouch did not stimulate acid secretion from a vagally innervated gastric fistula (15). Light peptic digestion of the albumin made it an effective stimulant of acid secretion, and dialysis of the peptic digest did not abolish the effect, indicating that polypeptides are effective. Unfortunately, these studies were done using acid secretion to monitor gastrin release and should be repeated with direct measurement of gastrin radioimmunoassay.

It has been known for some time that amino acids release gastrin, but the studies on the relative effectiveness of individual amino acids in stimulating gastrin release have given contradictory results. Strunz and co-workers (102) infused 300 ml of 100 mM solutions of 21 different amino acids into the stomach of dogs through a gastric fistula during a 30-min period. Only four amino acids evoked an increase in serum gastrin greater than that produced by saline: cysteine, phenylalanine, tryptophan, and hydroxyproline. Konturek and co-workers (65) found that of the 18 amino acids tested, only serine, valine, and tryptophan caused significant release of gastrin from a vagally denervated antral pouch in dogs. Both Strunz and co-workers (102) and Konturek and co-workers (65) found poor correlation between gastrin release and stimulation of acid secretion and suggested that amino acids might stimulate acid secretion by nongastrin mechanisms. In human sub-

TABLE 2. *Distention-induced gastric reflexes for gastrin release and acid secretion in dog*

Part distended	Vagi	Path	Target	Product	Effect of vagotomy
Oxyntic gland area	Intact	Vagovagal	Parietal cell	Acid	Decreased
			G cell	Gastrin	Abolished
	Cut	Intramural	Parietal cell	Acid	
Pyloric gland area	Intact	Vagovagal	Parietal cell	Acid	Abolished
			G cell	Gastrin	Decreased
	Cut	Intramural	G cell	Gastrin	

jects, Byrne and co-workers (7) instilled 600 ml of 100 mM solutions of 18 amino acids into the stomachs of human subjects and measured acid secretion by intragastric titration and serum gastrin by radioimmunoassay. Tryptophan and phenylalanine were strong gastrin releasers and strong stimulants of acid secretion. The other amino acids were weaker stimulants of acid secretion and did not cause significant increases in serum gastrin. Clearly, additional studies are needed to clarify the relative potency of individual amino acids in releasing gastrin. Dose-response studies should be done, and the different molecular species of gastrins should be measured separately.

The water extractives of meat, such as gravies, bouillon, liver extract, and peptone, are known to be strong stimulants of acid secretion and are frequently used as test meals. In a recent study (27) in gastric fistula dogs, liver extract and a mixture of free amino acids in the same molar ratio as found in liver extract were compared in dose-response fashion for stimulation of acid secretion and increase in serum gastrin concentration. The potencies of the amino acid mixture and the liver extract were not significantly different for gastrin release or acid secretion; within individual dogs, there was a strong correlation between increase in gastrin concentration and increase in acid secretion. Because of marked differences in individual sensitivity to gastrin, correlations between serum gastrin and acid secretion may not be evident between subjects, even when they are clearly present with subjects.

Another recent dose-response study using peptone in human subjects (67) showed strong correlation between increment of serum gastrin and increment of acid secretion within subjects. Thus there is no reason to discard the notion that increase in serum gastrin is the main and perhaps the sole mechanism by which chemical agents acting in the stomach stimulate acid secretion.

Before radioimmunoassay of gastrin was available and release of gastrin could be estimated only by its effect on acid secretion from denervated pouches, a case had been built, on pharmacological and physiological evidence, that release of gastrin was solely under cholinergic control (38). When the gastrin-producing G cell of the antral mucosa was anatomically identified and shown to have an apical microvillous surface exposed to the gastric lumen (94), it was postulated that chemical agents in the lumen could act directly on the G cell to release gastrin. Furthermore, the demonstration that atropine might enhance, inhibit, or have no effect on gastrin release (52), depending on the dose and the conditions of the study, weakened the case for exclusive cholinergic control of gastrin release. Release of gastrin appears to be controlled by a number of factors, including direct action of luminal agents on the G cell and both inhibitory and stimulatory cholinergic effects. A further discussion of the effects of atropine on gastrin release may be found in the chapter by Richardson.

When tested in isolated antral pouches, there is strong potentiation between distention and chemical stimuli in causing release of gastrin (15); in the intact stomach, however, peak gastrin release by chemical stimuli is attained with low pressures (101). This is in agreement with the relatively low effectiveness of distention as a gastrin releaser in the intact stomach.

The only recognized gastric reflexes are those initiated by distention. In principle, such reflexes could also be initiated by chemical agents, but no such evidence yet exists.

Debas and Grossman (16) reported that instillation of a 10% solution of liver extract at pH 8.0 into a Heidenhain pouch led to a marked increase in titratable acidity, which they interpreted as showing direct stimulation of HCl secretion by a chemical agent acting topically on the oxyntic gland area. Spenney (97) pointed out that solutions at high pH bathing the gastric mucosa could act as a sink for passage of gaseous CO_2 from the blood into the intragastric solution, where it would be transformed into bicarbonate at the high pH and thus be available for titration; thus it could be mistaken for secreted HCl. In unpublished studies, we have confirmed Spenney's prediction. Much of the titratable acid that accumulates in the pouch fluid when liver extract at pH 8.0 is introduced into a Heidenhain pouch is carbonic acid rather than HCl. Other studies (66) purporting to show stimulation of HCl secretion by chemical agents acting topically on the oxyntic gland area must now be reexamined for the possible participation of this same artifact. Until the contribution of this factor has been fully evaluated, the question of whether chemical agents acting on the oxyntic mucosa can stimulate HCl secretion remains unanswered.

Intestinal Phase

It was recognized as early as 1900 that the presence of food in the small intestine could stimulate gastric acid secretion (69). The recognized initiators of the intestinal phase (Table 1) are distention and the digestion products of protein (64). The same kinds of agents that are effective as chemical stimulants in the gastric phase, such as liver extract, peptone, and amino acid mixtures, are also effective as intestinal phase stimulants.

Acid secretion in response to food in the small intestine still occurs after all extrinsic nerves between the two organs have been severed (36); thus the mechanism is at least in part humoral. Konturek and co-workers (62) found that secretion of acid from a gastric fistula in response to infusing liver extract into the small intestine was increased by truncal vagotomy. The mechanism of this effect of vagotomy is not known, but it is clear that vagal innervation is not needed for the intestinal phase.

Estimates of the magnitude of the intestinal phase vary considerably. Kauffman and Grossman (59) found that the peak response to intraduodenal infusion of saline was about 3% of maximal response to histamine, and the peak response to liver extract was about 7% of maximum. By contrast, Konturek and co-workers (64) achieved 20% of maximum with saline and 50% with liver extract. In the latter studies, the mean basal rate of secretion was about 2 mmoles hr^{-1}, whereas in the former, it was about 0.2 mmoles hr^{-1}. Intestinal phase stimulation strongly potentiates the response to other stimuli, such as exogenous histamine and gastrin (18); thus the level of basal secretion could have a marked influence on the magnitude of the response.

Konturek and co-workers (62,64) have found an increase in serum gastrin concentration in association with the intestinal phase, but Kauffman and Grossman (59) did not. No increase in serum gastrin has been found in association with the intestinal phase in human subjects (53).

Since intravenously administered amino acids stimulate gastric acid secretion (68), at least part of the humoral mechanism of the intestinal phase is probably due to absorbed amino acids. Because the response to distention cannot be accounted for in this way, a hormone is probably involved. Crude extracts of intestinal mucosa with gastric acid stimulatory action have been prepared (78), but no information on the chemical nature of the active ingredient is yet available. The hypothetical hormone of the intestinal phase has been tentatively named entero-oxyntin (39) to distinguish it from gastrin, which is also present in intestinal mucosa in small amounts.

Table 1 summarizes the sites, initiators, paths to the parietal cell, and mediators at the parietal cell of the principal mechanisms for stimulation of acid secretion.

INHIBITION OF ACID SECRETION

As there are cephalic, gastric, and intestinal phases of stimulation of acid secretion, so too are there inhibitory mechanims that operate in each of these phases.

Cephalic Phase Inhibition

Preshaw's group (103) noted that despite the elevation of serum gastrin produced by sham feeding in dogs with vagally innervated antral pouches, acid secretion from Heidenhain pouches in these animals was not stimulated. Preshaw postulated that sham feeding might release an inhibitor of gastrin-stimulated acid secretion that was selectively active in vagally denervated oxyntic mucosa. To test this hypothesis, he stimulated acid secretion from Heidenhain pouches by infusion of pentagastrin and then sham fed the animals after a plateau of secretion had been established. The author found that sham feeding inhibited pentagastrin-stimulated acid se-

cretion from Heidenhain pouches (85). These findings were confirmed and extended by Sjodin (91) and co-workers who found that the inhibition produced by sham feeding was abolished by truncal vagotomy, thus indicating that vagal stimulation participated in the effect. In another study (92), they found that resection of the antrum and duodenal bulb abolished the inhibition produced by sham feeding. Accordingly, they postulated that vagal stimulation releases from the antrum and/or duodenal bulb an inhibitor of gastrin-stimulated acid secretion. The nature of this hypothetical substance has not been identified.

Another indication that vagal activity inhibits gastrin-stimulated acid secretion from Heidenhain pouches comes from the observation that the maximal response to gastrin is less than the maximal response to histamine in such pouches (79). Truncal vagotomy does not change the maximal response to histamine but increases the maximal response to gastrin; it is thus equal to the histamine maximum (24). This has been interpreted to mean that basal vagal activity releases a substance that inhibits gastrin-stimulated acid secretion from the Heidenhain pouch. Presumably, this could be the same agent released by sham feeding. Both hypothetical stubstances have been referred to as vagogastrone (39). Stening and Grossman (99) found that extragastric vagotomy was as effective as truncal vagotomy in increasing the maximal response of Heidenhain pouches to gastrin, thus suggesting that the source of the hypothetical vagogastrone was extragastric. This appears to differ from the results of Sjodin and Andersson (92), who found that antrectomy plus duodenal bulbectomy eliminated the inhibitory effect of sham feeding. It would be necessary to study both types of effects in the same animals before deciding whether this apparent discrepancy is real.

Maximal acid secretion in response to sham feeding in dogs is about equal to the maximum to histamine; whereas it is only about 40% in humans. This suggests that sham feeding has an inhibitory as well as a stimulatory effect on the vagally innervated oxyntic mucosa of man. It has not yet been possible to demonstrate such an effect by superimposing sham feeding on a background of stimulation, since such a procedure always leads to augmentation or no change rather than to inhibition (88).

Gastric Phase Inhibition

The most clearly established mechanism of gastric phase inhibition is inhibition of gastrin release by acid bathing the antral mucosa. Acidification of the antral mucosa inhibits gastrin release induced by sham feeding (103), by distention of an antral pouch (17), and by bathing the antral mucosa with chemical releasants, such as liver extract (20). An anomalous finding is that acidification of the gastric contents did not inhibit gastrin release in response to distention of the whole stomach in man (89). In most instances, the exact relationship between pH and degree of inhibition of gastrin release has not been carefully studied. In general, marked suppression is seen at pH 2, and complete abolition of release is usally found at pH 1. While acidification of antral mucosa suppresses the action of gastrin releasers, alkalinization of the antral mucosa does not act as a stimulus for gastrin release other than by withdrawing inhibition. Alkalinization alone, in the absence of a primary gastrin releaser, does not cause gastrin release (15).

Konturek and co-workers (63) have presented evidence to show that acidification of the oxyntic mucosa inhibits acid secretion in response to all stimuli, including gastrin and histamine. Repetition of these studies by Carter and Grossman (9), using a validated intrapouch titration system as well as volume markers and extrapouch titration, failed to show any effect of luminal pH on acid secretion in response to histamine or pentagastrin over the pH range 1 to 9.

Studies in both dogs (112) and humans (90) indicate that distention of the antrum can inhibit pentagastrin-stimulated acid secretion from the vagally innervated oxyntic mucosa. It is not know whether this effect is neurally or hormonally mediated. Thus antral distention, like sham feeding, produces both stimulatory and inhibitory effects. Which of these predominates will depend on the conditions under which the study is done.

Intestinal Phase Inhibition

Three agents that inhibit acid secretion when instilled into the small intestine have been identified: acid, fat, and hyperosmolar solutions.

When large amounts of unbuffered acid are introduced in such a way as to give it access to large areas of the small intestine, inhibition of acid secretion is probably mediated mainly by the secretin released by the acid. The following points of evidence support this conclusion: (a) acid in the intestine and exogenous secretin inhibit gastrin-stimulated acid secretion but are almost completely ineffective against histamine-stimulated secretion (54); (b) graded rates of infusion into the duodenum produce graded increases in pancreatic bicarbonate secretion and parallel graded increases in inhibition of gastrin-stimulated acid secretion, both of which can be mimicked by graded doses of exogenous secretin (83); and (c) the kinetics of inhibition by acid in the duodenum and by exogenous secretin are both noncompetitive (54).

When acid is confined to the duodenal bulb, it can still inhibit acid secretion. Under these circumstances, however, its effect cannot be accounted for by release of secretin, because it is not associated with an increase

in pancreatic bicarbonate secretion. Andersson and co-workers (1) showed that acid confined to a pouch of the duodenal bulb could inhibit acid secretion stimulated by sham feeding, a meal, or by infusion of gastrin but failed to inhibit histamine-stimulated secretion. The effect was at least in part hormonal, because it persisted when either or both the duodenal bulb and/or the oxyntic mucosa were extrinsically denervated. The name bulbogastrone was proposed for the hormone, and crude extracts were prepared (105); no recent work has been reported. Other work (61) indicated that acid bathing the duodenal bulbar mucosa inhibited acid secretion from a gastric fistula but not from a Heidenhain pouch, thus suggesting that the mechanism was neural. A possible explanation for the discrepancy is that Andersson (1) found it necessary to distend the bulbar pouch with acid to get inhibitory effects, whereas the workers who found effects only in vagally innervated stomach allowed the acid to flow over the bulbar mucosa without increased pressure. Perhaps both neural and hormonal mechanisms exist, and the latter can be elicited only with acid under pressure.

It has long been recognized that fat in the small intestine inhibits acid secretion (1). Early studies showed that the fat had to be in an absorbable form (fatty acid or monoglyceride) to be effective, and that only fatty acids with 10 or more carbons in the chain were effective. At an early stage, it was shown that the inhibitory effect of fat persisted after the extrinsic nerves to the stomach and intestine had been severed. This indicated that a humoral mechanism was at least in part responsible. The hypothetical hormonal agent was called enterogastrone; much effort was expended in attempting to isolate and identify it. Among the peptides from intestinal mucosa that have been isolated and sequenced, gastric inhibitory polypeptide (GIP) is the strongest candidate to be the enterogastrone released by fat. GIP is released by fat (6), and it inhibits gastrin-stimulated acid secretion in the Heidenhain pouch (81). However, it is a weak inhibitor of gastrin-stimulated acid secretion from the vagally innervated gastric fistula, whereas fat in the intestine inhibits secretion from the gastric fistula even more effectively than from the Heidenhain pouch (21). Therefore, either the main mechanism by which fat in the small intestine inhibits acid secretion is neural rather than hormonal, or the hormone responsible for the strong inhibition of the vagally innervated gastric fistula has not yet been isolated. It is difficult to devise experiments to distinguish between a purely neural mechanism and a hormonal mechanism that requires the permissive action of nerves.

Solutions that are hyperosmolar with respect to blood plasma produce inhibition of acid secretion when infused into the small intestine (1). The mechanism still operates when extrinsic nerves between the intestine and stomach have been severed; thus it is at least in part humoral. The relative importance of neural and humoral components has not been assessed. The mechanism by which hyperosmolar solutions in the small intestine inhibit acid secretion is unknown.

Catecholamines inhibit gastrin-stimulated acid secretion by both alpha- and beta-adrenergic effects (50). Electrical stimulation of the splanchnic nerves also strongly inhibits acid secretion (87). The alpha-adrenergic effects and the effects of splanchnic nerve stimulation are almost certainly caused by restriction of blood flow to the gastric mucosa. The degree to which these effects participate in the physiological regulation of gastric acid secretion is unknown. This pathway is probably utilized in the strong inhibition of gastric motility and secretion that occurs with severe pain or injury.

UNSOLVED PROBLEMS AWAITING FUTURE RESEARCH

One of the most remarkable aspects of the regulation of acid secretion is the phenomenon of potentiation, whereby two stimulants acting together can produce a greater effect than the sum of the individual respones. The mechanism of this effect is unknown. It does not occur at the second messenger stage (cyclic AMP for histamine and calcium for cholinergic agents; see chapter by Soll). There must be convergence before the final step of stimulation of H^+ secretion; it is at this point of convergence that the mechanism of potentiation can be expected to operate.

The mechanisms regulating the synthesis, storage, and release of histamine in the region of the parietal cells are not fully understood.

Vagal stimulation produces both stimulation and inhibition of both the G cell and the parietal cell, with stimulation usually predominating. Acetylcholine appears to be the main mediator for stimulation of the parietal cell and plays a major role in inhibition of the G cell, possibly by releasing yet another substance. The mediators for vagal inhibition of the parietal cell and for vagal stimulation of the G cell remain to be identified.

Although the stimulation of acid secretion and of gastrin release produced by a protein meal can be mimicked by a mixture of free amino acids similar to those found in the meal, we know very little about the relative potency of individual amino acids and of small peptides acting alone and in combinations.

Our greatest area of ignorance is the mechanisms by which substances in the intestine stimulate and inhibit acid secretion. The intestinal phase stimulatory hormone, entero-oxyntin, has not yet been isolated and sequenced. The mediators of the inhibitory effects of fat, acid, and hyperosmolar solutions are unknown.

Finally, little is known about the possible role in regulation of acid secretion of the many peptides found in

endocrine and neuronal cells of the gastric mucosa (see chapter by Walsh).

REFERENCES

1. Andersson, S. (1967): Gastric and duodenal mechanisms inhibiting gastric secretion of acid. In: *Handbook of Physiology. Section 6: Alimentary Canal. Volume 2, Secretion,* edited by C. F. Code, pp. 865–878. American Physiological Society, Washington, D.C.
2. Antia, F., Rosiere, C. E., Robertson, C., and Grossman, M. I. (1951): Effect of vagotomy on gastric secretion and emptying time in dogs. *Am. J. Physiol.,* 66:470–479.
3. Barreras, R. F. (1973): Calcium and gastric secretion. *Gastroenterology,* 64:1168–1184.
4. Brooks, F. P. (1954): Insulin hypoglycemia and gastric secretion. *Am. J. Dig. Dis.,* 10:737–741.
5. Broome, A., and Bergstrom, H. (1966): Selective surgery for duodenal ulcer based on preoperative acid production. *Acta Chir. Scand.,* 132:170–179.
6. Brown, J. C., Dryburgh, J. R., Ross, S. A., and Dupre, J. (1975): Identification and actions of gastric inhibitory polypeptide. *Recent Prog. Horm. Res.,* 31:487–532.
7. Byrne, W. J., Christie, D. L., Ament, M. E., and Walsh, J. H. (1977): The effect of individual L-amino acids on gastric acid secretion, serum gastrin release and gastric emptying time in man. *Clin. Res.,* 25:108A (Abstr.).
8. Cano, R., Isenberg, J. I., and Grossman, M. I. (1976): Cimetidine inhibits caffeine-stimulated gastric acid secretion in man. *Gastroenterology,* 78:1082–1084.
9. Carter, D. C., and Grossman, M. I. (1978): Effect of luminal pH on acid secretion from Heidenhain pouches evoked by topical and parenteral stimulants. *J. Physiol.,* 281:227–237.
10. Code, C. F. (1977): Reflections on histamine, gastric secretion and the H_2 receptor. *N. Engl. J. Med.,* 296:1459–1462.
11. Cohen, S., and Booth, G. H., Jr. (1975): Gastric acid secretion and lower-esophageal-sphincter pressure in response to coffee caffeine. *N. Engl. J. Med.,* 91:897–899.
12. Cooke, A. R. (1972): Ethanol and gastric function. *Gastroenterology,* 623:501–502.
13. Cooke, A. R., Chvasta, T. E., and Granner, D. E. (1974): Histamine, pentagastrin, methyl xanthines and adenyl cyclase activity in acid secretion. *Proc. Soc. Exp. Biol. Med.,* 147:674–678.
14. Davenport, H. W. (1967): Ethanol damage to canine oxyntic glandular mucosa. *Proc. Soc. Exp. Biol. Med.,* 126:657–662.
15. Debas, H. T., Csendes, A., Walsh, J. H., and Grossman, M. I. (1974): Release of antral gastrin. In: *Endocrinology of the Gut,* edited by W. Y. Chey and S. F. Brooks, pp. 222–212. Charles B. Slack, Thorofare, New Jersey.
16. Debas, H. T., and Grossman, M. I. (1975): Chemicals bathing the oxyntic gland area stimulate acid secretion in dog. *Gastroenterology,* 69:651–659.
17. Debas, H. T., Konturek, S. J., Walsh, J. H., and Grossman, M. I. (1974): Proof of a pyloro-oxyntic reflex for stimulation of acid secretion. *Gastroenterology,* 66:526–532.
18. Debas, H. T., Slaff, G. F., and Grossman, M. I. (1975): Intestinal phase of gastric acid secretion: Augmentation of maximal response of Heidenhain pouch to gastrin and histamine. *Gastroenterology,* 68:691–698.
19. Debas, H. T., Walsh, J. H., and Grossman, M. I. (1975): Evidence for oxyntopyloric reflex for release of antral gastrin. *Gastroenterology,* 68:691–698.
20. Debas, H. T., Walsh, J. H., and Grossman, M. I. (1975): Mechanisms of release of antral gastrin. In: *Gastrointestinal Hormones, A Symposium,* edited by J. C. Thompson, pp. 425–435. University of Texas Press, Austin.
21. Debas, H. T., and Yamagishi, T. (1977): Gastric inhibitory polypeptide (GIP) is not the primary mediator of the enterogastrone action of fat. *Gastroenterology,* 74:1118.
22. Elwin, C. E. (1969): Stimulation of gastric acid secretion by irrigation of the antrum with some aliphatic alcohols. *Acta Physiol. Scand.,* 75:1–11.
23. Emas, S., and Grossman, M. I. (1967): Effect of truncal va-

gotomy on acid and pepsin responses to histamine and gastrin in dogs. *Am. J. Physiol.,* 212:1007-1012.

24. Emas, S., and Grossman, M. I. (1969): Response of Heidenhain pouch to histamine, gastrin and feeding before and after truncal vagotomy in dogs. *Scand. J. Gastroenterol.,* 4:497-503.

25. Emas, S., Svensson, S.-C., Dorner, M., and Kaess, H. (1976): Gastric acid and serum gastrin responses to insulin and 2-deoxy-D-glucose in duodenal ulcer patients before and after partial gastrectomy. *Scand. J. Gastroenterol.,* 11:667-672.

26. Faroog, O., Walsh, J. H. (1975): Atropine enhances serum gastrin response to insulin in man. *Gastroenterology,* 68:622-666.

27. Feldman, E. J., and Grossman, M. I. (1980): Liver extract and its free amino acids equally stimulate acid secretion. *Am. J. Physiol.,* 239:G493-G496.

28. Feldman, M., Dickerman, R. M., McClelland, R. N., Cooper, K. A., Walsh, J. H., and Richardson, C. T. (1979): Effect of selective proximal vagotomy on food-stimulated gastric acid secretion and gastrin release in patients with duodenal ulcer. *Gastroenterology,* 76:926-931.

29. Feldman, M., Richardson, C. T., and Fordtran, J. S. (1980): Effect of sham feeding on gastric acid secretion in healthy subjects and duodenal ulcer patients: Evidence for increased basal vagal tone in some ulcer patients. *Gastroenterology,* 79:796-800.

30. Feldman, M., Richardson, C. T., Taylor, I. L., and Walsh, J. H. (1979): Effect of atropine on vagal release of gastrin and pancreatic polypeptide. *J. Clin. Invest.,* 63:294-298.

31. Feldman, M., Walsh, J. H., Wong, H. C., and Richardson, C. T. (1977): Role of gastrin heptadecapeptide in the acid secretory response to amino acids in man. *J. Clin. Invest.,* 61:308-313.

32. Gardner, J. D., Jackson, M. J., Batzri, S., and Jensen, R. T. (1978): Potential mechanisms of interaction among secretagogues. *Gastroenterology,* 74:348-354.

33. Gianturco, C. (1934): Some mechanical factors of gastric physiology. *Am. J. Roent. Rad. Ther.,* 31:745-749.

34. Gillespie, I. E., Clark, D. H., Kay, A. W., and Tankel, H. I. (1960): Effect of antrectomy, vagotomy with gastrojejunostomy and antrectomy with vagotomy on the spontaneous and maximal gastric acid output in man. *Gastroenterology,* 38:361-367.

35. Greenall, M. J., Lyndon, P. J., Goligher, J. C., and Johnston, D. (1975): Long term effect of highly selective vagotomy on basal and maximal acid output in man. *Gastroenterology,* 68:1421-1425.

36. Gregory, R. A., and Ivy, A. C. (1941): The humoral stimulation of gastric secretion. *Q. J. Exp. Physiol.,* 31:111-128.

37. Grossman, M. I. (1962): Secretion of acid and pepsin in response to distention of vagally innervated fundic gland area in dogs. *Gastroenterology,* 41:718-721.

38. Grossman, M. I. (1967): Neural and hormonal stimulation of gastric secretion of acid. In: *Handbook of Physiology. Section 6: Alimentary Canal. Volume 2, Secretion,* edited by C. F. Code, pp. 835-863. American Physiological Society, Washington, D.C.

39. Grossman, M. I. (1974): Candidate hormones of the gut. *Gastroenterology,* 67:1016-1019.

40. Grossman, M. I. (1979): Chemical messengers: A view from the gut. *Fed. Proc.,* 38:2341-2343.

41. Grossman, M. I. (1979): Neural and hormonal regulation of gastrointestinal function: an overview. *Ann. Rev. Physiol.,* 41:27-33.

42. Grossman, M. I. (1979): Vagal stimulation and inhibition of acid secretion and gastrin release: Which aspects are cholinergic? In: *Gastrins and the Vagus,* edited by J. F. Rehfeld and E. Andrup, pp. 105-113. Academic Press, London.

43. Grossman, M. I., and Konturek, S. J. (1974): Inhibition of acid secretion in dog and by metiamide, a histamine antagonist acting on H_2-receptors. *Gastroenterology,* 66:517-521.

44. Hirschowitz, B. L. (1968): Apparent kinetics of histamine dose-responsive gastric water and electrolyte secretion in the dog. *Gastroenterology,* 54:514-522.

45. Hirschowitz, B. (1975): Regulation of gastric secretion. In: *Functions of the Stomach and Intestine,* edited by M. H. F. Friedman, pp. 145-166. University Park Press, Baltimore.

46. Hirschowitz, B. I., and Hutchison, G. A. (1977): Long-term

47. Hirschowitz, B. I., Pollard, H. M., Hartwell, S. W., and London, J. (1956): The action of ethyl alcohol on gastric acid secretion. *Gastroenterology,* 30:244-253.

48. Hirschowitz, B. I., and Sachs, G. (1965): Vagal gastric secretory stimulation by 2-deoxy-D-glucose. *Am. J. Physiol.,* 209:452-460.

49. Hollander, F., and Weinstein, V. A. (1956): Causes of basal secretion of HCl in the dog. *Fed. Proc.,* 15:95.

50. Holton, P. (1973): Catecholamines and gastric secretion. In: *Pharmacology of Gastrointestinal Motility and Secretion,* edited by P. Holton, pp. 287-315. Pergamon Press, Oxford.

51. Impicciatore, M., Debas, H., Walsh, J. H., Grossman, M. I., and Bertaccini, G. (1974): Release of gastrin and stimulation of acid secretion by bombesin in dog. *Rend. Gastroenterol.,* 6:99-101.

52. Impicciatore, M., Walsh, J. H., and Grossman, M. I. (1977): Low doses of atropine enhance serum gastrin response to food in dogs. *Gastroenterology,* 72:995-996.

53. Isenberg, J. I., Ippoliti, A. F., and Maxwell, V. (1977): Perfusion of the proximal small intestine with peptone stimulates gastric acid secretion in man. *Gastroenterology,* 73:746-752.

54. Johnson, L. R., and Grossman, M. I. (1969): Characteristics of inhibition of gastric secretion by secretin. *Am. J. Physiol.,* 217:1401-1404.

55. Johnson, L. R. (1971): The control of gastric secretion: No room for histamine? *Gastroenterology,* 61:106-118.

56. Johnston, D., Wilkinson, A. R., Humphrey, C. S., Smith, R. B., Goligher, J. C., Kragelund, E., and Amdrup, E. (1973): Serial studies of gastric secretion in patients after highly selective (parietal cell) vagotomy without a drainage procedure for duodenal ulcer. *Gastroenterology,* 64:12-21.

57. Kadekaro, M., Timo-Iaria, C., Vicentini, M. L. M. (1977): Control of gastric secretion by the central nervous system. In: *Nerves and the Gut,* edited by F. P. Brooks and P. W. Evers, pp. 377-429. Charles B. Slack, Thorofare, New Jersey.

58. Kasbekar, D. (1967): Studies of resting isolated frog gastric mucosa. *Proc. Soc. Exp. Biol.,* 125:267-271.

59. Kauffman, G. L., Jr., and Grossman, M. I. j(1979): Serum gastrin during intestinal phase of acid secretion in dogs. *Gastroenterology,* 77:26-30.

60. Knutson, U., and Olbe, L. (1974): The effect of exogenous gastrin on the acid sham feeding response in antrum-bulb-resected duodenal ulcer patients. *Scand. J. Gastroenterol.,* 9:231-238.

61. Konturek, S. J., and Johnson, L. R. (1971): Evidence for an enterogastric reflex for the inhibition of acid secretion. *Gastroenterology,* 61:667-674.

62. Konturek, S. J., Llanos, O. L., Rayford, P. L., and Thompson, J. C. (1977): Vagal influence on gastrin and gastric acid responses to gastric and intestinal meals. *Am. J. Physiol.,* 232(6):E542-E546.

63. Konturek, S. J., Obtulowicz, W., and Tasler, J. (1975): Characteristics of gastric inhibition by acidification of oxyntic gland area. *J. Physiol.,* 251:699-709.

64. Konturek, S. J., Radecki, T., and Kwiecien, N. (1978): Stimuli for intestinal phase of gastric secretion in dogs. *Am. J. Physiol.,* 234(1):E64-E69.

65. Konturek, S. J., Tasler, J., Cieszowski, M., Dobranzanska, M., and Wunsch, E. (1977): Stimulation of gastrin release and gastric secretion by amino acids bathing pyloric gland area. *Am. J. Physiol.,* 233(3):E170-E174.

66. Konturek, S. J., Tasler, J., Obtulowicz, W., and Cieszkowski, M. (1976): Comparison of amino acids bathing the oxyntic gland area in the stimulation of gastric secretion. *Gastroenterology,* 70:66-69.

67. Lam, S. K., Isenberg, J. I., Grossman, M. I., Lane, W. H., and Walsh, J. H. (1980): Gastric acid secretion is abnormally sensitive to endogenous gastrin released after peptone test meals in duodenal ulcer patients. *J. Clin. Invest.,* 65:555-562.

68. Landor, J. H., and Ipapo, V. S. (1977): Gastric secretory effect of amino acids given enterally and parenterally in dogs. *Gastroenterology,* 73:781.

69. Leconte, P. (1900): Fonctions gastro-intestinales. *Cellule,* 17:285-318.

70. Levant, J. A., Walsh, J. H., and Isenberg, J. I. (1973): Stimulation of gastric secretion and gastrin release by single oral doses of calcium carbonate in man. *N. Engl. J. Med.,* 289:555-558.

71. MacGregor, I. L., Martin, P., and Meyer, J. H. (1977): Gastric emptying of solid food in normal man and after subtotal gastrectomy and truncal vagotomy with pyloroplasty. *Gastroenterology,* 72:206-211.

72. Marks, I. N., Komarov, S. A., and Shay, H. (1960): Maximal acid secretory response to histamine and its relation to parietal cell mass in the dog. *Am. J. Physiol.,* 199:579-588.

73. McGuigan, J. E., and Trudeau, W. J. (1968): Immunochemical measurement of elevated levels of gastrin in the serum of patients with pancreatic tumors of the Zollinger-Ellison variety. *N. Engl. J. Med.,* 278:1308-1313.

74. Meyer, J. H., Mandiola, S., Shadcher, A., and Cohen, M. (1977): Dispersion of solid food by the canine stomach. *Gastroenterology,* 72:1102 (Abstr.).

75. Moore, J. G., and Wolfe, M. (1973): The relation of plasma gastrin to the circadian rhythm of gastric acid secretion in man. *Digestion,* 9:97-105.

76. Nilsson, G., Simon, J., Yalow, R. S., and Berson, S. A. (1972): Plasma gastrin and gastric acid responses to sham feeding and feeding in dogs. *Gastroenterology,* 63:51-59.

77. Olbe, L. (1964): Potentiation of sham feeding response in Pavlov pouch dogs by subthreshold amounts of gastrin with and without acidification of denervated antrum. *Acta Physiol. Scand.,* 61:244-254.

78. Orloff, M. J., Guillemin, R. C. L., and Nakaji, N. T. (1977): Isolation of the hormone responsible for the intestinal phase of gastric secretion. *Gastroenterology,* 72:820.

79. Passaro, E. P., Jr., and Grossman, M. I. (1964): Effect of vagal innervation on acid and pepsin response to histamine and gastrin. *Am. J. Physiol.,* 206:1068-1076.

80. Pavlov, I. P. (1910): *The Work of the Digestive Glands,* 2nd edition, translated by W. H. Thompson. Griffin, London.

81. Pederson, R. A., and Brown, J. C. (1972): The inhibition of histamine-, pentagastrin-, and insulin-stimulated gastric secretion by pure gastric inhibitory polypeptide. *Gastroenterology,* 62:393-400.

82. Petersen, H., and Grossman, M. I. (1978): Stimulation of gastric acid secretion by dimaprit in unanesthetized rats. *Agents Actions,* 8:566-567.

83. Preshaw, R. M. (1969): Pancreas and liver. In: *Exocrine Glands,* edited by S. Y. Botelho, F. P., Brooks, and W. B. Shelley, pp. 247-252. University of Pennsylvania Press, Philadelphia.

84. Preshaw, R. M. (1970): Gastric acid output after sham feeding and during release or infusion of gastrin. *Am. J. Physiol.,* 219:1409-1416.

85. Preshaw, R. M. (1973): Inhibition of pentagastrin stimulated gastric acid output by sham feeding. *Fed. Proc.,* 32:410a.

86. Rangachari, P. K. (1975): Histamine release by gastric stimulants. *Nature,* 253:53-55.

87. Reed, J. D., Sanders, D. J., and Thorpe, V. (1971): The effect of splanchnic nerve stimulation on gastric acid secretion and mucosal blood flow in the anethetized cat. *J. Physiol. (Lond.),* 214:1-13.

88. Richardson, C. T., Walsh, J. H., Cooper, K. A., Feldman, M., and Fordtran, J. S. (1977): Studies on the role of cephalic-vagal stimulation in the acid secretory response to eating in normal human subjects. *J. Clin. Invest.,* 60:435-441.

89. Schiller, L. R., Walsh, J. H., and Feldman, M. (1980): Distention-induced gastrin release in man: effects of luminal acidification and intravenous atropine. *Gastroenterology (in press).*

90. Schoon, I. M., Bergegardh, S., Grotzinger, U., and Olbe, L. (1978): Evidence for a defective inhibition of pentagastrin-stimulated gastric acid secretion by antral distension in the duodenal ulcer patient. *Gastroenterology,* 75:363-367.

91. Sjodin, L. (1975): Inhibition of gastrin-stimulated canine acid secretion by sham-feeding. *Scand. J. Gastroenterol.,* 10:73-80.

92. Sjodin, L., and Andersson, S. (1977): Effect of resection of antrum and duodenal bulb on sham-feeding-induced inhibition of canine gastric secretion. *Scand. J. Gastroenterol.,* 12:43-47.

93. Sjodin, L., and Nilsson, G. (1975): Role of antrum and duodenum in the control of postprandial gastric acid secretion and plasma gastrin concentration in dogs. *Gastroneterology,* 69:928-934.

94. Solcia, E., Capella, C., Vassallo, G., and Buffa, R. (1975): Endocrine cells of the gastric mucosa. *Int. Rev. Cytol.,* 42:223-286.

95. Soll, A. H. (1978): Three-way interactions between histamine, carbachol, and gastrin on aminopyrine uptake by isolated canine parietal cells. *Gastroenterology,* 74:1146.

96. Soll, A. H., and Walsh, J. H. (1979): Regulation of gastric acid secretion. *Ann. Rev. Physiol.,* 41:35-53.

97. Spenney, J. G. (1979): Physical chemical and technical limitations to intragastric titration. *Gastroenterology,* 76:1025-1034.

98. Steinbach, J. H., Hines, J. C., and Code, C. F. (1979): Gastric acid secretion during the interdigestive myoelectric complex. *Fed. Proc.,* 38:884.

99. Stening, G. F., and Grossman, M. I. (1970): Gastric acid response to pentagastrin and histamine after extragastric vagotomy in dogs. *Gastroenterology,* 59:364-371.

100. Stenquist, B., Nilsson, G., Rehfeld, J. F., and Olbe, L. (1979): Plasma gastrin concentrations following sham feeding in duodenal ulcer patients. *Gastroenterology,* 14:305-312.

101. Strunz, U. T., and Grossman, M. I. (1978): Effect of intragastric pressure on gastric emptying and secretion. *Am. J. Physiol.,* 235(5):E552-E555.

102. Strunz, U. T., Walsh, J. H., and Grossman, M. I. (1978): Stimulation of gastrin release in dogs by individual amino acids. *Proc. Soc. Exp. Biol. Med.,* 157:440-441.

103. Tepperman, B. L., Walsh, J. H., and Preshaw, R. M. (1972): Effect of antral denervation on gastrin release by sham feeding and insulin hypoglycemia in dogs. *Gastroenterology,* 63:973-980.

104. Uvnas, B. (1942): The part played by the pyloric region in the cephalic phase of gastric secretion. *Acta Physiol. Scand. [Suppl. 13],* 4:1-85.

105. Uvnas, B. (1971): Role of duodenum in inhibition of gastric acid secretion. *Scand. J. Gastroenterol.,* 6:113-125.

106. Uvnas-Wallensten, K., and Andersson, H. (1977): Effect of atropine and metiamide on vagally induced gastric acid secretion and gastrin release in anesthetized cats. *Acta Physiol. Scand.,* 99:496-502.

107. Walsh, J. H., and Holmquist, A. L. (1976): Radioimmunoassay of bembesin peptides: Identification of bombesin-like immunoreactivity in vertebrate gut extracts. *Gastroenterology,* 70:948 *(abstr.).*

108. Weiss, A., and Sciales, W. J. (1961): The effect of tolbutamide on human basal gastric secretion. *Ann. Intern. Med.,* 55:406-415.

109. Woodward, E. R., Robertson, C., Ruttenberg, H. D., and Schapiro, H. (1957): Alcohol as a gastric secretory stimulant. *Gastroenterology,* 32:727-737.

110. Wormsley, K. G., and Grossman, M. I. (1965): Maximal histalog test in control subjects and patients with peptic ulcer. *Gut,* 6:427-435.

111. Wyrwicka, W., and Garcia, R. (1979): Effect of restraint on gastric secretion in cats. *Pavlov. J. Biol. Sci.,* 14:249-253.

112. Yamagishi, T., and Debas, H. T. (1977): Antral distension with acid inhibits gastric acid secretion. *Gastroenterology,* 72:1152.

Physiology of the Gastrointestinal Tract, edited by
Leonard R. Johnson. Raven Press, New York © 1981.

Chapter 24

Physiology of Isolated Canine Parietal Cells: Receptors and Effectors Regulating Function

Andrew H. Soll

This chapter considers regulation of gastric acid secretion by chemical transmitters from the vantage point of information gained from studies with isolated parietal cells and gastric glands. The evidence indicating the existence of specific receptors for secretagogues on the parietal cell is reviewed. The role of potentiating interactions between secretagogues in the regulation of parietal cell function is considered, as is the secondary effector mechanisms that may mediate secretagogue action. The rationale for the use of isolated cells and glands for studying these questions is that certain fundamental problems, particularly regarding the site of action of gastric secretagogues, have been difficult to unravel *in vivo* or by using intact gastric mucosa *in vitro*. Several factors contributed to these difficulties. As reviewed by Grossman elsewhere in this book (25), parietal cell function *in vivo* is affected by inputs from endocrine, paracrine, and neurocrine pathways, for which gastrin, histamine, and acetylcholine, respectively, are the best recognized transmitters. Not only does the parietal cell receive inputs from these three pathways, but their effects on parietal cell function are interdependent. This interdependence is most clearly evident in the apparent lack of specificity of the H_2 receptor antagonists and anticholinergic agents in their inhibition of acid secre-

tion *in vivo*. At similar concentrations, cimetidine inhibits not only histamine action but also stimulation by gastrin, vagal pathways, and food (24,25,47,54). Anticholinergic agents also show an apparent lack of specificity, inhibiting, in the same concentration range, stimulation by histamine, gastrin, and food, as well as by cholinomimetics (15,27). Interdependency between secretagogues has also been demonstrated *in vivo* by the administration of combinations of stimulants which, under certain circumstances, produce potentiation (24,25,59). To some extent, inhibition of acid secretion by vagotomy and antrectomy may also reflect interference with the interdependency between secretagogues. Thus there is little question that secretagogues are interdependent in their action on acid secretion *in vivo*. To further complicate *in vivo* studies, histamine, present in mast cells in the lamina propria (61), and acetylcholine, present in the mucosal nerves, are intimately associated with their target, the parietal cell. In the basal state, the parietal cell appears to be under the effects of this endogenous histamine and acetylcholine, since basal acid secretion is inhibited by both cimetidine (26) and anticholinergic agents (20). Thus *in vivo*, it is impossible to study the action of a single stimulant on acid secretion; removal of the parietal cell from the influences of these endogenous stimulants represents a major advantage of isolated cell studies. With isolated cells, since stimulants can be added alone or in combination, the specificty of receptors and potential mechanisms for secretagogue interdependence can be studied.

A second major advantage of isolated cell studies is the potential for cell separation. Gastric mucosa represents such a complex mixture of cell types that enrichment of various subpopulations becomes essential for certain studies, such as determining the cell responsible for stimulant effects on cyclic AMP generation or calcium influx.

TECHNIQUES FOR ISOLATING PARIETAL CELLS

A variety of techniques for dispersing gastric mucosal cells and gastric glands by enzyme digestion have been published. There is considerable similiarity in the several steps involved in these procedures, which have been developed for frog (10,43), rat (36,66), dog (17,50,53), rabbit (5,23,41), mouse (49), and guinea pig (3). In most procedures, the first step involves preparing the mucosa for digestion by bluntly separating the mucosa from the underlying tissue. Croft and Ingelfinger (17) emphasized the importance of separating the mucosa from the submucosa itself. They injected saline to raise a bleb of mucosa that could then be removed. A similar separation can also be achieved by blunt dissection (53). Mucosa can then be minced by scissors or chopped by use of a McIllwain tissue chopper (57). These steps are essential for adequate dispersion at low enzyme concentrations.

Berglindh et al. (5) prepare mucosa by intraarterial injection of saline under high pressure, followed by separation of the mucosa from submucosa. This perfusion step apparently facilitates preparation of intact gastric glands. In preliminary studies, low pressure perfusion of the gastric circulation with collagenase-containing medium appeared to enhance the yield of cells but not the degree of responsiveness to stimulation. Therefore, the gains did not appear to warrant the additional time required (A. H. Soll and J. Ferrari, *unpublished observations*). A rigorous comparison of these various methods would be worthwhile. In studies whith guinea pig, Batzri and Gardner (3) squeeze mucosa that has been stripped from submucosa through a stainless steel mesh. In rat, Lewin et al. (36) tie mucosa into an inverted sac, into which they inject pronase solutions.

The second step in dispersion involves treatment with enzymes. Pronase and crude collagenase have been most widely used. Crude collagenase is indeed crude; it is obtained from clostridia histolyticum and contains a variety of enzyme activities besides collagenase, including clostripain, proteases, and trypsin. At least some of these other components in collagenase are important for

dispersion; purified collagenase fails to disperse cells from fundic mucosa in concentrations that are effective in dispersing acinar cells from pancreas (T. Solomon and A. H. Soll, *unpublished observations*). Simply incubating fundic mucosa in collagenase does not readily disperse single cells but rather allows preparation of gasric gland fragments in both rabbit (5) and dog (61).

The incorporation of a calcium chelation step, adapted from the studies of Amsterdam et al. (1,2), greatly enhances the yield of single cells (53). By interspersing a calcium chelation step achieved with 1 to 2 mM EDTA, a yield of 35 to 80 $\times$ 10^6 cells/g canine fundic mucosa can be produced with collagenase concentrations of 0.25 mg/ml (53,57). There is little difference in either the cell yield or cell responsiveness to stimulation with use of any of the four types of crude collagenase made by Worthington Biochemicals (Freehold, New York) or crude collagenase I, available through Sigma (St. Louis, Missouri) (57). Since some variation between the lots of collagenase does exist, each lot should be tested before a large quantity is purchased. Conditions for storage of collagenase are important in that repeated freezing and thawing can have deleterious effects on enzyme activity. Sealing small aliquots of collagenase under nitrogen for low temperature storage is advisable.

Since treatment with collagenase, pronase, or EDTA is at least somewhat deleterious to cells, there is considerable advantage in reducing enzyme concentrations and avoiding unnecessarily rigorous calcium chelation. If digestion of the intercellular matrix or disruption of cell junctions is inadequate, however, vigorous and equally deleterious mechanical means may be necessary to produce isolated cells.

We do find that the ease of tissue dispersion varies among species and with the condition and age of the animals. The increased density of the collagen matrix in older animals may be a factor. Rabbit fundic mucosa appears to require less collagenase exposure than canine mucosa for equal degrees of digestion. Canine antrum is much more resistant to enzyme treatment than is canine fundic mucosa.

After enzyme digestion, most procedures incorporate a final mechanical step, such as repeated aspiration through a pipette, to enhance cell yield. In our studies with canine mucosal cells, at the end of the enzyme digestion, we have drawn the cell suspension into a 20-ml plastic syringe without a needle three times, followed by filtering through nylon mesh (53). The cells are then washed twice in fresh buffer using a disposable 5-ml pipette tip (53). We have not found that the yield is sufficiently enhanced by further mechanical steps to warrant the additional time. Even the syringe step described above adds only minimally to yield when the digestion is optimal. As mentioned above, these mechanical steps can be deleterious, particularly when they are done at low temperatures, which restrict membrane fluidity and thus may impair sealing of defects created by ripping apart cell junctions. Gentle handling of the cells is important, as bubble formation, with its attendant high surface tension, may damage cells. In general, it is best to avoid exposing cells to storage at 4° C, as the resultant shifts in ion composition may alter cell responsiveness; such effects, however, have not been particularly marked in our studies with parietal cells.

TECHNIQUES FOR CELL SEPARATION

The parietal cell contents of the unfractionated mucosal cell suspensions prepared from canine fundic mucosa range from 10 to 28% (53), although other investigators (3) have reported higher percentages. Parietal cells have been enriched by use of both velocity and density separation techniques. Velocity separation can be accomplished by unit gravity sedimentation (40,49), use of the elutriator rotor (53,57,71), and by brief, repeated centrifugation (52,64). Velocity separation is based on Stokes law,

$$SV = (2/9) \, r^2(\varrho_p - \varrho_m)g/\eta$$

in which SV is the sedimentation velocity, ϱ_p and ϱ_m, respectively, are the density of the cells and medium, r is the radius of the cell, η is the viscosity of the medium, and g is the gravitational field. Cell size is thus the major determinant of sedimentation velocity; with its larger size, the parietal cell sediments more rapidly than the other mucosal cells. The parietal cell, however, must be separated from persisting gastric gland fragments (57). The degree of enrichment of parietal cells achieved with these techniques ranges from 50 to 90%. Unit gravity sedimentation produces good separation of mucosal cells yet requires considerable time in the cold room for each run; thus it provides only a small yield of the enriched cell fractions. Repeated centrifugation (64) produces larger yields and does not require specialized equipment; however, reproducibile fractions of variable parietal cell content are difficult to prepare.

In our studies with canine mucosal cells, we have used the Beckman elutriator rotor (53,57,71). Separation in the elutriator rotor is based on the principle of counterflow centrifugation (42). A set of rotating seals allows continuous perfusion of the separation chamber during centrifugation. Flow within the funnel-shaped separation chamber is more rapid near the periphery, where the cross-sectional area is small, and slower near the center, where the cross-sectional area is greater. Cells equilibrate within the chamber as a function of their sedimentation velocity, with the smaller and thus slower cells near the center, and the larger, more rapidly sedimenting cells at the periphery. As flow rate is increased, successively larger cells are eluted. Since it has not been possible to prepare fractions with a pure subpopulation of a given type of mucosal cell, we have examined all the

fractions from the elutriator separation. The distribution among these fractions of parietal cells, chief cells, mucus cells, and histamine was determined (Fig. 1) (See refs. 53,57,61,63). Determining the distribution of such various markers in cell separation experiments is very important, since even minor contamination by an unidentified cell type can influence the properties of that cell fraction in a given study. In studies with rat fundic mucosa, we have found that histamine-containing cells have a light density, thus making it difficult to separate them from the parietal cells by density gradient separation only (62).

Density separations have been performed using a variety of media, including sucrose (36,37), albumin (61), Ficoll (23,41,67), and Percoll. Both step gradients (23,41,67) and linear gradients (36,37,61) have been used. Step gradients are much simpler technically and may provide a good yield of highly enriched cells; however, these gradients may not provide resolution of various subpopulations of mucosal cells. We have used linear gradients to separate the histamine-containing cells from canine fundic mucosa (61), but for routinely enriching parietal cells, we have not found density separation to have any advantage over separation in the elutriator rotor. The choice of media for density separation is important, because these media may have deleterious effects on cell viability. Lewin and co-workers (64) discontinued using sucrose because of such effects.

Conceptually, one can neatly separate velocity (isokinetic) and density (isopyknic) separations as techniques that separate on the basis of cell size or cell density, respectively. Separation in either case is a function of the sedimentation velocity. With velocity separations, density of the medium is kept low, and separation is a dynamic process that depends on the square of the

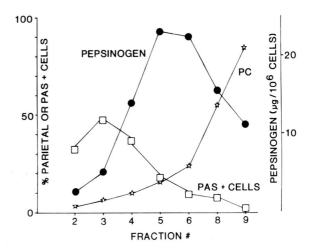

FIG. 1. Cell separation using the elutriator rotor. Isolated canine mucosal cells were separated using a Beckman elutriator rotor, as previously described (53,71). The distribution among the cell fractions of cells staining positively with PAS, of pepsinogen, and of parietal cells (PC) is noted. [This figure was adapted from an earlier publication (71).]

cell radius. On the other hand, isopyknic separations are equilibrium processes using a medium with a range of densities matching that of the cells to be separated. Cells are forced through the gravitational field until their sedimentation velocity reaches zero as they encounter a medium density equivalent to their own density. In practice, separations are often not so clearly of one type. If either the gravitational force or run time in a density separation is inadequate to force the cell to an equilibrium position, then the separation achieved will depend on both cell size and cell density. This combined velocity and density separation can be an advantage if the cell under study is both larger and more dense than the other cells present. The parietal cell is the largest of the mucosal cells and, because of its large complement of membranes, one of the lightest (A. H. Soll, *unpublished observations*). Thus a velocity separation in a medium of density approaching that of the parietal cell (1.045 to 1.055) would probably yield a poor result.

An additional factor than can complicate separation procedures is introduced when the osmolality differs from that normally encountered in extracellular fluid. A medium with a high osmolality, such as sucrose, will serve to increase the apparent cell density and thus shift the equilibrium position of the cells. Such separations in high osmolality will lead to overestimates of cell density (36). The use of high osmolality solutions may explain why previous studies (23,41,67) found parietal cells to pellet through rather than float in step density gradients made up of Ficoll in a standard balanced salt solution with a final density of 1.070. In our studies with canine mucosal cells, we used a combination of 20% bovine serum albumin and 9% Ficoll in distilled water to produce a medium with a density of about 1.085 and an osmolality of 290 to 300 mOsm Kg^{-1} (61). With a medium such as Percoll, it is possible to achieve densities in this range without risking high osmolality.

INDICES OF RESPONSE TO STIMULATION

In intact mucosa, the secretion of H$^+$ into the gastric lumen is accompanied by the simultaneous equimolar secretion of HCO$_3^-$ at the basal surface of the cell. With dispersion, this polarity is lost, and thus the secretion of H$^+$ per se is difficult to measure. Michelangeli (44), in his studies with isolated oxyntic cells from amphibian mucosa, demonstrated a transient acidification of the medium. Although these studies indicated that isolated oxyntic cells are capable of secreting hydrochloric acid, it is unlikely that the direct measurement of acid secretion will be a generally useful index of parietal cell response to stimulation, since the response is transient and blunted by the coupled secretion of bicarbonate. Stimulants have also been shown to increase chloride flux in isolated rabbit parietal cells that have been polarized by exposure to an electric field (23). This technique,

however, has not been widely used. Several other indirect indicies of parietal cell response to stimulation have been developed.

Oxygen Consumption

The secretion of acid is a highly energy-dependent process, as reflected by the high density of mitochondria in the parietal cell. In systems such as the *ex vivo* canine stomach preparation (33), where acid secretion and oxygen consumption can be measured simultaneously, there is a tight correlation between the effects of stimulants on these parameters. Michelangeli (43), using a Clark-type polarographic electrode, demonstrated that stimulants increased oxygen consumption by isolated amphibian cells. Using similar techniques, treatment with secretagogues increased the rate of oxygen consumption by parietal cells isolated from canine fundic mucosa (53). Berglindh et al. (5), using a Gilson respirometer, found that treatment with stimulants increases oxygen consumption by isolated gastric glands.

Morphological Transformation

With stimulation, the parietal cell *in vivo* undergoes a dramatic morphological transformation, characterized by the coalescence of the cytoplasmic tubulovesicles that fill the cytoplasm in the basal state into secretory canaliculi that drain into the gastric lumen. Parietal cells *in vitro* also may undergo a similar transformation (5,43,60). Figure 2 illustrates an isolated canine parietal cell which has been treated with a cholinomimetic agent with the appearance of secretory canaliculi lined with microvilli.

Aminopyrine Accumulation

Shore and co-workers (51) demonstrated that weak bases partitioned between the gastric circulation and gastric juice as a function of their pKa. This pH partition phenomenon formed the basis for the use of the clearance of weak bases, such as aminopyrine, as an index of mucosal blood flow (29). Berglindh et al. (5) found that their gastric gland preparation accumulated ^{14}C-aminopyrine (AP). The accumulation of AP serves as a handy index of the response of isolated canine parietal cells to stimulation (57). The accumulation of AP by isolated gastric glands was interpreted as possibly reflecting accumulation of acid in the lumen of the gland. We have shown that isolated canine parietal cells accumulate AP, indicating that accumulation was taking place within the cell itself. AP is a weak base, with a pKa of 5.0; at cytoplasmic pH, AP is thus un-ionized and highly permeable across plasma membranes. When AP diffuses into the acidified secretory canaliculi and tubulovesicles of the stimulated parietal cell, it picks up a H$^+$ and, being ionized, is thus locked in by the sur-

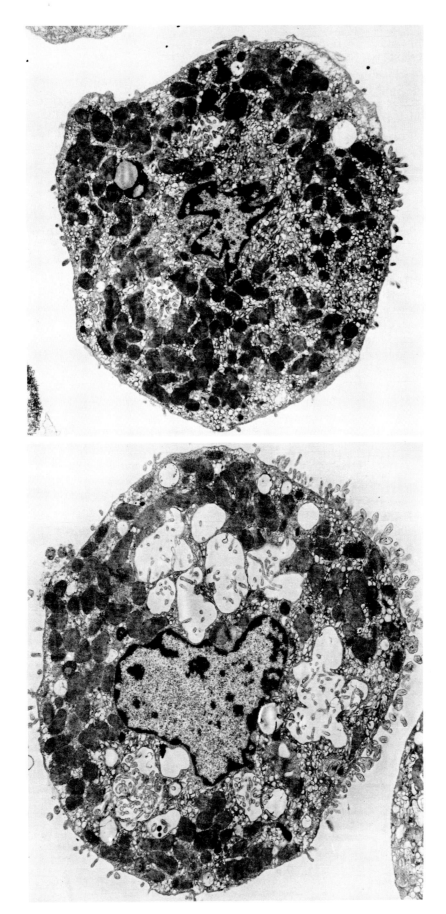

FIG. 2. Morphologic transformation of isolated canine parietal cells. Parietal cells were incubated in Earles balanced salt solution in the absence (**top**) or presence (**bottom**) of carbachol (100 μM). After 20 min, cells were fixed in 1% glutaraldehyde in cacodylate buffer (0.1 M, pH 7.4). Electron microscopy was then performed on Epon-embedded sections in collaboration with Dr. J. Lechago and B. Crawford.

rounding lipophilic barrier. It is important to recognize that the accumulation of AP does not serve as an index of the quantity of acid secreted but rather of the acid sequestered within the parietal cell. AP accumulation thus may not correspond exactly with other indicies of parietal cell response, such as oxygen consumption (57). Nonetheless, AP accumulation serves as a simple and reliable index of the response of parietal cells to stimulation.

THE EXISTENCE OF SPECIFIC RECEPTORS ON THE PARIETAL CELL

As discussed earlier, there is little question that histamine, gastrin, and cholinergic pathways stimulate acid secretion. The location and specificity of the receptors for these actions, however, has not been clarified by *in vivo* study. Two theories have been put forward to explain the actions and interdependence of the stimulants of acid secretion (Fig. 3). The first model, championed initially by MacIntosh (39) and further developed by Code (16) and Black et al. (9), represents a series concept wherein histamine is the final common mediator regulating parietal cell function, with acetylcholine and gastrin serving to release histamine from its fundic mucosal stores. According to this model, the parietal cell would have receptors only for histamine. This concept would thus fit with the ability of H_2 receptor antagonists to inhibit the action of acetylcholine and gastrin, but it would not explain the potentiating interactions demonstrated *in vivo* or the ability of anticholinergic agents to inhibit histamine action. According to the second theory, the parietal cell has specific receptors for histamine, gastrin, and acetylcholine. Furthermore, interactions occur between secretagogues in their action on the parietal cell itself. Studies with isolated parietal cells allow these two possibilities to be tested.

Histamine

Histamine stimulates parietal cell function, as evidenced by changes in oxygen consumption (5,43,53), AP accumulation (5,57), and morphologic transformation (5,60). With canine parietal cells, the action of histamine is relatively weak but is markedly enhanced by inhibition of the cyclic AMP-degrading enzyme phosphodiesterase by isobutylmethylxanthine (IMX) (Fig. 4) (53,57). In isolated parietal cells from rabbit, histamine stimulation of AP accumulation is 10- to 20-fold greater than that found with canine cells (Fig. 4). The reason for this difference has not been elucidated (see below).

There is little controversy regarding the notion that histamine is acting at an H_2 receptor on the parietal cell. H_2 blockers inhibit histamine action on oxygen consumption and AP accumulation by canine parietal cells (53,57) and rabbit isolated gastric glands (7,14). Cimetidine, in increasing concentrations, produced a progressive parallel shift of the dose response for histamine stimulation of AP accumulation (Fig. 5). The dissociation constant calculated from these data is 1 μM (57) and thus is similar to those found in guinea pig atrium and rat uterus (11). A somewhat different value was obtained in similiar studies with isolated rabbit gastric glands (14), but it is unlikely that this represents a significant difference. Atropine (10 μM) did not inhibit histamine stimulation of parietal cell function (Fig. 5), unless studied at very high concentrations (57).

H_1 receptor antagonists, such as mepyramine, also can inhibit histamine stimulation of isolated parietal cells (57). This effect was only found at mepyramine concentrations about 10μM; furthermore, it was not specific for histamine, since stimulation by carbachol and the cyclic AMP analog dibutyryl cyclic AMP was also blocked. Since these effects were found only with concentrations of H_1 antagonists 10^5-fold greater than the

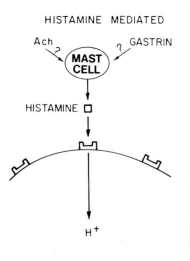
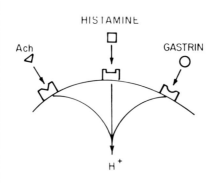

FIG. 3. Two possible models for interaction of stimulus on parietal cell function are illustrated. **Left:** Acetylcholine (Ach) and gastrin action is mediated by release of histamine, with only histamine acting directly on the parietal cell. **Right:** All three stimulants act directly on the parietal cell, with potentiating interactions accounting for the interdependency in their action.

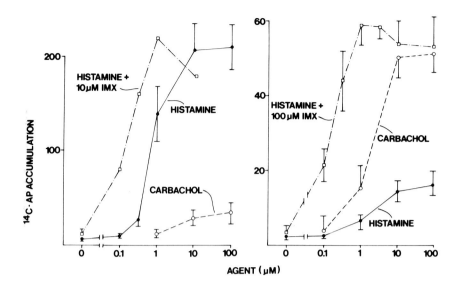

FIG. 4. Secretagogue stimulation of AP accumulation in rabbit **(left)** and canine **(right)** parietal cells. AP accumulation was determined as previously described (57); the data for canine parietal cells **(right)** are derived from these studies. Rabbit parietal cells **(left)** were prepared by similar techniques and enriched using the elutriator rotor to a mean parietal cell content of 58%. The data, the mean ± SE, are from four to five preparations of cells, with the exception of the data for the effects of histamine plus 10 μM IMX on rabbit cells, which represents data from two preparations.

range in which specific H_1 receptor blockade was found, these data should not be interpreted as reflecting an "H_1" action on the parietal cell. Rather, these findings highlight the importance of careful attention to the concentrations of agents used in studies of isolated cells. Erroneous conclusions can be easily drawn from the nonspecific actions found when agents are used in suprapharmacologic and/or supraphysiologic concentrations.

Cholinergic Receptors

Cholinomimetic agents stimulate parietal cell function, as evidenced by increases in oxygen consumption

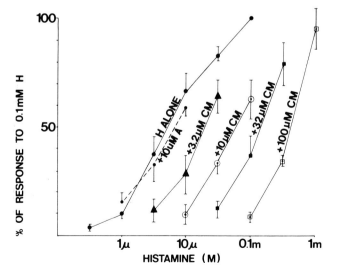

FIG. 5. H_2 receptor blockade of histamine-stimulated AP accumulation by isolated canine parietal cells. AP accumulation by canine parietal cells was determined as previously described (57) and expressed as a percentage of the response to 100 μM histamine (H). The responses to histamine alone and to histamine plus 10 μM atropine (A) and to histamine plus cimetidine (CM) at concentrations between 3.2 μM and 100 μM are illustrated as noted (Reproduced with permission from ref. 57.)

(5,43,53), AP accumulation (5,57), and morphologic transformation (Fig. 6). Berglindh et al. (5) noted a weak and transient stimulation of rabbit parietal cell function by cholinomimetic agents. With isolated parietal cells from rabbit, the response to carbachol is also found to be less than to histamine (Fig. 4). In contrast, with canine parietal cells, cholinergic agents produced sustained increases in both AP accumulation and oxygen consumption which were greater than those produced by histamine as a single stimulant, although histamine plus the phosphodiesterase inhibitor IMX produced a somewhat greater response than did carbachol (Fig. 4) (53,57). Thus even when parietal cells are isolated from rabbit and canine mucosa by identical techniques, there are differences in the relative potencies of histamine and cholinomimetics.

Anticholinergic agents inhibit carbachol action on oxygen consumption and AP accumulation (7,53,57). Atropine at concentrations between 3.2 and 100 nM produced a progressive, parallel, rightward shift of the dose response for carbachol stimulation of AP accumulation by isolated canine parietal cells, whereas cimetidine (10 μM) did not alter this dose-response relationship (57). The dissociation constant determined from this atropine effect was 1 nM, which is similar to that found for atropine inhibition of cholinergic stimulation in other tissues (57). Thus the isolated parietal cell, even after enzyme dispersion, retains pharmacologically typical muscarinic and H_2 receptors.

Gastrin

Although there is little controversy regarding the actions of histamine and cholinergic agents on isolated parietal cells, the effects of gastrin are disputed. With isolated canine parietal cells, gastrin produced a small but definite increase in both oxygen consumption (53) and AP accumulation (57). Gastrin caused a small increase in chloride flux by polarized parietal cells isolated from rabbit fundic mucosa (23). Pentagastrin, however, did not stimulate oxygen consumption by parietal cells isolated from amphibian mucosa (43), nor was stimulation of oxygen consumption or AP accumulation found in gastric glands from rabbit fundic mucosa (5,6).

The most convincing indication of direct action of gastrin on parietal cell function comes from its role in potentiating interactions with histamine (see below). Gastrin appears to be acting via a receptor that is distinct from muscarinic and histamine receptors in that neither atropine nor H_2 receptor antagonists block its action (53,57). In one study with rat mucosal cells, binding of ^{3}H-gastrin was found in fractions enriched in parietal cells (64). The [^{3}H]-gastrin, however, was of somewhat compromised biologic activity (21,38). Furthermore, the only effect of gastrin found in this preparation of cells was stimulation of adenylate cyclase in crude membrane fractions, an effect that may not be relevant to the action of gastrin on intact cells (63). Therefore, no correlation could be drawn between binding and biologic activity of gastrin to establish whether this binding represents interaction with the physiologically relevant gastrin receptor. Furthermore, the possibility has not been excluded that binding was to the histamine-containing cells in rat fundic mucosa, which are likely to have a gastrin receptor, since in rat, gastrin releases histamine and induces the activity of histidine decarboxylase (4).

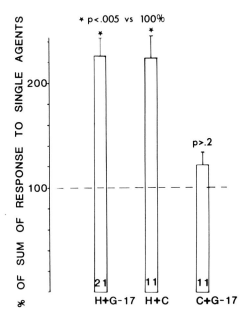

FIG. 6. Effects of combinations of agents on AP accumulation. Data for the effects of 10 μM histamine (H), 0.1 μM gastrin (G), and 1 μM carbachol (C) on AP accumulation have been expressed as a percentage of the maximal response to single agents. *Dashed line,* additive response equal to the sum of the individual responses. The statistical significance of the differences from this additive response is indicated. The number of preparations examined are indicated at the base of each column.

POTENTIATING INTERACTIONS BETWEEN SECRETAGOGUES

In vivo, the interdependence of secretagogue action is most clearly evident in the apparent nonspecificity of the effects of anticholinergic agents and H_2-receptor antagonists (see above). In contrast, with isolated parietal cells, these agents appear to be specific against cholinomimetics and histamine, respectively. This apparent contradiction may be explained by the existence of potentiating interactions, which are evident when parietal cells are treated with combinations of stimulants. For the purpose of this discussion, potentiating interactions are considered to exist when the response to a combination of agents is greater than the sum of the individual responses. The pattern of these potentiating interactions is similar whether assessed using AP accumulation or oxygen consumption as the index of response.

Treatment of isolated canine parietal cells with the combination of histamine and carbachol produced increases in both oxygen consumption (53) and AP accumulation (Fig. 6) that were greater than the sum of the response to single agents. Demonstration of this effect in canine parietal cells using oxygen consumption as the index of response required the presence of the phosphodiesterase inhibitor, IMX, probably because of the low sensitivity of measurement of oxygen consumption as an index of response. Monitoring AP accumulation, the degree of potentiation between histamine and carbachol was similar in the presence or absence of IMX (Fig. 6) (55). Potentiation between histamine and cholinergic agents was also found in studies with isolated rabbit gastric glands (6).

Furthermore, in isolated canine parietal cells, histamine potentiated the action of gastrin on both oxygen consumption (54) and AP accumulation (Fig. 6). In isolated rabbit gastric glands, however, the combination of histamine and gastrin did not produce greater stimulation of function than did histamine alone (6).

In contrast to the potentiating interactions found between histamine and gastrin and histamine and carbachol, the combination of carbachol and gastrin did not produce greater than an additive response by canine parietal cells (Fig. 6) (54). However, with a background of histamine, adding carbachol and gastrin together produced an increment in response that was greater than the sum of the increments in response produced by carbachol and by gastrin when added singly to the same background of histamine (55). Thus, under the conditions of these studies, it appears that there may be a three-way potentiation between these three stimulants.

When the effects of inhibitors are tested on these combinations of stimulants that produce potentiating interactions, an apparent nonspecificity is evident, reminiscent of that found *in vivo.* Thus, for example, if the response to gastrin is potentiated by interaction with histamine, this potentiated gastrin response is inhibited by H₂ receptor antagonists, presumably reflecting withdrawal of histamine potentiation of gastrin action (54). In contrast, atropine fails to inhibit the response, since there is no cholinergic component involved. Both atropine and cimetidine inhibited the response to the combination of histamine and carbachol, with the residual responses equivalent to those found with histamine or carbachol, respectively, as single agents (54). The effects of atropine and cimetidine on the combination of histamine, carbachol, and gastrin are of interest because they simulate a pattern found *in vivo*. When AP accumulation by isolated canine parietal cells was stimulated by this three-way combination of agents, treatment with cimetidine inhibited the response to a level similar to that produced by carbachol plus gastrin; treatment with atropine inhibited the response to that produced by histamine plus gastrin; and treatment with cimetidine and atropine simultaneously reduced the response to that found with gastrin alone (55).

In vivo, even in the basal state, the parietal cell appears to be under tonic influences from endogenous histamine and acetylcholine (see above). Thus the actions of any superimposed stimulant may be influenced by interactions with the effects of these endogenous secretagogues. When the effects of inhibitors *in vivo* are assessed, their actions may include blockade of the effects on endogenous histamine and acetylcholine. When gastrin is administered *in vivo*, therefore, its effects may involve interaction with endogenous histamine, and the net response may be influenced by histamine-acetylcholine interactions. The marked inhibition of gastrin action *in vivo* by H₂ receptor antagonists may reflect the fact that gastrin is an intrinsically weak stimulant of parietal cell function and requires potentiation by histamine for optimal effects. This possibility is of interest because of the parallel with the *in vitro* studies, in which gastrin was found to be a weak stimulant of the function of isolated canine parietal cells when acting alone, but its actions was markedly potentiated by histamine.

In vivo, cholinergic input appears to be of less importance to gastrin action on the parietal cell in that anticholinergics cause less inhibition of gastrin action than does cimetidine. Whether inhibition by atropine of gastrin action *in vivo* represents inhibition of a true potentiating interaction between gastrin and cholinergic inputs at the parietal cell remains unclear. These two stimulants may have interdependent actions at some other step in the integrated response of the fundic mucosa to stimulation, such as release of histamine, but there is no direct evidence for such a possibility. Alternatively, this inhibition may possibly reflect withdrawal of the interactions occurring in the basal state between endogenous acetylcholine and histamine, an effect that would impair the response of the parietal cell to any superimposed stimulus.

SECONDARY EFFECTOR MECHANISMS FOR SECRETAGOGUE ACTION

Cyclic AMP

The possibility that cyclic AMP may mediate secretagogue action on parietal cells has been studied extensively using intact mucosa; however, no clear picture of the role of cyclic AMP has emerged (19,30). This controversy regarding the effects of agents on cyclic AMP generation resulted largely from the difficulties of addressing this question using intact mucosa. There is little controversy regarding the effects of stimulants on cyclic AMP generation by isolated mucosal cells. Several groups have shown that histamine stimulates cyclic AMP generation by mucosal cells from dog (40,50,63,71), guinea pig (3), and rat (52,66) and isolated gastric glands from rabbit (14). In fractions prepared using the elutriator rotor, histamine stimulation of cyclic AMP production by canine fundic mucosal cells was found to correlate with the parietal cell content (Fig. 7). A similar pattern was evident in two other studies in which velocity cell separation was performed (40,52). In contrast to the ability of histamine to increase cyclic AMP production by parietal cells, treatment with cholinomimetics and gastrin did not alter cyclic AMP production under conditions in which stimulation of oxygen consumption and AP accumulation were found (Fig. 8). Gastrin may activate adenylate cyclase in broken cell preparations from rat fundic mucosa (38,64), but gastrin action in intact canine parietal cells does not appear to be linked to cyclic AMP generation.

Histamine stimulation of cyclic AMP production appears to be closely linked to stimulation of parietal cell function. In studies with canine parietal cells, a highly significant correlation was found between the effects of various combinations of histamine and IMX on rates of oxygen consumption and cyclic AMP production (63). Histamine stimulation of AP accumulation also occurred over the same concentration range in which stimulation of cyclic AMP generation was found, and with an IMX background of 10 μM, a linear correlation was found between histamine stimulation of AP accumulation and of cyclic AMP production. With a higher IMX background (100 μM), AP accumulation does not proportionately reflect the higher levels of stimulation found in the studies of oxygen consumption. Under these conditions, with canine parietal cells, little correlation was found between histamine stimulation of cyclic AMP formation and AP accumulation.

Histamine stimulation of cyclic AMP production by isolated rabbit parietal cells was of much greater mag-

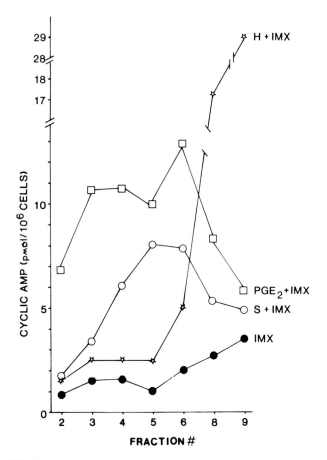

FIG. 7. Cellular distribution of hormone-stimulated cyclic AMP production. Canine fundic mucosal cells were separated by elutriation as noted in Fig. 1. Effects of prostaglandin E_2 (PGE$_2$, 100 μM), secretin (S, 0.1 μM) and histamine (H, 10 μM) on cyclic AMP production in the presence of 100 μM IMX were determined in each of the cell fractions. Data are the means of four preparations of cells and are expressed in picomoles of cyclic AMP generated per 10^6 cells during a 5-min incubation. (Reproduced with permission from ref. 71.)

nitude than that found with canine parietal cells (Fig. 9). With canine parietal cells, 10 μM histamine produced a twofold increase in cyclic AMP production, whereas this concentration of histamine increased cyclic AMP production by isolated rabbit parietal cells by 7.5-fold. The addition of the phosphodiesterase inhibitor IMX markedly potentiated the response in both rabbit and canine parietal cells (Fig. 9). The reason for the difference between canine and rabbit parietal cells is not known; differences in the activities of both adenylate cyclase and phosphodiesterase must be evaluated. With isolated gastric glands from rabbit, AP accumulation, oxygen consumption, and cyclic AMP generation were found to be closely correlated during histamine stimulation (14).

There is little question that histamine stimulates cyclic AMP production by reacting with an H$_2$ receptor, since H$_2$ receptor blockers have been shown to inhibit stimulation of cyclic AMP production in canine (50,63), rat (52), and guinea pig (3) parietal cells and in rabbit gastric glands (14). The dissociation constant determined for this effect of H$_2$ antagonists on histamine stimulation of cyclic AMP production (14,40) is similar to that found for stimulation of AP accumulation (see above) and for that found in other tissues. These latter findings are further evidence indicating that the action of histamine on cyclic AMP production is closely linked to its stimulation of parietal cell function.

In further support of this view linking cyclic AMP with histamine action, the 8-bromo and dibutyryl analog of cyclic AMP have been found to stimulate parietal cell function, as evidenced by increases in oxygen consumption (63), AP accumulation (57), and morphologic transformation (43). The corresponding analogs of cyclic

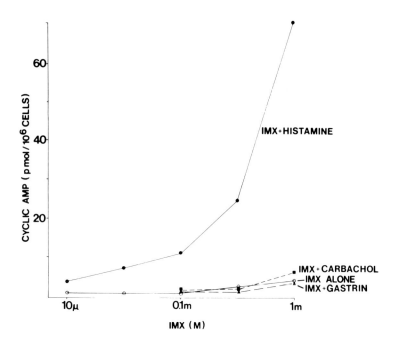

FIG. 8. Effects of histamine, carbachol, and gastrin on cyclic AMP production by isolated canine parietal cells. Cyclic AMP production by three preparations of enriched canine parietal cells was determined following treatment with histamine (10 μM), carbachol (100 μM), or gastrin (100 μM), each in the presence of the indicated concentration of IMX. [Data adapted from a previous report (63).]

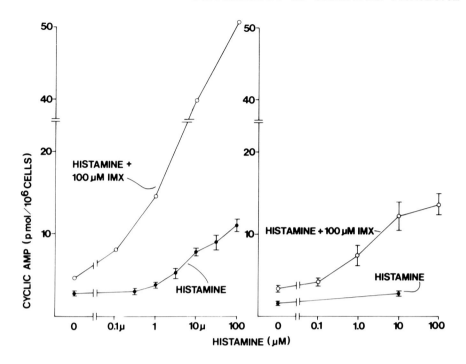

FIG. 9. Effects of histamine and IMX on cyclic AMP production by rabbit **(left)** and canine **(right)** parietal cells. Effects on cyclic AMP production of histamine with and without an IMX background were tested in four preparations of enriched rabbit parietal cells **(left)** and in five preparations of enriched canine parietal cells **(right)**. [Latter data adapted from a previous publication (63).]

GMP did not increase AP accumulation by canine parietal cells (57).

As mentioned above, the inhibition of phosphodiesterase activity potentiates the action of histamine on AP accumulation (Fig. 4) (14,57), oxygen consumption (53), and cyclic AMP production (Figs. 8 and 9) by isolated canine parietal cells. IMX and a second phosphodiesterase inhibitor Ro76398 were found to be equally potent in their effects on AP accumulation and cyclic AMP production, whereas effects of theophylline were found only at 100-fold higher concentrations (63). With rabbit gastric glands, the presence of IMX was found to shift the dose-response relationships for histamine stimulation of AP accumulation and oxygen consumption to the left, while not altering the concentration of histamine producing 50% stimulation of cyclic AMP production (14). Thus in the presence of IMX, a given concentration of cyclic AMP was found to produce a higher level of stimulation. These findings may reflect the possibility that cyclic AMP turnover at a specific site may be of greater importance than the total cell content of cyclic AMP. IMX, however, has been recognized to have actions independent of phosphodiesterase inhibition (13), which may explain the apparent discrepancy found in these studies with rabbit gastric glands.

IMX as a single agent stimulates oxygen consumption (53) and AP accumulation (57) by isolated canine parietal cell. These effects were inhibited by H_2 receptor antagonists. Similarly, in rabbit mucosa in culture, IMX stimulation of intrinsic factor secretion was also inhibited by cimetidine (31). The mechanisms by which IMX as a single agent stimulates parietal cell function and by which cimetidine inhibits this effect have not been elucidated.

Unfractionated canine gastric mucosal cells have a relatively high content of histamine, which is largely due to the mast cells present (61). Histamine is present in the supernate of the unenriched cell suspensions at concentrations above 0.1 μM (M. A. Beaven and A. H. Soll, *unpublished observations*). With elutriation, mast cells are eluted with the small cells (with fractions 2 and 3 in Fig. 1), and the content of histamine in the parietal cell fractions (8 and 9 in Fig. 1) is less than 1% of that found in these two fractions. However, these parietal cells have been incubated in the presence of 0.1 μM histamine during preparation, and this endogenous histamine may be occupying the parietal cell H_2 receptors even after enrichment. It is then possible that IMX stimulation of parietal cell function reflects enhancement of the action of this endogenous histamine. This hypothesis is reasonable because the threshold for IMX stimulation of parietal cell function occurs at IMX concentrations of between 32 and 100 μM (53,57); against these concentrations of IMX, the threshold for stimulation of both AP accumulation (57) and oxygen consumption (53) is found at histamine concentrations of 0.1 μM.

The hypothesis that the stimulation of parietal cell function by IMX as a single agent reflects enhancement of the action of residual endogenous histamine was tested by determining the effects of removing this histamine. Enriched parietal cell fractions (fraction 8 in Fig. 1) were initially incubated in the presence of 10 μM cimetidine and then washed extensively in cimetidine-free Earles balanced salt solution. These cimetidine-washed cells were then compared to cells that had been incubated in a similar fashion in the presence of 100 nM histamine and then washed. Cimetidine-washed cells from five preparations had a decreased AP accumulation in response to 0.1 and 1 mM IMX, when compared to control cells, whereas the response to 0.1 µM histamine with a 100 µM IMX background was not diminished (Fig. 10). Adding cimetidine (10 µM) caused further inhibition of AP accumulation in response to IMX in both groups (Fig. 10).

These data support the view that the action of IMX as a single stimulant on parietal cell function may reflect, at least in part, enhancement of the residual endogenous histamine that appears to be bound to parietal cell H_2 receptors. IMX may be acting through additional mechanisms (13), but these have yet to be defined in the parietal cell. The observation that cimetidine at concentrations as low as 1 µM inhibits IMX stimulation of AP accumulation favors the possibility that this inhibition reflects H_2 receptor blockade. Cimetidine may have actions on parietal cell function independent of H_2 receptor blockade, although none has thus far been established.

PROSTAGLANDINS AND CYCLIC AMP

One of the most convincing arguments against the role of cyclic AMP in the stimulation of acid secretion came from studies of the effects of prostaglandins on cyclic AMP production in intact mucosa. Prostaglandins were shown to inhibit acid secretion (48) and yet to stimulate cyclic AMP production and/or activate adenylate cyclase in intact mucosa (19,30,65). If prostaglandins were found to stimulate adenylate cyclase in the parietal cell itself, then few would argue for a positive link between cyclic AMP and parietal cell stimulation. Studies with isolated parietal cells have helped to clarify this issue; when mucosal cells are separated by velocity techniques, prostaglandin stimulation of cyclic AMP production has been found to correlate in-versely with the content of parietal cells (Fig. 7) (40,52,71).

Although none of these studies excludes an effect of prostaglandin on parietal cell cyclic AMP production, they do indicate that the effect will be minor compared to stimulation of cyclic AMP production in nonparietal cells. The cell separation data do not allow firm conclusions regarding the cell responsible for prostaglandin stimulation of mucosal cyclic AMP production but suggest an effect on both mucus and chief cells (Figs. 1 and 7). It must be stressed that stimulation of cyclic AMP production by prostaglandins in both isolated cells and intact mucosa occurs at concentrations above 1 µM (58,71). At much lower concentrations, more interesting effects of prostaglandins are found; these are more likely to be related to prostaglandin inhibition of parietal cell function.

Prostaglandins specifically inhibit histamine-stimulated AP accumulation by isolated canine parietal cells (Fig. 11) (58). This effect occurs at PGE_2 concentrations between 1 nM and 100 µM. Similar concentrations of PGE_2 did not inhibit stimulation of AP accumulation by carbachol, gastrin, or dibutyryl cyclic AMP (58). When the effects of either carbachol or gastrin were enhanced by interaction with histamine, however, PGE_2 did inhibit stimulation to the extent of withdrawing histamine enhancement of carbachol or gastrin action (Fig. 11). A similar inhibition of histamine-stimulated AP accumulation has been found in isolated rabbit parietal cells. With rabbit cells, but not with canine parietal cells (58), prostaglandin inhibition of histamine action was fully surmountable at higher concentrations of histamine (Fig. 12).

Since PGE_2 inhibited the action of histamine but not dibutyryl cyclic AMP, it would be expected to block histamine enhancement of cyclic AMP production. Two

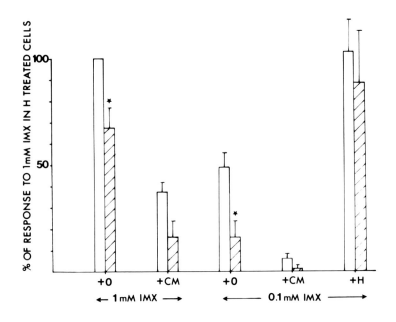

FIG. 10. Possible effects of residual endogenous histamine on IMX stimulation of parietal cell function. Five preparations of enriched parietal cells were preincubated for 10 min in Earles solution in the presence of either 100 µM cimetidine (*hatched bars*) or 0.1 µM histamine (*open bars*). After washing the cells three times in cimetidine-free Earles, AP accumulation was determined as described previously (57). The following treatment groups were examined: 1 mM IMX, 1 mM IMX plus 10 µM cimetidine (CM), 0.1 mM IMX, 0.1 mM IMX plus 10 µM cimetidine, and 0.1 mM IMX plus 0.1 µM histamine (H). The data were normalized to the AP accumulation ratio over basal produced in the histamine preincubated cells by 1 mM IMX, which was 37.7 ± 12.7. Statistical significance of the differences between the pretreatment groups is indicated by the star for $p < 0.05$.

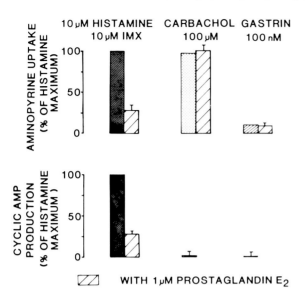

FIG. 11. Effects of prostaglandin E_2 on hormone stimulation of AP accumulation and cyclic AMP production by isolated canine parietal cells. AP accumulation was determined as previously described (57,58), with the data expressed as the percentage of the maximal response to histamine (10 μM) plus 10 μM IMX. The effects on AP accumulation of carbachol (100 μM) and gastrin (100nM) are also illustrated. Prostaglandin E_2 (1μM) inhibited histamine stimulation but not the effects of carbachol or gastrin. In the lower portion of the figure, the effects of these agents on cyclic AMP production are illustrated. Prostaglandin inhibited histamine stimulation of cyclic AMP production; neither gastrin nor carbachol altered cyclic AMP production.

studies with canine parietal cells have yielded similiar findings that prostaglandins of the E group at concentrations in the nanomolar range inhibit histamine-stimulated cyclic AMP production (Fig. 11) (40,58).

The above studies indicate that prostaglandins specifically inhibit histamine-stimulated parietal cell function and appear to exert this action by blocking cyclic AMP production. Prostaglandin inhibition of hormone-stimulated cyclic AMP production was first demonstrated by Butcher and Baird (12), who found PGE_1 inhibition of epinephrine-stimulated lipolysis and cyclic AMP production in isolated fat cells. Way and Durbin (69) proposed that prostaglandin inhibition of acid secretion may be mediated by specific inhibition of histamine-stimulated parietal cell function.

CALCIUM AND PARIETAL CELL ACTIVATION

The importance of increases in cytosol calcium in coupling stimulant action with cell response is well recognized in a variety of cell types (see refs. 8,18,46). This increased cytosol calcium may result from either enhanced calcium entry across the plasma membrane or mobilization of calcium from intracellular stores, such as mitochondria. The role of gating of extracellular calcium in stimulant action on isolated parietal cells has been studied by assessing the magnitude of the stimulation of AP accumulation in the presence of varying extracellular calcium concentrations (56). When extracellular calcium was decreased from the usual 1.8 mM to 0.1 mM, carbachol stimulation of AP accumulation was impaired by 92%, whereas histamine stimulation under similar conditions was impaired by only 28%. There was thus a highly significant difference in dependency on extracellular calcium between cholinergic and histamine stimulation. Decreasing extracellular calcium to 0.1 mM had an intermediate effect on the small response to gastrin, causing a 67% impairment.

A similar pattern of dependency on extracellular calcium was found in studies using lanthanum, a trivalent

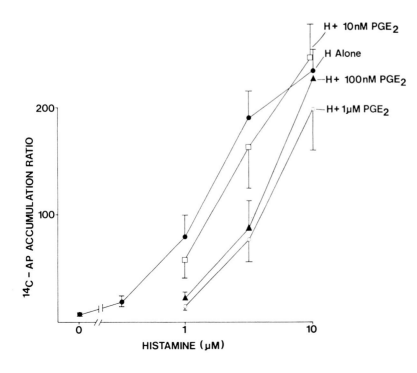

FIG. 12. Effects of prostaglandin E_2 on histamine-stimulated AP accumulation by isolated rabbit parietal cells. AP accumulation was determined for rabbit parietal cells prepared and enriched by previously described methods (57). The effects of three concentrations of PGE_2 were tested on stimulation by the indicated concentrations of histamine. Data are the mean ± SE for four preparations of cells. Note that prostaglandin inhibition of histamine action is fully surmountable, with the data suggesting a parallel rightward shift of the dose-response relationship.

cation that impairs calcium flux across plasma membranes and displaces surface bound calcium (34). Lanthanum (100 μM) impaired carbachol stimulation by 83%, while causing no significant impairment of histamine stimulation and a 40% decrease in gastrin stimulation. The impairment of cholinergic stimulation with calcium removal was rapidly restored by readdition of the extracellular calcium. These observations indicated that carbachol stimulation of parietal cell function depended on a rapidly exchangeable, lanthanum-accessible pool of calcium.

The possibility that cholinergic stimulation was mediated by gating of extracellular calcium across the plasma membrane was tested by determining the influx of $^{45}Ca^{2+}$. Calcium influx, tested from 1 to 20 min after cholinergic stimulation, was increased, and a highly significant correlation was found between cholinergic stimulation of calcium influx and stimulation of oxygen consumption. Neither histamine nor gastrin altered calcium influx from that found with untreated cells. In cell separation experiments, the magnitude of carbachol-stimulated calcium influx correlated with the parietal cell content of the fractions examined, indicating that parietal cells were the predominant cell type accounting for the observed changes in calcium influx. Enhanced calcium influx may be occurring in other cell types, but these studies did not provide evidence for this possibility.

These data indicate that cholinergic but not histaminic stimulation of parietal cell function is closely linked to enhanced influx of extracellular calcium. On the other hand, activation of parietal cell function by histamine but not carbachol is closely linked to stimulation of cyclic AMP generation. Although the data presented above indicate that gastrin action demonstrates some dependence on extracellular calcium, the data do not show that gastrin action is linked to calcium gating. Elucidation of the mechanisms involved in gastrin action requires further study.

RECEPTORS AND EFFECTORS FOR PARIETAL CELL FUNCTION

The available studies with isolated parietal cells generally support the following model for regulation of parietal cell function by chemical transmitters (Fig. 13). The parietal cell has specific receptors for histamine, gastrin, and acetylcholine. The histamine and acetylcholine receptors appear to be pharmacologically typical H_2 and muscarinic receptors, respectively. The specificity of the receptors on the parietal cell for these three stimulants is at odds with the apparent nonspecificity of H_2 and anticholinergic receptor antagonists in their action on acid secretion in vivo. This discrepancy may be explained by the existence of potentiating interactions between histamine and gastrin and histamine and

cholinergic agents in their actions on the parietal cell, but not between cholinergic agents and gastrin directly. Assuming that histamine and acetylcholine are continuously released at the parietal cell even in the basal state, such interactions will always be present in intact mucosa. In the presence of these potentiating interactions, H_2 and anticholinergic receptor antagonists display a cross-specificity reminiscent of that found in vivo and suggesting that interference with potentiating interactions may account for an important component of their actions in vivo.

The action of histamine but not cholinergic agents or gastrin is closely linked to enhanced generation of cyclic AMP. Prostaglandins specifically block histamine stimulation of parietal cell function by interfering with a step prior to generation of cyclic AMP. The action of cholinergic agents but not of histamine is closely related to enhanced influx of calcium across the plasma membrane. The mechanisms mediating activation by gastrin have not been elucidated.

The existence of potentiating interactions involving endogenous histamine and acetylcholine may be of great importance in vivo in modulating parietal cell sensitivity to superimposed stimulation. The mechanisms underlying these interactions have not been clarified, although it does appear that potentiation reflects the convergence of cyclic AMP-dependent and calcium-dependent path-

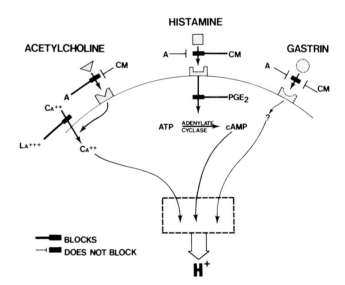

FIG. 13. A proposed model for the actions, interactions, and effectors for secretagogue stimulation of the function of isolated parietal cells. Receptors for acetylcholine, histamine, and gastrin are indicated, as are the proposed sites of action of atropine (A) and cimetidine (CM). The effect of acetylcholine on calcium influx is indicated, along with lanthanum inhibition of calcium influx. Although gastrin action appears to be linked to enhanced calcium influx or mobilization of intracellular calcium, the question mark indicates that solid data are lacking. Histamine stimulation of adenylate cyclase and the proposed site of action for inhibition by PGE_2 are also indicated. [This figure was adapted from one previously published (54).]

ways, as had been suggested for the pancreatic acinar cell (22). It is unlikely that potentiation occurs at the level of cyclic AMP generation in that the magnitude of histamine-stimulated cyclic AMP production is not affected by the presence of carbachol or gastrin under the same conditions that produce a potentiated parietal cell response. Carbachol stimulation of calcium influx is likewise not influenced by the presence of histamine, suggesting that the potentiation observed between these agents is not mediated by histamine enhancement of carbachol-stimulated calcium influx. Therefore, the only data available regarding the mechanisms of the potentiating interactions are negative, in that these interactions do not involve potentiation of either cyclic AMP generation or enhanced influx of calcium. Presumably, potentiation must involve some step at which the calcium and cyclic AMP paths converge before the final event of H^+ secretion.

RISK-BENEFIT CONSIDERATIONS IN STUDIES USING ISOLATED PARIETAL CELLS

The use of isolated parietal cells can facilitate certain lines of investigation regarding the factors regulating parietal cell function *in vivo*. The gains resulting from this approach have been outlined above and include removal of the parietal cell from the effects of endogenous transmitters, allowing the actions of single stimulants and the interactions between stimulants to be elucidated. Cells in suspension can be easily used for studies, such as examining cyclic AMP production or calcium influx. Cell separation can be performed, localizing certain effects, such as stimulation of cyclic AMP production, to specific cell types. There are many potential limitations which must be kept in mind while interpreting data obtained by such an approach.

Effects of Enzyme Treatment and Calcium Chelation

Treatment of cells with proteolytic enzymes can have deleterious effects on structural and functional sites on the cell surface. Exposure to a specific enzyme can selectively alter components of the surface membrane. For example, treatment with neuramidase cleaves siliac acid groups, which impairs calcium gating by myoblasts in culture (35). Trypsin impairs insulin binding by isolated adipocytes, an effect that is reversible with short-term culture (32). Pituitary cells are rendered nonfunctional by trypsin dispersion; with short-term culture, however, the cells recover the ability to release hormones upon exposure to hypothalamic releasing hormones (68). Considering the wide variety of enzyme activities in the crude collagenase used to disperse parietal cells, it is surprising that functional responses are retained at all, and that receptors for histamine and ace-

tylcholine retain their pharmacologic properties. Calcium removal has deleterious effects on cell integrity (1,2). The probability of altered cell function with dispersion must be kept in mind, along with the possibility that short-term culture may allow some reversal of these deleterious effects.

Loss of Intercellular Junctions and Communication and Cell Polarity

Intercellular connections are clearly of greater functional importance than simply holding cells together in the tissue they comprise. These cell connections allow communication between cells, which may include transport of molecules of a variety of sizes and may provide a low resistance pathway for ionic conductance (28). Pancreatic acinar cells show a greater release of amylase with stimulation (45,70) when studied as dispersed acini rather than as single cells. This probably reflects effects of both disrupted intercellular connections and disturbed cell polarity. Williams (70) has noted that isolated pancreatic acinar cells, while retaining overall polarity, have lost apical specialization, including the microfilament and microvillous complex.

In contrast to these dramatic effects of dispersion on pancreatic acinar cell function, single parietal cells function at least as well as parietal cells present in isolated gastric glands. Basal oxygen consumption in isolated canine gastric glands is about 8 μl/mg dry weight (5,14); assuming a 3:1 ratio of wet to dry weight, 4.2 μg DNA/mg wet weight, and 8.5 μg DNA/10^6 cells (71), basal oxygen consumption is roughly 5 μl/10^6 cells/hr in these glands. This estimate compares with a figure of 3 to 5 μl/10^6 cells/hr for isolated canine mucosal cells when enriched to a parietal cell content of 30 to 50% (53).

Stimulation of oxygen consumption in both the isolated glands from rabbit (5,14) and dispersed canine cells (53) ranges from 50 to 100% over basal levels. The accumulation of AP appears to be somewhat greater in canine parietal cells than in isolated canine gastric glands (Fig. 14). Although basal AP accumulation ratios obtained with isolated rabbit parietal cells (Fig. 4) are somewhat lower than those found with isolated glands (5,14), the stimulated ratios are at least threefold greater in isolated cells than in glands. With loss of apical connections with neighboring cells, the apical openings of the secretory canaliculi may close, thus allowing the canaliculi to dilate, providing larger volume for the accumulation of AP. Thus the loss of cell communications and cellular polarity has less pronounced effects on the function of parietal cells than of pancreatic acinar cells. It is unlikely that loss of cell polarity has no effect on the structure and function of the specialized apical and basolateral membranes of the parietal cells, but these influences are unclear.

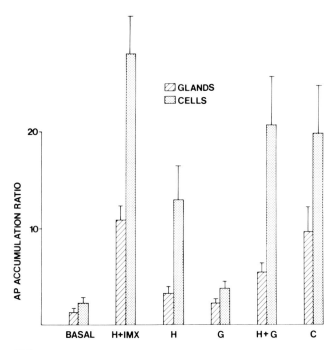

FIG. 14. Comparison between the responses of parietal cells and gastric gland fragments isolated from canine fundic mucosa. Parietal cells were prepared by techniques previously described (53). Gastric glands were prepared by similar techniques, with the exception of not exposing the tissue to EDTA. Glands were then separated by sedimentation at unit gravity (5). For calculation of the AP accumulation ratios for the glands. DNA values were determined by the Burton technique and converted to cell counts assuming 8.5 μg DNA/10^6 cells (71). Parietal cells were counted on hematoxylin and eosin stained sections prepared from paraffin blocks; glands were found to contain 32 $\pm$ 3% parietal cells. Data represent the mean $\pm$ SE for five preparations of cells and glands.

Loss of Integrative Functions Present in Intact Mucosa

Isolating the parietal cell has the advantage of removing the cell from endogenous influences which may alter cell function. This reductionistic approach obviates the possibility of demonstrating the relative importance of the inputs of the various chemical transmitters on parietal cell function *in vivo*. Studies with isolated parietal cells demonstrate that acetylcholine and gastrin may act by directly stimulating the parietal cell, and that the action of these two agents is potentiated by interaction with histamine. Acetylcholine and gastrin may also cause the release or enhance the formation of histamine as well, a possibility that has not been tested by the present studies. Furthermore, acetylcholine, in addition to stimulating the parietal cell, may trigger inhibitory pathways by such mechanisms as release of potential inhibitors, including somatostatin or glucagon. The relevance of knowledge gained by studying functional responses of isolated parietal cells will only become clear when these findings are integrated with the functional properties of other cell types, of the mucosal neural elements, and of the intact mucosa as a unit.

Interpretation of Negative Findings

Cell function may be impaired by the rigors of tissue dispersion and cell separation for many reasons. Caution is needed, therefore, in interpreting negative data, such as the failure of the parietal cell to respond to a given stimulus. The failure of rabbit gastric glands to respond to gastrin may reflect the absence of a gastrin receptor on the parietal cell (5,43), or it may reflect the loss of this receptor due to enzyme treatment or the selective loss of the capacity of the cell to respond to gastrin because of impairment of the specific effector systems involved. Calcium gating mechanisms may be sensitive to neuramidase treatment, probably reflecting the importance of critical siliac acid groups (35). It would not be surprising to see such functional groups selectively impaired during cell dispersion. Furthermore, minor structural variations among species in critical functional groups on the membrane may produce differing sensitivity to the rigors of the *in vitro* environment and may account for some of the variation in the pattern of responses to stimulants.

Physiologic, Pharmacologic, and Toxic Effects of Agents

Isolated cells can be treated with high concentrations of drugs and hormones, concentrations that would often be either toxic or obviously nonspecific in their actions *in vivo*. *In vitro*, toxicity and nonspecificity may not be readily apparent. Two clear examples are atropine and mepyramine. When studied in nanomolar concentrations, these agents are specific inhibitors for muscarinic cholinergic receptors and H_1 receptors, respectively. However, both agents inhibit the action of pharmacologically unrelated agonists when used in 10^6-fold higher concentrations (57). These actions of high concentrations of atropine and mepyramine are not necessarily related to specific receptor blockade. Affinity of an antagonist for a receptor is independent of the agonist used or the tissue studied; therefore, antagonist actions should be considered to reflect interaction with a specific receptor only when they are found in the same concentration range as that in which specific actions have been fully characterized (9). This comparison can best be done by determining the dissociation constants for drug action in a given system; this value should be the same for all actions of an antagonist reflecting blockade of a specific receptor. When a higher concentration of an agent is required to see an effect, the specificity of its action in that case should be suspect. Following similiar reasoning, in order for a given *in vitro* action of an agonist to be considered of potential physiological relevance, this action should be found in a similiar concentration range as that producing other physiological actions of agonist; a requirement for higher doses suggests an impaired response to the agent or a suprapharmacologic action.

Species Differences in Parietal Cell Responses to Stimulation

Although it is theoretically unsatisfying to resort to species differences to explain discrepancies in data, it appears that the *in vitro* behavior of isolated cells does depend on the species of origin. Thus, when compared under identical conditions to canine parietal cells, rabbit parietal cells show an attentuated response to cholinergic agents and no significant response to gastrin (Fig. 4). Furthermore, histamine produces a more pronounced stimulation of both AP accumulation and cyclic AMP production in rabbit parietal cells than in canine cells (Fig. 9). The explanation for these differences is not clear at present, but may relate to factors such as the sensitivity of certain receptors to dispersion by enzyme treatment, the delicate nature of effector systems that involve gating of extracellular calcium, or differences in the activity of enzymes, such as phosphodiesterase. The significance of such differences must be interpreted with great caution until an explanation becomes clear.

Species Differences in the Histamine-Storing Cells of the Fundic Mucosa.

Histamine is stored by mast cells in canine and human fundic mucosa (61) and by an enterochromaffin-like endocrine cell in the rat fundic mucosa (4,62). In the rat, but not the dog, gastrin has been shown to increase the activity of histidine decarboxylase, the enzyme that forms histamine (4). In the frog, pentagastrin causes release of histamine from gastric mucosa *in vitro* (45a). The content and turnover of histamine in the rat and amphibian fundic mucosa is thus influenced by gastrin, but the extent to which gastrin modulation of histamine formation and release serves as a major regulator of parietal cell function in these species *in vivo* remains unsettled. In order to establish a causal link between gastrin-induced liberation of histamine and gastrin-stimulated acid secretion, the release of histamine must be proportional to, and necessary for, gastrin stimulation of acid secretion. Furthermore, with histamine stored in gastrin-sensitive, endocrine-like cells in some species and in an *apparently* gastrin-resistant, mast-like cells in other species, it is possible that the role played by gastrin in the physiological regulation of parietal cell function will differ among these species. The cell responsible for histamine storage has not been established in several species, nor has the effect of gastrin on histamine storage and release. Recent studies suggest that histamine may be stored in an endocrine-like cell in both the frog (M. C. Landais and F. Michelangeli, *personal com-*

munication) and in the rabbit (7a) and that in both of these species gastrin serves to enhance histamine formation and release. Consideration of these important species differences regarding the storage, formation, and release of histamine is essential to sorting out the controversies regarding the regulation of parietal cell function.

Interpretation of Cell Separation Studies

Since cell separation techniques do not yet produce pure populations of a given cell type, interpretation of cell separation studies must always consider the effects of the cells present other than those under prime consideration. The potential influence of those other cells can be fully assessed only when those other cell types have been identified. Unfortunately, markers for every cell type may not be readily available or fully specific and sensitive. A gradient separation that allows correlation between a given activity and abundance of a given cell type in the separated cell fractions can be seductively convincing. It is possible, however, that two cell types may distribute in the gradient in a similiar fashion. In the absence of pure fractions and perfect markers, one must attempt to identify all pertinent cell types and interpret findings with appropriate caution.

Acknowledgments

This work was supported in part by NIAMDD grants AM-19984 and AM-17328 and by the Research Service of the Veterans Administration.

REFERENCES

1. Amsterdam, A., and Jamieson, J. D. (1974): Studies on dispersed pancreatic exocrine cells. I. Dissociation technique and morphologic characteristics of separated cells. *J. Cell Biol.,* 63:1037–1056.
2. Amsterdam, A., Solomon, T. E., and Jamieson, J. D. (1978): Sequential dissociation of the exocrine pancreas into lobules, acini, and individual cells. In: *Methods in Cell Biology, Vol. 20,* edited by R. M. Prescott, pp. 361–378. Academic Press, New York.
3. Batzri, S., and Gardner, J. D. (1978): Cellular cyclic AMP in dispersed mucosal cells from guinea pig stomach. *Biochim. Biophys. Acta,* 541:181–189.
4. Beaven, M. A. (1978): Histamine: its role in physiological and pathological processes. In: *Monographs in Allergy, Vol. 13,* edited by P. Kallos, p. 114. Karger, Basel.
5. Berglindh, T., Helander, H. F., and Obrink, K. J. (1976): Effects of secretagogues on oxygen consumption, aminopyrine accumulation, and morphology in isolated gastric glands. *Acta Physiol. Scand.,* 97:404–414.
6. Berglindh, T. (1977): Potentiation by carbachol and aminophylline of histamine-and db-cAMP-induced parietal cells activity in isolated gastric glands. *Acta Physiol. Scand.,* 99:75–84.
7. Berglindh, T. (1977): Effects of common inhibitors of gastric acid secretion on secretagogue-induced respiration and aminopyrine accumulation in isolated gastric glands. *Biochim. Biophys. Acta,* 464:217–233.
7a. Bergqvist, E., Waller, M., Hammar, L., and Obrink, K. J.

(1980): Histamine as the secretory mediator in isolated gastric glands. In: *Hydrogen Ion Transport in Epithelia*, edited by I. Shulz, G. Sachs, J. G. Forte, and K. J. Ullrich, pp. 429–437. Elsevier/North Holland Biomedical Press, New York.

8. Berridge, M. J. (1975): The interaction of cyclic nucleotides and calcium in the control of cellular activity. In: *Advances in Cyclic Nucleotide Research, Vol. 6*, edited by P. Greengard and G. A. Robison, pp. 1–98. Raven Press, New York.

9. Black, J. W., Duncan, W. A. M., Durant, C. J., Ganellin, C. R., and Parsons, E. M. (1972): Definition and antagonism of histamine H_2-receptors. *Nature*, 236:385–390.

10. Blum, A. L., Shah, G. T., Wiebelhaus, V. D., Brennan, F. T., Helander, H. F., Leballos, R., and Sachs, G. (1971): Pronase method for isolation of viable cells from necturus gastric mucosa. *Gastroenterology*, 61:189–200.

11. Brimblecombe, R. W., Duncan, W. A. M., Durant, G. J., Emmett, J. C., Ganellin, C. R., Leslie, G. B., and Parsons, M. E. (1978): Characterization and development of cimetidine as a histamine H_2-receptor antagonist. *Gastroenterology*, 74:339–347.

12. Butcher, R. W., and Baird, C. E. (1968): Effects of prostaglandins on adenosine 3′, 5′-monophosphate levels in fat and other tissues. *J. Biol. Chem.*, 243:1713–1717.

13. Chapman, R. A., and Miller, D. J. (1974): Structure-activity relations for caffeine: A comparative study of the inotropic effects of the methylxanthines, imidazoles and related compounds on the frog's heart. *J. Physiol.*, 242:615–634.

14. Chew, C. S., Hersey, S. J., Sachs, G., and Berglindh, T. (1980): Histamine responsiveness of isolated gastric glands. *Am. J. Physiol.*, 238:G312–320.

15. Code, C. F., Hightower, N. C., and Hallenbeck, G. S. (1951): Comparison of the effects of methantheline bromide (Banthine) and atropine on the secretory responses of vagally innervated and vagally denervated gastric pouches. *Gastroenterology*, 19:254–264.

16. Code, C. F. (1965): Histamine and gastric secretion: a later look, 1955-1965. *Fed. Proc.*, 24:1311–1321.

17. Croft, D. N., and Inglefinger, F. J. (1969): Isolated gastric parietal cells: Oxygen consumption, electrolyte content and intracellular pH. *Clin. Sci.*, 37:491–501.

18. Douglas, W. W. (1976): The role of calcium in stimulus-secretion coupling. In: *Stimulus-Secretion Coupling in the Gastrointestinal Tract*, edited by R. M. Case and H. Goebell, pp. 17–29. MTP Press, Lancaster, England.

19. Dousa, T. P., and Dozios, R. R. (1977): Interrelations between histamine, prostaglandins and cyclic AMP in gastric secretion: A hypothesis. *Gastroenterology*, 73:904–912.

20. Dotevall, G., Schroder, G., and Walan, A. (1955): The effect of poldine, glycopyrrolate and l-hyoscyamine on gastric acid secretion in man. *Acta Med. Scand.*, 177:169–174.

21. Gardner, J. D. (1979): Receptors for gastrointestinal hormones. *Gastroenterology*, 76:202–214.

22. Gardner, J. D., and Jackson, M. J. (1977): Regulation of amylase release from pancreatic acinar cells. *J. Physiol. (Lond.)*, 270:439–444.

23. Glick, D. M. (1974): Simulated chloride transport by isolated parietal cells. *Biochem. Pharmacol.*, 23:3283–3288.

24. Grossman, M. I. (1978): Control of gastric secretion. In: *Gastrointestinal Disease*, edited by M. H. Sleisenger and J. S. Fordtran, pp. 640–659. Saunders, Philadelphia.

25. Grossman, M. I. (1981): *This volume.*

26. Henn, R. M., Isenberg, J. I., and Maxwell, V. (1975): Inhibition of gastric acid secretion by cimetidine in patients with duodenal ulcer. *N. Engl. J. Med.*, 293:371–374.

27. Hirschowitz, B. I., and Sachs, G. (1969): Atropine inhibition of insulin, histamine, and pentagastrin stimulated gastric electrolyte and pepsin secretion in the dog. *Gastroenterology*, 56:693–702.

28. Iwatsuki, N., and Petersen, O. H. (1977): Pancreatic acinar cells: The acetylcholine equilibrium potential and its ionic dependency. *J. Physiol. (Lond.)*, 269:735–751.

29. Jacobson, E. D., Linford, R. H., and Grossman, M. I. (1966): Gastric secretion in relation to mucosal blood flow studied by a clearance technique. *J. Clin. Invest.*, 45:1–13.

30. Jacobson, E. D., and Thompson, W. J. (1976): Cyclic AMP and gastric secretion: The illusive second messenger. *Adv. Cyclic Nucleotide Res.*, 7:199–224.

31. Kapadia, C. R., Schafer, D. E., Donaldson, R. M., and Ebersole, E. R. (1979): Evidence for involvement of cyclic nucleotides in intrinsic factor secretion by isolated rabbit gastric mucosa. *J. Clin. Invest.*, 63:1044–1049.

32. Kono, T., and Barham, F. W. (1971): The relationship between the insulin-binding capacity of fat cells and the cellular response to insulin. *J. Biol. Chem.*, 246:6210–6216.

33. Kowalewski, K., and Kolodej, A. (1972): Relation between hydrogen ion secretion and oxygen consumption by *ex vivo* isolated canine stomach, perfused with homologous blood. *Can. J. Physiol. Pharmacol.*, 50:955–961.

34. Langer, G. A. (1976): Events at the cardiac sarcolemma: localization and movement of contractile-dependent calcium. *Fed. Proc.*, 35:1274–1278.

35. Langer, G. A., Frank, J. S., Nudd, L. M., and Seraydarian, K. (1976): Sialic acid: Effect of removal on calcium exchangeability of cultured heart cells. *Science*, 193:1013–1015.

36. Lewin, M., Cheret, A. M., Soumarmon, A., and Girodet, J. (1974): Methode pour l'isolement et le tri des cellules de la muqueuse fundique de rat. *Biol. Gastroenterol.*, 7:139–144.

37. Lewin, M., Cheret, A. M., Soumarmon, A., Girodet, J., Ghesquier, D., Grelac, F., and Bonfils, S. (1976): Isolated cells and a highly enriched population of parietal cells from rat gastric mucosa for the study of H^+ secretion mechanism. In: *Stimulus-Secretion Coupling in the Gastrointestinal Tract*, edited by R. M. Case and H. Goebell, pp. 371–375. MTP Press, Lancaster, England.

38. Lewin, M., Soumarmon, A., and Bali, J. P. (1976): Interaction of ^3H-labeled synthetic human gastrin I with rat gastric plasma membranes. Evidence for the existence of biologically reactive gastrin receptor sites. *FEBS Lett.*, 66:168–172.

39. MacIntosh, F. C. (1938): Histamine as a normal stimulant of gastric secretion. *Q. J. Exp. Physiol.*, 28:87–98.

40. Major, J. S., and Scholes, P. (1978): The localization of a histamine H_2-receptor adenylate cyclase system in canine parietal cells and its inhibition by prostaglandins. *Agents Action*, 8:324–331.

41. McDougual, W. S., and Decosse, J. J. (1970): Method for determining differential secretory function of isolated cells *in vitro*: Chloride movement in isolated parietal cells. *Exp. Cell. Res.*, 61:203–206.

42. McEwen, C. R., Stallard, R. W., and Julos, E. Th. (1968): Separation of biological particles by centrifugal elutriation. *Anal. Biochem.*, 23:369–377.

43. Michelangeli, F. (1976): Isolated oxyntic cells: Physiological characterization. In: *Gastric Hydrogen Ion Secretion*, edited by D. K. Kasbekar, G. Sachs, and W. S. Rehm, pp. 212–236. Marcel Dekker, New York.

44. Michelangeli, F. (1978): Acid secretion and intracellular pH in isolated oxyntic cells. *J. Membr. Biol.*, 38:31–50.

45. Peikin, S. R., Rottman, A. J., Batzri, S., and Gardner, J. D. (1978): Kinetics of amylase release by dispersed acini prepared from guinea pig pancreas. *Am. J. Physiol.*, 235:E743–749.

45a. Rangachari, P. K. (1975): Histamine release by gastric stimulants. *Nature*, 253:53–55.

46. Rasmussen, H., and Goodman, D. B. P. (1977): Relationships between calcium and cyclic nucleotides in cell activation. *Physiol. Rev.*, 57:421–509.

47. Richardson, C. R. (1978): Effect of H_2-receptor antagonists on gastric acid secretion and serum gastrin concentration. A review. *Gastroenterology*, 74:366–370.

48. Robert, A. (1976): Antisecretory, antiulcer, cytoprotective and diarrheogenic properties of prostaglandins. In: *Advances in Prostaglandin and Thromboxane Research, Vol. 2*, edited by B. Samuelsson and R. Paoletti, pp. 507–520. Raven Press, New York.

49. Romrell, L. J., Coppe, M. R., Munro, D. R., and Ito, S. (1975): Isolated and separation of highly enriched fractions of viable mouse gastric parietal cells by velocity sedimentation. *J. Cell Biol.*, 65:428–438.

50. Scholes, P. A., Cooper, A., Jones, D., Major, J., Walters, M., and Wilde, C. (1976): Characterization of an adenylate cyclase system sensitive to histamine H_2-receptor excitation in cells from dog gastric mucosa. *Agents Actions*, 6:677–682.

51. Shore, P. A., Brodie, B. B., and Hogben, C. A. M. (1957): The gastric secretion of drugs: A pH partition hypothesis. *J. Pharmacol. Exp. Ther.*, 119:361–369.

52. Sonnenberg, A., Hunziker, W., Koelz, H. R., Fischer, J. A., and Blum, A. L. (1978): Stimulation of endogenous cyclic AMP (cAMP) in isolated gastric cells by histamine and prostaglandin. *Acta Physiol. Scand. [Suppl.]*, 307–317.

53. Soll, A. H. (1978): The actions of secretagogues on oxygen uptake by isolated mammalian parietal cells. *J. Clin. Invest.,* 61:370–380.

54. Soll, A. H. (1978): The interaction of histamine with gastrin and carbamylcholine on oxygen uptake by isolated mammalian parietal cells. *J. Clin. Invest.,* 61:381–389.

55. Soll, A. H. (1978): Three-way interactions between histamine, carbachol, and gastrin on aminopyrine uptake by isolated canine parietal cells. *Gastroenterology,* 74:1146 (Abstr.).

56. Soll, A. H. (1981): Extracellular calcium and cholinergic stimulation of isolated canine parietal cells. *J. Clin. Invest. (in press).*

57. Soll, A. H. (1980): Secretagogue stimulation of ^{14}C-aminopyine accumulation by isolated canine parietal cells. *Am. J. Physiol.,* 238:G366–G375.

58. Soll, A. H. (1980): Specific inhibition by prostaglandins E$_2$ and I$_2$ of histamine-stimulated ^{14}C-aminopyrine accumulation and cyclic adenosine monophosphate generation by isolated canine parietal cells. *J. Clin. Invest.,* 65:1222–1229.

59. Soll, A. H., and Grossman, M. I. (1978): Cellular mechanisms in acid secretion. *Ann. Rev. Med.,* 29:495–507.

60. Soll, A. H., Lechago, J., and Walsh, J. H. (1976): The isolated mammalian parietal cell: Morphological transformation induced by secretagogues. *Gastroenterology,* 70:975 (Abstr.).

61. Soll, A. H., Lewin, K., and Beaven, M. A. (1979): Isolation of histamine-containing cells from canine fundic mucosa. *Gastroenterology,* 77:1283–1290.

62. Soll, A. H., Lewin, K. J., and Beaven, M. A. (1981): Isolation of histamine-containing cells from rat gastric mucosa: Biochemical and morphologic differences from mast cells. *Gastroenterology (in press).*

63. Soll, A. H., and Wollin, A. (1979): Histamine and cyclic AMP in isolated canine parietal cells. *Am. J. Physiol.,* 237:E444–E450.

64. Soumarmon, A., Cheret, A. M., and Lewin, M. J. M. (1978): Localization of gastrin receptors in intact isolated and separated fundic rat cells. *Gastroenterology,* 73:900–903.

65. Thompson, W. J., Chang, L. K., Rosenfeld, G. C., and Jacobson, E. D. (1977): Activation of rat gastric mucosal adenyl cyclase by secretory inhibitors. *Gastroenterology,* 72:251–254.

66. Thompson, W. J., Rosenfeld, G. C., Ray, T. K., and Jacobson, E. D. (1976): Activation of adenyl cyclase from isolated rat parietal cells by gastric secretagogues. *Clin. Res.,* 537A.

67. Walder, A. I., and Lunseth, J. B. (1963): A technique for separation of the cells of the gastric mucosa. *Proc. Soc. Exp. Biol. Med.,* 112:494–496.

68. Walker, A. M., and Hopkins, C. R. (1978): Stimulation of luteinising hormone release by luteinising hormone releasing hormone in the porcine anterior pituitary: Role of cyclic AMP. *Mol. Cell. Endocrinol.,* 10:327–341.

69. Way, L., and Durbin, R. P. (1969): Inhibition of gastric acid secretion *in vitro* by prostaglandin E$_1$. *Nature,* 221:874–875.

70. Williams, J. A. (1977): Effects of cytochalasin B on pancreatic acinar cell structure and secretion. *Cell Tissue Res.,* 179:453–466.

71. Wollin, A., Soll, A. H., and Samloff, I. M. (1979): Actions of histamine, secretion, and PGE$_2$ on cyclic AMP production by isolated canine fundic mucosal cells. *Am. J. Physiol.,* 237:E437–E443.

Physiology of the Gastrointestinal Tract, edited by
Leonard R. Johnson. Raven Press, New York © 1981.

Chapter 25

Gastric Acid Secretion in Humans

Mark Feldman and Charles T. Richardson

The normal human stomach contains approximately one billion parietal cells and under maximal stimulation can secrete 30 mmoles/hr or more hydrochloric acid. When a subject is fasting, the normal stomach secretes small amounts of acid relative to the secretory capacity; some subjects secrete no acid at all. When a meal is eaten, however, acid secretion is stimulated due to increased vagal activity, gastric distention, and chemical reactions of food with the gastrointestinal mucosa. As a result, acid secretion is stimulated to near maximal rates. In this chapter, we review the physiological mechanisms that lead to stimulation of acid secretion in humans and discuss the chemicals that mediate these responses. In addition, we discuss factors that determine the rate of basal acid secretion and the maximal secretory capacity. First, it is necessary to review methods of measuring human gastric acid secretion.

METHODS

Gastric Aspiration

Aspiration of gastric contents is the simplest and most widely used method of measuring acid secretion. Early studies of gastric physiology in humans were performed by aspirating gastric juice from stomachs of subjects with gastric fistulas. Because such subjects are rare, in most instances gastric juice is aspirated via a tube introduced into the stomach through the nose or mouth.

Ideally, gastric aspiration should withdraw each H^+ that the stomach has secreted. Accordingly, it is imperative that the aspirating ports of the tube be positioned, usually by fluoroscopy, in the most dependent portion of the stomach. Even when the tube has been positioned correctly, some acid (10 to 20%) escapes aspiration and empties through the pylorus into the duodenum (27,46).

Besides emptying from the stomach, a secreted H^+ may "escape" aspiration by diffusing back across the gastric mucosa or may be neutralized by alkaline secretions, such as duodenal juice, nonparietal gastric secretion, or saliva. All three mechanisms (pyloric losses, H^+ back diffusion, and neutralization) lead to an underestimation of gastric acid secretion. Despite these limitations, gastric aspiration is a useful method of measuring acid secretion. Basal acid secretion and maximal acid secretion in response to parenteral stimulants are commonly measured using this technique.

The H^+ concentration in a sample of aspirated gastric juice can be determined by one of two methods. First, the specimen can be titrated *in vitro* with a base (e.g., NaOH). Which pH to titrate to is arbitrary and controversial. The number of millimoles of base needed to titrate a volume of gastric juice to a pH endpoint (e.g., 7.0) represents the "titratable" acidity (in millimoles per liter) of the sample.

A second method of determining the H^+ concentration of a sample of gastric juice is to measure its pH with a glass electrode. Since the glass electrode measures

H^+ activity (a_{H^+}) and not concentration (c_{H^+}), it is necessary to convert a_{H^+} to c_{H^+} by the following equation:

$$c_{H^+} = \frac{a_{H^+}}{\gamma_{H^+}}$$

where γ is the activity coefficient for H^+ in gastric juice. Hydrogen ions have lower activity (i.e., are less apparent to the glass electrode) in polyionic solutions, such as gastric juice, than in pure HCl solutions (γ gastric juice $< \gamma$ pure HCl). Tables of activity coefficients for gastric juice have been developed by Moore (80). Although the glass electrode technique is simple, it is important that the electrode be calibrated daily with standardized solutions (e.g., pH 1.00, 4.01, and 7.00). If the pH of the specimen is near or lower than the lowest pH standard, the specimen should also be titrated with NaOH. Recently, a method has been developed that combines the glass electrode with *in vitro* titration (89).

In Vivo Intragastric Titration

The major limitation of gastric aspiration is that this method cannot accurately measure acid secretion while food is in the stomach. In 1973, Fordtran and Walsh (34) introduced a new technique—*in vivo* intragastric titration—for measuring food-stimulated gastric acid secretion. A double-lumen nasogastric tube is inserted into the stomach; then, either a meal is eaten in a normal manner, or a homogenized meal is infused into the stomach. Every 2 to 3 min, a sample of gastric contents (meal plus secreted fluid) is obtained through one lumen. If the pH of the specimen (determined by glass electrode) has fallen below the original pH of the meal as a result of acid secretion, a base, such as sodium bicarbonate, is infused into the stomach through the other lumen until the pH is restored to the original meal pH. For a given time period, the number of millimoles of base added to maintain pH constant is equal to the number of millimoles of acid secreted (34,119). This method was originally validated *in vitro* and has subsequently been validated *in vivo* (54) in patients with achlorhydria (while exogenous HCl was infused into the stomach to simulate acid secretion) and in animals with fundic pouches (11).

The major advantages of *in vivo* intragastric titration are: (a) applicability to studies with food in the stomach, (b) accuracy (between pH 5.5 and 2.5) (34,105,119), (c) reproducibility (34), and (d) the method is unaffected by gastric emptying (assuming good mixing of gastric contents with infused buffer). One criticism of *in vivo* titration is that intragastric pH is artifically held constant. However, it is possible to study the effect of intragastric pH on gastric acid secretory responses to food by performing *in vivo* titration studies at different intragastric pHs on separate days (119) or sequentially on the same day (112). Moreover, a constant intragastric pH is often desirable when gastrin release is being evaluated.

Recently, *in vivo* intragastric titration and gastric aspiration were compared as methods for measuring basal acid secretion in healthy human subjects (27). Saline was infused continously into the stomach during intragastric titration. Secretion rates were more than twofold as great when measured by titration than by aspiration. This is probably because when performing intragastric titration, even small amounts of fluid in the stomach cause gastric distention and stimulate acid secretion. Thus *in vivo* titration cannot be used to measure "basal" acid secretion in humans.

Indicator-Dilution Methods

In the early 1950s, Hunt and his colleagues (49) introduced the serial test meal, which contained sucrose and phenol red. From the dilution of the phenol red marker and the concentrations of acid and chloride, the authors calculated the acid secretory response to the liquid meal. This method cannot be used for meals that contain a buffer, such as protein.

Malagelada and co-workers (70) devised an indicator-dilution method which is applicable to liquid and solid meals. Using two markers (one gastric and one duodenal), they can calculate gastric acid secretion and gastric emptying simultaneously. Their methods are described in more detail elsewhere in this volume. Other workers (39) have used similar indicator-dilution methods.

CHEMICAL MEDIATORS OF ACID SECRETION IN HUMANS

Three endogenous substances—histamine, gastrin, and calcium—increase acid secretion when administered parenterally to humans. Since calcium releases gastrin (14), the effect of calcium on the parietal cell may be mediated through gastrin. Two other endogenous substances—acetylcholine and enkephalins—increase acid secretion in animals (62,90). In man, cholinergic agonist drugs cause little if any stimulation of acid secretion (97, 117), so there is little evidence that acetylcholine is a stimulant in humans. The effect of enkephalins on human acid secretion has not been reported.

It must be emphasized that an increase in acid secretion during parenteral infusion of an endogenous substance does not prove that the substance causes an increase in acid secretion under physiological conditions. Only when the concentration of the substance can be measured before and after a physiological stimulus (such as a meal) is it possible to determine whether the amount of mediator released is capable of causing the acid secretory response observed. This has been demonstrated only in the case of gastrin heptadecapeptide (G-17). The amount of G-17 released into the circula-

tion by an amino acid meal is sufficient to account for
the entire acid secretory response to the meal (33). Thus
there is evidence that gastrin plays a physiological role
in causing the increase in gastric acid secretion in response to a meal.

Studies using specific pharmacological antagonists
suggest that acetycholine, histamine, and enkephalins
play a role in acid secretion. Atropine (a muscarinic
antagonist), cimetidine (a histamine H_2 receptor antagonist), and naloxone (an opiate receptor antagonist) reduce acid secretion in the basal state and in response to
food and sham feeding (21,45,59,61,101,110; M. Feldman, *unpublished data*). Since these antagonists also
reduce gastrin-stimulated acid secretion (1,60; M. Feldman, *unpublished data*), acetylcholine, histamine, and
enkephalins may act in a permissive role to allow the parietal cell to more optimally respond to gastrin. Although
it is also possible that physiological stimuli release acetylcholine, histamine, and/or enkephalins into the circulation or in the vicinity of parietal cells, there is no
evidence to support this.

Calcium is another mediator that may play a permissive role in acid secretion. Individuals with severe hy-
pocalcemia are often achlorhydric (2,23). When serum
calcium concentrations are restored to normal, the parietal cells again secrete acid. Acutely elevating serum
calcium concentrations above normal increases acid secretion (14). It is unknown whether physiological events
that increase acid secretion, such as meals, increase the
amount of calcium near or in the parietal cell.

There are several endogenous substances capable of
reducing gastric acid secretion when infused exogenously. These include several gut peptides [secretin (19),
somatostatin (91), glucagon (13), gastric inhibitory peptide (73), and vasoactive intestinal peptide (69)] as well
as prostaglandins (95), dopamine (115), and magnesium
ions (14). It is uncertain whether any of these compounds play a physiological role in suppressing acid secretion.

H^+ within the gastric lumen also inhibit acid secretion
in response to all known physiological stimuli, e.g.,
food (119), sham feeding (31), and distention (20). This
inhibition by luminal acid is not due to a topical effect
on the parietal cells since the parietal cell response to
exogenous pentagastrin is unaffected by luminal pH
(11). The inhibitory effect of luminal acid on gastric
acid secretion is mediated by effects on gastrin release
and perhaps secretin release (see below).

In summary, many endogenous substances are capable of increasing or decreasing gastric acid secretion.
However, only G-17 has been shown to cause the acid
secretory response to a physiological stimulus. Histamine, acetylcholine, enkephalins, and calcium probably
play permissive roles; there is no evidence at present that
any of these compounds cause an increase in acid secretion in response to a physiological stimulus.

MAXIMAL SECRETORY CAPACITY AND PARIETAL CELL MASS

In addition to expressing acid secretion data in millimoles per unit time, it is often convenient to express
data as a fraction of the maximal secretory capacity of
the stomach. For clinical and research purposes, the
maximal secretory capacity can be estimated by the
maximal acid output (MAO) or peak acid output (PAO)
following administration of a maximal dose of histamine or gastrin pentapeptide (pentagastrin).[1] Since
MAO is thought to correlate with the number of parietal
cells present (10), the MAO and PAO are indirect estimates of parietal cell mass.

Figure 1 displays PAO for 105 healthy volunteers
studied consecutively in our laboratory. PAO varied
from 7.4 to 80.0 mmoles/hr. Based on the data of Card
and Marks (10), this range of PAO would correspond
to approximately 0.3 to 3.0 billion parietal cells. Unlike
the basal acid output (BAO), which varies considerably
from day to day (see below), the PAO remains relatively
constant over long periods of time (121).

PAO (and hence parietal cell mass) is a function of
sex, body weight, lean body mass, and age. Although
it is likely that PAO is determined by genetic factors,
there is little supporting evidence. Men have significantly higher mean PAOs than women of the same age
(40,122) (Fig 1). This difference is partly because men
weigh more and have larger lean body mass than women
(3). The fact that weight and lean body mass correlate
with PAO (3,48) suggests that larger individuals have
more parietal cells than smaller individuals. Although
children have lower PAOs than adults, PAOs in children are similar to adult values when expressed as millimoles per kilogram body weight per hour (15). In
adults, it is not certain whether PAO decreases in older
age groups (40,122).

There is evidence that the parietal cell mass and PAO
can increase under the trophic influence of gastrin. For
example, individuals with gastrin-producing tumors
(Zollinger-Ellison syndrome) may have PAOs of 100
mmoles/hr or more and have associated increases in
parietal cell mass (83). Removing the effect of gastrin
on parietal cells (by performing antrectomy) leads to
parietal cell atrophy (72) and to a decrease in PAO (7).
The parietal cell atrophy and the fall in PAO after antrectomy can be prevented at least in part with exogenous pentagastrin (7,53). These findings suggest that endogenous gastrin is trophic for parietal cells.

---

[1] In this chapter, we use PAO when referring to maximal secretory
capacity. This can be defined as the sum of the two highest consecutive 15-min acid outputs after parenteral administration of 6µg/kg
pentagastrin or 40 µg/kg histamine (both maximally effective doses).
This 30-min value is usually multiplied by 2 to express results in millimoles per hour. MAO represents the sum of the four 15-min acid
outputs after pentagastrin or histamine (4).

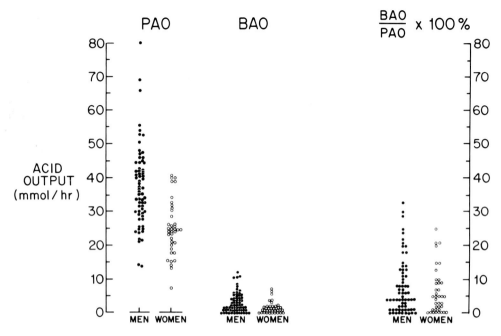

FIG. 1. PAO, BAO, and ratio of BAO to PAO in 105 healthy volunteers. *Closed circles,* men; *open circles,* women. Ages averaged 29 years for men (range 20 to 48) and 31 years for women (range 18 to 53).

There is experimental evidence that histamine (71), chronic hypercalcemia (perhaps through gastrin) (82), and electrical stimulation of the anterior hypothalamus (88) can increase parietal cell mass or density. Since patients with duodenal ulcer have higher mean PAO than control subjects (40), it is possible but unproved that some trophic factor (perhaps increased vagal activity) leads to the increase in parietal cell mass in these patients.

Following vagotomy in patients with duodenal ulcer, the PAO decreases by 50 to 60% (28,52,63). This occurs whether the antrum and duodenum are left innervated (selective proximal vagotomy) or are denervated (truncal vagotomy). Although the mechanism by which vagotomy reduces PAO is unclear, it is probably not due to a decrease in parietal cell mass because it occurs very quickly (within 24 hr) (87). In one study, PAO to histamine could be restored with mecholyl, suggesting that PAO falls after vagotomy because of loss of the permissive effect of acetylcholine (87). However, chronic anticholinergic therapy for several months does not reduce PAO to histamine (84). Moreover, in another study, PAO to pentagastrin after vagotomy could not be restored by carbacholine (96). It is likely that an intact vagus plays a permissive role in maximal acid secretion.

A recent study in dogs (37) reported that the reduced response to pentagastrin after vagotomy could be restored with the beta-adrenergic antagonist propranalol, suggesting that the fall in PAO after vagotomy may be due to unopposed adrenergic suppression of parietal cell function. The role of the adrenergic nerves on acid se-cretion in humans is poorly understood and must be studied in greater detail, especially in vagotomized individuals.

BASAL ACID SECRETION

Gastric acid secreted in the absence of all intentional and avoidable stimulation is called basal acid secretion. Since basal acid secretion is affected by such factors as thought, sight, and smell of food, basal acid secretion should be measured in a room that is devoid of food odors. In addition, the rate of basal acid secretion can be influenced by the emotional state of the individual. Anxiety, frustration, resentment, and guilt increase acid secretion (76).

The rate of basal acid secretion (usually called BAO) varies from hour to hour in the same individual and tends to follow a circadian pattern (78). The lowest secretory rates occur between 5 and 11 a.m., whereas the highest rates occur between 2 and 11 p.m. The cause for these cyclic variations in basal acid secretion is not known.

Even when measured at the same time of day in the same individual, BAO varies from day to day (Fig. 2). Among nine subjects studied five times over a 1.5- to 9-month period, BAOs varied considerably from each individual's mean BAO (coefficient of variation averaged 80%). It was not uncommon for a subject to secrete almost no acid on one day and more than 6 mmoles/hr on another day.

It is apparent from Fig. 2 that BAO varies considerably between individuals. In Fig. 1, BAO measure-

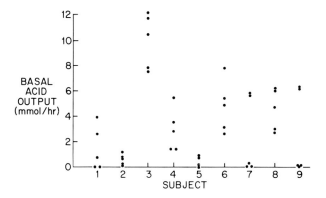

FIG. 2. BAO measured on five separate occasions in nine healthy subjects 1.5 to 9 months apart. The coefficient of variation ([SD ÷ mean] × 100%) averaged 80% and ranged from 22 to 131%. No subject was achlorhydric on any study.

ments are plotted in 105 healthy volunteers. BAO ranged from 0 to 12.8 mmoles/hr (mean 2.5, median 1.6 mmoles/hr). Despite the fact that males and females were age matched, males had a significantly higher mean BAO than females (3.0 versus 1.6 mmoles/hr).

If BAO were determined solely by the number of parietal cells present, the ratio of BAO and PAO should be nearly constant. As shown in Fig. 1 (right), however, BAO/PAO varies considerably from 0 to 32% (mean 7%, median 5%). Thus other factors beside PAO are responsible for the differences between subjects.

When basal serum gastrin concentrations and basal acid secretion are measured simultaneously, there is either no correlation (36) or a negative correlation (113). Moreover, there is no correlation between total immunoreactive serum gastrin levels and circadian changes in BAO (81). Similar studies measuring G-17 have not been performed. At present, there is no evidence that differences in basal acid secretion between subjects or in the same subject are attributable to changes in circulating gastrin levels.

A recent study found a correlation between changes in BAO and serum levels of pancreatic polypeptide (102). Since release of this hormone is thought to be under vagal control, the authors postulated that fluctuations in BAO represent fluctuations in basal vagal tone.

GASTRIC ACID SECRETION IN RESPONSE TO EATING

As discussed above, under basal conditions, the normal human stomach secretes acid at a rate that varies from 0 to approximately 30% of the maximal secretory capacity (PAO). When an appetizing meal is eaten, acid secretion increases and by 90 min is near the maximum that can be attained with exogenous histamine (34) (Fig. 3, top). Despite the fact that acid secretion increases rapidly during the first hour after a meal, the pH within the stomach remains relatively high (above 3.0) for at

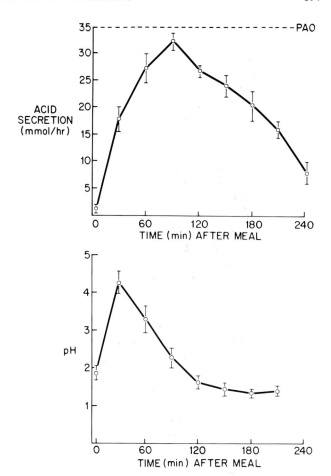

FIG. 3. Mean (± SE) acid secretion (**top**, $N = 6$) and intragastric pH (**bottom**, $N = 10$) following a sirloin steak meal in healthy subjects. On one day, after the meal was eaten, acid secretion was measured by intragastric titration to pH 5.5. On another day, intragastric pH was permitted to seek its natural level. The mean basal acid secretion rate and basal pH (prior to the meal) are shown at 0 min. The PAO is also indicated.

least 1 hr because food protein buffers secreted acid (70) (Fig. 3, bottom). During the second and third hours, the pH falls because much of the food buffer has emptied from the stomach.

The mechanisms that increase acid secretion after eating include: (a) cephalic-vagal stimulation, (b) gastrointestinal distention, and (c) chemical reactions of food with the gastrointestinal mucosa. Although these mechanisms are discussed separately, interactions between mechanisms occur, and it may be difficult to separate individual components. For example, it is impossible to study chemical reactions of food on the gastric mucosa without also distending the stomach.

Cephalic-Vagal Stimulation of Acid Secretion

Cephalic-vagal stimulation of acid secretion is activated by the thought, sight, smell, and taste of appetizing food. Afferent signals are sent to various centers within the brain (e.g. visual cortex, olfactory area). Efferent messages then travel downward through the hypothalamus, mesencephalon, and brainstem to the dorsal motor nuclei of the tenth cranial nerves (vagus nerves). The vagi contribute long, descending, preganglionic neurons, which travel to the stomach where axons terminate near short, postganglionic neurons, which innervate target cells (parietal cells in the fundus, gastrin cells in the antrum).

Since this reflex can be interrupted by vagotomy (26,28,56,86), it is assumed that the cephalic phase of acid secretion is mediated solely via the vagi. Although this concept has not been challenged, afferent signals activated by eating may also activate sympathetic pathways or release hormones from the brain which increase gastric acid secretion. If a nonvagal mechanism contributes to the cephalic phase of acid secretion, however, this putative mechanism also can be blocked by vagotomy.

Until recently, most information on the cephalic phase of gastric acid secretion in humans came from studies in rare patients with esophagostomies and gastrostomies. In 1973, Knutson and Olbe (55) described a new method for measuring acid secretion during sham feeding. Through a gastrostomy (which had been created at the time of surgical repair of a perforated duodenal ulcer), a rubber tube was introduced into the lower esophagus. Swallowed food was diverted from the stomach to the exterior through the rubber tube, and gastric acid output was measured by gastric aspiration from a separate tube placed into the stomach through the gastrostomy.

Mayer and associates (74) popularized a nonsurgical technique: "modified" sham feeding. During modified sham feeding, subjects chew and expectorate (rather than swallow) an appetizing meal, while gastric acid is aspirated through a nasogastric tube. This method leads to acid secretory responses comparable to conventional sham feeding (i.e., sham feeding that includes swallowing) (108). Because of its simplicity, modified sham feeding has been used recently to evaluate the cephalic phase of acid secretion in humans. Although small amounts of food sometimes are accidentally swallowed, this does not influence the results if the aspirated gastric juice is titrated to pH 7.0 (55). The use of the pH electrode to measure H^+ concentration may underestimate acid output during sham feeding if large amounts of swallowed food are present, since swallowed food can buffer acid and thus raise pH (M. Feldman and C. T. Richardson, *unpublished observations*).

Modified sham feeding leads to a rapid increase in gastric acid secretion (Fig. 4). Even after sham feeding ends, acid secretion remains elevated above basal levels for 1 hr or more. The maximal acid secretion rate in response to sham feeding ranges from 22 to 88% of the PAO (55-58,61,74,75,79,93,108); an average figure is 50%. Merely talking about appetizing food without seeing or smelling it increases acid secretion to approx-

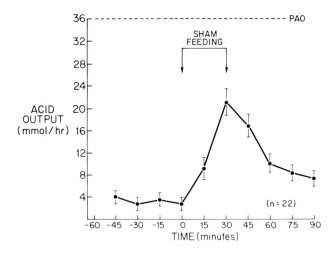

FIG. 4. Mean (± SE) acid output before, during, and after modified sham feeding in 22 healthy subjects. Sham feeding began at 0 min and lasted for 30 min (*arrows*). PAO for these subjects is shown.

imately 30% of PAO (29). Anticipation of an appetizing meal (including the sight and smell of food in preparation) elicited an acid response that was 55% of PAO in one study (79).

Why sham feeding-stimulated acid secretion rates do not approach PAO is unclear. One possibility is that not all parietal cells are vagally innervated. Another explanation is that vagal activation by sham feeding also may activate inhibitory mechanisms for acid secretion. For example, vagal stimulation may release a hormone ("vagogastrone") which inhibits gastric acid secretion. Evidence to support the existence of such a hormone has come from studies in dogs with vagally denervated fundic pouches (92,103). In these animals, sham feeding inhibited pentagastrin-stimulated acid secretion by 30 to 40%. Stenquist and his associates (107), attempting to demonstrate a similar mechanism in duodenal ulcer patients who had been treated by parietal cell vagotomy, found that sham feeding inhibited pentagastrin-stimulated acid secretion only slightly (16%) and briefly. Thus, at present, there is little evidence for vagal inhibition of acid secretion in humans.

Cephalic-Vagal Gastrin Release

Several experiments in animals (using electrical vagal stimulation, insulin-induced hypoglycemia, or sham feeding to activate vagal pathways) have demonstrated that vagal stimulation releases gastrin. When serum gastrin concentrations in response to sham feeding have been measured in humans, some investigators have reported significant gastrin rises (28-30,58,74), while others have not (61,75,79,93,109). To some extent, the discrepancies may be due to differences in patient selection, sham feeding methods, and gastrin radioimmunoassays. Results from studies in our laboratory are shown in Fig.

5 (left). Sham feeding led to a significant (15 ± 4 pg/ml) rise in serum gastrin concentrations.

For several reasons, it is likely that a rise in serum gastrin concentration on the order of 15 pg/ml could contribute to the cephalic phase of acid secretion. First, when human G-17 was infused into normal subjects, a plasma G-17 rise of 15 pg/ml led to an acid secretion rate that was about 30 to 40% of PAO (33). Thus seemingly small gastrin rises can lead to relatively high acid secretion rates. Second, when the gastrin response to sham feeding is blocked by antral acidification, the acid secretory response to sham feeding is reduced by 40 to 50% (31). Third, antrectomy reduces sham feeding-stimulated acid secretion more than antrectomy reduces PAO (58,85). Taken together, these observations suggest that gastrin contributes to the cephalic phase of acid secretion in humans.

Vagal stimulation may also potentiate the effect of gastrin on the parietal cell. Roland and co-workers (97) found that cholinergic agonist drugs lowered the dose of pentagastrin necessary to produce half-maximal acid secretion. Whether sham feeding would likewise shift the gastrin dose-response curve to the left has not been tested in humans, although this seems likely. Vagotomy, on the other hand, shifts the pentagastrin dose-response curve to the right (24,96). Thus, although sham feeding releases gastrin following parietal cell vagotomy (the antrum remains innervated), released gastrin does not elicit acid secretion, presumably because of decreased

sensitivity to gastrin as a result of denervation of the parietal cell area (28).

There is evidence that sham feeding not only activates pathways that release gastrin but also activates pathways that inhibit gastrin release (30). When atropine is administered prior to sham feeding, the ensuing gastrin response is enhanced (Fig. 5, left). Atropine also enhances the gastrin response to insulin-induced hypoglycemia (25). Since intragastric pH was kept constant (at 5.0) in these two studies, the enhancement of gastrin release by atropine could not have been caused by differences in gastric acidity. Blockade of a putative inhibitory cholinergic pathway by atropine would lead to unopposed stimulation of gastrin release by a separate, atropine-insensitive (and therefore probably noncholinergic) vagal pathway. The nature of the neurotransmitter that releases gastrin during sham feeding is speculative. Candidates include neuropeptides (e.g., bombesin) and catecholamines (e.g., norepinephrine).

Distention

Two methods have been used to measure acid secretory responses to gastric distention in humans. Either a balloon is used to selectively distend the fundus (41-44) or the antrum (6,100), and acid secretion is measured by aspiration; or a liquid test meal is used to distend the entire stomach, and acid secretion measured by indicator-dilution (18,49) or in vivo intragastric titration

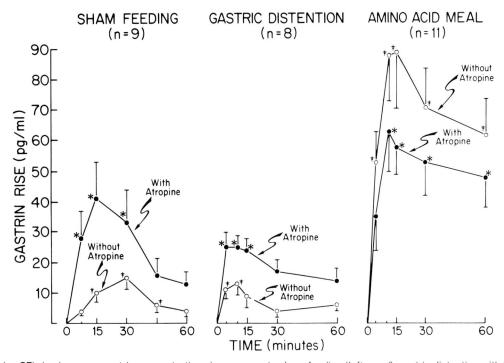

FIG. 5. Mean (± SE) rise in serum gastrin concentrations in response to sham feeding (*left panel*), gastric distention with 700 ml saline (*center panel*), or a 700 ml amino acid meal (*right panel*). Subjects were studied with and without a parenteral injection of 2.3 μg/kg atropine. In all studies, intragastric pH was held constant at 5.0 by *in vivo* intragastric titration. Significant gastrin rises above basal levels are shown as ‡. Significant differences between gastrin rises with and without atropine are shown as *. Atropine enhanced gastrin release in response to sham feeding and distention, whereas atropine inhibited the gastrin response to amino acids. It is apparent from this figure that intragastric amino acids are more potent stimulants of gastrin release than sham feeding or distention.

(27,99,104). Despite the differences in techniques, all studies have found that gastric distention stimulates acid secretion. On the other hand, unlike what occurs in dogs, distention of the duodenum and jejunum does not appear to increase acid secretion in humans (38).

There is controversy regarding the relationship between the volume or pressure to which the stomach is distended and the rate of acid secretion. In one study, distention with 100 ml saline elicited as much acid secretion as did 700 ml (27) (Fig. 6). In another study, distention with a mannitol solution at 5 cm H_2O pressure led to as much acid secretion as did distention at 10 or 15 cm H_2O (104). On the other hand, studies using balloons to distend the fundus have found a positive correlation between distending volume and acid output, with a maximal response occurring at 600 ml distention (41,42) (Fig. 7). Since a liquid meal is a transient stimulus which empties from the stomach, while a distended balloon is a constant stimulus, the apparent differences in dose-response studies may be purely technical. Nevertheless, studies with liquid meals have pointed out that even small distending volumes (50 to 100 ml) can stimulate acid secretion. The peak acid secretion rate in response to distention amounts to 20 to 50% of PAO.

Gastric distention stimulates acid secretion by activating both long vagovagal reflexes and short intramural reflexes. Balloon distention of the fundus elicits an acid secretory response without increasing serum gastrin concentrations, suggesting that there is an oxynto-oxyntic reflex but not an oxyntopyloric reflex in humans (44). The oxynto-oxyntic reflex is markedly reduced by atropine or by proximal gastric vagotomy (Fig. 7). Balloon distention of the antrum neither increases acid secretion nor increases serum gastrin concentrations in healthy subjects (100). Thus balloon studies have not demonstrated pyloro-oxyntic or pyloropyloric reflexes in normal humans.

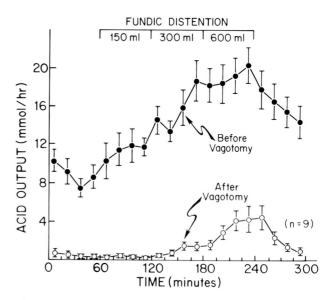

FIG. 7. Effect of fundic distention with a balloon on mean (± SE) acid output in nine patients with duodenal ulcer. The balloon was sequentially inflated to 150, 300, and 600 ml. Results are shown before and after parietal cell vagotomy. (Modified with author's permission from ref. 42.)

Distention may also activate reflexes that inhibit acid secretion. For example, antral distention with a 150-ml balloon inhibits pentagastrin-stimulated acid secretion by approximately 20% (100). In addition, fundic distention inhibits pentagastrin-stimulated acid secretion in some but not all healthy subjects and duodenal ulcer patients (43). Distention may be a relatively weak stimulant of acid secretion because distention activates both excitatory and inhibitory reflexes.

Distention-Induced Gastrin Release

Evidence suggests that distention of the entire stomach with liquid test meals activates both stimulatory and inhibitory reflexes regulating gastrin release (99). For example, when a small dose of atropine was given prior to gastric distention with 700 ml saline, the gastrin response was enhanced (Fig. 5, center). These studies suggest that distention activates atropine-sensitive (cholinergic) reflexes which normally (i.e., in the absence of atropine) suppress gastrin release. This may explain why a significant gastrin response to distention is difficult to demonstrate in the absence of atropine (8,93,94,99).

Chemical Reactions of Food With Gastrointestinal Mucosa

The acid secretory response to intragastric homogenized food (containing protein, carbohydrate, and fat) is much greater than the response to intragastric saline (94), reaching 60 to 70% of the PAO (Fig. 8). The difference between the response to food and the response

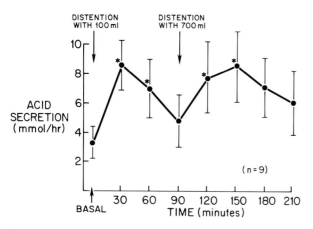

FIG. 6. Effect of gastric distention with 100 ml saline and then with 700 ml saline on mean (± SE) acid secretion in nine healthy subjects. Significant increases over basal secretion rates are shown as *. Distention with 700 ml led to no more acid secretion than distention with 100 ml.

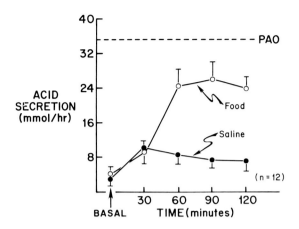

FIG. 8. Mean (± SE) acid secretion in response to 600 or 700 ml intragastric saline and in response to 600 ml intragastric food in 12 healthy subjects. Basal acid secretion is shown, as is PAO for these subjects.

to saline distention is presumably a result of chemical reactions of food constituents with the gastric and intestinal mucosa. Since food infused into the stomach empties into the small intestine, the acid secretory response to food is a net result of both gastric and intestinal mechanisms, some stimulatory and others inhibitory. In general, the stomach and upper small intestine have a net stimulatory role in acid secretion, whereas the distal jejunum and ileum play a net inhibitory role (16,17,38). The major effect of the small intestine is inhibitory, since small bowel resection leads to increased gastric acid secretion (35).

Role of Individual Food Constituents

Protein. The major constituent of food that stimulates acid secretion is protein. Undigested proteins, such as albumin, are weak stimulants of acid secretion if peptic digestion is prohibited by maintaining intragastric pH at 5.0 (94). Peptic digests of protein, such as polypeptides, peptones, and amino acids, are potent stimulants of acid secretion. Not all amino acids are equally effective in stimulating acid secretion, however. For example, phenylalanine is a potent stimulant, whereas a glycine solution is no more effective than an equal volume of saline (9).

Amino acids and peptides stimulate gastric acid secretion mainly by releasing G-17-I and G-17-II. The rises in plasma G-17 concentrations in response to a mixed amino acid meal are sufficient to account for the entire acid secretory response to the meal (33). Furthermore, when a series of peptone meals of different concentrations are infused into the stomach, there is a close correlation between plasma G-17 rise and increase in acid secretion in individual subjects (66). Thus G-17 appears to be the major physiological mediator of the acid secretory response to dietary protein. Amino acids and peptides also release big gastrins (G-34-I and G-34-

II) into the circulation (22). However, since G-34 is about one-sixth as potent as G-17 on a molar basis (118), it is unlikely that the amounts of G-34 released after a meal contribute substantially to food-stimulated acid secretion.

There are at least three other mechanisms by which meals containing amino acids and peptides could stimulate gastric acid secretion. First, amino acids within the gastric lumen might stimulate parietal cells directly; such a mechanism has not been demonstrated in humans. Second, once amino acids are absorbed from the intestine into the circulation, they are capable of stimulating acid secretion (51). In fact, intravenously infused amino acids are about as potent as equal amounts of intraduodenal amino acids, leading to a secretion rate that is 30 to 35% of PAO. This suggests that in humans, the stimulatory portion of the "intestinal" phase of acid secretion may be due largely to absorbed nutrients. Whether circulating amino acids stimulate parietal cells directly or release some other secretogogue is uncertain, although it is known that serum gastrin levels do not increase during intravenous amino acid infusion. A third mechanism by which amino acids could stimulate acid secretion is via release of a nongastrin secretogogue from the small intestine: entero-oxyntin.

Carbohydrate. Glucose solutions infused into the stomach stimulate acid secretion to approximately the same extent as equal volumes of saline, presumably via gastric distention (93). When glucose is infused intraduodenally or intravenously, however, acid secretion in response to food or sham feeding is inhibited significantly (68,77). The mechanism by which intraduodenal and intravenous glucose inhibits acid secretion is unclear.

Fat. Fat is an inhibitor of gastric acid secretion. Whether it is infused into the stomach (39) or into the jejunum (12), the acid secretory response to a protein meal is inhibited by 50 to 65% (Fig. 9). The mechanism by which fat inhibits acid secretion is unknown. Several gut peptides, including gastric inhibitory peptide (GIP),

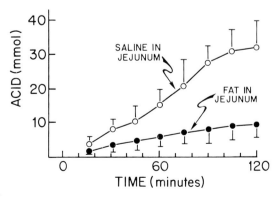

FIG. 9. Mean (± SE) cumulative acid secretion in response to an intragastric steak meal in seven healthy subjects. On one day, saline was infused into the jejunum; on another day, 20 g fat was infused into the jejunum. (Modified with permission from ref. 12.)

enteroglucagon, vasoactive intestinal polypeptide (VIP), and cholecystokinin (CCK), are released into the circulation by meals containing fat. It has not been shown, however, that rises in the circulating concentrations of any of these peptides are sufficient to account for the acid secretory inhibition observed (12). The inhibition of acid secretion by fat is not due to suppression of gastrin release (12,39,94).

Recent studies (116) indicate that intravenous fat can inhibit acid secretion stimulated by intravenous amino acids about as well as equal amounts of intraduodenal fat. In those studies, there was no rise in serum CCK or GIP during intravenous fat infusion. Thus, like other nutrients (amino acids, glucose), fat circulating in the human bloodstream is capable of affecting gastric acid secretion.

Calcium. Oral calcium stimulates acid secretion and gastrin release (67). Whether the acid secretory response to oral calcium is mediated solely via gastrin or whether calcium ions also stimulate parietal cells directly is not known. One study has demonstrated that decalcified milk stimulates less gastric acid secretion than milk containing calcium (50).

Caffeine. Caffeine stimulates acid secretion (98), although the exact mechanism is not known. Methylated xanthines, by inhibiting the enzyme phosphodiesterase, increase intracellular cyclic AMP concentrations. Whether increases in cyclic AMP in parietal cells are responsible for the increased acid secretion is unclear. Since decaffeinated coffee stimulates about as much acid secretion as does regular coffee, coffee also contains stimulants of acid secretion other than caffeine.

RELATIVE ROLES OF CEPHALIC—VAGAL STIMULATION, DISTENTION, AND CHEMICAL REACTIONS IN THE ACID SECRETORY RESPONSE TO EATING

When sham feeding and intragastric food infusion (both submaximal stimulants of acid secretion) are initiated simultaneously, normal eating is simulated. Acid secretion rates approach maximal, as all mechanisms (cephalic-vagal stimulation, distention, and chemical reactions) are activated (Fig. 10). The relative contributions of cephalic-vagal, distention, and chemical stimulation to this acid secretory response are shown in Table 1. During the first hour, cephalic-vagal stimulation accounts for approximately one-half of the response, while distention and chemical reactions account for approximately one-fourth each. During the second hour, however, chemical reactions account for almost one-half of the acid secreted, distention approximately one-fifth, and cephalic stimulation for only one-tenth. Thus, during the early part of a meal, cephalic-vagal stimulation is the most potent mechanism, whereas chemical stimulation, mainly via gastrin release, is more potent

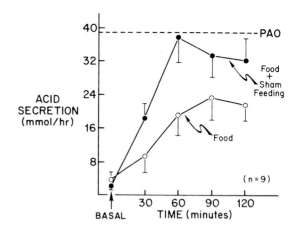

FIG. 10. Mean (± SE) acid secretion in response to 600 ml intragastric food or in response to 600 ml intragastric food plus sham feeding in nine healthy subjects. Basal acid secretion was measured (*arrows*), and food was then infused. Sham feeding began with food infusion and lasted 30 min. PAO for these subjects is shown. The food plus sham feeding study simulates what happens during normal eating (see Fig. 3).

later. The fact that acid secretion was higher when all mechanisms were activated simultaneously than the sum of the individual stimuli acting separately suggests that there may be potentiation between different mechanisms.

REGULATION OF GASTRIN RELEASE

Acid Inhibition

As already mentioned, the responsiveness of parietal cells is unaffected by luminal pH. Gastrin release in response to several physiological stimuli is inhibited, however, when the gastric lumen becomes acidified. This inhibition is associated with an inhibition of gastric acid secretion.

As shown in Fig. 11 (*top*), the gastrin response to sham feeding is completely abolished and the gastrin response to an amino acid meal is inhibited by luminal acidification to pH 2.5 (31,119). The acid secretory responses to these stimuli are also reduced at pH 2.5 (Fig. 11, *bottom*). Gastrin and acid secretory responses to gastric distention are relatively resistant to luminal acidification to pH 2.5 (99) (Fig. 11).

The mechanism by which luminal acid inhibits gastrin release is unclear. The presence of microvilli on the luminal surface of gastrin cells suggests that acid can directly suppress these cells. Atropine, however, can prevent acid inhibition of sham feeding-induced gastrin release, suggesting that a cholinergic pathway is involved in the inhibition (31). One possibility is that luminal acid releases somatostatin from antral D cells, and that somatostatin locally inhibits gastrin release (114). This hypothesis would require that the release of somatostatin or its action on the gastrin cell could be

TABLE 1. *Relative contributions of cephalic-vagal stimulation, gastric distention, and chemical reactions to acid secretory response to eating in nine normal human subjects*

Stimuli	Millimole acid secreted (%)[a]	
	First hour	Second hour
Cephalic-vagal stimulation	12.0 (47)	3.3 (11)
Distention	6.3 (25)	5.6 (19)
Chemical reactions	5.8 (23)	12.7 (42)
All stimuli acting simultaneously	25.6 (100)	30.0 (100)

[a]Represents basal-subtracted responses to cephalic-vagal stimulation by sham feeding; to gastric distention with 600 ml saline; to chemical reactions to 600 ml intragastric homogenized food; and to simultaneous sham feeding plus 600 ml intragastric food (all stimuli acting simultaneously). Acid secretion was measured by aspiration during cephalic-vagal stimulation and by intragastric titration to pH 5.0 in the other experiments. Response to distention has been subtracted from response to homogenized food to obtain response attributed to chemical reactions. Numbers in parentheses refer to responses to individual stimuli expressed as a percent of the response to all stimuli acting simultaneously. The fact that the response to all stimuli acting simultaneously was greater than the sum of the individual stimuli (especially in the second hour) suggests potentiation between stimuli (From ref. 93).

blocked by atropine. Whether atropine can prevent acid inhibition of food-stimulated gastrin release is not known.

Part of the inhibition of gastrin release (and acid secretion) by luminal acid may also be due to acid entering the small intestine, releasing inhibitory substances, including secretin. However, it is uncertain whether secretin or other inhibitors play a physiological role in inhibiting human gastrin release.

Vagal-Cholinergic Mechanisms

The roles of vagal and cholinergic mechanisms on chemically induced gastrin release are complex and incompletely understood. Many studies that have evaluated atropine permitted subjects to eat the food (activating cephalic-vagal as well as distention and chemical mechanisms) and also did not control intragastric pH (5,65,120). Furthermore, in several studies evaluating the effect of vagotomy on food-stimulated gastrin release, intragastric pH was not kept constant (47,64,106). Thus higher food-stimulated serum gastrin concentrations after atropine or vagotomy may have been caused by less acid inhibition of gastrin release. When amino acid solutions are infused directly into the stomach and intragastric pH held constant, 2.3 μg/kg atropine causes a small but significant reduction in gastrin release (Fig. 5, right). Higher doses of atropine (up to 25 μg/kg) do not reduce gastrin concentrations below control levels (59; L. R. Schiller and M. Feldman, *unpublished observations*). Thus amino acid-stimulated gastrin release appears to be different from sham feeding-induced and distention-induced gastrin release in that atropine does not enhance gastrin release in response to amino acids.

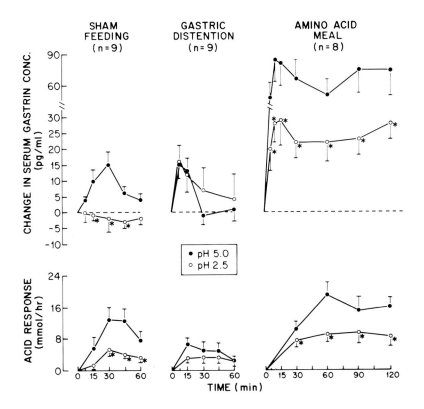

FIG. 11. Effect of intragastric pH on mean (± SE) change in serum gastrin concentration (**top**) and on acid response (**bottom**) to sham feeding, gastric distention with 700 ml saline, or a 700 ml amino acid meal. Intragastric pH was kept constant at either 5.0 (*closed circles*) or 2.5 (*open circles*) and acid secretion measured by intragastric titration. Significant differences are shown by *.

Following truncal (111) or parietal cell vagotomy (28), basal serum gastrin concentrations increase, and food-stimulated gastrin release is enhanced, even when intragastric pH is controlled (Fig. 12, top). Hypergastrinemia does not lead to hypersecretion of acid, however, because vagotomy also reduces the maximal capacity to secrete acid in response to exogenous pentagastrin (PAO) and presumably in response to endogenous gastrin (Fig. 12, bottom).

The mechanism by which vagotomy leads to elevated basal and food-stimulated serum gastrin concentrations is unclear. One possibility is that vagotomy destroys an inhibitory pathway for gastrin release. A second possibility is that the reduction in acid secretion after vagotomy, by chronically elevating intragastric pH, leads to gastrin cell hyperplasia (47).

SUMMARY

This chapter deals with the mechanisms that regulate acid secretion in humans. Although emphasis has been placed on gastrin, histamine, calcium, and vagal-cholinergic activity, it is likely that other substances, such as endogenous opiate-like peptides (enkephalins), prostaglandins, and somatostatin, also play physiological roles. Future investigation using specific antagonist compounds (e.g., opiate receptor antagonists) or compounds that block the synthesis or release of these

chemicals (e.g., prostaglandin synthesis inhibitors) may help clarify the function of these substances. Also, studies of isolated parietal cells may help determine whether receptors for these compounds are present on the human parietal cell.

REFERENCES

1. Aadland, E., Berstad, A., and Semb, L. S. (1977): Effect of cimetidine on pentagastrin-stimulated gastric secretion in healthy man. *Scand J. Gastroenterol.,* 12:501–506.
2. Babbott, F. L., Johnston, J. A., and Haskins, C. H. (1923): Gastric acidity in infantile tetany. *Arch. Dis. Child.,* 26:486–501.
3. Baron, J. H. (1969): Lean body mass, gastric acid, and peptic ulcer. *Gut,* 10:637–642.
4. Baron, J. H. (1970): The clinical use of gastric function tests. *Scand. J. Gastroenterol. [Suppl. 6],* 6:9–46.
5. Becker, H. D., Reeder, D. D., and Thompson, J. C. (1974): Effect of atropine on basal and food-stimulated serum gastrin levels in man. *Surgery,* 75:701–704.
6. Bergegårdh, S., and Olbe, L. (1975): Gastric acid response to antrum distention in man. *Scand. J. Gastroenterol.,* 10:171–176.
7. Bergegårdh, S., and Olbe L. (1976): The effect of long-term postoperative pentagastrin infusion on the maximal acid responses to pentagastrin in patients subjected to antrectomy. *Scand. J. Gastroenterol.,* 11.347–351.
8. Bloom, S. R., Sarson, D. L., Christofides, N. D., Albuquerque, R. H., Adrian, T. E., Ghatei, M. A., and Modlin, I. M. (1978): The release of gastrointestinal hormones following an oral water load and atropine in man. *Gastroenterology,* 74:1010.
9. Byrne, W. J., Christie, D. L., Ament, M. E., and Walsh, J. H. (1977): Acid secretory response in man to 18 individual amino acids. *Clin. Res.,* 25:108A.
10. Card, W. I., and Marks, I. N. (1960): The relationship between the acid output of the stomach following "maximal" histamine stimulation and the parietal cell mass. *Clin. Sci.,* 19:147–163.
11. Carter, D. C., and Grossman, M. I. (1978): Effect of luminal pH on acid secretion from Heidenhain pouches evoked by topical and parenteral stimulants. *J. Physiol.,* 281:227–237.
12. Christiansen, J., Bech, A., Fahrenkrug, J., Holst, J. J., Lauritsen, K., Moody, A. J., and Schaffalitzky de Muckadell, O. (1979): Fat-induced jejunal inhibition of gastric acid secretion and release of pancreatic glucagon, enteroglucagon, gastric inhibitory polypeptide, and vasoactive intestinal polypeptide in man. *Scand. J. Gastroenterol.,* 14:161–166.
13. Christiansen, J., Holst, J. J., and Kalaja, E. (1976): Inhibition of gastric acid secretion in man by exogenous and endogenous pancreatic glucagon. *Gastroenterology,* 70:688–692.
14. Christiansen, J., Rehfeld, J. F., and Stadil, F. (1975): Interaction of calcium and magnesium on gastric acid secretion and serum gastrin concentration in man. *Gastroenterology,* 68:1140–1143.
15. Christie, D. L., and Ament, M. E. (1976): Gastric acid hypersecretion in children with duodenal ulcer. *Gastroenterology,* 71:242–244.
16. Clain, J. E., Go, V. L. W., and Malagelada, J. -R. (1978): Inhibitory role of the distal small intestine on the gastric secretory response to meals in man. *Gastroenterology,* 74:704–707.
17. Clain, J. E., Malagelada, J. -R., Go, V. L. W., and Summerskill, W. H. J. (1977): Participation of the jejunum and ileum in postprandial gastric secretion in man. *Gastroenterology,* 73:211–214.
18. Cooke, A. R. (1970): Potentiation of acid output in man by a distention stimulus. *Gastroenterology,* 58:633–637.
19. Dalton, M. D., Eisenstein, A. M., Walsh, J. H., and Fordtran, J. S. (1976): Effect of secretin on gastric function in normal subjects and in patients with duodenal ulcer. *Gastroenterology,* 71:24–29.
20. Debas, H. T., Konturek, S. J., Walsh, J. H., and Grossman, M. I. (1974): Proof of a pyloro-oxyntic reflex for stimulation of acid secretion. *Gastroenterology,* 66:526–532.

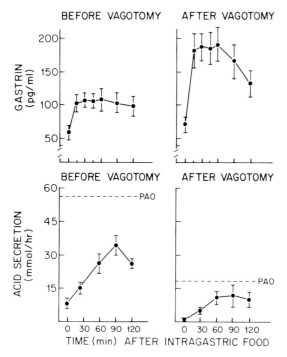

BEFORE VAGOTOMY   AFTER VAGOTOMY

BEFORE VAGOTOMY   AFTER VAGOTOMY

TIME (min) AFTER INTRAGASTRIC FOOD

FIG. 12. Mean (± SE) serum gastrin concentrations (**top**) and acid secretion (**bottom**) in eight patients with duodenal ulcer studied before (**left**) and 6 to 12 weeks after (**right**) parietal cell vagotomy. 600 ml homogenized food was infused at 0 min and acid secretion measured (and pH kept constant) by intragastric titration to pH 5.0. PAOs before and after vagotomy are also shown.

21. Deering, T. B., and Malagelada, J. -R. (1977): Comparison of an H$_2$-receptor antagonist and a neutralizing antacid on postprandial acid delivery into the duodenum in patients with duodenal ulcer. *Gastroenterology,* 73:11–14.

22. Dockray, G. J., and Taylor, I. L. (1976): Heptadecapeptide gastrin: Measurement in blood by specific radioimmunoassay. *Gastroenterology,* 71:971–977.

23. Donegan, W. L., and Spiro, H. M. (1960): Parathyroids and gastic secretion. *Gastroenterology,* 38:750–759.

24. Elder, J. B., Gillespie, G., Campbell, E. H. G., Gilliespie, I. E., Crean, G. P., and Kay, A. W. (1972): The effect of vagotomy on the lower part of the acid dose-response curve to pentagastrin in man. *Clin. Sci.,* 43:193–200.

25. Farooq, O., and Walsh, J. H. (1975): Atropine enhances serum gastrin response to insulin in man. *Gastroenterology,* 68:662–666.

26. Farrell, J. I. (1928): Contributions to the physiology of gastric secretion. The vagi as the sole efferent pathway for the cephalic phase of gastric secretion. *Am. J. Physiol.,* 85:685–687.

27. Feldman, M. (1979): Comparison of acid secretion rates measured by gastric aspiration and by in vivo intragastric titration in healthy human subjects. *Gastroenterology,* 76:954–957.

28. Feldman, M., Dickerman, R. M., McClelland, R. N., Cooper, K. A., Walsh, J. H., and Richardson, C. T. (1979): Effect of selective proximal vagotomy on food-stimulated gastric acid secretion and gastrin release in patients with duodenal ulcer. *Gastroenterology,* 76:926–931.

29. Feldman, M., and Richardson, C. T. (1981): ''Partial'' sham feeding releases gastrin in normal human subjects. *Scand. J. Gastroenterol. (in press).*

30. Feldman, M., Richardson, C. T., Taylor, I. L., and Walsh, J. H. (1979): Effect of atropine on vagal release of gastrin and pancreatic polypeptide. *J. Clin. Invest.,* 63:294–298.

31. Feldman, M., and Walsh, J. H. (1980): Acid inhibition of sham feeding-stimulated gastrin release and gastric acid secretion: Effect of atropine. *Gastroenterology,* 78:772–776.

32. Feldman, M., Walsh, J. H., and Taylor, I. L. (1980): Effect of naloxone and morphine on gastric acid secretion and on serum gastrin and pancreatic polypeptide concentrations in man. *Gastroenterology,* 79:294–298.

33. Feldman, M., Walsh, J. H., Wong, H. C., and Richardson, C. T. (1978): Role of gastrin heptadecapeptide in the acid secretory response to amino acids in man. *J. Clin. Invest.,* 61:308–313.

34. Fordtran, J. S., and Walsh, J. H. (1973): Gastric acid secretion rate and buffer content of the stomach after eating. *J. Clin. Invest.,* 52:645–657.

35. Frederick, P. L., Sizer, J. S., and Osborne, M. P. (1965): Relation of massive bowel resection to gastric secretion. *N. Engl. J. Med.,* 272:509–514.

36. Gedde-Dahl, D. (1974): Radioimmunoassay of gastrin. Fasting serum levels in humans with normal and high gastric acid secretion. *Scand. J. Gastroenterol.,* 9:41–47.

37. Gottrup, F., Örnsholt, J., and Andersen, D. (1979): Effects of two types of β-adrenergic blockade on gastric acid secretion during pentagastrin stimulation in non-vagotomized and in vagotomized gastric fistula dogs. *Scand. J. Gastroenterol.,* 14:857–864.

38. Grabner, P., Semb, L. S., and Myren, J. (1979): Comparison of gastric secretory response in man to duodenal and jejunal liver extract perfusion. *Scand. J. Gastroenterol.,* 14:385–388.

39. Gross, R. A., Isenberg, J. I., Hogan, D., and Samloff, I. M. (1978): Effect of fat on meal-stimulated duodenal acid load, duodenal pepsin load, and serum gastrin in duodenal ulcer and normal subjects. *Gastroenterology,* 75:357–362.

40. Grossman, M. I., Kirsner, J. B., and Gillespie, I. E. (1963): Basal and histalog-stimulated gastric secretion in control subjects and in patients with peptic ulcer or gastric cancer. *Gastroenterology,* 45:14–26.

41. Grötzinger, U., Bergegårdh, S., and Olbe, L. (1977): Effect of fundic distention on gastric acid secretion in man. *Gut,* 18:105–110.

42. Grötzinger, U., Bergegårdh, S., and Olbe, L. (1977): Effect of atropine and proximal gastric vagotomy on the acid response to fundic distention in man. *Gut,* 18:303–310.

43. Grötzinger, U., Bergegårdh, S., and Olbe, L. (1977): Effects of fundic distention of pentagastric-stimulated gastric acid secretion in man. *Gastroenterology,* 73:447–452.

44. Grötzinger, U., Rehfeld, J. F., and Olbe, L. (1977): Is there an oxyntopyloric reflex for release of gastrin in man? *Gastroenterology,* 73:753–757.

45. Henn, R. M., Isenberg, J. I., Maxwell, V., and Sturdevant, R. A. L. (1975): Inhibition of gastric acid secretion by cimetidine in patients with duodenal ulcer. *N. Engl. J. Med.,* 293:371–375.

46. Hobsley, M., and Silen, W. (1969): Use of an inert marker (phenol red) to improve accuracy in gastric secretion studies. *Gut,* 10:787–795.

47. Hughes, W. S., and Hernandez, A. J. (1976): Antral gastrin concentration in patients with vagotomy and pyloroplasty. *Gastroenterology,* 71:720–722.

48. Hume, R., and Melrose, A. G. (1967): Relation between maximal acid output of stomach and lean body mass. *Br. Med. J.,* 1:30–31.

49. Hunt, J. N., and MacDonald, I. (1952): The relation between the volume of a test-meal and the gastric secretory response. *J. Physiol.,* 117:289–302.

50. Ippoliti, A. F., Maxwell, V., and Isenberg, J. I. (1976): The effect of various forms of milk on gastric-acid secretion: Studies in patients with duodenal ulcer and normal subjects. *Ann. Int. Med.,* 84:286–289.

51. Isenberg, J. I., and Maxwell, V. (1978): Intravenous infusion of amino acids stimulates gastric acid secretion in man. *N. Engl. J. Med.,* 298:27–29.

52. Jepson, K., and Johnston, D. (1968): Effect of vagotomy on human gastric acid secretion stimulated by gastrin pentapeptide and by histalog. *Gastroenterology,* 55:665–669.

53. Johnson, L. R., and Chandler, L. R. (1973): RNA and DNA of gastric and duodenal mucosa in antrectomized and gastrin-treated rats. *Am. J. Physiol.,* 224:937–940.

54. Kaess, H., and Unger, W. (1975): Evaluation of a new method for the intragastric titration of gastric juice. *Acta Hepatogastroenterol.,* 22:242–248.

55. Knutson, U., and Olbe, L. (1974): Gastric acid response to sham feeding in the duodenal ulcer patient. *Scand. J. Gastroenterol.,* 8:513–522.

56. Knutson, U., and Olbe, L. (1973): The gastric acid response to sham feeding in duodenal ulcer patients after proximal selective vagotomy. *Scand. J. Gastroenterol. [Suppl. 20],* 8:16–17.

57. Knutson, U., and Oble, L. (1974): Gastric acid response to sham feeding before and after resection of antrum and duodenal bulb in duodenal ulcer patients. *Scand. J. Gastroenterol.,* 9:191–201.

58. Knutson, U., Olbe, L., and Ganguli, P. C. (1974): Gastric acid and plasma gastrin responses to sham feeding in duodenal ulcer patients before and after resection of antrum and duodenal bulb. *Scand. J. Gastroenterol.,* 9:351–356.

59. Konturek, S. J., Biernat, J., Oleksy, J., Rehfeld, J. F., and Stadil, F. (1974): Effect of atropine on gastrin and gastric acid response to peptone meal. *J. Clin. Invest.,* 54:593–597.

60. Konturek, S. J., Olesky, J., and Wysocki, A. (1968): Effect of atropine on gastric acid response to graded doses of pentagastrin and histamine in duodenal ulcer patients before and after vagotomy. *Am. J. Dig. Dis.,* 13:792–800.

61. Konturek, S. J., Kwiecien, N., Obtulowicz, W., Mikos, E., Sito, E., Oleksy, J., and Popiela, T. (1978): Cephalic phase of gastric secretion in healthy subjects and duodenal ulcer patients: Role of vagal innervation. *Gut,* 20:875–881.

62. Konturek, S. J., Tasler, J., Cieszkowski, M., Mikos, E., Coy, D. H., and Schally, A. V. (1980): Comparison of methionine-enkephalin and morphine in the stimulation of gastric acid secretion in the dog. *Gastroenterology,* 78:294–300.

63. Konturek, S. J., Wysocki, A., and Oleksy, J. (1968): Effect of medical and surgical vagotomy on gastric response to graded doses of pentagastrin and histamine. *Gastroenterology,* 51:392–400.

64. Korman, M. G., Hansky, J., and Scott, P. R. (1972): Serum gastrin in duodenal ulcer. III. Influence of vagotomy and pylorectomy. *Gut,* 13:39–42.

65. Korman, M. G., Soveny, C., and Hansky, J. (1971): Serum gastrin in duodenal ulcer. *Gut,* 12:899–902.

66. Lam, S. K., Isenberg, J. I., Grossman, M. I., Lane, W. H., and Walsh, J. H. (1980): Gastric acid secretion is abnormally sensitive to endogenous gastrin released after peptone test meals in duodenal ulcer patients. *J. Clin. Invest.*, 65:555–562.

67. Levant, J. A., Walsh, J. H., and Isenberg, J. I. (1973): Stimulation of gastric secretion and gastrin release by single oral doses of calcium carbonate in man. *N. Engl. J. Med.*, 289:555–558.

68. MacGregor, I. L., Deveney, C., Way, L. W., and Meyer, J. H. (1976): The effect of acute hyperglycemia on meal-stimulated gastric, biliary, and pancreatic secretion, and serum gastrin. *Gastroenterology*, 70:197–202.

69. Makhlouf, G. M., Zfass, A. M., Said, S. I., and Schebalin, M. (1978): Effect of synthetic vasoactive intestinal peptide (VIP), secretin and their partial sequences on gastric secretion. *Proc. Soc. Exp. Biol. Med.*, 157:565–568.

70. Malagelada, J. -R., Longstreth, G. F., Summerskill, W. H. J., and Go, V. G. W. (1976): Measurement of gastric functions during digestion of ordinary solid meals in man. *Gastroenterology*, 70:203–210.

71. Marks, I. N. (1957): The effect of prolonged histamine stimulation on the parietal cell population and the secretory function of the guinea-pig stomach. *Q. J. Exp. Physiol.*, 42:180–189.

72. Martin, F., Macleod, I. B., and Sircus, W. (1970): Effect of antrectomy on the fundic mucosa of the rat. *Gastroenterology*, 59:437–444.

73. Maxwell, V., Shulkes, A., Brown, J. C., Solomon, T. E., Walsh, J. H., and Grossman, M. I. (1980): Effect of gastric inhibitory polypeptide on pentagastrin-stimulated acid secretion in man. *Dig. Dis. Sci.*, 25:113–116.

74. Mayer, G., Arnold, R., Feurle, G., Fuchs, K., Ketterer, H., Track, N. S., and Creutzfeldt, W. (1974): Influence of feeding and sham feeding upon serum gastrin and gastric acid secretion in control subjects and duodenal ulcer patients. *Scand. J. Gastroenterol.*, 9:703–710.

75. Mignon, M., Galmiche, J. P., Accary, J. P., and Bonfils, S. (1974): Serum gastrin, gastric acid and pepsin responses to sham-feeding in man. *Gastroenterology*, 66:856.

76. Mittelmann, B., and Wolff, H. G. (1942): Emotions and gastroduodenal function. Experimental studies on patients with gastritis, duodenitis and peptic ulcer. *Psychosom. Med.*, 4:5–61.

77. Moore, J. G., and Crespin, F. (1980): Influence of glucose on cephalic-vagal-stimulated gastric acid secretion in man. *Dig. Dis. Sci.*, 25:117–122.

78. Moore, J. G., and Englert, E. (1970): Circadian rhythm of gastric acid secretion in man. *Nature*, 226:1261–1262.

79. Moore, J. G., and Motoki, D. (1979): Gastric secretory and humoral response to anticipated feeding in five men. *Gastroenterology*, 76:71–75.

80. Moore, E. W., and Scarlata, R. W. (1965): The determination of gastric acidity by the glass electrode. *Gastroenterology*, 49:178–188.

81. Moore, J. G., and Wolfe, M. (1973): The relation of plasma gastrin to the circadian rhythm of gastric acid secretion in man. *Digestion*, 9:97–105.

82. Neely, J. C., and Goldman, L. (1962): Effect of calciferol-induced chronic hypercalcemia on the gastric secretion from Heidenhain pouch. *Ann. Surg.*, 155:406–411.

83. Neuberger, P., Lewin, M., Recherche, C., and Bonfils, S. (1972): Parietal and chief cell populations in four cases of the Zollinger-Ellison Syndrome. *Gastroenterology*, 63:937–942.

84. Norgaard, R. P., Polter, D. E., Wheeler, J. W., and Fordtran, J. S. (1970): Effect of long-term anticholinergic therapy on gastric acid secretion, with observations on the serial measurement of peak histolog response. *Gastroenterology*, 58:750–755.

85. Noring, O. (1951): The cephalic phase of gastric secretion following partial gastrectomy. *Gastroenterology*, 19:118–125.

86. Pavlov, I. P. (1910): The centrifugal (efferent) nerves to the gastric glands and of the pancreas. In: *The Work Of The Digestive Glands*, 2nd edition, translated by W. H. Thompson, pp. 48–59. Charles Griffin, Philadelphia.

87. Payne, R. A., and Kay, A. W. (1962): The effect of vagotomy on the maximal acid secretory response to histamine in man. *Clin. Sci.*, 22:373–382.

88. Pearl, J. M., Ritchie, W. P., Gilsdorf, R. B., Delaney, J. P., and Leonard, A. S. (1966): Hypothalamic stimulation and feline gastric mucosal cellular populations. *JAMA*, 195:281–284.

89. Peeters, T. L., and Vantrappen, G. (1978): Why gastric acidity must be determined by titration, and how. *Gastroenterology*, 74:1139.

90. Pevsner, L., and Grossman, M. I. (1955): The mechanism of vagal stimulation of gastric acid secretion. *Gastroenterology*, 28:493–499.

91. Phillip, J., Domschke, S., Domschke, W., Urbach, H. -J., Reiss, M., and Demling, L. (1977): Inhibition by somatostatin of gastrin release and gastric acid responses to meals and pentagastrin in man. *Scand. J. Gastroenterol.*, 12:261–265.

92. Preshaw, R. M. (1973): Inhibition of pentagastrin stimulated gastric acid output by sham feeding. *Fed. Proc.*, 32:410.

93. Richardson, C. T., Walsh, J. H., Cooper, K. A., Feldman, M., and Fordtran, J. S. (1977): Studies on the role of cephalic-vagal stimulation in the acid secretory response to eating in normal human subjects. *J. Clin. Invest.*, 60:435–441.

94. Richardson, C. T., Walsh, J. H., Hicks, M. I., and Fordtran, J. S. (1976): Studies on the mechanisms of food-stimulated gastric acid secretion in normal human subjects. *J. Clin. Invest.*, 58:623–631.

95. Robert, A., Nezamis, J. E., and Phillips, J. P. (1967): Inhibition of gastric secretion by prostaglandins. *Dig. Dis.*, 12:1073–1076.

96. Roland, M., Berstad, A., and Liavag, I. (1974): Acid and pepsin secretion in duodenal ulcer patients in response to graded doses of pentagastrin or pentagastrin and carbacholine before and after proximal gastric vagotomy. *Scand. J. Gastroenterol.*, 9:511–518.

97. Roland, M., Berstad, A., and Liavag, I. (1975): Effect of carbacholine and urecholine on pentagastrin-stimulated gastric secretion in healthy subjects. *Scand. J. Gastroenterol.*, 10:357–362.

98. Roth, J. A., and Ivy, A. (1944): The effect of caffeine on gastric secretion in the dog, cat and man. *Am. J. Physiol.*, 141:454–461.

99. Schiller, L. R., Walsh, J. H., and Feldman, M. (1980): Distention-induced gastrin release. Effects of luminal acidification and intravenous atropine. *Gastroenterology*, 78:912–917.

100. Schoon, I. M., Bergegärdh, S., Grötzinger, U., and Olbe, L. (1978): Evidence for a defective inhibition of pentagastrin-stimulated gastric acid secretion by antral distention in the duodenal ulcer patient. *Gastroenterology*, 75:363–367.

101. Schoon, I. M., and Olbe, L. (1978): Inhibitory effect of cimetidine on gastric acid secretion vagally activated by physiological means in duodenal ulcer patients. *Gut*, 19:27–31.

102. Schwartz, T. W., Steinquist, B., Olbe, L., and Stadil, F. (1979): Synchronous oscillations in the basal secretion of pancreatic-polypeptide and gastric acid. *Gastroenterology*, 76:14–19.

103. Sjodin, L. (1975): Inhibition of gastrin-stimulated canine acid secretion by sham feeding. *Scand. J. Gastroenterol.*, 10:73–80.

104. Soares, E. C., Zaterka, S., and Walsh, J. H. (1977): Acid secretion and serum gastrin at graded intragastric pressures in man. *Gastroenterology*, 72:676–679.

105. Spenney, J. G. (1979): Physical chemical and technical limitations to intragastric titration. *Gastroenterology*, 76:1025–1034.

106. Stadil, F., Rehfeld, J. F., Christiansen, P. M., and Kronborg, O. (1974): Gastrin response to food in duodenal ulcer patients before and after selective or highly selective vagotomy. *Br. J. Surg.*, 61:884–888.

107. Stenquist, B., Knutson, U., and Olbe, L. (1978): The vagogastrone mechanism in man. *Scand. J. Gastroenterol.*, 13:895–901.

108. Stenquist, B., Knutson, U., and Olbe, L. (1978): Gastric acid responses to adequate and modified sham feeding and to insulin hypoglycemia in duodenal ulcer patients. *Scand. J. Gastroenterol.*, 13:357–362.

109. Stenquist, B., Nilsson, G., Rehfeld, J. F., and Olbe, L. (1979): Plasma gastrin concentrations following sham feeding in duodenal ulcer patients. *Scand. J. Gastroenterol.*, 14:305–311.

110. Stenquist, B., Rehfeld, J. F., and Olbe, L. (1979): The effect of proximal gastric vagotomy and anticholinergics on the acid and gastrin responses to sham feeding in duodenal ulcer patients. *Gut*, 20:1020–1027.

111. Thompson, J. C., Lowder, W. S., Peurifoy, J. T., Swierczek, J. S., and Rayford, P. L. (1978): Effect of selective proximal vagotomy and truncal vagotomy on gastric acid and serum gastrin responses to a meal in duodenal ulcer patients. *Ann. Surg.,* 188:431–437.

112. Thompson, J. C., and Swierczek, J. S. (1977): Acid and endocrine responses to meals varying in pH in normal and duodenal ulcer subjects. *Ann. Surg.,* 186:541–548.

113. Trudeau, W. L., and McGuigan, J. E. (1971): Relations between serum gastrin levels and rates of gastric hydrochloric acid secretion. *N. Engl. J. Med.,* 284:408–412.

114. Uvnäs-Wallenstein, K., Efendic, S., and Luft, R. (1977): Vagal release of somatostatin into the antral lumen of cats. *Acta. Physiol. Scand.,* 99:126–128.

115. Valenzuela, J. E., Defilippi, C., Diaz, G., Navia, E., and Merino, Y. (1979): Effect of dopamine on human gastric and pancreatic secretion. *Gastroenterology,* 76:323–326.

116. Varner, A. A., Isenberg, J. I., Elashoff, J. D., Lamers, C. B. H. W., and Shulkes, A. A. (1979): Intravenous fat inhibits amino acid (AA) stimulated gastric acid secretion (GAS) in man. *Gastroenterology,* 76:1264.

117. Vatn, M. H., Schrumpf, E., and Myren, J. (1975): The effect of carbachol and pentagastrin on the gastric secretion of acid, pepsin, and intrinsic factor (IF) in man. *Scand. J. Gastroenterol.,* 10:55–58.

118. Walsh, J. H., Isenberg, J. I., Ansfield, J., and Maxwell, V. (1976): Clearance and acid-stimulating action of human big and little gastrins in duodenal ulcer subjects. *J. Clin. Invest.,* 57:1125–1131.

119. Walsh, J. H., Richardson, C. T., and Fordtran, J. S. (1975): pH dependence of acid secretion and gastrin release in normal and ulcer subjects. *J. Clin. Invest.,* 55:462–468.

120. Walsh, J. H., Yalow, R. S., and Berson, S. A. (1971): The effect of atropine on plasma gastrin response to feeding. *Gastroenterology,* 60:16–21.

121. White, W. D., and Juniper, K. (1973): Repeatability of gastric analysis. *Dig. Dis.,* 18:7–13.

122. Wormsley, K. G., and Grossman, M. I. (1965): Maximal histalog test in control subjects and patients with peptic ulcer. *Gut,* 6:427–435.

Physiology of the Gastrointestinal Tract, edited by
Leonard R. Johnson. Raven Press, New York © 1981.

Chapter 26

Physiology of the Gastric Circulation

Paul H. Guth and Kathryn W. Ballard

The past two decades have witnessed a significant increase in our knowledge of the physiology of the gastric circulation. Improvements in techniques to measure gastric mucosal blood flow and total gastric blood flow have played the major role in this advance. Other techniques have better defined the anatomic organization of the gastric microvasculature. These techniques have been successfully employed to determine the effect of various factors, such as gastrointestinal hormones, histamine, and prostaglandins on gastric blood flow. The purpose of this chapter is to review the current status of our knowledge of gastric circulatory physiology.

This chapter is organized as follows: First, the anatomic organization of both the gross and microscopic vascular supply to the stomach is described, including a delineation of areas of controversy and areas where knowledge is deficient. Next, the major techniques used to study the gastric circulation, and the principles underlying each, are described. The factors controlling gastric blood flow are presented. Finally, the role of blood flow in gastric physiology, including acid secre-

tion, and pathophysiology, including mucosal injury, is discussed.

ANATOMY

Supplying Vessels

The celiac artery (axis), which arises from the front of the aorta between the 12th thoracic and first lumbar vertebrae, provides the principal arterial supply to the stomach. This short major vessel gives rise to the left gastric, hepatic, and splenic arteries. Classic descriptions, such as those of Michels (118), and the more recent angiographic studies (127), agree that these vessels or branches from them comprise the six main arteries supplying blood to the stomach, i.e., the left and right gastric, the left and right gastroepiploic, the short gastric branches of the splenic, and small branches from the gastroduodenal arteries. Six other secondary arteries have also been described as frequently sending branches to the stomach. These are the superior pancreaticoduodenal, the supraduodenal artery of Wilkie, which supplies the pylorus and duodenum, the retroduodenal, which frequently gives off one or more pyloric branches, the transverse pancreatic, the dorsal pancreatic, and the left inferior phrenic arteries. All the supplying vessels anastomose extensively among themselves and with vessels arising from the superior mesenteric artery. Atypical vascular patterns often occur. Some of these have been described in detail by Michels (118) in human cadaver studies and by others (126) in angiographic studies.

The typical pattern of arterial supply to the stomach is diagrammed in Fig. 1. The left gastric artery reaches the lesser curvature at the level of the cardia, where it turns downward and branches into vessels that supply the anterior and posterior surfaces of the body and fundus of the stomach. The branch to the lesser curvature descends to the right toward the pylorus and anastomoses with the right gastric artery. The right gastric artery is smaller than the left. It is a branch of the hepatic artery and courses along the lesser curvature from the pylorus toward the left. The right and left gastric arteries, as they traverse the lesser curvature, send branches at intervals to the anterior and posterior walls of the antrum. The right gastroepiploic (a branch from the gastroduodenal artery) and left gastroepiploic (a branch from the splenic artery) arteries traverse the greater curvature and send branches at intervals to the anterior and posterior walls of the antrum and corpus. The short gastric arteries arise from the splenic artery as it passes behind the greater curvature of the fundus and supply branches to the anterior and posterior walls of the stomach in this region.

Microvessels

Muscle

There is no definitive description of the vascular supply of the muscle layer of the stomach. Our current knowledge is based on *in vivo* studies of the rat gastric microcirculation (60) and vascular injection studies of human postmortem material (137).

In vivo microscopic studies of the rat gastric microcirculation revealed that as the branches from the supplying arteries pierce the muscle coat, they send branches to the muscle (60). These in turn branch and ultimately divide into capillaries, which course in the superficial and deep muscle layers. There is free communication between the capillaries in the same plane, as well as between capillaries in different planes. Although the terminal arteriole usually divides into capillaries, thoroughfare channels were seen in rare instances. This type of communication differs from the short arteriovenous anastomosis. The thoroughfare channel is formed by an arteriole that has reached near capillary size (metarter-

iole) but continues for some distance to terminate in a venule, thereby short-circuiting the capillary bed. The capillary network drains into venules accompanying the arterioles. These in turn drain into veins emerging from the submucosal plexus. In vascular injection studies of human stomachs, Piasecki (137) described the presence of a subserosal and a deep muscle vascular plexus.

Submucosa

After piercing the muscle coat, the supplying arteries pass to the outer portion of the submucosa and form primary arterial arcades by anastomosing among themselves (13,60). These provide smaller anastomosing branches, which form successively smaller arteriolar arcades. Ultimately, the smaller arcades give rise to mucosal arterioles, which pierce the muscularis mucosae (Fig. 2). Deep in the mucosa, they divide into two to four branches, which enter the capillary plexus in the mucosa.

The lesser curvature in the rat appears to have a much less extensive arterial anastomotic network than the other gastric regions. The mucosal arterioles arise from the primary arcade. Barlow et al. (13) and Piasecki (137), in the lesser curvature of the human stomach, described end arteries, i.e., some mucosal arterioles coming directly from the branches of the right and left gastric arteries.

The submucosal veins follow the pattern of the arteries. Collecting veins, which pass perpendicularly through the mucosa, carry blood from the mucosa to the submucosa. They drain into veins that are larger than their respective arteries to form the venous submucosal plexus. In turn, this plexus drains into veins that follow the same course as the primary arterial branches to the stomach. As with the arterial supply, just before the veins leave the muscle, they receive branches from veins draining the muscle layer.

Arteriovenous anastomoses.

Based on intravascular dye injection studies of human stomachs, Barlow et al. (13) described the presence of arteriovenous anastomoses or shunts in the submucosa. This structural arrangement offered a possible mechanism for the control of blood flow to the mucosa. On the basis of glass microsphere studies in the dog, Walder (177) concluded that mucosal blood flow is a function of mucosal arteriolar resistance and shunt resistance. In studies of the gastric circulation, the role of submucosal arteriovenous anastomoses has frequently been used to explain experimental results. More recently, however, considerable physiologic and anatomic data have been published which question the existence of shunts.

The anatomic description of the arteriovenous anas-

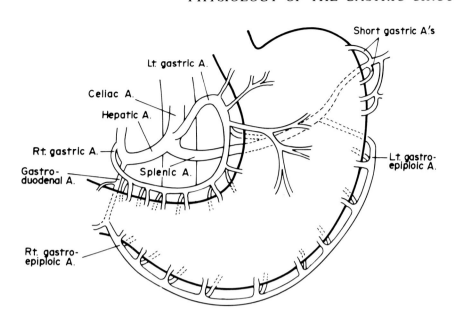

FIG. 1. Diagrammatic representation of the arterial supply of the stomach.

tomoses is based on injection studies, such as those of Barlow et al. (13). There are several factors that may lead to misinterpretation of these specimens. Staubesand and Hammersen (162) demonstrated that overlapping vessels may appear to be anastomosing. An apparent arteriovenous anastomosis must be viewed from various angles to avoid this error. In addition, pressure-flow relationships and anatomy are distorted by injection techniques, as a result of either the injection pressure or the injection material occluding vessels.

Similarly, the conclusions drawn from microsphere studies, such as those of Walder (177), have been questioned by more recent investigations with improved, accurately sized microspheres with radioactive labels. These permit quantitative estimates of shunt flow. In studies in the baboon, dog, and rat (4,25,154,187), shunt flow was reported as 0 to 5.2% of total flow.

Thus if shunt flow does exist, it is relatively insignificant, accounting for no more than 5% of total flow. *In vivo* microscopic studies in the rat (60,75) and cat (66) also have failed to reveal evidence of shunts. Utilizing a fluorescent *in vivo* microscopy technique in the rat, Guth and Moler (59) were able to follow the flow of fluoroscein-labeled albumen through the submucosal arterioles to mucosal capillaries and did not see any flow directly from submucosal arterioles to submucosal venules. Finally, in an injection study of human stomachs similar to that of Barlow et al. (13), Piasecki (137) was unable to confirm the presence of submucosal arteriovenous anastomoses in the human stomach.

In conclusion, although there are some recent studies using injection (72) or dye dilution (16) techniques that suggest the presence of shunts, the predominance of current evidence is strongly against their presence.

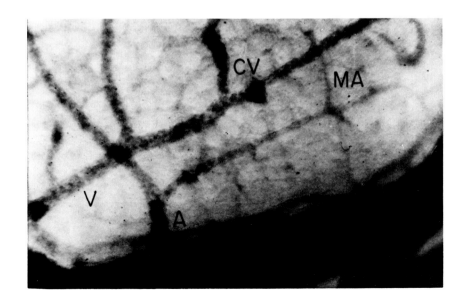

FIG. 2. *In vivo* photomicrograph of the rat gastric submucosal vascular bed. The characteristic submucosal arterial (A) and venous (V) plexi are seen. The venous network can be distinguished by the larger diameter of its vessels and the presence of collecting veins (CV), seen in cross-section, which drain into the venous anastomotic network. An arterial arcade gives rise to a mucosal arteriole (MA), which divides and enters the capillary network. This mucosal arteriole appears to be entering a vein; in actuality, it goes beneath the vein to enter the mucosa. The honeycomb-like appearance of the mucosal capillary bed is barely visible (original magnification, × 100). (From ref. 63, by permission of Williams & Wilkins.)

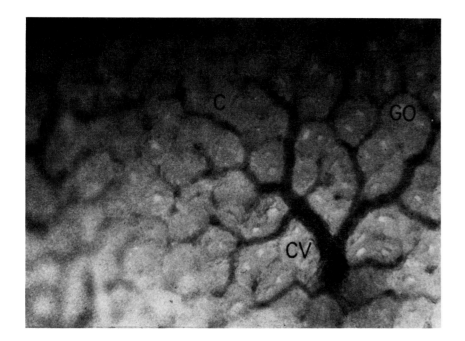

FIG. 3. *In vivo* photomicrograph of the surface of the rat gastric mucosa. The honeycomb-like appearance of the capillaries (C) surrounding the glands and ultimately draining into collecting veins (CV) is clearly seen. The orifices (GO) of the glands in the center of surrounding capillaries can be seen in some areas (original magnification, × 100). (From ref. 63, by permission of Williams & Wilkins).

Mucosa

The mucosal arterioles pierce the muscularis mucosa and enter the mucosa (13,41,60). Each mucosal arteriole divides into several branches, each of which in turn breaks up into several capillaries in the base of the mucosa. The mucosal arterioles are interconnected by slender anastomosing channels, but there are no direct anastomoses with mucosal veins. The capillaries pass perpendicularly to the mucosal surface where they branch into loops around the gland openings (13,60,63) (Fig. 3). Most glands are supplied by two to three capillaries. The capillaries run between and parallel to the glands but interconnect by short channels at right angles to the axis of the gland tubules (13). Some investigators (129) claim the arterioles also course through the mucosa parallel to the glands, but others (60) found the arterioles do not extend beyond the base of the mucosa. Blood from the capillary bed drains into collecting veins distributed throughout the mucosa. These course perpendicularly from the superficial mucosa to the submucosa, where they enter the submucosal venous plexus.

Antral-Body Portal System

Taylor and Torrance (170) studied the direction of blood flow from the gastric mucosa of the antrum of the rat stomach by the injection of [86]RbCl. Radioactivity was shown to be transported via the bloodstream from the antrum to the parietal cell mass without first passing through the general circulation. The authors suggested a "portal" or direct transport system from antral mucosa to the body of the stomach. This claim has not been studied by others, and vascular anatomic studies have not revealed such a portal system.

Comment

The gastric circulation can be regarded as a multicompartmental circuit organized as series-coupled and parallel-coupled sections (Fig. 4). The submucosa and mucosa contain series-coupled submucosal arteries, mucosal arterioles, mucosal capillaries, mucosal collecting veins, and submucosal veins. The muscle also contains series-coupled arterioles, capillaries, venules, and veins. Since the main supplying artery sends a branch to the muscle layer and then continues to the submucosa to form the submucosal arterial plexus, however, the muscle vascular bed is in parallel with the submucosa-mucosa vascular bed. This arrangement provides an anatomic explanation for the changes in distribution of flow between muscle and submucosa-mucosa under certain experimental conditions (which are presented in subsequent sections). The main supplying artery, which continues to the submucosa, and its branch to the muscle layer may respond differently to vasoactive agents or experimental procedures. This arrangement also explains the importance of the submucosal arteriolar network in controlling blood flow to the mucosa. Constriction of these vessels decreases, and dilatation increases, mucosal flow. No submucosal arteriovenous anastomoses are present.

TECHNIQUES FOR MEASURING GASTRIC BLOOD FLOW

Gross Flow

The oldest method for measuring blood flow in an organ is by collection of the venous effluent. This technique, which assumes that venous drainage reflects ar-

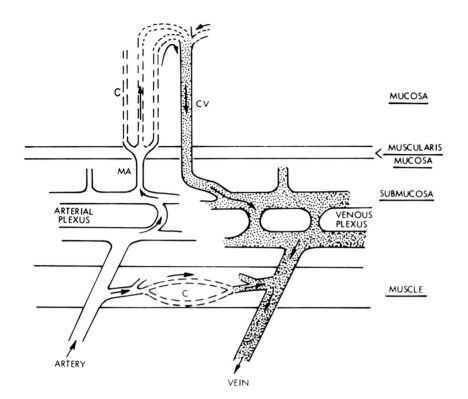

FIG. 4. Diagrammatic representation of the gastric microcirculation. MA, mucosal arteriole; C, capillary; CV, collecting vein. The microvasculature of the muscle layer is in parallel with that of the mucosa, while the microvasculature of the submucosa is in series with that of the mucosa. There are no arteriovenous anastomoses. (From ref. 56, by permission of Grune & Stratton.)

terial inflow, necessitates the surgical isolation of a vein, e.g., the gastrosplenic, in which case complete splenectomy often is performed. In some instances, the omentum also is removed. Scrupulous attention must be paid to the ligation of all drainage channels other than the one from which effluent is to be collected. It is especially difficult to isolate gastric blood flow from that of the pancreas and duodenum. The most obvious disadvantage of this technique is the surgical trauma to the experimental animal. In addition, venous pressure must be lowered to zero or less to collect the blood.

A less traumatic technique is the use of the electromagnetic flow meter, developed by Kolin (95). When a conducting fluid, i.e., one with ions, such as blood, moves through a magnetic field, an electromagnetic force is created, which is proportional to the flow rate. In practice, a cuff transducer is placed around the vessel to pick up the electrical signal for amplification and recording. The electromagnetic flow meter is virtually insensitive to the velocity profile[1] in the vessel, which is a distinct advantage for this method.

Although there is surgical trauma during placement of the cuff, the incision can be closed and the animal allowed to recover (81). In earlier models of electromagnetic flow meters, the vessels had to be repeatedly oc-

cluded to determine baseline or zero flow; this is achieved electronically, without occlusion, in newer models.

Mucosal Blood Flow

Clearance Techniques

The gastric mucosa receives approximately 70% of total gastric blood flow. Several methods have been developed to measure gastric mucosal blood flow. Gastric clearance techniques, based on principles described by Shore et al. (156) and developed by Jacobson et al. (82), are widely employed. They can be used on either anesthetized or unanesthetized animals after full recovery from the trauma of the surgical preparation. Both gastric secretion and blood flow can be measured simultaneously. The method is based on the principle that diffusion of weak organic compounds, such as weak bases, through lipid membranes depends on the degree of ionization of the compound. Lipid membranes are selectively permeable to the undissociated form of the molecule. The cell membrane, which separates plasma and gastric juice, is a lipid barrier; at the pH of blood, the unionized base diffuses freely through the membrane. When it comes in contact with the markedly lower pH of the gastric juice, the base dissociates; no longer being so lipid soluble, it cannot diffuse back into the blood. This marked difference in pH accounts for the difference in concentration of the ionized molecule in the gastric juice and plasma phases; the extent of this difference depends on the pKa of the compound.

---

[1] If it is assumed that each particle of liquid flowing in a tube moves parallel to the axis of the tube with a constant velocity, the liquid may be thought of as cylindric layers (laminas) moving at velocities which are a function of their radii. In blood vessels, the lamina in contact with the vessel wall is relatively stationary. Velocity increases inward to the central axis, where it is greatest. The velocity profiles thus form a parabola.

According to the model of Shore et al. (156), bases administered parenterally would be expected to be concentrated in the gastric juice. Thus, using a derivation of the Henderson-Hasselbalch equation,

$$R = \frac{1 + 10 \, (pKa-pH_{gastric\,j})}{1 + 10 \, (pKa-pH_{plasma})}$$

R is the ratio of the concentration of weak base in gastric juice to that in plasma. Drugs with a pKa of 5 to 10 will be transported from the plasma and accumulate in the gastric juice. The pKa of aminopyrine is 5. If we take the pH values for gastric juice and plasma to be 1 and 7, respectively, then $R = (1 + 10^4)/(1 + 10^{-2}) = 10^4$; i.e., the predicted ratio is about 10,000:1. The observed R for aminopyrine was 40 (156). This suggested that the clearance of aminopyrine was limited by blood flow. Assuming that the mucosa completely clears the drug from the circulation on a single passage through that tissue which is exposed to acid gastric juice, this clearance technique can be used to estimate blood flow. Although this assumption cannot be tested directly since venous blood from the stomach drains nonmucosal structures as well as the mucosa, Jacobson et al. (82) have presented good evidence that this assumption is acceptable. Thus, for example, although plasma aminopyrine concentrations varied between experiments over the range of 15 to 53 μg/ml, at maximal secretory rates, nearly all R values fell in the range of 30 to 40, indicating a fairly constant extraction ratio across the gastric mucosa. In addition, the amount of aminopyrine in the gastric content in 1 hr (concentration in gastric juice $\times$ volume rate of secretion/hr) was found to be approximately the same as the amount cleared from the circulation (arteriovenous difference of aminopyrine for the gastric circulation $\times$ blood flow/hr). In contrast to the small intestine, kidney, brain, heart, and lungs, or forelimb, the stomach was the only organ that consistently extracted aminopyrine in concentrations higher than that in the plasma. These and other considerations of the validity of the method have been discussed in detail by Jacobson (78).

The studies by Jacobson et al. (82) were performed in unanesthetized dogs with vagally denervated gastric fundic (Heidenhain) pouches. A loading dose of aminopyrine was followed by a continuous intravenous infusion of a maintenance dose throughout the experiment to stabilize plasma aminopyrine concentration. Various agents were infused intravenously. Gastric juice samples from the pouch were collected every 15 min, and the volume, H^+concentration, and aminopyrine concentration were determined. Venous blood samples were taken every hour and analyzed for aminopyrine concentration. The clearance, which represents pouch mucosal plasma flow, was calculated from the equation $C =$ GV/P, where C is the clearance (ml/min), G and P are gastric juice and plasma aminopyrine concentrations (mg/ml), and V is the gastric secretory rate (ml/min). The ratio of G/P, designated as R, tells us how much plasma flow in the mucosa occurred per unit of secretory volume (substituting R for G/P in the clearance equation yields $C = RV$ or $R = C/V$).

Cowley et al. (34) demonstrated that, by the intragastric instillation of exogenous acid, aminopyrine clearance could be used to measure gastric mucosal blood flow in the nonsecreting state. Rudick et al. (146) also substantiated that gastric clearance of aminopyrine is dependent not on the secretion of H^+, but on an acid milieu in the gastric lumen.

Jacobson (79) has shown that the ratio of clearance to secretory rate (R, or the ratio of aminopyrine concentration in gastric content to that in plasma) is a helpful guide to the mechanism of gastric secretory inhibition. With an agent known to constrict blood vessels and to inhibit acid secretion, such as norepinephrine, R values, as well as secretion and blood flow, were depressed. Thus the primary effect of norepinephrine was on the circulation, so that blood flow became a limiting factor for secretion. In contrast, with prostaglandin E_1 (PGE$_1$), both secretion and blood flow fell, but R either did not change or increased. Thus PGE$_1$ decreased acid secretion by some mechanism other than inhibition of blood flow; the decreased blood flow was secondary to the declining secretory activity. This interpretation of R is widely used in analyzing the mechanism of secretory inhibition by various agents. Questions about its validity have been raised (G. L. Kauffman, Jr., *personal communication*). For example, in their original publication describing the aminopyrine clearance technique, Jacobson et al. (82) observed that vasopressin, a known vasoconstrictor, decreased both secretion and blood flow, but R rose slightly.

Because of bone marrow toxicity, the large doses of aminopyrine required to give serum concentrations that can be readily measured spectrophotometrically make the technique unacceptable for human studies. Tague and Jacobson (166) studied ^{14}C-aminopyrine clearance as a measure of gastric mucosal blood flow in the dog. Only trace amounts of the agent were needed. An excellent correlation between the standard spectrophotometric and the radiometric clearance of aminopyrine was found ($r = 0.99$). In human studies, Guth et al. (57) presented data indicating that ^{14}C-aminopyrine clearance is probably a valid measure of mucosal blood flow. As in studies of Jacobson et al. (82), R decreased as secretion increased, varying between 15 and 45 at maximal rates of secretion. There was a positive relationship between gastric secretion and blood flow.

Other compounds that have been used to measure gastric clearance include ^{14}C-aniline, ^{99}technetium (^{99}Tc), and neutral red. Aniline is a weak base that does not affect acid secretion. In the rat, cat, and dog, radio-aniline clearance compared favorably with that of aminopyrine (27,36,156). Because of its tendency to become bound to plasma, aniline has a measured R about 20% less than that for aminopyrine. [99]Tc clearance in rats was found to be 15% less than ^{14}C-aminopyrine (167); in humans, it was significantly less than aminopyrine clearance in the dog (19). Furthermore, gastric back-diffusion of ^{99}Tc can occur if it is allowed to accumulate in the stomach; reabsorption occurs if it reaches the duodenum (167).

Neutral red is a basic dye with a pKa of 6.5. Using a sensitive spectrofluorometric method to measure neutral red, Aures et al. (9) found that, in the dog, the clearance of neutral red from blood to gastric juice was indistinguishable from that of aminopyrine. In humans, however, these same investigators (10) found that a metabolite of neutral red was formed that was poorly cleared into gastric juice and interfered with the accurate measurement of neutral red clearance. Knight and McIsaac (89) modified the extraction procedure in order to extract only diffusible neutral red from plasma. With this modification, neutral red clearance appears to be a valid measure of gastric mucosal blood flow in humans, R averaging 22 and clearance increasing with acid secretion. Knight and his colleagues (89–92) have carried out numerous studies with this technique in humans.

Indicator-Dilution (Fractional Extraction) Technique

^{42}K and ^{86}Rb technique.

The indicator-dilution technique, using ^{42}K or ^{86}Rb, has been used to determine gastric blood flow and its distribution under basal and experimental conditions (38,39,55,148,153,185). This technique is based on the assumption that the fraction of the injected isotope in an organ 30 to 60 sec after injection of a small bolus of the isotope is equal to the fraction of the cardiac output perfusing that organ. Theoretically, all the ^{42}K or ^{86}Rb in the blood flowing through an organ exchanges with intracellular K in a single passage through the organ. By multiplying cardiac output by the fraction of injected isotope in an organ, one obtains the blood flow of that organ.

Radioactive-labeled microsphere technique.

The radioactive-labeled microsphere technique is a form of the indicator-dilution method. Microspheres of a uniform size are injected into the left ventricle. The spheres are distributed to the different organs according to the fraction of the cardiac output going to the respective organs. The microspheres are trapped in vessels less than the diameter of the spheres. From the radioactivity of the tissue in which the investigator is interested, the total amount of radioactivity injected, and the cardiac output, the flow in milliliters per minute to that tissue can be calculated. The critical assumption of the microsphere is different from that of the ^{42}K and ^{86}Rb methods. For the microspheres, the question is whether or not they distribute at arterial bifurcations in proportion to blood flow. The questionable assumption in the ^{42}K or ^{86}Rb technique is that all tissues have the same extraction ratio for the isotope. For the microspheres, all vessels less than the diameter of the spheres should extract 100% of those entering; in the absence of significant arteriovenous shunt flow, all tissues would have equal extractions for the spheres. Delaney and Grim (38) found close agreement between the mean distribution in the mucosa, submucosa, and muscularis of the dog stomach of 16- or 10-μm diameter microspheres and ^{42}K.

Advantages and disadvantages. An advantage of the microsphere technique over the isotope technique is that microspheres with different labels, e.g., ^{85}Sr, ^{141}Ce, and ^{51}CR, can be injected at different times during an experiment (with determination of cardiac output each time by obtaining an integrated blood sample from the aorta using a withdrawal pump at a constant rate for a short period of time). When the animal is killed at the end of the experiment, the organ blood flow at the different times during the course of the study is obtained from the organ concentration of the different labels and the cardiac output for the time the label was injected.

Greenway and Murthy (54) have raised serious questions about the validity of the microsphere technique in assessing distribution of blood flow when the blood vessels of the area studied are in series rather than in parallel. In a study of the distribution of blood flow in the intestine, the authors found that the distribution of microspheres between the mucosa and submucosa depended on the size of the microspheres. The smaller the spheres, the more were found in the mucosa, e.g., 47.4% of 12-μm spheres as compared with 26.3% of 17-μm spheres. It also depended on the state of the vascular bed. When given during an infusion of vasopressin, the mucosa-submucosa distribution of 17-μm spheres was 20.9 to 79.1%. A subsequent infusion of isoprenaline resulted in movement of some of the spheres from the submucosa into the mucosa, the distribution becoming 44.4 to 55.6%. Their data suggested that the intestine consists of two parallel-coupled sections, one to the muscle and the other through the submucosa to the mucosa. The vessels in the submucosa are in series with those in the mucosa, and submucosal shunts do not exist. On the basis of *in vivo* microscopic studies, the same is true of the microvascular bed of the stomach (see Fig. 4).

Comparison with aminopyrine clearance. Archibald et al. (3) have used the labeled microsphere technique in a comparative study with aminopyrine clearance technique in anesthetized dogs prepared with a chambered segment of the greater curvature of the stomach. Paired flow measurements were made in dogs secreting in response to intravenous histamine, in nonsecreting dogs given intravenous isoproterenol, and in dogs given no drugs (resting state). Isotonic HCl was maintained on the mucosal surface during all experiments. While there was a reasonably close relationship between the two methods in estimating mucosal perfusion during histamine stimulation (clearance averaged 90% of the microsphere value), during isoproterenol infusion and in the resting state, clearance averaged only 38 and 46%, respectively, of the microsphere value. The authors conclude that aminopyrine clearance reflects only a small fraction of mucosal blood flow in the nonsecreting stomach, even in the presence of exogenous acid. They speculate that externally applied acid in the resting stomach may not provide as effective a pH gradient for cells lining the glands as when they are continuously exposed to a fresh supply of acid in the secreting stomach. An alternative explanation is that the aminopyrine clearance technique may be measuring blood flow only in the superficial gastric mucosa.

Thus there are advantages and disadvantages of each method. The number of flow measurements obtainable with the aminopyrine clearance technique is unlimited, and results are less sensitive to chance fluctuations in flow than are microsphere-determined blood flows. Furthermore, aminopyrine clearance is less expensive and does not require killing the animal. The microsphere method permits a limited number of fairly accurate, instantaneous flow measurements to be made.

Heat Clearance Technique

Mucosal blood flow has been measured in unanesthetized animals by a heat clearance technique (18) and with a thermocouple (49,52,93,164). These methods are based on the assumption that change in blood flow in a tissue will result in altered thermal conductivity of the tissue. In the heat clearance technique, a small heater coil is affixed to the mucosal wall and maintained there by continuous suction of about 5 mm Hg. The coil contains a thermistor to measure temperature within the coil. Energy is supplied to the heater at constant rate, and changes in blood flow result in altered thermal conductivity. A second, remote thermistor picks up the ambient tissue temperature. Thermal conductivity (flow) is given by:

$$\lambda = KI^2/\phi$$

where λ = thermal conductivity (flow), K = instrument constant, ϕ = temperature difference between the two thermistors, and I^2 = current supplying the heater coil. Since I^2 is constant, for any particular instrument, flow $(\lambda) = 1/\phi$. Although this technique can

be used in conscious animals with appropriate chronic gastric pouches, it has several disadvantages: (a) measurements are only qualitative; i.e., results are expressed in units such as millivolts and not milliliters per minute; (b) the suction required to attach the device to the mucosa may interfere with flow; and (c) gastric contractions interfere with the record and cause electrical interference.

Indicator Washout Technique

Indicator washout of inert gases, e.g., ^{85}Kr or ^{133}Xe, has also been used to estimate blood flow (17,104). These gases are lipid soluble and pass rapidly across the blood-tissue interface, being limited only by blood flow. They are almost completely eliminated by the lungs in one passage, so that practically no recirculation occurs. A bolus of known concentration of indicator is injected intraarterially or, alternatively, is placed in the gastric lumen and the disappearance of the isotope (dQ/dt) recorded. The radioactive decay rate versus time is plotted on similog paper. For a single compartment vascular bed, the curve is monoexponential. Most organs (including the stomach), however, are heterogeneous, and more than one flow rate to different compartments occurs. The resulting multiexponential curve must be analyzed by a curve peeling procedure, which makes the assumption that the components of the curve each have exponential washout curves that can be added for the total curve.

Results of actual blood flow measurements with the various techniques, in terms of ml blood flow min^{-1}g^{-1}, distribution of blood flow among tissue layers, and milliliters per minute as measured by the aminopyrine clearance techniques are presented in Table 1, 2, and 3, respectively.

Other Techniques for Studying the Gastric Microvasculature

In Vivo *Microscopy*

Recent advances in *in vivo* study of microcirculation have led to methods for observing the gastric circulation in the living animal (60,75,142). A fasted rat is anesthetized, the abdomen opened, and the stomach exteriorized. An incision is made in the duodenum just distal to the pylorus, and a clad fiberglass rod is passed retrograde into the stomach. Transillumination of the gastric wall is achieved by passing light from a high-intensity light source through the rod. Removal of the muscle and serosal layers from a small area on the anterior wall permits visualization of blood flow through the submucosal arterial network, down to the deep layer of mucosa, and back through mucosal venules to the submucosal venous network (Fig. 2). The area under study is kept

TABLE 1. *Gastric blood flow*[a]

Species	Total blood flow		Mucosal blood flow		Method	Ref.
	Resting	Stimulated	Resting	Stimulated		
Dog	0.54	0.73 (Hist) 1.07 (Epi)	1.13	—	[42]K clearance	38,39
Dog	0.32 (Antr)	0.47 (Hist) 1.12 (Epi)	—	—	[42]K clearance	38,39
	0.61 (Corp)	0.83 (Hist) 1.04 (Epi)	—	—		
Dog	0.61 (Antr) 0.53 (Corp)	—	—	—	[42]K clearance	38
Dog	0.40	—	—	—	[42]K clearance	148
Dog	0.52–0.56	—	0.68	—	[86]Rb clearance	50,119
Dog	0.41 (Antr) 0.56 (Corp)	—	—	—	[86]Rb clearance	37
Rat	—	—	3.24 (Antr)	7.15 (Pentagast) 12.84 (Hist)	[86]Rb clearance	168
			2.35 (Corp)	6.65 (Pentagast) 7.52 (Hist)		
Rat	0.40–0.41	—	—	—	[86]Rb clearance	55,163
Dog	—	—	0.94	—	[85]Kr clearance	17
Dog	0.178–0.60	—	0.31–0.36	—	Microspheres	22,29,103,155
Dog	—	—	0.44 (Antr) 1.14 (Corp) 0.91 (Fund)	—	Microspheres	151
Dog	0.60	1.18 (Eating)	0.36	0.92 (Eating)	Microspheres	22
Cat	—	—	0.37–0.43 0.27	— 0.52 (Pentagast)	Microspheres	158
Swine	—	—	0.16 (Antr) 0.16 (Corp) 0.14 (Fund)	— — —	Microspheres	103
Dog	0.31	—	—	—	Flow meter (splenic vein)	116
Cat	1.80	—	—	—	Venous effluent	110

[a] Expressed as ml/min × g tissue^{-1}.

moist and warm by bathing it continuously with Krebs' solution.

The superficial mucosa can be visualized with a different preparation. A long incision is made in the anterior wall of the forestomach just proximal to the "rumenal ridge." Part of the adjacent posterior wall of the

TABLE 2. *Distribution of gastric blood flow*[a]

Species	Muscle	Submu-cosa	Mu-cosa	Method	Ref.
Dog	15	13	72	[42]K Clearance	39
Rat	—	—	51	[86]Rb clearance	55
Ba-boon	—	—	77	Microspheres	187
Dog	29.8	20.3	49.9	Microspheres	29
Dog	—	—	72	Microspheres	30
Dog	21.7	10.2	68.1	16 μm Spheres	3
Dog	20.9	34.5	44.8	26 μm Spheres	3

[a] Percent of total blood flow.

gradular stomach is then everted through the incision, thus exposing the mucosa to direct visualization. The fiberglass rod is placed beneath the serosa of the everted portion of the stomach. The flow of red blood cells through the capillaries around the mouth of the gastric glands and into the collecting veins can be seen clearly in this preparation (Fig. 3).

In vivo fluorescence microscopy has been developed for the study of vascular permeability—the movement of large molecules across microvessels (125,180). A microscope with a vertical illuminator and appropriate filters is employed. Fluorescein isothiocyanate conjugated to serum albumin is injected intravenously. A closed circuit television system using extremely light-sensitive silicon intensifier target video camera permits video monitoring and videotaping of the flow of the fluorescent conjugate through the microvessels, and, under appropriate experimental conditions, diffusion out of the vessels into the interstitium. This technique has recently been adapted for the study of gastric microcirculation (59).

TABLE 3. *Mucosal blood flow measured by aminopyrine clearance technique*

Species	Resting blood flow (ml/min)	Stimulated blood flow (ml/min)	Type of preparation	Ref.
Human	50.0	150 (Pentagast)	Intact	57
Dog	3.00	—	Vascular pedicle	31
Dog	1.00	13 (Hist)	Vascular pedicle	123
Dog	4.30	12.1 (Hist)	Whole stomach	125
Dog	10.00	—	Whole stomach	176
Dog	1.80–30.3	—	Heidenhain pouch	8,34,94,165
Dog	0.40	10.5 (Hist)	Heidenhain pouch	166
Dog	2.00	8.9 (Hist)	Fundic pouch (chambered)	171
Dog	2.90	—	Fundic pouch (chambered)	30
Cat	2.76	3.50 (Meat extract in antral pouch)	Fundic pouch (chambered)	20
Dog	1.16 (ml/min/g Mucosa)	—	Heidenhain pouch	33

Injection and Fixation Techniques

Injection and fixation of the vascular bed has been attempted since before Harvey's discovery of circulation (71). Barlow (12) injected radio-opaque substances at 150 mm Hg pressure into one of the gastric or gastro-epiploic arteries of stomachs excised at surgery or removed from cadavers. Bismuth oxychloride was used to fill the larger, and silver iodide the smaller vessels. Piasecki (137,138) injected India ink in 2% gelatin or a barium sulfate suspension in his studies of canine and human gastric vasculature. The tissues were fixed in formaline and sectioned, or were cleared (Spalteholz technique) and examined under a dissecting microscope.

To preserve the living vascular geometry, silicone elastomer microvascular filling techniques have been used (26,72,160). These room temperature, vulcanizing silicone rubbers are infused at normal systemic pressure. Special care is taken to maintain pressure relationships until the cast is hardened. The specimen is then cleared in glycerol, or the parenchymal tissue dissolved with caustic, e.g., KOH, and embedded in plastic.

It is difficult to completely fill the capillary bed with injected material. The viscosity, surface tension, and size of particles of the filling agent must be considered. Injection at nonphysiologic pressures can distort the true geometry of the vessels.

In Vitro *Arterial Strips*

In vitro preparations of arteries and veins for studies of vascular reactivity to various stimuli have been used widely. The vessels can be cut into ring segments 2 to 5 mm in length or into helical strips, or they can be incised in intact, unbranched lengths of several centimeters (173). The ring segments are suitable for smaller vessels. They can be cannulated with small stainless steel wires and coupled to a force transducer for measurement of tension development. Larger vessels can be studied by cutting helical strips and suspending them between the transducer and a fixed hook. The method is unsatisfactory for very small vessels due to the trauma to intramural nerves and to the vascular smooth muscle. Most large and medium-sized vessels are suitable for *in vitro* perfusion. A cannula with a T-connection coupled to the pressure transducer can be tied into the lumen of the vessel. If the preparation is then perfused at constant flow, the contraction of the vessel will be reflected in the changes in perfusion pressure. If it is undesirable to have the effluent enter the bath, an outlet cannula can be tied into the outflow end of the vessel.

CONTROL OF GASTRIC BLOOD FLOW

Neural

Central Nervous System

> In. . .predisposition, from whatever cause. . .fear, anger, or whatever depresses or disturbs the nervous system—the villous coat (of the stomach) becomes sometimes red and dry, at other times pale and moist, and loses its smooth and healthy appearance; . . .

This description by Beaumont (14), based on observations of the exposed gastric mucosa of his patient St. Martin in the early 19th century, is probably the first evidence that the central nervous system plays a role in gastric function, including blood flow. Observations of this nature were extended by Wolf (184) in the study of the gastrostomy of his patient, Tom. The author described two opposing patterns of gastric reaction to emotional conflicts. One, an arousal pattern, was characterized by vascular engorgement of the mucosa, increased secretion of HCl, and increased motor activity. The other, marked by a general attitude of withdrawal, was characterized by pallor of the mucosa and a decrease in acid secretion and motor activity.

Using a stereotactic method to implant electrodes in dogs, Leonard and his colleagues (102) studied the effect of anterior and posterior hypothalamic stimulation on left gastric artery blood flow (via an electromagnetic flow meter probe) and acid secretion. Low frequency stimulation (25 cps) of the anterior hypothalamus resulted in a parasympathetic vascular and secretory pattern, i.e., increased blood flow and acid secretion. Vagotomy abolished this effect, and stimulation of the distal end of the cut vagus nerve increased blood flow. Stimulation of the posterior hypothalamus resulted in a sympathetic vascular acid and secretory pattern, i.e., marked decrease in gastric blood flow, and inhibition of histamine-stimulated acid secretion. Celiac ganglionectomy abolished the gastric blood flow change.

Osumi et al. (131) studied changes in gastric mucosal blood flow, using the aminopyrine clearance technique, and acid secretion following electrical stimulation of the lateral hypothalamic area in the rat. Repetitive stimulation at 10 cps for 10 min elicited a significant, reproducible increase in both gastric mucosal blood flow and acid output. Because the injection of norepinephrine into the lateral ventricle blocked these increases, the authors also speculated that a central noradrenergic inhibitor mechanism is involved in the regulation of gastric mucosal blood flow and acid secretion.

The results of the preceding studies can be accepted only with reservation, pending confirmation by other investigators. There have been many more studies on the effect of central nervous stimulation on gastric acid secretion than on blood flow; the results are highly discrepant. Thus Sen and Anand (152), like Porter et al. (139), reported that anterior hypothalamic stimulation increased acid secretion, while posterior stimulation did not; Feldman et al. (45) reported that posterior stimulation increased gastric acid secretion, while anterior stimulation did not; Porter et al. (139) observed an increase in acid secretion with both anterior and posterior stimulation, although the posterior response was a delayed one; finally, both Smith and McHugh (159) and Zukoskie et al. (188) reported no change in acid secretion with either anterior or posterior hypothalmic stimulation.

Autonomic Nervous System

Sympathetic.

The sympathetic nerve supply to the stomach is derived from the sixth to the 10th spinal nerves and terminates in the celiac ganglia. From here, postganglionic fibers reach the stomach as discrete nerves, as nerves mixed with vagal fibers, or as nerves accompanying the arteries. Using a fluorescent histochemical method,

Furness (47) found that the arteries to the stomach were richly supplied by adrenergic nerves, as were those penetrating the musculature. There was a profusion of heavily innervated arteries in the submucosa.

On histologic section, the adrenergic nerves were seen at the outer edge of the media of the arteries. The smaller branches (mucosal arteries), which crossed the muscularis mucosae to supply the mucosal capillaries, also were accompanied by adrenergic axons. The capillaries were almost exclusively without adrenergic innervation. The veins within the stomach wall were sparsely innervated. In the submucosa, a few of the larger veins (100 to 200 μm) had adrenergic fibers with them, but veins of less than 100 μm were generally not innervated. The smaller veins carrying blood away from the stomach were all innervated but less densely than the accompanying arteries. As the veins become larger, their density of innervation becomes greater but still less so than the adjacent artery. These studies by Furness (47) were performed in the guinea pig, rat, cat and rabbit. Similar findings were reported by Jacobowitz (76), in that blood vessels in the submucosa and basal parts of the mucosa were fairly densely innervated, while those in the superficial parts of the mucosa were almost devoid of adrenergic fluorescence.

Electrical stimulation of the sympathetic fibers to the stomach resulted in decreased total blood flow (venous outflow measurement) (84), celiac (66) and gastroepiploic (135) artery flow (electromagnetic flow probe), and gastric mucosal blood flow (aminopyrine clearance technique) (21,141). Using a study of histologic sections of stomachs following intravascular injection of colored dyes or India ink, Schnitzlein (149) observed that stimulation of the celiac ganglion caused contraction of the arterioles and relative ischemia of the gastric mucosa. Arabehety et al (2) observed that splanchnic section resulted in a marked increase in filling of gastric mucosal capillaries with India ink. Thus several independent investigators, using different techniques, came to the same conclusion; i.e., stimulation of the sympathetic fibers to the stomach decreases both total and mucosal blood flow of the stomach.

Jansson et al. (84) observed that when stimulation of sympathetic fibers was prolonged, blood flow, following the initial fall, increased and reached a new steady-state flow level within 3 to 4 min. This phenomenon has been termed autoregulatory escape from vasoconstrictor influence. This term was suggested by Ross (143) to avoid confusion with autoregulation (maintenance of blood flow to a tissue despite alterations in perfusion pressure), and since the escape phenomenon occurs with adrenergic agents but not with vasopressin. Originally the escape was attributed to a flow redistribution in the stomach wall due to the opening of submucosal arteriovenous anastomoses during sympathetic stimulation (46). Both *in vitro* arterial segment studies (44) and *in vivo* microscopic observations (61,64), however, indicate that escape is due to relaxation of initially constricted vessels and not to the opening of shunts.

The *in vivo* microscopic studies also demonstrated the important role of constriction and dilatation of submucosal arterioles in regulating gastric mucosal blood flow in the rat (63) and cat (66). Stimulation of the left splanchnic nerve for 3 min caused an initial constriction of submucosal arterioles followed by partial escape. No arteriovenous anastomoses were seen either in the resting state or during nerve stimulation. *In vivo* microscopic observations of the superficial mucosal blood flow during splanchnic nerve stimulation revealed a slowing of flow with progressively fewer red blood cells present in the capillaries and in the collecting veins into which they feed. Finally, there was a complete cessation of flow with no red blood cells seen in the majority of capillaries, and the mucosa appeared blanched. After a while, even though splanchnic stimulation was continuing, escape occurred with a partial return of flow. There was no statistically significant difference between the mean time to maximum constriction of submucosal arterioles and to maximum blanching of the mucosa, or between time to escape in the two areas. Thus the submucosal arterioles appear to be the vascular segment controlling gastric mucosal blood flow, constriction of these arterioles decreasing and dilatation increasing mucosal blood flow.

Parasympathetic.

The parasympathetic supply to the stomach is via the vagus nerves. Martinson (111) and Jansson (83) demonstrated that in the cat, the vagus nerves may be divided into low and high threshold groups of fibers (duration of electrical stimulus, less than or greater than 0.5 msec). Stimulation of the low threshold set induced an atropine-resistant, nonadrenergic relaxation of the stomach. Martinson (110) showed that stimulation of the vagal relaxatory fibers caused a concomitant augmentation of gastric blood flow (venous outflow measurement) and secretion. Atropine reduced the blood flow increase and completely abolished the secretory response.

These observations led Jansson et al. (85) to conclude that the blood flow increase to the stomach during vagal stimulation is largely secondary to an augmented secretion. Careful scrutiny of graphs published by Martinson (110), however, shows a prompt (within 1 min) increase in blood flow with the onset of vagal stimulation. This suggests a direct dilator effect of vagal stimulation preceding acid secretion (which takes several minutes), as well as the increase in blood flow initiated by the increase in acid secretion.

Bell and Battersby (17) used a ^{85}Kr clearance technique to measure gastric mucosal blood flow in the dog.

Vagotomy caused a statistically significant reduction in gastric mucosal blood flow in 10 of 12 dogs. The reduction in mucosal flow regularly occurred within 5 min of nerve section (the earliest measurement made), suggesting a direct vagal effect on the vasculature.

An *in vivo* microscopy technique in the rat was used by Guth and Smith (63) to study the possible direct vascular effect of vagal nerve stimulation. Gastric submucosal arteriolar diameter was measured immediately before and after vagal nerve stimulation (8 V, 2 msec duration, 6 ips). In 45 or 51 stimulation episodes in 11 rats, the arterioles dilated within 10 sec of beginning stimulation and constricted within 10 sec of cessation of stimulation. These changes were significant at $p < 0.001$. Similar results were obtained in the cat (66). The findings of immediate submucosal arteriolar dilatation with vagal stimulation and constriction on cessation of stimulation are compatible with a direct dilator effect of vagal stimulation on the vascular smooth muscle of these vessels. This does not deny the important role of other factors secondary to augmented acid secretion in enhancing blood flow to the stomach. The immediate "on-off" response observed in the *in vivo* microscopic study, however, is too rapid to be explained by factors secondary to acid secretion.

Nakamura et al. (125) used the aminopyrine clearance technique to study gastric mucosal blood flow and the venous outflow procedure to measure total blood flow in the dog before and after vagotomy. The authors found a decrease in both total and gastric mucosal blood flow during the immediate postvagotomy period. This reduction was maintained in dogs studied 3 months after vagotomy. Although there is a consensus concerning the early effects of vagotomy on gastric mucosal blood flow, there is controversy concerning the long-term effects. Bell and Shelley (18) reported that no long-term effect of vagotomy was found on mucosal blood flow as measured by the heat clearance technique. Similarly, Delaney (37), using the radiorubidium indicator-dilution technique, found no significant change in corpus blood flow 4 to 6 weeks after truncal vagotomy; gastric antral flow was increased. The authors speculate that either the decrease in antral muscle tonus following denervation or reflux of duodenal content through the pyloroplasty might account for the increase in antral blood flow. Analogous findings in *in vivo* microscopic studies in the rat for up to 1 hr after vagotomy were described by Hunter et al. (75). There was decreased submucosal blood flow in the corpus but increased flow in the antral submucosal microvessels.

Parasympathetic-Sympathetic Interaction.

Evidence for cholinergic inhibition of adrenergic neurotransmission in the canine gastric artery has been presented by Van Hee and Vanhoutte (173). In dog gastric artery strips studies, they found that the contractile response to electrical stimulation was abolished by tetrodotoxin and phenoxybenzamine, indicating that the contractions were induced by release of endogenous norepinephrine from adrenergic nerve endings. Acetylcholine, which by itself had no effect on basal tension, inhibited the response to electrical stimulation. This suggests that there are muscarinic receptors on the sympathetic nerve endings, the activation of which mediates inhibition of adrenergic neurotransmission.

Left gastric artery perfusion studies were performed in the intact dog. Vagal stimulation depressed the vasoconstrictor response to sympathetic (celiac plexus) nerve stimulation significantly more than those induced by exogenous norepinephrine. These data indicate that, in the blood vessels of the stomach, endogenously released acetylcholine exerts an inhibitor modulatory influence on adrenergic neurotransmission. In the resting state, vagal stimulation caused a prompt decrease in perfusion pressure, consistent with the data presented in the previous section of a direct vascular dilatatory effect of vagal stimulation.

Biogenic Amines

Catecholamines

The literature concerning the effect of catecholamines on gastric blood flow presents markedly discrepant findings. Using bubble flow meters, Cumming et al. (35) found epinephrine to be a dilator and norepinephrine a constrictor of the canine gastric circulation when infused intravenously over a dose range of 1 to 8 $\mu g/kg^{-1}min^{-1}$. In the cat stomach, Thompson and Vane (172) observed dilator responses when epinephrine was infused intravenously at a rate of 2 $\mu g/kg^{-1}min^{-1}$ but constrictor responses when infused at 10 $\mu g/kg^{-1}min^{-1}$. Using the ^{42}K indicator-dilution technique in the dog, Delaney and Grim (39) found that epinephrine (1 $\mu g/kg^{-1}min^{-1}$ i.v.) increased and norepinephrine (2 $\mu g/kg^{-1}min^{-1}$ i.v.) decreased gastric perfusion. Nicoloff et al. (128) measured left gastric and splenic arterial blood flows electromagnetically and observed vasoconstriction in response to the intravenous infusion of norepinephrine but dilatation in some dogs and constriction in others with the same dose of epinephrine. Using the aminopyrine clearance technique, Jacobson et al. (82) showed a reduction in gastric mucosal blood flow by intravenous epinephrine during gastrin stimulation, Cowley and Code (33) found an increase in the nonsecreting canine pouch.

Variations in the method of measuring blood flow, dose, route, and duration of drug administration, type of anesthesia, species, and animal preparation may be responsible for these differing findings with the intravenous administration of vasoactive agents. The direct effect of the agents on the gastric circulation is confounded by their effects on cardiac output and other vascular beds. *In vitro* studies of the effect of agents on arterial strips, *in vivo* microscopic study of the topical application of agents, and the close intra-arterial infusion of agents permit study of the direct gastric vascular effects of the agents.

Van Hee and Vanhoutte (173) performed *in vitro* studies on isolated helical strips of canine gastric arteries. Contractile responses were obtained to increasing concentrations (10^{-5} to 10^{-9} M) of both epinephrine and norepinephrine. Epinephrine produced a greater maximal tension, but there was no significant difference between the dose-response curves for the two catecholamines when the results were expressed as percentage of the maximal response obtained with each catecholamine. The adrenergic blocking agent phenoxybenzamine caused dose-dependent inhibition of the response to both epinephrine and norepinephrine. The β-agonist isoproterenol did not cause a significant change in tension and did not significantly affect the contractile response to 10^{-6} M norepinephrine. The direct constricting effect of both catecholamines was also demonstrated in the intact animal in *in vivo* microscopic studies in the rat (58,62). Application of 10^{-6} M epinephrine (62) and 10^{-5} to 10^{-7} M norepinephrine (58) to the intact, exposed gastric submucosal vascular bed produced prompt constriction of the arterioles.

Zinner et al. (186) studied the effects of the close intra-arterial injection of adrenergic agents on the gastric circulation in anesthetized dogs. Blood flow through the right and left gastric arteries was measured electromagnetically, and the agents studied were infused via catheters in these vessels. Epinephrine and norepinephrine induced constriction followed by dilatation (escape from adrenergic constriction) in both circulations. The constrictor components were attenuated or abolished by α-adrenergic blockade with phenoxybenzamine, and the dilator components were attenuated by β-adrenergic blockage with propranolol. The β-agonist isoproterenol produced vasodilatation of both right and left gastric circulations; this effect was attenuated by β-adrenergic blockade. The constrictor response was similar in both circulations, but the dilator response was greater in the left gastric circulation. With epinephrine (0.5 $\mu g/kg^{-1}min^{-1}$), the dilator response following the initial constriction in the left gastric artery resulted in a blood flow after 3 min that was significantly greater than control flow. This might explain the dilator effect of epinephrine infusions reported by several investigators.

Zinner et al. (187) also studied the effect of close intra-arterial injection of epinephrine (0.5 $\mu g/kg^{-1}min^{-1}$) in the baboon. Total gastric blood flow was measured electromagnetically, and radioactive microspheres (15 ± 5 μm) were used to determine regional distribution. Control flow was 55 ml/min^{-1}, with 77% of flow going to the gastric mucosa and 2% of injected spheres appearing in the liver. In contrast to the dog studies, epinephrine infusion resulted in a sustained vasoconstriction, with no escape from adrenergic constriction. There was neither redistribution of flow (change in percent flow to the gastric mucosa) nor change in arteriovenous shunting (percent spheres appearing in the liver).

The above *in vitro and in vivo* microscopic and close intra-arterial injection studies indicate that both norepinephrine and epinephrine initially constrict gastric arteries and decrease gastric blood flow. In the dog but not in the baboon, the close intra-arterial studies suggest that both are "mixed" adrenergic agonists, with an α-adrenergic constricting effect and a β-adrenergic dilating effect. The β-adrenergic dilating effect is much more pronounced with epinephrine. Isoproterenol is a "pure" β-adrenergic agonist and increases gastric blood flow.

Histamine.

The importance of considering route of administration and dosage in studying the effects of agents on the gastric circulation is clearly demonstrated by histamine. More than 15 years ago, Peter et al. (136) and Jacobson (77) found that histamine dilates the gastric circulation and increases gastric blood flow when it is infused locally under circumstances in which it has no effect on systemic arterial pressure, or when it is infused systemically in small doses. In contrast, Menguy (114) observed that the administration of large amounts of histamine by a systemic route can cause abrupt hypotension and presumably a sympathetic discharge resulting in constriction and a decreased blood flow to the stomach.

Histamine acts via two types of receptors: first, those blocked by the older antihistamine agents, such as mepyramine (e.g., the receptors mediating bronchial constriction), termed H_1 (6), and second, those not blocked by mepyramine (e.g., the receptors mediating gastric acid secretion), termed H_2 (20). The recently developed H_2 antagonists (20) block the latter receptors.

Main and Whittle (109) studied the types of histamine receptors in the gastric mucosa using the ^{14}C-aniline clearance technique to measure gastric mucosal blood flow. When acid secretion was inhibited by the histamine H_2 receptor antagonists burimamide and metiamide, histamine still increased gastric mucosal blood flow. The selective histamine H_1 receptor agonist 2-pyridylethylamine had no effect on acid output but increased resting mucosal blood flow. These results suggested that histamine H_2 receptors, primarily concerned with acid secretion, and H_1-receptors, concerned with vasodilatation, are both present in the gastric mucosa.

Guth and Smith (67) studied the types and functions of histamine receptors in the submucosal arterioles of the corpus and antrum of cat and rat stomachs using an *in vivo* microscopy technique. Change in arteriolar diameter in response to superfusion of the exposed submucosal vascular bed with histamine with and without the H_1 antagonist mepyramine and the H_2 antagonist metiamide was measured by an image-splitting technique. H_1 and H_2 histamine receptors subserving vasodilatation were demonstrated in both areas in both species. In a subsequent study (68), the authors demonstrated similar vasodilatation of gastric submucosal arterioles in response to superfusion with the H_1 agonists 2-pyridylethylamine and 2-thiazole-ethylamine and the H_2 agonist dimiprit. These studies indicate that histamine increases gastric blood flow by stimulating both H_1 and H_2 histamine receptors on the gastric submucosal arterioles.

In contrast to the findings of Main and Whittle (109) in the rat, Konturek et al. (100) observed that with metiamide in the dog, inhibition of histamine-stimulated acid secretion was always associated with a marked reduction in mucosal blood flow. R, the ratio of aminopyrine concentration in the gastric juice to that in plasma, was not significantly changed by metiamide. Since this ratio expresses milliliters of plasma flow required for the formation of 1 ml gastric juice, this indicates that the reduction in gastric mucosal blood flow was secondary to an inhibition of gastric secretion. One possible explanation for the discrepancy in findings between the rat and dog studies, besides species difference, is a difference in experimental design. Main and Whittle (109) infused metiamide first to study its effect on resting flow (no effect) and then added the histamine infusion and obtained an increase in mucosal flow but not acid secretion. Konturek et al. (100) first infused histamine to obtain a marked rise in acid secretion and mucosal blood flow and then added metiamide, with a resultant decrease in both parameters. Since resting blood flow and acid secretion were not measured, they could not be compared with the histamine plus metiamide measurements.

The H_2 receptor antagonists have no effect on resting mucosal blood flow in the anesthetized animal. This was studied in the rat (109) and cat (70) with metiamide using the ^{14}C-aniline or aminopyrine clearance technique and in the rat (133) and dog (40) with cimetidine using a radiolabeled microsphere technique.

The effect of H_2 receptor antagonists on gastric mucosal blood flow in animals subjected to ulcerogenic procedures is controversial. Cimetidine treatment reduced gastric ischemia in hemorrhagic shock in miniature pigs (103) but not in rats (133), and metiamide reduced gastric ischemia in rats subjected to restraint stress (150). The reason for these discrepant findings is not clear.

An interaction between histamine and sympathetic

nerve stimulation has been described. McGrath and Shepherd (112) found that histamine inhibited norepinephrine release and constriction caused by sympathetic nerve stimulation in isolated blood vessels. This effect was blocked by metiamide and mimicked by an H_2 receptor agonist. In the isolated, perfused gracilis muscle, Powell (140) observed that histamine reduced vasoconstriction caused by sympathetic nerve stimulation but not norepinephrine infusion. This effect was prevented by treatment with metiamide and mimicked by dimaprit, an H_2 agonist. These results indicate that, in some vascular beds, histamine can modulate sympathetic vasoconstriction by a prejunctional mechanism through an interaction with H_2 receptors. This could be of pathophysiologic significance because of the high quantities of histamine contained in sympathetic nerves and vascular tissue. Analagous studies have not been performed in the gastric vasculature.

Tepperman et al. (171) have challenged the concept of the specificity of the gastric histamine receptors. The intra-arterial injection of tripilennamine, an H_1 receptor antagonist, inhibited the stimulation of acid secretion by histamine, and the H_2 antagonist metiamide inhibited the vasodilatory response to the H_1 receptor agonist, 2-methylhistamine. These findings have been questioned, however, because of the large dose of tripellennamine required to inhibit histamine-stimulated acid secretion; and 2-methylhistamine is not a pure H_1 agonist (132).

Gastrointestinal Hormones

It has been clearly demonstrated in a number of investigations that both gastrin and pentagastrin are potent stimulants of gastric acid secretion; and, secondary to the increase in acid secretion, there is an increase in gastric mucosal blood flow. This has been found in dog (82), cat (69), rat (106), and man (57,89). The evidence that the increase in blood flow is secondary to the increase in acid secretion is based on the finding that the ratio of gastric mucosal blood flow to acid secretion remains constant as both increase in response to increasing doses of pentagastrin. Jacobson and Chang (80) compared histamine and gastrin effects (using aminopyrine clearance) and found the ratio to be greater for histamine. This suggested that the increased mucosal flow due to histamine, in contrast to that due to gastrin, represented both a direct dilating property and an indirect metabolic effect secondary to secretion. This was confirmed by *in vivo* microscopic observations in the cat by Guth and Smith (65). The close intra-arterial infusion of histamine but not pentagastrin in doses approximating 3% of the intravenous D_{50} dose for stimulation of acid secretion caused prompt dilation of gastric submucosal arterioles.

Using the aminopyrine clearance technique in the

dog, Konturek et al. (97) found that both vasoactive intestinal peptide (VIP) and secretin decreased pentagastrin-stimulated acid secretion. This was accompanied by a fall in gastric mucosal blood flow. In another study (96), these investigators found that norleucine motilin decreased pentagastrin-stimulated acid secretion and mucosal blood flow. The ratio of blood flow to acid secretion remained unchanged, indicating that the fall in blood flow with all three hormones was secondary to the inhibition of acid secretion.

Vasopressin decreased gastric blood flow in the baboon (electromagnetic blood flow measurement) (187), the dog (aminopyrine clearance) (82), and the cat (radiolabeled microspheres) (157). Also, angiographic studies in humans (7) revealed marked constriction of the gastric arteries in response to the close intraarterial infusion of vasopressin. In the studies in baboons and humans, evidence for escape from vasopressin vasoconstriction was sought, but none was found.

Glucagon decreased pentagastrin- and histamine-stimulated acid secretion and mucosal blood flow in the dog (105). The ratio of blood flow to acid secretion remained unchanged.

In dogs with gastric fistulas and Heidenhain pouches, somatostatin inhibited acid and pepsin responses to pentagastrin, urecholine, and a peptone meal (99). The inhibition of pentagastrin-induced gastric secretion was associated with a marked reduction in mucosal blood flow. The ratio of aminopyrine concentration in gastric juice and blood plasma was not significantly changed, indicating that the reduction in mucosal blood flow was secondary to an inhibition of gastric secretion. A similar inhibition of gastric secretion and blood flow was obtained in cats with chronically implanted gastric fistulas (1).

The immediate effect of close intra-arterial infusion of hormones on cat gastric submucosal arterioles was studied by Guth and Smith (65) using *in vivo* microscopic technique. Glucagon had no effect. Natural but not synthetic secretin caused dilatation, suggesting the presence of a contaminating vasoactive agent in the former (both secretin preparations studied were potent stimulants of canine pancreatic secretion). The octapeptide of cholecystokinin, in a dose that could be considered physiologic (3% of the intravenous D_{50} for pancreatic secretion), caused vasodilatation.

Prostaglandins

Prostaglandins (PGs) are primarily local hormones (5). They produce their effects close to their site of release and usually are metabolized before they reach the arterial circulation (174). PGs synthesized intramurally in blood vessels can act directly to modify vascular smooth muscle tension (53). They also act indirectly, either by altering vessel responsiveness to other vasoactive substances (74,181) or by changing amounts of adrenergic neurotransmitter released from sympathetic nerve endings (73).

PGs are products of arachidonic acid metabolism (122), (Fig. 5). Arachidonic acid is released from cell membranes by the action of the enzyme phospholipase A_2. A cyclo-oxygenase then generates cyclic endoperoxides, PGG_2 and PGH_2, from this precursor. The endoperoxides are enzymatically (PG synthetase) converted to a variety of products: by an isomerase and by a reductase to PGE_2, PGD_2, and $PGF_{2\alpha}$; by thromboxane synthetase to thromboxane $A_2(TxA_2)$, which contracts blood vessels and aggregates platelets; or by 6,9-oxycyclase into prostacyclin (PGI_2), which relaxes most blood vessels and inhibits platelet aggregation. Whereas TxA_2 is the major metabolite of arachidonic acid in platelets, PGI_2 is the major metabolite in vessel walls. PGI_2 formation, followed by spontaneous breakdown to 6-oxo-$PGF_{1\alpha}$, is also the major route of endoperoxide metabolism in the rat stomach. Drugs, such as aspirin, and indomethacin inhibit the cyclooxygenase enzyme and thus inhibit the production of endoperoxides and all their derivatives.

It has been demonstrated that PGI_2 is not only formed by vascular tissue (120) but is avidly generated by the gastric mucosa of all species tested (121): rat, rabbit, cat, dog, guinea pig, and mouse. PG-metabolizing enzymes have been demonstrated in human biopsy specimens of the esophagus, gastric fundus, gastric corpus, gastric antrum, and duodenum (134). Using an immunohistofluorescence procedure, PG-forming cyclooxygenase was demonstrated in the lamina propria of the mucosa and in blood vessels of the submucosa, muscularis externa, and serosa of the porcine stomach (15).

Using a ^{14}C-aniline clearance technique to measure gastric mucosal blood flow in the rat, Main and Whittle (108) observed that indomethacin, in doses sufficient to inhibit PG formation, significantly reduced resting gastric mucosal blood flow. Similarly, Kauffman et al. (86) found that indomethacin decreased basal gastric mucosal blood flow in the conscious dog. In *in vivo* microscopic studies in the rat, indomethacin decreased the diameter of gastric submucosal arterioles, the vessels controlling blood flow to the mucosa (58). These findings indicate that endogenous PGs may determine, in part, basal gastric mucosal blood flow.

In the rat, PGI_2 increased resting mucosal blood flow (^{14}C-aniline clearance technique); and, during PGI_2 inhibition of pentagastrin-induced acid secretion, the ratio of mucosal blood flow to acid output increased (183). The breakdown product of PGI_2, 6-oxo-$PGF_{1\alpha}$, had no significant effect on gastric acid secretion or mucosal blood flow. Previously, Main and Whittle (107) demonstrated that PGs of the E and A series, which inhibit gastric acid secretion, also have a direct vasodilator action on the rat gastric mucosa. In *in vivo* microscopic studies, Guth and Moler (58) observed that superfusion of the exposed submucosal vascular bed with PGE_2 resulted in a dose-related dilatation of the submucosal arterioles. In the dog, Konturek et al. (98) reported that PGI_2 but not PGE_2 increased resting gastric mucosal blood flow. With inhibition of pentagastrin-induced gastric acid secretion, both PGI_2 and PGE_2 decreased mucosal blood flow, probably as a consequence of the inhibition of the secretory process (R remained constant). In the totally isolated *ex vivo* canine stomach, Kowalewski and Kolodej (101) found that PGE_2 had a potent vasodilator action on the gastric circulation; it reduced the gastric peripheral resistance and the gastric arterial perfusion pressure. Cheung and Lowry (30) studied the effect of the intraarterial infusion of PGE_1 on gastric total and mucosal blood flow (as measured by venous outflow and radiolabeled microspheres) and acid secretion in an exteriorized, chambered preparation of canine fundic stomach. PGE_1 completely inhibited histamine-stimulated acid secretion. This was accompanied by a significant increase in both total and mucosal blood flow.

Recently, a stable 5-6-dihydro analog of PGI_2, $6\beta PGI_1$, has been developed. In studies in the dog, Kauffman et al. (87) observed an inhibition of acid

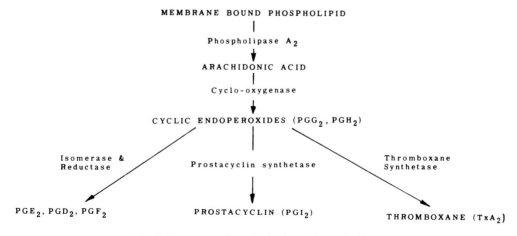

FIG. 5. Pathways of arachidonic acid metabolism.

secretion with both PGI_2 and $6\beta PGI_1$; whereas the ratio of mucosal blood flow to acid secretion during inhibition of secretion remained constant with PGI_2, however, it rose significantly with $6\beta PGI_1$. Furthermore, whereas PGI_2 caused a marked fall in arterial pressure, only a slight decrease occurred with $6\beta PGI_1$.

The demonstration of PG generation by gastric as well as vascular tissue and the potent effect of PGs on gastric acid secretion and blood flow strongly suggest an important role for locally synthesized PGs as modulators of gastric function. In a study in the anesthetized dog, Gerkins et al. (48) obtained data favoring such a hypothesis. Aspirin (100 mg/kg^{-1} i.v.) and indomethacin (8 mg/kg^{-1} i.v.) each decreased (a) resting left gastric artery blood flow (electromagnetic flow probe measurement), (b) sodium arachidonate-stimulated increased blood flow, and (c) the increase in flow associated with pentagastrin-stimulated acid secretion. Study of the distribution of blood flow using radiolabeled microspheres revealed that 90% of flow was to the mucosa-submucosal layer. Both the increase in flow accompanying pentagastrin infusion and the decrease in flow with indomethacin were entirely due to reduction in mucosal flow, the muscle layer flow remaining unaltered. Both aspirin and indomethacin potentiated pentagastrin-stimulated acid output while decreasing gastric blood flow. These data suggest that pentagastrin increases the output of vasodilatory and acid-inhibiting PGs.

Effect of Pulse Pressure

With the increasing use of cardiopulmonary bypass, the importance of an arterial pulse pressure in the regulation of organ blood flow and cardiac output distribution has come under investigation. Results have been contradictory. An increase in peripheral vascular resistance with nonpulsatile cardiopulmonary bypass has been demonstrated by some investigators (42) and a decrease by others (23). Shoor et al. (155) studied the effect of nonpulsatile arterial perfusion on gastric blood flow and intraorgan flow distribution in anesthetized dogs using radiolabeled microspheres. Total gastric blood flow, as well as the partitioning of that flow between antrum and corpus and mucosa and muscle layers, was not significantly altered by nonpulsatile arterial perfusion.

Effect of Gastric Motility

Chou and Grassmick (32) investigated the effect of increasing motility and intraluminal pressure on blood flow distribution within the wall of the dog stomach using radiolabeled microspheres. The infusion of physostigmine markedly elevated small intestine lumen pressure with only a few small fluctuations, indicating that the motility response was a tonic contraction. Total flow to the gastric body decreased, solely because of a significant decrease in blood flow to the mucosa-submucosa; the muscularis-serosa escaped the mechanical compression of increased wall tension. This is probably attributable to an active (exercise) hyperemia in the muscularis, as has been shown for skeletal muscle (11).

ROLE OF GASTRIC BLOOD FLOW IN GASTRIC PHYSIOLOGY

Acid Secretion

The relationship of secretion to blood flow was studied by Jacobson et al. (82) using the aminopyrine clearance technique in anesthetized dogs. During both histamine- and gastrin-stimulated acid secretion, aminopyrine clearance rose; R fell from high values (70 to 100) at low secretory rates to a steady plateau value of 30 to 40 at maximal secretory rates. Vasopressin infusion during background stimulation with histamine inhibited acid secretion and was associated with a parallel decline in clearance. Infusion of isoproterenol at a low dose (1.2 mg/hr^{-1}) did not affect histamine-stimulated secretion but markedly increased aminopyrine clearance.

These findings indicate that when the stomach is stimulated to secrete, mucosal blood flow increases. If blood flow to the stomach is reduced sufficiently, secretion decreases. However, the converse is not true. Increasing blood flow, as by low dose isoproterenol, does not increase secretion. Thus mucosal blood flow plays a supportive and permissive role in gastric secretion.

These results were confirmed by Harper et al. (69), who measured both total (venous effluent collection) and mucosal (aminopyrine clearance) blood flow in the anesthetized cat. With increase in acid secretion in response to either gastrin or histamine, there was a parallel increase in total and mucosal blood flow. The increase in total flow was a direct reflection of the increased mucosal flow. Similar increases in gastric mucosal blood flow with increases in acid secretion have been observed in the rat (109) and human (57,89). In studies in the conscious dog, Jacobson et al. (81) demonstrated that vagal (insulin or 2-deoxy-D-glucose) as well as histamine- and gastrin-stimulated acid secretion was accompanied by an increase in mucosal blood flow. In contrast to the findings of Harper et al. (69), however, there was no significant change in total blood flow. Under the conditions of their study, a redistribution of the circulation from nonmucosal tissues to the mucosa apparently accompanied the increased secretion. Gerkins et al. (48) provided evidence that the increase in gastric blood flow accompanying pentagastrin-stimulated acid secretion is related to the release of vasodilatory PGs. In their study, the increase in total blood flow was entirely due to an increase in mucosal blood. Some of the reported discrepancies in blood flow could be related to whether the studies were performed on conscious or anesthetized animals.

Mucosal Integrity

Prevention of Mucosal Injury

In recent years, experimental evidence has accumulated that mucosal blood flow plays an important role in the prevention of injury to the gastric mucosa. Two lines of evidence have been developed in support of this concept.

First, decreased mucosal blood flow is needed for gastric mucosal injury. Mersereau and Hinchey (117) observed that while 150 mmoles HCl caused no gastric damage in the normotensive rat, the gastric mucosa in the hypotensive rat was ischemic, and as little as 50 mmoles HCl produced erosions. In both the dog (144) and rat (182), bile salt-induced gastric lesions were significantly increased by reduction of gastric mucosal blood flow with either vasopressin or indomethacin. Cheung and Chang (28) observed that the topical barrier breaker *p*-chloromercuribenzene sulfonate did not cause gross damage unless mucosal ischemia, produced by hemorrhagic shock, was present. There appeared to be a critical relationship between the level of mucosal perfusion and the rate of H^+ back-diffusion; lesion formation occurred only when there was a marked reduction in the ratio of mucosal blood flow to H^+ loss.

Second, increased mucosal blood flow protects against gastric mucosal injury. Increasing gastric mucosal blood flow by the intraarterial infusion of isoproterenol significantly decreased gastric damage produced by either topical bile salts plus shock (145) or topical aspirin (113). Whittle (182) observed that the administration of a PG analog increased mucosal blood flow and protected rats against lesions produced by bile salts + acid + indomethacin. This suggests that one means by which PG may exert its cytoprotective effect is by increasing gastric mucosal blood flow.

Menguy and Masters (115) demonstrated that the gastric mucosa is extremely sensitive to a deficit in energy metabolism. In rats subjected to hemorrhagic shock, a greater decrease in energy substrates developed in the gastric mucosa than in other organs. This energy deficit could result in cell death with formation of mucosal lesions. These findings suggest that mucosal blood flow, by maintaining adequate tissue oxygenation, plays an important role in preventing mucosal injury.

On the other hand, using an intramucosal pH probe, Kivilaakso et al. (88) demonstrated a profound drop in intramucosal pH following hemorrhagic shock in the rabbit. The authors suggested that the critical determinant of ulceration during shock is not tissue anoxia but an impaired capacity of the mucosa to remove or buffer the influx of acid. Similarly, Moody et al. (124) postulated that increasing blood flow protects against mucosal damage by topical barrier breakers by disposing of H^+ ions "by buffer, dilution, or other processes that allow the surface cells to withstand increased penetration by H^+ ion."

Effect of Disruption of the Gastric Mucosal Barrier to Acid Back-Diffusion

Augur (8) observed that gastric mucosal blood flow (aminopyrine clearance) increased when the gastric mucosa of the canine Heidenhain pouch was damaged by aspirin or ethanol. In contrast, O'Brien and Silen (130) found that both aspirin and sodium taurocholate caused a reduction in aminopyrine clearance. Ritchie (144), using the aminopyrine clearance technique in the dog, and Whittle (182), using the ^{14}C-aniline clearance technique in the rat, observed an increase in mucosal blood flow in response to the topical application of sodium taurocholate. Since the validity of aminopyrine clearance as a measure of mucosal blood flow when flow is low has been questioned (3), Cheung et al. (31) restudied this question using both aminopyrine clearance and radiolabeled microspheres to measure mucosal flow and venous outflow to measure total flow in a canine gastric chamber preparation. Aspirin, sodium taurocholate, and ethanol caused a significant increase in both total venous flow and microsphere-measured mucosal blood flow. Aminopyrine clearance increased to a much smaller extent with aspirin and taurocholate injury but did not increase with ethanol injury. These results suggest that aminopyrine clearance is unreliable in quantitating mucosal blood flow changes in the presence of mucosal injury. The authors also noted that aspirin-induced erosions occur at discrete sites and are usually preceded by focal pallor, suggesting focal ischemia. They postulate that the increase in overall gastric mucosal blood flow may be a secondary defensive response to damage.

Bruggeman et al. (24) studied this problem using a perfused isolated segment of dog stomach. Bathing the mucosal surface with salicylic acid in 160 m_N HCl resulted in a prompt fall in vascular resistance (increase in flow). Salicylic acid alone had no effect, but subsequent replacement of the bathing solution with 160 m_N HCl caused an immediate fall in resistance. Back-diffusion of acid, therefore, was the proximate cause of vasodilatation. Pretreatment with pyrilamine plus cimetidine (an H_1 and an H_2 receptor antagonist, respectively) largely blocked the fall in resistance, suggesting that mucosal histamine liberated during acid back-diffusion mediated the vasodilatation. Since the block was not complete, back-diffusing acid acting directly on resistance vessels might also play a role.

Eating

Bond et al. (22) employed a radiolabeled microsphere technique to study the effect of feeding on blood flow to the different tissue layers of the stomach of conscious dogs. Flow measurements were obtained 45 min after ingestion of a high-protein meal, at which time the bulk of the meal was in the stomach and jejunum. Following feeding, blood flow to the whole stomach wall increased significantly. This increase was entirely due to increased flow to the mucosa. The submucosa-muscularis flow remaining unchanged. Taylor et al. (169) determined the effect of fasting on gastric mucosal blood flow using the ^{86}RbCl indicator-dilution technique in the rat. Food in the stomach markedly increased antral as well as corpus blood flow. With progressive starvation, the antral:corpus flow ratio decreased.

Changes in Gastric Blood Flow With Age

Varga and Csaky (175) studied changes in blood supply to various parts of the rat gastrointestinal tract with age using the ^{86}Rb indicator-dilution technique. Cardiac output, in relative values, ml/min^{-1}kg^{-1}, decreased with age. The total weight of the alimentary tract as a percent of body weight declined with age from 6.6% in 25- to 28-day-old rats to 1.9% in 240-day-old-rats. The proportional weight of the various parts of the gastrointestinal tract was the same in all age groups, with the exception of the cecum, which increased. Blood flow to the glandular stomach rose from 0.228 ml/min^{-1}g^{-1} in 25- to 28-day-old rats to 0.424 in 29- to 34-day-old rats and then progressively fell to 0.177 and 0.114 ml/min^{-1}g^{-1} in 45- to 66- and 240-day-old rats.

Effect of Local and Systemic Hypothermia

Iced water or iced saline gastric lavage is widely used to arrest bleeding from acute erosive gastritis. Controlled clinical studies to evaluate the effectiveness of this procedure have not been performed. Several animal experimental studies have been performed, and the results are conflicting. In the normal canine stomach, gastric iced water lavage but not lavage with water at body temperature reduced gastric blood flow by approximately 65%, as measured by venous outflow technique (147,178) or the electromagnetic flow meter technique (179). In contrast, in cats in which acute gastritis had been induced by the gastric instillation of 10% acetic acid, neither iced water nor warm water gastric lavage significantly affected blood flow to the mucosa or muscle layer, as measured by the radiolabeled microsphere technique (161). The latter study suggests the possibility that local hypothermia may not affect the gastric circulation in stomachs with acute gastritis.

Total body hypothermia has also been used to control massive upper gastrointestinal hemorrhage in humans (51). The effect of lowering body temperature to 31 °C on gastric blood flow was studied in normal dogs using the radiorubidium clearance technique (43). There was a significant reduction (approximately 60%) in blood flow to all layers of the corpus but not to the antrum. In this study, the authors state, without presenting data, that intragastric cooling to 10° to 15 °C produced similar results.

REFERENCES

1. Albinus, M., Blair, E. L., Case, R. M. Coy, D. H., Gomez-Pan, A., Hirst, B. H., Reed, J. D., Schally, A. V., Shaw, B., Smith, P. A., and Smy, J. R. (1977): Comparison of the effect of somatostatin on gastrointestinal function in the conscious and anesthetized cat and on the isolated cat pancreas. *J. Physiol. (Lond.)*, 269:77–91.
2. Arabehety, J. T., Dolcini, H. A., and Gray, S. J. (1959): Sympathetic influences on circulation of the gastric mucosa of the rat. *Am. J. Physiol.*, 197:915–922.
3. Archibald, L. H., Moody, F. G., Simons, M. A. (1975): Comparison of gastric mucosal blood flow as determined by aminopyrine clearance and γ-labeled microspheres. *Gastroenterology*, 69:630–635.
4. Archibald, L. H., Moody, F. G., and Simons, M. (1975): Measurement of gastric blood flow with radioactive microspheres. *J. Appl. Physiol.*, 38:1051–1056.
5. Armstrong, J. M., Dusting, G. J., Moncada, S., and Vane, J. R. (1978): Cardiovascular actions of prostacyclin (PGI$_2$), a metabolite of arachidonic acid which is synthesized by blood vessels. *Circ. Res. [Suppl. 1]*, 43:112–119.
6. Ash, A. S. F., and Schild, H. O. (1966): Receptors mediating some actions of histamine. *Br. J. Pharmaco.*, 27:427–439.
7. Athanasoulis, C. A., Baum, S., Waltman, A. C., Ring, E. J., Imbembo, A., and VanderSalm, T. J. (1974): Control of acute gastric mucosal hemorrhage. Intra-arterial infusion of posterior pituitary extract. *N. Engl. J. Med.*, 290:603–610.
8. Augur, N. A. (1970): Gastric mucosal blood flow following damage by ethanol, acetic acid or aspirin. *Gastroenterology*, 58:311–320.
9. Aures, D., Guth, P. H., and Grossman, M. I. (1975): Use of neutral red to measure gastric mucosal blood flow. *Gastroenterology*, 68:1057.
10. Aures, D., Baumann, H., Guth, P. H., and Grossman, M. I. (1976): A metabolite of neutral red that interferes with its use in measuring gastric mucosal blood flow in man. *Gastroenterology*, 70:965.
11. Barcroft, H. (1963): Circulation in skeletal muscle. In: *Handbook of Physiology: Circulation*, sect. 2, vol. 11, chapt. 40. Am. Physiol. Soc., Washington, D.C.
12. Barlow, T. E. (1952): Vascular patterns in the alimentary canal. In: *Ciba Symposium: Visceral Circulation*, edited by G. E. W. Wolstonholme, pp. 21–35. Churchill, London.
13. Barlow, T. E., Bentley, F. H., and Walder, D. N. (1951): Arteries, veins and arteriovenous anastomoses in the human stomach. *Surg. Gynecol. Obstet.*, 93:657–671.
14. Beaumont, W. (1833): *Experiments and Observations on the Gastric Juice and the Physiology of Digestion*. Dover Publications, New York.
15. Bebiak, D. M., Miller, E. R., Huslig, R. L., and Smith, W. L. (1979): Distribution of prostaglandin-forming cyclooxygenase in the porcine stomach. *Fed. Proc.*, 38:884.
16. Bell, P. R. F. (1967): Gastric arterio-venous shunts. An investigation using a dye dilution technique. *Scand. J. Gastroenterol.*, 2:59–67.
17. Bell, P. R. F., and Battersby, C., (1968): Effect of vagotomy on gastric mucosal blood flow. *Gastroenterology*, 54:1032–1037.
18. Bell, P. R. F., and Shelley, T. (1968): Gastric mucosal blood

flow and acid secretion in conscious animals measured by heat clearance. *Am. J. Dig. Dis.*, 13:685–696.

19. Bickel, J. G., Witten, T. A., and Killian, M. D. (1972): Use of pertechnate clearance in the study of gastric physiology. *Gastroenterology*, 63:60–66.

20. Black, J. W., Duncan, W. A. M., Durant, C. J., Ganellin, C. R., and Parsons, M. E. (1972): Definition and antagonism of histamine H_2-receptors. *Nature*, 236:385–390.

21. Blair, E. L., Grund, E. R., Reed, J. D., Sanders, D. J., Sanger, G., and Shaw, B. (1975): The effect of sympathetic nerve stimulation on serum gastrin, gastric acid secretion and mucosal blood flow responses to meat extract stimulation in anesthetized cats. *J. Physiol.*, 253:493–504.

22. Bond, J. H., Prentiss, R. A., and Levitt, M. D. (1979): The effects of feeding on blood flow to the stomach, small bowel, and colon of the conscious dog. *J. Lab. Clin. Med.*, 93:594–599.

23. Boucher, J. K., Rudy, L. W., and Edmunds, H. (1974): Organ blood flow during pulsatile cardiopulmonary bypass. *J. Appl. Physiol.*, 36:86–90.

24. Bruggeman, T. M., Wood, J. G., and Davenport, H. W. (1979): Local control of blood flow in the dog's stomach: vasodilatation caused by acid back-diffusion following topical application of salicylic acid. *Gastroenterology*, 77:736–744.

25. Buchin, R. F., and Edlich, R. F. (1969): Quantitation of gastric arteriovenous blood flow by the microsphere clearance technique. *Arch. Surg.*, 99:579–581.

26. Bulkley, G., Goldman, H., Trencis, L., and Silen, W., (1970): Gastric microcirculatory changes in hemorrhagic shock. *Surg. Forum*, 21:27–30.

27. Chahal, P., Holton, P., and King, J. A. (1976): Comparison of neutral red and other markers used for the estimation of gastric mucosal blood flow. *J. Physiol.*, 256:29P.

28. Cheung, L. Y., and Chang, N. (1977): The role of gastric mucosal blood flow and H^+ back-diffusion in the pathogenesis of acute gastric erosions. *J. Surg. Res.*, 22:357–361.

29. Cheung, L. Y., Chang, F., and Moody, F. G. (1976): Canine gastric blood flow and its distribution during hemmorhagic shock. *Clin. Res.*, 24:104A.

30. Cheung, L. Y., and Lowry, S. F. (1978): Effects of intra-arterial infusion of prostaglandin E_1 on gastric secretion and blood flow. *Surgery*, 83:699–704.

31. Cheung, L. Y., Moody, F. G., and Reese, R. S. (1975): Effect of aspirin, bile salt, and ethanol on canine gastric mucosal blood flow. *Surgery*, 77:786–792.

32. Chou, C. C., and Grassmick, B., (1978): Motility and blood flow distribution within the wall of the gastrointestinal tract. *Am. J. Physiol.*, 235:H34–H39.

33. Cowley, D. J., and Code, C. F., (1970): Effects of secretory inhibitors on mucosal blood flow in the nonsecreting stomach of conscious dogs. *Am. J. Physiol.*, 218:270–274.

34. Cowley, D. J., Code, C. F., and Fiasse, R., (1969): Gastric mucosal blood flow during secretory inhibition by gastrin pentapeptide and gastrone. *Gastroenterology*, 56:659–665.

35. Cumming, J. D., Haigh, A. L., Harries, E. H. L., and Nutt, M. E. (1963): A study of gastric secretion and blood flow in the anesthetized dog. *J. Physiol.*, 168:219–233.

36. Curwain, B. P., and Holton, P. (1973): The measurement of dog gastric mucosal blood flow by radioactive aniline clearance compared with aminopyrine clearance. *J. Physiol.*, 229:115–131.

37. Delaney, J. P. (1967): Chronic alterations in gastrointestinal blood flow induced by vagotomy. *Surgery*, 62:155–158.

38. Delaney, J. P., and Grim, E. (1964): Canine gastric blood flow and its distribution. *Am. J. Physiol.*, 207:1195–1202.

39. Delaney, J. P., and Grim, E. (1965): Experimentally induced variations in canine gastric blood flow and its distribution. *Am. J. Physiol.*, 208:353–358.

40. Delaney, J. P., Michel, H. M., and Bond, J. (1978): Cimetidine and gastric blood flow. *Surgery*, 84:190–193.

41. Doran, F. S. A. (1951): Aetiology of chronic gastric ulcer. Observations on the blood supply of the human gastric mucosa with a note on the arteriovenous shunt. *Lancet*, 1:199–202.

42. Dunn, J., Kirsh, M., Harness, J., Carroll, M., Straker, J., and Sloan, H. (1974): Hemodynamic, metabolic, and hematologic effects of pulsatile cardiopulmonary bypass. *J. Thorac. Cardiovasc. Surg.*, 68:138–147.

43. Edlich, R. F., Borner, J. W., and Wangensteen, O. H. (1970): Gastric blood flow: Its distribution during systemic hypothermia. *Am. J. Surg.*, 120:38–40.

44. Fara, J. W., and Ross, G. (1972): Escape from drug-induced constriction of isolated arterial segments from various vascular beds. *Angiologica*, 9:27–33.

45. Feldman, S., Birnbaum, D., and Behar, A. J. (1961): Gastric secretion and acute gastroduodenal lesions following hypothalamic and preoptic stimulation. *J. Neurosurg.*, 18:661–670.

46. Folkow, B., Lewis, D. H., Lundgren, O., Mellander, S., and Wallentin, I. G., (1964): The effect of graded vasoconstrictor fiber stimulation on the intestinal resistance and capacitance vessels. *Acta Physiol. Scand.*, 61:445–457.

47. Furness, J. B. (1971): The adrenergic innervation of the vessels supplying and draining the gastrointestinal tract. *Z. Zellforsch.*, 113:67–82.

48. Gerkins, J. F., Shand, D. G., Flexner, C., Nies, A. S., Oates, J. A., and Data, J. L. (1977): Effect of indomethacin and aspirin on gastric blood flow and acid secretion. *J. Pharmacol. Exp. Ther.*, 203:646–652.

49. Gibbs, F. A. (1933): A thermoelectric blood flow recorder in the form of a needle. *Proc. Soc. Exp. Biol. Med.*, 31:141–146.

50. Goodhead, B. (1969): Blood flow in different areas of the gastrointestinal tract in the anesthetized dog. *Can. J. Physiol. Pharmacol.*, 47:787–790.

51. Gowen, G. F., and Lindemuth, W. W. (1961): General hypothermia for managing gastrointestinal hemmorhage. A report of 3 cases in which total body hypothermia was used to control massive gastrointestinal hemmorrhage. *JAMA*, 175:29.

52. Grayson, J. (1952): Internal calorimetry in the measurement of blood flow. *J. Physiol.*, 118:54–72.

53. Greenberg, R. A., and Sparks, H. V. (1969): Prostaglandins and consecutive vascular segments of the canine hind limb. *Am. J. Physiol.*, 216:567–571.

54. Greenway, C. V., and Murthy, V. S. (1972): Effects of vasopressin and isoprenaline infusions on the distribution of blood flow in the intestine: Criteria for the validity of microsphere studies. *Br. J. Pharmacol.*, 46:177–188.

55. Guth, P. H. (1972): Gastric blood flow in restraint stress. *Am. J. Dig. Dis.*, 17:807–813.

56. Guth, P. H. (1977): The gastric microcirculation and gastric mucosal blood flow under normal and pathological conditions. In: *Progress in Gastroenterology, Vol. III*, edited by G. B. J. Glass, pp. 323–347.

57. Guth, P. H., Baumann, H., Grossman, M. I., Aures, D., and Elashoff, J. (1978): Measurement of gastric mucosal blood flow in man. *Gastroenterology*, 74:831–834.

58. Guth, P. H., and Moler, T. L. (1979): Endogenous prostaglandins in the regulation of the rat gastric microcirculation. *Microvasc. Res.*, 17:S15.

59. Guth, P. H., and Moler, T. L. (1979): In vivo fluorescence microscopy of the gastric microcirculation. *Gastroenterology*, 76:1147.

60. Guth, P. H., and Rosenberg, A. (1972): In vivo microscopy of the gastric microcirculation. *Am. J. Dig. Dis.*, 17:391–398.

61. Guth, P. H., Ross, G., and Smith, E. (1976): Changes in intestinal vascular diameter during norepinephrine vasoconstrictor escape. *Am. J. Physiol.*, 230:1466–1468.

62. Guth, P. H., and Smith, E. (1974): Vasoactive agents and the gastric microcirculation. *Microvasc. Res.*, 8:125–131.

63. Guth, P. H., and Smith, E. (1975): Neural control of gastric mucosal blood flow in the rat. *Gastroenterology*, 69:935–940.

64. Guth, P. H., and Smith, E. (1975): Escape from vasoconstriction in the gastric microcirculation. *Am. J. Physiol.*, 223:1893–1895.

65. Guth, P. H., and Smith, E. (1976): The effect of gastrointestinal hormones on the gastric microcirculation. *Gastroenterology*, 71:435–438.

66. Guth, P. H., and Smith, E. (1977): Nervous regulation of the gastric microcirculation. In: *Nerves and the Gut*, edited by F. P. Brooks and P. W. Evers, pp. 365–373. Charles B. Slack, New York.

67. Guth, P. H., and Smith, E. (1978): Histamine receptors in the gastric microcirculation. *Gut*, 19:1059–1063.

68. Guth, P. H., Smith, E., and Moler. T. (1981): H_1 and H_2 receptors in rat gastric submucosal arterioles. *Microvasc. Res. (in press)*.

69. Harper, A. A., Reed, J. D., and Smy, J. R. (1968): Gastric blood flow in anesthetized cats. *J. Physiol.*, 194:795-807.

70. Harris, D. W., Smy, J. R., Reed, J. D., and Venables, C. W. (1975): The effects of burimamide and metiamide on basal gastric function in the cat. *Br. J. Pharmacol.*, 53:293-297.

71. Harvey, W. (1628): *Movement of the Heart and Blood in Animals. An Anatomical Essay*, translated by K. J. Franklin (1957). Blackwell, Oxford.

72. Hase, T., and Moss, B. J. (1973): Microvascular changes in the development of stress ulcer in rats. *Gastroenterology*, 65:224-234.

73. Hedquist, P. (1973): Autonomic neurotransmission. In: *The Prostaglandins*, edited by P. W. Ramwell, pp. 101-131. Plenum Press, New York.

74. Holmes, S. W., Horton, E. W., and Main, I. H. M. (1963): The effect of prostaglandin E_1 on responses of smooth muscle to catecholamines, angiotensin and vasopressin. *Br. J. Pharmacol.*, 21:538-543.

75. Hunter, G. C., Goldstone, J., Villa, R., and Way, L. W. (1979): Effect of vagotomy upon intragastric redistribution of microvascular flow. *J. Surg. Res.*, 26:314-319.

76. Jacobowitz, D. (1965): Histochemical studies of the autonomic innervation of the gut. *J. Pharmacol. Exp. Ther.*, 149:358-364.

77. Jacobson, E. D. (1963): Effects of histamine, acetylcholine and norepinephrine on gastric vascular resistance. *Am. J. Physiol.*, 204:1013-1017.

78. Jacobson, E. D. (1968): Clearance of the gastric mucosa. *Gastroenterology*, 54:434-448.

79. Jacobson, E. D. (1970): Comparison of prostaglandin E_1 and norepinephrine on the gastric mucosal circulation. *Proc. Soc. Exp. Biol. Med.*, 113:516-519.

80. Jacobson, E. D., and Chang, A. C. K. (1969): Comparison of gastrin and histamine on gastric mucosal blood flow. *Proc. Soc. Exp. Biol. Med.*, 130:484-486.

81. Jacobson, E. D., Eisenberg, M. M., and Swan, K. G. (1966): Effects of histamine on gastric blood flow in conscious dogs. *Gastroenterology*, 51:466-472.

82. Jacobson, E. D., Linford, R. H., and Grossman, M. I. (1966): Gastric secretion in relation to mucosal blood flow studied by a clearance technique. *J. Clin. Invest.*, 45:1-13.

83. Jansson, G. (1969): Extrinsic nervous control of gastric motility. *Acta Physiol. Scand. [Suppl. 326]*, 76:1-42.

84. Jansson, G., Kampp, M., Lundgren, O., and Martinson, J. (1966): Studies on the circulation of the stomach, *Acta Physiol. Scand. [Suppl. 277]*, 68:91.

85. Jansson, G., Lundgren, O., and Martinson, J. (1970): Neurohormonal control of gastric blood flow. *Gastroenterology*, 58:425-429.

86. Kauffman, G. L., Jr., Aures, D., and Grossman, M. I. (1979): Indomethacin decreases basal gastric mucosal blood flow. *Gastroenterology*, 76:1165.

87. Kauffman, G. L., Jr., Whittle, B. J. R., Aures, D., Vane, J. R., and Grossman, M. I. (1979): Effects of prostacyclin and a stable analogue, 6_β-PGI_1, on gastric acid secretion, mucosal blood flow, and blood pressure in conscious dogs. *Gastroenterology*, 77:1301-1306.

88. Kivilaakso, E., Fromm, D., and Silen, W. (1978): Relationship between ulceration and intramural pH of gastric mucosa during hemorrhagic shock. *Surgery*, 84:70-78.

89. Knight, S. E., and McIsaac, R. L. (1977): Neutral red clearance as an estimate of gastric mucosal blood flow in man. *J. Physiol.*, 272:62-63P.

90. Knight, S. E., McIsaac, R. L., and Fielding, L. P. (1977): The effect of the histamine-H_2-antagonist cimetidine on gastric mucosal blood flow. *Gut*, 18:A948.

91. Knight, S. E., McIsaac, R. L., and Fielding, L. P. (1977): Comparison of gastric mucosal blood flow (GMBF) in normal subjects and patients with duodenal ulcer. *Br. J. Surg.*, 64:864.

92. Knight, S. E., McIsaac, R. L., and Fielding, L. P. (1978): The effect of highly selective vagotomy on the relationship between gastric mucosal blood flow and acid secretion in man. *Br. J. Surg.*, 65:721-723.

93. Koch, H., and Demling, L. (1976): The value of the thermocouple in the measurement of the gastric mucosal blood flow. *Res. Exp. Med. (Berl.)*, 167:71-84.

94. Koch, H., Domschke, S., Behohlavek, D., Domschke, D., Wunsch, E., Jaeger, E., and Demling, L. (1976): Gastric mucosal blood flow and pepsin secretion in dogs-stimulation by 13-nle-motilin. *Scand. J. Gastroenterol.*, 11:93-96.

95. Kolin, A. (1960): Blood flow determination by electromagnetic method. *Med. Phys.*, 3:141-155.

96. Konturek, S. J., Dembinski, A., Krol, R., and Wunsch, E. (1977): Effect of 13-Nle-motilin on gastric secretion, serum gastrin level and mucosal blood flow in dogs. *J. Physiol. (Lond.)*, 264:665-672.

97. Konturek, S. J., Dembinski, A., Thor, P., and Krol, R. (1976): Comparison of vasoactive intestinal peptide (VIP) and secretin in gastric secretion and mucosal blood flow. *Pfluegers Arch.*, 361:175-181.

98. Konturek, S. J., Lancaster, C. Hanchar, A. J., Nezamis, J. E., and Robert, A. (1979): The influence of prostacyclin on gastric mucosal blood flow in resting and stimulated canine stomach. *Gastroenterology*, 76:1173.

99. Konturek, S. J., Tasler, J., Cieskowski, M., Coy, D. H., and Schally, A. V. (1976): Effect of growth hormone release-inhibiting hormone on gastric secretion, mucosal blood flow, and serum gastrin. *Gastroenterology*, 70:737-741.

100. Konturek, S. J., Tasler, J., Obtulowicz, W., and Rehfeld, J. F. (1974): Effect of metiamide, a histamine H_2-receptor antagonist, on mucosal blood flow and serum gastrin level. *Gastroenterology*, 66:982-986.

101. Kowalewski, K., and Kolodej, A. (1974): Effect of prostaglandin-E_2 on gastric secretion and on gastric circulation of totally isolated *ex vivo* canine stomach. *Pharmacology*, 11:85-94.

102. Leonard, A. S., Long, D., French, L. A., Peter, E. T., and Wangensteen, O. H. (1964): Pendular pattern in gastric secretion and blood flow following hypothalamic stimulation—origin of stress ucler? *Surgery*, 56:109-120.

103. Levine, B. A., Schwesinger, W. H., Sirinek, K. R., Jones, D., and Pruitt, B. A. (1978): Cimetidine prevents reduction in gastric mucosal blood flow during shock. *Surgery*, 84:113-119.

104. Levitt, M. D., and Levitt, D. G. (1973): Use of inert gases to study the interaction of blood flow and diffusion during passive absorption from the gastrointestinal tract of the rat. *J. Clin. Invest.*, 52:1852-1862.

105. Lin, T. M., and Warrick, M. W. (1971): Effect of glucagon on pentagastrin-induced gastric acid secretion and mucosal blood flow in the dog. *Gastroenterology*, 61:328-331.

106. Main, I. H. M., and Whittle, B. J. R. (1973): Gastric mucosal blood flow during pentagastrin- and histamine-stimulated acid secretion in the rat. *Br. J. Pharmacol.*, 49:534-542.

107. Main, I. H. M., and Whittle, B. J. R. (1973): The effects of E and A prostaglandins on gastric mucosal blood flow and acid secretion in the rat. *Br. J. Pharmacol.*, 49:428-436.

108. Main, I. H. M., and Whittle, B. J. R. (1975): Investigation of the vasodilator and antisecretory role of prostaglandins in the rat gastric mucosa by use of non-steroidal anti-inflammatory drugs. *Br. J. Pharmacol.*, 53:217-224.

109. Main, I. H. M., and Whittle, B. J. R. (1976): A study of the vascular and acid-secretory responses of the rat gastric mucosa to histamine. *J. Physiol.*, 257:407-418.

110. Martinson, J. (1965): The effect of graded vagal stimulation on gastric motility, secretion and blood flow in the cat. *Acta Physiol. Scand.*, 65:300-309.

111. Martinson, J. (1965): Studies on the efferent vagal control of the stomach. *Acta Physiol. Scand. [Suppl. 255]*, 65:1-24.

112. McGrath, M. A., and Shepherd, J. T. (1976): Inhibition of adrenergic neurotransmission in canine vascular smooth muscle by histamine. *Circ. Res.*, 39:566-573.

113. McGreavy, J. M., and Moody, F. G. (1977): Protection of gastric mucosa against aspirin-induced erosions by enhanced blood flow. *Surg. Forum*, 28:357-359.

114. Menguy, R. (1962): Effects of histamine on gastric blood flow. *Am. J. Dig. Dis.*, 7:383-393.

115. Menguy, R., and Masters, Y. F. (1974): Gastric mucosal energy metabolism and "stress ulceration." *Ann. Surg.*, 180:538-548.

116. Meredith, J. H., and Khan, J. (1967): Gastric blood flow measurement by technetium clearance technic. *Am. J. Surg.*, 33:969–972.

117. Mersereau, W. A., and Hinchey, E. J. (1973): Effect of gastric acidity on gastric ulceration induced by hemorrhage in the rat, utilizing a gastric chamber technique. *Gastroenterology*, 64:1130–1135.

118. Michels, N. A. (1955): *Blood Supply and Anatomy of the Upper Abdominal Organs.* J. B. Lippincott, Philadelphia.

119. Molina, J. E., Edlich, R. F., Borgen, L., Borner, J., and Wangensteen, O. H. (1972): Study of the gastric microcirculatory changes during vagal nerve stimulation. *Surg. Gynecol., Obstet.*, 135:422–428.

120. Moncada, S., Gryglewski, R., Bunting, S., and Vane, J. R. (1976): An enzyme isolated from arteries transforms prostaglandin endoperoxides to an unstable substance that inhibits platelet aggregation. *Nature*, 663–665.

121. Moncada, S., Salmon, J. A., Vane, J. R., and Whittle, B. J. R. (1977): Formation of prostacyclin (PGI$_2$) and its product, 6-oxo-PGF$_{1\alpha}$, by the gastric mucosa of several species. *J. Physiol.*, 275: 4–5P.

122. Moncada, S., and Vane, J. R. (1979): The role of prostacyclin in vascular tissue. *Fed. Proc.*, 38:66–71.

123. Moody, F. G. (1967): Gastric blood flow and acid secretion during direct intraarterial histamine administration. *Gastroenterology*, 52:211–224.

124. Moody, F. G., McGreavy, J., Zalewsky, C., Cheung, L. Y., and Simons, M. (1977): The cytoprotective effect of mucosal blood flow in experimental erosive gastritis. *Acta. Physiol. Scand.* [*Special Suppl.*], 35–43.

125. Nakamura, K., Ishi, K., Kusano, M., and Hayashi, S. (1974). Acute and long-term effects of vagotomy on gastric mucosal blood flow. In: *Vagotomy. Latest Advances with Special Reference to Gastric and Duodenal Ulcer*, edited by F. Halle and S. Andersson, pp. 109–111. Springer-Verlag, New York.

126. Nakamura, Y., and Wayland, H. (1975): Macromolecular transport in the cat mesentery. *Microvasc. Res.*, 9:1–21.

127. Nebesar, R. A., Kornblith, P. L., Pollard, J. J., and Michels, N. A. (1969): *Celiac and Superior Mesenteric Arteries. A Correlation of Angiograms and Dissections.* Little, Brown, Boston.

128. Nicoloff, D. M., Peter, E. T., Stone, N. H., and Wangesteen, O. H. (1964): Effects of catecholamines on gastric secretion and blood flow. *Ann. Surg.*, 159:32–36.

129. Nylander, G., and Olerud, S. (1961): The vascular pattern of the gastric mucosa of the rat following vagotomy. *Surg. Gynecol. Obst.*, 112:475–480.

130. O'Brien, P., and Silen, W. (1973): Effects of bile salts and aspirin on the gastric mucosal blood flow. *Gastroenterology*, 64: 246–253.

131. Osumi, Y., Aibara, S., Sakae, K., and Fujiwara, M. (1977): Central noradrenergic inhibition of gastric mucosal blood flow and acid secretion in rats. *Life Sci.*, 20:1407–1416.

132. Owen, D. A. A. (1975): The effects of histamine and some histamine-like agonists on blood pressure in the cat. *Br. J. Pharmacol.*, 55:173–179.

133. Owen, D. A. A., Parsons, M. E., Farrington, H. E., and Blackmore, R. (1979): Reduction by cimetidine of acute gastric hemorrhage caused by reinfusion of blood after exposure to exogenous acid during gastric ischemia in rats. *Gastroenterology*, 77:979–985.

134. Peskar, B. M. (1978): Regional distribution of prostaglandin-metabolizing enzymes in the mucosa of the human upper gastrointestinal tract. *Acta Hepatogastroenterol.*, 25:49–51.

135. Peter, E. T., Nicoloff, D. M., Leonard, A. S., Walder, A. I. and Wangensteen, O. H. (1963): Effect of vagal and sympathetic stimulation and ablation on gastric blood flow. *JAMA*, 183: 1003–1005.

136. Peter, E. T., Nicoloff, D. M., Sosin, H., Walder, A. I., and Wangesteen, O. H. (1962): Relationship between gastric blood flow and secretion. *Fed. Proc.*, 21:264.

137. Piasecki, C. (1974): Blood supply to the human gastroduodenal mucosa with special reference to the ulcer-bearing areas. *J. Anat.*, 118:295–335.

138. Piasecki, C. (1975): Observations on the submucous plexus and

139. mucosal arteries of the dog's stomach and first part of the duodenum. *J. Anat.*, 119:133–148.

139. Porter, R. W., Movius, H. J., and French, J. D. (1953): Hypothalamic influences on hydrochloric acid secretion of the stomach. *Surgery*, 33:875–880.

140. Powell, J. R. (1979): Effects of histamine on vascular sympathetic neuroeffector transmission. *J. Pharmacol. Exp. Ther.*, 208:360–365.

141. Reed, J. D., Sanders, D. J., and Thorpe, V. (1971): The effect of splanchnic nerve stimulation on gastric acid secretion and mucosal blood flow in the anesthetized cat. *J. Physiol.*, 214: 1–13.

142. Rosenberg, A., and Guth, P. H. (1970): A method for the in vivo study of the gastric microcirculation. *Microvasc. Res.*, 2: 111–112.

143. Ross, G. (1971): Escape of mesenteric vessels from adrenergic and nonadrenergic vasoconstriction. *Am. J. Physiol.*, 221: 1217–1222.

144. Ritchie, W. P., Jr. (1975): Acute gastric mucosal damage induced by bile salts, acid, and ischemia. *Gastroenterology*, 68: 699–707.

145. Ritchie, W. P., Jr., and Shearburn, E. W., III (1977): Influence of isoproterenol and choleystyramine on acute gastric mucosal ulcerogenesis. *Gastroenterology*, 73:62–65.

146. Rudick, J., Werther, J. L., Chapman, M. L., Dreiling, D. A., and Janowitz, H. D. (1969): Mucosal blood flow in canine antral and fundic pouches. *Fed. Proc.*, 28:687.

147. Salmon, P. A., Griffin, W. O., and Wangensteen, O. H. (1959): Effect of intragastric temperature changes upon gastric blood flow. *Proc. Soc. Exp. Biol. Med.*, 101:442–444.

148. Sapirstein, L. A. (1967): The indicator fractionation technique for the study of regional blood flow: *Gastroenterology*, 52: 365–371.

149. Schnitzlein, H. N. (1957): Regulation of blood flow through the stomach of the rat. *Anat. Rec.*, 127:735–754.

150. Schwille, P. O., Lang, G., and Hofmann, P. (1977): Rat gastric secretion and mucosal blood flow during restraint stress-effect of a low dose metiamide. *Res. Exp. Med.*, 171:205–210.

151. Seitz, W., Grimm, W., and Badenheim, W. (1979): Histamine stimulated gastric mucosal blood flow after selective proximal vagotomy. *Microvasc. Res.*, 17:S16.

152. Sen, R. N., and Anand, B. K. (1957): Effect of electrical stimulation of the hypothalamus on gastric secretory activity and ulceration. *Indian J. Med. Res.*, 45:507–513.

153. Setchell, B. P., and Linzell, J. L. (1974): Soluble indicator techniques for tissue blood flow measurement using ^{86}RbCl, urea, antipyrine (phenazone) derivatives of ^{3}H-water. *Clin. Exp. Pharmacol. Physiol. [Suppl.]*, 1:15–29.

154. Shoemaker, C. P., Jr., and Powers, S. R., Jr. (1966): The absence of large functional arteriovenous shunts in the stomach of the anesthetized dog. *Surgery*, 60:118–126.

155. Shoor, P. M., Griffith, L. D., Dilley, R. B., and Bernstein, E. F. (1979): Effect of pulseless perfusion on gastrointestinal blood flow and its distribution. *Am. J. Physiol.*, 236:E28–E32.

156. Shore, P. A., Brodie, B. B., and Hogben, C. A. M. (1957): The gastric secretion of drugs: A pH partition hypothesis. *J. Pharmacol. Exp. Ther.*, 119:361–369.

157. Skarstein, A. (1978): Effect of vasopressin on blood flow distribution in the stomach of cats with gastric ulcer. *Scand. J. Gastroenterol.*, 13:783–788.

158. Skarstein, A., Svanes, K., Soreide, O., and Varhaug, J. E. (1977): Effect of pentagastrin on blood flow distribution in the stomach of cats with gastric ulcer. *Scand. J. Gastroenterol.*, 12:71–76.

159. Smith, G. P., and McHugh, P. R. (1967): Gastric secretory response to amygdaloid or hypothalamic stimulation in monkeys. *Am. J. Physiol.*, 213:640–644.

160. Sobin, S. S. (1966): Vascular injection methods. In: *Methods in Medical Research*, edited by C. A. Weiderhielm. pp. 233–238, Yearbook Medical Publishers, Chicago.

161. Soreide, O., Svanes, T., Varhaug, J. E., and Svanes, K. (1978): Acute gastritis in cats. Effect of water lavage and local hypothermia on gastric blood flow. *Digestion*, 18:248–260.

162. Staubesand, J., and Hammersen, F. (1956): Zur Problematik

des Nachweises arterio-venöser Anastomosen im Injektionspräparat. I. Beobachtungen an Menschlichen Nierenbecken. *Z. Anat.*, 119:365-370.

163. Steiner, S. H., and Meuller, G. C. E. (1961): Distribution of blood flow in the digestive tract of the rat. *Circ. Res.*, 9:99-102.

164. Stow, R. W. (1965): Thermal measurement of tissue blood flow. *Trans. N.Y. Acad. Sci.*, 27:748-758.

165. Swan, K. G., and Jacobson, E. D. (1967): Gastric blood flow and secretion in conscious dogs. *Am. J. Physiol.*, 212:891-896.

166. Tague, L. L., and Jacobson, E. D. (1976): Evaluation of ^{14}C-aminopyrine clearance of determination of gastric mucosal blood flow. *Proc. Soc. Exp. Biol. Med.*, 151:707-710.

167. Taylor, T. V., Pullan, B. R., Elder, J. B., and Torrance, B. (1975): Observations of gastric mucosal blood flow using ^{99}Tc^m in rat and man. *Br. J. Surg.*, 62:788-791.

168. Taylor, T. V., Pullan, B. R., Goddard, J., and Torrance, B. (1978): Effect of secretogogues on mucosal blood flow in the antrum and corpus of the stomach. *Gut*, 19:14-18.

169. Taylor, T. V., Pullan, B. R., and Torrance, B. (1976): Effect of fasting on mucosal blood flow in antrum and corpus of the stomach. *Eur. Surg. Res.*, 8:227-235.

170. Taylor, T. V., and Torrance, B. (1975): Is there an antral-body portal system in the stomach? *Gut*, 16:781-784.

171. Tepperman, B. L., Tague, L. I., and Jacobson, E. D. (1978): Inhibition of canine gastric acid secretion by an H$_1$-receptor antagonist to histamine. *Dig. Dis.*, 23:801-808.

172. Thompson, J. E., and Vane, J. R. (1953): Gastric secretion induced by histamine and its relationship to the rate of blood flow. *J. Physiol.*, 121:433-444.

173. Van Hee, R. H., and Vanhoutte, P. M. (1978): Cholinergic inhibition of adrenergic neurotransmission in the canine gastric artery. *Gastroenterology*, 74:1266-1270.

174. Vane, R. (1969): The release and fate of vasoactive hormones in the circulation. *Br. J. Pharmacol.*, 35:209-242.

175. Varga, F., and Csaky, T. Z. (1976): Changes in the blood supply of the gastrointestinal tract in rats with age. *Pfluegers Arch.*, 364:129-133.

176. Varro, V., Dobronte, Z., and Sagi, I. (1978): Interrelation between gastric blood flow and HCl secretion in dogs. *Acta Med. Acad. Sci. Hung.*, 35:1-20.

177. Walder, D. N. (1952): Arteriovenous anastomoses of the human stomach. *Clin. Sci.*, 11:59-71.

178. Wangensteen, O. H., Salmon, P. A., Griffen, W. O., Paterson, J. R. S., and Fattah, F. (1959): Studies of local gastric cooling as related to peptic ulcer. *Ann. Surg.*, 150:346-358.

179. Waterman, N. G., and Walker, J. L. (1974): Effect of a topical adrenergic agent on gastric blood flow. *Am. J. Surg.*, 127:241-243.

180. Wayland, H., Fox, J. R., and Elmore, M. D. (1975): Quantitative fluorescent tracer studies in vivo. *Bibl. Anat.*, 13:61-64.

181. Weiner, R., and Kaley, G. (1969): Influence of prostaglandin E$_1$ on the terminal vascular bed. *Am. J. Physiol.*, 217:563-566.

182. Whittle, B. J. R. (1977): Mechanisms underlying gastric mucosal damage induced by indomethacin and bile salts, and the actions of prostaglandins. *Br. J. Pharmacol.*, 60:455-460.

183. Whittle, B. J. R., Boughton-Smith, N. K., Moncada, S., and Vane, J. R. (1978): Actions of prostacyclin (PGI$_2$) and its product 6-oxo-PGF$_1$ on the rat gastric mucosa in vivo and in vitro. *Prostaglandins*, 15:955-968.

184. Wolf, S. (1965): *The Stomach*, pp. 179-193. Oxford University Press, New York.

185. Wood, E. H., editor (1962): Symposium on use of indicator-dilution techniques in the study of the circulation. *Circ Res.*, 10:377-581.

186. Zinner, M. J., Kerr, J. C., and Reynolds, D. J. (1975): Adrenergic mechanisms in canine gastric circulation. *Am. J. Physiol.*, 229:977-982.

187. Zinner, M. J., Kerr, J. C., and Reynolds, D. G. (1976): Distribution and arteriovenous shunting of gastric blood flow in the baboon: Effect of epinephrine and vasopressin infusions. *Gastroenterology*, 71:299-302.

188. Zukoski, C. F., Lee, H. M., and Hume, D. M. (1963): Effect of hypothalamic stimulation on gastric secretion and adrenal function in the dog. *J. Surg. Res.*, 3:301-306.

Physiology of the Gastrointestinal Tract, edited by
Leonard R. Johnson. Raven Press, New York © 1981.

Chapter 27

Gastric Mucosal Barrier

David Fromm

That the gastric mucosa behaves as a semipermeable membrane that allows acid secreted into the lumen to diffuse back into the mucosa was reported by Teorell in 1933 (142). Since then, several investigators have emphasized the existence of an ion diffusion barrier, but it was not until the publication of Davenport's experiments in 1964 (26,36) that the concept of a gastric mucosal barrier aroused new interest and subsequently assumed clinical significance. A diverse number of topically applied agents are known, or at least have been reported, to increase mucosal permeability (32); these range from cobra venom (35) to clinically significant agents, such as salicylates, alcohol, duodenal contents, and hypertonic solutions.

Until recently, the gastric mucosal barrier was primarily thought of in terms of passive permeability. Its restrictive nature allows the lumen of the stomach to maintain its high concentration of acid without digesting itself. It is generally believed that an increase in spontaneous permeability to acid results in mucosal damage. Newer data, however, are beginning to illustrate the complexity of the mechanisms whereby gastric mucosa protects itself against its own secreted acid and how certain agents alter the mucosa.

METHODS

A number of *in vivo* and *in vitro* methods have been used to study the effects of various chemicals and altered physiologic conditions on permeability and other properties that may alter the ability of the gastric mucosa to protect itself against acid diffusion.

In Vivo

The majority of *in vivo* studies have been primarily concerned with the effects of various agents and conditions on changes in permeability. The design of these studies essentially involves placing a known solution into the stomach and analyzing the changes in ionic flows over a period of time. The solution is placed in either a gastric pouch (26) or on a mucosal flap with intact blood supply (104), or the solution is continuously perfused through the stomach (137) (Fig. 1). The solution usually contains a relatively low concentration of Na^+ and a relatively high concentration of H^+, which mimics normal circumstances and favors the movement of these ions along their concentration gradients. In many studies, the transmural electrical potential difference

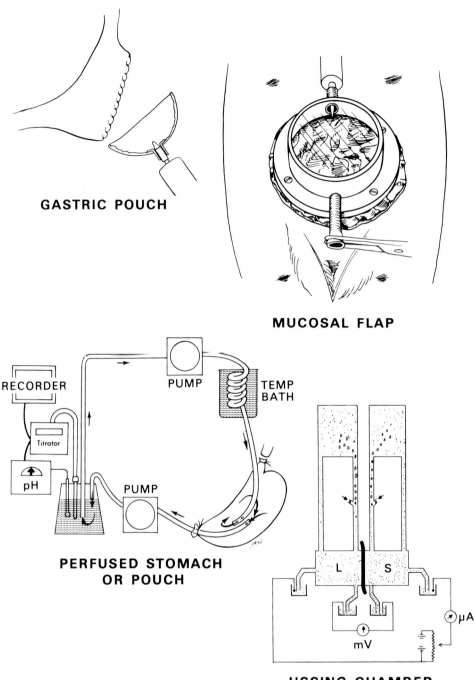

FIG. 1. Frequently used methods for studying the effects of various agents or conditions on the gastric mucosa. (Modified from refs. 48,104,137.) Combinations and variations of these methods are common. The gastric pouch is not in continuity with the gastrointestinal tract and may be reused. The mucosal flap with its blood supply intact is seated in a chamber. In the continuous perfusion model (*lower left*) the pH meter is connected to an automatic titrator and recorder which represents a pH stat apparatus. This titrates the pH of the effluent sample container at a preset value. The Ussing chamber is an *in vitro* perfusion apparatus divided into a luminal (L) and serosal (S) half by the mucosa (*dark stipled bar*). The two central salt agar bridges are in contact with reference electrodes connected to a volt meter (mV). The two peripheral salt agar bridges communicate with Ag-$AgCl_2$ electrodes connected to a DC source (μA) from which a current can be passed to short-circuit the tissue. *Arrows*, gas inlets which are a part of a gas-lift circulating system.

(PD) has been measured as well. An increase in the rate of luminal loss of H^+ associated with an increase in the rate of luminal gain of Na^+ and K^+ in conjunction with a decrease in the PD has been considered to indicate an increase in mucosal permeability, or what has been termed disruption of the gastric mucosal barrier. Such changes must be interpreted with caution, however, since other factors may cause similar changes in the absence of an increase in mucosal permeability.

A limitation of *in vivo* studies using the above methods involves the difficulty of differentiating between the passive and active unidirectional flows of various ions. In the presence of a semipermeable membrane, such as the gastric mucosa, ions can move out of the lumen (from the luminal to the serosal side of the mucosa) or into the lumen (from the serosal to the luminal side of the mucosa) not only by diffusional but also by active transport processes. The former are largely concentration dependent and therefore passive, whereas the latter are related to energy consumption allowing transfer of ions against their concentration gradients.

An example of passive ion transport is the diffusion of H^+ from the gastric lumen into the mucosa, which has been frequently referred to as back-diffusion. An example of active transport is H^+ secretion. Most *in vivo* studies have investigated net ionic flow, which is the arithmetic difference between the unidirectional luminal-to-serosal and unidirectional serosal-to-luminal flows. Unidirectional flows, or fluxes, have been measured in a few *in vivo* investigations, but no distinction between active and passive components of such ion flows has been made. The importance of this distinction is apparent upon considering, for example, H^+ diffusion out of the lumen (Fig. 2). This is a net flux dependent on the luminal-to-serosal (passive) and serosal-to-luminal (active) H^+ fluxes. Thus inhibition of H^+ secretion alone would cause an apparent increase in back-diffusion. In this circumstance, however, normally occurring back-diffusion is simply unmasked, and thus the change in net H^+ flux does not necessarily imply a change in permeability. The net H^+ flux also can be influenced by the flow of HCO_3^-, which may originate from the cells of the gastric mucosa (56) and/or a transmural source (53) (e.g., blood). Thus, because of the complexity of ion transport, measurement of net fluxes alone may lead to erroneous interpretations (48,49).

Following the induction of an apparent increase in permeability, a fall in the PD has been almost routinely

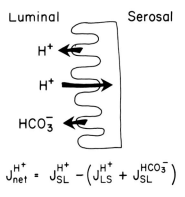

$$J_{net}^{H^+} = J_{SL}^{H^+} - \left(J_{LS}^{H^+} + J_{SL}^{HCO_3^-}\right)$$

FIG. 2. Relationship of unidirectional luminal (L)-to-serosal (S) flux (J_{LS}) and unidirectional S-to-L flux (J_{SL}) of H^+ and HCO_3^- to net H^+ flux ($J_{net}^{H^+}$). Negative $J_{net}^{H^+}$ indicates real or apparent luminal loss of acid.

observed. The PD has been suggested to be a sensitive index of mucosal integrity (58); but its usefulness in this regard has been overemphasized. In the majority of instances, corrections have not been made for liquid junction potentials, which are considerable in the presence of a high concentration of acid in the lumen (121) (Fig. 3). Also, a decrease in PD may result not only from an alteration of passive ion transport but also from alterations of active ion transport (49). Furthermore, a change in the magnitude of the spontaneous PD may also influence the magnitude of passive ion flows (145). A solution to the latter problem involves nullifying, or short-circuiting, the PD to zero and correlating the ion flux changes with the change in tissue electrical conductance. There are difficulties in the application of this experimental technique to tissues *in vivo* (123).

That increases in ionic flows are in fact related to an increase in mucosal permeability has in some instances been substantiated by the observation of an increase in plasma protein in the gastric lumen. Another way to solve the problem of distinguishing between major changes in active and passive components of ionic fluxes

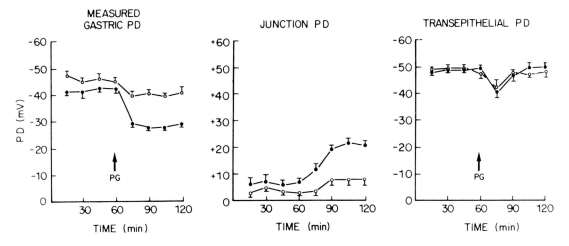

FIG. 3. Importance of liquid junction potentials. (From ref. 121.) The gastric PD (**left**) was obtained with flowing saline (*solid circles*) or KCl (*open circles*) electrodes in patients before and after administration of pentagastrin (PG). The junction PD (**middle**) was determined by calculation and the transepithelial PD was obtained by subtracting the junction from measured PD (mean ± SEM).

during apparent alterations of mucosal permeability is to use an independent permeability probe; lithium has been proposed. In a canine model, the luminal-to-serosal flux of Li^+ has been reported to share a constant relationship to the diffusion of H^+ (22). Li^+ has been used as a marker in studies of gastric mucosal permeability in humans (60,136). This avoided the potential danger of placing a relatively high concentration of HCl in the lumen and some of the assumptions used to calculate the back-diffusion of H^+ in this situation (112,135). The use of Li^+ as an indicator of mucosal permeability in both dogs and humans has been questioned (71,130); the controversy may be related to a number of experimental variables.

In Vitro

Several of the interpretative problems in alterations of ion flows across the gastric mucosa *in vivo* can be resolved by *in vitro* techniques. The latter more readily permit distinction between unidirectional and net ion transport processes and permeability changes. Although *in vitro* experiments involve artificial circumstances, several of the basic concepts of ion transport by the gastric mucosa have been derived from studies made under isolated conditions. In many instances, observations both *in vivo* and *in vitro* have been complementary. An advantage of *in vitro* techniques is that they permit isolation of the tissue from extramucosal effects (e.g., alterations in blood flow, release of certain humoral agents) and electrical and chemical gradients which may influence ion transport processes. The most frequently used method involves placement of the gastric mucosa in an Ussing-type chamber (145) which allows separate perfusion of the luminal and serosal surfaces of the tissue (Fig. 1).

GENERAL ASPECTS OF PERMEABILITY ALTERATIONS AND ACID DIFFUSION

Permeability Pathway

Permeability and electrical measurements of amphibian fundic mucosa suggest that, at most, 20% of ionic conductance normally is paracellular (140). This implies that under spontaneous conditions, a major portion of H^+ diffusion from the lumen occurs by cellular pathways. In contrast, the paracellular pathway accounts for 80% of the tissue conductance of amphibian antral mucosa under spontaneous conditions (139). Under conditions of increased permeability, however, the paracellular route may be affected to a greater degree than the cellular one (129). Studies of isolated gastric mucosa using permeability probes suggest that a major change occurs in the paracellular pathway when ethyl alcohol (37, 50), salicylate (6,44), and bile salts (6) are topically ap-

plied to the gastric mucosa. *In vivo* studies in which the source of an increase in luminal protein has been determined after mucosal contact with a few agents (e.g., ethyl alcohol, acetylsalicylic acid) also suggest that a major alteration occurs in the paracellular permeability pathway (21,29,35,74).

Some agents that increase mucosal permeability (e.g., urea), disrupt the tight intercellular junctions (42). On the other hand, the tight junctions remain intact, despite an increase in mucosal permeability and variable and sometimes extensive cellular damage after mucosal exposure to acetylsalicylic acid (4,65,69,113), bile salt (43), and ethyl alcohol (42). Thus disruption of the junctional complex is neither essential for the occurrence nor a necessary consequence of an increase in mucosal permeability to H^+.

Morphologic Changes

There is a surprising uniformity of ultrastructural damage to the mucosa after exposure to agents that presumably increase permeability by different mechanisms. Most of the morphologic studies have been directed at the effects of salicylate. In the presence of a low pH, damage of the surface mucus cells is evident within minutes of exposure of acetylsalicylic acid (4,69,119). This initial involvement of the surface mucus cells also has been observed after topical exposure to ethyl alcohol (42) and bile salts (43,134). Changes are first noted within the cell, without prior detectable changes in the cell membrane. Various degrees of damage to surface mucus cells have also been observed in humans (4,62,69), but the luminal pH has not been controlled in these studies. Cell death, slough, and erosions occur rapidly. Intracellular changes of parietal cells also occur (4,62,119, 155) and are more evident in those cells situated in the mid-upper regions of the gastric pits (119). After exposure to topically applied agents, repair begins rapidly (39,81,151,155), and the extensive initial damage noted contrasts with the paucity and focal nature of erosions noted a few hours later (69).

Mucus

A number of drugs and bile salts that increase the permeability of the gastric mucosa also are associated with a decrease in the synthesis, secretion (82,97,118,146), or quality of mucus (95). It has been postulated that alterations of gastric mucus may lead to ulceration (97), but the protective role of mucus against luminal H^+ (which is required for ulceration to occur) is believed to be minimal. Mucus has a limited buffering capacity (152), and concentrated films of mucus interfere with the diffusion of HCl to only a limited extent (67). Solubilization of gastric mucus using *n*-acetylcysteine does not appear to alter mucosal permeability *in vivo* (34), and some drugs that decrease mucus secretion (97) do not increase mucosal permeability (24). Even though mucus may add an unstirred layer (67,152) possibly containing a rather steep pH gradient (67), it is generally believed that mucus affords little protection.

Pepsin Secretion

The secretion of pepsin is increased when gastric mucosal permeability is increased by topically applied agents in HCl (45,74). Although there is a linear correlation between pepsin output and the extent of lesions caused by acetylsalicylic acid in HCl, addition of pepsin to a solution of acetylsalicylic acid in HCl does not significantly affect the severity of the resulting lesions (61). Furthermore, irrigation of the gastric mucosa with pepsin does not aggravate the permeability changes caused by acetylsalicylic acid (27). Intramucosal activation of pepsinogen to pepsin also does not occur following par-

enteral administration of acetylsalicylic acid, which results in gross mucosal damage (93).

An increase in gastric mucosal permeability in the absence of luminal acid (e.g., caused by ethyl alcohol) is not associated with a stimulation of pepsin secretion. Acid must be present for such stimulation to occur (74) (Fig. 4). Thus acid is a stimulant of pepsin secretion in the presence of increased mucosal permeability (74), but the resulting increased amount of pepsin in gastric juice does not appear to aggravate the mucosal injury.

Histamine Release

Increased quantities of histamine have been shown to be present in the lumen (73) and venous effluent (75) (Fig. 5) of stomach exposed to salicylate and acetic acid, which increase mucosal permeability. It has been postulated that this increased availability of histamine results in the stimulation of H^+ secretion, thereby increasing

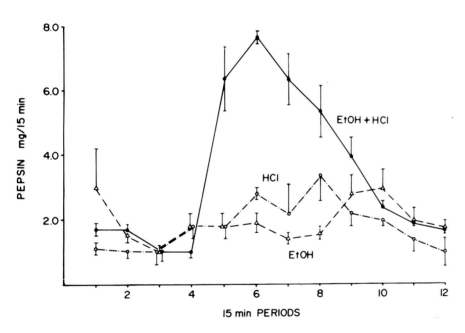

FIG. 4. Effect of 15% ethyl alcohol in 100 mm HCl on pepsin secretion by vagally denervated canine gastric pouches. The pouch pH was 7.5 during periods 1–4 and 9–12 (mean ± SEM). (From ref. 74.)

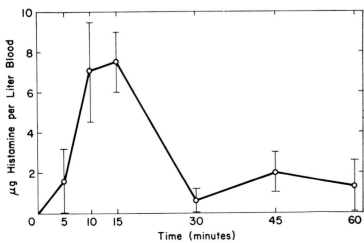

FIG. 5. Change in gastric venous histamine concentration during salicylic acid irrigation of canine stomach. (From ref. 75.) The concentration of histamine found during a control period was subtracted from that found at each time interval after instillation of salicylic acid, 20 mm at zero time. An increased concentration of histamine was also found in the salicylic acid irrigating solution within 5 min (mean ± SEM).

existing tissue damage (29). Histamine release, however, is not a necessary consequence of an increase in permeability (37,40).

The effects of histamine on gastric mucosal permeability to acid *in vivo* are controversial. For normal gastric mucosa, histamine has been reported to decrease (153) or have no effect (1,106) on the diffusion of H^+ into the mucosa. Data from isolated gastric mucosa of the rabbit suggest that histamine decreases mucosal permeability to H^+ in both the absence and presence of salicylate (54). Histamine also does not stimulate acid secretion by isolated gastric mucosa continuously exposed to salicylate. Thus data from isolated mucosa suggest that histamine may exert a protective effect in the presence of permeability alterations of rabbit stomach induced by salicylate. On the other hand, *in vivo* studies of the rabbit stomach suggest that histamine, in contrast to isolated conditions, does not substantially affect mucosal permeability (83).

Active Ion Transport

In addition to increasing mucosal permeability, several agents (e.g., salicylate, ethyl alcohol, and bile salt) also alter active ion transport processes to varying degrees (47,50,52) (Fig. 6). The predominant effect is a reduction or inhibition of various active transport processes (H^+, Na^+, Cl^-). This does not imply, however,

that an increase in permeability is necessarily associated with or results from inhibition of active transport. Inhibition of active ion transport (e.g., by ouabain) is not associated with an increase in mucosal permeability (50, 53). Ethyl alcohol still increases mucosal permeability after active transport has been inhibited by ouabain (50), (Fig. 7). Exposure of the mucosa to a relatively low concentration of salicylate causes a decrease in active transport as well as an increase in permeability, but subsequent exposure to ouabain, which completely inhibits active transport, does not result in a further increase in permeability (47).

Inhibition of active ion transport is not a necessary consequence of H^+ diffusing from the lumen into the tissue, since at neutral luminal pH, inhibition of active transport can occur upon exposure to agents that increase permeability in the absence of luminal H^+ (50, 52). In the case of fundic mucosa, it might be argued that H^+ could diffuse from the parietal cells into the tissue in the absence of luminal H^+, but this argument does not hold for similar effects of agents on antral mucosa. Studies with pyridine compounds also suggest that H^+ diffusion does not necessarily inhibit active ion transport (55). Pyridine alone decreases the spontaneous diffusion of acid into isolated antral mucosa without altering active ion transport; yet a relatively low concentration of pyridine containing a carboxyl group (nicotinic acid), which also decreases spontaneous H^+

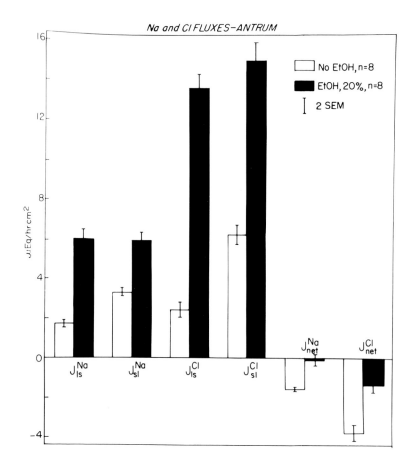

FIG. 6. Effects of 20% ethyl alcohol on ion transport across isolated antral mucosa of rabbits. (Modified from ref. 50.) Both unidirectional isotopic fluxes of Na and Cl increase after exposure to ethyl alcohol. However, ethyl alcohol reduced the net secretion of Na and Cl. J_{ls}, unidirectional luminal (l)-to-serosal (s) flux; J_{sl}, unidirectional s-to-l flux; J_{net}, net flux ($J_{ls} - J_{sl}$).

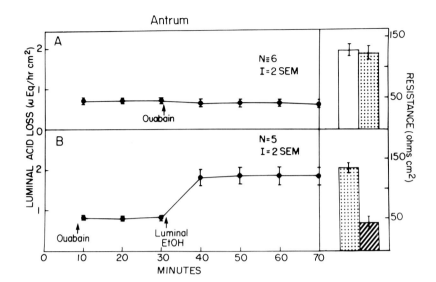

FIG. 7. Effects of 20% ethyl alcohol on luminal acid loss by isolated antral mucosa of rabbits. (Modified from ref. 50.) Inhibition of net Na and Cl transport by ouabain did not alter the effect of ethyl alcohol. Ethyl alcohol decreased the tissue electrical resistance (or increased total conductance), which is associated with an increase in permeability.

diffusion into the tissue, alters active transport by antral mucosa (Fig. 8).

Although inhibition of active transport is not necessarily associated with an increase in gastric mucosal permeability, the H^+ secretory (an active transport process) state of the mucosa appears to play an important role in the mucosal defense against H^+ diffusing into the tissue. When a physiologic concentration (120 mM) of HCl is placed in the lumen of rabbit stomach, erosions of the mucosa occur (137). This is probably due to the fact that

the spontaneous permeability of rabbit fundic mucosa is greater than that of most other species (51,83,137).[1] The erosions occurring in the presence of luminal H^+ usually can be prevented by stimulating H^+ secretion with histamine, but histamine is ineffective in preventing

---

[1] That spontaneous gastric ulcerations are rarely seen in healthy rabbits probably is due to the fact that rabbits retain food (and hence buffer) in their stomachs even after prolonged periods of fasting.

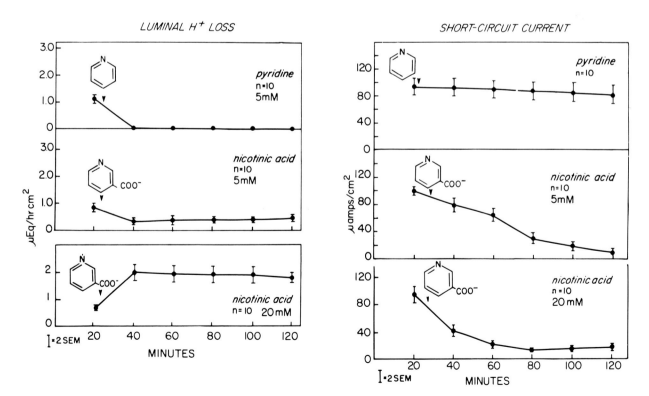

FIG. 8. Effects of pyridine compounds on luminal acid loss and short-circuit current (I_{sc}) of isolated antral mucosa of rabbits. (Modified from ref. 55.) Pyridine (**top**) inhibits luminal acid loss without affecting I_{sc}, which is a reflection of net ion transport. Nicotinic acid, 5 mM (**middle**), also decreases the rate of luminal acid loss but in addition decreases I_{sc}. A fourfold increase in nicotinic acid (**bottom**) increases luminal acid loss and decreases I_{sc} (see text).

these lesions if the rabbits are pretreated with a H_2 receptor antagonist, which inhibits acid secretion (83, 137). The protective effect of histamine in stimulating acid secretion is related to its effect on the intramural pH of the mucosa.

Intramural pH

In some experimental models, an increase in rate of luminal H^+ loss appears to be a prerequisite for the occurrence of gross mucosal damage (38,126,149). On the other hand, mucosal ulceration also has been observed in the absence of an increase in the spontaneous rate of luminal H^+ loss (20,105,156). Nevertheless, there is almost universal agreement that the luminal presence of H^+ is a necessary requirement for gross mucosal damage. These observations suggest that the critical determinant of microscopic or gross mucosal damage does not appear to be the absolute amount of H^+ entering the tissue (133), even though the net loss of H^+ from the lumen varies linearly with the luminal concentration of H^+ (23). A more crucial factor in the process of ulceration is related to the ability of the mucosa to neutralize diffusing H^+.

An increase in luminal H^+ loss from rabbit stomach is associated with a significant decrease in the intramural pH of the mucosa, and a linear relationship exists between the rate of luminal acid loss and intramural pH (83) (Fig. 9). This decrease in intramural pH, which occurs in unstimulated stomach, is associated with the occurrence of ulcerations. On the other hand, stimulation of acid secretion by histamine, which prevents ulceration, is associated with an insignificant change in intramural pH (Fig. 10). The less permeable antral mucosa of rabbits exposed to HCl does not ulcerate, and the decrease in intramural pH is less than that observed for fundic mucosa (83). These data suggest that the H^+ se-

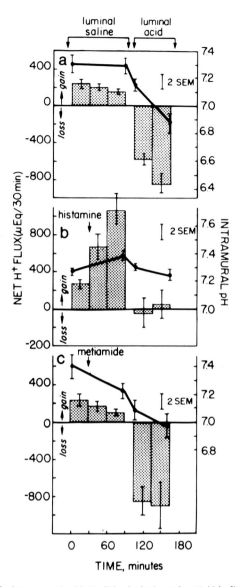

FIG. 10. Intramural pH (*solid circles*) and net H^+ fluxes in spontaneously secreting (**a**), histamine-stimulated (**b**), and metiamide-inhibited (**c**) fundic pouches of rabbits exposed to luminal saline and then luminal H^+, 120 mM. (From ref. 83.)

cretory state of the mucosa can influence its ability to withstand diffusing H^+ by modifying the buffering ability of the tissue. The most likely source of the additional buffer during histamine stimulation is the so-called alkaline tide. An increase in blood flow induced by histamine also may contribute by delivering more buffer to the tissue (90) or by washing away excessive quantities of H^+.

Although a major increase in H^+ diffusion from the lumen into the tissue probably does not occur during hemorrhagic shock, in this circumstance the capacity of the mucosa to dispose of H^+ also is compromised (84). A decrease in intramural pH occurs, caused by both H^+ diffusing from the lumen and systemic acidosis (85). This inability of rabbit fundic mucosa to dispose of H^+

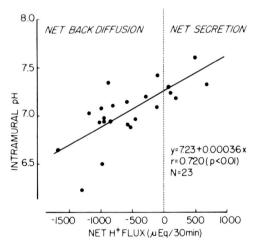

FIG. 9. Relationship between intramural pH and net H^+ flux in rabbit fundus *in vivo*. (From ref. 83.)

probably is related to a decrease in H⁺ secretion and blood flow as a consequence of shock. In contrast to rabbits, the intramural pH of the less permeable canine fundic mucosa decreases at a slower rate during hemorrhagic shock, which may account for the paucity of ulcers in this situation (85). When canine fundic mucosal permeability is increased during shock by the addition of bile salt to the H⁺ luminal content, however, the decrease in intramural pH is more rapid and profound. In this circumstance, extensive gross mucosal damage occurs.

Blood Flow

Mucosal blood flow responses to agents that increase mucosal permeability are somewhat contradictory when measured by the aminopyrine clearance method (3,108). This method reflects only a small fraction of mucosal blood flow compared to the use of gamma-labeled microspheres (2). Data from gamma-labeled microsphere studies used to measure blood flow indicate that salicylate, bile salt, and ethyl alcohol cause a significant increase in mucosal blood flow (18) (Fig. 11). It is believed that this response is due to mucosal injury rather than to effects of the injurious agent per se, because the degree of change in blood flow appears to be proportional to the gross mucosal injury (18). It is recognized, however, that current methods for measuring blood flow do not measure focal alterations. For example, focal pallor of the mucosa precedes the appearance of superficial erosions induced by salicylate, even though measurements indicate an increase in total blood flow of the mucosa (18).

A pharmacologically induced increase in mucosal circulation has been shown to prevent ulceration induced by bile salt in the gastric lumen of animals subjected to hemorrhagic shock, even though the diffusion of H⁺ from the lumen is not significantly different from that observed in the absence of the pharmacologic stimulation of blood flow (127). A decrease in mucosal blood flow alone is not necessarily injurious to the gastric mucosa. It is remarkable that when only HCl (80 to 160 mM) is present in the gastric lumen during severe (40 mm

Hg) and prolonged (4 hr) hemorrhagic shock in monkeys and dogs, there is no significant alteration in net ion fluxes or visible damage of the mucosa (38,125). On the other hand, fundic mucosa of rabbits subjected to hemorrhagic shock will develop ulcerations, but this contrasting effect probably is attributable to the apparently unique permeability property of rabbit gastric mucosa. Thus tissue anoxia alone *in vivo* is not associated with an increase in gastric mucosal permeability. Severe anoxia for less than 1.5 hr *in vitro* also is not associated with an increase in permeability (8,53).

Differences Between Fundic and Antral Mucosa

Agents that affect fundic mucosal permeability and active transport processes also affect antral mucosa in a similar way; in some situations, subtle differences have been shown to occur, or the differences are ones of degree of change. For example, mucosal damage associated with shock usually is more intense in the proximal stomach than in the antrum. Aside from considerations of pH and pooling of gastric contents in the fundus of a supine animal or patient, metabolic differences between the parietal cell bearing and the antral mucosa also may contribute to the difference in degrees of damage. In both active and resting states, the oxygen demand of the proximal stomach is greater than that of the antrum (131). The parietal cell-bearing mucosa lacks glycogen and has a relative inability to utilize anaerobic glycolysis as an alternate source of energy (98). Under conditions of complete ischemia, dephosphorylation of the adenylate pool is less marked in the antrum than in the more proximal stomach (99). An additional difference is that the breakdown of high energy phosphates is less marked in the antrum than in the proximal mucosa during hemorrhagic shock (100).

There also are spontaneous permeability differences between antral and fundic mucosa, but species differences may exist. In dogs, the permeability of antral mucosa appears to be greater than that of fundic mucosa (41,149). In contrast, rabbit antral mucosa is less permeable than fundic mucosa (47,51-53,83,85).

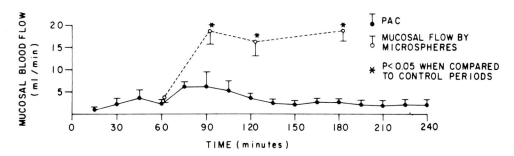

FIG. 11. Mucosal blood flow response of canine mucosal flap preparation to taurocholate (40 mM) applied from 60 to 120 min. PAC, mucosal blood flow measured by aminopyrine clearance (mean ± SEM). (Modified from ref. 18.)

The Barrier

The "barrier" often has been used in the generic sense to refer to the property of the stomach that prevents H^+ in its lumen from damaging the mucosa. Most studies dealing with the barrier have equated "disruption of the barrier" with an increase in mucosal permeability to the common cations H^+, Na^+, and K^+. Thus the barrier has been used by most investigators to refer to the passive permeability characteristics of the mucosa. Consideration of H^+ diffusion only in terms of permeability is restrictive, however, and has led to some confusion concerning damage to the mucosa. Injury may occur in the presence of luminal H^+, even though the rate of H^+ diffusion into the tissue does not increase. In this circumstance, the buffering ability of the mucosa may be compromised, even though the permeability characteristics of the mucosa remain intact. Thus it is no longer proper to refer to the barrier as a single entity, because there are at least two barriers; one is related to permeability and the other to the buffering ability of the mucosa. Simple reference to permeability or buffering would avoid confusion and allow stricter definition while leaving room for description of other mechanisms by which the mucosa protects itself against its own secreted acid.

EFFECTS OF SOME SPECIFIC AGENTS

Duodenal Contents

Bile Salts

The effect of bile or bile salts on mucosal permeability is both pH and concentration dependent (7,9,52,134). The severity of the permeability change is directly related to the concentration of bile salt. Although the presence of H^+ is not essential for the change in permeability caused by bile salts, there is an inverse association between the severity of this change and the pH of the luminal content. The more H^+ present, the greater is the diffusion gradient for mucosa made more permeable by bile salt (or any other agent that increases permeability). Another effect of H^+ relates to the solubility of the various bile salts. When the luminal pH is much below the pKa of a given bile salt, it will precipitate and decrease the effect of that bile salt on the mucosa (43,66,134). For example, taurine-conjugated bile salts (pKa around 1.8) cause a greater degree of damage at a low pH, whereas deconjugated or dehydroxylated bile salts, with a much higher pKa (around 5), cause less damage at a low pH than at a high pH (43,66,134). The pH of the luminal contents also determines the amount of bile salt absorbed, the un-ionized form being absorbed to a

greater degree (23,43). The importance of bile salt absorption in causing permeability change, however, has not been firmly established.

The permeability change induced by bile salt is believed to be related to its detergent, or lipid-disrupting, quality. Dissolution of mucosal phospholipid (143) and release or leakage of acid hydrolases (147) occur. The latter has been observed with gallbladder bile, but only in the presence of H^+. Bile alone also minimally alters the specific activity of lysosomal enzymes of antral mucosa, but in the presence of H^+ the specific activity of antral lysosomal enzymes increases (68). Whether these enzymatic changes are due to absorption of bile salts or acid, or both, is not clear.

Lysolecithin and Pancreatic Juice

Lysolecithin is formed in the presence of bile salts and Ca^{2+} when pancreatic phospholipase A hydrolyses the lecithin in bile. Phospholipase A and pancreatic juice do not appear to alter mucosal permeability (34), but lysolecithin increases permeability (33,84). This effect does not require the presence of H^+ and is related to the concentration of lysolecithin (33,84).

Alcohol

Alcohol increases the permeability of the gastric mucosa, but the presence of H^+ (as in the case of bile salt and lysolecithin) is not required for this effect (30,42,50, 74). Straight chain alcohols are more damaging to the mucosa on a mole for mole basis than their branched isomers (25). The damaging effects of alcohol also are related to its carbon chain length (25,148), lipid solubility (148), and concentration (25,81,148). Concentrations of ethyl alcohol less than about 10% do not appear to alter mucosal permeability (30,39), even though concentrations of ethyl alcohol of 5.5% interfere with some mucosal metabolic processes (59).

Some of the effects of ethyl alcohol may be related to its osmotic activity, but specific osmotic effects have not been clearly separated from the enzymatic effects of alcohol (77,107,115,116,132,141,154). Isotonic ethyl alcohol approximates only 1.6% v/v (42). The damaging effects of ethyl alcohol appear to depend more on the concentration in contact with the mucosa than on the quantity absorbed (30). The effects of ethyl alcohol, however, are not exactly duplicated by other osmotically active agents (5,40,42). The osmolar limits required for a change in permeability to occur have not been precisely established but appear to be greater than 1,100 mOsm/kg (46).

Salicylate

Salicylate must be present in an acid medium in order to damage the gastric mucosa. A relatively low pH is required to maintain salicylate predominantly in its unionized, lipid-soluble form, which readily permeates the cellular lipoprotein mosaic facing the lumen. As this occurs, alterations in the mucosa permit an increase in the diffusion of H^+ from the lumen into the tissue, causing cellular damage (26–28,31). As salicylate enters cells, the relatively high intracellular pH causes the drug to exist predominantly in its ionized form, which has been postulated to interfere with intracellular metabolism (94). Many data are consistent with most of these concepts.

Under isolated conditions in the absence of luminal H^+, salicylate selectively alters ion permeability by increasing the flow of cations and decreasing the flow of anions through antral mucosa (47). These changes also initially occur in the presence of H^+ but subsequently give way to a nonspecific increase in permeability to both cations and anions (Fig. 12). The flux of paracellular permeability probes is not increased during the ion selective phase but does increase during the nonspecific permeability phase. These data suggest that the subsequent nonspecific increase in permeability caused by salicylate is attributable to the mucosa becoming overwhelmed by the diffusing H^+.

In theory, the salicylate anion should not permeate the mucosa at neutral pH. Thus the ion selective effects of salicylate at neutral pH suggest that the initial effect of the drug is related to an alteration of electrical field strength rather than to absorption of the anion. However, the fact is that salicylate is absorbed at pH near neutrality, and the rate of this absorption is not negligible, even though it is less than that occurring at lower pH values (31). Salicylate may also initially act as a cation carrier, which is consistent with the observation that the increase in diffusion of H^+ requires the continual presence of low concentrations of salicylate in the lumen (52). Other investigators, however, have postulated that the metabolic alterations associated with salicylate absorption account for the increase in mucosal permeability.

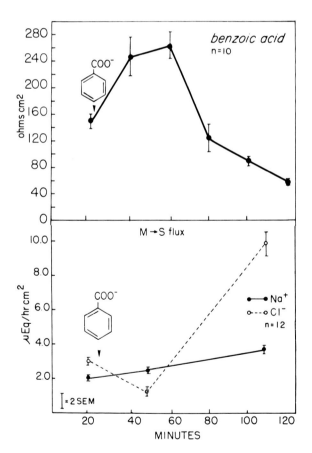

FIG. 12. Effects of 5 mM benzoic acid on tissue electrical resistance and the passive unidirectional mucosal (M) (or luminal)-to-serosal (S) fluxes of Na and Cl across isolated antral mucosa of rabbits. (Modified from ref. 55.) Ion selective effects occur during the high resistance phase. Effects of benzoic acid are identical to those observed for sodium salicylate.

Metabolic Effects

Salicylate is known to affect intermediary metabolism, but the relationship of this to alterations of permeability or the ability of the mucosa to handle acid diffusion induced by salicylate (or other agents) is unclear. Like bile salts (88), the ATP content of gastric mucosa is reduced after exposure to acetylsalicylic acid (78,89,138). Salicylate also inhibits protein synthesis by the gastric mucosa; the magnitude of this effect appears to be related to the concentration of the drug (102).

It is well established that salicylate interferes with oxidative phosphorylation (11,14,17,72,76,78,144). Most believe this is an uncoupling phenomenon, which may be concentration dependent. Low concentrations of salicylic acid have been reported to uncouple and higher concentrations to inhibit mitochondrial respiration after a brief period of uncoupling (138). That the gastric mucosal effects of relatively low or high concentrations of salicylate are not simply due to uncoupling of oxidative phosphorylation is suggested by the observation that another uncoupler of oxidative phosphorylation, dinitrophenol, has different effects on permeability and ion transport (86,124). Both salicylate and dinitrophenol inhibit active transport processes, but dinitrophenol, unlike salicylate, does not increase mucosal permeability. Furthermore, acetylsalicylic acid and dinitrophenol have different effects on Na^+ uptake by a mixed population of isolated gastric mucosal cells (86).

Salicylates, like ethyl alcohol, also affect cyclic AMP activity of the gastric mucosa (92,103). Acetylsalicylic acid has been reported to increase adenylate cyclase activity (92) and inhibit phosphodiesterase activity (114) of mucosal homogenates. The significance of these changes is unclear, especially since isolated gastric mucosa exposed to salicylate is resistant to stimulation of acid secretion by exogenous cyclic adenosine monophosphate as long as salicylate is present in the bathing medium (54).

Carboxyl Group

Even though salicylate has complex effects on the gastric mucosa, the chemical structure of salicylate is relatively simple: a hydroxyl and a carboxyl group attached to a benzene ring. Neither the benzene nor the phenolic components mimic the effects of the intact salicylate molecule (55). A free (e.g., formic acid) or exposed (e.g., benzoic acid) carboxyl group in sufficient concentration, however, mimics the effects of salicylate (Fig. 12). These data, in addition to the ion selective effects of salicylate, implicate the carboxyl group as being essential to its damaging effects on the stomach. Close analogs of salicylates, such as salicylamide ($R:CONH_2$) and methylsalicylate ($R:COOCH_3$), which are readily absorbed by the mucosal cells but do not have an exposed carboxyl group, do not cause morphologic damage to the gastric mucosa (69,87). Many of the nonsteroidal, anti-inflammatory, nonsalicylate compounds also contain an exposed carboxyl group, which is believed to be associated with the damaging effects of these agents on the gastric mucosa (63,117,120). The carboxyl group of salicylate, in addition to being associated with an increase in mucosal permeability, has been implicated in the inhibitory effects of salicylate on active ion transport, which appears to occur independently of the increase in diffusing H^+ (55).

Parenteral Salicylate

Acetylsalicylic acid given parenterally also damages the gastric mucosa. Large doses may increase the permeability of the mucosa to acid (111). Small doses also result in ulceration, but this is not associated with the permeability changes observed after intraluminal instillation of the drug (15). The presence of H^+ in the lumen is required for the occurrence of ulcers (64,79). On the one hand, these data suggest that parenteral acetylsalicylic acid may interfere with the ability of the mucosa to buffer spontaneously diffusing H^+; on the other hand, a different mechanism may play a role. It has been reported that sodium salicylate, in contrast to acetylsalicylic acid, grossly injures rat mucosa only when in direct contact (that is, luminally) with the mucosa (12,13). Whether these different effects of the two forms of salicylate are relatively specific for certain species or are related to prostaglandin metabolism is unsettled.

Steroids

Direct contact of the gastric mucosa with various adrenal corticosteroids does not alter permeability (24). Treatment with prednisolone parenterally for up to 3 months also does not alter the permeability of canine fundic pouches (23). It has been reported, however, that parenteral administration of prednisolone for 2 weeks potentiates the effects of acetylsalicylic acid and taurocholate on mucosal permeability (23). It has been postulated that this facilitating effect of prolonged parenteral steroid administration is attributable to a decrease in the rate of cellular turnover (23). The relationship of cellular turnover to changes in permeability, however, is not entirely clear. Various drugs (e.g., acetylsalicylic acid and phenylbutazone) increase the exfoliation of surface epithelial cells (96), but phenylbutazone does not appear to alter mucosal permeability (24).

PROTECTORS

Amino Acids

Various amino acids (e.g., L-glutamine, L-lysine, L-arginine) placed in the gastric lumen have been reported to decrease the injury caused by acetylsalicylic acid and bile salt (70,91,109,110). In many instances, this "protective" effect may be attributed to the alkaline pH of the amino acid solution (110) or to the amino acids acting as weak buffers (91).

Prostaglandins

Various prostaglandin compounds confer striking protection of the gastric mucosa to several harmful agents in a variety of animal models. While prostaglandins inhibit H^+ secretion, these compounds still exert a protective effect in nonantisecretory doses and in the presence of luminal H^+. Robert (128) has proposed calling this property of prostaglandins cytoprotective. The mechanism of this is unclear, but several of the effects of prostaglandins are known (101). In addition to inhibition of H^+ secretion, prostaglandins have been shown to increase cyclic AMP activity, active Na^+ transport, HCO_3^- secretion (57,80), blood flow, and mucus secretion and to stabilize lysosomal membranes. Because of the luminal accumulation of fluid which occurs with prostaglandins, the absorption of injurious agents might be decreased. However, it has been shown that 16,16-dimethyl prostaglandin E_2 does not reduce the salicylate content of the gastric mucosa (10).

Histamine Receptor Antagonism

Although the combined use of H_1 and H_2 receptor antagonists has been reported to protect the stomach against bile salt (122), this has not been shown to be the case in another study (19) or for salicylate (10). H_2 receptor antagonism alone will prevent damage, but the mechanism is controversial. Under certain circumstances, the protective effect appears to be related to the inhibition of H^+ secretion (16). In other situations, cimetidine appears to exert a protective effect independent of its ability to inhibit H^+ secretion (10,79), but the mechanism of this protective effect is not known.

ACKNOWLEDGMENTS

This work was supported in part by research grant AM-25227 from the National Institutes of Health, United States Public Health Service.

REFERENCES

1. Altamirano, M. (1970): Backdiffusion of H^+ during gastric secretion. *Am. J. Physiol.,* 218:1–6.
2. Augur, N. A. (1970): Gastric mucosal blood flow following damage by ethanol, acetic acid or aspirin. *Gastroenterology,* 58:311–320.
3. Archibald, L. H., Mood, F. G., and Simons, M. A. (1975): Comparison of gastric mucosal blood flow as determined by aminopyrine clearance and γ-labeled microspheres. *Gastroenterology,* 69:630–635.
4. Baskin, W. N., Ivey, K. J., Krause, W. J., Jeffrey, G. E., and Gemmell R. T. (1976): Aspirin-induced ultrastructural changes in human gastric mucosa. *Ann. Int. Med.,* 85:299–303.
5. Biggerstaff, R. J., and Leitch, G. J. (1977): Effects of ethanol on electrical parameters of the in vivo rat stomach. *Am. J. Dig. Dis.,* 22(12):1064–1068.
6. Birkett, D., and Silen, W. (1973): Alteration of physical pathways through gastric mucosa by bile and ASA. *Gastroenterology,* 64:701.
7. Birkett, D., and Silen, W. (1974): Alteration of the physical pathways through the gastric mucosa by sodium taurocholate. *Gastroenterology,* 67:1131–1138.
8. Birkett, D., and Silen, W. (1975): Effect of severe anoxia on the permeability of gastric mucosa. *Proc. Soc. Exp. Biol. Med.,* 148:256–260.
9. Black, R. B., Hole, D., and Rhodes, J. (1971): Bile damage to the gastric mucosal barrier: The influence of pH and bile acid concentration. *Gastroenterology,* 61:178–184.
10. Bommelaer, G., and Guth, P. H. (1979): Protection by histamine receptor antagonists and prostaglandin against gastric mucosal barrier disruption in the rat. *Gastroenterology,* 77:303–308.
11. Bosund, I. (1957): The effect of salicylic acid, benzoic acid and some of their derivatives on oxidative phosphorylation. *Acta Chem. Scand.,* 11:541–544.
12. Brodie, D. A., and Chase, B. J. (1967): Role of gastric acid in aspirin-induced gastric irritation in the rat. *Gastroenterology,* 53:604–610.
13. Brodie, D. A., Hooke, P. L. D., and K. F. (1971): Effects of route of administration on the production of gastric hemorrhage in the rat by aspirin and sodium salicylate. *Am. J. Dig. Dis.,* 16:985–989.
14. Brody, T. M. (1956): Action of sodium salicylate and related compounds on tissue metabolism *in vitro. J. Pharmacol. Exp. Ther.,* 117:39–51.
15. Bugat, R., Thompson, M. R., Aures, D., and Grossman, M. I. (1976): Gastric mucosal lesions produced by intravenous infusion of aspirin in cats. *Gastroenterology,* 71:754–759.
16. Carmichael, H. A., Nelson, L. M., and Russell, R. I. (1978): Cimetidine and prostaglandin: Evidence for different modes of action of the rat gastric mucosa. *Gastroenterology,* 74:1229–1232.
17. Charnock. J. S., Opit, L. J., and Hetzel, B. S. (1962): An evaluation of the effect of salicylate on oxidative phosphorylation in rat-liver mitochondria. *Biochem. J.,* 83:602–606.
18. Cheung, L. Y., Moody, F. G., and Reese, R. S. (1975): Effect of aspirin, bile salt and ethanol on gastric mucosal blood flow. *Surgery,* 77:786–792.
19. Cheung, L. Y., and Porterfield, G. (1978): Is histamine a mediator in bile-induced gastric mucosal injury? *J. Surg. Res.,* 24:272–276.
20. Cheung, L. Y., Stephenson, L. W., Moody, F. G., et al. (1975): Direct effects of endotoxin on canine gastric mucosal permeability and morphology. *J. Surg. Res.,* 18:417–425.
21. Chowdhury, A. R., Malmud, L. S., and Dinoso, V. P., Jr. (1977): Gastrointestinal plasma protein loss during ethanol ingestion. *Gastroenterology,* 72:37–40.
22. Chung, R. S. K., Field, M., and Silen, W. (1973): Permeability of gastric mucosa to hydrogen and lithium. *Gastroenterology,* 64:593–598.
23. Chung, R. S. K., Field, M., and Silen, W. (1978): Effects of methylprednisolone on hydrogen ion absorption in the canine stomach. *J. Clin. Invest.,* 62:262–270.
24. Chvasta, T. E., and Cooke, A. R. (1972): The effect of several ulcerogenic drugs on the canine gastric mucosal barrier. *J. Lab. Clin. Med.,* 79:302–315.
25. Cooke, A. R., and Kienzle, M. G. (1974): Studies of anti-inflammatory drugs and aliphatic alcohols on antral mucosa. *Gastroenterology,* 66:56–62.
26. Davenport, H. W. (1964): Gastric mucosal injury by fatty and acetylsalicylic acids. *Gastroenterology,* 46:245–253.
27. Davenport, H. W. (1965): Damage to the gastric mucosa: Effects of salicylate and stimulation. *Gastroenterology,* 49:189–196.
28. Davenport, H. W. (1965): Potassium fluxes across the resting and stimulated gastric mucosa: Injury by salicylate and acetic acids. *Gastroenterology,* 49:238–245.
29. Davenport, H. W. (1966): Fluid produced by the gastric mucosa during damage by acetic and salicylic acids. *Gastroenterology,* 50:487–499.
30. Davenport, H. W. (1967): Ethanol damage to canine oxyntic glandular mucosa. *Proc. Soc. Exp. Biol. Med.,* 126:657–662.
31. Davenport, H. W. (1969): Gastric mucosal hemorrhage in dogs: Effects of acid, aspirin and alcohol. *Gastroenterology,* 56:439–449.
32. Davenport, H. W. (1970): Backdiffusion of acid through the gastric mucosa and its physiological consequences. In: *Progress in Gastroenterology,* edited by G. B. J. Glass, pp. 48. Grune & Stratton, New York.
33. Davenport, H. W. (1970): Effect of lysolecithin digitonin, and phospholipase A upon the dog's gastric mucosal barrier. *Gastroenterology,* 59:505–509.
34. Davenport, H. W. (1971): Protein-losing gastropathy produced by sulfhydryl reagents. *Gastroenterology,* 60:870–879.
35. Davenport, H. W. (1974): Plasma protein shedding by the canine oxyntic glandular mucosal induced by topical application of snake venoms and ethanol. *Gastroenterology,* 67:264–270.
36. Davenport, H. W., Warner, H. A., and Code, C. F. (1964): Functional significance of gastric mucosal barrier to sodium. *Gastroenterology,* 47:142–152.
37. Dawson, D. C., and Cooke, A. R. (1978): Parallel pathways for ion transport across rat gastric mucosa: Effect of ethanol. *Am. J. Physiol.,* 235:E7–E15.
38. DenBesten, L., and Hamza, K. N. (1972): Effect of bile salts on ionic permeability of canine gastric mucosa during experimental shock. *Gastroenterology,* 62:417–424.
39. Dinoso, V. P., Chey, W. Y., Siplet, H., and Lorber, S. H. (1970): Effects of ethanol on the gastric mucosa of the Heidenhain pouch of dogs. *Am. J. Dig. Dis.,* 15:809–817.
40. Dinoso, V. P., Chuang, J., and Murthy, N. S. (1976): Changes in mucosal and venous histamine concentrations during instillation of ethanol in the canine stomach. *Am. J. Dig. Dis.,* 21:93–97.

41. Dyck, W. P., Werther, J. L., Rudick, J., and Janowitz, H. D. (1969): Electrolyte movement across canine antral and fundic gastric mucosa. *Gastroenterology,* 56:488-495.

42. Eastwood, G. L., and Kirchner, J. P. (1974): Changes in the fine structure of mouse gastric epithelium produced by ethanol and urea. *Gastroenterology,* 67:71-84.

43. Eastwood, G. L. (1975): Effect of pH on bile salt injury to mouse gastric mucosa. *Gastroenterology,* 68:1456-1465.

44. Flemström, G., and Marsden, N. V. B. (1973): Dextran permeability, electrical properties, and H^+ secretion in isolated frog gastric mucosa after acetylsalicylic acid. *Gastroenterology,* 64:278-284.

45. Frenning, B. (1971): The disappearance of acetylsalicylic acid (ASA) in aqueous solution from the cat stomach and its influence on the transmucosal ion transport in the innervated non-secreting stomach. *Acta Physiol. Scand.,* 83:235-246.

46. Frenning, B. (1974): The effects of large osmolarity variations on the gastric mucosal ion permeability. *Acta Physiol. Scand.,* 90:1-13.

47. Fromm, D. (1976): Ion selective effects of salicylate on antral mucosa. *Gastroenterology,* 71:743-749.

48. Fromm, D. (1978): Gastric mucosal defense mechanisms: Effects of salicylate and histamine. *Am. J. Surg.,* 135:379-384.

49. Fromm, D. (1979): Gastric mucosal "barrier." *Gastroenterology,* 77:396-398.

50. Fromm, D., and Robertson, R. (1976): Effects of alcohol on ion transport by isolated gastric and esophageal mucosa. *Gastroenterology,* 70:220-225.

51. Fromm, D., Schwartz, J. H., and Quijano, R. (1975): Transport of H^+ and other electrolytes across isolated gastric mucosa of the rabbit. *Am. J. Physiol.,* 228:166-171.

52. Fromm, D., Schwartz, J. H., and Quijano, R. (1976): Effects of salicylate and bile salt on ion transport by isolated gastric mucosa of the rabbit. *Am. J. Physiol.,* 230:319-326.

53. Fromm, D., Schwartz, J. H., Robertson, R., and Fuhro, R. (1976): Ion transport across isolated antral mucosa of the rabbit. *Am. J. Physiol.,* 231:1783-1789.

54. Fromm, D., Silen, W., and Robertson, R. (1976): Histamine effects on H^+ permeability by isolated gastric mucosa. *Gastroenterology,* 70:1076-1081.

55. Fuhro, R., and Fromm, D. (1978): Effects of compounds chemically related to salicylate on isolated antral mucosa of rabbits. *Gastroenterology,* 75:661-667.

56. Garner, A., and Flemström, G. (1978): Gastric HCO_3-secretion in the guinea pig. *Am. J. Physiol.,* 234:E535-E541.

57. Garner, A., and Heylings, J. R. (1979): Stimulation of alkaline secretion in amphibian-isolated gastric mucosa by 16,16-dimethyl PGE_2 and $PGF_{2\alpha}$. *Gastroenterology,* 76:497-503.

58. Geall, M. G., Phillips, S. F., and Summerskill, D. M. (1970): Profile of gastric potential difference in man. *Gastroenterology,* 58:437-443.

59. Glowacka, D., Kopacz-Jodczyk, T., Mazurkiewica-Kilczewska, D., and Gindzienski, A. (1974): Effect of ethyl alcohol on the biosynthesis of glucosamine and galactosamine in the human gastric mucosal tissue in vitro. *Biochem. Med.,* 11:194-204.

60. Gordon, M. J., Skillman, J. J., Zervas, N. T., et al. (1973): Divergent nature of gastric mucosal permeability and gastric acid secretion in sick patients with general surgical and neurosurgical disease. *Ann. Surg.,* 178:285-294.

61. Guth, P. H., Aures, D., and Paulsen, G. (1979): Topical aspirin plus HCl gastric lesions in the rat. Cytoprotective effect of prostaglandin cimetidine, and probanthine. *Gastroenterology,* 76:88-93.

62. Hahn, K-J., Krischkofski, D., Weber, E., et al. (1975): Morphology of gastrointestinal effects of aspirin. *Clin. Pharmacol. Ther.,* 17:330-338.

63. Halvorsen, L., Dotevall, G., and Sevelius, H. (1973): Comparative effects of aspirin and naproxen on gastric mucosa. *Scand. J. Rheumatol. [Suppl.],* 2:43-47.

64. Hansen, D. G., Aures, D., and Grossman, M. I. (1978): Histamine augments gastric ulceration produced by intravenous aspirin in cats. *Gastroenterology,* 74:540-543.

65. Harding, R. K., and Morris, G. P. (1976): Pathological effects of aspirin and of haemorrhagic shock on the gastric mucosa of the rat. Scanning electron microscopy (Part V). In: *Proceedings of the Workshop on Advances in Biomedical Applications of the SEM,* pp. 253-262. ITT Research Institute, Chicago.

66. Harmon, J. W., Doong, T., and Gadacz, T. R. (1978): Bile acids are not equally damaging to the gastric mucosa. *Surgery,* 84:79-86.

67. Heatley, N. G. (1959): Mucosubstance as a barrier to diffusion. *Gastroenterology,* 37:313-317.

68. Himal, H. S., Boutros, M., and Weiser, M. (1974): The relationship between bile and hydrochloric acid in the pathogenesis of acute gastric erosions. *Am. J. Gastroenterol.,* 62:405-409.

69. Hingson, D. J., and Ito, S. (1971): Effect of aspirin and related compounds on the fine structure of mouse gastric mucosa. *Gastroenterology,* 61:156-177.

70. Hung, C. R., Takeuchi, K., Okabe, S., Murata, T., and Takagi, K. (1976): Effects of L-glutamine on acetylsalycylic acid induced gastric lesions on acid back diffusion in dogs. *Jpn. J. Pharmacol.,* 26:703-709.

71. Ivey, K. J., Parsons, C., and Gray, C. (1974): Failure of lithium to provide a marker for gastric hydrogen ion back-diffusion in man. *Gastroenterology,* 66:69-72.

72. Jeffrey, S. W., and Smith, M. J. H. (1959): Some effects of salicylate on mitochondria from rat liver. *Biochem. J.,* 72:462-465.

73. Johnson, L. R. (1966): Histamine liberation by gastric mucosa of pylorus-ligated rats damaged by acetic or salicylic acids. *Proc. Soc. Exp. Biol. Med.,* 121:384-386.

74. Johnson, L. R. (1972): Pepsin secretion during damage by ethanol and salicylic acid. *Gastroenterology,* 62:412-416.

75. Johnson, L. R., and Overholt, B. F. (1967): Release of histamine into gastric venous blood following injury by acetic or salicylic acid. *Gastroenterology,* 52:505-509.

76. Jörgensen, T. G., Weis-Fogh, U. S., Nielsen, H. H., and Olesen, H. P. (1976): Salicylate- and aspirin-induced uncoupling of oxidative phosphorylation in mitochondria isolated from the mucosal membrane of the stomach. *Scand. J. Clin. Lab. Invest.,* 36:649-654.

77. Karppanen, H., Puurunen, J., Kairaluoma, M., and Larmi, T. (1976): Effects of ethyl alcohol on the adenosine 3′,5′-monophosphate system of the human gastric mucosa. *Scand. J. Gastroenterol.,* 11:603-607.

78. Kasbekar, D. K. (1973): Effects of salicylate and related compounds on gastric HCl secretion. *Am. J. Physiol.,* 225:521-527.

79. Kauffman, G. L., Jr., and Grossman, M. I. (1978): Prostaglandin and cimetidine inhibit the formation of ulcers produced by parenteral salicylates. *Gastroenterology,* 75:1099-1102.

80. Kauffman, G. L., and Grossman, M. I. (1979): Gastric alkaline secretion: Effect of topical and intravenous 16-16 dimethyl prostaglandin E_2. *Gastroenterology,* 76:1165.

81. Kawashima, K., and Glass, G. B. J. (1975): Alcohol injury to gastric mucosa in mice and its potentiation by stress. *Am. J. Dig. Dis.,* 20:162-172.

82. Kent, P. W., and Allen, A. (1968): The biosynthesis of intestinal mucins. *Biochem. J.,* 106:645-658.

83. Kivilaakso, E., Fromm, D., and Silen, W. (1978): Effect of the acid secretory state on intramural pH of rabbit gastric mucosa. *Gastroenterology,* 75:641-648.

84. Kivilaakso, E., Fromm, D., and Silen, W. (1978): Effects of lysolecithin on isolated gastric mucosa. *Surgery,* 84:616-621.

85. Kivilaakso, E., Fromm, D., and Silen, W. (1978): Relationship between ulceration and intramural pH of gastric mucosa during hemorrhagic shock. *Surgery,* 84:70-78.

86. Koelz, H. R., Fischer, J. A., Sachs, G., and Blum, A. L. (1978): Specific effect of acetylsalicylic acid on cation transport of isolated mucosal cells. *Am. J. Physiol.,* 235:E16-E21.

87. Kumar, R., and Ballimoria, J. D. (1978): Gastric ulceration and the concentration of salicylate in plasma in rats after administration of ^{14}C-labelled aspirin and its synthetic triglyceride, 1,3-dipalmitoyl-2 (2′-cetoxy-[14C] carboxylbenzoyl) glycerol. *J. Pharm. Pharmacol.,* 30:754-758.

88. Kuo, Y. J., and Shanbour, L. L. (1976): Inhibition of ion transport by bile salts in canine gastric mucosa. *Am. J. Physiol.,* 231:1433-1437.

89. Kuo, Y. J., and Shanbour, L. L. (1976): Mechanism of action of aspirin on canine gastric mucosa. *Am. J. Physiol.,* 230:762-767.

90. Lee, J. S., and Silverberg, J. W. (1976): Effect of histamine on

intestinal fluid secretion in the dog. *Am. J. Physiol.*, 231: 793-798.

91. Lim, J. K., Napang, P. K., Overman, D. O., and Jacknowitz, A. I. (1979): Beneficial effects of methionine and histidine in aspirin solutions on gastric mucosal damage in rats. *J. Pharm. Sci.*, 68:295-298.

92. Mangla, J. C., Kim, Y. M., and Rubulis, A. A. (1974): Adenyl cyclase stimulation by aspirin rat gastric mucosa. *Nature*, 250:61-62.

93. Mangla, J. C., Kim, Y. M., and Turner, M. D. (1974): Are pepsinogens activated in gastric mucosa after aspirin-induced injury? *Experientia*, 15:727-729.

94. Martin, B. K. (1963): Accumulation of drug anions in gastric mucosal cells. *Nature*, 198:896-897.

95. Martin, G. P., Marriott, C., and Kellaway, I. W. (1978): Direct effect of bile salts on phospholipids on the physical properties of mucus. *Gut*, 19:103-107.

96. Max, M., and Menguy, R. (1970): Influence of adrenocorticotropin, cortisone, aspirin, and phenylbutazone on the rate of exfoliation and the rate of renewal of gastric mucosal cells. *Gastroenterology*, 58:329-336.

97. Menguy, R. (1969): Gastric mucus and the gastric mucous barrier. *Am. J. Surg.*, 117:806-812.

98. Menguy, R., Desbaillets, L., and Masters, Y. F. (1974): Mechanism of stress ulcer: Influence of hypovolemic shock on energy metabolism in the gastric mucosa. *Gastroenterology*, 66:46-55.

99. Menguy, R., and Masters, Y. F. (1974): Mechanism of stress ulcer. II. Differences between the antrum, corpus, and fundus with respect to the effects of complete ischemia on gastric mucosal energy metabolism. *Gastroenterology*, 66:509-516.

100. Menguy, R., and Masters, Y. F. (1974): Mechanism of stress ulcer. III. Effects of hemorrhagic shock on energy metabolism in the mucosa of the antrum, corpus, and fundus of the rabbit stomach. *Gastroenterology*, 66:1168-1176.

101. Miller, T. A., and Jacobson, E. D. (1979): Gastrointestinal cytoprotection by prostaglandins. *Gut*, 20:75-87.

102. Mitznegg, P., Estler, C. J., Loew, F. W., and van Seil, J. (1977): Effect of salicylates on cyclic AMP in isolated rat gastric mucosa. *Acta Hepatogastroenterol.*, 24:372-376.

103. Mizek, S., and Spenney, J. G. (1978): Protein synthesis in aspirin injured gastric mucosa. *Clin. Res.*, 26:50A.

104. Moody, F. G., and Durbin, R. P. (1965): Effects of glycine and other instillates on concentration of gastric acid. *Am. J. Physiol.*, 209:122-126.

105. Moody, F. G., and Aldrete, J. S. (1971): Hydrogen permeability of canine gastric secretory epithelium during formation of acute superficial erosions. *Surgery*, 70:154-160.

106. Moody, F. G., and Davis, W. L. (1970): Hydrogen and sodium permeation of canine gastric mucosa during histamine and sodium thiocyanate administration. *Gastroenterology*, 59:350-357.

107. Newsome, L. R., and Leitch, G. J. (1978): Direct inhibition of gastrointestinal carbonic anhydrase by ethanol. *Digestion*, 17:370-373.

108. O'Brien, P., and Silen, W. (1973): Effect of bile salts and aspirin on the gastric mucosal blood flow. *Gastroenterology*, 64:246-253.

109. Okabe, S., Hung, C. R., Takeuchi, K., and Takagi, K. (1976): Effects of L-glutamine on acetylsalicylic acid or taurocholic acid-induced gastric lesions and secretory changes in pylorus-ligated rats under normal or stress conditions. *Jpn. J. Pharmacol.*, 26:455-460.

110. Okabe, S., Takeuchi, K., Honda, K., and Takagi, K. (1976): Effects of various amino acids on gastric lesions induced by acetylsalicylic acid (ASA) and gastric secretion in pylorus-ligated rats. *Drug Res.*, 26:534-537.

111. Overholt, B. F., Brodie, D. A., and Chase, B. J. (1969): Effect of the vargus nerve and salicylate administration on the permeability characteristics of the rat gastric mucosal barrier. *Gastroenterology*, 56:651-658.

112. Overholt, B. F., and Pollard, H. M. (1968): Acid diffusion into the human gastric mucosa. *Gastroenterology*, 54:182-189.

113. Pfeiffer, C. J., and Weibel, J. (1973): The gastric mucosal

114. Puurunen, K. H., and Kairaluoma, M. (1975): Effects of nonsteroidal anti-inflammatory drugs on cyclic nucleotide phosphodiesterase activities of the human gastric mucosa. *Scand. J. Rheumatol.*, 4:50.

115. Puurunen, J., and Karppanen, H. (1975): Effects of ethanol on gastric acid secretion and gastric mucosal cyclic AMP in the rat. *Life Sci.* 16:1513-1520.

116. Puurunen, J., Karppanen, H., Kairaluoma, M., and Larmi, T. (1976): Effects of ethanol on the cyclic AMP system of the dog gastric mucosa. *Eur. J. Pharmacol.*, 38:275-279.

117. Rainsford, K. D. (1978): Structure-activity relationships of nonsteroid anti-inflammatory drugs. 1. Gastric ulcerogenic activity. *Agents Actions.* 8/6:587-605.

118. Rainsford, K. D. (1978): The effects of aspirin and other nonsteroid anti-inflammatory/analgesic drugs on gastro-intestinal mucus glycoprotein biosynthesis in vivo. Relationship to ulcerogenic actions. *Biochem. Pharmacol.*, 27:877-885.

119. Rainsford, D. K., and Brune, K. (1978): Selective cytotoxic actions of aspirin on parietal cells: A principal factor in the early stages of aspirin-induced gastric damage. *Arch. Toxicol.*, 40:143-150.

120. Rainsford, K. D., and Whitehouse, M. W. (1976): Gastric irritancy of aspirin and its congeners: Anti-inflammatory activity without this side-effect. *J. Pharm. Pharmacol.*, 28:599-601.

121. Read, N. W., and Fordtran, J. S. (1979): The role of intraluminal junction potentials in the generation of the gastric potential difference in man. *Gastroenterology*, 76:932-938.

122. Rees, W. D. W., Rhodes, J., Wheeler, M. H., Meek, E. M., and Newcombe, R. G. (1977): The role of histamine receptors in the pathophysiology of gastric mucosal damage. *Gastroenterology*, 72:67-71.

123. Rehm, W. S. (1968): An analysis of the short-circuiting technique applied to *in vivo* tissues. *J. Theor. Biol.*, 20:341-354.

124. Rehm, W. S., and LeFevre, M. E. (1965): Effect of dinitrophenol on potential, resistance and H^+ rate of frog stomach. *Am. J. Physiol.*, 208:922-930.

125. Ritchie, W. P., Jr. (1974): Effect of hemorrhage on electrical and pH gradients in the intact stomach of the subhuman primate. *Gastroenterology*, 67:25-263.

126. Ritchie, W. P., Jr. (1975): Acute gastric mucosal damage induced by bile salts, acid, and ischemia. *Gastroenterology*, 68:699-707.

127. Ritchie, W. P., Jr., and Shearburn, E. W., III (1977): Influence of isoproterenol and cholestyramine on acute gastric mucosal ulcerogenesis. *Gastroenterology*, 73:62-65.

128. Robert, A. (1976): Antisecretory, antiulcer, cytoprotective and diarrheogenic properties of prostaglandins. In: *Advances in Prostaglandins and Thromboxane Research, Vol. 2*, Edited by B. Samuelsson and R. Paoletti, pp. 507-521. Raven Press, New York.

129. Sachs, G., Hirschowitz, B. I., and Shoemaker, R. L. (1972): Microelectrode studies of aspirin damage to gastric mucosa. *Gastroenterology*, 62:804.

130. Saik, R. P., and Brown, D. (1978): Lithium: not a sensitive indicator of hydrogen ion diffusion. *J. Surg. Res.*, 25:163-165.

131. Sato, N., Kamada, T., Kawano, S., Abe, H., and Hagihara, B. (1978): Oxidative and phosphorylative activities of the gastric mucosa of animals and humans in relation to the mechanism of stress ulcer. *Biochim. Biophys. Acta*, 538:236-243.

132. Sernka, T. J., and Jackson, A. F. (1975): Hyperosmotic instillation of rat stomach. *Life Sci.*, 17:435-442.

133. Silen, W. (1977): New concepts of the gastric mucosal barrier. *Am. J. Surg.*, 133:8-12.

134. Silen, W., and Forte, J. G. (1975): Effects of bile salts on amphibian gastric mucosa. *Am. J. Physiol.*, 228:637-644.

135. Skillman, J. J., Gould, S. A., Chung, R. S. K., and Silen, W. (1970): The gastric mucosal barrier: Clinical and experimental studies in critically ill and normal man, and in the rabbit. *Ann. Surg.*, 172:564-584.

136. Smith, B. M., Skillman, J. J., Edwards, B. G., and Silen, W. (1971): Permeability of the human gastric mucosa. *N. Engl. J. Med.*, 285:716-721.

response to acetylsalicylic acid in the ferret: An ultrastructural study. *Am. J. Dig. Dis.*, 18:834-846.

137. Smith, P., O'Brien, P., Fromm, D., and Silen, W. (1977): Secretory state of gastric mucosa and resistance to injury by exogenous acid. *Am. J. Surg.*, 133:81–85.

138. Spenney, J. G., and Brown, M. S. (1977): Effect of acetylsalicylic acid on gastric mucosa. II. Mucosal ATP and phosphocreatine content, and salicylate effects on mitochondrial metabolism. *Gastroenterology*, 73:995–999.

139. Spenney, J. G., Flemstrom, G., Shoemaker, R. L., and Sachs, G. (1975): Quantitation of conductance of pathways in antral mucosa. *J. Gen Physiol.*, 65:645–662.

140. Spenney, J. G., Shoemaker, R. L., and Sachs, G. (1974): Microelectrode studies of fundic gastric mucosa: Cellular coupling and shunt conductance. *J. Membr. Biol.*, 19:105–128.

141. Tague, L. L., and Shanbour, L. L. (1974): Effects of ethanol on gastric mucosal adenosine 3′ 5′ monophosphate (cAMP). *Life Sci.*, 14:1065–1073.

142. Teorell, T. (1933): Untersuchungen uber die magensaftsekretion. *Scand. Arch. Physiol.*, 66:225–230.

143. Thomas, A. J., Nahrwold, D. L., and Rose, R. C. (1972): Detergent action of sodium taurocholate on rat gastric mucosa. *Biochim. Biophys. Acta*, 282:210–213.

144. Thompkins, L., and Lee, K. H. (1969): Studies on the mechanism of action of salicylates IV: Effect of salicylates on oxidative phosphorylation. *J. Pharm. Sci.*, 58:102–105.

145. Ussing, H. H., and Zerahn, K. (1951): Active transport of sodium as the source of electric current in the short-circuited frog skin. *Acta Physiol. Scand.*, 23:110–127.

146. Waldron-Edward, D., DeCaens, C., Robert, A., Bader, J. P., Robert, L., and Labat-Robert, J. (1978): The effect of drugs and secretagogues on the biosynthesis of gastric mucins. *Biochem. Pharmacol.*, 27:2775–2780.

147. Wassef, M. K., Lin, Y. N., and Horowitz, M. I. (1978): Phospholipid-deacylating enzymes or rat stomach mucosa. *Biochim. Biophys. Acta*, 528:318–330.

148. Weisbrodt, N. W., Kienzie, M., and Cooke, A. R. (1973): Comparative effects of alipathic alcohols on the gastric mucosa. *Proc. Soc. Exp. Biol. Med.*, 142:450–454.

149. Werther, J. L. Janowitz, H. D. Dyck, W. P. Chapman, J. L. and Rudick, J. (1970): The effect of bile on electrolyte movement across canine gastric antral and fundic mucosa. *Gastroenterology*, 59:691–697.

150. Werther, J. L., and Horowitz, I. (1970): The effect of stress on the gastric mucosal barrier in rats. *Proc. Soc. Exp. Biol. Med.*, 154:415–417.

151. Willems, G., Vansteenkiste, Y., and Smets, P. H. (1971): Effects of ethanol on the cell proliferation kinetics in the fundic mucosa of dogs. *Am. J. Dig. Dis.*, 16:1057–1063.

152. Williams, S. E., and Turnberg, L. A. (1978): Gastric mucus: Studies of its "protective" properties. *Gut*, 19:A434.

153. Wlodek, G. K., and Leach, R. K. (1967): The Effect of histamine stimulation on the net ionic fluxes of Heidenhain and Pavlov fundic pouches. *Can. J. Surg.*, 10:47–52.

154. Wollin, A., Barnes, L. D., Hui, Y. S., and Dousa, T. P. (1975): Activation of protein kinase in the guinea pig fundic gastric mucosa by histamine. *Life Sci.* 17:1303–1306.

155. Yoemans, N. D. (1976): Electron microscopic study of the repair of aspirin-induced gastric erosions. *Dig. Dis.*, 21:533–541.

156. Zinner, M. J., Turtinen, B. A., and Gurll, N. J. (1975): The role of acid and ischemia in production of stress ulcers during canine hemorrhagic shock. *Surgery*, 77:807–816.

Physiology of the Gastrointestinal Tract, edited by
Leonard R. Johnson. Raven Press, New York © 1981.

Chapter 28

Electrophysiology of Exocrine Gland Cells

O. H. Petersen

Electrophysiology is important when considering ion transports across membranes and cells, since these depend on both chemical and electrical gradients. The superior resolution of modern methods has offered the opportunity to probe individual cells and apply substances at specific locations; it has made these microelectrophysiological techniques indispensable for a detailed examination of stimulus-secretion coupling modes in exocrine gland cells. This chapter deals quantitatively with the resting properties of the exocrine gland cell membranes and the effects of a variety of substrates, neurotransmitters, and peptide hormones. There are many different secretory cell types throughout the alimentary canal, and no attempt is made to deal with all of these. Most electrophysiological investigations have been carried out on various salivary glands, the stomach, the exocrine pancreas, and the liver. Since the electrophysiology of the stomach is dealt with in the chapter by Sachs, only results relating to salivary glands, pancreas, and liver are discussed here.

RESTING MEMBRANE PROPERTIES

Resting Membrane Potential

The resting membrane potential is measured as the electrical potential difference between the tip of a glass microelectrode inserted into a cell and a reference electrode in contact with the extracellular fluid space. Inevitably, a leak is created in the plasma membrane around the shaft of the inserted microelectrode. The success of the measurement depends essentially on the ability of the plasma membrane to seal the leak (85). As microelectrode techniques have improved, the magnitude of gland cell resting potentials has increased. Table 1 shows a set of recent values for the major salivary glands, the pancreas, and the liver. A detailed discussion of the evaluation of and the criteria for correct membrane potential measurements has been published (85).

TABLE 1. *Resting membrane potentials in some exocrine glands*

Cell	Ref.	Membrane potential (mV)
Mouse parotid acinar	74	− 69
Mouse submaxillary acinar	72	− 57
Rat submaxillary acinar	104	− 57
Rat parotid acinar	21	− 73
Mouse pancreas acinar	71	− 40
Rat pancreas acinar	71	− 36
Mouse liver parenchymal	81	− 39

Resting Input Resistance

Applying a square wave current pulse (I) across a cell membrane results in a membrane potential change (V_1) (Fig. 1). If the current pulse is long enough, a steady state is reached. The membrane potential displacement at steady state is related to the intensity of the applied current by Ohm's law:

$$V = RI$$

R is the input resistance. For salivary gland, pancreatic, and liver parenchymal cells the input resistance is relatively low, varying from about 0.6 MΩ in the mouse liver (26) to about 7 MΩ in the rat pancreas (71). Before anything was known about cell to cell communication, one might have assumed that individual cells were electrically isolated; in the pancreas, where the surface area of an acinar cell is about 582 μm^2 (4), the input resistance of 7 MΩ might have been thought to represent a specific membrane resistance of about 40 Ωcm^2. In fact, such low values were reported for both salivary glands (65) and liver (105). In view of our current knowledge on cell to cell communication, such low values are obviously wrong. It is now clear that the low input resistance in gland cells is not due to leakiness of the plasma membranes but to the extensive coupling networks. Variations in input resistance between different tissues are probably largely due to variations in the extent of these communication networks. Calculation of specific membrane resistance requires an evaluation of the cable properties of the tissues.

Cell to Cell Coupling

When two separate microelectrodes are inserted into neighboring cells and current pulses injected through one of the microelectrodes, electrotonic potential changes are recorded not only from the current injection cell but also from the neighbor (Fig. 1). Such current spread to adjacent cells was described for *Chironomus* salivary glands by Loewenstein (60) and for mammalian liver by Penn (75). In mammalian pancreas and salivary

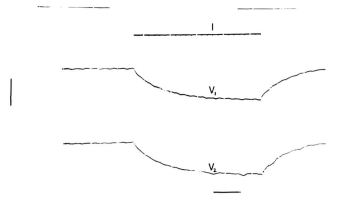

FIG. 1. Electrical coupling between two cells within the same mouse pancreatic acinus. A rectangular hyperpolarizing current pulse (I) was injected into cell 1 resulting in an electrotonic potential change (V_1) not only in the same cell but also in a neighboring cell (V_2). Calibration: Horizontal, 20 ms; vertical, 2 nA and 10 mV.

glands, cell to cell communication was first described some years later (82,93,103). In addition to electrical communication, it has also been shown that various organic fluorescent probes can pass directly from cell to cell. This demonstration was again first done on *Chironomus* salivary glands (62) but has recently been confirmed for mammalian pancreas (39,49) and salivary glands (31,54). In the pancreas, both fluorescein (MW, 332) and procion yellow (MW, 697) could be observed to move from the injection cell to adjacent neighboring cells (Fig. 2).

Cable Properties

In the liver, current spreads out in a regular three-dimensional network. The quantitative nature of the spatial distribution of electrotonic potentials due to a current point source has been investigated by Graf and Petersen (26) in superfused mouse liver segments. Figure 3 shows the steady-state amplitude of electrotonic potentials as a function of linear distance from the current source. In this situation, we are dealing with a two-dimensional infinite network having a finite thickness (d) of approximately 200 μm (26). Over short distances, the relationships shown (Fig. 3) are best described by the equation for three-dimensional current spread:

$$V_r = (R_i I_o / 4\pi r)\exp(-r/\lambda_3)$$

where r = radial distance from the current source, λ_3 = space constant, I_o = applied current, R_i = R_i'/f + $R_o/(1 - f)$, R_i' = intracellular resistivity, R_o = extracellular resistivity, and f = intracellular fraction of tissue volume.

The larger r becomes relative to the thickness (d), the more horizontal spread will predominate. The voltage distribution is best described by the equation for a two-dimensional system:

$$V_r = (R_i'I_0/2\pi d)K_0(r/\lambda_2)$$

where K_0 is a Bessel function.

An equation adequately describing the voltage distribution in the liver segments over a wide range of radial distances has been given (26):

$$V_r = 2 \sum_{N=1}^{\infty} \frac{I_0R_ie^{-\sqrt{r^2+(nd)^2}/\lambda_3^2}}{4\pi\sqrt{r^2+(nd)^2}} + \frac{I_0R_ie^{-r/\lambda_3}}{4\pi r}$$

The lines in Fig. 3 represent the theoretical relationship as calculated by this equation for d = 200 μm and space constants (λ_3) of 390, 455, 440, and 290 μm for control, sucrose, methylsulfate, and high K solutions, respectively.

In the mouse pancreas, the spatial voltage distribution caused by a current point source has also been investigated. Because of the irregular structure of this gland, there is no regular network as in the liver. Voltage fields were mapped by measuring electrotonic potentials from microelectrode puncture sites, as observed under a phase contrast microscope (47). It was discovered that within one acinus, there was virtually no decrement in the size of electrotonic potentials; i.e., the coupling coefficient (the ratio V_2/V_1, in which V_2 is the electrotonic potential change in cell 2 due to current injection in cell 1, while V_1 is the electrotonic potential change in cell 1, the current injection cell) remained 1 (Fig. 1). Neighboring acini belonging to the same cluster were also coupled, generally with relatively high coupling coefficients (> 0.5). Different clusters of acini were totally electrically isolated from each other. It was estimated that about 500 cells constitute one electrical unit.

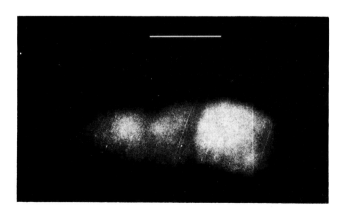

FIG. 2. Photograph taken through microscope (dark field) of the edge of mouse pancreas fragment placed in the perspex bath. A microelectrode filled with procion yellow is inserted into the cell to the right. Bar: 20 μm. ($\times$ 830.) Photograph taken 6 min after start of procion yellow ionophoresis (10 nA, 1/sec). The procion yellow has clearly spread from the injected cell to two cells to the left. (From Iwatsuki and Petersen, ref. 49.)

Resting Specific Membrane Resistance and Capacitance

Having obtained some quantitative information on the cable properties of the mouse liver and pancreas (26,47), it is possible to make approximate calculations of the specific membrane resistance.

In the mouse liver, the space constant for intracellular current spread ($\lambda_3 + \sqrt{R_m/XR_i}$) was 390 μm under control conditions. R_i, a measure including the intracellular resistivity and the junctional resistance, was found to be 1.4 kΩcm. From these values and an estimate of cell membrane density (X) obtained by Blouin et al. (3) and Weibel et al. (108), the specific membrane resistance was calculated to be 5.1 kΩcm^2 (26).

In the mouse exocrine pancreas, the mapping of voltage fields allowed the approximation that the tissue consisted of sphere-shaped units with a diameter of 110 μm and that current injected would spread uniformly over the entire electrical unit. The stereological work of Bolender (4) has yielded information on average acinar cell volume, cell density, and surface plasma membrane area from which the experimentally obtained value for the input resistance of about 5 MΩ could be calculated to represent a specific membrane resistance of about 14 kΩcm^2 (47).

The rising phase of current-evoked electrotonic membrane potential changes (Fig. 1) always followed an equation of the form:

$$V = RI(1 - e^{-t/RC})$$

where V is the potential change, R the input resistance, and C the capacitance; RC is termed the time constant. In the mouse pancreas, RC is about 15 msec. This allows calculation of C; again using the morphometric data of Bolender (4), a value for the specific membrane capacitance of 1.1 μF/cm^2 was calculated (47). Since the specific membrane capacitance can be regarded as a biological constant with a value close to 1 μF/cm^2 (11,18), this is a convenient check and indicates that the assumptions underlying these calculations are not unreasonable.

The resting specific membrane resistance values calculated for mouse liver and pancreas are of the same order of magnitude as those recently arrived at for *Necturus* gall bladder and urinary bladder (19,20).

Electrodiffusional Control of the Membrane Potential

The membrane potential is sensitive to changes in extracellular K concentration ($[K]_o$). As expected, those gland cells having high membrane potentials (salivary glands) are most sensitive to changes in $[K]_o$. In the parotid, the slope of the linear curve relating membrane potential to $\log[K]_o$ is about 50 mV per 10-fold increase in $[K]_o$ (above $[K]_o$ = 10 mM) (74). This is high but less than the theoretically expected 61 mV per 10-fold in-

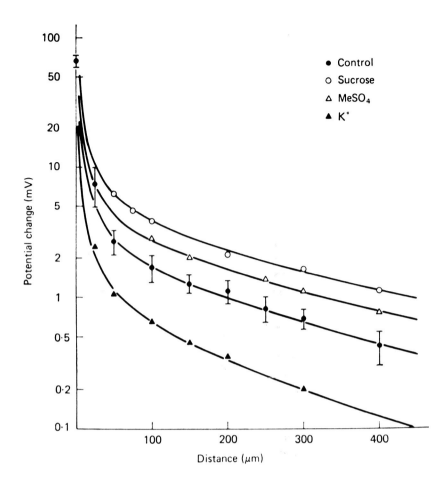

● Control
○ Sucrose
△ MeSO₄
▲ K⁺

FIG. 3. Relationship between the distance from the cell into which current was injected to the cell where the potential was measured and the steady state amplitude of electrotonic potential changes (logarithmic scale). *Filled circles,* mean values obtained from 38 preparations under control conditions; the other values were obtained from single preparations during superfusion with solutions of altered ionic composition. Current: 10^{-7} A. *Open circles,* NaCl replaced by sucrose (156 mM), $[Na^+]_o = 38.7$ mM, $[Cl^-]_o = 12.4$ mM. *Open triangles,* Cl^- replaced by methylsulfate, $[Cl^-]_o = 7.7$ mM. *Filled triangles,* Na^+ replaced by K^+, $[Na^+]_o = 46.4$ mM, $[K^+]_o = 100$ mM. The filled circle on the ordinate represents an extrapolated value obtained from input resistance measurements where current pulses generally smaller than 10^{-7} A were used. The lines represent the theoretical relationship calculated by the equation for a thickness of the layer of electrically coupled cells of 200 μm and space constants (λ_3) of 390, 455, 440, and 290 μm for control, sucrose, methylsulfate, and high K^+ solutions, respectively. Electrically coupled cells were occasionally encountered deeper than 200 μm from the superfused tissue surface. Curves calculated for d = 250 μm would fit the experimental data for control conditions if $\lambda_3 = 410$ μm and $R_i = 1.58$ kΩcm. (From Graf and Petersen, ref. 26.)

crease in $[K]_o$ for a K-selective membrane. Even the relatively high resting potential of -70 mV for the parotid is clearly less than the calculated K equilibrium potential (E_K):

$$E_K = 61.5 \log \frac{3.3}{116} \text{ mV} = -95 \text{ mV}$$

where 116 mM represents the intracellular K activity as measured directly in superfused mouse salivary gland segments by Poulsen and Oakley (99) and 3.3 mM represents the extracellular K activity (at a concentration of 4.7 mM, assuming an activity coefficient of 0.7). The membrane permeability, therefore, is predominated by K but with a contribution of other ions. In the mouse liver, Graf and Petersen (26) measured specific membrane resistance under various ionic conditions (Table 2). Two important pieces of information were obtained. The Cl conductance (G_{Cl}) of the membrane is very high, and the K conductance depends on $[K]_o$, i.e., increases with increasing $[K]_o$. The resting membrane ion conductance can be considered to consist of essentially three components: G_{Cl}, G_K, and G_{Na}. The results indicate that $G_{Cl} > G_K > G_{Na}$ (26). Although G_{Cl} is relatively high, Cl in the steady state does not influence the level of the resting potential (E_m); at least in the liver and the pancreas, Cl is passively distributed (85). The main

TABLE 2. *Specific membrane resistance ($k\Omega cm^2$) in mouse liver segment during exposure to saline solutions with different ionic concentrations[a]*

Saline solution	Specific membrane resistance ($K\Omega cm^2$)
Control (normal Krebs solution)	5
Low Cl (methylsulfate)	10
Low Na (choline)	7
Low NaCl (sucrose)	14
High K (100 mM)	0.6

[a]Values from Graf and Petersen (26).

reason for E_m being less negative than E_K would be a substantial Na contribution. In fact, in the liver, replacement of Na by choline caused a clear increase in specific membrane resistance (Table 2).

Role of Electrogenic Pump

The most dramatic demonstration of a direct pump contribution to the membrane potential can be achieved by reactivating maximally a previously blocked Na-K pump. Experimentally, this was achieved by exposing superfused pancreatic fragments to K-free solutions for more than 1 hr. This arrests the Na-K pump, since extracellular K is required for the operation; therefore, intracellular K is lost and Na accumulates. The resting potential becomes very low (Fig. 4). Readmitting, K to the extracellular solution in the normal concentration (4.7 mM) results in an immediate marked hyperpolarization, which is blocked by the specific inhibitor of the Na-K pump ouabain (80) (Fig. 4). It has further been shown that (a) ouabain added during the K-induced hyperpolarization immediately abolished the potential change (80); (b) the K-induced hyperpolarization is not accompanied by a resistance change (73); (c) a K-induced initial hyperpolarization can be seen even when K is admitted in such a high concentration that the K equilibrium potential is less negative than the membrane potential at the time of readmission (25); and (d) the K-induced hyperpolarization occurs much quicker than the reestablishment of a normal intracellular [K] (99). There is now abundant direct evidence for the electrogenic character of the Na-K pump in mammalian gland cell membranes.

During normal resting conditions, however, the direct pump contribution to the resting potential is relatively small. Thus in both the pancreas and liver, ouabain application causes only an immediate depolarization of a few millivolts (25,80). Thus it is only under conditions of extreme intracellular Na loading that a direct pump contribution to the resting potential becomes dominant.

Linear Properties of Resting Membrane

If the plasma membrane behaved as an Ohmic resistor, there would be direct proportionality between mem-

brane potential change and intensity of applied current; i.e., the current-voltage (I/V) relationship would be linear. The resistance of the membrane, however, is made up of conductance pathways for various ions. For an individual ion, x, the following equation must apply (36):

$$I_x = G_x (E_m - E_x)$$

where I is current, G, conductance, E_m the membrane potential, and E_x the equilibrium potential for ion x. The current flow is clearly zero when the electrochemical potential gradient ($E_m - E_x$) is zero. Applying the Goldman-Hodgkin-Katz equation (24,37) to the I/V relationship for individual ions, it can be predicted that for K and Cl there is an outward going rectification (membrane passes outward current in preference to inward current), while for Na the opposite applies. Since the membranes are dominated mainly by K and Cl, we might expect the I/V relationship to be slightly curved, corresponding to outward going rectification (85). In practice, however, certainly for the pancreas, salivary glands, and liver (26,42,73,104), the relationship between membrane potential and current appears to be approximately linear within a limited range of membrane potentials (Fig. 5).

MEMBRANE EFFECTS OF STIMULANTS

The exocrine pancreas is by far the best investigated gland in the digestive tract with respect to stimulant-evoked changes in membrane potential and resistance. The pancreatic acinar cells are discussed first, since

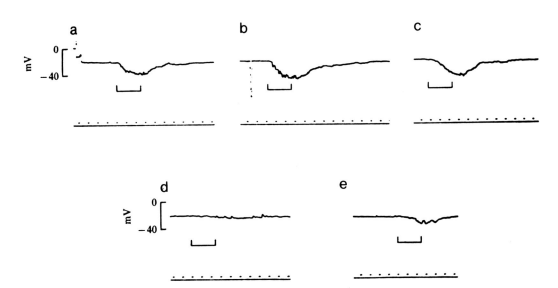

FIG. 4. Effect of short periods of K (4.7 mM) readmission (indicated by the horizontal bars) to a K-free solution on the pancreatic acinar cell membrane potential. All tracings are from the same cell. The time interval between consecutive tracings is 20 min. **a:** Impalement of cell (70 min after beginning superfusion with potassium-free solution. **b:** A 50-mV calibration signal (in steps of 10 mV) was applied. **a,b,c:** K readmission effects in the absence of any drug. **d:** Strophanthin-G (ouabain) (10^{-3} M) was present (introduced 5 min before the readmission of K) was shown. **e:** Recovery after removal of ouabain. Distance between time markings is 1 min. (From Petersen, ref. 80.)

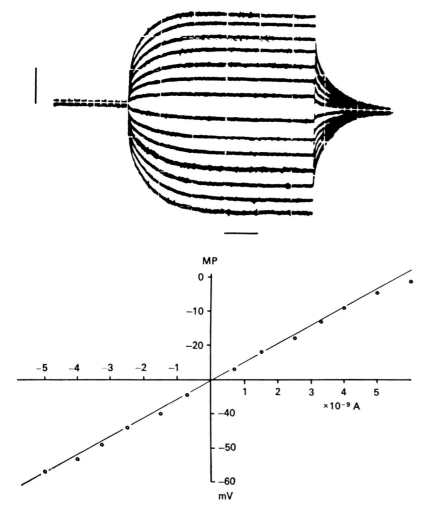

FIG. 5. Current-voltage relationship from resting mouse pancreatic acinus. Oscilloscope picture (**top**) shows electrotonic potential changes in response to rectangular de- or hyperpolarizing current pulses (not shown). Calibration: Horizontal, 20 msec; vertical 10 mV. **Bottom:** plot of the steady-state current-voltage relationship using the data from the oscilloscope picture. MP, membrane potential. (From Iwatsuki and Petersen, ref. 42.)

many points are likely to be valid also when considering the salivary glands and the liver.

Pancreatic Acini

Electrophysiological Characterization of Membrane Recognition Sites

The exocrine pancreas is stimulated to secrete by vagal nerve stimulation and by a variety of hormones (see chapters in this volume by Wood, Walsh, Gardner, and Meyer). Electrophysiological studies carried out on the rat pancreas *in vivo* have shown acinar cell membrane depolarization and resistance reduction in response to electrical stimulation of the cervical vagal nerves and to local as well as intravenous application of cholecystokinin (CCK), gastrin, and acetylcholine (ACh), while secretin has no effect (13,92). Detailed characterization of hormone receptor sites cannot be carried out in an *in vivo* preparation. In superfused isolated segments of mouse or rat pancreas, it is possible to define separate activation sites, their location, and the time course of cell activation.

Effects of nerve stimulation.

The best technique for nerve stimulation in the *in vitro* preparation is to use electrical field stimulation (FS) (12,70). FS evoked membrane depolarization, as did local microionophoretic application of ACh. Both effects were blocked by atropine. In the presence of atropine, FS never evoked any membrane effects. Effects were obtained at stimulation frequencies (2 to 5 Hz) likely to occur under physiological conditions, although maximal responses were obtained only at 20 or 40 Hz. The pancreatic acinar cells were never responsive to single shocks. At a stimulation frequency of, for example, 5 Hz, it was necessary to continue the stimulation for 5 to 10 sec to be able to observe a depolarization. The minimum latency for FS-evoked depolarization (at 40 Hz) was about 500 msec—a value of the same order of magnitude as for local ionophoretic ACh application (73).

Effects of FS were abolished by tetrodotoxin (TTX) (specific blocker of Na channels) (Fig. 6), indicating that FS works by exciting nerves in the pancreatic tissues. Spontaneous miniature depolarizations, fre-

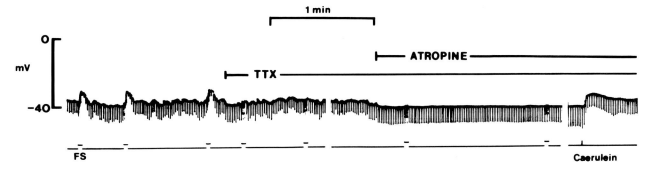

FIG. 6. Effects of TTX (10^{-6} M) and atropine (1.4×10^{-6} M) on mouse pancreatic acinar cell membrane potential and resistance. FS at marker signals indicates electric shocks of 10 V strength and 2 msec duration at a frequency of 40 Hz. The field stimulus was applied through two extracellular platinum electrodes placed on the surface of the pancreatic tissue. Throughout this recording, intracellular current pulses (1 nA, 100 msec) were repetitively applied, giving rise to the short vertical bars (electronic potentials) indicating input resistance. At marker signal labeled cerulein, one drop of 20 µg/ml cerulein solution was applied directly into the bath. The two breaks in the record represent 2 and 4 min intervals, respectively. (From Davison et al., ref. 12.)

quently observed in acini, were not affected by TTX (Fig. 6). That these depolarizations were also blocked by atropine (Fig. 6) indicates the existence of spontaneous transmitter release from nerve endings surrounding the acini. Indeed, Ca deprivation abolished both FS-evoked effects and spontaneous miniature depolarizations. All acinar cells investigated responded to FS. Since there is an extensive coupling network in the pancreas consisting of several neighboring acini, this need not indicate innervation of each acinar cell. Clearly, the innervation is less impressive than in, for example, the salivary glands, where single shock stimulation (also when applied as FS) is effective in eliciting a membrane potential change.

ACh released from nerve endings acts on the outside of the acinar cell membrane. The long delay of cell activation (0.5 sec), even when ACh is added by microionophoresis from the tip of a pipette located only a few microns from the acinar membrane (Fig. 7), made it imperative to consider a possible intracellular action of ACh. Iwatsuki and Petersen (41), however, showed that ACh evoked membrane depolarization only when added to the outside of the acinar membrane and not when injected intracellularly.

Effect of stimulation with peptides belonging to the gastrin and bombesin families.

Gastrin, pentagastrin, tetragastrin, CCK, and the amphibian skin peptide cerulein are peptides that share a common C-terminal tetrapeptide (28) (see Chapter 3 by Walsh). All evoke acinar cell depolarization and resistance reduction (40,46,71,89a,92). This membrane effect is not blocked by atropine. The relative potency of the various gastrin-like peptides in producing electrical effects is similar to their relative potency in evoking enzyme secretion. More recently, it has been shown that another amphibian skin peptide, bombesin, and its nonapeptide derivative, structurally quite different from the group of

gastrin-like peptides, also evoke membrane effects indistinguishable from those seen after ACh or nerve stimulation. Bombesin effects are also observed when ACh effects have been blocked by atropine (46,90). The minimum delay for cell activation by even close local extracellular peptide application (microionophoresis) is about 0.5 sec, i.e., similar to that shown for nerve stimulation or local ACh administration (Fig. 7).

Although the effects of gastrin-like peptides and bombesin peptides are indistinguishable, they are mediated by two different receptors. As seen in Fig. 8, dibutyryl-cyclic guanosine monophosphate (db-cGMP) applied externally will block the actions of cerulein (and also those of CCK and gastrin) without affecting the response to bombesin stimulation. Although there have been reports of penetration of peptide hormones into the intracellular space of several target tissues, injection of secretagogue peptides into acinar cells failed to evoke the characteristic potential and conductance changes observed following extracellular applications (97).

Lack of effect on acinar cells of stimulation with secretin and vasoactive intestinal peptide. Petersen and Ueda (92) showed that secretin in doses highly effective in eliciting fluid and bicarbonate secretion had no effect on acinar cell membrane potential and resistance. Cells not responsive to secretin always responded normally to subsequent stimulation with ACh or CCK. Secretin also had no effect on ACh- or CCK-evoked membrane effects. Similarly, the related vasointestinal peptide (VIP) failed to evoke any acinar membrane effects (G.T. Pearson, *unpublished*). Greenwell (27) has shown that certain cells in the mouse pancreas not responding to ACh or CCK stimulation (presumably ductal) react to secretin with hyperpolarization. This phenomenon has not been studied further.

Effects of amino acids.

A number of amino acids, e.g., alanine, valine, serine, and proline, evoke acinar cell membrane depolar-

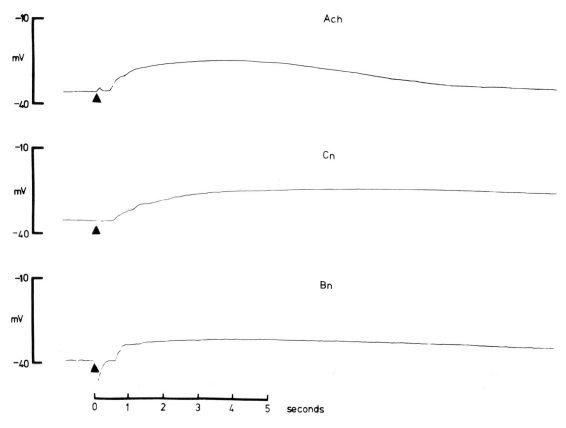

FIG. 7. Measurement of cell latency responses to ionophoretic application of acetylcholine (ACh), cerulein (Cn), and bombesin nonapeptide (Bn). **Upper trace:** ACh stimulation. A positive ejection current of 100 nA for 100 msec was applied through the ACh micropipette onto the surface of the pancreatic tissue and close to the impaled cell. *Arrow,* beginning of the stimulus artifact. **Middle trace:** Recording of acinar cell membrane potential from another mouse pancreas. A negative current pulse was passed through the cerulein micropipette (100 nA, 100 msec duration) to eject cerulein near the surface of the impaled cell. **Lower trace:** Bombesin ionophoresis (1,000 nA positive ejection current, 100 msec duration) near an impaled acinar cell. During the cerulein and bombesin ionophoresis experiments, the tissues were superfused with Krebs solution containing atropine (10^{-6} M). (From Petersen and Philpott, ref. 90.)

izentation and resistance reduction. Superficially, the depolarization in response to a pulse of local microionophoretic L-alanine application looks similar to ACh-evoked depolarization. Whereas the effect of ACh is blocked by atropine, however, the amino acid response persists. A number of transported L-amino acids are effective in evoking depolarization, but the D-isomers evoke only small responses. While the secretagogue-evoked membrane effects are characterized by a substantial delay of about 0.5 sec (Fig. 7), the depolarizing responses to local microionophoretic L-amino acid applications are virtually immediate (Fig. 9) (52).

Control of Membrane Resistance

Effects of stimulants on plasma membrane and junctional membrane resistance.

Exploiting the experimental fact that neighboring acinar cells within an acinus are so closely electrically coupled that there is no measurable resistance between them, one can treat different cells within an acinus as if

they were parts of one cell. Inserting two microelectrodes into the same acinus makes it possible to obtain measurements of ACh-evoked membrane resistance changes (Fig. 10). Application of short pulses of ACh (by microionophoresis) causes a marked reduction in membrane resistance and time constant of electrotonic potentials. The electrical time constant (RC) is reduced by the action of ACh in proportion to the reduction in resistance (R), indicating a constant capacitance (C) (surface plasma membrane area). Using slightly larger pulses of extracellular ACh application, an additional membrane effect is apparent.

Figure 11 shows an experiment in which simultaneous recordings from two coupled neighboring acini were made. A short ACh pulse evoked only the already described surface membrane resistance reduction. A larger one, after the initial resistance reduction, was seen to cause a substantial increase in the magnitude of electrotonic potentials in the current injection acinus, while the electrotonic potentials virtually disappeared in the neighboring acinus. The increase in size of R was not accompanied by a corresponding increase in RC, indi-

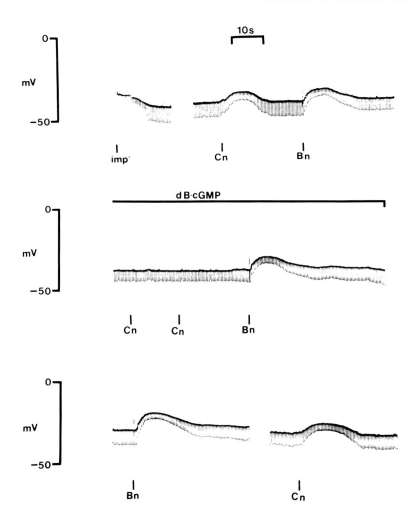

FIG. 8. Effect of cerulein (Cn) and bombesin nonapeptide (Bn) on membrane potential and resistance in pancreatic acinus. db-cGMP (1 mM) blocks reversibly the action of cerulein without interfering with the response to bombesin. The consecutive traces shown are all excerpts from the same continuous recording. imp, Cell impalement by microelectrode. Intervals between traces are from 5 to 23 min. Bombesin and cerulein were applied from two separate extracellular micropipettes by microionophoresis. (From Philpott and Petersen, ref. 96.)

cating a reduction of C. It is clear that this is a stimulant-evoked electrical uncoupling of neighboring acini. It is also possible to cause uncoupling of cells within an acinus; but this requires even larger and longer ACh pulses (43,44,47,88). ACh evokes a range of membrane effects: decrease of plasma membrane resistance, electrical uncoupling of neighboring acini (acinar-duct cell uncoupling), and electrical uncoupling of neighboring acinar cells (within individual acini). Secretagogues belonging to the gastrin and bombesin families have an identical range of effects (46,47,88).

Application of transported L-amino acids to the outside of pancreatic acini also evokes reduction of plasma membrane resistance; in relation to the size of the evoked depolarization, the resistance change is modest, as compared with the effects of secretagogues. Amino acids never evoked electrical uncoupling of neighboring acini or neighboring cells within one acinus (52).

Dose-response curves for plasma membrane depolarization and resistance reduction.

The existence of two different types of membrane resistance changes (surface membrane and junctional membrane) complicates the presentation of dose-response curves for secretagogue-evoked reduction in plasma membrane resistance. As demonstrated in Fig. 11, however, the two processes have different time courses. The reduction in input resistance accompanied by reduction of electrical time constant always precedes the increase in input resistance caused by the uncoupling. Dose-response curves were obtained by superfusing fragments of tissue with solutions containing known concentrations of secretagogue.

Figure 12 shows an example of the effects evoked by 10^{-10} M cerulein. Maximal depolarization and minimum resistance were attained after about 1 min exposure to cerulein. Thereafter, the input resistance increased because of uncoupling. For the purpose of constructing dose-response curves for the surface membrane effect, the values for potential and resistance obtained 1 min after start of stimulation would be used. Examples of such dose-response curves compared to a dose-response curve for amylase secretion is shown in Fig. 13. Clearly, bombesin is effective in regulating plasma membrane resistance and potential over the same concentration range that controls amylase secretion. Similar findings have been made for ACh and gastrin-like peptides (85).

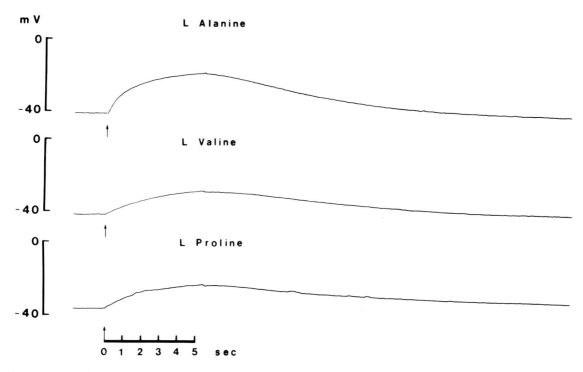

FIG. 9. Measurement of cell latency responses to ionophoretic application of L-alanine, L-valine, and L-proline. At marker signals, positive currents of 800 nA strength for 5 sec were applied through extracellular micropipettes filled with 1 M L-alanine, 0.5 M L-valine, or L-proline, respectively.

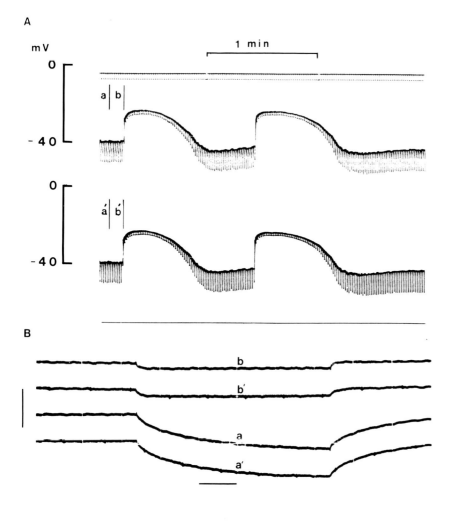

FIG. 10. Effect of local ACh application (microionophoresis) on pancreatic acinar membrane potential and resistance. **A:** Continuous pen recordings. Two simultaneous membrane potential measurements are shown. Current pulses (2 nA, 100 msec) were repetitively injected through the microelectrode recording the lower of the two potential traces. The current pulses evoked electrotonic potential changes (short-lasting potential deflections) in both injection cell (*lower trace*) and neighboring cell (*upper trace*). ACh was applied by microionophoresis from an extracellular micropipette (80 nA, 500 msec) at marker signals in bottom event-marker trace. **B:** Time course of the electrotonic potentials before (a, a′, taken at time indicated in **A**) and during stimulation (b, b′, taken at time indicated in **A**) is shown in the oscilloscope picture. Calibration in **B** is: Horizontal, 20 msec; vertical, 10 mV. (From Iwatsuki and Petersen, ref. 47.)

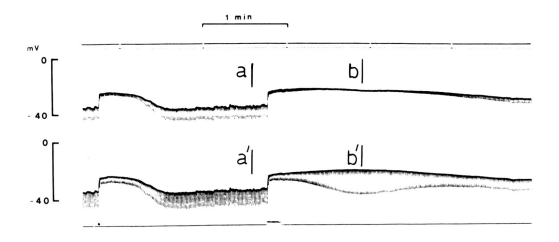

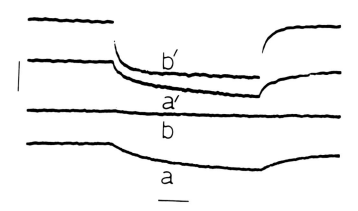

FIG. 11. Membrane potential and resistance measurements from two neighboring acini. The microelectrode recording the potential represented by the lower of the two traces in the pen recording was also used for repetitively passing hyperpolarizing current pulses (2.5 nA, 100 msec). For the duration of the marker signals in the bottom pen recording trace, ejecting current was passed through an extracellular AChCl-filled micropipette (60 nA, retaining current: 20 nA). The time course of the electrotonic potential changes before (a, a', at time indicated in pen recording) and during the action of ACh (b, b', at time indicated in pen recording) is shown in the oscilloscope picture. Calibration: Horizontal, 20 msec; vertical, 10 mV. (From Iwatsuki and Petersen, ref. 47.)

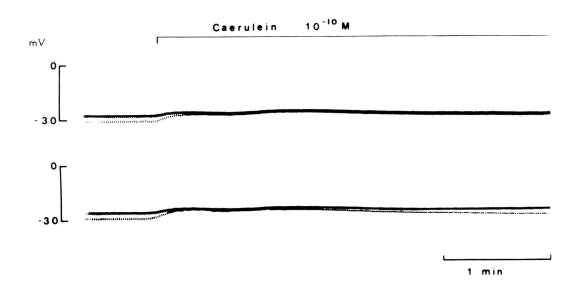

FIG. 12. Effect of cerulein (0.1 nM) on membrane potential, resistance, and cell-to-cell coupling. Current pulses (2 nA, 100 msec) injected through electrode recording lower potential trace. Note gradual increase in size of electrotonic potential changes in current-injection cell. (From Iwatsuki and Petersen, ref. 47.)

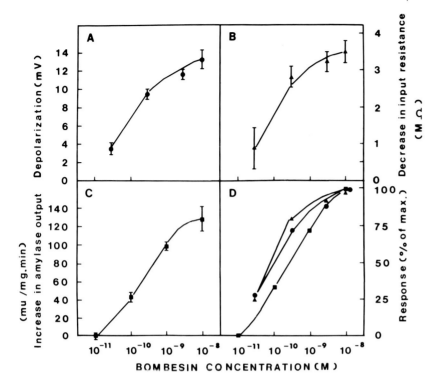

FIG. 13. Effect of bombesin on rat pancreatic acinar cell membrane potential, membrane resistance, and amylase secretion. Each point is mean ± SE. (N, 3 to 11). **A** and **B**: Data from the same cells of the same glands. **C**: Maximal increase in amylase output, expressed as milliunits amylase activity per milligram pancreatic tissue (wet weight) per minute. **D**: Results shown in **A**, **B**, and **C** are plotted together to enable comparison. (From Iwatsuki and Petersen, ref. 46.)

For L-alanine, small depolarizations were observed at 0.1 mM, with maximal effects occurring at 10 mM (52). Thus, while the peptide secretagogues are effective in evoking membrane resistance reduction at nanomolar or picomolar concentrations, the amino acids evoke effects only at millimolar concentrations.

Ionic mechanism of stimulant-evoked plasma membrane resistance reduction and depolarization.

The best way to determine the ion selectivity of the membrane channels opened by the action of an agonist is to determine the null (equilibrium or reversal) potential. The value of the null potential itself gives important information on ion channel permeability, and more can be learned by observing its ionic dependency. Figure 14 shows that the ACh null potential (E_{ACh}) in mouse pancreatic acini is about -15 mV. The null potential of nerve stimulation-induced effects (E_{FS}) is similar to E_{ACh} (12). At the null potential, the stimulant does not evoke any net current through the opened pathways. Therefore, the Goldman-Hodgkin-Katz equation can be used:

$$E = 61.5 \log \frac{P_K[K]_o + P_{Na}[Na]_o + P_{Cl}[Cl]_i}{P_K[K]_i + P_{Na}[Na]_i + P_{Cl}[Cl]_o} \qquad [1]$$

P_K, P_{Na}, etc., represent the permeabilities of the ACh-opened channels. Normally, only the contributions of the major monovalent ions are considered; this is indeed a reasonable approach (42,91). By measuring E_{ACh} also

during steady-state exposure to a Cl-free sulfate solution, it has been possible to calculate the relative permeabilities of the channels opened by ACh for Na, K, and Cl. P_{Cl} is about five time higher than P_K, while P_{Na} is approximately 2.5 times higher than P_K. At the ACh null potential, where the sum of the current flow through the transmitter-operated channels is 0, it is also possible to calculate the relative sizes of the Na, K, and Cl currents. $I_{Na}/I_K = 2.6$, while $I_{Cl}/I_K = 1.6$. The Na current is inward, while the Cl and K currents are outward. This means that ACh mainly causes an influx of NaCl with only a small K outflux.

The null potentials for the action of hormones belonging to the gastrin-CCK group and for peptides belonging to the bombesin group are identical to that determined for the action of ACh (46,90). Although a detailed ionic analysis has not been carried out for the action of the peptides, they probably operate the same ion channels as ACh.

In contrast, the action of the amino acids is completely different. The null potential for the action of L-alanine ($E_{alanine}$) is about $+40$ mV. This is very close to the calculated value of E_{Na}, indicating that the amino acid-evoked depolarization is caused by opening of conductance pathways selectively permeable to Na (52).

A common messenger may exist for secretagogues belonging to three different groups (ACh, gastrin, and bombesin) whose interactions with three different receptor sites operate the same ionic channels. Since all the secretagogues evoking membrane conductance changes also evoke marked changes in ^{45}Ca efflux from pre-

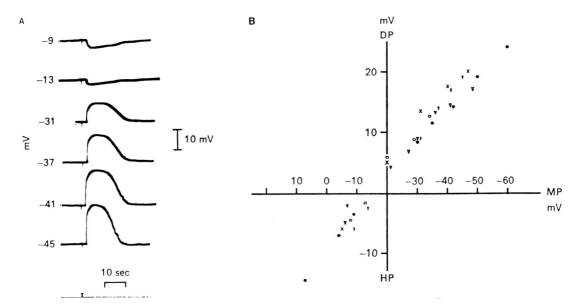

FIG. 14. Measurement of ACh null potential (E$_{ACh}$) in mouse pancreatic acinus. **A:** Family of traces showing effect of microionophoretic ACh application (bottom trace marker signal) at different resting membrane potentials (values written to the left of individual traces). The membrane potential was shifted by applying direct current through a separate intracellular microelectrode. **B:** Plot of data from six different mouse pancreatic acini. Crosses represent the results from **A**. DP or HP, ACh-evoked de- or hyperpolarization; MP, membrane potential. (From Iwatsuki and Petersen, ref. 42.)

labeled tissue (23,67), the internal messenger could be Ca. Intracellular Ca application specifically evokes membrane depolarization and resistance reduction (Fig. 15). The null potential for this action of Ca is about −16 mV, i.e., a value similar to that obtained for the secretagogue actions (43,87). Furthermore, it has been shown recently (89) that intracellular EGTA (Ca chelating agent) injection inhibits secretagogue-evoked membrane depolarization and resistance reduction. It seems likely, therefore, that Ca is the intracellular mediator of the secretagogue-evoked, but of course not the amino acid-evoked, membrane effects.

Membrane depolarizations evoked by short pulses of ACh application are not sensitive to even prolonged exposure of the tissue to Ca-free solutions. In contrast, it is possible to show a clear Ca dependence of the secretagogue-evoked membrane effects during sustained stimulation (58). While sustained stimulation (over 10 to 20 min) causes sustained membrane depolarization and resistance reduction in a normal ionic milieu, only a transient effect was observed in the absence of external Ca, despite continued stimulation. If, during sustained stimulation, Ca is removed, the membrane response is abolished. The effect is reversible upon readmission of Ca (Fig. 16). Clearly, Ca in the initial phase must come from an internal source (most likely the plasma membrane), while in the sustained phase Ca enters from the interstitial fluid. Although external Ca is critical for sustained secretagogue-evoked membrane depolarization, the ion is not essential for amino acid-induced depolarization. Thus during sustained depolarization evoked

by continued amino acid exposure, removal of external Ca has virtually no effect (89).

Salivary Gland Acini

Electrophysiological Characterization of Membrane Recognition Sites

Salivary gland secretion is regulated mainly by parasympathetic and sympathetic nerves through release of the transmitters ACh and norepinephrine. Both transmitters stimulate secretion. ACh mainly causes secretion of fluid, whereas norepinephrine also has a marked effect on release of protein. More recently, it has been shown that substance P (SP) and related peptides can evoke salivation.

Effects of parasympathetic nerve stimulation.

The classic work of Lundberg (64) showed that electrical stimulation of the chorda tympani caused a characteristic membrane potential change in acinar cells, which was blocked by atropine. All acinar cells responded to stimulation. The innervation appeared dense since it was common to obtain membrane responses to single shock stimulation. Similar findings have been made by Kagayama and Nishiyama (53).

A more detailed study of the effects of nerve stimulation has been carried out using an isolated *in vitro* preparation in which electrical FS can excite nerves within the tissue (22). In the mouse parotid, at least, FS

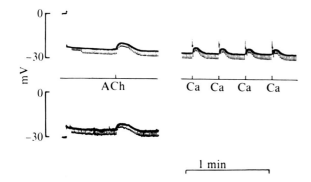

FIG. 15. Mouse pancreatic acinus; action of extracellular ACh and intracellular Ca^{2+} on membrane potential and resistance. **Left:** Effect of a short pulse of ionophoretic ACh application $(6 \times 10^{-8}$ A, 0.5 sec, retaining current 2×10^{-8} A) on membrane potential and resistance in two electrically coupled acinar cells. *Upper trace,* potential measured by an intracellular KCl electrode through which hyperpolarizing rectangular current pulses $(2 \times 10^{-9}$ A, 100 msec duration) were injected repeatedly. *Lower trace,* membrane potential of a neighboring cell recorded with a $CaCl_2$ electrode. At the point of interruption of the tracings, the $CaCl_2$ electrode was disconnected from the recording system and connected to a stimulator so that current could be injected through the electrode. At the marker signals labeled Ca^{2+}, 5 nA, 0.5 sec depolarizing current pulses were applied through the Ca^{2+} electrode. (From Iwatsuki and Petersen, ref. 43.)

results in effects mediated by cholinergic nerves. All membrane effects evoked by FS are blocked by atropine. The FS effects are attributable to induction of action potentials in nerves, since TTX specifically blocks the responses. Figure 17 shows membrane potential changes in response to single electrical shocks. The minimal latency for FS-evoked responses was between 180 and 300 msec. With repetitive stimulation at low frequencies, a sequence of separate depolarizations could be observed. At somewhat higher frequencies, these fused to a continued depolarization. At high stimulation

frequencies, cessation of stimulation was associated with an initial marked hyperpolarization before the potential returned to the prestimulation control level (Fig. 18).

Effects of local microionophoretic ACh application were similar to those seen after FS (Fig. 19). The response to microionophoretic ACh application was also blocked by atropine. The minimal latency of the potential change evoked by close microionophoretic application was similar to that observed with FS. The effects of FS were not inhibited by catecholamine antagonists, such as phentolamine and propranolol. The major difference between FS and local microionophoretic ACh application is that in the absence of Na or Ca, FS quickly ceases to have any effect, whereas the responses to local ACh application are retained, although in a somewhat altered form. The Na dependence of FS-evoked responses is attributable to the failure of nerve transmission in the absence of Na, whereas the Ca dependence is explained by the Ca requirement for ACh secretion from nerve terminals (22).

Effects of sympathetic nerve stimulation.

Lundberg (64) demonstrated acinar cell potential changes in response to stimulation of cervical sympathetic nerves. Kagayama and Nishiyama (53) studied this phenomenon further. In contrast to parasympathetic stimulation, single electrical shocks never evoked cell responses. Following repetitive stimulation, responses similar to those obtained after parasympathetic stimulation were obtained. The minimal latency for cell depolarizations evoked by sympathetic nerve stimulation were about 500 msec, a long latency compared to the 180 msec seen with parasympathetic nerve stimulation.

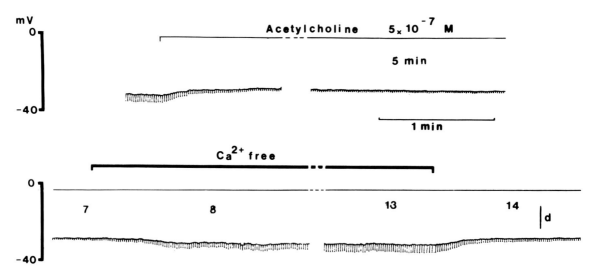

FIG. 16. Mouse pancreatic acinus; effect of omitting and readmitting Ca (2.6 mM) on membrane potential and resistance during sustained ACh stimulation. Current pulses (2 nA, 100 msec) were injected into a neighboring coupled cell. Time (minutes) refers to the start of ACh stimulation, which was sustained throughout the period represented by this trace. (From Laugier and Petersen, ref. 58.)

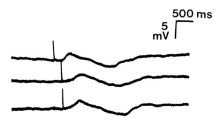

FIG. 17. Oscilloscope picture showing membrane potential responses to single shock stimuli (2 msec, 15 V). The three responses are from the same parotid acinar cell. The resting membrane potential is −65 mV in each case, although they have been displaced on the screen for presentation. Vertical bars preceding each response are the stimulus artifacts. (From Gallacher and Petersen, ref. 22.)

The effects of sympathetic nerve stimulation could be mimicked by epinephrine or norepinephrine. Unfortunately, nerve stimulation experiments have not been carried out *in vitro* since the effects of electrical FS, at least in the isolated mouse parotid, were mediated by parasympathetic nerves (22).

The technique of local microionophoretic drug application *in vitro* has been extensively used to characterize the membrane response to catecholamines. As seen in Fig. 19, epinephrine causes a membrane electrical response similar to that evoked by local ACh application. This response is caused by the interaction with α-adrenoceptors, since it is blocked by phentolamine in a concentration (10^{-5} M) that does not interfere with isoproterenol-evoked enzyme secretion (22,86). While the epinephrine-evoked potential and conductance change disappear after phentolamine addition, a small, delayed depolarization not associated with any clear conductance change appears. This effect is abolished by β-adrenergic blockade (propranolol).

In the mouse parotid, ionophoretic application of isoproterenol evokes a response similar to that seen after epinephrine in the presence of phentolamine, namely, a small, delayed (minimal latency 4 sec) depolarization not accompanied by a resistance change (104). The β-component in the epinephrine response is generally inconspicuous, but in some cases it is possible to observe a slight modification of the epinephrine-evoked potential change after propranolol. Phenylephrine (α-agonist) evokes membrane responses similar to those seen after epinephrine application. The minimal latency for epinephrine-evoked depolarization is 300 to 400 msec (22,104).

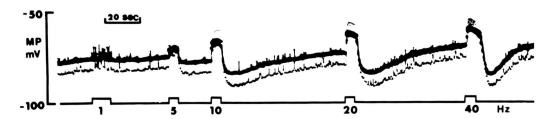

FIG. 18. Continuous recording of parotid acinar membrane potential and input resistance (current pulses 1.5 nA hyperpolarizing, 100 msec). Note the spontaneous miniature depolarizations and fluctuations in input resistance. The response to electrical FS (1 msec 15 V) at 1, 5, 10, 20, and 40 Hz is shown. At 1 Hz, the response is a train of spikes identical to the miniature depolarizations. At 5 Hz, the response is a sustained depolarization with a reduction in input resistance. At 10 to 40 Hz, the initial depolarization is followed by a delayed hyperpolarization, increasing in magnitude with frequency, during which the input resistance returns to normal. (From Gallacher and Petersen, ref. 22.)

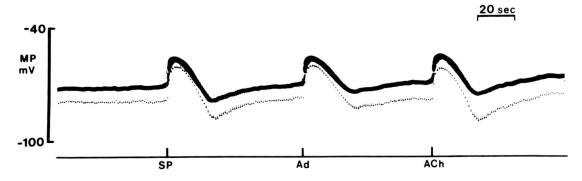

FIG. 19. Recording of membrane potential and input resistance from acinar cell of rat parotid; responses to ionophoretic application of SP, epinephrine (Ad), and ACh. The SP micropipette contained 3.5 mM of peptide in 20 mM acetic acid (pH 5 to 7). The ejection current was 200 nA applied for 500 msec. Responses were recorded to ejection charges as low as 10 nC. Ionophoresis of a control solution (20 mM sodium acetate acidified to pH 5.7) never evoked any response. Epinephrine ionophoresis was achieved at 500 nA for 200 msec, ACh at 100 nA for 1 sec. Hyperpolarizing current pulses (2 nA, 100 msec) were repetitively injected through the recording microelectrode to obtain input resistance. (From Gallacher and Petersen, ref. 21.)

Effects of stimulation with substance P. Bertaccini and De Caro (2) demonstrated that physalemin and eledoisin are powerful sialogogues. Later it was shown that hypothalamic extracts also evoked salivary secretion (59). Using saliva formation as a bioassay for the extract, Chang and Leeman (8) and Chang et al. (9) isolated a peptide of 11 amino acids in pure form and also determined the amino acid sequence. This peptide has exactly the same properties as Euler and Gaddum's (16) SP. SP evokes a membrane potential and conductance change in salivary acinar cells almost indistinguishable from the responses to ACh or epinephrine (Fig. 19); however, the SP-evoked response persists in the presence of full cholinergic and adrenergic blockade (21). The minimal latency of SP-evoked effects in the presence of the autonomic blocking agents is 1.7 sec, which is somewhat longer than the minimum latencies to cholinergic and adrenergic stimulation.

Control of Membrane Resistance

ACh, epinephrine, and SP all evoke marked reductions in input resistance (Fig. 19). Recording with two separate indwelling microelectrodes showed that the resistance reduction occurs to the same extent in two neighboring cells, directly demonstrating that it is due to a decrease in plasma membrane resistance (103). In many cases, the resistance decrease is so dramatic that the electrotonic potential changes set up by current injection virtually disappear (21,104). Figure 19 shows that following the initial membrane resistance reduction and depolarization, there is a hyperpolarization not associated with any marked resistance change. This component seems to be mediated not by opening of membrane channels but by activating an electrogenic pump (see below).

Ionic mechanism of stimulant-evoked membrane resistance and potential change.

The null potential for the action of ACh, epinephrine (E_{Epi}), and SP (E_{SP}) can be determined in a way similar to that already described for the action of secretagogues on the pancreatic acinar cells. The null potentials for the three secretagogues are the same (21), with a value of about -60 to -65 mV in both the mouse and rat parotid (21,22,103,104). This value is more negative than that found in the pancreatic acinar cells (-15 to -20 mV) and indicates that the ion selectivity of channels operated by secretagogues differs markedly in the salivary glands and the pancreas. The relatively negative null potential in the salivary glands indicates a marked permeability of the receptor-operated channels to K. An ACh-evoked increase in K permeability (P_K) has been suggested by Yoshimura and Imai (38,110) and Petersen (76,77); but more convincing evidence was produced by Nishiyama

and Petersen (72) and, most definitively, by Roberts et al. (103).

During exposure of tissue to a Cl-free solution, E_{ACh} attained a mean value of about -80 mV. In individual cases, values of -90 mV were observed. In this condition, $E_{ACh} = E_K$. The slope of the linear curve representing the membrane potential as a function of $[K]_o$ during ACh stimulation is also close to the theoretically expected value for a K-selective electrode (72). Since E_{ACh} under normal ionic conditions is somewhat less negative than E_K, the receptor-operated channels must also be permeable to one or several ions other than K. The analysis favors permeability to Na; but it cannot yet be ruled out that there is also a certain permeability to Cl (103).

That E_{ACh}, E_{Epi}, and E_{SP} (-60 to -65 mV) are so close to the resting membrane potential (E_m) (-65 to -75 mV) explains that the potential changes in response to stimulation sometimes are inconspicuous, even in cases with dramatic resistance reduction. It is also now clear why stimulation-evoked hyperpolarizations are readily seen when low resting potentials due to cell damage are obtained.

Ionic mechanism of stimulant-evoked secondary hyperpolarization.

While the initial stimulant-evoked potential change can be adequately explained by opening of ion channels in the plasma membrane, this is not so for the delayed hyperpolarization (Figs. 18 and 19). As seen in Fig. 18, the hyperpolarization associated with short periods of stimulation does not start until the stimulus has ceased. For the somewhat longer stimulation periods, there is a trend toward hyperpolarization during the continued stimulation, particularly at high frequencies; but as soon as the stimulation is discontinued, the membrane begins to hyperpolarize at a much steeper rate. This dramatic increase in rate of hyperpolarization following cessation of stimulation occurs simultaneously with a marked increase in resistance. It has proved impossible to reverse this secondary hyperpolarization by hyperpolarizing the plasma membrane prior to a stimulus; rather, the secondary hyperpolarization increases in magnitude as the resting potential becomes more negative (104). Furthermore, the secondary hyperpolarization is specifically blocked by ouabain and exposure to Na-free or K-free perfusion solutions (103). All these findings can be explained only by the secondary hyperpolarization being due to activation of the electrogenic Na-K pump. Since the receptor-operated channels are permeable to Na in addition to K, and the opening of these channels will cause K release and Na uptake (76–79,98,102), the pump is clearly being activated by the stimulant-evoked increase in intracellular Na concentration ($[Na]_i$).

That interactions with three different membrane receptor sites (cholinergic, α-adrenergic, and peptidergic) evoke identical membrane potential and conductance changes suggests a common mediator. Analogous to the conclusion obtained from work on the pancreatic acinar cells, it is tempting to suggest that Ca may be acting as the "second messenger" for the opening of the ion channels. In the lacrimal gland, where ACh and epinephrine evoke membrane changes almost identical to those seen in the salivary glands (45), intracellular Ca application evokes similar changes even in the presence of full autonomic blockade (48). Furthermore, in the salivary glands, Putney and co-workers (30,101,102) have demonstrated that the stimulant-evoked K release and Na uptake is Ca-dependent and can be mimicked by the divalent cation ionophore A23187 together with Ca. Although complete evidence of the kind established for the pancreatic cells is lacking, indirect evidence suggests that the salivary gland acini function in a way similar to the pancreatic acini, except that the ion selectivities of the receptor-operated channels are somewhat different.

Liver Parenchymal Cells

Electrophysiological Characterization of Membrane Recognition Sites

Membrane potential changes have been observed in response to α- and β-adrenergic agonists and glucagon (Fig. 20) (26,33,34,81). The membrane potential change in response to a specific β-adrenergic agonist, such as isoproterenol, is less sharp in onset than that to epinephrine (26). The glucagon receptor is specific for this hormone since a chemically related hormone, secretin, has no electrical effect on the liver cells (81).

Control of Membrane Resistance and Potential

Both catecholamines and glucagon cause marked hyperpolarization and clear reduction of membrane resis-

tance. Haylett and Jenkinson (33) showed that the norepinephrine-induced potential change depended markedly on extracellular K concentration ($[K]_o$). In the extreme case of increasing $[K]_o$ to 146 mM, it was even possible to reverse the polarity of the norepinephrine-evoked potential change. This information, together with the information that norepinephrine causes an increase in ^{42}K efflux from liver cells and reduces tissue K concentration, indicates that norepinephrine acts on the liver cell membrane by increasing P_K, as has been discussed extensively for the salivary glands. To exclude the possibility that norepinephrine hyperpolarized liver cells by activating an electrogenic Na-K pump (25), it was shown that ouabain in a concentration blocking the hyperpolarization caused by K readmission to K-free solution (33) did not reduce the norepinephrine-induced hyperpolarization. The effect of norepinephrine on membrane potential and resistance is mainly due to α-adrenoceptor activation (34), as in the salivary glands.

In the guinea pig, isoproterenol normally has little effect on the membrane potential, but an effect can be clearly demonstrated if isoproterenol is applied shortly after excitation of α-receptors. The same is true of isoproterenol effects on K release (34,35). In the rat and mouse, isoproterenol has a clear effect on the membrane potential (Fig. 20) (81,107), but the effect is much slower to develop than that of epinephrine. Epinephrine would be expected to excite both α- and β-adrenoceptors, whereas isoproterenol would mainly activate β-receptors. Therefore, α-adrenoceptor activation results in a rapid hyperpolarization mediated at least in part by an increase in potassium conductance (G_K), while isoproterenol causes a slower change in potential, the mechanism of which is yet unknown. Since exogenous cAMP also causes membrane hyperpolarization (81,107), the isoproterenol effect probably is mediated

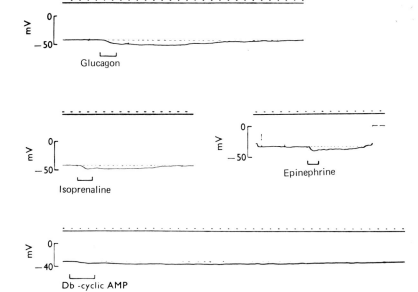

FIG. 20. Cell membrane potential recordings from superfused mouse liver segments. Effect of glucagon (10^{-7} M), isoproterenol and epinephrine (adrenaline) (10^{-6} M), and db-cAMP (10^{-3} M). In the time marker trace, pulses occur every minute. (From Petersen, ref. 81.)

by a rise in intracellular cAMP concentration. In agreement with this is the finding that epinephrine added during superfusion of mouse liver fragments with db-cAMP caused only the initial rapid effect and that isoproterenol has no effect in the presence of exogenous cAMP (26). Using three-dimensional cable analysis of current spread in the liver (Fig. 3), it is possible to calculate the specific membrane resistance and the effect of epinephrine. Graf and Petersen (26) have shown that epinephrine (10^{-5} M) reduces the specific membrane resistance of the mouse liver cell membrane by about 2 $k\Omega cm^2$.

In the perfused dog liver, epinephrine causes membrane depolarization rather than hyperpolarization. It has been suggested that this is due mainly to an increase in Na conductance (57). In guinea pig liver slices, norepinephrine causes an increase in tissue Na content simultaneously with a decrease in K content (33). It cannot be excluded that norepinephrine, in addition to causing an increase in P_K, increases P_{Na}. In the salivary gland, as already described, ACh and epinephrine increase both P_K and P_{Na}.

Glucagon effects on liver cell membrane potential were first demonstrated by Somlyo et al. (107), using a statistical multiple impalement technique. The first continuous recordings obtained with an indwelling microelectrode displaying glucagon effects were obtained by Petersen (81) (Fig. 20). Glucagon, like epinephrine, decreases the amplitude of electrotonic potential changes caused by current injection into a cell some distance away. Glucagon (10^{-7} M) causes a decrease in specific membrane resistance of about 2 $k\Omega cm^2$ (26). This conductance change is not impressive compared to the marked effects of peptide hormones, such as gastrin or bombesin, on pancreatic acinar cells and also requires much higher concentrations. It is doubtful that the hyperpolarizing effect of glucagon can be entirely accounted for by an increase in cell membrane conductance (most probably an increase in P_K). It may be important in this context to realize that several components were observed in the membrane potential

responses to glucagon (26,81). The conductance change is apparent only in the initial phase. Therefore, an electrogenic pump component may be involved in the later phase (26).

The hormone-induced increase in G_K may be mediated by an increase in $[Ca^{2+}]_i$, as discussed in connection with the salivary glands. Norepinephrine, for example, causes a marked increase in ^{45}Ca efflux from prelabeled liver slices (32), as earlier demonstrated for salivary glands (69).

RELATIONSHIP BETWEEN MEMBRANE ELECTRICAL CHANGES AND SECRETION OF FLUID AND ENZYMES

Only in the salivary glands and the pancreas is it possible to discuss the relationship between membrane electrical changes and secretion of fluid and enzymes. In the liver, for instance, the major secretagogues are bile acids, yet we have no information on the membrane electrical action of these compounds.

Pancreatic Acinar Cells

The pancreatic acinar cells secrete both digestive enzymes and fluid (94,109). These secretory processes are under the control of secretagogues whose electrical effects are reasonably well characterized.

Correlations Between Membrane Conductance Changes, Changes in Intracellular Messenger Concentrations, and Secretion

Table 3 summarizes qualitatively some of the key results obtained. Physiologically, the major acinar secretagogues are vagal nerve stimulation (ACh) and hormones belonging to the gastrin family, especially CCK. These secretagogues, in addition to causing cell

TABLE 3. *Effects of secretagogues on the pancreas*

Secretagogue	Membrane electro-physiological changes[a]	Increase in ^{45}Ca outflux	Increase in cellular cAMP concentration	Ca^{2+}-dependent secretion
ACh (and other cholinergic agents)	Yes (71,83)	Yes (67)	No (63)	Yes (93)
CCK (cerulein, gastrins)	Yes (46,71,92)	Yes (67)	No (63)	Yes (84,109)
Bombesin (bombesin nonapeptide)	Yes (46)	Yes (14)	No (14)	Yes (84)
Calcium ionophore A23187	Yes (100)	Yes (10)	?	Yes (100)
Secretin (VIP)	No (92)	No (23)	Yes (63)	No (109)
db-cAMP	No (92)	No (56)	Yes	No (109)

[a]Numbers in parentheses are references.

membrane conductance, increase, and depolarization, increase ^{45}Ca efflux from prelabeled tissue fragments, isolated cells, or acini; they do not increase cellular cAMP levels. Peptides belonging to the bombesin family clearly fall into the same category as ACh and CCK. On the other hand, secretin and VIP, secretagogues that have no effects on the electrophysiological properties, markedly increase cellular cAMP but have no effects on Ca metabolism. Whereas ACh-, CCK-, or bombesin-evoked enzyme and fluid secretion is acutely Ca dependent, secretion evoked by secretin and VIP does not depend markedly on extracellular Ca. There is at least a qualitative correlation between situations in which changes in membrane conductance and changes in cellular Ca metabolism occur. However, there does not seem to be any correlation between changes in cAMP and membrane conductance.

The dose-response curves for ACh-evoked membrane depolarization and increase in ^{45}Ca efflux have been shown to be almost identical (67). As already discussed, intracellular Ca application mimics the secretagogue action, whereas intracellular EGTA injection inhibits ACh and hormone-evoked membrane electrical actions. There is obviously more than a correlation, both qualitatively and quantitatively, between changes in cellular Ca metabolism and membrane conductance changes; the two phenomena are causally related.

The Ca that is involved in stimulus-secretion coupling is probably the same Ca that is also involved in stimulus-permeability coupling. For both secretion and membrane electrical changes, there is an initial phase after start of stimulation that is relatively independent of extracellular Ca (58,93). These phenomena seem to occur within the same time frame as the stimulant-evoked increase in ^{45}Ca efflux (67), i.e., about the initial 10 to 20 min. Thereafter, both secretion and high membrane conductance require the presence of extracellular Ca (58,84,93).

Finally, it should be mentioned that at high doses of ACh or CCK, amylase secretion from isolated pancreatic acini decreases with increasing concentration. The hormone concentrations at which the inhibition begins to be noticeable also correspond to the concentrations at which reduction in cell to cell coupling have been observed, i.e., about 10^{-5} M ACh or 10^{-9} M cerulein (88). Unfortunately, it is not possible to obtain good dose-response curves for the electrical uncoupling phenomenon, since this would require an approach with many intracellular electrodes from which recordings were made simultaneously and some way of integrating the response as seen from several cells. At present, it is possible only to speculate that there may be some relationship between electrical uncoupling and inhibition of secretion; yet it is still difficult to see a causal relationship between these two phenomena.

Importance of Secretagogue-Evoked Membrane Conductance and Potential Change for Secretion

The secretagogue-evoked conductance changes cause movements of ions across the acinar cell membrane. The main result is influx of Na and Cl and a smaller efflux of K. Since one of the important secretory processes in the pancreas is formation of fluid, the membrane ion fluxes may be involved in this process.

In the rat pancreas, juice secreted in response to cerulein or CCK (octapeptide) has a HCO_3 concentration of only 30 mM, whereas the Na concentration is 133 mM and the K concentration 4.9 mM (106). In both the rat and the mouse, micropuncture work has shown the composition of the acinar fluid secretion. The data of Mangos et al. (66) show that the acinar fluid obtained during cholinergic stimulation (pilocarpine) is isotonic with plasma, having a plasma-like Na concentration and a Cl concentration (114 mM) even higher than in plasma (102 mM). The HCO_3 concentration (36 mM), although somewhat higher than in plasma (25 mM), is much lower than the Cl concentration. The acinar fluid secretion thus appears to be mainly an isotonic NaCl solution.

From work done on the isolated perfused rat pancreas (94,109), it is clear that fluid secretion stimulated by ACh or cerulein, as well as basal fluid secretion, is absolutely dependent on the presence of Na and Cl in the perfusion fluid; however, the presence of HCO_3, crucial for secretin-evoked fluid secretion, is of no significance. While both Na and Cl are needed, the data suggest a special role for Na. Readmission of Na to a Na-free solution, either in the absence of stimulation or in the presence of ACh or cerulein, results invariably in a transient enhancement of fluid secretion above the level observed prior to Na deprivation (94). This type of response does not occur with Cl.

The acinar fluid secretion is clearly not a necessary and passive consequence of enzyme secretion, since ouabain can markedly reduce cerulein-evoked fluid secretion (to about 50% of control) without reducing enzyme (amylase) output (94). The fact that ouabain, the specific inhibitor of the Na-K pump, can markedly reduce or even abolish fluid secretion demonstrates the great importance of the transmembrane Na gradient for fluid secretion.

These data from secretory studies point to the crucial importance for Na and Cl in the process of secretion and to the necessity of having a Na gradient across the plasma membrane. The data strongly suggest an important role in fluid secretion for the secretagogue-evoked increase in Na and Cl permeability.

The secretagogue-evoked increase in Na and Cl permeability is mediated by an increase in ionized cytosol Ca concentration. In the sustained phase of hormone-evoked secretion, the necessary Ca comes from the extracellular fluid. If the hormone-evoked membrane conductance changes were important for fluid secretion, one would anticipate that hormone-evoked fluid secretion should be Ca dependent, and such is the case. During sustained stimulation with cerulein, fluid secretion is acutely and reversibly blocked by removal of extracellular Ca. Furthermore, the effect is specific for the neutral fluid secretion evoked by the acinar secretagogues, since there is no such Ca-dependence for secretin-evoked fluid secretion (109).

Figure 21 shows a simplified scheme, based on presently available evidence, accounting for stimulus-premeability and stimulus-secretion coupling. A link is supposed to exist between Na and Cl influx at the baso-lateral acinar cell membrane and fluid secretion, but the precise nature of this link is not yet clear. A model, based on findings made in dogfish rectal glands (17), has been suggested (88) in which Na flowing into the cell due to Ca-opening of Na channels is pumped out into the interstitial fluid by the Na-K pump and enters the lumen through the intercellular spaces and tight junctions while Cl proceeds through the cell. However fluid secretion operates, the importance of Na for Cl transfer is obvious. Since Cl appears to be in equilibrium across the acinar cell membrane in the resting state, an increase in Cl permeability itself will not cause Cl uptake. For this to take place, depolarization is necessary, which is brought about by the increase in Na conductance. The increase in Na conductance is important for both Na and Cl influx. The crucial importance of the Na-K pump is also clear from this model. Without the pump, there would be no Na gradient, and stimulation could not cause Cl uptake.

The importance of the reduction in cell to cell communication is less clear than the importance of changes in plasma membrane conductance. Petersen and Iwat-

suki (88) suggested that the decrease in interacinar coupling probably reflects uncoupling of acinar cells from duct cells and that this might be useful in order to avoid intermixing of different stimulus-secretion coupling mechanisms (Ca in the acinar cells, cAMP in the duct cells). Also, the uncoupling response may be linked to the pancreatic growth response (see Chapter 34). According to an attractive theory for control of tissue growth (61) (the asynchronous, dilution model), a reduction of the coupling network in a tissue should produce a growth response. Clearly, the secretagogue-evoked uncoupling phenomenon is poorly understood, and more research is necessary to clarify all its implications.

Salivary Gland Acinar Cells

Correlations Between Membrane Conductance Changes, Ion Fluxes, and Secretion

Table 4 summarizes qualitatively some of the key results obtained. It is apparent that activation of three different receptor sites—cholinergic, α-adrenergic, and peptidergic (SP)—evoke exactly the same effects, whereas β-adrenergic activation results in different cellular changes. The analogy with the pancreatic results (Table 3) is clear. Those receptors coupled to the Ca system (102) are also coupled to marked membrane conductance changes and ion flux changes, whereas those receptors coupled to adenylcyclase are not linked to such membrane events.

The electrophysiological data already described have shown that the marked conductance increase is attributable to increases in Na and K permeability. Secretagogue-evoked K release from salivary gland cells was demonstrated as early as 1956 (6) and has since

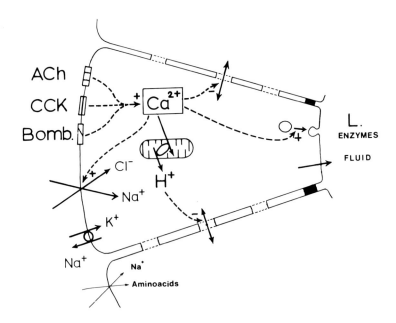

FIG. 21. Schematic diagram showing intracellular events after excitation of ACh, CCK, and bombesin receptors in pancreatic acinar cells. Some of the more important membrane transport pathways are shown.

TABLE 4. *Effects of secretagogues on salivary glands*

Secretagogue	Membrane conductance increase	Increase in ^{45}Ca influx and efflux	Increase in cellular cAMP concentration	K release or ^{86}Rb release	Ca-dependent secretion
ACh	Yes (72,77,104)	Yes (30,55,69)	No (7)	Yes (6,76,101)	Yes (95,102)
α-Adrenergic agonists	Yes (104)	Yes (30,55,69)	No (1,7)	Yes (76,101)	Yes (95,102)
β-Adrenergic agonists	No (104)	No (55)	Yes (7,29,111)	No (7,102)	No (95,102)
Substance P	Yes (21)	Yes (30,102)	No (7)	Yes (30,102)	Yes (102)

repeatedly been shown for a variety of salivary glands (102). An increase in Na uptake was indirectly shown by Petersen (76,77) and directly demonstrated by Poulsen (98) and Putney (102). It was also demonstrated long ago that following the initial stimulant-evoked K release, there was active accumulation of K, a process mediated by the Na-K pump and inhibited by ouabain (76,78). This latter phase is manifest in the electrical recordings as a secondary hyperpolarization not associated with a conductance change (103,104).

From the work of Putney (102) and his collaborators, it is now clear that the Na and K ion flux changes evoked by secretagogues are mediated by an increase in intracellular ionized Ca concentration in complete analogy with the original proposal for the pancreas. Unfortunately, technical problems have prevented the demonstration of this phenomenon with electrical techniques.

Nielsen and Petersen (69) first assessed stimulant-evoked changes in cellular Ca metabolism. Both ACh and epinephrine markedly and immediately accelerate the release of ^{45}Ca from prelabeled perfused submaxillary gland and also caused a delayed increase in ^{45}Ca uptake. Koelz et al. (55) subsequently showed that isoproterenol does not evoke this effect. Putney (101,102) demonstrated that the initial change in stimulant-evoked K permeability is independent of external Ca, whereas a sustained phase of K release is entirely dependent on external Ca. The initial phase in stimulus-permeability coupling is supposed to be mediated by Ca released from inside the cells. These two phases of Ca dependency are similar to that which has been described for the pancreas. No electrical studies with sustained stimulation have been carried out.

Importance of Secretagogue-Evoked Membrane Conductance Changes for Secretion

Figure 22 shows a schematic diagram relating the electrophysiological phenomena resulting in K release and Na uptake to the secretory events in the acinar cells. By far the most dramatic protein secretion can be obtained by β-adrenergic stimulation, while fluid secretion is stimulated to a much greater extent by cholinergic or α-adrenergic stimulation. As outlined in Fig. 22, there

are two pathways to protein secretion: one involving cAMP and one involving Ca. With respect to fluid secretion, it is still not clear exactly how cellular transports work together to produce the isotonic Na- and Cl-rich primary acinar secretion. The Na-K pump, as indicated in Fig. 22, seems to be located on the basolateral rather than the luminal membrane (5,68). It is known that ouabain-sensitive Na-K pumping and fluid secretion can be dissociated, at least in the short term (minutes) (78); but we are ignorant about what happens at the luminal membrane.

As discussed in relation to pancreatic acinar fluid secretion, there is probably a link between secretagogue-evoked fluid secretion and Na influx (102). It is interesting to note that while the fluid secretion process in the pancreas and the salivary glands in both cases results in an isotonic NaCl-rich fluid, the basolateral ion flux changes are different. In the pancreas, secretagogues open channels permeable mainly to Na and Cl with resulting NaCl influx; whereas in the salivary glands, the

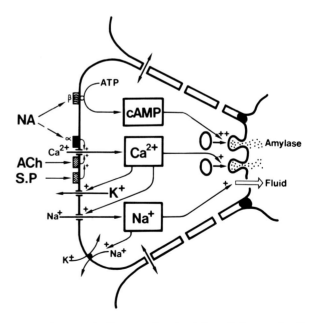

FIG. 22. Schematic diagram showing intracellular events after excitation of cholinergic, α- and β-adrenergic, and peptidergic receptors in parotid acinar cells. Some of the more important pathways are shown. NA, norepinephrine.

channels seem to be Na and K permeable with resulting Na influx and K efflux. In both cases, the role of the Na-K pump is apparently to maintain the Na gradient across the plasma membrane. For the salivary glands, there is clearly a problem in regard to Cl. Cl concentration intracellularly is considerably higher than expected on the basis of a passive distribution (85), indicating the existence of some primary or secondary active Cl accumulation. The role of such a mechanism in fluid secretion remains to be determined.

CONCLUSION

Electrophysiology of secretory cells in the alimentary canal has helped to map a number of important electrolyte transport pathways. Because of the good time resolution of electrophysiological methods and the opportunity to probe continuously individual gland cell units at the same time as injecting agonists or messengers inside or outside cells, precise data important to our understanding of stimulus-secretion coupling have been gained. For the pancreatic acinar cells (where relatively complete sets of data exist) the electrophysiological approach has been useful in defining receptor sites, cell to cell coupling, and secretagogue-evoked opening of specific membrane conductance pathways. Further electrophysiological work also in other gland cells may help to clarify the secretory processes and their control mechanisms.

REFERENCES

1. Batzri, S., Amsterdam, A., Selinger, Z., Ohad, I., and Schramm, M. (1971): Epinephrine-induced vacuole formation in parotid gland cells and its independence of the secretory process. *Proc. Natl. Acad. Sci. USA*, 68:121–123.
2. Bertaccini, G., and De Caro, G. (1965): The effect of physalaemin and related polypeptides on salivary secretion. *J. Physiol. (Lond.)*, 181:68–81.
3. Blouin, A., Bolender, R. P., and Weibel, E. R. (1977): Distribution of organelles and membranes between hepatocytes and non-hepatocytes in the rat liver parenchyma. A stereological study. *J. Cell Biol.*, 72:441–455.
4. Bolender, R. P. (1974): Stereological analysis of the guinea pig pancreas. *J. Cell Biol.*, 61:269–287.
5. Bundgaard, M., Møller, M., and Poulsen, J. H. (1977): Localization of sodium pump sites in cat salivary glands. *J. Physiol. (Lond.)*, 273:339–353.
6. Burgen, A. S. V. (1956): The secretion of potassium in saliva. *J. Physiol. (Lond.)*, 132:20–39.
7. Butcher, F. R. (1978): Calcium and cyclic nucleotides in the regulation of secretion from the rat parotid by autonomic agonists. *Adv. Cyclic Nucleotide Res.*, 9:707–721.
8. Chang, M. M., and Leeman, S. E. (1970): Isolation of a sialogogic peptide from bovine hypothalamic tissue and its characterization as substance P. *J. Biol. Chem.*, 245:4784–4790.
9. Chang, M. M., Leeman, S. E., and Niall, H. D. (1971): Amino-acid sequence of substance P. *Nature*, 232:86–87.
10. Christophe, J. P., Frandsen, E. K., Conlon, T. P., Krishna, G., and Gardner, J. D. (1976): Action of cholecystokinin, cholinergic agents, and A-23187 on accumulation of guanosine 3':5'-monophosphate in dispersed guinea pig pancreatic acinar cells. *J. Biol. Chem.*, 251:4640–4645.
11. Cole, K. S. (1928): Electric impedance of suspension of spheres. *J. Gen. Physiol.*, 12:29–36.
12. Davison, J. S., Pearson, G. T., and Petersen, O. H. (1980): Pancreatic acinar cells: Effects of electrical field stimulation on membrane potential and resistance. *J. Physiol. (Lond)*, 301:295–305.
13. Davison, J. S., and Ueda, N. (1977): Depolarization of rat pancreatic acinar cells by cervical vagal stimulation. *J. Physiol. (Lond.)*, 266:39–40P.
14. Deschodt-Lanckman, M., Robberecht, P., de Neef, M. L., and Christophe, J. (1976): In vitro action of bombesin and bombesin-like peptides on amylase secretion, calcium efflux, and adenylate cyclase activity in the rat pancreas. *J. Clin. Invest.*, 58:891–898.
15. Douglas, W. W., and Poisner, A. M. (1963): The influence of calcium on the secretory response of the submaxillary gland to acetylcholine or to noradrenaline. *J. Physiol. (Lond.)*, 165:528–541.
16. Euler, U. S. von, and Gaddum, H. J. (1931): An unidentified depressor substance in certain tissue extracts. *J. Physiol. (Lond.)*, 72:74–87.
17. Eveloff, J., Kinne, R., Kinne-Saffran, E., Murer, H., Silva, P., Epstein, F. H., Stoff, J., and Kinter, W. B. (1978): Coupled sodium and chloride transport into plasma membrane vesicles prepared from dogfish rectal gland. *Pfluegers Arch.*, 378:87–92.
18. Fricke, H. (1923): The electric capacity of cell suspensions. *Physiol. Rev.*, 21:708–709.
19. Frömter, E. (1972): The route of passive ion movement through the epithelium of *Necturus* gallbladder. *J. Membr. Biol.*, 8:259–301.
20. Frömter, E., and Gebler, B. (1977): Electrical properties of amphibian urinary bladder epithelia. III. The cell membrane resistances and the effect of amiloride. *Pfluegers Arch.*, 371:99–108.
21. Gallacher, D. V., and Petersen, O. H. (1980): Substance P increases membrane conductance in parotid acinar cells. *Nature*, 283:393–395.
22. Gallacher, D. V., and Petersen, O. H. (1980): Electrophysiology of parotid acini: Effects of electrical field stimulation and ionophoresis of neurotransmitters. *J. Physiol. (Lond.)*, 305:43–57.
23. Gardner, J. D., Conlon, T. P., Klaeveman, H. L., Adams, T. D., and Ondetti, M. A. (1975): Action of cholecystokinin and cholinergic agents on calcium transport in isolated pancreatic acinar cells. *J. Clin. Invest.*, 56:366–375.
24. Goldman, D. E. (1943): Potential, impedance and rectification in membranes. *J. Gen. Physiol.*, 27:37–60.
25. Graf, J., and Petersen, O. H. (1974): Electrogenic sodium pump in mouse liver parenchymal cells. *Proc. R. Soc. [B.]*, 187:363–367.
26. Graf, J., and Petersen, O. H. (1978): Cell membrane potential and resistance in liver. *J. Physiol. (Lond.)*, 284:105–126.
27. Greenwell, J. R. (1975): The effects of cholecystokinin-pancreozymin, acetylcholine and secretin on the membrane potentials of mouse pancreatic cells *in vitro*. *Pfluegers Arch.*, 353:159–170.
28. Gregory, R. A. (1974): The gastrointestinal hormones: a review of recent advances. *J. Physiol. (Lond.)*, 241:1–32.
29. Guidotti, A., Weiss, B., and Costa, E. (1972): Adenosine 3',5'-monophosphate concentrations and isoproterenol induced synthesis of deoxyribonucleic acid in mouse parotid gland. *Mol. Pharmacol.*, 8:521–530.
30. Haddas, R. A., Landis, C. A., and Putney, J. W. (1979): Relationship between calcium release and potassium release in rat parotid gland. *J. Physiol. (Lond.)*, 291:457–465.
31. Hammer, M. G., and Sheridan, J. D. (1978): Electrical coupling and dye transfer between acinar cells in rat salivary glands. *J. Physiol. (Lond.)*, 275:495–505.
32. Haylett, D. G. (1976): Effects of sympathomimetic amines on ^{45}Ca efflux from liver slices. *Br. J. Pharmacol.*, 57:158–160.
33. Haylett, D. G., and Jenkinson, D. H. (1972): Effects of noradrenaline on potassium efflux, membrane potential and electrolyte levels in tissue slices prepared from guinea-pig liver. *J. Physiol. (Lond.)*, 225:721–750.

34. Haylett, D. G., and Jenkinson, D. H. (1972): The receptors concerned in the actions of catecholamines on glucose release, membrane potential and ion movements in guinea-pig liver. *J. Physiol. (Lond.),* 225:751-772.

35. Haylett, D. G., and Jenkinson, D. H. (1973): Actions of catecholamines on the membrane properties of liver cells. In: *Drug Receptors,* edited by H. P. Rang, pp. 15-28. Macmillan, London.

36. Hodgkin, A. L. (1964): *The Conduction of the Nervous Impulse.* Liverpool University Press, Liverpool.

37. Hodgkin, A. L., and Katz, B. (1949): The effect of sodium ions on the electrical activity of the giant axon of the squid. *J. Physiol. (Lond.),* 108:37-77.

38. Imai, Y. (1965): Study of the secretion mechanism of the submaxillary gland of dog. Part 2. Effects of exchanging ions in the perfusate on salivary secretion and secretory potential, with special reference to the ionic distribution in the gland tissue. *J. Physiol. Soc. Jpn.,* 27:313-324.

39. Iwatsuki, N. (1978): Direct demonstration of cell-to-cell communication in mammalian pancreatic acini: transfer of fluorescent probe molecults. *J. Physiol. (Lond.),* 285:1-2P.

40. Iwatsuki, N., Katoh, K., and Nishiyama, A. (1977): The effects of gastrin and gastrin analogues on pancreatic acinar cell membrane potential and resistance. *Br. J. Pharmacol.,* 60:147-154.

41. Iwatsuki, N., and Petersen, O. H. (1977): Pancreatic acinar cells: localization of acetylcholine receptors and the importance of chloride and calcium for acetylcholine-evoked depolarization. *J. Physiol. (Lond.),* 269:723-733.

42. Iwatsuki, N., and Petersen, O. H. (1977): Pancreatic acinar cells: The acetylcholine equilibrium potential and its ionic dependency. *J. Physiol. (Lond.),* 269:735-751.

43. Iwatsuki, N., and Petersen, O. H. (1977): Acetylcholine-like effects of intracellular calcium application in pancreatic acinar cells. *Nature,* 268:147-149.

44. Iwatsuki, N., and Petersen, O. H. (1978): Pancreatic acinar cells: Acetylcholine-evoked electrical uncoupling and its ionic dependency. *J. Physiol. (Lond.),* 274:81-96.

45. Iwatsuki, N., and Petersen, O. H. (1978): Membrane potential, resistance and intercellular communication in the lacrimal gland: effects of acetylcholine and adrenaline. *J. Physiol. (Lond.),* 275:507-520.

46. Iwatsuki, N., and Petersen, O. H. (1978): In vitro action of bombesin on amylase secretion, membrane potential, and membrane resistance in rat and mouse pancreatic acinar cells. A comparison with other secretagogues. *J. Clin. Invest.,* 61:41-46.

47. Iwatsuki, N., and Petersen, O. H. (1978): Electrical coupling and uncoupling of exocrine acinar cells. *J. Cell Biol.,* 79:533-545.

48. Iwatsuki, N., and Petersen, O. H. (1978): Intracellular Ca²⁺ injection causes membrane hyperpolarization and conductance increase in lacrimal acinar cells. *Pfluegers Arch.,* 377:185-187.

49. Iwatsuki, N., and Petersen, O. H. (1979): Direct visualization of cell to cell coupling: Transfer of fluorescent probes in living mammalian pancreatic acini. *Pfluegers Arch.,* 380:277-281.

50. Iwatsuki, N., and Petersen, O. H. (1979): Pancreatic acinar cells: The effect of CO_2, NH_4Cl and acetylcholine on intercellular communication. *J. Physiol. (Lond.),* 291:317-326.

51. Iwatsuki, N., and Petersen, O. H. (1979): Does exocytosis influence membrane resistance in parotid acini? *J. Physiol. (Lond.),* 292:81-82P.

52. Iwatsuki, N., and Petersen, O. H. (1980): Amino acids evoke short-latency membrane conductance increase in pancreatic acinar cells. *Nature,* 283:492-494.

53. Kagayama, M., and Nishiyama, A. (1974): Membrane potential and input resistance in acinar cells from cat and rabbit submaxillary glands in vivo: Effects of autonomic nerve stimulation. *J. Physiol. (Lond.),* 242:157-172.

54. Kater, S. B., and Galvin, N. J. (1978): Physiological and morphological evidence for coupling in mouse salivary gland acinar cells. *J. Cell Biol.,* 79:20-26.

55. Koelz, H. R., Kondo, S., Blum, A. L., and Schulz, I. (1977): Calcium ion uptake induced by cholinergic and α-adrenergic stimulation in isolated cells of rat salivary glands. *Pfluegers Arch.,* 370:37-44.

56. Kondo, S., and Schulz, I. (1976): Ca²⁺ fluxes in isolated cells of rat pancreas. Effects of secretagogues and different Ca²⁺ concentration. *J. Membr. Biol.,* 29:185-203.

57. Lambotte, L. (1973): Effect of activation of α and β adrenergic receptors on the hepatic cell membrane potential in perfused dog liver. *J. Physiol. (Lond.),* 232:181-192.

58. Laugier, R., and Petersen, O. H. (1980): Pancreatic acinar cells: Electrophysiological evidence for stimulant-evoked increase in membrane calcium permeability in the mouse. *J. Physiol. (Lond.),* 303:61-72.

59. Leeman, S. E., and Hammerschlag, R. (1967): Stimulation of salivary secretion by a factor extracted from hypothalamic tissue. *Endocrinology,* 81:803-810.

60. Loewenstein, W. R. (1966): Permeability of membrane junctions. *Ann. N.Y. Acad. Sci.,* 137:441-472.

61. Loewenstein, W. R. (1979): Junctional intercellular communication and the control of growth. *Biochim. Biophys. Acta,* 56:1-65.

62. Loewenstein, W. R., and Kanno, Y. (1964): Studies on an epithelial (gland) cell junction. I. Modifications of surface membrane permeability. *J. Cell Biol.,* 22:565-586.

63. Long, B. W., and Gardner, J. D. (1977): Effects of cholecystokinin on adenylate cyclase activity in dispersed pancreatic acinar cells. *Gastroenterology,* 73:1008-1014.

64. Lundberg, A. (1955): The electrophysiology of the submaxillary gland of the cat. *Acta Physiol. Scand.,* 35:1-25.

65. Lundberg, A. (1957): The mechanism of establishment of secretory potentials in sublingual gland cells. *Acta Physiol. Scand.,* 40:35-58.

66. Mangos, J. A., McSherry, N. R., Nousia-Arvanitakis, S., and Irwin, K. (1973): Secretion and transductal fluxes of ions in exocrine glands of the mouse. *Am. J. Physiol.,* 225:18-24.

67. Matthews, E. K., Petersen, O. H., and Williams, J. A. (1973): Pancreatic acinar cells: acetylcholine-induced membrane depolarization, calcium efflux and amylase release. *J. Physiol. (Lond.),* 234:689-701.

68. Nakagaki, I., Goto, T., Sasaki, S., and Imai, Y. (1978): Histochemical and cytochemical localization of (Na^+-K^+)-activated adenosine triphosphatase in the acini of dog submandibular glands. *J. Histochem. Cytochem.,* 26:835-845.

69. Nielsen, S. P., and Petersen, O. H. (1972): Transport of calcium in the perfused submandibular gland of the cat. *J. Physiol. (Lond.),* 223:685-697.

70. Nishiyama, A., Katoh, K., Saitoh, S., and Wakui, M. (1980): Effect of neural stimulation on acinar cell membrane potentials in isolated pancreas and salivary gland segments. *Membr. Biochem.,* 3:49-66.

71. Nishiyama, A., and Petersen, O. H. (1974): Pancreatic acinar cells: Membrane potential and resistance change evoked by acetylcholine. *J. Physiol. (Lond.),* 238:145-158.

72. Nishiyama, A., and Petersen, O. H. (1974): Membrane potential and resistance measurement in acinar cells from salivary glands in vitro: effect of acetylcholine. *J. Physiol. (Lond.),* 242:173-188.

73. Nishiyama, A., and Petersen, O. H. (1975): Pancreatic acinar cells: ionic dependence of acetylcholine-induced membrane potential and resistance change. *J. Physiol. (Lond.),* 244:431-465.

74. Pedersen, G. L., and Petersen, O. H. (1973): Membrane potential measurement in parotid acinar cells. *J. Physiol. (Lond.),* 234:217-227.

75. Penn, R. D. (1966): Ionic communication between liver cells. *J. Cell Biol.,* 29:171-174.

76. Petersen, O. H. (1970): Some factors influencing stimulation-induced release of potassium from the cat submandibular gland to fluid perfused through the gland. *J. Physiol. (Lond.),* 208:431-447.

77. Petersen, O. H. (1970): The dependence of the transmembrane salivary secretory potential on the external potassium and sodium concentration. *J. Physiol. (Lond.),* 210:205-215.

78. Petersen, O. H. (1971): Formation of saliva and potassium transport in the perfused cat submandibular gland. *J. Physiol. (Lond.),* 216:129-142.

79. Petersen, O. H. (1971): Initiation of salt and water transport in

mammalian salivary glands by acetylcholine. *Philos. Trans. R. Soc. Lond. [Biol.],* 262:307–314.

80. Petersen, O. H. (1973): Electrogenic sodium pump in pancreatic acinar cells. *Proc. R. Soc. [B.],* 184:115–119.

81. Petersen, O. H. (1974): The effect of glucagon on the liver cell membrane potential. *J. Physiol. (Lond.),* 239:647–656.

82. Petersen, O. H. (1975): Electrical coupling between pancreatic acinar cells. *J. Physiol. (Lond.),* 250:2–4P.

83. Petersen, O. H. (1976): Electrophysiology of mammalian gland cells. *Physiol. Rev.,* 56:535–577.

84. Petersen, O. H. (1978): Calcium dependence of bombesin-evoked pancreatic amylase secretion. *J. Physiol. (Lond.),* 285:30–31P.

85. Petersen, O. H. (1980): *Electrophysiology of Gland Cells.* Academic Press, New York.

86. Petersen, O. H., Gray, T. A., and Hall, R. A. (1977): The relationship between stimulation-induced potassium release and amylase secretion in the mouse parotid. *Pfluegers Arch.,* 369:207–211.

87. Petersen, O. H., and Iwatsuki, N. (1978): The role of calcium in pancreatic acinar cell stimulus-secretion coupling: An electrophysiological approach. *Ann. N.Y. Acad. Sci.,* 307:599–617.

88. Petersen, O. H., and Iwatsuki, N. (1979): Hormonal control of cell to cell coupling in the exocrine pancreas. In: *Hormonal Receptors in Digestion and Nutrition,* edited by G. Rosselin, pp. 191–202. Elsevier/North-Holland, Amsterdam.

89. Petersen, O. H., and Laugier, R. (1980): Receptor-mediated control via the calcium effector of membrane ion permeability in pancreatic acinar cells. *Biochem. Soc. Trans.,* 8:268 270.

89a. Petersen, O. H., and Matthews, E. K. (1972): The effect of pancreozymin and acetylcholine on the membrane potential of the pancreatic acinar cells. *Experientia,* 28:1037–1038.

90. Petersen, O. H., and Philpott, H. G. (1979): Pancreatic acinar cells: Effects of microionophoretic polypeptide application on membrane potential and resistance. *J. Physiol. (Lond.),* 290:305–315.

91. Petersen, O. H., and Philpott, H. G. (1980): Pancreatic acinar cells: The anion selectivity of the acetylcholine-opened chloride pathway. *J. Physiol. (Lond.),* 306:481–492.

92. Petersen, O. H., and Ueda, N. (1975): Pancreatic acinar cells: Effect of acetylcholine, pancreozymin, gastrin and secretin on membrane potential and resistance *in vivo* and *in vitro. J. Physiol. (Lond.),* 257:461–471.

93. Petersen, O. H., and Ueda, N. (1976): Pancreatic acinar cells: The role of calcium in stimulus-secretion coupling. *J. Physiol. (Lond.),* 254:583–606.

94. Petersen, O. H., and Ueda, N. (1977): Secretion of fluid and amylase in the perfused rat pancreas. *J. Physiol. (Lond.),* 264:819–835.

95. Petersen, O. H., Ueda, N., Hall, R. A., and Gray, T. A. (1977): The role of calcium in parotid amylase secretion evoked by excitation of cholinergic, α- and β-adrenergic receptors. *Pfluegers Arch.,* 372:231–237.

96. Philpott, H. G., and Petersen, O. H. (1979): Separate activation sites for cholecystokinin and bombesin on pancreatic acini. An electrophysiological study employing a competitive antagonist for the action of CCK. *Pfluegers Arch.,* 382:263–267.

97. Philpott, H. G., and Petersen, O. H. (1979): Extracellular but not intracellular application of peptide hormones activates pancreatic acinar cells. *Nature,* 281:684–686.

98. Poulsen, J. H. (1974): Acetylcholine-induced transport of Na^+ and K^+ in the perfused cat submandibular gland. *Pfluegers Arch.,* 349:215–220.

99. Poulsen, J. H., and Oakley, B. II (1979): Intracellular potassium ion activity in resting and stimulated mouse pancreas and submandibular gland. *Proc. R. Soc. Lond. [B.],* 204:99–104.

100. Poulsen, J. H., and Williams, J. A. (1977): Effects of the calcium ionophore A23187 on pancreatic acinar cell membrane potentials and amylase release. *J. Physiol. (Lond.),* 264:323–339.

101. Putney, J. W. (1976): Biphasic modulation of potassium release in the rat parotid gland by carbachol and phenylephrine. *J. Pharmacol. Exp. Ther.,* 198:375–384.

102. Putney, J. W. (1979): Stimulus-permeability coupling: Role of calcium in the receptor regulation of membrane permeability. *Pharmacol. Rev.,* 30:209–245.

103. Roberts, M. L., Iwatsuki, N., and Petersen, O. H. (1978): Parotid acinar cells: Ionic dependence of acetylcholine-evoked membrane potential changes. *Pfluegers Arch.,* 376:159–167.

104. Roberts, M. L., and Petersen, O. H. (1978): Membrane potential and resistance changes induced in salivary gland acinar cells by microiontophoretic application of acetylcholine and adrenergic agonists. *J. Membr. Biol.,* 39:297–312.

105. Schanne, O., and Coraboeuf, E. (1966): Potential and resistance measurements of rat liver cells *in situ. Nature,* 210:1390–1391.

106. Sewell, W. A., and Young, J. A. (1975): Secretion of electrolytes by the pancreas of the anaesthetized rat. *J. Physiol. (Lond.),* 252:379–396.

107. Somlyo, A. P., Somlyo, A. V., and Friedmann, N. (1971): Cyclic adenosine monophosphate, cyclic guanosine monophosphate, and glucagon: Effects on membrane potential and ion fluxes in the liver. *Ann. N.Y. Acad. Sci.,* 185:108–114.

108. Weibel, E. R., Stäubli, W., Gnägi, H. R., and Hess, F. A. (1969): Correlated morphometric and biochemical studies on the liver cell. *J. Cell Biol.,* 42:68–91.

109. Ueda, N., and Petersen, O. H. (1977): The dependence of caerulein-evoked pancreatic fluid secretion on the extracellular calcium concentration. *Pfluegers Arch.,* 370:179–183.

110. Yoshimura, H., and Imai, Y. (1967): Studies on the secretory potential of acinal cell of dog's submaxillary gland and the ionic dependency of it. *Jpn. J. Physiol.,* 17:280–293.

111. Young, J. A., and van Lennep, E. W. (1979): Transport in salivary and salt glands. In: *Membrane Transport in Biology, Vol. 4, Transport Organs,* edited by G. Giebisch, pp. 563–692. Springer, Berlin.